VOL XIII, NO 1 MARCH 1986

Seminars in Oncology

Brain Tumors

William R. Shapiro, *Guest Editor*

Contributors

William R. Shapiro
Joan Rankin Shapiro • Peter C. Burger
Joseph Ransohoff • Patrick Kelly • Edward Laws
Diane F. Nelson • Raul C. Urtasun • William M. Saunders • Philip H. Gutin
Glenn E. Sheline • Ronald G. Blasberg • Dennis R. Groothuis • David J. Brooks
Ronald P. Beaney • David G.T. Thomas • Dennis E. Bullard
G. Yancey Gillespie • M. Stephen Mahaley • Darell D. Bigner
Jeffrey C. Allen • Julian Bloom • Inta Ertel • Audrey Evans
Denman Hammond • Helen Jones • Victor Levin
Derek Jenkin • Richard Sposto
William Wara

Grune & Stratton, Inc.
Harcourt Brace Jovanovich, Publishers

Seminars in Oncology

Brain Tumors

VOL XIII, NO 1 **MARCH 1986**

Table of Contents

Introduction: Brain Tumors .... *William R. Shapiro* 1

Biology of Gliomas: Heterogeneity, Oncogenes, Growth Factors .... *Joan Rankin Shapiro* 4

Malignant Astrocytic Neoplasms: Classification, Pathologic Anatomy, and Response to Treatment .... *Peter C. Burger* 16

The Role of Intracranial Surgery for the Treatment of Malignant Gliomas *Joseph Ransohoff, Patrick Kelly, and Edward Laws* 27

Therapy of Adult Malignant Brain Tumors: What Have the Clinical Trials Taught Us? *William R. Shapiro* 38

Recent and Current Investigations of Radiation Therapy of Malignant Gliomas *Diane F. Nelson, Raul C. Urtasun, William M. Saunders, Philip H. Gutin, and Glenn E. Sheline* 46

Principles of Brain Tumor Chemotherapy .... *William R. Shapiro and Joan R. Shapiro* 56

Chemotherapy of Brain Tumors: Physiological and Pharmacokinetic Considerations *Ronald G. Blasberg and Dennis R. Groothuis* 70

The Role of Positron Emission Tomography in the Study of Cerebral Tumors *David J. Brooks, Ronald P. Beaney, and David G.T. Thomas* 83

Immunobiology of Human Gliomas .... *Dennis E. Bullard, G. Yancey Gillespie, M. Stephen Mahaley, and Darell D. Bigner* 94

Brain Tumors in Children: Current Cooperative and Institutional Chemotherapy Trials in Newly Diagnosed and Recurrent Disease .... *Jeffrey C. Allen, Julian Bloom, Inta Ertel, Audrey Evans, Denman Hammond, Helen Jones, Victor Levin, Derek Jenkin, Richard Sposto, and William Wara* 110

Subject Index 123

POINT OF VIEW

Hospice: The Game is Not Over .... *Robert E. Enck* 128

Erratum 130

Given the choice:

A More Cons

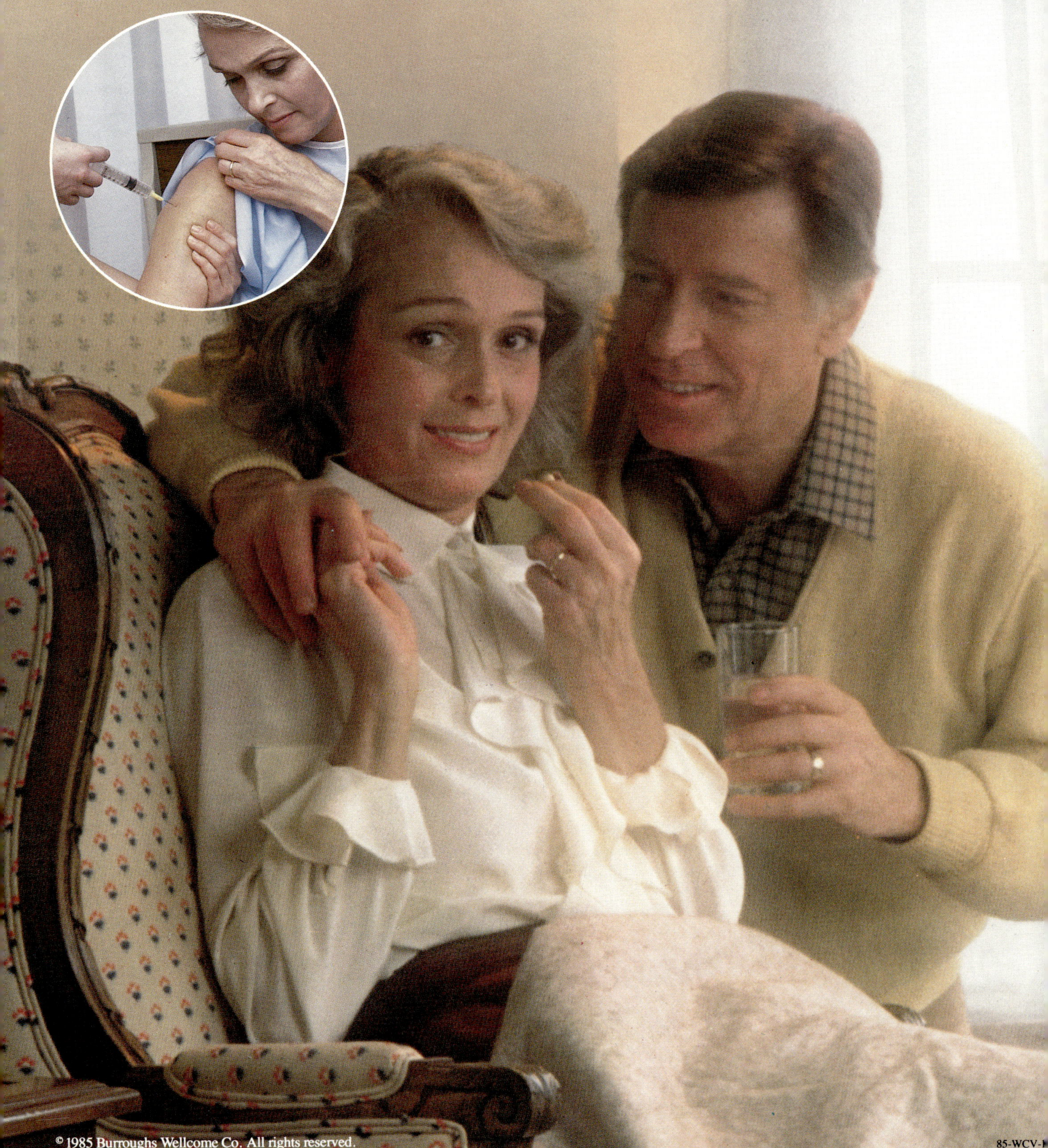

Seminars in Oncology

Biological Response Modifiers

VOL XIII, NO 2 **JUNE 1986**

Table of Contents

INTRODUCTION

Biological Response Modifiers .... *Carl M. Pinsky* 131

Clinical Development of Biological Response Modifiers: Comparison With Cytotoxic Drugs
Michael J. Hawkins, Daniel F. Hoth, and Robert E. Wittes 132

IMMUNOMODULATORS

Local Administration of Immunomodulators .... *Carl M. Pinsky* 141

Biologic Response Modifiers as Adjuncts to Other Therapeutic Modalities .... *Ernest C. Borden and Michael J. Hawkins* 144

SEROLOGY

Immunochemical Characterization of Human Tumor Antigens .... *Ralph A. Reisfeld* 153

Monoclonal Antibodies: Potential Applications to the Treatment of Cancer.... *Alan N. Houghton and David A. Scheinberg* 165

Active Immunotherapy Against Cancer: Present Status .... *Donald L. Morton* 180

CELL-MEDIATED IMMUNITY

The Immunoaugmenting Effects of Cancer Chemotherapeutic Agents .... *M.J. Mastrangelo, D. Berd, and H. Maguire, Jr.* 186

Effects of Biological Response Modifiers on Effector Cells With Cytotoxic Activity Against Tumors .... *Ronald B. Herberman* 195

The Adoptive Immunotherapy of Cancer Using the Transfer of Activated Lymphoid Cells and Interleukin-2 .... *Steven A. Rosenberg* 200

(Continued on following page)

CYTOKINES

Interferons and Interferon Inducers in Cancer Treatment .... *Susan E. Krown* 207

Lymphokines: From Conjecture to the Clinic .... *Steven Gillis, Paul J. Conlon, David Cosman, Thomas P. Hopp, Steven K. Dower, Virginia Price, Diane Y. Mochizuki, and David L. Urdal* 218

Differentiation Factors .... *Janice L. Gabrilove* 228

FUTURE PERSPECTIVES

Future Perspectives for Biological Response Modifiers: A Viewpoint .... *E. Mihich* 234

Subject Index 255

Seminars in Oncology

Plasma Cell Myeloma and the Myeloma Proteins

VOL XIII, NO 3 **SEPTEMBER 1986**

Table of Contents

INTRODUCTION

Plasma Cell Myeloma and the Myeloma Proteins: Introduction and Dedication *Mehdi Farhangi* 259

The Structure of Immunoglobulins and Their Genes, DNA Rearrangement and B Cell Differentiation, Molecular Anomalies of Some Monoclonal Immunoglobulins *Steven M. Rosen, Joel N. Buxbaum, and Blas Frangione* 260

Plasmacytomas in Mice .... *Michael Potter* 275

Immunosuppression and Infection in Multiple Myeloma .... *Daniel R. Jacobson and Susan Zolla-Pazner* 282

Bone Destruction and Hypercalcemia in Plasma Cell Myeloma .... *Gregory R. Mundy and Donald R. Bertolini* 291

Staging and Kinetics of Multiple Myeloma .... *Brian G.M. Durie* 300

Laboratory Monitoring of Myeloma Proteins .... *Robert A. Kyle and John P. Garton* 310

Chemotherapy of Previously Untreated Multiple Myeloma Patients: An Analysis of Recent Treatment Results .... *Jonathan R. Sporn and O. Ross McIntyre* 318

Treatment of Refractory Multiple Myeloma and Considerations for Future Therapy *Robert A. Kyle, Philip R. Greipp, and Morie A. Gertz* 326

Interferons in the Treatment of Multiple Myeloma .... *M. Robert Cooper and Charles E. Welander* 334

Clinical Implications of Monoclonal Light Chains .... *Alan Solomon* 341

Monoclonal Immunoglobulins With Antibody Activity in Myeloma, Macroglobulinemia and Related Plasma Cell Dyscrasias .... *Giampaolo Merlini, Mehdi Farhangi, and Elliott F. Osserman* 350

The Clinical Implications of Monoclonal Immunoglobulins .... *Mehdi Farhangi and Giampaolo Merlini* 366

Index 380

Controls delayed N&V for hours in the cancer outpatient

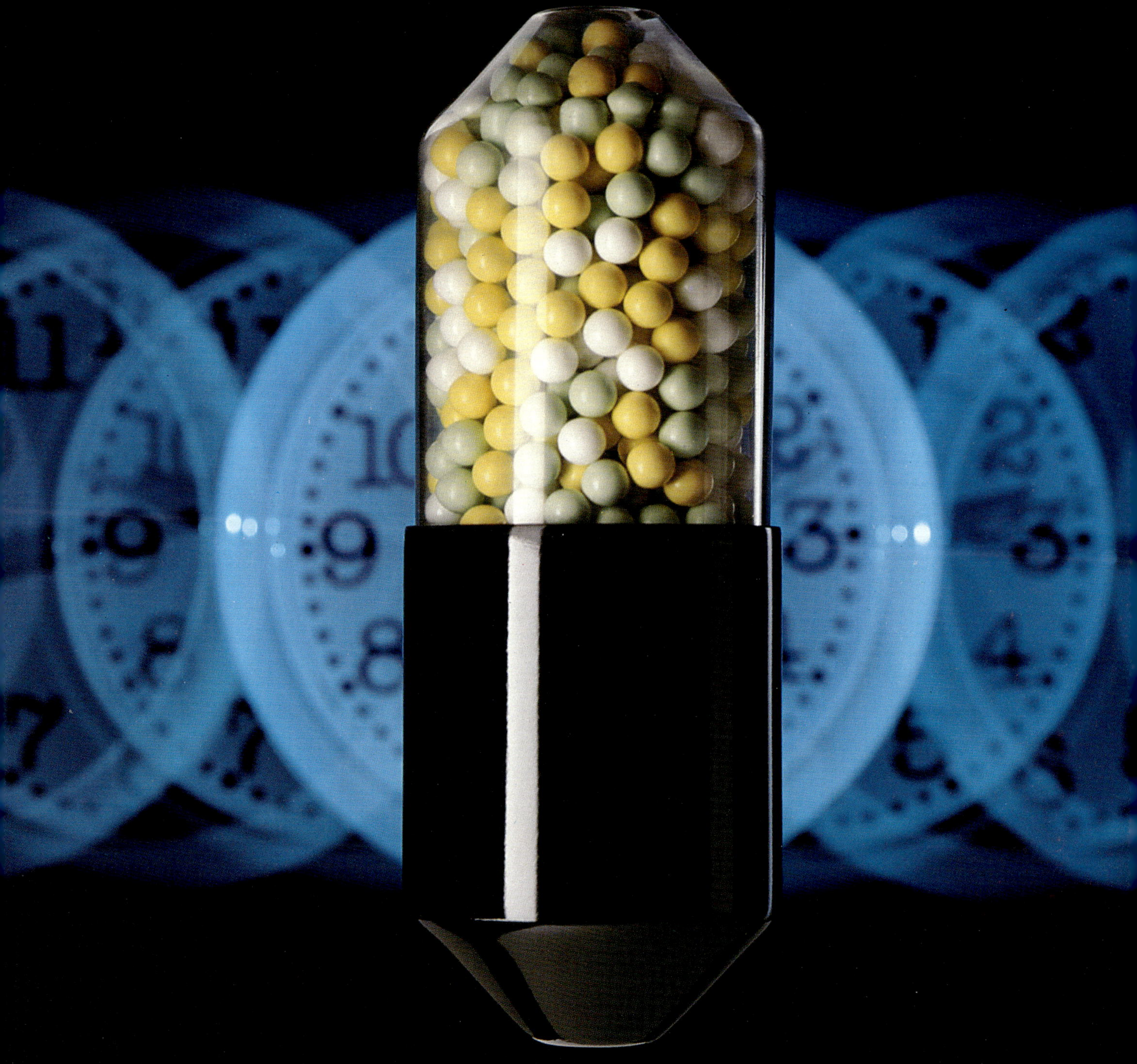

Seminars in Oncology

Breast Cancer
Part I

VOL XIII, NO 4 **DECEMBER 1986**

Table of Contents

Introduction: Breast Cancer .... *Gianni Bonadonna* 383

Minimal Breast Cancer: A Clinically Meaningful Term? .... *G. Saccani Jotti, J.Y. Petit, and G. Contesso* 384

Monoclonal Antibodies and Breast Cancer .... *Ann Thor, Maureen O. Weeks, and Jeffrey Schlom* 393

The Role of New Imaging Modalities in Staging and Follow-up of Breast Cancer *Stephen A. Feig* 402

The Clinical Investigator and the Evolution of the Treatment of Primary Breast Cancer *Paul P. Carbone and Douglass C. Tormey* 415

Conservative Surgery: The American Experience .... *Bernard Fisher and Norman Wolmark* 425

Conservative Surgery and Radiation Therapy for Early Breast Cancer: Results, Controversies, and Unsolved Problems .... *Abram Recht, James L. Connolly, Stuart J. Schnitt, Blake Cady, Susan Love, Robert T. Osteen, W. Bradford Patterson, Robert Shirley, William Silen, Steven Come, I. Craig Henderson, Barbara Silver, and Jay R. Harris* 434

Indexes 450

Seminars in Oncology

Seminars in Oncology

Vol XIII, No 1 **March 1986**

Introduction: Brain Tumors

NEOPLASMS frequently affect the nervous system. Primary tumors of the central nervous system are the second most common cancer in children, and in adults are more common than systemic Hodgkin's disease. In 1984 in the United States, there were approximately 12,000 new cases of primary central nervous system cancer, representing about 2% of the cancer "problem." Nevertheless, such patients have not been considered to be "oncology patients." They are often referred to neurosurgeons and neurologists, and initial therapy is almost always operative. The radiation therapist has then been responsible for the bulk of the remaining therapy. However, in recent years substantial numbers of patients with malignant brain tumors have been offered chemotherapy, and with the advent of chemical treatment has come increasing involvement of the community of oncological physicians in the care of these patients. This clinical interest has combined with recent developments in cellular and genetic molecular biology to foster a new scientific interest in brain tumors. A number of new discoveries about the biology of brain tumor growth have resulted. Further research has been aided by several new techniques of diagnosis and therapy that allow more direct study of patients, including positron emission tomography, magnetic resonance imaging, stereotactic laser surgery, and interstitial radiotherapy.

With this increasing interest in the biology and therapy of brain tumors, it seems highly appropriate to review some of these recent developments. By such a review, it should be possible to iterate both the state of the art for the care of such patients and the basis for hope of better care in the future.

When a patient develops systemic cancer, his body must deal with a cancer burden consisting of a population of neoplastic cells in the blood or bone marrow (leukemia) or in a solid, single mass or in multiple or metastatic masses (carcinoma or sarcoma). For the average adult, it is thought that a one-kilogram burden of systemic tumor is lethal. In contrast, a brain tumor shares its space in the skull with the brain, which already occupies 1,200 cc, and in this confined space 100 grams of tumor and surrounding edema is lethal. By the time a patient develops neurologic symptoms, the tumor is usually 30 to 60 grams in size. Low-grade neuroectodermal tumors are slow growing, with few mitoses, no necrosis, and no vascular proliferation. Malignant tumors are characterized by more rapid growth, invasiveness, frequent mitotic figures, necrosis, vascular proliferation, and endothelial hyperplasia. However, benign brain tumors that cannot be entirely excised will be lethal, and malignant brain tumors rarely metastasize out of the central nervous system. Thus, the distinction between benign and malignant is less important for intracranial tumors than for systemic cancer.

Laboratory investigations have determined that most phenotypic expressions examined in human malignant gliomas, eg, DNA content, immunology, or metabolic phenomena, are heterogeneous. In her chapter on the genetics of brain tumors, Dr Joan Rankin Shapiro reviews these investigations. She describes the heterogeneous cell types in gliomas, identified by their karyotypes, and relates abnormal numbers of specific chromosomes to several important phenotypic characteristics, including rapid growth. Such abnormal chromosomes carry genes that are involved with growth factors, growth factor receptors, and gene products of proto-oncogenes. In addition to their role in the etiology of gliomas, these factors may also be important in resistance to chemotherapeutic agents.

Dr Peter Burger argues convincingly that the three-tiered system of classifying astrocytomas used by most of the Cooperative Group studies is preferable to the four-tiered system of Kernohan because it more accurately correlates with prognosis. He also reviews the pathological findings after radiation therapy and chemotherapy, including both the nature and topography of recurrent tumor and some of the toxic changes in the brain.

Intracranial tumors differ from systemic cancers in several ways. The microenvironment of tumors in the brain, the blood-brain barrier, influences both diagnosis and therapy. The blood-brain barrier in a normal brain retards entry of many compounds, including radiologic contrast agents and chemotherapeutic agents. The blood-brain barrier appears to be intact in most low-grade neuroectodermal tumors, but it becomes progressively disrupted in malignant brain tumors. The breakdown of the barrier allows the entry of contrast agents and radioisotopes that permit the tumor to be perceived separately from the brain in scanning techniques. Both experimental and clinical studies suggest that some disruption of the barrier in malignant tumors also permits the entry of chemotherapeutic agents. It is not yet clear to what degree the blood-brain barrier breaks down, especially at the growing edge of an infiltrative malignant brain tumor or within very small brain tumors; in both circumstances, the barrier may be only minimally disrupted. A second factor that distinguishes brain tumors from systemic cancer is the absence of a lymphatic system in the brain. Fluid that accumulates from leaking capillaries within the brain tumor cannot be removed except via slow diffusion toward the cerebrospinal fluid pathways. This fluid, or cerebral edema, itself produces symptoms by adding to the mass effect of tumors. Central nervous system tumors are also distinguished from systemic cancer by the rarity with which they metastasize to the rest of the body. Instead, they tend to infiltrate within the brain, and some have a predilection to spread along cerebrospinal pathways, producing obstruction and hydrocephalus. This is especially true of medulloblastomas. Perhaps the most important difference between central nervous system neoplasms and systemic cancer is that cancer operations are not possible in the brain. Removing generous margins of normal tissue along with such visceral tumors as lung or colonic cancer interferes with normal function to only a moderate degree. On the other hand, attempting to remove normal tissue margins in a brain tumor can produce irreparable neurologic dysfunction. The surgeon removing visceral cancer operates in the surrounding normal tissue. The neurosurgeon attempting to remove a primary neuroectodermal tumor must stay within the confines of the tumor if he is to spare brain tissue. Often, he must leave tumor-infiltrated brain tissue because its removal would produce unacceptable neurologic dysfunction. Such considerations weigh heavily in the management of patients with brain tumors.

In this symposium, the section on therapy begins with a review by Dr Ransohoff and his colleagues of the diagnosis and initial surgical therapy of gliomas. They present the view that a full resection within the confines of the tumor is worthwhile. They then offer initial data on two new forms of surgical treatment, stereotactic laser surgery and hematoporphyrin/laser therapy. Dr William Shapiro then reviews data from the Brain Tumor Study/Cooperative Group on large scale clinical trials of multimodality therapy of malignant gliomas. Dr Nelson and her colleagues introduce newer forms of radiation therapy: Radiation plus radiosensitizers, hyperfractionation, heavy particles, interstitial brachytherapy, and hyperthermia plus brachytherapy. While it is too early to report results from many of these protocols, they offer conceptually exciting new therapeutic programs. Two major problems important in the chemotherapy of malignant gliomas are identified by Drs William and Joan Shapiro as heterogeneity of the tumor cells and restrictions to drug entry imposed by the blood-brain barrier. They present evidence that the small near-diploid glioma cell is probably resistant to chemotherapeutic agents, while the hyperdiploid, unstable cell is sensitive. Several new experimental approaches to these problems are presented along with a review of the characteristics of many drugs in use for brain tumors.

The complexity of blood-brain and blood-tumor barrier phenomena can now be analyzed by techniques that permit the precise measurement of capillary permeability and blood flow in submacroscopic regions of experimental animal brain tumors. The methods—quantitative autoradiography—and the implications of the results for brain tumor chemotherapy are presented by Dr Blasberg and Dr Groothuis. Modern technology also permits regional studies in humans of brain tumor metabolism, blood flow, and capillary permeability. Dr Brooks and his colleagues present some of their results using positron emission tomography, and suggest how this technique can be used to study chemotherapeutic drug entry.

Whereas immunobiology of brain tumors is one of the oldest fields in brain tumor research, the advent of monoclonal antibodies has also made it one of the newest. Immunobiology of brain tumors is treated in detail by Dr Bullard and his colleagues, who also review attempts at immunotherapy.

As noted above, the second commonest tumor in children is the brain tumor. Problems of its therapy are reviewed by Dr Allen who is joined by many of the physicians responsible for cooperative group and institutional clinical trials for this disease. Their presentation is a clear exposition of the current status of such treatment.

In organizing this symposium, I became aware of how much progress had been made in this field in the last 20 years. Because of clinical research, patients are living a little longer, usually with a better quality of life. Fundamental research has expanded rapidly, both because of the advent of new techniques in molecular genetics and because of the entry into the field of a critical mass of interested new scientists. It is the clinical and experimental researchers who offer the hope that over the next 20 years, brain tumors will become better understood and better treated. Many of these people took valuable time from their busy schedules to offer the view of the future represented by this written symposium. For this generosity, I offer my grateful thanks.

William R. Shapiro, MD
Department of Neurology
Memorial Sloan-Kettering Cancer Center
Cornell University Medical College
New York

Biology of Gliomas: Heterogeneity, Oncogenes, Growth Factors

Joan Rankin Shapiro

CANCER CELLS exhibit a vast array of phenotypes that distinguish them from their normal cellular counterparts. Although it is clear that cancer cells have altered DNA, the nature and location of the lesion amid the myriad of base sequences remain unknown. Recently, a group of genes was identified that can produce cellular transformation. They are called oncogenes and, like other genes, they code for proteins used in the cell's structure or in the regulation of its biochemistry. It appears that only a small number of oncogenes reside within the genome and that they have remained highly conserved throughout eukaryotic evolution. When such genes are activated they free the host cell from the normal constraints of cellular growth and/or differentiation, thereby directing the normal cell into malignant progression.

The first part of this paper will review the research leading to the identification of oncogenes and mechanisms of their activation. The second part will relate these findings to current investigations in human primary central nervous system tumors.

ONCOGENES AND PROTO-ONCOGENES

Within vertebrate organisms, a group of proto-oncogenes has remained highly conserved throughout evolution. If these proto-oncogenes are inappropriately expressed (oncogenes) they will induce and/or maintain a malignant state.

Two disciplines, one involving the transfer of genetic material from one cell to another (gene transfer), the second dedicated to the study of a family of RNA tumor viruses (retroviruses), identified a group of genes (oncogenes) that were capable of transforming a normal cell into a malignant cell. At first there appeared to be two sets of oncogenes; one was discovered by gene transfer methods (transfection), the other by viralogical techniques. In fact, these two groups are related; oncogenes detected by gene transfer are homologous to the transforming genes found in retroviruses. For example, the Kirsten murine sarcoma virus contains a v-onc gene (Ki-ras) that is homologous (similar base sequences) to the c-onc gene detected by transfection of DNA from human lung and colon carcinomas.[1] A second retrovirus that is related to the Kirsten strain is the Harvey murine sarcoma virus. The transforming gene of this virus, v-Ha-ras, is homologous to the c-onc gene detected in the transfection of DNA isolated from the human EJ/24 bladder carcinoma cell line.[2,3] To date, about 18 cellular proto-oncogenes have been identified[4] and only a few appear not to have a viral counterpart.

Two hypotheses have been proposed to explain the mechanisms that cause the activation of proto-oncogenes, the mutation hypothesis and the gene dosage hypothesis, although they are not mutually exclusive. Mechanisms that involve virus integration result in the amplification or over-production of the gene product. This may be accomplished when a retrovirus carrying a v-onc gene integrates in the host DNA, or by the insertion of a viral promoter and/or enhancer that turns on a c-onc gene.[4,5]

The other mechanisms do not appear to involve a virus but rather an alteration of the host DNA. Three groups of structural chromosome abnormalities are recognized in human cancer: reciprocal translocations, deletions, and duplications,[6] and each has been identified with the aberrant expression of a proto-oncogene. Since 1960, specific chromosome alterations have been described for certain malignancies,[7,8] although we have only recently begun to explore their probable meaning at the molecular level.[9] Burkitt's lymphoma involves a specific non-random chromosomal change, usually involving the translocation of a portion of human chromosome 8 to chromosome 14. Variant forms have also been identified that involve chromosome 8 translocated to chromosomes 2 or 22.[10–13] Klein hypothesized that in Burkitt's lymphoma a normal c-myc gene (chromosome 8) is translocated

From the George C. Cotzias Laboratory of Neuro-Oncology, Department of Neurology, Memorial Sloan-Kettering Cancer Center, Cornell University Medical College, New York.

Address reprint requests to Joan Rankin Shapiro, PhD, Department of Neurology, Memorial Sloan-Kettering Cancer Center, 1275 York Ave, New York, NY 10021.

0093–7754/86/1301–0002$05.00/0

into the chromosome region of a transcriptionally active immunoglobulin gene (heavy chain genes chromosome 14, kappa light chains chromosome 2, and lambda light chains chromosome 22) whose promoter now controls the transcription of c-myc.[9] The gene product is functionally normal but its expression is altered.

Deletions and duplications can include whole chromosomes, segments of chromosomes, or individual genes. Deletions involving small portions of a chromosome are features of several tumors that occur primarily in children and young adults. These include retinoblastoma,[14] Wilms' tumor[15] and neuroblastoma.[16] It is presumed that deletions found in these tumors remove normal control mechanisms placed on proto-oncogenes, thus promoting the malignant phenotype.[12,13] Cloning the breakpoints of such translocated chromosomes should provide information on the rearrangement of DNA base sequences by techniques similar to those used to study the translocation involving chromosomes 14 and 18.[17]

Duplications of genes are frequently reported in the form of homogeneous staining regions (HSRs) and double minutes (DMs), both in long term lines and freshly resected material.[18] These features are associated with amplification of a c-onc gene,[19-21] although the mechanisms involved in their activation and how they initiate the transformation phenotype are unknown.

The loss or gain of chromosomes during cell division (segregational errors) are one of several mechanisms that produce the aneuploid chromosomal complements associated with malignant cells. The role of numerical abnormalities in the amplification of onc gene products is the least understood aspect of the gene dosage hypothesis. Evidence to support chromosome ploidy as a form of gene amplification comes from investigations using somatic cell genetics in which a normal cell is fused with a tumor cell to form a hybrid cell.[22-24] In these studies the malignant phenotype appears to act as a recessive trait in that the hybrid cell is usually not malignant unless either there are too many "malignant" genes or too few "normal" genes. When the chromosomes' coding for the malignant phenotype are overrepresented, the hybrid cell becomes malignant.[22] Presumably the addition of these extra recessive genes permits the malignant phenotype to override the normal constraints placed on these genes. When the chromosomes coding for the normal phenotype are lost, the hybrid cell also becomes malignant.[24] In these hybrids the expression of the malignant phenotype is thought to occur because chromosomes that have the ability to suppress these genes are lost.

Recently, investigations on human tumor cells suggest that the ploidy of a given chromosome may also be a form of gene amplification. Alitalo et al[25] demonstrated in a colon carcinoma cell line that the overrepresentation of a marker chromosome was associated with a 10-fold increase in c-myb expression. The amplification of c-myb has not been found in other colon carcinoma lines and therefore is not an oncogene normally amplified in this tumor.

Alterations in DNA can also occur by point mutation (a single base sequence change), which then lead to the synthesis of an abnormal polypeptide. The ras gene family was identified in several human carcinomas, sarcomas and some hematopoietic malignancies.[1-3,26-34] In each of the malignancies where the base sequence of the ras gene was analyzed, a mutation occurred in only two positions of the polypeptide, amino acid residues 12 and 61, suggesting that there are "hot spots" in the ras coding region.[26] How such alterations change the conformation of the protein from its normal function remains to be determined.

ONCOGENES AND MALIGNANCY AS A MULTISTEP PROCESS

Despite the growing evidence that oncogenes are involved in cellular transformation, a direct role is difficult to assign, in part because transformation (spontaneous or induced) is a multistep process requiring both initiation and promotion.[35] Cellular transformation, induced by a ras gene, however, appears to be a single event.[4] This apparent discrepancy may be due to the type of cells used in the transfection assay, specifically the NIH 3T3 mouse fibroblast cells. These cells are not normal although they possess certain normal cellular phenotypes, eg, contact inhibition. They will, however, form spontaneous malignant colonies, suggesting that they are already primed (initiated) and a single event such as the introduction of an activated oncogene (ras) could promote cellular transformation. Therefore, the introduction of an oncogene may represent one step in a multistep process, since normal diploid cells cannot be transformed by ras alone.[4]

In support of this hypothesis, several recent investigations demonstrated that oncogenes work in concert with one another to produce the transformed phenotype.[36] The earliest work to suggest this possibility was that of Cooper and Neiman, who demonstrated that transformation of fibroblasts required two oncogenes; the activated myc gene could not by itself transform these cells.[37] They identified the transforming gene by the transfection assay and discovered that it belonged to a new family of oncogenes they designated as B-lym. Since then, other studies demonstrated that co-transfection of several oncogenes is required for transformation of normal primary cells. Further, transformation can also occur from the co-transfection of two RNA retroviruses[34,38–41] or a DNA and an RNA virus.[42]

Emerging with these investigations on cooperativity of oncogenes is the concept that some genes immortalize cells while others confer tumorigenic properties, and together they produce the transformed phenotype.[41] Genes that fall into one or the other complementation groups may share a number of similarities as to structure (base sequence) and/or location within the cell,[4,32,43] suggesting that some oncogenes transform cells via a common pathway.

ONCOGENES AND GLIOMAS

To date, most brain tumor research has focused on phenotypic differences between normal and malignant glia[44]; only recently have investigations begun to detail events at the genotypic level. The previous discussion dealt with the discovery of oncogenes and their role in the multistep process of tumorigenesis. Exactly how oncogenes implement the transformation phenotype is still incompletely known, although some are known to be involved with two key cellular functions, phosphorylation and cell proliferation. In the following discussion we shall review some of the laboratory investigations on gliomas, which implicate several oncogenes in the initiation of uncontrolled cell growth.

It is evident that malignant gliomas are heterogeneous, and that such heterogeneity is complex.[45] It can occur at the cellular level in which two neighboring cells within the same region are different, eg, large nucleated cell *v* a small nucleated cell, or it can occur as a regional phenomenon in which two distant areas of the tumor differ[46] (Figs 1–5). Histopathologically, glioblastomas are described as heterogeneous, ie, pleomorphic with many diverse cell types.[47] Proliferative fields of cells are intermingled amid giant multinucleated cells or cells with various sized nuclei and/or cytoplasmic contents. Still other features, eg, vascularization, necrosis, and satellitosis, add to the tumor's complex pattern. The question is, how does this heterogeneity affect the behavior of the tumor?

There are many ways to approach the analysis of cellular heterogeneity. One approach is cytogenetic analysis of the chromosomal complement of tumor cells. The metaphase chromosomes are

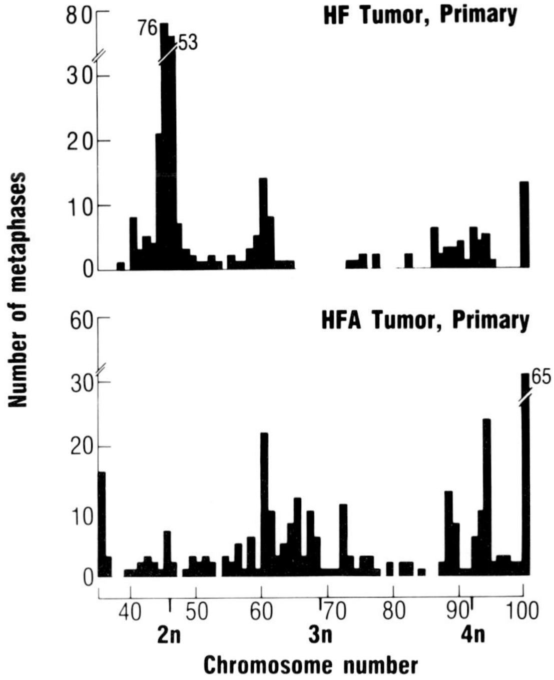

Fig 1. The two histograms HF and HFA illustrate the distribution of chromosome numbers found in metaphase cells. The freshly resected glioblastoma tumor was removed from a female patient and was dissected into two regions at the interface of what appeared grossly to be normal cortex (HF) adjacent to tumor (HFA). Each region was dissociated into a pool of single cells and subjected to cytogenetic analysis within 72 hours post-plating.[56] Over two hundred cells were counted for each region. Region HF was predominantly near-diploid (2n) in chromosome number while region HFA was primarily hyperdiploid with the majority of cells having triploid (3n) and tetraploid (4n) chromosomal complements.

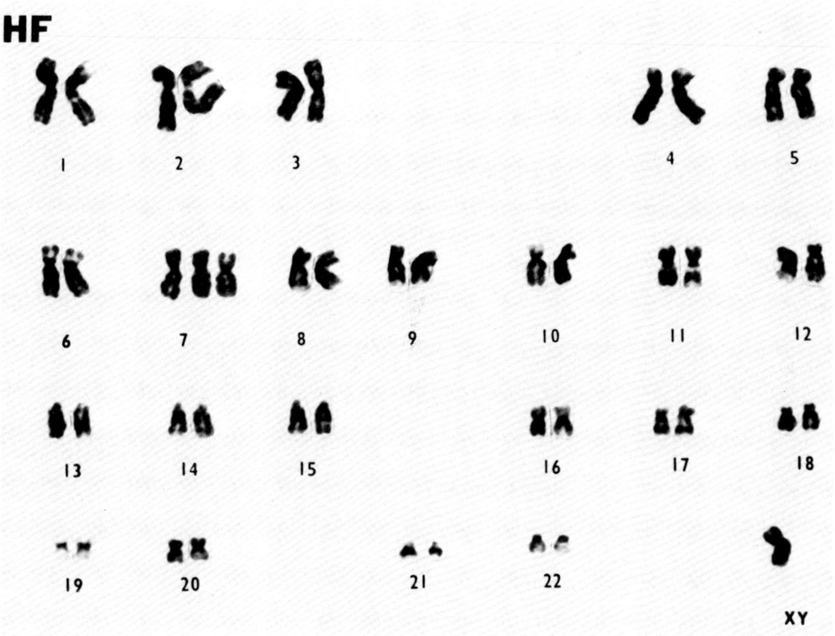

Fig 2. A metaphase cell prepared from the suspension cultures of the HF region. This karyotype contains 46 chromosomes and is representative of tumors that are primarily near-diploid in chromosome number. It is monosomic for a sex chromosome and trisomic for chromosome 7. The Giemsa bands (G-Bands) appear normal for all chromosomes. X1,100.

collected and arranged into a karyotype that can be likened to a "fingerprint" of the genomic content of each cell. The chromosome number and rearrangements of chromosomes in the karyotype (translocations, deletions, and duplications) are important elements in such an analysis. The karyotype is also a marker that can be used to follow malignant evolution, with each analysis being a window at some point in the malignant progression. Chromosomal diversity of freshly resected gliomas was recognized before chromosome banding was possible.[48–52] Stem lines and sidelines found in each tumor were delineated by modal chromosome number and/

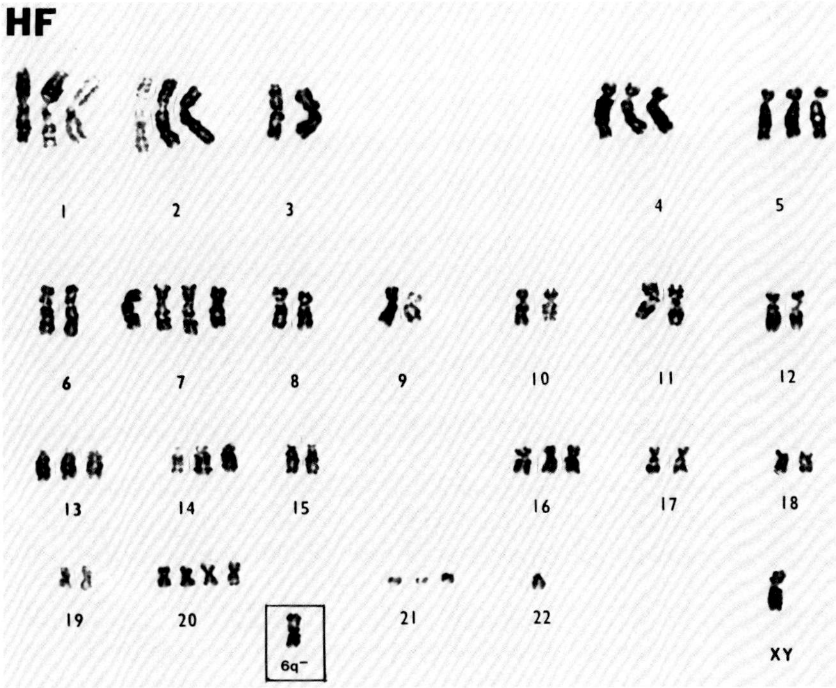

Fig 3. A metaphase cell prepared from the suspension cultures of the HF region. This karyotype contains 56 chromosomes with normal G-bands and one marker chromosome designated 6q- in which the lower portion of the q arm is deleted (enclosed area). The 6q-deletion was the only marker chromosome seen more than once and therefore represents a clonal subpopulation within this region. Cells carrying marker chromosomes represented less than 2% of the total cells analyzed in this region. In addition to the marker chromosome this cell has undergone numerous segregational errors; chromosomes 7 and 20 are tetrasomic, chromosomes 1, 2, 4, 5, 13, 14, 16, and 21 are trisomic and chromosomes 22 and the sex chromosome are monosomic.

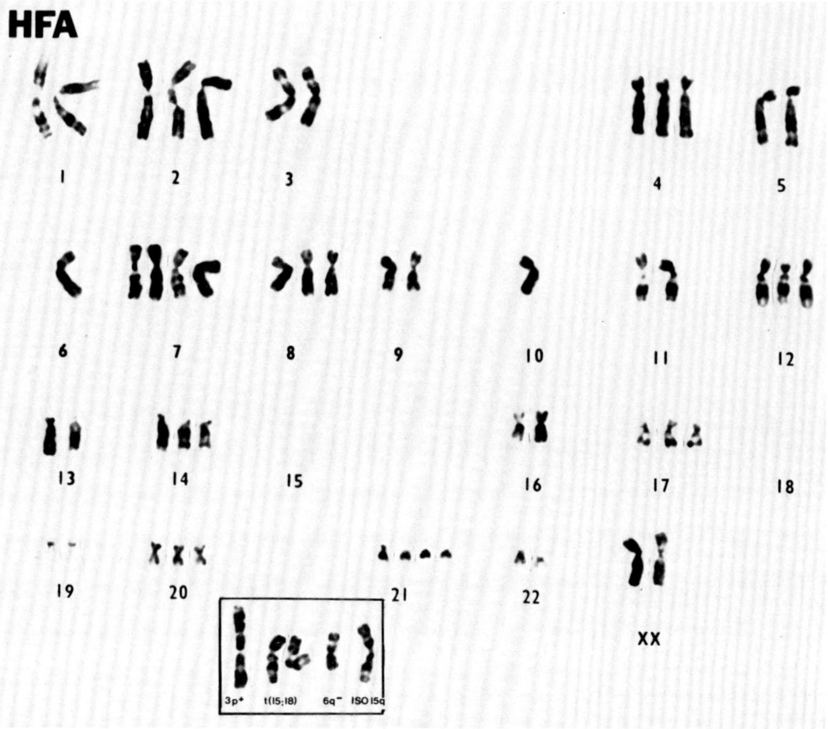

Fig 4. This karyotype was prepared from the suspension cultures of the HFA region. It is a cell with 56 chromosomes, five of which are marker chromosomes (enclosure). This cell is representative of this region in that several markers were found in most of the metaphases analyzed. One marker (6q-) is identical to the marker in Fig 3 and suggests that some of the cells from this clonal subpopulation have undergone additional karyotypic evolution. Chromosomes 15 and 18 are now represented as a translocation chromosome, t(15;18) and chromosome 3 has additional chromatin added to the p arm (3p+), and chromosome 6 has split horizontally at the centromere to form an isochromosome, i(6p).

or aberrant marker chromosomes.[52,53] With advances in chromosome banding techniques, a greater resolution of each metaphase chromosome was possible. Using these techniques, several studies confirmed and elaborated on the extensive heterogeneity characteristic of malignant gliomas.[54–60]

We have previously discussed the relationship between abnormal chromosome structure and/or number and the activation of proto-oncogenes. To datc, a single structural rearrangement has not been identified in any of the primary cytogenetic analyses of human gliomas,[54–60] suggesting that this is a secondary event in the evolution of this tumor system. There are, however, a specific pattern of chromosome gains and losses found in both astrocytomas and malignant gliomas.[61] These non-random karyotypic changes are best illustrated by our recent analysis of eight astrocytomas.[62] The chromosome data support the histopathological findings of the relative homogeneity of the low-grade astrocytoma compared to the glioblastoma multiforme.[47] Most of the cells contained near-diploid chromosome numbers (42–50 chromosomes/metaphase). Structural chromosome rearrangements occurred in less than 1% to 2% of the cells analyzed; they were usually present in only one karyotype and were therefore not a clonal subpopulation of the tumor. The most common karyotypic feature was the loss or gain of chromosomes, but many karyotypes had a normal 46 G-banded pattern. Whether these cells were normal reactive astrocytes or tumor cells with DNA lesions undetectable by this type of analysis, remains to be determined. Investigations in human breast cancer suggest that many normal G-banded cells in mammary tumors are not normal and exhibit invasive properties in the appropriate assay.[63,64] The most consistent feature in our study[62] and those reported by others,[54,55,58] was a cellular subpopulation containing 45 chromosomes, in which a single sex chromosome (the x in the female and the y in the male) was missing. In five of eight tumors from our study, there was a second cell population with 45 chromosomes that was missing chromosomes 22 and a sex chromosome but was trisomic for chromosome 7. All eight of these tumors had a small proportion of hyperdiploid cells (57 to several hundred chromosomes/metaphase). These cells appeared to originate by endoreduplication[59] since most chromosome numbers were represented by four homologues. Although random chromosome loss

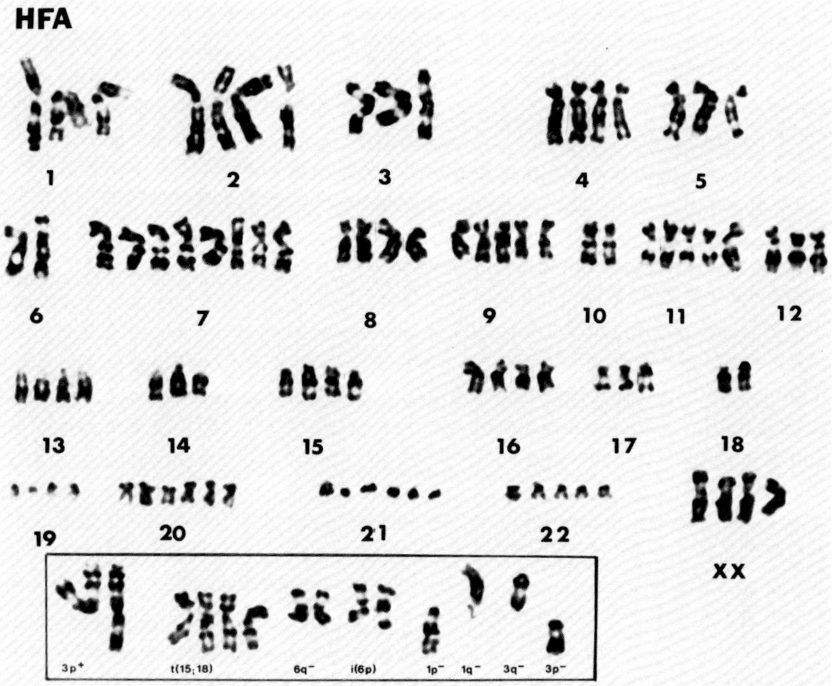

Fig 5. A karyotype of a metaphase cell with 106 chromosomes, which was obtained from the short-term cultures of the HFA region. This cell may have arisen by endoreduplication because four of the eight marker chromosomes are duplicated. In addition to the four markers seen in Fig 4, chromosomes 1 and 3 have other rearrangements involving the loss of either the p or q arm of the chromosomes. One chromosome is notably overrepresented (chromosome 7), which is typical of cells in advanced stages of karyotypic evolution. Regions containing cells with hyperploidy of chromosome 7 may in fact represent the areas that have amplified levels of receptor kinase activity,[104,105] while regions of a tumor such as seen in Fig 2 will have near-normal activity.

for any one chromosome number was high in this group of cells, chromosome 22 and one sex chromosome continued to be underrepresented.

In comparison to these findings in astrocytomas, cytogenetic analysis of most high-grade tumors demonstrates extensive heterogeneity with numerous subpopulations and isolated cell types.[56,60] There is both a greater range of chromosome numbers (35 to 200 chromosomes/metaphase) and more chromosome rearrangement than in low-grade tumors. In addition to aberrant chromosome numbers, high-grade tumors have one to five marker chromosomes/metaphase and such cells may represent more than 50% of the total cells analyzed. However, the pattern of gain and loss is similar to that in low grade tumors; chromosome 7 is overrepresented and chromosome 22 and the sex chromosome are underrepresented. Thus, there appears to be a link between astrocytomas and malignant gliomas and the difference between the two groups is the additional chromosome involvement in the high-grade tumors. For example, in our study, there was an overrepresentation of chromosomes 1 and 20 and an underrepresentation of chromosomes 10 and 19 in high-grade tumors.[60]

Occasionally, tumor biopsies classified as high-grade malignant gliomas demonstrated few chromosome abnormalities in their karyotypes. Such karyotypes had chromosomal complements similar to those found in low-grade tumors. One possible explanation for this discrepancy is that the surgical specimen represented only a part of the tumor and that regions elsewhere might show greater chromosomal abnormalities. Figure 1 illustrates the distribution of tumor cells, by chromosome number, in two different regions of the same tumor. Figures 2–5 illustrate the karyotypic differences and evolution of cell types in these two regions. Several studies such as those depicted in this set of figures led to our study of regional heterogeneity in gliomas that confirmed this hypothesis.[47] Cytogenetic results from one low-grade astrocytoma and three glioblastomas multiforme resected almost in toto demonstrated karyotypic homogeneity in the low-grade tumor and regional heterogeneity in the malignant gliomas. The low-grade astrocytoma was relatively homogeneous with each region composed of near-diploid (2n) cells in which the sex chromosome was the most frequently missing chromosome in all regions. Chromosomes 7, 20, and 22 were diploid for most karyotypes except for one region. In this region, many of the cells were monosomic for chromosome 22 and trisomic or tetrasomic for chromosome 7; chromosome 20 was diploid in about half of the cells in this region and triploid in the other half. In two of the three glioblastomas multiforme, distinct differences occurred among the regions. In general, regions adjacent to each other had cells with similar karyotypic patterns and marker chromosomes, but regions distant from each other contained cells with different chromosome numbers and different marker chromosomes. The third tumor had karyotypic characteristics of both low- and high-grade gliomas. Two regions were primarily near-diploid in chromosome number (45,XO cells missing a y chromosome). A third region contained both a near-diploid population and a hyperdiploid population (3n to 4n chromosome numbers). A small proportion of the near-diploid cells was only monosomic for the sex chromosome, but the majority was trisomic for chromosomes 1, 7, and 20, and monosomic for 10, 22, and the sex chromosome. A fourth region contained mostly 46,Xy normal G-banded karyotypes and a small representation of cells with a chromosome number of 45 or less.

Regional examination of gliomas emphasizes several aspects of this tumor. The first is that regional heterogeneity is a consistent finding in glioblastoma multiforme and many of these regions are quite different from each other. Second, near-diploid cell populations may be found in some malignant gliomas; their karyotypes may be similar to those found in low-grade tumors, but other regions usually contain morc abnormal karyotypic patterns. Third, specific chromosome patterns of over- or underrepresentation do not occur in every region, but may be seen when the entire tumor specimen is examined. The pattern of chromosome abnormalities that we observed in gliomas, including overrepresentation of chromosome 7 and underrepresentation of chromosome 22, is similar to that demonstrated in other neoplasms. Such findings are consistent with Mitelman's hypothesis[65] that only a few chromosomes are likely to be involved in the neoplastic process.

The mechanisms by which abnormalities of chromosomes 7 and 22 relate to glial malignancies may reside in the proto-oncogenes mapped to these chromosomes: c-erb-B to chromosome 7[66,67] and c-sis to chromosome 22.[68,69] Several lines of investigation support such a hypothesis. The first observation identified the two receptors, the platelet-derived growth factor (PDGF) receptor and epidermal growth factor (EGF) receptor, on both normal glia and glioma cells.[70–72] The second was the discovery that the proto-oncogene sis (c-sis) encodes for one of the polypeptides of PDGF[73–76] and the proto-oncogene c-erb-B encodes for 3 of the 4 domains of EGF receptor.[77] Both of these proto-oncogenes are directly involved in stimulating cell division in normal glial cells; the c-sis gene product by virtue of binding to the PDGF receptor and the c-erb-B gene product which is a truncated form of the EGF receptor. Each of these receptors has a cytoplasmic protein kinase domain that is responsible for the phosphorylation of cellular proteins, which in itself is an important factor in gene regulation.[78]

The sis gene was first known as a viral transforming gene (v-sis) of the Simian Sarcoma Virus (SSV),[79] then later found to be derived from a closely related cellular gene (c-sis) that produced PDGF.[73–75] The protein encoded by v-sis in malignant or SSV transformed cells is called p28. This processed molecule is both structurally and immunologically similar to cellular (c-sis) PDGF.[76] More recently, the viral gene product was found to be secreted into the culture medium in a biologically active form, and its properties were identical to cellular PDGF,[80] suggesting that the gene products of both v-sis and c-sis behave similarly in the way they transform cells.

Because most human solid tumors are not associated with viruses, the amplification of sis-related mRNAs in solid tumors (some of which were gliomas),[81] suggests that these proto-oncogenes were activated. Conditioned medium and cell lysates prepared from several human tumor cells lines demonstrated a PDGF-like polypeptide that was capable of inducing DNA synthesis in a manner identical to that of human PDGF.[82–88] Although we do not know what activates this proto-oncogene, once it is activated it has the ability to transform normal cells in culture.[89]

Growth factors circulate as normal components of blood serum. They are potent mitogens that bind to their respective cell-surface receptors. The message is internalized, stimulating DNA synthesis and finally cell division. The intracellular pathways are not well defined and many cellular proteins involved in this pathway are uncharacterized.[90] Temin recognized that in comparison to normal cells, the requirement for serum supplement in tumor cell cultures was substantially reduced.[91] Sporn and Todaro identified tumor cells that produced a growth factor to which the cell itself was responsive.[92] This observation led them to propose the autocrine growth stimulation model of tumor cell proliferation. Investigations on cell lines whose growth appears to be auto-regulatory offer clues as to how the gene product of v-sis or c-sis can initiate the transformation of normal cells. Tumor lines from several different sarcomas and gliomas[82–88,93] secrete a PDGF or PDGF-like molecule and appear to be autocrine tumor systems. These investigations have been hampered because cell lines known to secret PDGF-like molecules often lack or have reduced numbers of receptors on producer cells.[93] Betsholtz and coworkers attempted to circumvent this problem by isolating a clone of the osteosarcoma line U-2 that produced low levels of PDGF-like molecule while also expressing functional PDGF receptors.[86] Exogenously added PDGF antibodies did not suppress the complete growth of these cells, as would be expected if the plasma membrane were the only site of interaction between the endogenously produced molecule and the PDGF receptor. The authors suggested several reasons for these results: (1) the autocrine model does not apply to this aberrant growth factor synthesis, (2) the compartmentalization of the receptor sequestered it from the effects of the antibody, (3) the PDGF-like molecules are secreted close to the receptor minimizing diffusion and therefore inhibition by antibody, or (4) the PDGF-like molecule and receptor were allowed to interact during the secretory process, thereby eliminating the need for PDGF-like molecules to be secreted.

Glioma lines that secrete a PDGF molecule or a PDGF-like molecule were described by several groups.[84,85,87,88,94] Nister reported[85,87] the secretion of a PDGF-like molecule in a clonal isolate of a long-term glioma cell line U-343. The secreted molecule was structurally and immunologically related to PDGF and was capable of stimulating DNA synthesis. In a commentary on PDGF, Antoniades[94] alluded to as yet unpublished work demonstrating the production of a PDGF-like molecule by human gliomas. Neither of these studies however, implied that either chromosome rearrangement or ploidy of chromosome 22 was present in the cells they examined.

In our laboratory hyperploidy of chromosome 22 was associated with the PDGF or PDGF-like expression of the molecule.[88] In the development of several BCNU drug resistant lines, the overrepresentation of chromosome 22 was correlated with the stimulation of DNA synthesis using cell lysates and conditioned medium prepared from these drug treated cells. The DNA stimulation was limited only to cells that had PDGF receptors (normal glia, human fibroblasts, and NIH 3T3 cells), while no such stimulatory activity was observed in PDGF receptor-negative cells (epithelial-derived cells). Parallel cultures of normal glia and controls showed no stimulation of DNA synthesis above or equal to that produced by 20% fetal calf serum. Further, the cells that emerged in the drug resistant lines were similar in karyotype to a small population of cells found in the primary cytogenetic analysis of the freshly resected tumors.

The second proto-oncogene of importance in gliomas is the amplification of the c-erb-B gene encoding a truncated form of the EGF receptor. The transforming protein (v-erb-B) of avian erythroblastosis virus (AEV)[95] induces erythroid leukemia and sarcoma in chickens, and is enhanced by another gene in the viral genome called v-erb-A. In normal human cells the EGF receptor is a 170 kilodalton glycoprotein with four domains, an external EGF binding domain and a transmembrane domain that links two cytoplasmic domains.[96,97] The cytoplasmic domains are important in phosphorylating intracellular proteins, specifically on the tyrosine residue.[97,98] The product of the c-erb-B gene is a truncated form of this molecule. The role that this alteration plays in the function of the receptor and the amplification of the receptor kinase activity is not yet known.[99–101] Several investigations on different human tumor lines are now helping to provide that information.

In the human epidermoid carcinoma line A431, an excessive number of EGF receptors was identified on the cell surface.[99–101] Only low concentrations of the growth factor ligand, EGF, are needed to stimulate proliferation, while EGF concentrations that are mitogenic for many other tumor cell lines actually inhibit A431 cells.[102,103] In general, and dependent upon the A431 clone being analyzed, the expression of the c-erb-B gene at the mRNA level seems to correlate with the amplified EGF receptor.[99–101] However, this tumor is a long-term line and may possess characteristics that are unique. In this respect, the findings of Libermann and coworkers[104,105] are extremely important. These investigators demonstrated that four of ten freshly resected human glioma tumors all had amplified EGF receptor kinase activity similar to the amplified levels found in the A431 tumor. Receptor kinase activity measured in oligodendrogliomas, meningiomas, and autopsed brain specimens was not amplified. It is also possible that the failure to find amplified receptor kinase activity in the other six gliomas was attributed to the regional differences described previously.

Of further interest are mitogens secreted by some virally transformed lines and human tumor lines that compete for the EGF receptor. These factors identified as alpha- and beta-transforming growth factor (alpha- and beta-TGFs) are synergistic with EGF.[106] This might explain why some conditioned medias from transformed cells are so mitogenic to non-transformed cells. More importantly, gene products like the TGFs and those yet uncharacterized may have mitogenic roles within the intracellular milieu.

The number of EGF receptors and the overrepresentation and rearrangement of chromosome 7 in the A431 suggests they are involved in the amplification of this receptor.[67] It is also possible that the abnormal chromosome patterns in gliomas involving chromosomes 7 (carrying c-erb-B) and 22 (carrying c-sis) are directly involved in the malignant process. For chromosome 7, the overrepresentation is consistent with gene amplification. For c-sis there is an apparent contradiction in the underrepresentation of chromosome 22 and the amplification of the PDGF or PDGF-like product. It is possible that chromosome 22 is not completely deleted, but is involved in a yet undetected translocation. Such a translocated chromosome in which c-sis is involved might explain how the PDGF molecule could be altered from that of the normal gene product of c-sis, and/or be removed from the cells' normal constraints governing the expression of the gene. The breaking and reinsertion of DNA can alter the normal base sequence arrangement and/or place the gene under the control of another actively transcribing gene such as Klein proposed for the activation of the c-myc gene in Burkitt's lymphoma.[9]

One important therapeutic question relating to oncogenes is whether their products can be potential therapeutic targets. The drug resistance studies suggest this could be a possibility. In our studies BCNU killed the majority of hyperdiploid cells, leaving only the near-diploid resistant population.[107] If the near-diploid cell population that remained is amplified for chromosome 22, both its growth factor product and/or growth factor receptor could be blocked. Such a therapeutic modality is an appropriate target for future research.

CONCLUSION

Much work remains, but this is an era when we are now beginning to understand cancer at the molecular level. There are several known links between oncogenes and tumorigenesis. The genes described above give rise to products that are crucial in the control of cell growth and differentiation. In some transformed cells the products of these oncogenes are similar if not identical to the normal cellular gene product, while in others they are aberrant. In either case the overproduction of a normal gene product or of its mutant form means that normal cells can be transformed into malignant cells. This also produces targets for new therapeutic approaches when the detailed knowledge of both their structure and function are known.

REFERENCES

1. Der C, Krontiris T, Cooper GM: Transforming genes of human bladder and lung carcinomas are homologous to the ras genes of Harvey and Kirsten sarcoma viruses. Proc Natl Acad Sci USA 79:3637–3640, 1982

2. Parada LF, Tabin CJ, Shih C, et al: Human EJ bladder carcinoma oncogene is homologous to Harvey sarcoma virus ras gene. Nature 297:474–478, 1982

3. Santas E, Tronick S, Aaronson SA, et al: T24 human bladder carcinoma oncogene is an activated form of the normal human homologue of Balb- and Harvey-MSV transforming genes. Nature 298:343–347, 1982

4. Land H, Parada LF, Weinberg RA: Cellular oncogenes and multistep carcinogenesis. Science 222:771–778, 1983

5. Payne GS, Bishop JM, Varmus HE: Multiple arrange-

ments of viral DNA and an activated host oncogene in bursal lymphomas. Nature 295:209–214, 1982

6. Gilbert F: Chromosomes, genes and cancer: A classification of chromosome abnormalities in cancer. J Natl Cancer Inst 71:107–1114, 1983

7. Nowell PC, Hungerford DA: A minute chromosome in human chronic granulocytic leukemia. Science 132:1497, 1960

8. Sandberg AA: The Chromosomes in Human Cancer and Leukemia, New York, Elsevier, 1980

9. Klein G: Specific chromosomal translocations and the genesis of B-cell–derived tumors in mice and men. Cell 32:311–315, 1983

10. Manolor G, Manolova Y: Marker bands in one chromosome 14 from Burkitt lymphoma. Nature 237:33–34, 1972

11. Lenoir GM, Preud'homme JL, Bernheim A, et al: Correlation between immunoglobulin light chain expression and variant translocation in Burkitts lymphoma. Nature 298:474–476, 1982

12. Rowley JD: Human oncogene locations and chromosome aberrations. Nature 301:290–291, 1983

13. Yunis JJ: The chromosomal basis of human neoplasia. Science 221:227–236, 1983

14. Balaban G, Gilbert F, Nichols W, et al: Abnormalities of chromosome 13 in retinoblastomas from individuals with normal constitutional karyotypes. Cancer Genet Cytogenet 6:213–221, 1982

15. Riccardi VM, Sujansky E, Smith AC, et al: Chromosomal imbalance in aniridia-Wilms' tumor association. Pediatrics 61:604–610, 1978

16. Gilbert F, Feder M, Balaban G, et al: Human neuroblastomas and abnormalities of chromosomes 1 and 17. Cancer Res 44:5444–5449, 1984

17. Tsujimoto Y, Finger LR, Yunis J, et al: Cloning of the chromosome breakpoint of neoplastic B cell with the t(14;18) chromosome translocation. Science 226:1097–1099, 1984

18. Cowell JK: Double minutes and homogeneously staining regions: Gene amplification in mammalian cells. Annu Rev Genet 16:21–60, 1982

19. Alitalo K, Schwab M, Lin CC, et al: Homogeneously staining chromosomal regions contain amplified copies of an abundantly expressed cellular oncogene (c-myc) in malignant neuroendocrine cells from a human. Proc Natl Acad Sci USA 80:1701–1711, 1983

20. Kohl NE, Kanda N, Schreck RR, et al: Transposition and amplification of oncogene-related sequences in human neuroblastomas. Cell 35:359–367, 1983

21. Schwab M, Alitalo K, Kempnauer KH, et al: Amplified DNA domain with limited homology to the myc cellular oncogenes is shared by human neuroblastoma cell lines and a human neuroblastoma tumor. Nature 305:245–248, 1983

22. Klein G: The role of gene dosage and genetic transpositions in carcinogenesis. Nature 294:313–318, 1981

23. Rowley JD: Mapping of human chromosomal regions related to neoplasia: evidence from chromosome 1 and 17. Proc Natl Acad Sci USA 74:5729–5733, 1977

24. Benedict WF, Weissman BE, Mark C, et al: Tumorigenicity of human HT 1080 fibrosarcoma X normal fibroblast hybrids: chromosome dosage dependency. Cancer Res 44:3471–3479, 1984

25. Alitalo K, Winguist R, Lin CC, et al: Aberrant expression of amplified c-myb oncogene in two cell lines from a colon carcinoma. Proc Natl Acad Sci USA 81:4534–4538, 1984

26. Yuasa Y, Gol RA, Chang A, et al: Mechanism of activation of an N-ras oncogene of SW-1271 human lung carcinoma cells. Proc Natl Acad Sci USA 81:3670–3674, 1984

27. Goldfarb M, Shimizu K, Perucho M, Wigler M: Isolation and preliminary characterization of a human transforming gene from T24 bladder carcinoma cells. Nature 296:404–409, 1982

28. Shih C, Weinberg RA: Isolation of a transforming sequence from a human bladder carcinoma cell line. Cell 29:161–169, 1982

29. Pulciani S, Santos E, Lauver AV, et al: Oncogenes in solid human tumors. Nature 300:539–542, 1982

30. Eva A, Tronick SR, Gol RA, et al: Transforming genes of human hematopoietic tumors: Frequent detection of ras-related oncogenes whose activation appears to be independent of tumor phenotype. Proc Natl Acad Sci USA 80:4926–4930, 1983

31. Shimizu K, Goldfarb M, Perucho M, et al: Isolation and preliminary characterization of the transforming gene of a human neuroblastoma cell line. Proc Natl Acad Sci USA 80:383–387, 1983

32. Shimizu K, Goldfarb M, Suard Y, et al: Three human transforming genes are related to the viral ras oncogenes. Proc Natl Acad Sci USA 80:2112–2116, 1983

33. Hall A, Marshall CJ, Spurr NK, et al: Identification of the transforming gene in two human sarcoma cell lines as new member of the ras gene family located on chromosome 1. Nature 303:396–400, 1983

34. Murray MJ, Cunningham JM, Parada LF, et al: The HL-60 transforming sequence: A ras oncogene coexisting with altered myc genes in hematopoietic tumors. Cell 33:749–757, 1983

35. Farber E: The multistep nature of cancer development. Cancer Res 44:4217–4223, 1984

36. Assoian RK, Grotendorst GR, Miller DM: Cellular transformation by coordinated action of three peptide growth factors from human platelets. Nature 309:804–806, 1984

37. Cooper GM, Neiman PE: Two distinct candidate transforming genes of lymphoid leukosis virus-induced neoplasms. Nature 292:857–858, 1981

38. Land H, Parada LF, Weinberg RA: Tumorigenic conversion of primary embryo fibroblasts requires at least two cooperating oncogenes. Nature 304:596–602, 1983

39. Eliyahu D, Raz A, Gruss P, et al: Participation of p53 cellular tumor antigen in transformation of normal embryonic cells. Nature 312:646–649, 1984

40. Parada LF, Land H, Weinberg RA, et al: Cooperation between gene encoding p53 tumour antigen and ras in cellular transformation. Nature 312:649–651, 1984

41. Jenkins JR, Rudge K, Currie GA: Cellular immortalization by a cDNA clone encoding the transformation-associated phosphoprotein p53. Nature 312:651–654, 1984

42. Ruley HE: Adenovirus early region 1A enables viral and cellular transforming genes to transform primary cells in culture. Nature 304:602–606, 1983

43. Ralston R, Bishop JM: The protein products of the

myc and myb oncogenes and adenovirus Ela are structurally related. Nature 306:803–806, 1984

44. Ponten J, Westermark B: Properties of human malignant glioma cells in vitro. Medical Biology 56:184–193, 1978

45. Bigner DD: Biology of gliomas: Potential clinical implications of glioma cellular heterogeneity. Neurosurgery 9:320–326, 1981

46. Shapiro JR, Pu P-Y, Mohamed AN, et al: Regional heterogeneity in high grade gliomas. Proc Amer Assn Cancer Res 25:375, 1984

47. Rubinstein LJ: Current concepts in neuro-oncology, in Thomas RA, Green JR (eds): Advances in Neurology. New York, Raven, 1976, pp 1–25

48. Bicknell JM: Chromosome studies of human brain tumors. Neurology 17:485–490, 1967

49. Lubs HA, Salmon JH: The chromosomal complement of human solid tumors II. Karyotypes of glial tumors. J Neurosurg 23:160–168, 1965

50. Hansteen I-L: Chromosome studies in glial tumors. Europ J Cancer Clin Oncol 3:183–191, 1967

51. Wilson CB, Kaufmann L, Barker M: Chromosome analysis of glioblastoma multiforme. Neurology 20:821–828, 1970

52. Mark J: Chromosomal characteristics of neurogenic tumours in adults. Hereditas 68:61–100, 1971

53. Mark J: Chromosomic patterns in benign and malignant tumors in the human nervous system, in German JL (ed): Chromosomes and Cancer. New York, Wiley, 1974, pp 481–495

54. Saadi AA, Latimer F: Non-random chromosomal abnormalities in human brain tumors. Am J Hum Genet 32:61A, 1980

55. Yamada K, Kondo T, Yoshioka M, et al: Cytogenetic studies in twenty human brain tumors: association of no. 22 chromosome abnormalities with tumors of the brain. Cancer Genet Cytogenet 2:293–307, 1980

56. Shapiro JR, Yung W-KA, Shapiro WR: Isolation, karyotype and clonal growth of heterogeneous subpopulations of human malignant gliomas. Cancer Res 41:2349–2359, 1981

57. Rey JA, Bello MJ, de Campos JM, et al: Chromosome studies in two human brain tumors. Cancer Genet Cytogenet 8:159–165, 1983

58. Bigner SH, Mark J: Chromosomes and chromosomal progression of human gliomas in vivo, and in athymic nude mice, in Rosenblum ML, Wilson CB (eds): Progress in Experimental Tumor Research: Brain Tumor Biology. Basel, Karger, 1984, pp 67–82

59. Shapiro JR, Shapiro WR: The subpopulations and isolated cell types of freshly resected high-grade human gliomas: Their influence on the tumor's evolution in vivo and behavior and therapy in vitro. Cancer Metastasis Rev 4:107–124, 1985

60. Shapiro JR, Pu P-Y, Mohamed AN, et al: Specific karyotypic changes in 11 glioblastomas multiforme. Cancer Genet Cytogenet (submitted for publication)

61. Shapiro JR, Mohamed AN, Pu P-Y, et al: Identical non-random karyotypic changes seen in the primary cytogenetic analysis of low-grade and high-grade gliomas. Proc Am Assoc Cancer Res 26:32, 1985

62. Shapiro Jr, Mohamed AN, Pu P-Y, et al: Karyotypic deviations seen in 8 low-grade astrocytomas. Cancer Genet Cytogenet (submitted for publication)

63. Smith H, Liotta LA, Hancock MC, et al: Invasiveness and ploidy of human mammary carcinoma in short-term culture. Proc Natl Acad Sci USA 82:1805–1809, 1985

64. Wolman SR, Smith H, Stampfer M, et al: Growth of diploid cells from breast cancers. Cancer Genet Cytogenet (in press)

65. Mitelman F: Restricted number of chromosomal regions implicated in aetiology of human cancer and leukemia. Nature 310:325–327, 1984

66. Davies RL, Grosse VA, Kucherlapati R, et al: Genetic analysis of epidermal growth factor action: Assignment of human epidermal growth factor receptor gene to chromosome 7. Proc Natl Acad Sci USA 77:4188–4192, 1980

67. Shimizu N, Kondo I, Gamou S, et al: Genetic analysis of hyperproduction of epidermal growth factor receptors in human epidermoid carcinoma A431 cells. Somatic Cell Mol Genet 10:45–53, 1984

68. Dalla-Favera RC, Gallo RC, Giallongo A, et al: Chromosomal localization of the human homolog (c-sis) of the simian sarcoma virus onc gene. Science 218:686–688, 1982

69. Swan DC, McBride OW, Robbins KC, et al: Chromosomal mapping of the simian sarcoma virus onc gene analogue in human cells. Proc Natl Acad Sci USA 79:4691–4695, 1982

70. Westermark B, Wasteson A: A platelet factor stimulating human normal glial cells. Exp Cell Res 98:170–174, 1976

71. Simpson DL, Morrison R, de Vellis J, et al: Epidermal growth factor binding and mitogenic activity on purified populations of cells from the central nervous system. J Neurosci Res 8:453–462, 1962

72. Heldin C-H, Westermark B, Wasteson A: Specific receptors for platelet-derived growth factor on cells derived from connective tissue and glia. Proc Natl Acad Sci USA 78:3664–3668, 1981

73. Doolittle RF, Hunkapiller MW, Hood LE, et al: Simian sarcoma virus onc gene, v-sis, is derived from the gene (or genes) encoding a platelet-derived growth factor. Science 221:275–277, 1983

74. Waterfield MD, Scrace GT, Whittle N, et al: Platelet-derived growth factor is structurally related to the putative transforming protein p28 sis of simian sarcoma virus. Nature 304:35–39, 1983

75. Devare SG, Reddy EP, Law D, et al: Nucleotide sequence of the simian sarcoma virus genome: Demonstration that its acquired cellular sequences encode the transforming gene product. Proc Natl Acad Sci USA 80:731–735, 1983

76. Robbins KC, Antoniades HN, Devare SG, et al: Structural and immunological similarities between simian sarcoma virus gene product(s) and human platelet-derived growth factor. Nature 305:605–608, 1983

77. Downward J, Yarden Y, Mayes E, et al: Close similarity of epidermal growth factor receptor and v-erb-B oncogene protein sequences. Nature 307:521–527, 1984

78. Bishop JM: Cellular oncogenes and retroviruses. Annu Rev Biochem 52:301–354, 1983

79. Thielen GJ, Gould D, Fowler M, et al: c-Type virus in

tumor tissue of a woolly monkey (Lagothrix spp.) with fibrosarcoma. J Natl Cancer Instit 47:881–889, 1971

80. Owen AJ, Pantazis P, Antoniades HN: Simian sarcoma virus-transformed cells secrete a mitogen identical to platelet-derived growth factor. Science 225:54–56, 1984

81. Eva A, Robbins KC, Andersen PR, et al: Cellular gene analogous to retroviral onc genes are transcribed in human tumour cells. Nature 295:116–119, 1982

82. Heldin C-H, Westermark B, Wasteson A: Chemical and biological properties of a growth factor from human-cultured osteosarcoma cells: Resemblance with platelet-derived growth factor. J Cell Physiol 105:235–246, 1980

83. Graves DT, Owen AJ, Antoniades HN: Evidence that a human osteosarcoma cell line which secretes a mitogen similar to platelet-derived growth factor requires growth factors present in platelet-poor plasma. Cancer Res 43:83–87, 1983

84. Betsholtz C, Heldin C-H, Nister M, et al: Synthesis of a PDGF-like growth factor in human glioma and sarcoma cells suggests the expression of the cellular homologue to the transforming protein of simian sarcoma virus. Biochem Biophys Res Commun 117:176–182, 1983

85. Nister M, Heldin C-H, Wasteson A, et al: A platelet-derived growth factor analog produced by a human clonal glioma cell line. Ann NY Acad Sci 397:25–33, 1982

86. Betsholtz C, Westermark B, Ek B, et al: Coexpression of a PDGF-like growth factor and PDGF receptors in a human osteosarcoma cell line: Implications for autocrine receptor activation. Cell 39:447–457, 1984

87. Nister M, Heldin C-H, Wasteson A, et al: A glioma-derived analog to platelet-derived growth factor: Demonstration of receptor competing activity and immunological cross-reactivity. Proc Natl Acad Sci USA 81:926–930, 1984

88. Mohamed AN, Pu P-Y, Shapiro WR, et al: Correlation of BCNU resistance in human glioma cells with over-representation of chromosome 22 and production of a factor resembling platelet-derived growth factor (PDGF). Proc Am Assoc Cancer Res 26:32, 1985

89. Gazit A, Igarashi H, Chiu I-M, et al: Expression of normal human sis/PDGF-2 coding sequence induces cellular transformation. Cell 39:89–97, 1984

90. Stiles CD: The molecular biology of platelet-derived growth factor. Cell 33:653–655, 1983

91. Temin HM, Pierson RW, Dulak NC: The role of serum in the control of multiplication of avian and mammalian cells in culture, in Rosenblat GH, Cristofalo R (eds): Growth, Nutrition and Metabolism of Cells in Culture. Orlando, Fla, Academic, 1972, pp 49–81

92. Sporn MB, Todaro GJ: Autocrine secretion and malignant transformation of cells. N Engl J Med 303:878–880, 1980

93. Bowen-Pope DF, Vogel A, Ross R: Production of platelet-derived growth factor-like molecules and reduced expression of platelet-derived growth factor receptors accompany transformation by a wide spectrum of agents. Proc Natl Acad Sci USA 81:2396–2400, 1984

94. Antoniades HN: Commentary: Platelet-derived growth factor and malignant transformation. Biochem Pharmacol 33:2823–2828, 1984

95. Yamamoto T: The erb-B gene of avian erythroblastosis virus is a member of the src gene family. Cell 35:71–78, 1983

96. Carpenter S, Cohen S: Epidermal growth factor. Annu Rev Biochem 48:193–216, 1979

97. Hunter T: The epidermal growth factor receptor gene and its product. Nature 311:414–416, 1984

98. Hunter T, Cooper JA: Epidermal growth factor induces rapid tyrosine phosphorylation of proteins in A431 human tumor cells. Cell 24:741–752, 1981

99. Ullrich A, Coussens L, Hayflick JS, et al: Human epidermal growth factor receptor cDNA sequence and aberrant expression of the amplified gene in A431 epidermoid carcinoma cells. Nature 309:418–425, 1984

100. Lin CR, Chen WS, Kruiger W, et al: Expression cloning of human EGF receptor complimentary DNA: Gene amplification and three related messenger RNA products in A431 cells. Science 224:843–848, 1984

101. Xu Y-H, Ishii S, Clark AJL, et al: Human epidermal growth factor receptor cDNA is homologous to a variety of RNAs overproduced in A431 carcinoma cells. Nature 309:806–810, 1984

102. Gill GN, Lazar CG: Increased phosphotyrosine content and inhibition of proliferation of EGF-treated A431 cells. Nature 293:305–307, 1981

103. Kawamoto T: Growth stimulation of A431 cells by epidermal growth factor: Identification of high-affinity receptors for epidermal growth factor by an anti-receptor monoclonal antibody. Proc Natl Acad Sci USA 80:1337–1341, 1983

104. Libermann TA, Razon N, Bartal AD, et al: Expression of epidermal growth factor receptors in human brain tumors. Cancer Res 44:753–760, 1984

105. Libermann TA, Nusbaum HR, Razon N, et al: Amplification, enhanced expression and possible rearrangement of the EGF receptor gene in primary human brain tumors of glial origin. Nature 313:144–147, 1984

106. Todaro GT, Marquardt H, Twardzik DR, et al: Transforming growth factors produced by tumor cells, in Owens AH, Coffey DS, Baylin SB (eds): Tumor Cell Heterogeneity: Origin and Implications. Orlando, Fla, Academic, 1982, pp 205–224

107. Shapiro JR, Pu P-Y, Shapiro WR: Resistant cell types in human gliomas, in Salmon S, Trent JM (eds): Tumor Cell Cloning. Orlando, Fla, Grune & Stratton, 1984, pp 133–142

Malignant Astrocytic Neoplasms: Classification, Pathologic Anatomy, and Response to Treatment

Peter C. Burger

MALIGNANCY in a human glioma is dependent on the lesion's anatomic position, infiltrative properties, responsiveness to therapeutic agents, and proliferative potential of neoplastic cells surviving treatment. Any of these factors can produce clinical malignancy, independent of the neoplasm's histologic composition. In general usage, however, the term "malignant" is usually reserved for lesions with both clinical and histological evidence of malignancy, the latter in the form of cellular atypia, pleomorphism, and mitotic activity. So defined, most malignant gliomas belong to the large group of fibrillary astrocytic neoplasms that frequent the cerebral hemispheres, the brain stem, and the spinal cord.[1] This discussion focuses on malignant fibrillary astrocytic neoplasms in the cerebral hemispheres since they are by far the most numerous, and are a major topic in this volume.

CLASSIFICATION

In spite of the fact that fibrillary astrocytic neoplasms are so common, there are continuing differences of opinion about their classification. Such differences relate to the number of grades to which lesions can be assigned, and to the histologic criteria used to make those assignments.

The classic, four-tiered Broders system, widely used in general pathology, was first applied to astrocytic neoplasms at the Mayo Clinic in 1949.[2,3] This classification, which now eponymously honors Dr Kernohan, places lesions in one of four grades in proportion to the degree of a neoplasm's histologic malignancy. The glioblastoma is subdivided into lesions of lesser and greater histologic malignancy, astrocytoma grade 3 and 4, respectively. Shortly after this classification was formulated, Ringertz proposed a three-tiered system that recognized a well differentiated astrocytoma at one end, and the glioblastoma at the other.[4] An intermediate lesion completed the scheme. Presently, both the four- and the three-tiered systems are in general use, although the weight of opinion appears to be shifting in favor of the latter, since there is some skepticism concerning the utility of subdividing the glioblastoma, or at least subdividing the glioblastoma as it is defined today.[1,5–7]

Two recent studies from large cooperative oncology groups support the value of a three-tiered system and underscore the importance of stratifying patients with malignant astrocytic neoplasms into two groups. A study by Nelson et al from the Radiation Therapy Oncology Group (RTOG) and Eastern Cooperative Oncology Group (ECOG),[7] and another by ourselves from the National Brain Tumor Study Group (BTSG)[8] reviewed the survivals of patients with malignant astrocytic neoplasms previously classified as either (1) an anaplastic, malignant, or "atypical" astrocytoma or (2) a glioblastoma multiforme. Patients with the third grade of fibrillary astrocytic lesion, the well differentiated astrocytoma, were not considered. In both studies, the original review of slides had been done without clinical information such as the age of the patient or the location of the lesion. Similar results were obtained, when, subsequently, the post-randomization survivals were compared to the histological diagnoses. For the RTOG-ECOG, the percentage of 18-month survivals for the glioblastoma and anaplastic astrocytoma were 15% and 62%, respectively. For the BTSG, the 24-month survivals for patients with the glioblastoma were 8% and 12% in two phase III studies, while the 24-month survivals in patients with the anaplastic astrocytomas in the same phase III studies were 38% and 50%.

Both study groups evaluated also the utility of the four-tiered system. Nelson et al compared the survivals of patients whose glioblastoma had been classified by the referring pathologists as grade 4 with those classified as grade 3. No

From the Department of Pathology, Duke University Medical Center, Durham, North Carolina.

Supported in part by Grant U10-CA36005-01 from the Division of Cancer Treatment, National Institutes of Health, Department of Health and Human Services.

Address reprint requests to Peter C. Burger, MD, Box 3712, Department of Pathology, Duke University Medical Center, Durham, NC 27710.

0093–7754/86/1301–0003$05.00/0

significant difference was noted. We investigated the prognostic values of 9 histologic variables in 184 patients with glioblastomas, and found no criterion, or set of criteria, to subdivide glioblastoma into grades 3 and 4, except possibly for a rare giant cell glioblastoma which seemed to have a longer survival.[9] Of course, neither of these studies invalidates a four-tiered system, but authors who use it are well advised to define the histologic criteria utilized. Because this is often not done, it is difficult to interpret many published clinical and radiographic studies of malignant gliomas that include no description of how, or by whom, lesions were graded. The issue frequently comes to a focus on grade III lesions, which are glioblastomas by the Kernohan system and an anaplastic astrocytoma by the three-tiered system.

CLINICOPATHOLOGIC FEATURES

Anaplastic Astrocytoma

In accord with Kernohan's findings that, in a population of patients, the histological grades of the fibrillary astrocytic neoplasms increases with patient age, the anaplastic astrocytoma in the cerebral hemispheres occurs in patients intermediate in age between that of the well differentiated astrocytoma and the glioblastoma.[2,3] For three combined Phase III trials from the BTSG, the mean age of 175 patients with an anaplastic astrocytoma was 46 years, and for 1,265 patients with a glioblastoma was 56 years.[8]

The macroscopic features of the lesion also emphasize the anaplastic astrocytoma's intermediate position in the astrocytic neoplasms since it is better circumscribed than the astrocytoma but less discrete than the glioblastoma. Radiographically, the anaplastic astrocytoma is usually noted as a mass lesion of low density that is less likely to contain contrast enhancement than a glioblastoma (Figs 1A and 1B).[10,11]

Microscopically, the anaplastic astrocytoma is a lesion of fibrillary astrocytes in which cellularity and nuclear pleomorphism are prominent. The cells, which are usually less numerous than in a glioblastoma, are more evenly distributed and frequently infiltrate over a wide zone in which preexisting neurons and glia are entrapped (Figs 1C and 1D).[12] We accept some vascular proliferation in this lesion, but, as is discussed below, we do not accept necrosis, which to us indicates a glioblastoma.

Glioblastoma Multiforme

Patients with the glioblastoma are usually older than those with the anaplastic astrocytoma and usually have been symptomatic for a shorter period.[2,3] In the BTSG study cited above, the average duration of preoperative symptoms was 5.4 months, in contrast to 15.7 months for patients with the anaplastic astrocytoma.

By computerized tomography, the classic glioblastoma is an expansile lesion with three distinct zones: (1) a low density center, (2) a distinct rim of contrast enhancement, and (3) a corona of low-density white matter (Fig 2A). The macro- and microscopic counterparts of these zones are: (1) a central area of soft variegated necrotic tissue, (2) a gray fleshy rim of hypercellular neoplasm, and (3) yellow "edematous" white matter with focal infiltrating neoplastic glia (Figs 2B and 2C).[10–13]

Histologically, a remarkable feature of the glioblastoma's cellular composition is the inter- and intratumoral heterogeneity. The scope of this heterogeneity has made morphologic subclassification of the glioblastoma difficult, although it is possible to define certain general cell types. For a recent study, we defined six cells, recognizing that such categorization does not do justice to this lesion's heterogeneity. We found that in 43 surgically excised lesions, 21 contained one cell type, 20 contained 2 cell types, and 2 contained 3 cell types.[14]

In addition to its cytologic composition, the glioblastoma multiforme is noted for two secondary features, namely, vascular proliferation and necrosis, the latter often surrounded by a distinctive and diagnostic aggregation ("pseudopalisading") of nuclei (Fig 2D). Both our classification, as well as that by Nelson et al referred to above, employ necrosis, with or without the pseudopalisading, as an important feature differentiating the glioblastoma from the anaplastic astrocytoma.[7,8]

TOPOGRAPHY

It has been apparent for many years that there is a relation between the degree of cellular differentiation of the fibrillary astrocytic neoplasms and the degree of macroscopic circumscrip-

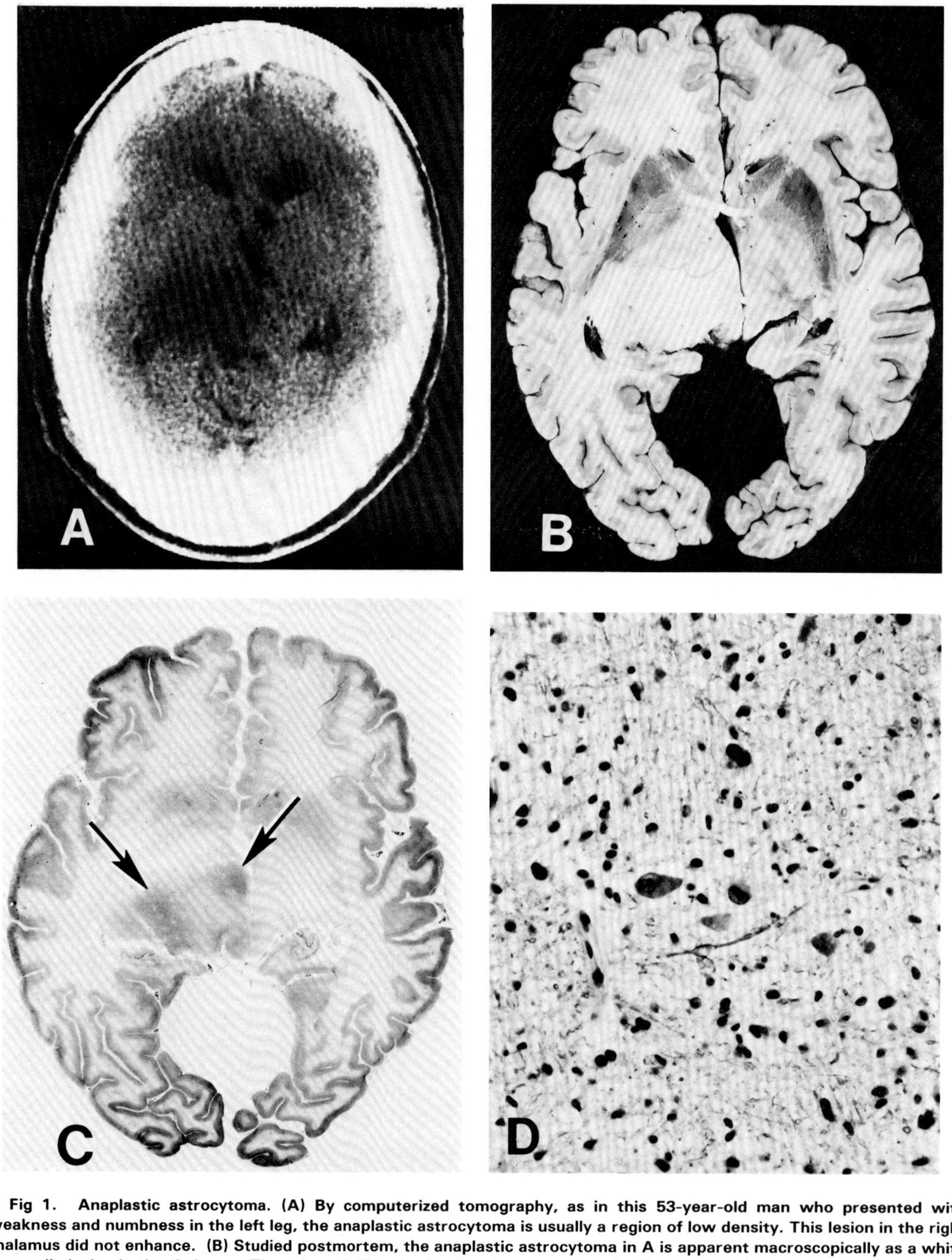

Fig 1. Anaplastic astrocytoma. (A) By computerized tomography, as in this 53-year-old man who presented with weakness and numbness in the left leg, the anaplastic astrocytoma is usually a region of low density. This lesion in the right thalamus did not enhance. (B) Studied postmortem, the anaplastic astrocytoma in A is apparent macroscopically as a white expansile lesion in the thalamus. There is an infiltrative border along the posterior limb of the internal capsule. (C) A whole mount histologic section discloses the darkly-stained region of neoplasm (arrows). In contrast to the glioblastoma multiforme, there is no central area of necrosis (Cresyl Fast Violet). (D) The microscopic characteristics of anaplastic astrocytoma include large, angulated, hyperchromatic nuclei and infiltration of the surrounding tissue. Here, large thalamic neurons have been incorporated (hematoxylin-eosin; original magnification × 400).

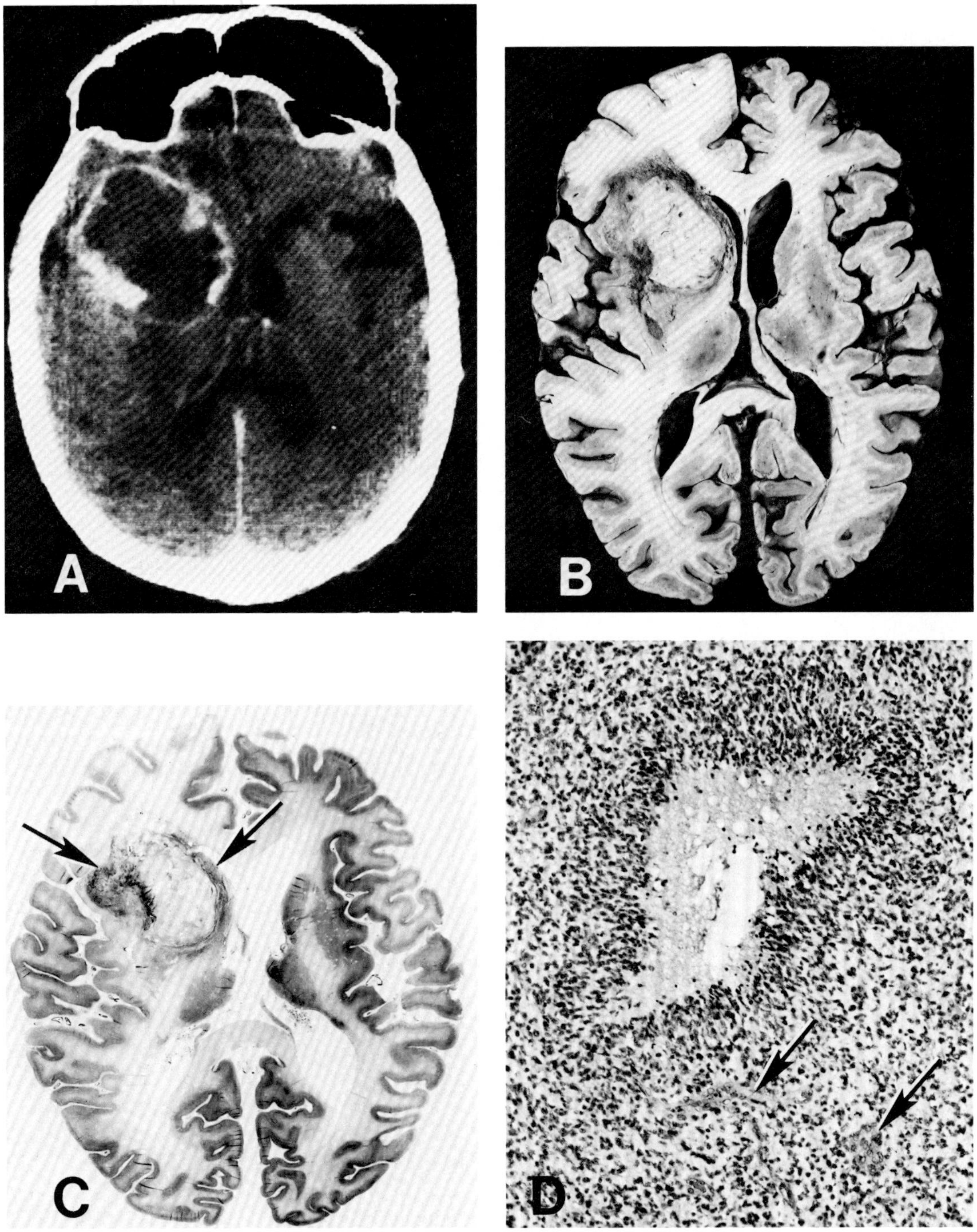

Fig 2. Glioblastoma multiforme. (A) As in this 73-year-old male who presented with a change in mental status, the glioblastoma usually contains a contrast-enhancing ring that circumscribes a central area of low density, and is surrounded by white matter of low density. The patient expired before radiation therapy could be administered. (B) The specimen from A emphasizes the macroscopic discreteness that characterizes many glioblastoma multiformes. The central white area is necrosis. (C) In a whole mount histologic section, the darkly-staining, and therefore markedly cellular, ring of tumor (arrows) corresponds to the ring of contrast enhancement as seen in A (Cresyl Fast Violet). (D) Microscopically, the ring of the glioblastoma multiforme is highly cellular and frequently contains small foci of necrosis with peripheral pseudopalisading (top). Abnormal blood vessels such as those with endothelial proliferation (arrows) are often seen (hematoxylin-eosin; original magnification × 100).

tion.[3,15] Thus, the well differentiated astrocytoma is diffusely infiltrating, whereas the glioblastoma multiforme is macroscopically better circumscribed. In 1940 Scherer suggested that anatomical features favoring radical surgical extirpation were present in about 20% of glioblastomas.[15] The CT scan has reemphasized these features and depicts the glioblastoma as a rather discrete lesion because of its ring of contrast enhancement. From these images a reasonably localized quality to the lesion has been inferred. For example, it has been suggested that in most cases all of the neoplasm resides within 2 cm of the enhancing rim.[16]

It would appear to be simple to confirm the above deductions by pathologic studies, but such has not been the case. For the purposes of a conference on stereotactic biopsy, we quantitated the size of the three zones of the untreated glioblastoma in six brains studied postmortem.[12] We found that in each of the six specimens, the minimum thickness of this infiltrating rim was generally less than 1 mm and the maximum thickness ranged from 4 to 33 mm. The 33 mm infiltrating rim was present in a very large, advanced lesion, but in the five smaller neoplasms in patients who died earlier in the course of the disease, the region of infiltration was 15 mm or less. These calculations were based on the abnormality that we felt could be diagnosed as neoplastic in a small specimen such as that obtained by a needle biopsy, and understates the thickness of the infiltrating rim as determinable by the study of larger histologic sections. Boethius and his colleagues studied the histological features of the glioblastoma in stereotactic biopsies and correlated those findings with the site of the biopsy as determined by computerized tomography.[17] In five typical glioblastomas, the surrounding area of local density or edema contained only edematous parenchyma. No tumor was seen. These findings in regard to the localization of the glioblastoma may appear to reinforce the perceived discreteness of this lesion; however, the interpretation of these data should be tempered by the realization that most glioblastomas contain a predominant component of small anaplastic cells whose nuclei are frequently as small as 20–25 microns in cross-sectional area.[18] They are therefore similar in size to those of normal glia and vascular endothelial cells from which they can be difficult, or impossible, to distinguish. Such a distinction is not problematic in the enhancing rim or proximal zone of infiltration where the neoplastic cells are present in large numbers (Figs 3A and 3B). In more distant regions, however, where the issue is more critical, it becomes difficult to establish the neoplastic nature of isolated small cells (Figs 3C and 3D).

Thus, the critical issue concerning the extent of the glioblastoma remains unsolved. If the lesion is confined within a reasonably narrow geographic zone, perhaps less than 2 cm from the enhancing rim, then local therapies such as interstitial irradiation[19] may effect long survival and even cure. If the lesion extends significantly beyond such a limit, life may be prolonged by aggressive local therapy, but late recurrence in more peripheral zones may be anticipated.

RESPONSE TO THERAPY

Remission

Following surgical resection and radiotherapy, the glioblastoma frequently enters a stage of "remission" or "quiescence" during which it regresses in size and symptomatic expression.[13] Such lesions can be found in individuals dying of causes unrelated to the neoplasm, such as pulmonary embolism and myocardial infarction. Studies of such specimens define the glioblastoma in this phase as well circumscribed, heavily collagenized, frequently calcified, extensively necrotic, and often cystic (Figs 4A, 4B, and 4C).[13,14] When compared to the microscopic appearance of the original surgical specimen, the histologic features of such lesions record the effects of radiotherapy. Such comparisons make it clear that radiotherapy is often remarkably effective in depopulating the glioblastoma of the smaller anaplastic elements that frequently predominate before treatment (Fig 4D). Such a depopulation unmasks less radiosensitive elements such as fibrillary and gemistocytic astrocytes.[14] Large bizarre glia are often uncovered or, more likely, induced by radiotherapy (Fig 4E). The effect of chemotherapy alone is unknown. We found no apparent effects in a small number of brains examined postmortem.[20]

Recurrence

In spite of the optimism one can derive from studying the lesion in remission, malignant gliomas, as treated presently by as much as 6,000

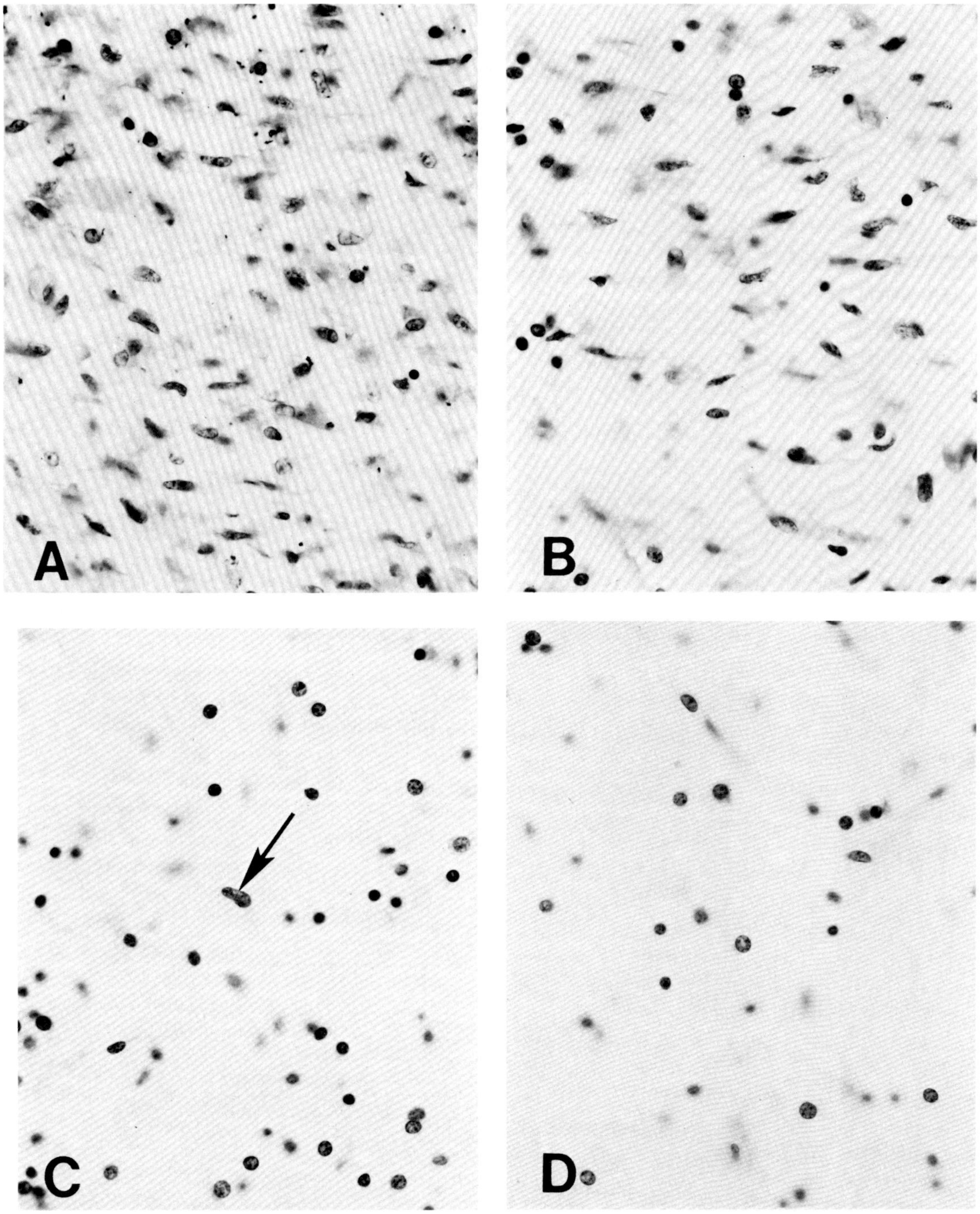

Fig 3. Glioblastoma multiforme. Sections taken at 0, 0.2, 1.0, and 2.0 cm from the hypercellular rim of an untreated glioblastoma underscore the difficulty in localizing the extent of this lesion. (A) In this section from the hypercellular ring, the neoplastic nature of the tissue is apparent from the cytologic characteristics of the cells, but also by their density (Cresyl Fast Violet; original magnification × 400). (B) At 0.2 cm from the outer edge of the rim, the lesion is less cellular than in A, but still sufficiently cellular to make the neoplastic nature of the lesion clear (Cresyl Fast Violet; original magnification × 400). (C) One cm from the edge of the rim, normal, round-to-slightly-oval nuclei of astrocytes and oligodendroglia are scattered across the field. In addition, there is one elongated, slightly larger nucleus (arrow). Although this nucleus shares cytologic features with those of the neoplastic cells seen in A and B, it is difficult to establish the neoplastic nature of such an isolated cell and therefore to determine the extent of the glioblastoma (Cresyl Fast Violet; original magnification × 400). (D) At 2.0 cm from the edge of the enhancing area, the field apparently contains only astrocytes, oligodendrocytes, and scattered vascular endothelial cells. It is clearly difficult, however, to exclude the possibility that scattered neoplastic cells are also present in this or adjacent fields (Cresyl Fast Violet; original magnification × 400).

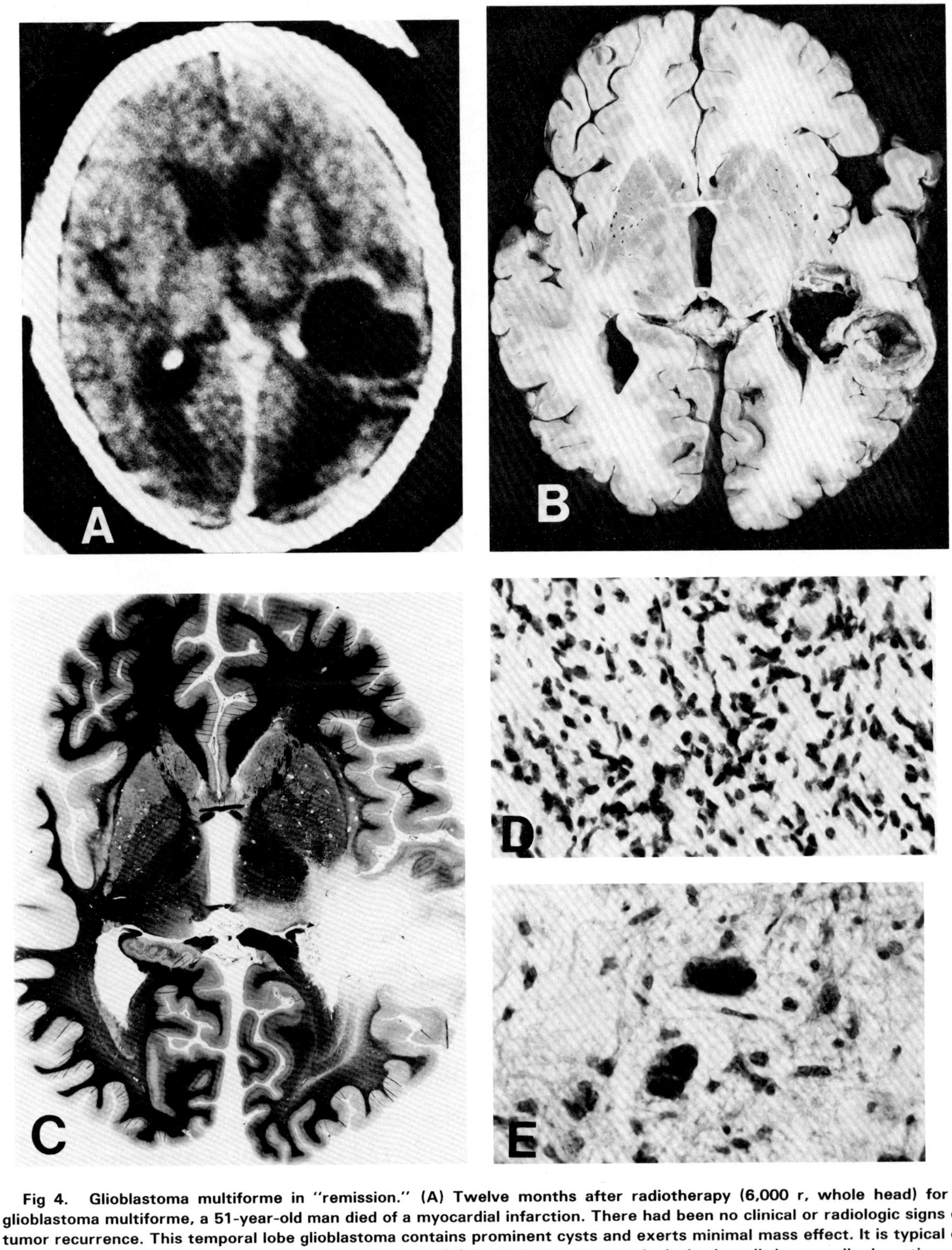

Fig 4. Glioblastoma multiforme in "remission." (A) Twelve months after radiotherapy (6,000 r, whole head) for a glioblastoma multiforme, a 51-year-old man died of a myocardial infarction. There had been no clinical or radiologic signs of tumor recurrence. This temporal lobe glioblastoma contains prominent cysts and exerts minimal mass effect. It is typical of many malignant gliomas in "quiescence" or "remission." (B) Studied postmortem, the lesion is well circumscribed, cystic, and contains a fibrotic wall. In contrast to the initial lesion whose mass effect was documented by computerized tomography, it now produces minimal displacement of adjacent structures. (C) A whole brain section in the same horizontal plane as A and B discloses the multiloculated cystic cavity and the paucity mass effect of the glioblastoma in "remission" (Hematoxylin and Eosin/Luxol Fast Blue). (D and E) The two photomicrographs compare the lesion in this patient before and after radiotherapy. In D, is the highly cellular neoplasm seen in the operative specimen (hematoxylin-eosin; original magnification × 250). In E, the postmortem specimen is less cellular and contains bizarre giant cells (hematoxylin-eosin; original magnification × 400).

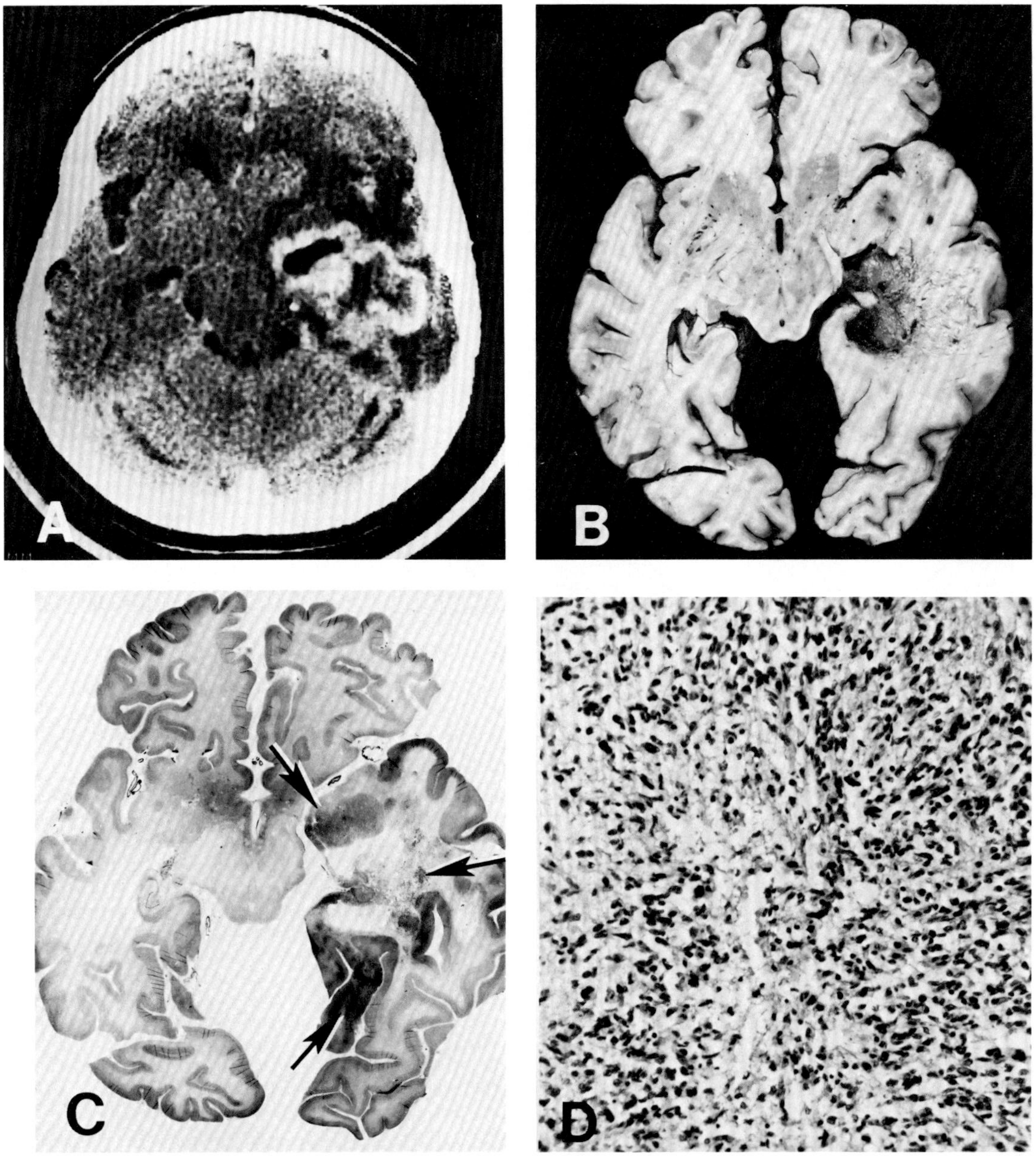

Fig 5. Glioblastoma multiforme in recurrence. (A) As is typical of recurrence in a glioblastoma, it has occurred in the margins of the previous resection in this 59-year-old woman. The ring shaped area of enhancement is associated with considerable mass effect and surrounding low density. (B) The patient expired as a consequence of the lesion's mass effect. In horizontal section, the neoplasm is necrotic and focally fleshy. (C) A whole mount histologic section emphasizes the hypercellular neoplasm (arrows) congruent with the contrast enhancement in A. An area of central necrosis is also seen (Cresyl Fast Violet). (D) As in this case, the recurrent glioblastoma is often composed of small anaplastic cells (hematoxylin-eosin; original magnification × 170).

rads of whole head radiation, recur. This is apparent as new or increased clinical symptoms, enlargement of the lesion by CT scan, or both (Figs 5A, 5B, and 5C). This recurrence usually occurs within one year of surgery, although there is considerable variation in the timing of this event. Pathologic studies of recurrent neoplasms disclose that recurrence usually repopulates a lesion's small anaplastic cells so as to reconstitute the quiescent lesion into one similar to the original neoplasm (Fig 5D). Such a repopulation begins in the immediate environs of the original lesion.[13-15] Since local therapy has been also advocated for recurrent lesions, the topography

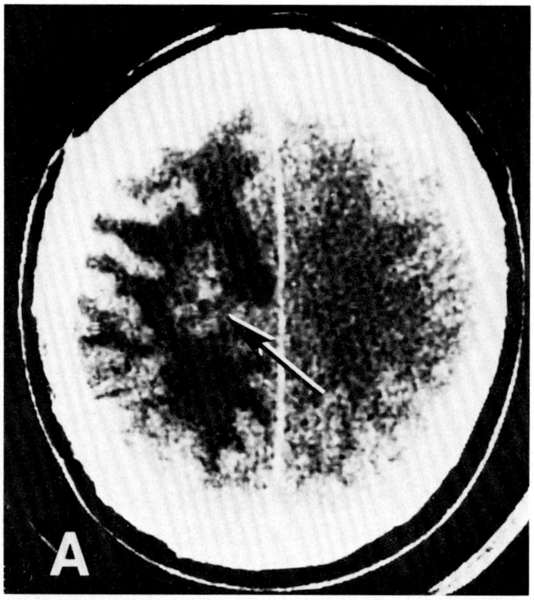

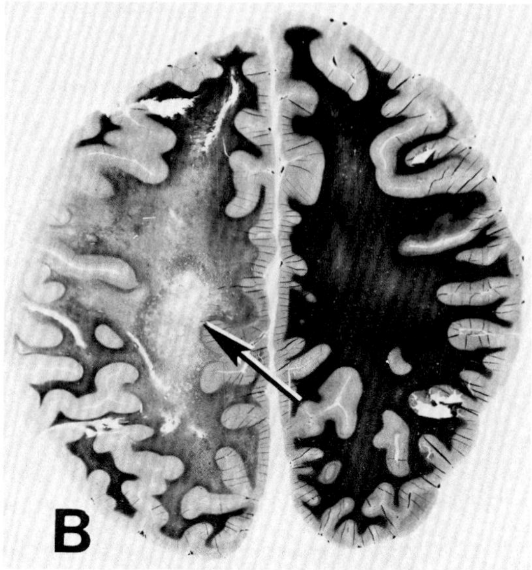

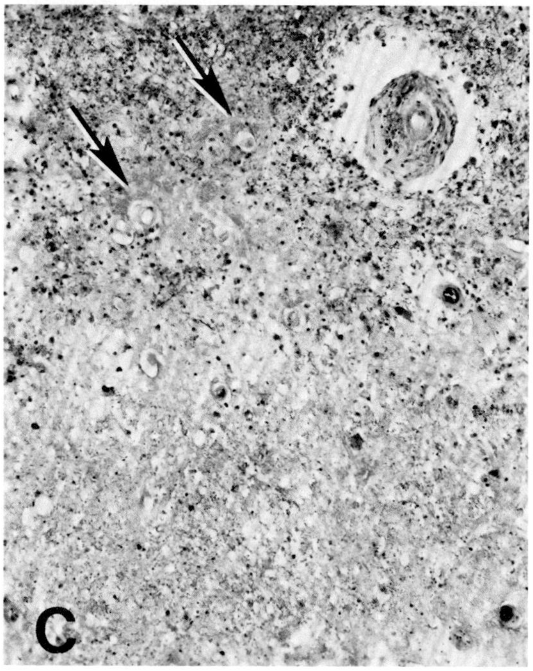

Fig 6. Radionecrosis. (A) Five months after administration of 6,000 rads for an anaplastic astrocytoma of the left frontal lobe, this patient developed increased symptoms and an area of contrast enhancement (arrow) surrounded by extensive low density of the white matter. (B) In a whole mount histologic section, the region corresponding to the area of contrast enhancement has a coagulative character and spares the overlying gray matter. Both are typical, although not diagnostic, of radionecrosis. Note the marked pallor of the white matter congruent with the region of low density on the CT scan (hematoxylin-eosin/Luxol Fast Blue). (C) Histologically, the area of necrosis at the arrow in B is amorphous coagulated parenchyma (bottom) surrounded by blood vessels with fibrinoid necrosis (arrows). Neoplastic astrocytes were present at the anterolateral edge of the necrotic mass, emphasizing that neoplasm and radionecrosis can coexist (hematoxylin-eosin/Luxol Fast Blue; original magnification × 68).

of such lesions is of considerable interest. It has been our experience that recurrent lesions that have run their course and killed the patient freely infiltrate the cerebrum, and, often, neoplastic cells can be found in the opposite cerebral hemisphere, cerebellum, and brain stem.

COMPLICATIONS OF THERAPY

It has been recognized for many years that therapeutic radiotherapy carries a risk of cerebral delayed radionecrosis.[21] The entity was best defined in patients treated for extracranial disease in whom there were no compounding variables, such as an adjacent brain tumor, to complicate interpretation of the microscopic findings in and around the necrotic area. In such a setting, the classic white matter coagulative necrosis, fibrinoid vascular necrosis, endothelial cell abnormalities, telangiectasis, and vascular hyalinization emerged as clear consequences of the therapy.

Recently, however, cerebral radionecrosis has been increasingly a sequela of therapy for an intracranial mass lesion, after a dose of 5,000 rads or greater and after approximately a year or more post-therapy.[21] It has been difficult to assess the incidence of this phenomenon since it mimics the clinical and radiographic expressions of recurrent neoplasia (Figs 6A, 6B, and 6C). It can even be difficult to define the scope of this problem pathologically by study of biopsy material since radionecrosis and recurrent neoplasm can coexist. Thus, the presence of radionecrosis in a surgical specimen does not establish it as a cause of the symptoms, nor does the finding of neoplastic cells exclude the possibility of radionecrosis nearby. It has also been difficult to assess the incidence in postmortem specimens because of the difficulty in acquiring a sufficient number of randomly selected brains.

Radionecrosis is often assumed to occur only as a large, symptomatic, generally fatal lesion, but pathologic postmortem studies define it as more common, but often clinically less important, than supposed.[13,14] Peritumoral necrosis and vascular changes characteristic of radionecrosis may also occur sooner than the typical one-year or more interval. One hopes that new techniques such as positron emission tomography and nuclear magnetic resonance imaging will be helpful in defining the incidence of radionecrosis and distinguishing it from recurrent neoplasm.

An additional state in patients with treated malignant gliomas is a progressive neurologic deterioration associated with large ventricles and low density white matter. Such findings have been noted in the "long term" survivors of the glioblastoma and raise concern that it is a consequence of therapy, particularly radiotherapy.[22] Like radionecrosis, the incidence of this "entity" has not been determined.

In conventional doses, administered systemically, chemotherapy for malignant gliomas has not been blamed solely for specific intracranial lesions, although some lesions seen in brain tumor patients are those which have been associated with the combination of chemo- and radiotherapy.[13,18] However, when given systemically in large doses, BCNU has been associated with multiple cerebral and spinal lesions with many similarities to radionecrosis.[23] One would suspect that intracarotid delivery of chemotherapeutic agents such as BCNU may be associated with lesions of the brain parenchyma, particularly if radiotherapy is administered concurrently. Such lesions have already been reported.[24]

CONCLUSION

From all of the above, it is clear that there are many unresolved important issues in regard to the localization of malignant gliomas before and after treatment, the nature of lesions producing clinical "recurrence," the beneficial effects of therapy, and the complications of treatment. In light of the aggressive new treatments, such as local radiation and intracarotid delivery of drugs, the resolution of these issues is increasingly important. Postmortem studies have been instrumental in the past and have much to offer in the future. A plea is made to study malignant gliomas postmortem.

REFERENCES

1. Burger PC, Vogel FS: Surgical Pathology of the Nervous System and Its Coverings (ed 2). Wiley, New York, 1982, pp 226–266

2. Svien HJ, Mabon RF, Kernohan JW: Astrocytomas. Proc Staff Mtg Mayo Clinic 24:54–64, 1949

3. Kernohan JW, Sayre GP: Tumors of the central nervous system. Armed Forces Institute of Pathology, Washington, DC, 1952

4. Ringertz N: "Grading" of gliomas. Acta Pathol Microbiol Immunol Scand 27:51–64, 1950

5. Russell DS, Rubinstein LJ: Pathology of tumours of the nervous system. Williams and Wilkins, Baltimore, 1977, pp 146–172, 226–244

6. Zülch KJ: Histological typing of tumours and the central nervous system. World Health Organization, Geneva, 1979, pp 43–45, 50

7. Nelson JS, Tsukada Y, Schoenfeld D, et al: Necrosis as a prognostic criterion in malignant supratentorial astrocytic gliomas. Cancer 52:550–554, 1983

8. Burger PC, Vogel FS, Green SB, et al: Glioblastoma multiforme and anaplastic astrocytoma: Pathologic criteria and prognostic implications. Cancer 56:1106–1112, 1985

9. Burger PC, Vollmer RT: Histologic factors of prognostic significance in the glioblastoma multiforme. Cancer 46:1179–1186, 1980

10. Steinhoff H, Lanksch W, Kazner E, et al: Computed tomography in the diagnosis and differential diagnosis of glioblastomas. A qualitative study of 295 cases. Neuroradiology 14:193–200, 1977

11. Lilja A, Bergstrom K, Spannare B, et al: Reliability of computed tomography in assessing histopathological features of supratentorial gliomas. J Comput Assist Tomogr 5:625–636, 1981

12. Burger PC: Pathologic anatomy and CT correlations

in the glioblastoma multiforme. Appl Neurophysiol 46:180–187, 1983

13. Burger PC, DuBois PJ, Schold SC Jr, et al: Computerized tomographic and pathologic studies of the untreated, quiescent, and recurrent glioblastoma multiforme. J Neurosurg 58:159–169, 1983

14. Giangaspero F, Burger PC: Correlation between cytologic composition and biologic behavior in the glioblastoma multiforme. A postmortem study of 50 cases. Cancer 52:2320–2333, 1983

15. Scherer HJ: The forms of growth in gliomas and their practical significance. Brain 63:1–35, 1940

16. Hochberg FH, Pruitt A: Assumptions in the radiotherapy of glioblastoma. Neurology 30:907–911, 1980

17. Boethius J, Collins VP, Edner G, et al: Stereotactic biopsies and computer tomography in gliomas. Acta Neurochi 40:223–232, 1978

18. Giangaspero F, Muhlbaier LH, Burger PC: The glioblastoma and the metastatic carcinoma: A morphometric study of nuclear size and shape. Appl Pathol 2:160–167, 1984

19. Gutin PH, Phillips TL, Wara WM, et al: Brachytherapy of recurrent malignant brain tumors with removable high-activity iodine-125 sources. J Neurosurg 60:61–68, 1984

20. Burger PC, Mahaley MS Jr, Dudka L, et al: The morphologic effects of radiation administered therapeutically for intracranial gliomas. A postmortem study of 25 cases. Cancer 44:1256–1272, 1979

21. Sheline GE, Wara WM, Smith V: Therapeutic irradiation and brain injury. Int J Radiat Oncol Biol Phys 6:1215–1228, 1980

22. Lieberman AN, Foo SH, Ransohoff J, et al: Long term survival among patients with malignant brain tumors. Neurosurgery 10:450–453, 1982

23. Burger PC, Kamenar E, Schold SC Jr, et al: Encephalomyelopathy following high-dose BCNU therapy. Cancer 48:1318–1327, 1981

24. Kleinschmidt-DeMasters BK: Intra-carotid BCNU leukoencephalopathy. J Neuropathol Exp Neurol 43:293, 1984

The Role of Intracranial Surgery for the Treatment of Malignant Gliomas

Joseph Ransohoff, Patrick Kelly, and Edward Laws

THE ROLE of intracranial surgery in the management of malignant gliomas has changed considerably in the last decade. Improvements in diagnostic techniques, particularly the advent of CT scanning, and more recently magnetic resonance imaging (MRI), the development of programs for improved radiation therapy and the advent of multiple chemotherapies for the treatment of brain tumors have all led to a more positive approach to these neoplasms and pari passu a more aggressive and definitive surgical attitude. There is no longer a real justification for the small craniotomy or "biopsy" followed by no definitive therapy; in a sense, sending the patient home to die. There is no longer justification for a large external decompression achieved by removing a segment of skull and leaving the dura widely open, which did prolong life, but resulted in cerebral herniation at the decompression site and often the eventual development of cerebral fungus. Even the more recent practice of the removal of large amounts of normal brain tissue (lobectomy) in order to provide for internal decompression is rarely warranted unless perioperative brain swelling would otherwise prevent reconstitution of the cranial vault. As survival times have lengthened, the long-term effects of radiation therapy and chemotherapy have been found to be associated with progressive cerebral atrophy and the loss of higher integrative functions, hence the need to spare normal tissue.

Surgery in the management of malignant gliomas must be justified on the basis of good surgical principles as well as on sound oncological concepts. Aggressive tumor resection is unquestionably the most effective method of rapid reduction of tumor burden. In the case of the tumor under consideration, not only is tumor burden reduced, but so also is the hypoxic core area, known to contain those cells most resistant to radiation therapy and least available to chemotherapy delivered via the vascular system. This region also contains the necrotic areas that cannot be cleared by the brain, lacking as it does an effective lymphatic system. The surgical aims must include the reduction of the mass effect of the tumor, including the shift of brain structures, and the relief of increased intracranial pressure. Postoperative neurological deficits should be minimal for both focal and diffuse signs, as the patient's post surgical functional status has been shown to correlate significantly with survival time.

Stereotactic CT guided biopsy can now be safely performed on deep lesions, if it is deemed advisable, to establish a definitive diagnosis and thus initiate appropriate chemotherapy as well as radiation therapy. Small superficial subcortical lesions can be accurately localized with intraoperative ultrasound and safely removed in order to establish the diagnosis.

In summary then, intracranial surgery in the management of malignant brain tumors should be based on the neurosurgical principles of elimination of symptoms and the preservation of normal anatomy, and on the oncological principles of reducing tumor burden and eliminating hypoxic cells and necrotic tissue.

DIAGNOSIS

Malignant astrocytoma has its peak incidence between the ages of 40 and 60 and affects males more commonly than females in a ratio of 3 to 2. While they may occur anywhere in the central nervous system, they are most common in the supratentorial white matter. Malignant gliomas arising in the pons, cerebellum and spinal cord constitute less than 5% of these tumors in adults.[1] About 5% are multifocal, usually showing either macroscopic or microscopic continuity with other tumors. Approximately 2% are truly multicentered with no continuity between or among tumor centers.[2]

Signs and symptoms of intracranial gliomas are about equally divided among phenomena related to diffuse cerebral dysfunction, focal

From the Department of Neurosurgery, New York University Medical Center, New York and the Mayo Clinic, Rochester, Minn.

Address reprint requests to Joseph Ransohoff, MD, New York University Medical Center, Department of Neurosurgery, 550 First Ave, New York, NY 10016.

0093-7754/86/1301-0004$05.00/0

neurological deficits, and convulsive seizures. Complaints related to increased intracranial pressure include headache, obtundation, and finally nausea and vomiting. Diffuse signs of cerebral dysfunction, which are often subtle at the onset, include difficulty with short-term memory, mild personality changes, and lack of attention to personal hygiene. The onset of hemiparesis, a visual field defect and even a mild speech disturbance, are at times not recognized for several weeks, and in the older age group are often attributed to cerebral vascular disease. Tumors arising in the nondominant temporal lobe, frontal lobes, or corpus callosum can often be subtle in terms of the development of symptoms and may grow to considerable size before the patient is suspected of harboring a brain tumor. A generalized or focal seizure is a dramatic event and usually leads to early definitive diagnostic evaluation.

CT scanning with and without contrast enhancement particularly with the newer high resolution equipment, is highly suggestive of the diagnosis of a single intracranial malignant tumor. A mass lesion surrounded by white matter edema with solid or so-called "ring" (Fig 1) enhancement is seen in malignant glioma; the differential diagnosis is that of a single intracranial metastatic tumor or on rare occasions, a brain abscess. The single metastasis cannot be distinguished from a malignant glioma by neuroradiologic studies. The radionuclide scan of brain abscess will often demonstrate a ring-like image, in contrast to the solid image seen in the malignant gliomas. The CT ring enhancement in brain abscess often thins in the deeper tissues, at times the site of perforation into the ventricular system (Fig 2). Double-dose contrast enhancement studies, as well as delayed scanning, can be useful if multiple lesions are suspected. Radionuclide scanning still remains an important study from two aspects. The technetium 99 scan can, at times, demonstrate multiplicity of lesions not seen on the earlier generation CT scanners. Secondly, lower grade gliomas tend to show on CT studies as a non-enhancing mass (Fig 3) with negative radionuclide brain scan.

Magnetic Resonance Imaging (MRI) is valuable in the diagnosis of low grade gliomas where the non-enhancing CT area may be mistaken for an infarct, yet is clearly visible on MRI as a mass lesion (Fig 4). The MRI is probably more accurate than CT for definition of multiple small lesions and in tumors of the brain stem and

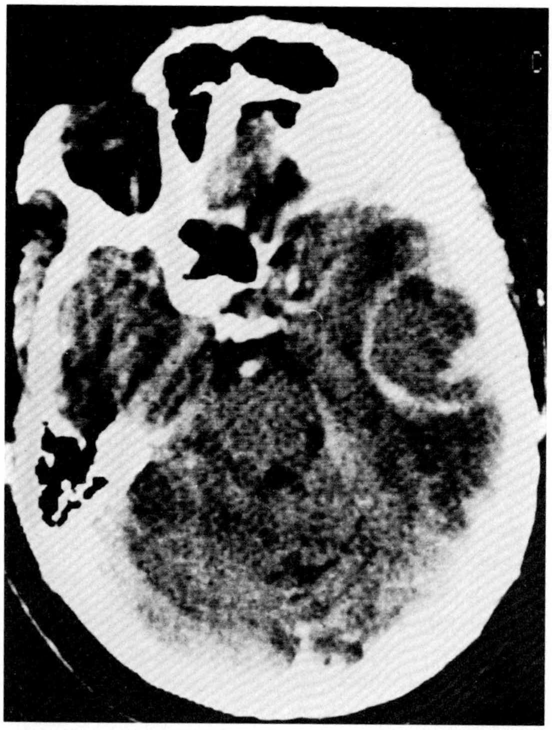

Fig 1. **Ring enhancement on contrast CT scan characteristic of malignant glioma.**

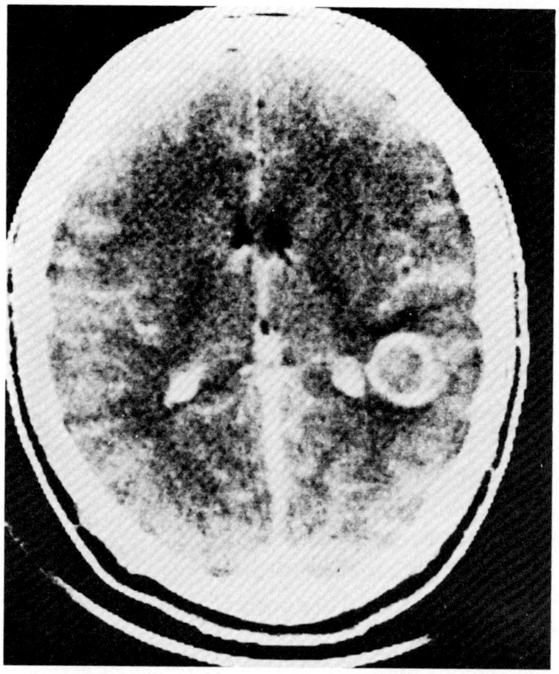

Fig 2. **Contrast CT scan of brain abscess.**

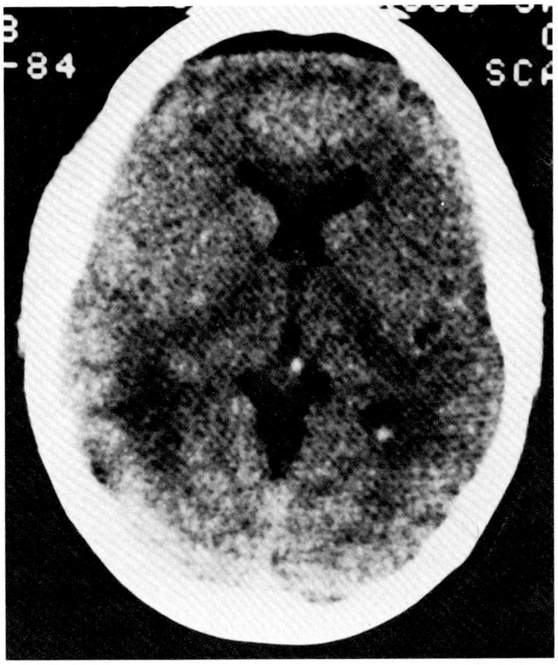

Fig 3. CT scan of low grade glioma showing nonenhancing temporal lesion.

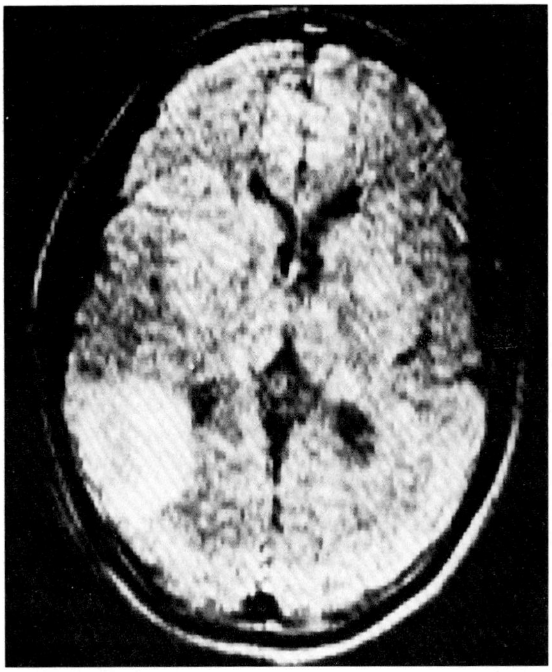

Fig 4. MRI—same patient as in Fig 3, demonstrating extent of low grade glioma.

posterior fossa. MRI is unquestionably becoming a very important technique in the diagnosis and management of brain tumors.

Cerebral angiography will often demonstrate typical neovascularity producing the so-called tumor stain in malignant gliomas. An "early draining vein" may be visible in malignant tumors, but also occurs with brain abscesses. Angiography should be selective, ie, separate internal and external carotid injections via a femoral catheter technique. Extensive supply to an otherwise malignant-appearing tumor from the external carotid vasculature is much more likely to represent a meningioma or other nonectodermal tumor. Lumbar puncture is not indicated and ventriculography and pneumoencephalography are rarely performed. Digital intravenous angiography (DIVA) is a rapidly developing technique that carries relatively low risk. With further refinements it will likely become a substitute for conventional angiography.

In one study 96% of all clinically symptomatic gliomas were detected by CT scan versus 76% detected by brain scan, 75% by angiogram, and 80% by clinical assessment.[3] Four percent of malignant gliomas were not detected by CT scanning. Rarely false positive scans were noted when artifacts were interpreted as tumors. In another study, the CT scan was able to differentiate among different histological grades of gliomas with reasonable accuracy.

In summary, the combination of an enhancing CT scan with neovascularity, and early draining veins demonstrated on selective angiography, is almost diagnostic of a malignant glioma or a single intracranial metastasis. In the absence of a tumor stain on angiography, a positive radionuclide scan has almost equal diagnostic significance. MRI will become increasingly important in diagnosis as the technique becomes more available.

PREOPERATIVE MANAGEMENT

The preoperative management of the patient with malignant glioma includes 48 hours of anticonvulsant therapy (Dilantin, Parke-Davis, Morris Plains, NJ, 100 mg tid and phenobarbital, 30 mg bid). Corticosteroids are employed throughout the operative period to reduce pre- and postoperative edema. In patients with significant neurological deficits, the response to large doses of preoperative steroids will aid in the decision as to how extensive a surgical resection should be attempted. Corticosteroids do not have an oncolytic effect in brain tumors, hence the clearing of a neurological deficit suggests that the deficit is due to peritumoral edema rather than tumor infiltration and destruction. The response to steroids may therefore predict the expected result of radical tumor debulking.

The CT scan will demonstrate the relationship of the tumor mass to the adjacent ventricular system and is of greater value than the angiogram in operative planning. A tumor, which on the basis of vascular displacement might be considered to be arising within the thalamus, may be seen on CT scan to displace the ventricular system medially and upward, particularly the temporal horn, indicating that it is surgically accessible. However, a tumor stain on angiography surrounding critical vasculature such as the middle cerebral artery and fed by thalamoperforating vessels, can predict a poor surgical result. Extremely hypervascular gliomas, except those located in polar positions, that is, the tip of the frontal, the temporal or occipital lobe, can also indicate difficult surgical problems and may mitigate against surgical intervention. Corpus callosum or so-called butterfly gliomas, particularly those arising in the posterior half of this structure, are rarely good candidates for surgical resection. Frontal lobe gliomas that appear to invade the corpus callosum are not necessarily excluded from surgical management.

The decision, therefore, for primary surgical intervention is based upon the patient's neurological status before and after the use of high dose corticosteroids, and the CT scan and angiographic demonstration of the exact location of the tumor mass. The goal of primary surgical therapy is that of achieving a radical removal of tumor tissue with preservation of normal brain and restoration or maintenance of good neurological function. Attempted surgical resection is generally excluded in patients with tumors located directly within the areas subserving speech, tumors arising within the thalamus on either side, or in the corpus callosum, particularly the posterior half of this structure. These patients are generally considered for radiation therapy and chemotherapy as a primary mode of treatment and surgery is reserved for the occasional delayed intervention. Stereotactic biopsy is recommended prior to therapy if there is any question as to the pathological nature of the tumor. The criterion for delayed surgery and surgery of recurrent tumors will be discussed in a subsequent section of this article.

SURGICAL RESECTION

Once the most important surgical decision has been reached, that is, to carry out primary surgical removal, and careful preoperative planning has been undertaken, all patients are given 250 mg of methylprednisolone intravenously the night before surgery and again the following morning. Anticonvulsant dosages are doubled for the 12 hours preoperatively and 500 cc of 20% mannitol is given intravenously via a previously placed central line after induction of anesthesia. Details of the surgical technique are beyond the scope of this chapter, but certain surgical principles will be reviewed.

If possible, the scalp incision should be placed behind the hairline, although cosmetic considerations are of secondary importance particularly since high dose radiation therapy produces severe hair loss. A large free bone flap is developed, centered over the area of tumor planned for elective excision. If the tumor does not present on the brain surface, ultrasound is useful in determining the most direct route to the lesion while avoiding areas of critical brain function. Many gliomas have a pseudocapsule and can be removed grossly by dissecting in the plane between tumor and edematous brain. Tumor resection should be carried out, wherever possible, to the CT predetermined limits, whether the lateral wall of the ventricle, the medial margin of the tentorium, or other clearly identifiable neuroanatomical structures. The operating microscope is used as needed in tumor dissection. The CUSA (Cooper-Cavitron, Stamford, Conn) surgical instrument removes tumor by ultrasound, the tip vibrating 20,000 times a minute accompanied by suction and aspiration, and is invaluable in achieving radical tumor removal. This technique has enabled surgeons to dissect neoplastic tissue from adjacent critical brain areas such as speech and motor centers without producing a major neurological deficit. The CUSA produces neither heat nor traction on surrounding tissues and, hence, it is particularly useful for removing areas of firm tumor tissue.

Once the planned resection has been achieved,

careful hemostasis is carried out with the use of the two point cautery, which coagulates small vessels between its tips. Because the electrical current does not pass through adjacent structures, the instrument can be used along the brainstem or other critical areas. The tumor cavity is then lined with a thin layer of oxidized (absorbant) cotton or gauze to prevent oozing of blood that might occur in the postoperative period. The greatest risk of postoperative hemorrhage occurs in those situations where tumor tissue has been incompletely removed, because bleeding from friable and abnormal capillaries is much more difficult to control than that from normal brain vasculature. Following hemostasis, the dura is closed as completely as possible and the free bone flap wired in place. There is rarely, if ever, any indication for leaving the dura open and discarding the bone flap. The brain should be well relaxed following the completion of tumor removal and if this is not the case, either a deep hemorrhage or inadequate tumor removal must be suspected and additional brain tissue may need to be removed in order to achieve relaxation. Parenthetically, it has been demonstrated that a so-called external decompression reduces cerebral tissue pressure and invites the occurrence of overwhelming brain edema.[4]

In the postoperative period, corticosteroids are continued at high dosage (1 g methylprednisolone qd in divided doses) for 48 to 72 hours, and then gradually tapered as tolerated over the subsequent week to ten days. Anticonvulsants are continued at a maintenance level on a permanent basis. A noncontrast CT scan should be obtained early in the postoperative period to document the amount of postoperative brain shift and the presence of any significant hematoma, either in the tumor bed or in the subdural or epidural spaces. The amount of demonstrable residual tumor can be determined one month after surgery with a contrast enhanced scan (Fig 5).

In summary, the preoperative planning, the operative techniques and the postoperative care must be carried out in a meticulous fashion in order to achieve an accepted morbidity and mortality rate in the conduct of radical glioma surgery. In patients who have been in good condition prior to surgery, the mortality and/or serious morbidity rate should be that of all elective

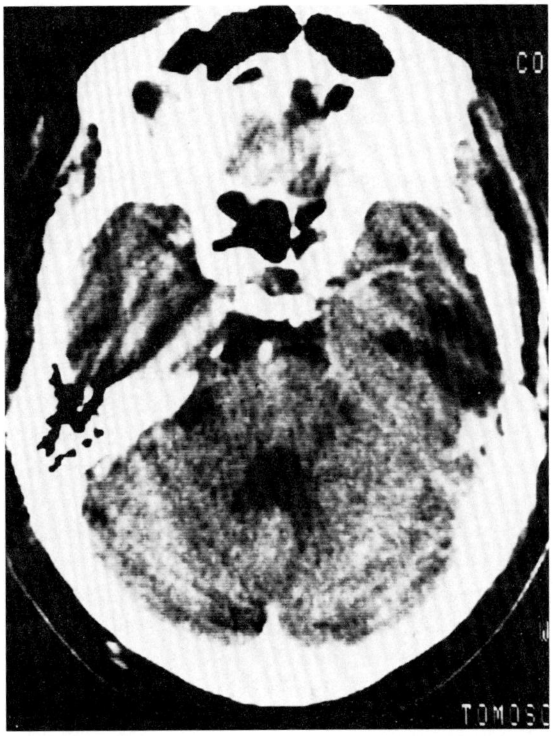

Fig 5. CT scan of residual tumor, same patient as in Fig 1.

neurosurgery, 7% to 10%. Review of the past 200 patients at NYU Medical Center with glioblastoma, whose preoperative Karnofsky Scales were 70 or better, revealed a 3% mortality and 8% morbidity rate (K Scale below 60). Postoperative radiation therapy and chemotherapy can be initiated within a week to ten days following surgical removal. Patients who have been maintained on corticosteroids for a prolonged period of time prior to surgery may demonstrate cerebral steroid dependency and require a slower steroid taper, particularly with the use of early postoperative radiation therapy.

A series of 115 patients was evaluated by comparison of their preoperative and postoperative CT scans correlating this information with survival time. A residual tumor burden of less than 45 mm in diameter was an important prognostic factor in long-term survival.[5]

STEREOTACTIC LASER SURGERY

When intra-axial tumors are deeply located in neurologically vital brain tissue, surgeons tend to be conservative in their resections, with the inevitable result that a kinetically significant amount of tumor tissue is left behind. A surgeon's three dimensional orientation decreases the deeper the procedure extends below the cortical surface. However, stereotactic methodology can provide mechanical control in three dimensional space and can be used to maintain surgical orientation during resection of tumors from subcortical areas. The carbon dioxide laser can be incorporated into the stereotactic instrumentation and its beam directed stereotactically for precision resection of defined tumor volumes located in three dimensional space.[6,7] Imaging modalities such as CT scanning, provide a three dimensional data base from which the target volume may be reconstructed.[7–9]

Patients undergo contrast-enhanced CT scanning with their head fixed in a CT compatible stereotactic holder.[10] Attached to the head holder is a CT localization system consisting of three localizing devices; one on each side of the head. The localization system produces a series of nine artifacts on each CT slice. The vertical height of the CT slice above the base ring is related to the distance of the reference mark corresponding to the middle (oblique) bar, from those corresponding to the verticals on each localization set. These describe three points in space which define a plane in relationship to the stereotactic instrument (Fig 6).

Following CT scanning, the patient is taken to the operating room and placed under general anesthesia. The archived data tape is read into a computer system located in the operating room.

The CT slices are displayed on a Ramtek (Santa Clara, Calif) raster scan display terminal in the operating room. The central pixel of each of the nine location artifacts is automatically digitized by an intensity detection program. The surgeon then digitizes multiple points along the outline of the tumor on each CT slice utilizing the terminal cursor and trackball (Fig 7). An interpolation program creates intermediate slices at one millimeter intervals, and each slice is given a thickness of one millimeter within the computer matrix. Thus, a solid volume in space is reconstructed (Fig 8). The tumor volume within the computer matrix may then be sliced orthogonally to any specified surgical viewline and the slices displayed on an operating room computer video monitor.

A stereotactic instrument (Fig 9) has been developed, which allows access to any intracranial target point and is interactive with the operating room computer system.

The tumor is approached through nonessential brain tissue via a linear scalp incision, a 2½ to 3 inch cranial trephine and circumferential dural opening. The white matter incision is made and deepened with the CO_2 laser as the laser and

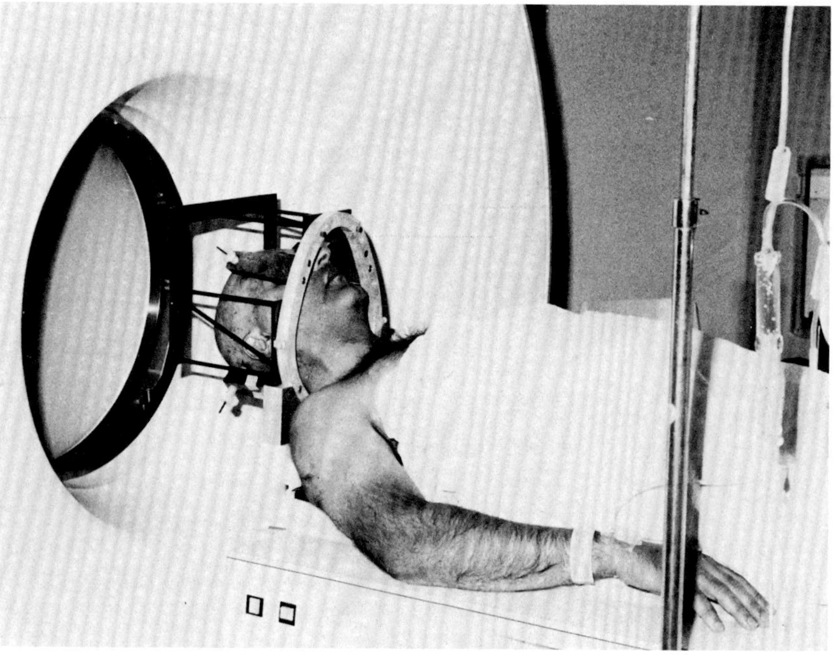

Fig 6. CT compatible stereotactic head holder.

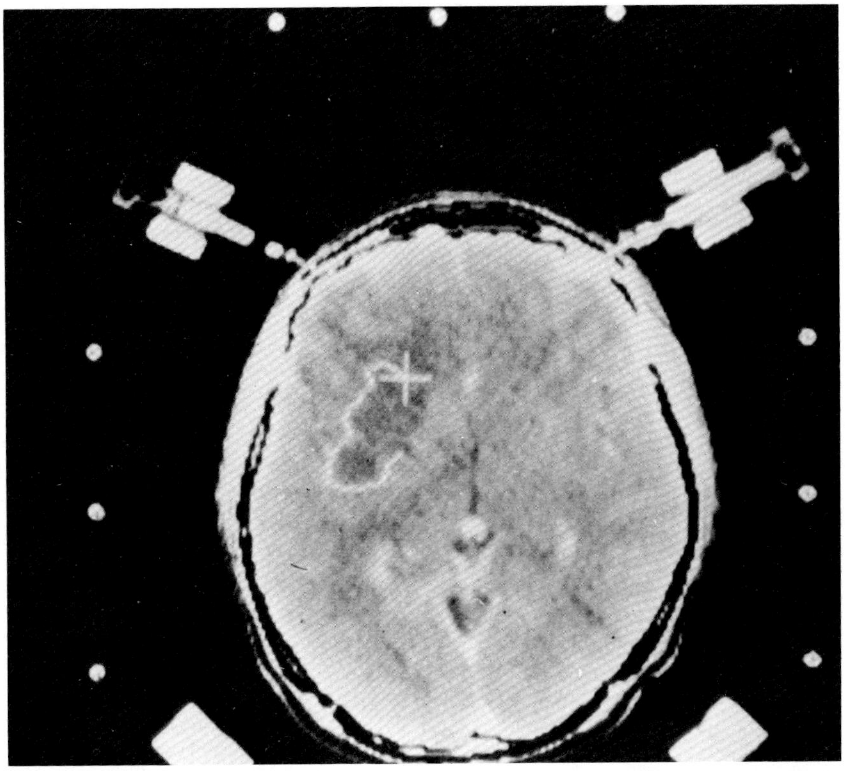

Fig 7. Outline of tumor on CT scan.

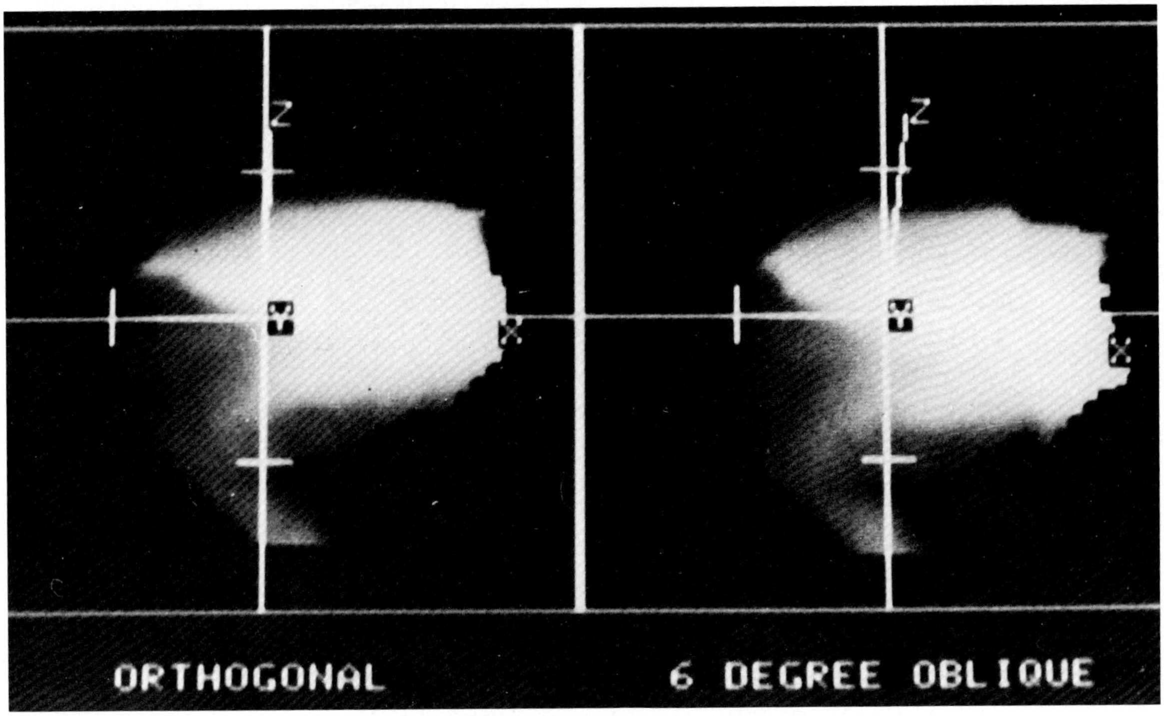

Fig 8. Reconstruction of tumor volume.

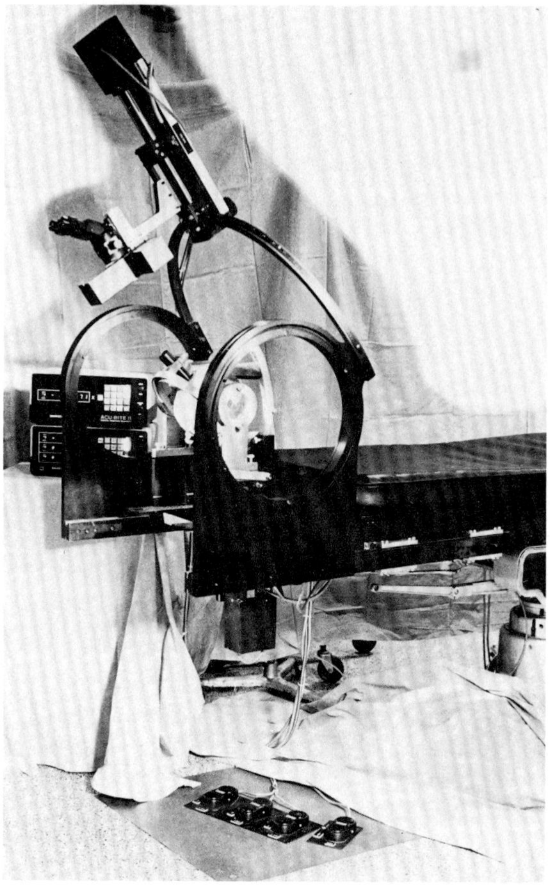

Fig 9. Stereotactic instrument.

microscope are directed toward the focal point of the stereotactic frame. At the outer border of the tumor (the position of which is calculated along the viewline by the computer) the incision is undercut by reflecting the laser beam with a stainless steel mirror. A self-retaining stereotactic retractor is then inserted.

The tumor is vaporized slice by slice utilizing 65 to 85 watts of defocused laser power in a continuous mode, progressing from the most superficial slice to the deepest. The position of the laser beam is monitored by the surgeon on the computer graphics terminal in reference to the tumor outline that has been reformatted from CT data. The reference stainless steel balls placed prior to surgery (Fig 10) confirm the depth of the surgical procedure as they are encountered. Ultimately, a cavity is produced which conforms to sagittal and coronal reconstructions of the tumor from CT scanning data.

Thirty-six patients have undergone 41 computer assisted stereotactic laser microsurgical procedures. Post-operative CT scanning revealed no evidence of residual tumor in 32 patients. However, some residual tumor was noted in the remaining nine patients. Four of these patients underwent a second procedure to remove residual tumor. An additional patient underwent a subsequent stereotactic laser procedure for a recurrent sarcomatous meningioma.

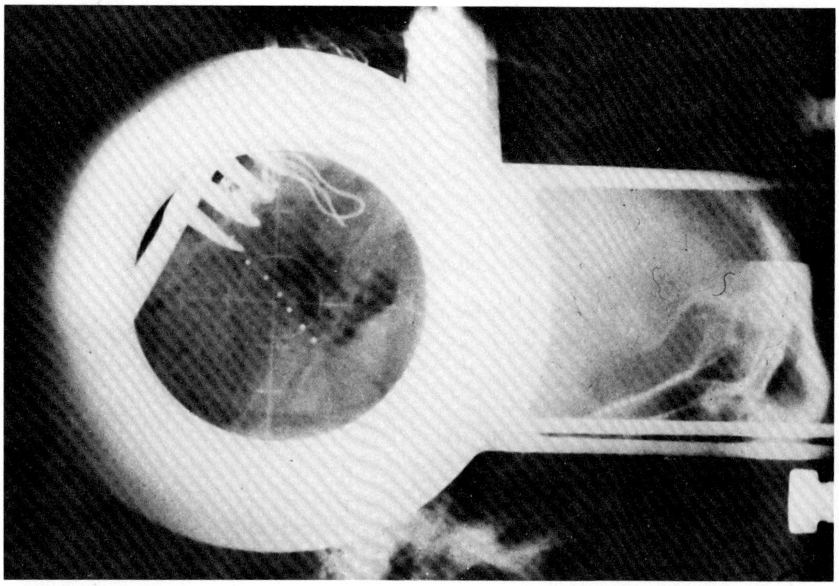

Fig 10. CT scan during stereotactic laser tumor removal.

Although the post-operative CT scan had demonstrated no tumor in 10 of the 13 patients with glioblastomas, nine had recurrence of their tumor on follow-up CT scan 3 to 11 months following their surgical procedure. Two patients with Grade III astrocytomas, one located in the posterior medial right frontal area extending into the corpus callosum, and the other located in the thalamus, have remained free of disease on CT scanning, three years and 26 months, respectively, following surgery. So far, no patient with metastatic tumor has had local intracranial recurrence following stereotactic laser resection of the tumor.

Our preliminary results (P.K.) indicate that deepseated lesions may be resected with satisfactory postoperative neurologic results, since controlled removal of the neoplasm can be accomplished with minimal trauma to surrounding brain tissue. The amount of actual tissue destruction produced by the CO_2 laser is limited to the spot size of the laser (about 0.8 mm) and a zone of thermal necrosis of 200 to 300 microns on either side of a laser incision. For this reason, tumors in neurologically critical areas, such as the thalamus, can theoretically be removed without significant damage to important normal adjacent tissue.

THE USE OF HEMATOPORPHYRIN AND ARGON LASER

The fact that certain fluorescent chemical compounds can be activated by exposure to light has been known for more than 100 years. Such compounds have been used biologically for detection of tumors of various kinds; many of these agents concentrate in a variety of neoplasms as well as other rapidly growing tissues.

Hematoporphyrin is one such agent that shares these characteristics. For practical purposes it is used as a hematoporphyrin derivative (HpD), prepared by acetylation of the parent compound. HpD can be given intravenously, is concentrated well in neoplasms, fluoresces red when activated by blue light, and, when activated by light of adequate intensity and proper wavelength, can produce a substantial cytotoxic reaction. This reaction is the basis of the clinical disorder protoporphyria II, wherein the skin is sensitized and damaged by light. Skin sensitivity and burns evoked by strong light are the major types of clinical adverse effects observed when HpD is used for therapy of tumors.

The use of HpD and its activation by light has been termed photoradiation therapy (PRT). This concept is currently under intense investigation in the laboratory and also in limited clinical trials. As a treatment modality it has great appeal, since it does not interfere with prior or subsequent therapy using other methods. Laboratory studies have confirmed many favorable aspects of the use of HpD for the management of brain tumors. In most animals and in man, the blood brain barrier effectively excludes HpD from entry into normal brain tissue. Brain tumor tissue readily absorbs the HpD, and peak concentrations are reached in 4 hours after intravenous administration; high concentrations may be maintained for as long as four days.[11]

Although cytotoxic activation of HpD in tumor cells is most efficient with blue light (405 nm), this wavelength has limited penetration capability in brain and tumor tissue. Red light (633 nm) produces a less efficient cytotoxic effect, but has the virtue of deeper effective penetration (up to 8 mm). Red light can be conveniently generated by an argon-dye laser or by a high intensity filtered lamp. This compromise of activating HpD with red light has been utilized in many of the clinical trials.

The basis of the cytotoxic effect is thought to be the release of free radicals in the cytoplasm of the tumor cells with ensuing damage to the cell membrane. Singlet oxygen (O) is thought to be the primary toxic agent. Heat inactivates this photodynamic effect, making it important to monitor the temperatures generated in tissue by the activating light.

Currently two concepts of PRT treatment of malignant tumors in humans have been utilized. Deep tumors can be treated stereotactically by implantation of one or more fiberoptic probes through needles. The tip of the fiberoptic probe acts as a point source of light generating a sphere of photoactivation. The second concept involves the surgical resection of an accessible lesion, and the treatment of the tumor bed with light of appropriate wavelength and intensity. In either case, the patient is given HpD, 5 mg/kg intravenously 4 to 48 hours prior to surgery. Following the injection of the drug, the patient must be protected from exposure to sunlight or high intensity artificial light for three to four weeks.

Experience at the Mayo Medical School includes laboratory investigations and clinical experience with 25 patients harboring malignant brain tumors. A Phase I study has been completed, and no major toxicity or adverse reaction has occurred. Evaluation of the Phase II study is difficult because of the short follow-up and the desperate nature of the patients treated. The results are not discouraging, and further efforts are under way to improve the methodology.

Laboratory efforts are under way to evaluate new combinations of activating light and photoactivated drugs. Methods for improving light delivery using cooling and diffusion media have been developed and are under trial. Techniques for enhancing the longevity and effectiveness of free radical generation are being investigated. With a number of groups working on this problem, one can anticipate further progress and more effective management of malignant brain tumors.

SURGERY OF RECURRENT GLIOMAS

Surgical removal of recurrent gliomas can be considered in patients who have had early satisfactory results and in whom regrowth of tumor can be documented on CT scan. One would hesitate to consider a patient for reoperation short of nine months to a year following the initial surgery and only in those patients in whom meaningful existence has been provided by the initial treatment regime. The tumor should be strictly localized to its original site and if evidence of extension across the midline to the other hemisphere or into deeper brain structures, including the thalamus or brainstem, can be documented on CT scan, surgery is not applicable. A greater number of patients are being seen with local tumor recurrence, undoubtedly as a result of the more rigorous use of radiation therapy and chemotherapy, than previously had been the case. At the time of repeat surgery these tumors are often well demarcated from surrounding brain. The postoperative CT scan may often be clean of any signs of gross tumor. In carefully selected patients a significant prolongation of useful life can be achieved, particularly if additional chemotherapy is applicable, following the removal of tumor regrowth.

Secondary surgery can be considered in patients who were initially deemed to be inoperable because of tumor location or in whom for other reasons, radiation and chemotherapy had been the initial treatment of choice. If good response was seen with significant reduction of tumor size, and regrowth is documented, tumor removal is often as easy as that following tumor recurrence. Tumor vascularity is significantly reduced, particularly in those lesions that were hypervascular on initial angiography, and the sharp demarcation between tumor and surrounding tissue makes the consideration of later secondary surgery in selected cases a reasonable option. Once again, the use of the ultrasonic surgical aspirator and the CO_2 laser have proven to be invaluable in terms of approaching relatively critical brain areas.

CONCLUSIONS

The current status of classical surgical therapy of malignant gliomas can be summarized as follows. With the correlative information available from CT scanning, radio nuclide scanning, cerebral angiography as well as that obtained from the general medical workup, surgery is rarely needed to establish the diagnosis of a malignant glioma. When indicated, a carefully controlled biopsy can be obtained through a burr hole needle biopsy, localization being achieved with the use of CT scanning. A carefully planned and executed surgical approach to these tumors can often achieve a near total removal of grossly recognizable tumor tissue as documented on postoperative CT scans. Mortality and morbidity rates in these highly malignant tumors can be kept at acceptable levels. Clearly, radiation therapy and chemotherapy have made a significant impact on long-term survival in the treatment of this cancer, however, surgery still remains the single most effective method for achieving a rapid reduction of tumor burden. In addition, one reduces increased intracranial pressure and relieves neurological signs and symptoms, hence, avoiding the complications of long-term corticosteroid therapy. Following surgery, the other antitumor programs have the best chance of achieving a significant increment of tumor cell kill.[12] Surgical therapy, therefore, has a distinct role to play in the multidisciplinary approach to the treatment of these difficult and highly aggressive neoplasms.

ACKNOWLEDGMENT

I am indebted to Dr Edward Laws of the Mayo Clinic for the section on the use of the argon laser and hematoporphyrin, to Dr Patrick Kelly of the Mayo Clinic for the section on stereotactic laser surgery, and to Drs Messina and Lieberskind of New York City for the MRI scans.

Part of this work was supported by Contract Number NO-CM-17473 from the National Cancer Institute.

REFERENCES

1. Russell DS, Rubinstein LJ: Pathology of the nervous system (ed 4). Baltimore, Williams & Wilkins, 1977, pp 147–282
2. Jellinger K: Glioblastoma multiforme: Morphology and biology, Acta Neurochir 42:5–32, 1978
3. Ambrose J, Gooding HR, Richardson AR: An assessment of the accuracy of computerized transverse axial scanning (EMI scanning) in the diagnosis of intracranial tumor: A review of 366 patients. Brain 98:569, 1975
4. Cooper PR, Rovit RL, Ransohoff J: Hemicraniectomy in the treatment of acute subdural hematoma: A reappraisal. Surg Neurol 5:25–30, 1976
5. Lieberman A, Foo SH, Ransohoff J, et al: Long term survival among patients with malignant brain tumors. Neurosurgery 10:450–453, 1982
6. Kelly PJ, Alker GJ Jr: A stereotactic approach to deep-seated CNS neoplasms using the carbon dioxide laser. Surg Neurol 15:331–334, 1981
7. Kelly PJ, Alker GJ Jr, Goerss S: Computer assisted stereotactic laser microsurgery for the treatment of intracranial neoplasms. Neurosurgery 10:324–331, 1982
8. Kelly PJ, Kall B, Goerss S, et al: Precision resection of intra-axial CNS lesions by CT-based stereotactic craniotomy and computer monitored CO_2 laser. Acta Neurochir 68:1–9, 1983
9. Kelly PJ, Kall B, Goerss S: Transposition of volumetric information derived from computed tomography scanning into stereotactic space. Surg Neurol 21:465–471, 1984
10. Goerss S, Kelly PJ, Kall B, et al: A computerized tomographic stereotactic adaptation system. Neurosurgery 10:375–379, 1982
11. Wharen RE Jr, Anderson RE, Laws ER Jr: Quantitation of hematoporphyrin derivative in human gliomas, experimental central nervous system tumors, and normal tissue. Neurosurgery 12:446–450, 1983
12. Ransohoff J, Lieberman A: Surgical therapy of primary malignant brain tumors. Clin Neurosurg 25:403–411, 1978

Therapy of Adult Malignant Brain Tumors: What Have the Clinical Trials Taught Us?

William R. Shapiro

UNTIL RECENTLY, malignant glioma, the most common of which is glioblastoma multiforme, was characterized by a rapidly fatal course with 50% mortality within six months and 90% mortality within 1½ years.[1] This grim picture has improved with the advent of vigorous multimodality therapy aimed at reducing tumor burden.[2] Multimodality therapy for malignant gliomas—cytoreductive surgery, radiation therapy, chemotherapy—has been under investigation by cooperative groups and individual institutions for the past 20 years. While most of these studies have yielded definitive data, the claim has been made that their results have been of little real value in that the therapies they have tested have extended survival only minimally and have not offered a major breakthrough that would more substantially improve therapy. Furthermore, clinical trials are expensive, and their results should be good enough to justify diverting funds away from more fundamental research. Unfortunately, we must treat our patients now; we do not have the luxury of waiting for a fundamental advance in therapy. The question is: Given the difficulty and expense of clinical research, are the results good enough to warrant continuing to place patients on protocol rather than treating them on an ad hoc basis? In this article, I shall try to show that the best of the clinical trials have substantially improved the way we treat our patients and have offered clues to several important biologic and therapeutic questions. I shall conclude that such research must continue pari passu with basic research if clinically relevant new therapeutic modalities are to be developed and implemented.

From the Department of Neurology, Memorial Sloan-Kettering Cancer Center, Cornell University Medical College, New York.

Address reprint requests to William R. Shapiro, MD, Department of Neurology, Memorial Sloan-Kettering Cancer Center, 1275 York Ave, New York, NY 10021.

0093-7754/86/1301-0005$05.00/0

ON THE NATURE OF CLINICAL TRIALS FOR BRAIN TUMORS

Clinical trials are of two types, phase III and phase II studies.* Phase III studies are controlled prospective trials that compare results in patients receiving experimental therapy with those in control groups who receive standard therapy. Phase II studies compare experimental groups to historic controls. The use of historic controls assumes that nothing significant has occurred in the natural history of the disease that could affect survival. That such an assumption may be incorrect can be concluded by observing the influence of computerized tomographic (CT) scanning on the earlier diagnosis of brain tumor, and therefore when treatment is initiated. Phase III trials have the advantage of a concurrent control group for comparison.

End points used in clinical studies include survival, "time-to-recurrence" or "disease-free survival," and various measures of the size of the brain tumor itself, including the CT scan and other imaging techniques. Survival studies have the advantage of a definite end point that usually relates to the size of the tumor and less to transient treatments like corticosteroid hormones. However, if small gains are to be appreciated in survival studies, large numbers of patients must be accrued. This need for many patients spawned the cooperative group studies, the one with the most experience being the National Cancer Institute—sponsored Brain Tumor Study Group (BTSG)—now the Brain Tumor Cooperative Group (BTCG). Other cooperative groups that have conducted prospective, controlled brain tumor therapy trials are the Radiation Therapy Oncology Group/Eastern Cooperative Oncology Group (RTOG/ECOG) and the Southwest Oncology Group in the

*A third type of study, phase I, is designed to evaluate toxicity of new therapeutic modalities; it measures therapeutic results only incidentally. Brain tumor patients are not usually included in phase I studies.

United States and several European and Japanese groups. The Northern California Oncology Group (NCOG) has conducted primarily phase II studies, which have often yielded clues that other groups have followed in designing phase III trials.

While most observers agree that group studies yield reliable data, the claim has been made that their results have not produced a "breakthrough." Furthermore, it is thought that their response time is slower than individual institutional studies, which are more flexible than those of the groups. The claim is often made that individual institutional investigations are more imaginative and innovative in their approaches, and therefore are more likely to make the sought-after breakthroughs. Unfortunately, the variability inherent in the natural history of malignant glioma makes it difficult to evaluate small studies, precisely because they include too few patients; indeed, it may be difficult to recognize any breakthroughs they may produce.

Because cooperative groups trials, primarily those of the BTSG, have most reliably established the state-of-the-art for therapy of malignant gliomas, I shall utilize their data in this article to assess the impact of clinical research on the management of gliomas.

PRINCIPLES OF EXPERIMENTAL THERAPY: CYTOREDUCTION

The goal of trials in brain tumor therapy is cytoreduction; that is, the decrease of the total tumor mass to a size that the body's immune system might suppress and eventually kill—approximately 0.0001 g or 1×10^5 cells.[2] Brain tumors can produce symptoms when they are quite small (usually seizures), but most patients presenting with neurologic symptoms usually have tumors 30 to 60 g in size (3 to 6×10^{10} cells). The neurosurgeon may be able to remove between 20% and 90% of the tumor, depending on its location (see Ransohoff et al, this issue). More commonly he can resect less than 50%, thus leaving a residual tumor burden of 1 to 5×10^9 cells. Subsequent radiation therapy (RT) might kill two additional logs of cells, reducing the tumor to about 1×10^7 cells. Chemotherapy must then kill two additional logs to reduce the cell burden to the desired 1×10^5 cells. However, the currently available chemotherapeutic agents produce a net cell kill of only about 1 log, and thus the tumor grows despite the drug. These considerations imply that present-day multimodality therapy can treat infiltrative brain tumors, but can rarely cure them. Nevertheless, vigorous therapy permits many patients to live longer with a better quality of life than is possible without such intervention.

PHASE III STUDIES

The results of four BTSG adjuvant RT/chemotherapy studies are summarized in Table 1. In the 6901 study, the median survival time following resection alone without postoperative RT or chemotherapy was only 14 weeks,[3] while surgery plus RT improved the median to at least 36 weeks. Chemotherapy with BCNU alone did not add significantly to postoperative survival, although a significant proportion of patients treated with RT plus BCNU survived 18 months (19% *v* only 4% for RT or BCNU alone). In the 7201 study, BCNU added to surgery and RT produced a median survival of 51 weeks ($P = .072$ *v* surgery plus RT) and an 18-month survivorship of 27%.[4] In the 7501 trial, surgery plus RT plus BCNU produced a median survival of 50 weeks ($P = .009$ *v* surgery plus RT plus methylprednisolone).[5] Trial 7702 demonstrated median survivorship between 42.0 and 45.5 weeks and 18-month survivorship between 13 and 23%.[6]

Each of these trials was designed to answer a specific question in brain tumor therapy. Trials 6901 and 7201 proved by controlled prospective examination that RT substantially improved survivorship over surgery plus either supportive care alone or supportive care and a single drug, BCNU. This result was of such importance that by trial 7501, it was elected to include RT in each of the study arms. There was the suggestion in trial 7201 that BCNU added to the survival afforded by surgery plus RT, but it was not until trial 7501 that the effectiveness of BCNU was confirmed (Fig 1). Trial 7501 also tested the value of a high-dose corticosteroid hormone as a chemotherapeutic agent. Corticosteroid hormones (eg, dexamethasone, methylprednisolone, prednisone) are crucial in treating patients with brain tumor. They act by reducing cerebral

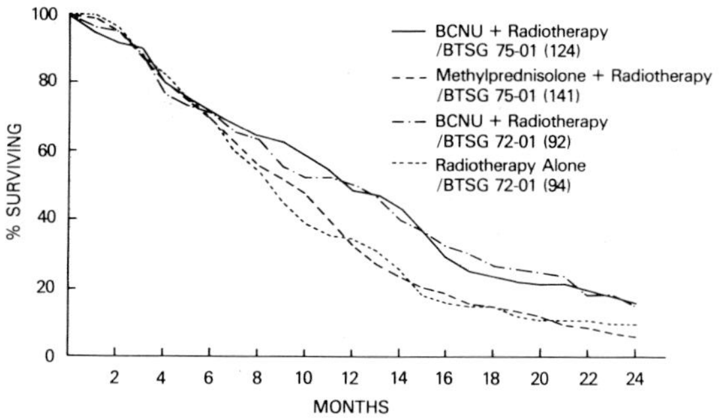

Fig 1. Comparison of selected survival curves for valid study group patients from BTSG study 72-01 and 75-01 Numbers of patients are shown in parentheses. It is evident that BCNU adds substantially to the survival of patients treated otherwise with surgery and radiation therapy. Reproduced from Cancer Treat Rep.[5]

edema, often improving neurologic symptoms. Because steroids prolong survival in experimental animal brain tumors and because they are chemotherapeutic in some leukemias and lymphomas, it was considered to be important to determine their chemotherapeutic effectiveness when used in brain tumor trials that tested new drugs. In trial 7501, patients were given high-dose corticosteroid hormones—methylprednisolone 400 mg/m^2/d for seven days of every 28—as part of a chemotherapeutic study. As noted in Table 1, methylprednisolone did not increase survival over that afforded by surgery plus RT alone; indeed, there was a suggestion that high-dose corticosteroid hormones increased the incidence of infections in patients receiving RT plus BCNU. In all subsequent trials, corticosteroids were used as needed to control neurologic symptoms without the concern that they would in themselves prolong survival.

In a similar trial, the RTOG/ECOG studied RT without or with chemotherapy in malignant glioma.[7] Four treatment protocols were tested in a randomized prospective trial: (1) daily fraction whole-brain RT to a total of 6,000 rad, (2) whole-brain RT to 6,000 rad plus 1,000 rad tumor boost, (3) 6,000 rad whole-brain RT plus BCNU, and (4) 6,000 rad whole-brain RT plus methyl-CCNU and DTIC. While there were no statistical differences in survival between the various groups, for the 40- to 60-year-old cohort survival was significantly prolonged by the chemotherapeutic agents over RT alone, although the two-drug regimen was quite toxic. The RT boost to the tumor did not make a difference. The finding that age is important in prognosis confirms BTSG observations (see below).

BTCG trial 7702 attempted to examine two new techniques in RT: hypoxic cell sensitizers and hyperfractionated RT. In the first method, misonidazole, a second-generation radiation sen-

Table 1. Results of Brain Tumor Study Group Phase III Trials of Postoperative Therapy

Treatment	No. of Patients	MST (wk)	18-Mo Survivorship (%)	Comments	Reference
Trial 6901	222				
Support		14	0	RT and RT + BCNU significantly	
BCNU		19	4	better than support	3
RT		36	4		
RT + BCNU		35	19		
Trial 7201	358				
Methyl-CCNU		24	10	RT, RT + BCNU, and RT + meth-	
RT		36	15	yl-CCNU significantly better	
RT + methyl-CCNU		42	23	than methyl-CCNU	4
RT + BCNU		51	27		
Trial 7501	527				
RT + Medrol		40	15	RT + BCNU and RT + procarba-	
RT + procarbazine		47	29	zine significantly better than	
RT + BCNU		50	24	RT + Medrol	5
RT + BCNU + Medrol		41	23		
Trial 7702	557				
RT + BCNU		44	16	No significant difference among	
Fraction RT + BCNU		45	25	the four arms	6
RT + misonidazole + BCNU		40	16		
RT + streptozotocin		43	25		

Abbreviation: MST, median survival time.

sitizer, was administered twice weekly so as to take advantage of four of the five RT treatments per week. In the other arm, the number of fractions over which the radiation was given was increased from the usual once per day to twice daily with approximately the same total ret dose (1,700 ret). Streptozotocin, a water-soluble sugar-containing nitrosourea previously tested in BTSG phase II studies, was also examined. As summarized in Table 1, no substantial difference in survival was noted among the four arms, suggesting that neither fractionated RT nor misonidazole contributed significantly to survival in such patients. An important consideration in this study was the use of misonidazole at a dose schedule (1.5 g/m^2 twice weekly) that was higher than that used previously, leading to concern about potential increased incidence of peripheral neuropathy. In fact, peripheral neuropathy occurred primarily in patients whose total misonidazole dose exceeded 10 g/m^2 and was rarely sufficiently severe to preclude completion of the course. (See Sheline et al, this issue, for further discussion about radiation sensitizers and hyperfractionation RT.)

In their most recent investigation (trial 8001), the BTSG examined several new issues. The study consists of three arms, all with RT: one arm with BCNU, a second with BCNU sequenced every two months with procarbazine, and a third arm combining BCNU with hydroxyurea and sequencing every two months with procarbazine plus VM-26. The rationale for this study relates to the question of heterogeneous chemosensitivity in malignant brain tumors (see W.R. Shapiro and J.R. Shapiro, this issue) and thus used multiple-drug combination chemotherapy. A second question relates to the need for whole-brain RT *v* focal RT. Studies by the BTSG[8,9] and by others[10] suggested that patients surviving three or more years following high-dose whole-brain RT might develop a syndrome of progressive dementia, enlarging ventricles, and pathologic changes suggesting diffuse radiation damage. Both the incidence of this disease and its pathogenesis are unknown (see Burger, this issue). A recent investigation utilizing CT scans suggests that a large proportion of gliomas tends to recur within 2 cm of the original tumor margins.[11] To examine the question of the need for whole-brain RT *v* focal RT, it was elected to modify the protocol to reduce the whole-brain RT component. After the accrual of the first 250 patients, subsequent patients were randomly assigned to one of two radiation protocols; half of these received standard whole-brain 6,000 rad RT; the remaining received partial whole-brain RT followed by a coned-down boost. The purpose of the protocol was to determine if coned-down RT reduced the efficacy of whole-brain RT, and if the coned-down RT could reduce the incidence of post-RT brain damage. While it is too early to evaluate the long-term results, it is already apparent that there is no difference in survival between patients treated with whole-brain RT only and those who receive partial whole-brain RT plus coned-down focal RT to the tumor.

A number of other phase III studies in malignant brain tumors have been reported, testing a variety of chemotherapeutic agents singly and in combination (reviewed elsewhere[12]). Among the chemotherapeutic agents tested, none appeared to have a specific therapeutic advantage. Thus, there are no substantial differences in the therapeutic effectiveness of BCNU, methyl-CCNU, procarbazine, and streptozotocin as tested in BTSG studies. While CCNU itself was not compared with the other nitrosoureas, it appears about as effective as BCNU and methyl-CCNU. Most of the combinations have not produced evidence of synergism; indeed, many have not even been additive because of the increased toxicity of the combinations.

PHASE II STUDIES

The purpose of phase II studies is to identify treatments (usually drugs) that may be effective in brain tumor therapy and should be tested in more definitive trials. In this respect, the purpose is the same as that of phase II studies for chemotherapy of any cancer. The criteria for evaluation for the phase II studies usually differ from those used to evaluate phase III studies. The BTSG has used overall survival from entry as the major end point for its phase II trials. While survival represents an excellent end point in phase III trials, it may not be the best end point for phase II studies. Drugs may not be effective enough by themselves to prolong overall survival, yet may be good enough to reduce the tumor's size or prolong disease-free survival. Furthermore, a method of evaluation that also includes a measure of tumor size gives more information than that evaluating survival only.

As noted above, a major problem with phase II trials is that the number of patients accrued is usually too small to draw a definitive conclusion about its efficacy unless the agent turns out to be a "silver bullet." If a drug improves survival by 50% or better or reduces the size of the visible tumor by 50%, it is likely to be identified by such studies. However, most of the available agents are clearly not that effective, and such trials must include enough patients to detect lesser efficacies.

Many agents have been tested in phase II trials and the interested reader is referred to several reviews.[12,13] While some of these studies have identified important new effective regimens, others have served the important function of identifying those drugs with little value in the treatment of brain tumors. In BTSG phase II trials, Adriamycin (Adria, Dublin, Ohio) proved to be ineffective, while hydroxyurea, VM-26, procarbazine, and several combinations were effective enough to be advanced into phase III trials. Phase II trials from other centers also contribute to BTSG studies; the pioneering work of the NCOG led to a new BTCG study using BCNU plus 5-FU, and several European studies led to the evaluation of combination chemotherapy with VM-26.

Table 2. The Influence of Prognostic Variables on Death Rate in Patients With Malignant Gliomas

Variable	Category	Death Rate*
Age	<45	0.36
	45–54	0.63
	55–64	0.89
	≥64	1.27
Histopathology	Glioblastoma	0.76
	Anaplastic astrocytoma	0.43
	90–100	0.44
	70-80	0.66
Performance status	50-60	0.96
(Karnofsky post-op)	10–40	1.31
Duration of symptoms	≤6	0.81
(mo)	>6	0.41
Level of consciousness	Normal	0.64
(post-op)	Abnormal	1.28
Blood type	B, O	0.62
	A, AB	0.84
Pretreatment WBC count		0.59
($\times$ 1,000/mm^3)	5.5–8.5 other	0.79
	≤200	0.99
Pretreatment platelet	201–300	0.79
count ($\times$ 1,000/mm^3)	>300	0.63

Adapted from trial 7501.[5] Each variable (and eight others) significantly correlated with survival. These eight were retained in a multivarate analysis after a "step-down" procedure.

*Death rates are expressed as the number of deaths per ten patient-months.

PROGNOSTIC VARIABLES

It is evident from BTSG studies and others[7] that certain patient characteristics can be related to the patient's prognosis—the so-called prognostic variables. Clinical characteristics that have proven to be prognostically important include the patient's age, his postoperative performance status (Karnofsky rating), the occurrence of seizures as part of the presentation of the brain tumor, possibly the tumor's location within the brain, and certain neurologic signs on initial examination.

The first detailed evaluation of prognostic factors was undertaken in the BTSG 7201 study[4] and identified 16 variables,[5] among which eight were used both for a Cox proportional hazards model[14] and a Weibull regression model to examine their effects on prognosis (Table 2). Young patients lived significantly longer than elderly patients; the death rate for patients under 45 was one third that of patients aged 65 or more. Patients with highly malignant glioblastoma multiforme survived half as long as those harboring less malignant gliomas. Postoperative Karnofsky rating was very important; patients with ratings of 90 to 100 had one third the death rate of patients with ratings of 40 or below. Similarly, the duration of symptoms was important; patients whose symptoms exceeded six months had a death rate half that of patients whose symptoms were less than six months. A long duration of symptoms correlated with the occurrence of seizures; the presence of seizures was a good prognostic sign, and their absence was a bad prognostic sign. An abnormal level of consciousness after surgery was associated with twice the death rate of that following a normal level of consciousness. Factors that were not so easily explained included blood types—B or O indicating a better prognosis than A or AB, elevated pretreatment WBC count, which carried a poor prognosis, as did relative thrombocytopenia.

To demonstrate the importance of prognostic variables, the patient data were divided into three risk groups on the basis of the percentage of patient survival at 24 months as predicted by the Weibull model. One hundred twenty-three patients with a predicted 24-month survival >25% constituted group 1; 271 patients with predicted survival between 2.5% and 25.0% were included in group 2; and 126 patients with predicted survival <2.5% were included in group 3. A plot of the actuarial survival curves for these three groups along with the predicted curves from the model is shown in Fig 2. The model provides a good fit to the data.

As noted above, the RTOG/ECOG study on adjuvant RT/chemotherapy also found that certain patient and tumor characteristics influence outcome.[7] Indeed, age was so important in their study that statistical improvement in survival occurred only in patients in the 40 to 60-year age range. Other prognostic variables in order of importance were histologic grade of tumor, initial performance status, time since initial symptoms, previous surgery, speech impairment, visual disturbance, presence or absence of seizures, and mental status. It is clear that many prognostic variables in combination influence survival at least as much as does combination multimodality therapy.

Two obvious conclusions follow from these data. The first is that a sufficient number of patients must be included in any trial to permit their even distribution among the treatment arms according to their prognostic variables; occasionally, this may require stratification. The

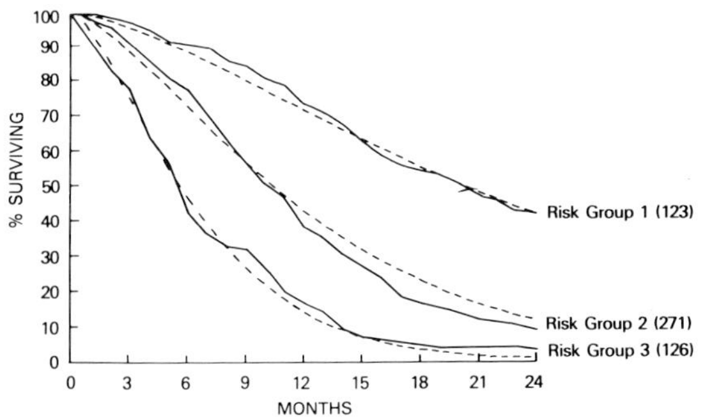

Fig 2. Survival curves for risk groups as defined in the text. Solid lines represent observed life-table survival rates, dashed lines represent predicted survival rates from the Weibull model. Numbers of patients are shown in parentheses. Reproduced from Cancer Treat Rep.[6]

need for an adequate number of patients is especially true for phase II trials; Eagan and Scott[15] demonstrated that prognostic variables profoundly affect the interpretation of therapeutic trials. Second, a search for the biologic reasons for the prognostic variables is likely to yield information useful in understanding tumors and their therapy.

QUALITY OF LIFE

In any discussion of clinical therapeutic research, an important consideration is whether the additional survival is purchased at the cost of so much toxicity that the patient's predictably foreshortened life is made even more miserable by his physician's ministrations. For patients with brain tumors, the problem is compounded by the fact that nervous system disease is often more incapacitating than systemic disease. The effects of the tumor on the brain, the initial surgical manipulation, and the subsequent radiation and chemotherapy must all be considered in evaluating quality of life.

Physicians actively engaged in clinical research find such considerations both troublesome and difficult to assess. Quantifying the quality of a patient's daily life is just as important as quantifying his survival, but far more difficult. Many schemes have been developed to measure quality of life, the most popular of which is the Karnofsky performance status. In studies at Memorial Sloan-Kettering Cancer Center, we attempted to quantify the effect of therapy on quality of life. In a study of surgery, we found that a tumor resection was more likely to alleviate existing symptoms than to produce additional ones.[2] In 82 patients assessed for abnormalities in speech, personality, or visual, sensory, or motor function, 80% of the abnormalities were improved or unchanged postoperatively, with 20% worsened, and there were new abnormalities in 13% of the functional areas examined. In a chemotherapy study,[16] we found that patients maintained their best postoperative performance status for about 75% of their remaining lifespan, and that the performance status was not adversely affected by the treatments. Thus, a patient's quality of life is far more dependent on the effects of the tumor than it is on the effects of the therapy. All treatment involves a judgment of potential gain *v* potential loss. For malignant glioma, therapy improves both quantity and quality of life.

CONCLUSIONS

Controlled prospective clinical trials of the BTSG and others have produced four noteworthy results that now influence the management of patients with malignant gliomas. (1) Radiation therapy significantly prolongs survival; the combination of whole-brain RT plus a focal tumor boost to a total tumor dose of 6,000 rad is the most effective. (2) Chemotherapy with BCNU produces a statistically significant increase in survival; the agents procarbazine, methyl-CCNU, CCNU, and streptozotocin are about as effective as BCNU. The number of long-surviving patients (those living longer than 18 months) is specifically related to the use of chemotherapy. (3) High-dose corticosteroid hormones are not chemotherapeutic. (4) Individual patient prognostic variables are identifiable that may provide guidelines to the use of available therapeutic modalities. In addition, controlled clinical trials have demonstrated that many agents are ineffective and have also shown that modifying RT with the radiation sensitizer misonidazole or twice-daily fractions does not improve survival beyond that achieved with standard RT.

It is clear that continued large-scale prospective trials are required to examine new treatment modalities in the most definitive manner. Phase II trials are also required if we are to test proposed modalities for their potential efficacy. In contrast to what has been promulgated by some, patients do not suffer from participation in clinical trials; in our experience, patients actually do better than those not participating. If possible, a patient should be placed in a clinical trial setting, either by referral to a center doing such research, or by the direct participation of the patient's physician in one of the several outreach programs associated with research centers.

For patients who cannot participate in clinical trials, the data presented here make it is possible to present guidelines for current care. The management of malignant gliomas should be based on the rationale of cytoreduction through multimodality therapy, including surgery, irradiation, and chemotherapy. Surgical resection of as much tumor as is neurologically safe should be the initial step. After surgery, patients should receive radiation therapy to a full tumor dose of 6,000 rad and about 4,500 rad to the remainder of the brain. Chemotherapy should be administered. There is no clearcut choice among a number of agents, although BCNU has been studied in greatest detail.

In 1970, the median survival of patients harboring malignant glioma using available surgical techniques and undefined radiation therapy was approximately six months. Prospective clinical trials over the last 15 years have demonstrated that median survival can be improved to a year or more and 25% to 30% of patients survive 18 months or longer. Newer therapeutic modalities have been suggested by recent laboratory investigations and hold the promise of improving survival further. It is evident that malignant neuroectodermal tumors should be treated vigorously using a multimodality approach.

REFERENCES

1. Jelsma R, Bucy PC: Glioblastoma multiforme, its treatment and some factors affecting survival. Arch Neurol 20:161–171, 1969

2. Shapiro WR: Treatment of neuroectodermal brain tumors. Ann Neurol 12:231–237, 1982

3. Walker MD, Alexander E Jr, Hunt WE, et al: Evaluation of BCNU and/or radiotherapy in the treatment of anaplastic gliomas: A cooperative clinical trial. J Neurosurg 49:333–343, 1978

4. Walker MD, Green SB, Byar DP, et al: Randomized comparisons of radiotherapy and nitrosoureas for the treatment of malignant glioma after surgery. N Engl J Med 303:1323–1329, 1980

5. Green SB, Byar DP, Walker MD, et al: Comparisons of carmustine, procarbazine, and high-dose methylprednisolone as additions to surgery and radiotherapy for the treatment of malignant glioma. Cancer Treat Rep 67:121–132, 1983

6. Green SB, Byar DP, Strike TA, et al: Randomized comparisons of BCNU, streptozotocin, radiosensitizer, and fractionation of radiotherapy in the postoperative treatment of malignant glioma (Study 7702). Proc Am Soc Clin Oncol 3:260, 1984

7. Chang CH, Horton J, Schoenfeld D, et al: Comparison of postoperative radiotherapy and combined postoperative radiotherapy and chemotherapy in the multidisciplinary management of malignant gliomas. Cancer 52:997–1007, 1983

8. Burger PC, Mahaley MS Jr, Dudka J, et al: The morphologic effects of radiation administered therapeutically

for intracranial gliomas. A postmortem study of 25 cases. Cancer 44:1256–1272, 1979

9. Burger PC, Dubois PJ, Schold SC Jr, et al: Computerized tomographic and pathologic studies of the untreated, quiescent, and recurrent glioblastoma multiforme. J Neurosurg 58:159–169, 1983

10. Schiffer D, Giordana MT, Paoletti P, et al: Pathology of human malignant gliomas after radiation and chemotherapy. Acta Neurochir (Wien) 53:205–216, 1980

11. Hochberg FH, Pruitt A: Assumptions in the radiotherapy of glioblastoma. Neurology 30:907–911, 1980

12. Hiesiger EM, Shapiro WR: Brain tumors, in Pinedo HM, Chabner BA (ed): Cancer Chemotherapy 1984. The EORTC Cancer Chemotherapy Annual 6. Amsterdam, Elsevier, 1984, pp 450–466

13. Edwards MS, Levin VA, Wilson CB: Brain tumor chemotherapy. An evaluation of agents in current use for phase II and III trials. Cancer Treat Rep 64:1179–1205, 1980

14. Cox DR: Regression models and life tables. J R Stat Soc [B] 34:187–202, 1972

15. Eagan RT, Scott M: Evaluation of prognostic factors in chemotherapy of recurrent brain tumors. J Clin Oncol 1:38–44, 1983

16. Shapiro WR, Young DF: Chemotherapy of malignant glioma. A controlled study of chemotherapy and irradiation. Arch Neurol 33:494–500, 1976

Recent and Current Investigations of Radiation Therapy of Malignant Gliomas

Diana F. Nelson, Raul C. Urtasun, William M. Saunders, Philip H. Gutin, and Glenn E. Sheline

THIS PAPER presents several new approaches to improving the efficacy of radiation therapy of malignant gliomas. It reviews experience with radiation sensitizers, unconventional fractionation schemes, heavy particle radiotherapy, interstitial brachytherapy, and hyperthermia. These techniques are directed toward improving the local control rate achievable by radiotherapy. Hopefully, one of these approaches, a combination thereof, or an outgrowth therefrom will eventually contribute to improved therapy of these diseases which, to date, have such a dismal prognosis.

RADIATION SENSITIZERS

The grim outlook for patients with malignant gliomas is due to the failure to control local disease. Local persistence after radiotherapy has often been attributed, at least in part, to the presence of hypoxic cells. Regions of coagulation necrosis present in glioblastoma multiforme are likely to contain cells that are hypoxic but still viable. Hypoxic cells are up to three times more resistant to radiation than well-oxygenated cells, hence, they require much larger photon doses to produce the same degree of cell kill as do well-oxygenated cells. Attempts to offset the effects of hypoxia have included utilization of hyperbaric oxygen during radiation, hypoxic cell radiation sensitizers, and high linear energy transfer (LET) radiation such as neutrons. Breathing oxygen under several atmosphere's pressure allows oxygen to diffuse greater distances from capillaries into tumor, thereby decreasing the number of hypoxic cells. Electron affinic compounds mimic the sensitizing effect of oxygen by acting as scavengers of free radicals, thus preventing the repair of sublethal DNA damage caused by radiation. Hypoxic cell sensitizers that have been used to treat malignant gliomas are the nitroimidazoles metronidazole, and misonidazole (MISO) (1-(2-nitro-1-imidazole)-2-methoxy-2-propanol).

The pyrimidine analogues such as 5-bromo-2-deoxyuridine (BUdR) are radiosensitizers that appear to act independently of the oxygen effect. When BUdR is incorporated into the DNA prior to irradiation it increases the radiation effect 2 to 3-fold. A differential effect between tumor and normal cells is possible because the glioma cells are dividing rapidly relative to the very slowly dividing endothelial and stromal cells, and relative to the nondividing normal glial cells. Furthermore, the blood-brain barrier tends to protect normal brain tissue, at least that which is not immediately adjacent to the tumor.

Hyperbaric Oxygen (HBO) as a Radiation Sensitizer

Breathing oxygen at three or four atmospheres of pressure increases the partial pressure of oxygen in the arterial blood up to 20-fold.[1] HBO also influences cerebral blood flow. It has been suggested by Chang[2] and Wende et al[3] that HBO causes normal cerebral vessels to constrict without effecting tumor vessels, thereby allowing increased blood flow to the tumor. Chang[2] reported a nonrandomized pilot clinical trial that utilized five different fractionation schedules with HBO in 38 patients (Table 1). There was no difference in survival for the 38 patients treated with HBO compared with the 42 controls: 66% *v* 62% at six months, 37% *v* 31% at one year, and 13% *v* 7% at two years. For the 18 patients who received HBO and 60 Gy (1 Gy equals 100 rad) in six weeks, the median survival was 46 weeks which may be compared to 55 weeks for patients who received 60 Gy plus BCNU in large randomized studies such as RTOG 79-18. Differences in the distribution of age, Karnofsky performance status, histology, and extent of surgery could account for the observed differences in survival. HBO has been abandoned in favor of the electron

From the Department of Radiation Therapy, University of Pennsylvania; the Division of Radiation Oncology, University of Alberta; the Department of Radiation Oncology, University of California, San Francisco; and the Department of Neurological Surgery, University of California, San Francisco.

Address reprint requests to Diana F. Nelson, MD, Department of Radiation Therapy, Hospital of the University of Pennsylvania, 3400 Spruce St, Philadelphia, PA 19104.

0093-7754/86/1301-0006$05.00/0

Table 1. Dose-Fractionation Schemes of Hyperbaric Oxygen-Treated Group v Controls[2]

	Group	
Dose	Oxygen	Control
36.00 Gy/9F/3 wk	8	10
40.00 Gy/10F/3⅓ wk	4	4
44.00 Gy/11F/3⅔ wk	2	5
50.00 Gy/15F/5 wk	6	8
60.00 Gy/30F/6 wk	18	15
Total	38	42

affinic compounds that serve the same function in radiation reactions but are not metabolized as they diffuse from capillaries through the tissues.

Electron Affinic Sensitizers

Metronidazole. Metronidazole (Flagyl) was the first sensitizer tested in a randomized trial in Grade IV supratentorial astrocytomas.[4] Six g/m^2 were administered four hours before a 3.35 Gy dose of radiation. This schedule was repeated three times per week (tiw) for three weeks in 16 patients. The control group received the same radiation dose and fractionation schedule without the sensitizer. The median survival rate without metronidazole was unusually short, being 15 weeks as compared to 26 weeks with metronidazole. This study showed that metronidazole could offset the poor median survival times associated with this particular dose-fractionation schedule, and indirectly tended to confirm the presence of hypoxic cells and their significance in Grade IV gliomas when such an accelerated fractionation is used. It remains to be seen whether or not hypoxic cells significantly contribute to the inability of conventional fractionation to control glioblastoma multiforme, as conventional fractionation allows more time for reoxygenation. A second trial by Urtasun[5] compared metronidazole (6 g/m^2) plus radiation (4.33 Gy tiw to a total of 39 Gy/9F/3W)* and with radiation alone (1.93 Gy daily to 58 Gy/30F/6W). There were approximately 17 patients in each treatment arm; the median survival was 24 to 25 weeks for each arm.

Misonidazole. MISO is a more effective sensitizer than metronidazole on an equal molar basis. Peak plasma levels are attained one to four hours after oral ingestion. The serum half-life ranges from nine to 17 hours.[6] Drug concentrations in the central nervous system (CNS) and in brain tumors is 76% to 92% of plasma values.[7,8] The chief dose-limiting toxicity is peripheral neuropathy which is predominantly sensory, but can be motor as well. The toxicity is associated with peripheral nerve demyelination and axonal degeneration.[9] Neurotoxicity limited the total MISO dose to 10 to 12 g/m^2[10] until it was observed that patients on phenytoin and/or dexamethasone had a lower incidence of MISO associated neurotoxicity.[11,12] Phenytoin is a microsomal–enzyme-inducing drug that shortens the plasma half-life of MISO without altering the peak or four hour plasma MISO levels.[13,14] Dexamethasone does not appear to alter the metabolism of MISO,[11] but has been associated with a decrease in peripheral neuropathy.[15] This decrease may be related to its membrane stabilizing characteristics.[11]

The use of MISO in the treatment of malignant gliomas has been evaluated by clinical trials that utilize hypofractionation (a small number of large sized fractions), conventional fractionation, and hyperfractionation (a large number of small fractions). Because larger enhancement ratios have been obtained in the laboratory with larger fractions of radiation and larger individual doses of MISO, the majority of studies have been with hypofractionation and have utilized larger than conventional daily doses of radiation in the range of 3 to 5 Gy.

In the Cambridge Trial,[16] 2.94 Gy were delivered on Mondays and Wednesdays, and 5.0 Gy on Fridays to a total dose of 43.52 Gy/4 weeks. In the sensitizer arm, 17 patients received 3 g/m^2 MISO four hours before the Friday dose of 5.0 Gy. One control group of 18 patients received the same "unconventional" fractionation schedule without MISO while a second control group of 20 patients was treated by conventional fractionation to 56.56 Gy/28 F/5.5 W. The median survival for the MISO arm was 39 weeks. This was not different than 38 weeks for conventional fractionation and not significantly better than 31 weeks for the altered fractionation control.

The Vienna Study Group[17] utilized a fractionation schedule of 4.0 Gy on Mondays and Thursdays during the first, second, and eighth (last) weeks of treatment while delivering conventional

*In this paper the total radiation dose–fractionation scheme will be donoted by total dose (Gy)/number of fractions (F)/total time in weeks (W) or days (D).

fractionation at 1.70 Gy/d five days per week during the third through seventh weeks of treatment to a total dose of 66.5 Gy/8 W. The MISO dose administered prior to each 4.0 Gy fraction was 4.5 g (ie, 2.1 to 2.7 g/m^2). Compared to the control group the MISO arm had a significantly increased median survival of 57.1 *v* 35.1 weeks ($P = 0.02$). The improved survival was limited to those patients who had undergone subtotal surgical resection. There was no difference between treatment arms in patients who had undergone "complete" surgical resection. The mean age of the MISO treatment group was ten years younger than the controls (50 *v* 60 years). The median survival of the MISO group was no different than that of irradiated-only control arms of other large randomized trials such as RTOG 79-18, suggesting that known prognostic factors such as age and performance status may have contributed to the observed difference. In a recent update[18] relative to a total of 40 patients with a minimum follow-up of 12 months, the median survival for the MISO group was 15.5 months *v* 8.7 months for the controls. However, median age for patients receiving MISO was younger, 51 *v* 56 years, and the number of patients entered into this study is small.

The Radiation Therapy Oncology Group (RTOG)[19] evaluated a fraction schedule of 4.0 Gy on Mondays and 1.50 Gy on Tuesdays, Thursdays, and Fridays for the first six weeks, combined with MISO 2.5 g/m^2 four hours preceeding the 4.0 Gy dose. During the seventh week the radiation dose was 1.8 Gy/fraction/d for five days. This radiation fractionation schedule was estimated to be equivalent radiobiologically to that used for the control group; namely, a total of 60.0 Gy delivered by 1.7 to 2.0 Gy/F five days per week. In both arms of the study, patients received 80 mg/m^2 BCNU intravenously on days 3, 4, and 5; this was repeated every eight weeks for two years. This study was closed to patient accrual with 285 evaluable patients followed a minimum of 9.9 months. At randomization into the study all patients were stratified by age, Karnofsky performance status, and histology, and these prognostic variables were thought to have been evenly distributed between the treatment arms. The extent of surgery was also equally distributed. The final statistical analysis revealed that the median survival time for the radiation plus BCNU arm was 55.0 weeks and that for the MISO plus radiation plus BCNU arm was 46.0 weeks. This difference was not statistically significant and can be explained by small differences in distribution of prognostic variable, especially histology. For the subgroup of 50 patients with anaplastic astrocytoma, survival with radiation plus BCNU was significantly longer than that for MISO plus radiation plus BCNU: 132.0 weeks *v* 57.5 weeks. It appears that MISO combined with this fractionation scheme adversely affected survival for patients with anaplastic astrocytoma. To determine whether it is the fractionation scheme, the MISO sensitization, or the combination that is responsible would require a study that is not warranted ethically.

The European Organization for Research on Treatment of Cancer (EORTC) is conducting a Phase III trial to evaluate accelerated fractionation with and without MISO. Conventional fractionation of 60 Gy/30 F/6 W is being compared to 30 Gy/15 F/5 D, followed by a two-week rest and another 30 Gy/15 F/5 D with or without MISO 1.2 g/m^2/d two hours before the first daily fraction. This Phase III trial opened in April 1981 after 122 patients had been entered into a Phase II trial.[20] In the preliminary Phase II trial 88 patients received MISO. All patients completed therapy according to schedule. No side effects occurred in 17% of the patients while severe side effects occurred in 18%. Because of differences in prognostic factors between the various treatment groups of the Phase II trial, the value of MISO cannot be evaluated on the basis of that portion of the EORTC studies. Results of the ongoing Phase III trial are awaited.

The Brain Tumor Study Group (BTSG)[21] evaluated 1.5 g/m^2 MISO twice weekly to a total dose of 18 g/m^2 combined with 60.0 Gy delivered by conventional fractionation at 1/7 to 2.0 Gy/F/d, plus BCNU 80 mg/m^2 for three days every eight weeks. With 140 patients in both the MISO arm and the non-MISO control arm, the survival curves are virtually superimposable with a median survival of 40 to 45 weeks.

The use of MISO with hyperfractionation was evaluated by Fulton et al.[22] The conventional fractionation (CF) control arm consisted of 58.0 Gy/30F/6W. The hyperfractionation control arms received 61.41 Gy/69F/4.5W delivered by 0.89 Gy/F three times per day with four hours between fractions. All patients received CCNU at time of recurrence. The median survival for 37 patients treated with CF was 27 weeks, for 36 patients treated with hyperfraction alone, 57 weeks, and for 35 patients treated with hyperfractionation and MISO, 49 weeks. MISO did not significantly alter the survival. The survival of patients who received conventional radiotherapy was significantly worse than either hyperfractionation arm and shorter than control arms in larger randomized trials such as those of the BTSG and RTOG where comparable radiation regimens were used. Perhaps a clustering of worse prognostic variables is responsible for this difference.

Based on these studies with MISO, it appears that if radiosensitizers are to be of significant clinical benefit, a less toxic, more effective electron affinic radiosensitizer is needed. One promising new compound, SR-2508, has been tested in animals. It does not cause the neurotoxic symptoms produced by MISO and desmethymisonidazole, but does appear to have some striated muscle toxicity. It is at least seven times less toxic than MISO on a mg-per-mg basis. It is a low lipophilic compound with a partition coefficient of 0.046, one-tenth that of MISO. It produces a brain-to-plasma concentration ratio of only 0.08. However, because the blood-brain barrier generally is broken in malignant gliomas, it might successfully enter into, and sensitize glioma cells while not sensitizing normal brain distant from tumor. More human studies are needed to evaluate SR-2508, both in Phase I-II trials and in determining its concentration in brain and brain tumors before it should be tested in a Phase III trial for the treatment of gliomas.

Halogenated Pyrimidines

Radiation sensitization by continuous intravenous infusion of BUdR concomitant with radiation therapy is being studied by the Northern California Oncology Group (NCOG). During each week of a six-week course of radiation therapy, a 96-hour infusion is delivered. Initially, 1.5 $g/m^2/24$ hours was administered, but this dose has been decreased to 0.8 $g/m^2/24$ hours because of thrombocytopenia and leukopenia.[23] At 0.8 $g/m^2/24$ hours, the only toxicity noted has been a rash in some patients (personal communication, Victor Levin, May 23, 1984). Intermittent infusion of BUdR[24] concomitant with radiotherapy also has been studied at the National Cancer Institute: with BUdR doses of 0.65 to 0.7 $g/m^2/12$ hours for two weeks, BUdR enhancement ratios greater than 1.5 were obtained with the human bone marrow CFUC assay. However, a maculopapular rash occurred in one-half of the patients. As a result of this, other schedules of BUdR and infusion with IUdR (iododeoxyuridine) are being investigated. Continuous infusion with BUdR 1 $g/m^2/24$ hours for two weeks has been found to be tolerable.[25] Further Phase I and Phase II testing is required for both BUdR and IUdR.

In summary, clinical trials using MISO have all been negative with the exception of the Vienna Study Group trial in which the observed differences may be due to an unequal distribution of prognostic variables between treatment groups. Neurotoxicity has limited the dose of MISO that could be administered. More effective, less toxic electron affinic sensitizers that can penetrate CNS tumors need to be developed before further testing is warranted in gliomas. Intravenous infusion of the halogenated pyrimidines is promising. However, results of current Phase I–II testing need to be evaluated before Phase III trials are initiated.

HYPERFRACTIONATION—CNS RADIATION TOLERANCE

Evidence for a radiation dose response in malignant gliomas has been presented by Walker et al[26] in a retrospective analysis covering several clinical protocols of the BTSG. Survival time for these patients was related to the radiation dose; survival time increased with increasing total dose up to 60 Gy fractionated over five days per week for a period of about six weeks. The major obstacle to the delivery of radiation doses higher than 60 Gy has been normal brain tissue tolerance, particularly late radiation damage. Late damage is related not only to the total dose of radiation and dose-per-individual fraction, but also to the volume of normal brain irradiated.[27,28] Thus, decreasing dose per fraction or the amount of brain included in the high-dose volume might be expected to increase tolerance and permit delivery of higher, more effective doses.

Improving CNS Tolerance by Reducing Volume Irradiated

Hochberg and Pruitt demonstrated[29] that radiotherapy failures in patients with malignant glioma are related to the delivery of insufficient doses of radiation to the known tumor volume rather than missing tumor extension beyond the main mass. In their computed tomography (CT) study failure within the known tumor volume plus a two centimeter margin represented approximately 80% of the failures. Tumor would have been missed because of multicentric presentation in only 5% to 6%. With the present use of CT for treatment planning in almost all patients and the probable increased use of MRI (magnetic resonance imaging) in the not too distant future, the likelihood of missing multicentric tumors or underestimating tumor volume has been significantly reduced. A logical change in the planning of treatment of these patients would be, therefore, to discontinue the current use of whole-brain irradiation, reducing the volume to a generous field including three quarters or less of the brain volume. This should increase the tolerance of the normal brain to radiation and decrease the volume of brain at risk.

Improving CNS Tolerance by Increasing Number of Radiation Fractions

There is evidence for both monkeys and humans that with conventional fractionation increasing the total dose of radiation beyond 60 Gy (even with a reduced volume) may lead to late brain damage with coalescing necrosis.[30,31] For a given total dose, however, the incidence of necrosis is inversely related to the number of individual fractions. It seems reasonable, therefore, to explore the use of a larger number of smaller individual fractions of radiation.[32,33–35]

The radiation tolerance of the normal glial and vascular tissues determines to a large extent the amount of radiation that can be delivered to malignant brain tumors. These tissues are in a slow or nonproliferative state while viable malignant glioma cells have a more rapid turnover of three to six days.[32] The glioma cells going through proliferation are at a higher risk of being exposed to radiation during the most sensitive part of their cell cycle (G2 and G1-S). This likelihood is increased by delivering small fractions of radiation at frequent intervals during a 24-hour period. It is also expected that with an increased number of smaller fractions, the less proliferative normal glial cells would gain more in terms of increased capacity for repair of sublethal radiation injury than would glioma tissues. Furthermore, since the dependence of radiation effect on the presence of oxygen falls with decreasing dose per fraction, radio-resistant hypoxic tumor cells should be more susceptible to small multiple daily fractions of radiation than to conventional single daily fractions. Thus increasing the number of fractions might be expected to result in increasing the difference between the survival of normal and tumor cells.

Reported clinical results for hyperfractionation in patients with malignant gliomas are conflicting. Payne et al[36] and the BTSG[21] found no improvement in the overall median survival; however, in both of these studies the total doses were relatively low, hence, the concept of hyperfractionation was not fully tested. On the other hand, Douglas et al[37] and Fulton et al[38] have demonstrated a significant increase in both time-to-tumor regrowth and overall survival for patients treated with hyperfractionated radiation. Preliminary Phase II studies conducted by the RTOG and reported by Nelson[39] also are encouraging. The last two groups have designed their further studies to test the concept of hyperfractionation at doses gradually escalating upward until normal tissue tolerance is reached and, therefore, will be able to assess clinically the advantages of hyperfractionation.

HEAVY PARTICLE RADIOTHERAPY

Another promising approach to the problem of local control of malignant brain tumors involves treatment with beams of heavy subatomic particles instead of standard photon beams (x-rays or gamma rays). In this section, the term "standard beam" refers to x-ray or gamma ray beams and "heavy particle" refers to subatomic particles heavier than electrons such as neutrons, protons, and heavier nuclei, and negative pi mesons (pions).

Heavy particle beams offer varying combinations of two types of advantage relative to standard beams.[40] First, heavy particle beams, except neutrons, give a superior localization of radiation dose to the defined target volume, thereby decreasing the dose to nearby tissues and organs. This is a result of the Bragg peak effect for charged particle beams. The charged particle beam penetrates a definite and controllable distance in tissue and most of the radiation dose is deposited in the stopping region, called the Bragg peak. This is in sharp distinction to standard beams for which the dose is continuously and exponentially decreasing after a variable region of dose build up (Fig 1). By placing the Bragg peak of a heavy particle beam in the tumor, a higher dose can be delivered to the tumor, with the same or lower dose given to the nearby normal tissues. Clinically, it is hoped that this will be reflected in a higher rate of local control, with an acceptably low rate of normal tissue damage.

Second, most heavy particle beams have biological superiority in terms of the killing of tumor cells. Several subsets of tumor cells have been identified that are relatively resistant to x-ray beams, eg, hypoxic cells and cells in the S phase of the mitotic cycle. For certain heavy particle beams these effects are significantly smaller. In addition, recovery of tumor cells by repair of sublethal or potentially lethal radiation damage is much less likely for some of the heavy particle beams than for the standard beams.

The heavy particle beams that have been used to date in clinical trials are neutrons, protons, helium ions, pions, and heavier ions such as neon. Since neutrons are not charged particles, they do not exhibit a Bragg peak effect and have no dose localization advantage relative to the standard beams. They are being tested clinically solely because of their biological advantages. On the other hand, protons and helium ions, the lightest of the ion beams, have a very sharp Bragg peak but little or no biological advantage. They are being tested, therefore, only for their excellent dose localization properties. Pions and ions heavier than helium are of particular interest clinically since they have both the dose localization and biological advantages.

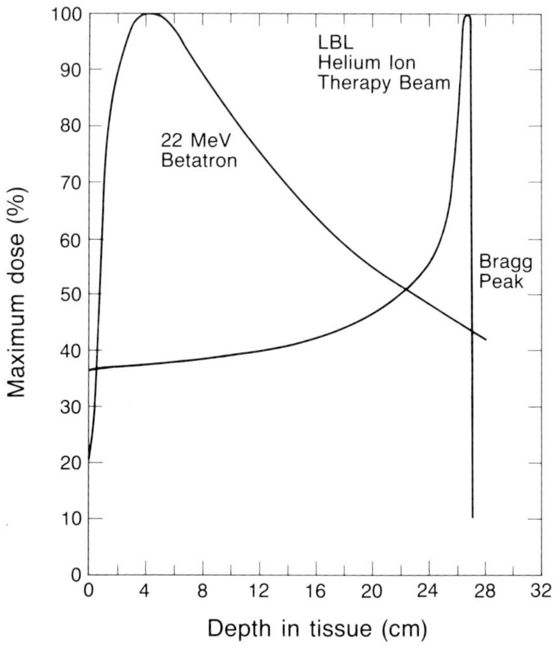

Fig 1. Depth—dose curve for x-ray beam from 22 MeV Betatron and helium ion beam from Lawrence Berkeley Laboratory 184" synchrocyclotron. (Reprinted from Radiat Phys Chem, vol 24, Saunders W, "Radiation oncology: The use of beam photons or particles for the treatment of tumors," 1984, Pergamon Press, Ltd, with permission.)

Clinical Results

To date, the main thrust of all heavy particle trials for malignant gliomas has been to establish the optimal dose and fractionation pattern to maximize tumor response and minimize normal tissue morbidity. The largest experience to date is with neutron therapy. Neutrons were the first heavy particle tested for radiotherapy, and many more facilities are available to test neutrons clinically than any of the other heavy particles. Early trials investigating the efficacy of neutron radiotherapy for malignant gliomas were carried out in Hammersmith Hospital[41] in London and at the University of Washington in Seattle.[42] Both groups have reported similar results: for presumably biologically equivalent radiation doses, patient survival was similar for neutrons and standard beams. Autopsy findings, however, revealed in the neutron-treated patients an apparently high rate of local tumor control and an unexpectedly high rate of diffuse degenerative changes in the white matter within the high-dose volume, probably due to underestimating the relative biological effectiveness (RBE) of neutrons. It is hoped that a dose may be found that will retain the tumor control rate at a high level, but avoid the lethal normal tissue damage. Currently in the United States a dose-searching protocol is being carried out by the RTOG in an attempt to find such an optimal dose. In this trial, patients are randomly assigned to one of six neutron doses given as a boost in conjunction with whole-brain photon irradiation.

Pions have dose distribution characteristics significantly superior to those for neutrons. The biological properties of this beam, while better than those of standard beams, are somewhat inferior to those of neutron beams. The largest series to date assessing the efficacy of pions for malignant gliomas was treated at the Los Alamos Meson Physics Facility (LAMPF). The LAMPF reported on 28 patients with glioblastoma multiforme with a median survival of ten months and 14 patients with Grade III astrocytoma with a median survival of 22 months.[43] A group of 17 patients with either glioblastoma multiforme or Grade III astrocytoma was treated with a pion boost after whole-brain radiotherapy with standard beams. As of the time of the report, the median survival for that group had not been reached, but the overall survival curve was very similar to that for patients with Grade III astrocytoma. Although the Los Alamos program has been terminated, the patients are still being followed and reports with long-term follow-up will be forthcoming. In the meantime, pion radiotherapy programs at the TRIUMF cyclotron in Vancouver, Canada, and at the Swiss Institute for Nuclear Research have come into clinical operation. Both groups are conducting pilot trials of pion therapy for malignant glioma, building upon the LAMPF experience.

At the Lawrence Berkeley Laboratory clinical trials of heavy-particle radiotherapy are being carried out in collaboration with the Radiation Oncology Department at the University of California, San Francisco.[44] To date, two types of particle beam have been used to treat malignant gliomas: helium ion beams and neon ion beams. Helium ion beams have an excellent dose distribution, but the biological properties are comparable to those of a 250 kVp x-ray beam. Since this beam was available for clinical trial several years earlier than heavier ion beams, it was tested earlier than neon for its efficacy for malignant gliomas. A group of 11 patients with anaplastic astrocytoma or glioblastoma multiforme was treated with helium, either solely or as a boost after whole-brain radiotherapy. Total doses ranged from 60 to 66 Gy Equivalents (GyE) (1 GyE delivered with a heavy particle beam has the same biological effect as 1 Gy delivered with Cobalt 60). The six patients with glioblastoma multiforme survived an average of nine months, and the five patients with an anaplastic astrocytoma survived an average of 33 months. These results suggested that a major improvement over results obtainable with standard beams was unlikely.

Subsequently, neon ion beams became available. Since a neon ion beam combines an excellent dose distribution with good biological properties, comparable to those of a neutron beam, the next (ongoing) pilot trial utilized a neon ion beam. Because of the radiation damage to CNS white matter encountered in the early neutron radiotherapy trials, it was decided that the initial patients in the neon trial would be treated with a conservative dose, and that the dose would be escalated if no morbidity was encountered. The dose selected to start the trial was 48 GyE, delivered in 16 fractions in four weeks. Eight patients, four with glioblastoma multiforme and four with anaplastic astrocytoma, received this dose. Their survival was not different from that expected with standard radiotherapy: those with glioblastoma survived a mean of eight months and those with astrocytomas a mean of 17 months. Autopsy results showed none of the white matter damage seen with neutrons, so the dose was escalated. These patients currently are receiving 54.0 GyE in 16 fractions in four weeks. Clinical results are not yet available at this dose level.

In summary, heavy particle radiotherapy is a promising modality for the treatment of malignant gliomas. Dose-searching trials are being carried out for neutron, pion, and neon beams. Radiobiological data support the hope that for one or more of these beams a dose and fractionation schedule can be found that will significantly increase the cure rate with an acceptably low complication rate.

INTERSTITIAL BRACHYTHERAPY

Rationale

Because radiation therapy has been the most effective modality against malignant brain tumors[45] but the possibility of necrosis prevents delivery of much more than 60 Gy by external radiation techniques, the use of high dose focal irradiation, brachytherapy, is under investigation. Intensive local therapy seems particularly rational in light of increasing evidence that malignant gliomas recur locally rather than diffusely.[29]

Techniques

Several radioactive isotopes have been used for brain tumor brachytherapy,[46] however, in recent years, Iodine-125 and Iridium-192 have been the most frequently implanted.[47–50] In most cases the radioactive sources are afterloaded in a removeable catheter that has been inserted into the malignant brain tumor; the central zones of such tumors are often soft in consistency which predispose to source movement unless held in a fairly rigid container. Interstitial implantation of brain tumors usually is done using a CT-directed stereotaxic technique.[51,52] CT stereotaxy allows careful treatment planning and superior implant accuracy. Computer programs are available for stereotaxic treatment planning, yielding implant coordinates for optimal isodose coverage.

Results

Interstitial brachytherapy has been used as a treatment for recurrent malignant gliomas and in primary therapy as adjuvant treatment for "boosting" the radiation dose to the tumor bed. The response rate for Iodine-125 implants in recurrent tumors is about 70%, but criteria of response (CT scan, neurological exam) are perturbed by local radiation necrosis.[50] Patients with recurrences treated by brachytherapy and who show progression of the disease or failure to respond as judged by traditional criteria may, nevertheless, do well in terms of overall survival. About half of the patients receiving such treatment have required reoperation and resection of necrotic material, which otherwise serves as a nidus for cerebral edema. Among these patients reoperated for necrosis are several in whom no active tumor could be identified in the surgical specimen and who have shown long-term survival (some nearly six years) after treatment for their recurrent glioblastomas. In some instances, however, the treatment, with the induction of focal necrosis, has proved neurologically devastating. Rather than attempting to salvage patients with recurrent tumors it, obviously, would be preferable to have a more effective primary therapy. A protocol is underway through the Northern California Oncology Group that tests the efficacy in patients with malignant gliomas of an adjuvant Iodine-125 implant "boost" of 60 Gy given in addition to an external radiation dose of 60 Gy. The implant dose is calculated at the outer edge of the CT-enhancing zone. The radiation sources are afterloaded in removable catheters; application time is around five to six days. It is too early to evaluate the results of this treatment plan.

HYPERTHERMIA IN CONJUNCTION WITH BRACHYTHERAPY

The greatest obstacles to the success of brain tumor brachytherapy are the relatively high incidence of focal brain injury and the occurrence of tumor regrowth peripheral to the intensely irradiated field. It may be that local tumor hyperthermia can ameliorate these problems by allowing a reduction in the radiation dose required for local tumor control.

Heat, at nonlethal temperatures, is known to sensitize cells to radiation.[53,54] Thermal enhancement of radiation is accentuated when radiation is delivered at low-dose rates in the range of those used in conventional interstitial brachytherapy.[55,56] Manning et al effectively treated advanced head and neck, gynecological, breast, and other tumors with radiation and hyperthermia.[56] The best responses were seen when interstitial heat was combined with interstitial brachytherapy.

The most effective current methods of delivering heat to a deep tumor target involve interstitially implanted microwave antennae or localized current field needle electrodes. Fewer implants probably will be required for effective heating with the microwave system; hence, this would seem to be the method of choice for brain tumor treatment. Since radioactive sources contained in catheters can be implanted into brain tumors using CT stereotaxic technique, and the methodology has been well established, it is relatively easy to extend the technique to the implantation of catheters that also hold heating antennae. Strohbehn and his coworkers have developed an interstitial microwave hyperthermia system operated at 915 MHz.[57,58] A few patients with brain tumors have been treated with hyperthermia, but because of the many technical problems in heating brain tumors and the unknown effects of heat on normal brain tissue, most studies to date have concentrated on canine models.[51] Such studies are underway at the University of California, San Francisco.

ADDENDUM: HYPERFRACTIONATION UPDATE—JANUARY 1986

Results of the Edmonton Hyperfractionation trial are given in Fig 2. The Edmonton group is presently treating patients at total tumor doses of 8,000 cGy in 80 fractions in an overall time of 5½ weeks using three 100 cGy fractions per day at intervals of four to six hours. We will, therefore, within a short period of time, be able to assess clinically its theoretical and experimental advantages.

Preliminary results from the RTOG Hyper-

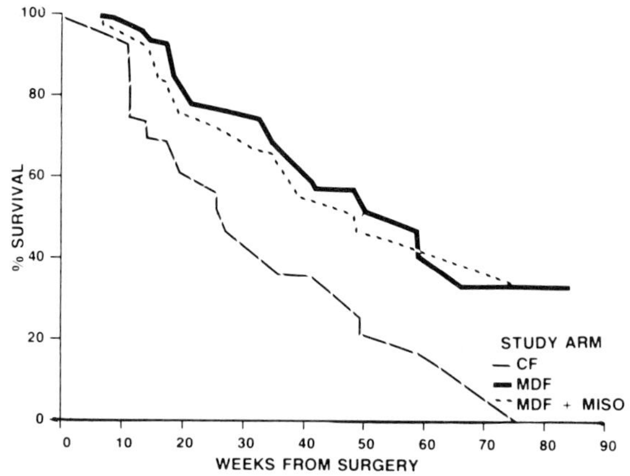

Fig 2. Survival after surgery. Survival experience in a randomized study of patients with malignant glioma treated with hyperfractionated radiation —, ---, total 101 patients. The conventional radiation control arm shows an inferior survival (CF — — —), 38 patients. P = .001. Hyperfractionated arms = 6,142 cGy in 64 fractions of 89 cGy in an overall time of 4½ weeks, three fractions per day at intervals of four hours; with or without Misonidazole, 1.25 g/M² every other day for the first 3 weeks. Control arm = 5,800 cGy in 30 fractions, in an overall time of 6 weeks. Abbreviations: MDF, multiple daily fractionation; CF, conventional fractionation.

fractionation protocol (RTOG 83-02) demonstrate no significant difference in survival between the treatment arms with an overall median of 44 weeks. Two hundred patients have been randomized among the treatment arms of 64.60 Gy, 72.00 Gy, and 76.80 Gy delivered in 1.2 Gy fractions twice daily, separated by four to six hours. There is equal distribution of prognostic variables between treatment arms. There is no apparent difference in toxicity between the treatment arms. Therefore, a higher dose arm of 81.60 Gy has been opened.

REFERENCES

1. Lamphier EH: Determinants in oxygenation, in Boerema I (ed): Clinical Application of Hyperbaric Oxygen. Amsterdam, Elsevier, 1964, pp 227–283

2. Chang CH: Hyperbaric oxygen as a radiation sensitizer in treatment of malignant gliomas, in Chang CH, Housepian EM (eds): Tumors of the Central Nervous System: Modern Radiotherapy in Multidisciplinary Management. New York, Mason Publishing, 1982, pp 23–30

3. Wende S, Zieler E, Nakayama N: Cerebral Magnification Angiography. New York, Springer-Verlag, 1974

4. Urtasun RC, Band P, Chapman JD, et al: Radiation and high-dose metronidazole in supratentorial glioblastomas. N Engl J Med 294:1364–1367, 1976

5. Urtasun RC, Feldstein ML, Partingor JP: Hypoxic cell sensitizers and radiotherapy for malignant gliomas, in Chang CH, Jousepian EM (eds): Tumors of the Central Nervous System: Modern Radiotherapy in Multidisciplinary Management. New York, Mason Publishing, 1982, pp 31–37

6. Marques RA, Stafford B, Flynn N, et al: Determination of metronidazole and misonidazole and their metabolites in plasma and urine by high performance liquid chromatography. J Chromatogr 146:163–166, 1978

7. Urtasun RC, Chapman JD, Band P, et al: Clinical phase I study of high-dose metronidazole: A specific in vivo and in vitro radiosensitization of hypoxic cells. Radiology 117:129–133, 1975

8. Urtasun RC, Band P, Feldstein ML, et al: Clinical phase I study of the hypoxic cell radiosensitizer Ro-07-0582, a 2-nitroimidazole derivative. Radiology 122:801–804, 1977

9. Urtasun RC, Chapman JD, Feldstein ML, et al: Peripheral neuropathy related to misonidazole: Incidence and pathology. Br J Cancer 37:271, 1978 (suppl)

10. Wasserman TH, Phillips TL, Johnson RJ, et al: Initial United States clinical and pharmacologic evaluation of misonidazole (RO-07-0587), an hypoxic cell radiosensitizer. Int J Radiat Oncol Biol Phys 5:775–786, 1979

11. Urtasun RC, Tanasichuk H, Fulton D, et al: High-dose misonidazole with dexmethasone rescue: A possible approach to circumvent neurotoxicity. Int J Radiat Oncol Biol Phys 8:365–369, 1982

12. Wasserman TH, Stetz J, Phillips TL: Clinical trials of misonidazole in the United States. Cancer Clin Trials 4:7–16, 1981

13. Bleehan NM: The Cambridge glioma trial of misonidazole and radiation therapy with associated pharmacokinetic studies. Cancer Clin Trials 3:267–273, 1980

14. Workman P, Bleehan NM, Wiltshire CR: Phenytoin shortens the half-life of the hypoxic cell radiosensitizer misonidazole in man: Implications for possible reduced toxicity. Br J Cancer 41:302, 1980

15. Nelson DF, Gillespie BW, Diener MD, et al: Is misonidazole neurotoxicity altered by the use of phenytoin and/or dexamethasone in RTOG 79-18 and RTOG 79-16? Int J Radiat Oncol Biol Phys 10:1731–1734, 1984

16. Bleehan NW, Wiltshire GR, Plowman PN, et al: A randomized study of misonidazole and radiotherapy for grade 3 and 4 cerebral astrocytoma. Br J Cancer 43:436–442, 1981

17. Kogelnik HD, Karcher KH, Szepesi T, et al: High-dose irradiation and misonidazole in the treatment of malignant gliomas. A preliminary report, in Karcher KH (ed): Progress in Radio-Oncology II. New York, Raven Press, 1982, pp 189–195

18. Stadler B, Karcher KH, Kogelnik HD, et al: Misonidazole and irradiation in the treatment of glioblastoma multiforme: Preliminary report of the Vienna study group. Int J Radiat Oncol Biol Phys (in press)

19. Nelson DF, Schoenfeld D, Weinstein AS, et al: A randomized comparison of misonidazole sensitized radiotherapy plus BCNU for treatment of malignant glioma after surgery: Preliminary results of an RTOG study. Int J Radiat Oncol Biol Phys 9:1143–1151, 1983

20. Ang KK, van der Schueren E, Notter G, et al: Split course multiple daily fractionated radiotherapy schedule combined with misonidazole for the management of grade III and IV gliomas: A pilot feasibility study of the radiotherapy group of the EORTC. Int J Radiat Oncol Biol Phys 8:1657–1664, 1982

21. Green SB, Byar DP, Strike TA, et al: Randomized comparisons of BCNU, streptozotocin, radiosensitizer, and fractionation of radiotherapy in the postoperative treatment

of malignant glioma (study 7702). Proc Amer Soc Clin Oncol 3:260, 1984 (abstr)

22. Shin KH, Urtasun RC, Fulton D, et al: Multiple daily radiation and misonidazole in the management of malignant astrocytoma. A preliminary report. Cancer 56:758–760, 1985

23. Phuphanich S, Levin E, Levin V: Phase I study of intravenous bromodeoxyuridine used concomitantly with radiation therapy in patients with primary malignant brain tumors. Int J Radiat Oncol Biol Phys 10:1769–1772, 1984

24. Kinsella TJ, Russo A, Mitchell JB, et al: A phase I study of intermittent intravenous bromodeoxyuridine (BUdR) with conventional fractionated irradiation. Int J Radiat Oncol Biol Phys 10:69–76, 1984

25. Kinsella TJ, Russo A, Mitchell JB, et al: The use of prolonged constant intravenous infusions of bromodeoxyuridine (BUdR) as a radiosensitizer. J Clin Oncol 2:1144–1150, 1984

26. Walker MD, Strike TA, Sheline GE: An analysis of dose-effect relationship in the radiotherapy of malignant gliomas. Int J Radiat Oncol Biol Phys 5:1725–1731, 1979

27. Van Der Kogel AJ: Radiation tolerance of the rat spinal cord: Time-dose relationships. Radiology 122:505–509, 1977

28. Hornsey S, White A: Iso-effect curve for radiation myelopathy. Br J Radiol 53:168–169, 1980

29. Hochberg FH, Pruitt A: Assumptions in the radiotherapy of glioblastoma. Neurology 30:907–911, 1980

30. Caveness WF: Pathology of radiation damage to the normal brain of the monkey, in Modern Concepts in Brain Tumor Therapy. National Cancer Institute Monograph 46:57–76, 1977

31. Sheline GE, Wara WM, Smith V: Therapeutic irradiation and brain injury. Int J Radiat Oncol Biol Phys 6:1215–1228, 1980

32. Hoshino T, Barker M, Wilson CB, et al: Cell kinetics of human gliomas. J Neurosurg 37:15–26, 1972

33. Fowler JF: La ronde—radiation sciences and medical radiology. Radio Oncol 1:1–22, 1983

34. Withers HR, Peters LJ, Thames HD, et al: Hyperfractionation. Int J Radiat Oncol Biol Phys 8:1807–1809, 1982

35. Peters LJ, Withers RH, Thames HD, et al: The problem, tumor radioresistance in clinical radiotherapy. Rome symposium. Int J Radiat Oncol Biol Phys 8:101–108, 1982

36. Payne DG, Simpson WJ, Keen C, et al: Malignant astrocytoma, hyperfractionated and standard radiotherapy with chemotherapy in a randomized prospective clinical trial. Cancer 50:2301–2306, 1982

37. Douglas BG, Worth AJ: Superfractionation in glioblastoma multiforme—results of a phase II study. Int J Radiat Oncol Biol Phys 8:1787–1794, 1982

38. Fulton DS, Urtasun RC, Shin KJ, et al: Misonidazole combined with hyperfractionation in the management of malignant glioma. Int J Radiat Oncol Biol Phys 10:1709–1712, 1984

39. Nelson D: Personal communication, 1984

40. Raju MR: Heavy Particle Radiotherapy. New York, Academic Press, 1980

41. Catterall M, Bloom HJG, Ash DV, et al: Fast neutrons compared with megavoltage x rays in the treatment of patients with supratentorial glioblastoma: A controlled pilot study. Int J Radiat Oncol Biol Phys 6:261–266, 1980

42. Parker RG, Berry HC, Gerdes AJ, et al: Fast neutron radiotherapy of glioblastoma multiforme. Am J Roentgenol 127:331–335, 1976

43. Bush SE, Smith AE, Zink SR: Pion radiotherapy at LAMPF. Int J Radiat Oncol Biol Phys 8:2181–2186, 1982

44. Castro JR, Saunders WM, Tobias CA, et al: Treatment of cancer with heavy charged particles. Int J Radiat Oncol Biol Phys 8:2191–2198, 1982

45. Walker MD, Alexander E Jr, Hung WE, et al: Evaluation of BCNU and/or radiotherapy in the treatment of anaplastic gliomas: A cooperative clinical trial. J Neurosurg 49:333–343, 1978

46. Bernstein M, Gutin PH: Interstitial irradiation of brain tumors: A review. Neurosurg 9:741–750, 1981

47. Mundinger F, Birg W, Osterag CB: Treatment of small cerebral gliomas with CT-aided stereotaxic curietherapy. Neuroradiology 16:564–567, 1978

48. Kelly PJ, Olsen MH, Wright AE: Stereotaxic implantation of iridium 192 into CNS neoplasms. Surg Neurol 10:349–354, 1978

49. Gutin PH, Phillips TL, Hosobuchi Y, et al: Permanent and removable implants for the brachytherapy of brain tumors. Int J Radiat Oncol Biol Phys 7:1371–1381, 1981

50. Gutin PH, Phillips TL, Wara WM, et al: Brachytherapy of recurrent malignant brain tumors with removable high-activity iodine-125 sources. J Neurosurg 60:61–68, 1984

51. Gutin PH, Domandy RH Jr: A coaxial catheter system for afterloading radioactive sources for the interstitial irradiation of brain tumors: Technical note. J Neurosurg 56:734–735, 1982

52. Heilbrun MP, Roberts TS, Apuzzo MLJ, et al: Preliminary experience with the Brown-Roberts-Wells (BRW) computerized tomographic stereotaxis guidance system. J Neurosurg 59:217–222, 1983

53. Westra A, Dewey WC: Variation in sensitivity to heat shock during the cell cycle of Chinese hamster cells in vitro. Int J Radiat Biol 19:467–477, 1971

54. Dewey WC, Hopwood LE, Sapareto SA, et al: Cellular responses to combinations of hyperthermia and radiation. Radiology 123:463–474, 1977

55. Gerner EW, Oval JH, Manning MR, et al: Dose-rate dependence of heat sensitization. Int J Radiat Oncol Biol Phys 9:1401–1404, 1983

56. Manning MR, Cetas TC, Miller RC, et al: Clinical hyperthermia: Results of a phase I trial employing hyperthermia alone or in combination with external beam or interstitial radiotherapy. Cancer 49:205–216, 1982

57. Strohbehn JW, Bowers E, Walsh J, et al: An invasive microwave antenna for locally induced hyperthermia for cancer therapy. J Microwave Powers 14:181–186, 1979

58. Coughlin JCT, Couple EB, Strohbehn JW, et al: Interstitial hyperthermia in combination with brachytherapy. Radiology 148:285–288, 1983

59. Lyons BE, Britt RH, Strohbehn JW: Localized hyperthermia in the treatment of malignant brain tumors using an interstitial microwave antenna array. IEEE-BME 31:53–62, 1984

Principles of Brain Tumor Chemotherapy

William R. Shapiro and Joan R. Shapiro

CHEMOTHERAPY of systemic cancers has been hampered by lack of therapeutic specificity, development of cellular resistance, and excessive toxicity to normal tissue. The chemotherapy of malignant brain tumors has the same difficulties, and, in addition, must contend with problems related to drug delivery, ie, low tumor blood flow and the blood-brain barrier. Furthermore, the initial treatment of brain tumors is much less successful than that of a number of systemic cancers. The kind of "cancer operation" possible in breast or colon cancer is impossible in brain tumors. There is no "surplus" tissue that can be removed from around a brain tumor so as to assure that a "total resection" has been done; the surrounding tissue is brain, which cannot regenerate itself. In a sense, malignant brain tumors share with oat-cell lung cancer and with leukemia the problem of the need to produce a "remission"; unfortunately, few remissions are yet possible in brain tumor therapy. The problem of cerebral edema adds to the difficulties of the chemotherapist, both because edema affects drug entry and because the effect of the chemotherapeutic agents on the tumor must be distinguished from that of corticosteroid hormone treatment of the edema, especially since steroids are so effective.

In this review we shall first examine aspects of the tumor that affect the way chemotherapeutic agents interact with the tumor cells. We shall next examine the influence of the blood-brain barrier and the problems of drug entry. We shall then review the drugs that have been used in brain tumor chemotherapy, and examine several new approaches currently being used clinically. Finally, we shall touch on several assay systems that are under development to help predict clinical response to treatment.

From the George C. Cotzias Laboratory of Neuro-Oncology, Department of Neurology, Memorial Sloan-Kettering Cancer Center, Cornell University Medical College, New York.

Address reprint requests to William R. Shapiro, MD, Department of Neurology, Memorial Sloan-Kettering Cancer Center, 1275 York Ave, New York, NY 10021.

0093-7754/86/1301-0007$05.00/0

CELLULAR ASPECTS OF BRAIN TUMOR CHEMOTHERAPY

Recent observations from the laboratory indicate that human malignant gliomas are not homogeneous in cellular composition but rather are composed of heterogeneous cell populations.[1] Heterogeneity of human brain tumors is suggested by their pleomorphic histological appearance. The term "glioblastoma multiforme" emphasizes the remarkable diversity of cells that morphologically comprise that tumor. Many malignant gliomas contain fields of benign-appearing tumor, reflecting the frequent clinical progression from a slowly to a rapidly growing neoplasm. Recent studies from our laboratory have confirmed that human gliomas are regionally heterogeneous, with great diversity of karyotypes from one area to another.[2] These regional cellular differences are also reflected in differences in chemosensitivity of the cells from each area. No one area of tumor is very representative of other areas, and conclusions from small biopsies about cellular composition, chemosensitivity, and even degree of malignancy must be drawn with considerable caution.

That heterogeneity (and especially regional heterogeneity) is important in the chemotherapy of brain tumors can readily be demonstrated by the differences in chemosensitivity of clonal populations isolated by early passage techniques.[3] Figure 1 illustrates dose-response curves of clones grown from a freshly resected human malignant glioma and treated with BCNU. The curves significantly differ, although the differences are not large. Figure 2 shows dose-response curves of clones treated with cisplatin; again small but significant differences were present. These cells were taken from a tumor in a patient who had not been previously treated with drug, and their response represents intrinsic chemotherapy sensitivity to clinically achievable blood concentrations of the drugs. In our study of regional glioma heterogeneity, we found that

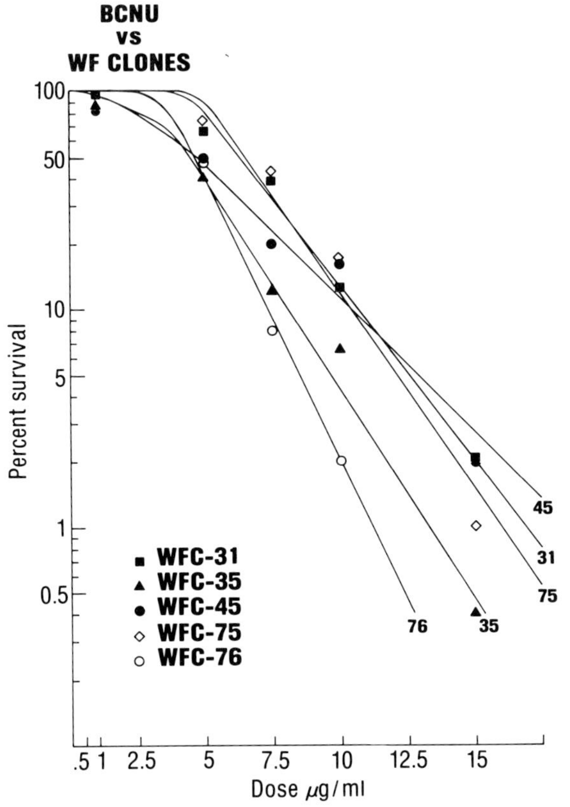

Fig 1. Semilog dose-response curves determined by colony-forming assay for 5 clones from tumor WF treated with BCNU at passage 12. A prominent shoulder effect is apparent in the response of the tumor clones. The ED_{50} doses ranged from 4.5 μg/mL (WFC-35) to 7.0 μg/mL (WFC-75). By log-probit analysis the ED_{50} doses among several of the clones differed significantly. (Adapted from Yung et al[3] with permission.)

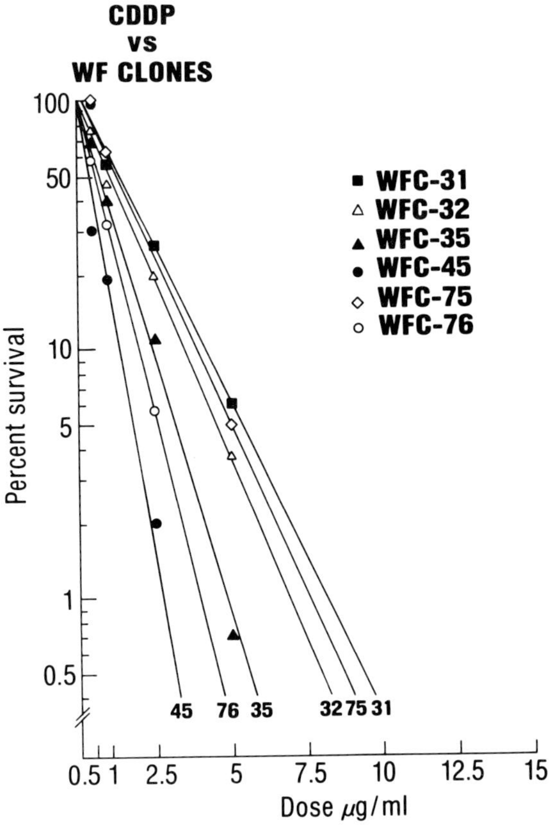

Fig 2. Semilog dose-response curves determined by colony-forming assay for 6 clones from tumor WF treated with cisplatin at passage 12. The ED_{50} doses ranged from 0.35 μg/mL (WFC-45) to 1.40 μg/mL (WFC-31). By log-probit analysis the ED_{50} doses among several of the clones differed significantly. (Adapted from Yung et al[3] with permission.)

mixed cell populations from different regions had different chemosensitivities, again reflecting intrinsic cellular resistance.[2]

Cellular chemosensitivity (and resistance) tends to be associated with a limited number of phenotypic and genotypic characteristics. Rapidly growing cells are often more sensitive to drugs than are slower growing cells. The chromosomes of rapidly growing cells are often unstable in tissue culture, ie, their daughter cells differ in karyotype, and these cells are often hyperploid. Such cells tend to be more sensitive to chemotherapeutic agents. In contrast, the more normal the cell's karyotype, the more stable it tends to be, and the more resistant it also tends to be.[4]

We have studied intrinsic and acquired resistance to chemotherapeutic agents among glioma cell populations and clones.[5] To test intrinsic resistance of cells from freshly resected tumors, the cells were exposed to BCNU and the genotype of the resistant cells compared to that of nontreated controls. The procedure was as follows: the surgical specimen was dissociated into single cells that were aliquoted for drug testing. The cells were incubated with BCNU in serum-free medium for 1 hour; control cells were incubated identically except they received no drug. The cells were plated, permitted to grow, and the number of colonies at 3 weeks in the treated plates was compared to the number in the controls. Other plates prepared and treated in parallel were cloned and each colony expanded for determination of modal chromosome number 10 to 15 generations after their isolation. The cells that survived doses of BCNU at levels greater than 7.5 μg/mL were primarily near-diploid in chromosome number, while cells that were hyperdiploid with chromosome numbers greater than 60 were sensitive to BCNU. The resistant phenotype was unstable, however; if these same lines were maintained in culture without treatment for any period of time, the results could be completely reversed.

To test acquired resistance, the cells were treated with a daily exposure of a single concentration of BCNU for 3 consecutive days. This was followed by a recovery period, with each subsequent exposure at a higher drug concentration than the previous treatment. The parental line and several clones were developed over 1 to 2 years. The chromosome pattern seen in Fig 3 illustrates how the majority of the surviving cells were near-diploid cells, especially at the highest drug concentrations, while serially maintained control cultures developed increased modal chromosome numbers. When the treated cultures were maintained in vitro without treatment for 3 to 4 months, then rechallenged with the last concentration of BCNU, they retained a small portion of resistant cells but the chromosome number became hyperdiploid instead of near-diploid. Structural rearrangements also emerged

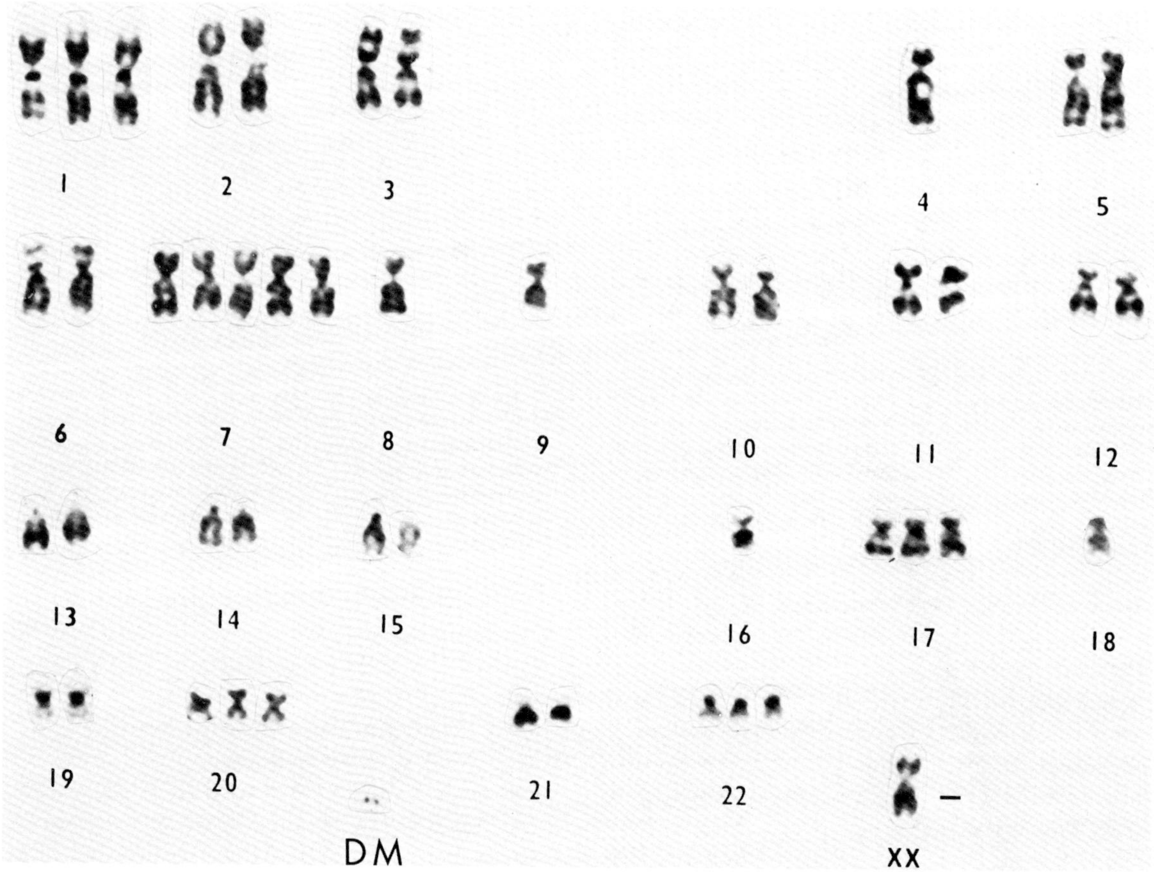

Fig 3. A representative near-diploid karyotype (47,XO) prepared from the BCNU drug-resistant (70 μg/mL) population of tumor EI. The chromosomes in this karyotype have normal standard Giemsa-banded patterns. The aberrant features include a single double minute (DM) and the overrepresentation of chromosomes 1, 7, 17, 20, and 22; and the underrepresentation of chromosomes 4, 8, 9, 16, 18, and the X. Analysis of many such karyotypes demonstrate that chromosomes 7, 20, and 22 are consistently overrepresented while only the X chromosome is underrepresented. Control cultures carried parallel to drug-treated cultures also illustrated an overrepresentation of chromosomes 7 and 20 while chromosome 22 was underrepresented, as was the X chromosome. The increased retention of chromosome 22 suggested that genes contained on this chromosome might be amplified in their expression. Crude extracts and concentrated medium prepared from this culture stimulated DNA synthesis on platelet-derived growth factor (PDGF) receptor-positive cells while their controls did not. Neither the drug-treated cultures nor their controls stimulated epidermal-derived cells (PDGF receptor-negative cells), suggesting that such cells were amplified in their expression of a PDGF or PDGF-like molecule (see JR Shapiro, this issue).

in these cultures that were not found in the cytogenetic analysis of the primary cells.

These data indicate that the most resistant cell in the freshly resected glioma is near-diploid, while hyperdiploid cells tend to be sensitive. Several other human tumors have shown similar results. In rhabdomyosarcomas, Houghten and Houghten[6] have found that a sensitive parental line was hyperdiploid in chromosome number and a drug-resistant line developed from these cells was diploid with a normal-appearing karyotype. Look and coworkers[7] had a similar finding in infants one year of age or younger who developed neuroblastoma. Using flow cytometry to determine the DNA content of each tumor sample, they found that the near-diploid tumors were resistant while the hyperdiploid tumors were sensitive to the currently used protocols. These findings in solid tumors appear to mimic results in leukemia and lymphoma studies; the malignant clones most resistant to therapy appear to be hypodiploid or near-diploid in chromosome number.[8]

THE BLOOD-BRAIN BARRIER AND THE PHARMACOKINETICS OF BRAIN TUMOR CHEMOTHERAPY

The blood-brain barrier (BBB) is the term applied to the relatively restricted transport between blood and the central nervous system (CNS) of certain molecules, usually water soluble, ionized and larger than about 200 daltons. The anatomic substrate of the BBB appears to reside in the endothelial cells of brain capillaries, which differ from capillaries in the rest of the body (except perhaps the testis) in that they are jointed together by tight intercellular junctions and are devoid of fenestrae. One consequence of the existence of the BBB is that the brain's extracellular or interstitial fluid also differs from that of other tissues in being an ultrafiltrate essentially identical to cerebrospinal fluid (CSF), instead of the transudate found elsewhere. In addition, the brain lacks a lymphatic system to return the ultrafiltrate to the blood stream, and relies instead on the relatively inefficient CSF pathways. For the physician the BBB represents the first problem in pharmacologic therapy of CNS disease; many drugs simply do not cross the barrier sufficiently to be effective.

For some time it was thought that the BBB also prevented entry of chemotherapeutic agents into CNS neoplasms. Thus, in 1962, Rall and Zubrod identified pharmacologic characteristics necessary for a drug to cross the barrier, because the barrier was thought to be intact in meningeal leukemia.[9] The situation appeared to be different for brain tumors. In patients with brain tumor, radioisotopes and radiocontrast materials readily cross into the tumor while failing to enter the surrounding brain tissue. Such penetration represents the mechanism by which the brain tumor is perceived separately from the brain. Laboratory evidence appeared to support the absence of a significant BBB in brain tumors. Vick et al[10] found endothelial abnormalities in the blood vessels of an autochthonous viral-induced experimental astrocytoma in the rat, which allowed the passage of high molecular weight horseradish peroxidase into the extracellular space of the tumor. Ausman et al[11] similarly found that the barrier was broken in the bulk of a choriocarcinoma in the brain of a monkey. It is clear, however, that the BBB is not completely broken in a brain tumor because water-soluble drugs found to be effective against tumors in extracranial sites in animals and man are much less effective when the tumor is in the CNS. The question remains quantitative as to how much the BBB is broken, or more precisely, what is the physiologic nature of the blood-tumor barrier (BTB)?

Quantitative definition of BTB has been attempted by a number of investigators.[12,13] Recently, new techniques utilizing quantitative autoradiography (QAR) have permitted detailed measurements of BBB, BTB, blood flow, and chemotherapeutic drug entry in and around experimental brain tumors in regions as small as $50 \times 50 \times 20\ \mu m$.[14] These techniques permit us to model blood-CNS transport in precise mathematical terms and thus promise to help resolve questions of drug entry into brain tumor.

As reviewed elsewhere in this issue, Blasberg et al[14] have performed QAR measurements on a number of animal brain tumor models and have presented convincing evidence of a variable breakdown of the BTB in different tumors and in different regions of the same tumor. They have also found that the blood flow in these tumors is lower than that in the surrounding brain. Using these measurements they have modeled drug entry, predicting certain kinds of behavior depending on the tumor studied and on its relative size and degree of anaplasia. Our laboratory has confirmed many of these observations and has attempted to study drug entry directly using radiolabelled chemotherapeutic agents. We also attempted to modify the BTB to determine if we could increase drug entry.

We began by investigating the entry of ^{14}C-MTX into the rat brain tumors. We used two inoculated tumors: Walker 256, a rat carcinosarcoma derived from a breast cancer and representative of metastatic brain tumors,[15] and C_6 glioma, a tumor originally induced as a rat brain tumor[16] and used here as representative of a primary brain tumor. As part of the project, we purposely opened the BBB using intracarotid (IC) hyperosmolar mannitol and modelled ^{14}C-AIB and ^{14}C-IAP with and without mannitol.[17] After determining the effect of opening the BBB on AIB and IAP, we again used IC mannitol and measured ^{14}C-MTX after IC administration in tumor, brain, and brain-adjacent-to-tumor (BAT) on the side of the drug administration and on the opposite side where a tumor was also implanted.[18] Thus we could compare intravenous (IV) with IC drug administration and IC alone with IC plus mannitol to open the barrier. The concentration $\times$ time (C $\times$ T) for the MTX was determined.

The IC mannitol had no effect on blood flow as measured by the ^{14}C-IAP. The capillary permeability was measured by the ^{14}C-AIB entry and expressed as K, a unidirectional blood-brain transfer rate constant. The results confirmed previous observations by Neuwelt et al[19] that IC hyperosmolar mannitol opens the BBB in the cortex of the rat to a marked, albeit variable degree. ^{14}C-AIB entry was increased in the cortical regions by mannitol from 49-fold at 1.37 mol/L (1.6 molal) mannitol to 105-fold in C_6 glioma rats at 1.6 mol/L (2.0 molal) mannitol. The effect of the mannitol on the brain tumors was considerably less marked and differed between the two tumors and between the two mannitol concentrations.[17] In the Walker 256 experiments, 1.37 mol/L mannitol failed to increase capillary permeability in the tumor, but 1.6 mol/L mannitol increased permeability 13-fold. In the C_6 glioma experiments, 1.37 mol/L mannitol failed to increase capillary permeability in the tumor, but a small increase (1.7-fold) occurred at the 1.6 mol/L mannitol concentration. The two tumors differed in the degree of capillary permeability prior to the mannitol. C_6 glioma was the more permeable with K values of 28 to 36 times greater than K values in the cortex, a substantial "breakdown" of the BBB, or more precisely, the BTB, and 3 times the K values of Walker 256. Thus, Walker 256 had "more room" to open its barrier further than did C_6 glioma, although opening the barrier required a substantial osmotic load (1.6 mol/L). The effect of the mannitol on the BAT depended both on the tumor type and on the mannitol concentration. However, some increased permeability occurred in all cases, the maximum increase occurring at 1.6 mol/L in the Walker 256 tumor series.

Recently, Nakagawa, et al[20] reported measurements of ^{14}C-AIB entry into rat RG-2 brain tumors after IC hyperosmolar mannitol. Mannitol in concentrations of 0.8 to 1.8 molal failed to increase capillary permeability in the tumor, while increasing permeability in the brain in a graded fashion—greater ^{14}C-AIB entry with greater mannitol osmolality. We measured entry of ^{14}C-MTX in sets of rats inoculated with C_6 glioma at time intervals of 5 to 90 minutes.[18] Both the mean concentration and the C $\times$ T over the 90 minutes was determined under several experimental conditions. IC delivery of the ^{14}C-MTX increased the C $\times$ T over IV delivery for cortex, tumor, and peritumoral brain (BAT) by 70%, 141%, and 99%, respectively. IC hyperosmolar mannitol increased the MTX C $\times$ T over arterial delivery without mannitol for cortex by 685%, tumor by 121%, and BAT by 216%. Thus, the largest drug increase in tumor with the smallest increase in brain followed IC drug delivery without mannitol.

These data are relevant to the clinical use of IC hyperosmolar mannitol in brain tumor chemotherapy. The efficacy of this technique in a given patient would depend on the BTB characteristics of that patient's individual tumor. In the animals, 1.6 mol/L mannitol, a greater concentration than the 1.37 mol/L used clinically, was required to open the barrier in the Walker 256 tumor. Specifically with respect to the MTX entry, one can utilize the ratio of the drug exposure (C $\times$ T) of the tumor to that of the cortex to express a kind of therapeutic index in which the tumor exposure is considered therapeutic and the cortical exposure toxic. In the IV treated rats, the therapeutic index was 1.77 while for the IC group it was 2.5; when mannitol was added, the ratio fell to 0.7. Thus, the largest increase in drug concentration in tumor with the smallest concomitant increase in cortical drug concentration follows IC drug delivery without mannitol. The effects of exposing normal brain to higher concentrations of potentially neurotoxic drugs must be weighed against their possible benefits in treating invariably lethal intracranial neoplasms.

AGENTS IN USE FOR BRAIN TUMOR CHEMOTHERAPY

Chemotherapeutic agents are cellular poisons, the actions of which are not specific to tumors but also affect normal cells. They may be cell cycle specific, ie, effective only during certain phases of the cell's life cycle, usually when DNA is synthesized, or cell cycle nonspecific, ie, the drug may be effective both during DNA synthesis and at other times during the cycle period. Some drugs such as BCNU that are cell cycle nonspecific are known to be more effective during DNA synthesis, however.[21] Modifying the growth fraction of a tumor with cell cycle nonspecific agents, radiation, or surgery may improve the efficacy of cell cycle–specific agents because the number of cells in active division may be increased. This may be especially valuable in combination chemotherapy where cell cycle–specific agents can be combined with cell cycle–nonspecific agents in order to reduce the total cell population and increase the percentage of cells in active division.

Chemotherapeutic agents have been chosen for use against brain tumors for a variety of reasons, but usually not because they were thought to be specific for such tumors. Some were tried because they were found to cross the BBB (nitrosoureas) or because they act in the brain (procarbazine is a mild monoamine oxidase inhibitor like certain antidepressants). Most were tried in one or another animal model of brain tumors and, if effective, were moved into the clinic. Table 1 lists some of the biochemical characteristics of several chemotherapeutic agents used against brain tumors. The results of clinical trials using these drugs are reviewed elsewhere in this issue (see Shapiro WR).

Nitrosoureas

The nitrosoureas are small, lipid-soluble drugs whose mechanism of action is thought to be alkylation. Several possess carbamoylating activ-

Table 1. Examples of Chemotherapeutic Agents Used for Primary Brain Tumors*

Agent	Molecular Weight	Solubility Log P†	Mechanism of Action	Toxicity
Nitrosoureas		Lipid	Alkylating	Myelosuppression
BCNU (Carmustine)	214	1.53		Also: pulmonary
CCNU (Lomustine)	233.7	2.85		hepatic
Methyl-CCNU (Semustine)	247.7	3.30		renal
PCNU	262.7	0.37		
Procarbazine	258	Water	Unknown	Myelosuppression
Cisplatin	300	Water	DNA X-link	Renal, auditory, neuropathy
Epipodophyllotoxin (VM-26)	656	Lipid‡	Spindle poison	Myelosuppression
Hydroxyurea	76	Water‖	Ribonucleoside reductase inhibitor	Myelosuppression
5-Fluorouracil (5-FU)	130	Water‖	Thymidylate synthetase inhibitor	Myelosuppression

*The clinical use of these and other drugs alone and in combination is reviewed elsewhere (Shapiro WR, this issue).
†Log P = 1-octanol/water partition coefficient.
‡Crosses BBB poorly.
‖Crosses BBB easily.

ity (through an isocyanate portion), which may impede repair of sublethal DNA damage caused by ionizing irradiation.[22] BCNU is a bifunctional alkylating agent with two chloroethyl moieties, and can therefore crosslink DNA.[23] The drug rapidly biotransforms and/or spontaneously decomposes, with a plasma half-life of less than 15 minutes in mice, which is probably similar to that in humans.[24] The dose-limiting toxicity is myelosuppression, which tends to be delayed with thrombocytopenia and leukopenia occurring at 3 to 4 weeks and lasting 1 to 3 weeks. Long-term usage of BCNU, especially in cumulative doses exceeding 1,500 mg/m^2, may induce pulmonary fibrosis, especially in patients with previous pulmonary disease or exposure to toxins, including tobacco.[25] Hepatic function tests often become abnormal, but usually normalize on discontinuing the drug. BCNU is usually administered intravenously, but in recent experimental trials, has been given intraarterially (see below). CCNU and methyl-CCNU are similar to BCNU in mechanism of action and metabolism; they are administered orally. Methyl-CCNU has rarely been associated with renal failure.[26] PCNU is an interesting drug because it most closely fits the model lipid-soluble compound predicted by the work of Hansch and others to be ideal as a chemotherapeutic agent on the basis of its Log P of 0.37.[27,28] Levin et al[29,30] has since suggested that its pharmacological behavior in humans may prevent it from fulfilling this prediction. However, results in Brain Tumor Cooperative Group (BTCG) trials suggests that PCNU may be quite effective.[31]

Procarbazine

Procarbazine is a water-soluble N-methylhydrazine. Its mechanism of action is unknown, but it appears to produce chromosomal breakage as well as inhibit protein synthesis and it therefore resembles an alkylating agent.[32] Despite its water solubility, it readily crossed the BBB and may produce mild CNS toxicity. Its major toxicity is myelosuppression, but it often causes nausea and vomiting and may rarely cause a severe rash.[33]

Cisplatin

Cisplatin is a water-soluble planar inorganic compound that appears to act through intrastrand and interstrand crosslinking of DNA in a manner similar to the bifunctional alkylating agents.[34] The electrically neutral compound diffuses into cells where the chloride ions are lost by hydrolysis. Two reactive ligand sites are then formed at which covalent linkages occur with nucleic acids or proteins. Cisplatin is primarily nephrotoxic and must be used with additional hydration.[35] It is also ototoxic, especially in the elderly, and may produce peripheral neuropathy.[36] Cisplatin is usually administered intravenously, but is under investigation as an intraarterial agent (see below).

Epipodophyllotoxin

Epipodophyllotoxin (VM-26) is a semisynthetic podophyllotoxin of large size that is highly lipophilic. The drug is a mitotic spindle poison like the vinca alkaloids. It has been found to be taken up by cells by passive diffusion and binds to high- and low-affinity binding sites.[37] VM-26 binds to tubulin, a microtubule subunit and in vitro causes a premitotic delay with cells irreversibly accumulating in the G_2-phase of the cell cycle.[38,39] It is a cell cycle–specific drug. Despite its high lipophilicity, only minimal amounts cross the BBB,[40] although the drug has been reported effective against some malignant gliomas in Phase II trials.[41] The major dose-limiting toxicity of VM-26 is hematologic, though this is not cumulative.

Hydroxyurea

Hydroxyurea is a cell cycle–specific drug that interferes with DNA synthesis through inhibition of ribonucleoside diphosphate reductase.[42] This enzyme catalyzes the reductive conversion of ribonucleotides to deoxyribonucleotides, which are necessary for DNA synthesis. It readily crosses the BBB despite its water solubility.[40]

5-Fluorouracil

5-Fluorouracil (5-FU) is a pyrimidine analog differing from uracil by a fluorinated 5 carbon. By acting as a false pyrimidine, 5-FU competes with uracil for the enzyme thymidylate synthetase and thereby inhibits production of thymidine. Thymidylate synthetase catalyzes the transfer of a methyl group from methylene tetrahydofolate to deoxyuridylic acid to form deoxythymidylic acid. Prior to binding with thymidylate synthetase, 5-FU must be converted to the corresponding ribonucleoside and ribonucleotide. RNA synthesis is also disturbed since 5-FU competes with uracil in the production of RNA. 5-FU is a cell cycle–specific drug since it blocks DNA synthesis. It is a small molecule and is water soluble, yet readily crosses the BBB.[44] Its use in brain tumor chemotherapy followed the observation that it acts synergistically with BCNU against the rat 9L gliosarcoma.[45]

NEWER METHODS IN BRAIN TUMOR CHEMOTHERAPY

Increasing Tumor Drug Concentrations

As noted above, an important problem in brain tumor chemotherapy is the development of resistance by tumor cells subjected to sublethal doses of cytotoxic drugs. We have found that human glioma cells in culture rapidly become more resistant to BCNU during repeated exposure to doses of 1 μg/mL.[46] One possible aim in brain tumor chemotherapy is to increase the concentration of drug in the tumor enough so as to kill "all" the cells and prevent the development of resistance. Three techniques to increase intratumor drug concentration have been introduced. The first uses very high-dose intravenous BCNU administration followed by autologous bone marrow transplantation to block the associated severe myelosuppression.[47] While the marrow is fairly well protected by this technique, the lungs are not and the patients may develop pulmonary toxicity. The second technique to increase drug concentration is to administer the drug regionally. By this method, the chemotherapeutic agent is infused via one of the arteries feeding the brain on the side of the tumor. Third, an attempt may be made to increase brain tumor drug concentration by purposely opening the BBB as described above in the rat experiments. We shall review briefly the last two techniques as they apply to humans.

Intraarterial chemotherapy. While IV BCNU has been the mainstay of chemotherapy of patients with malignant glioma, it is clearly not curative. Laboratory evidence suggested that higher concentrations of drug may be achieved in brain by "regional" chemotherapy using intraarterial (IA) infusion.[48] We found MTX C $\times$ T exposure in a rat brain tumor doubled when the drug was administered via the carotid artery in comparison to concentrations after IV administration.[18] Since the systemic arterial concentration is dependent on total drug dose, reducing the dose by regional administration would lower systemic exposure. Fenstermacher and Cowles[49] and Fenstermacher and Gazendam,[50] using a mathematical model, predicted that IC drug administration would produce as high as a tenfold greater drug concentration in brain tissue than would IV administration, while bone marrow levels of drug were predicted to be equivalent to those after IV administration. Madajewicz et al,[51] Greenberg et al,[52] Cascino et al,[53] and Hochberg et al[54] administered BCNU via the carotid artery in patients with primary or metastatic brain tumors. The results were variable, but several good responses were obtained. There was at least one instance of a response on the side of the infusion in a patient with bifrontal metastatic brain tumors whose tumor on the other side then responded when its ipsilateral carotid artery was infused.[53] A major limitation of this approach has been the occurrence of both eye and brain toxicity on the side of the infusion.[52] At least in part this is dose-dependent and its incidence is reduced when the dose is lowered. Attempting to prevent the toxicity by dissolving the BCNU in less alcohol appears to reduce the available drug because of diminished solubility.[55] Despite such potential difficulties, the concept of increasing drug concentration by this technique is sufficiently attractive that the BTCG has mounted a Phase III trial to compare IA with IV BCNU.

Another drug that might be more effective when administered regionally than by its usual IV route is cisplatin. Cisplatin has been under investigation for several years for the chemotherapy of brain tumors. One BTCG study found it to be minimally effective. However, the drug is attractive because it is relatively marrow sparing. Three recent reports describe IC cisplatin administration in patients with primary or metastatic brain tumor.[56–58] Of 70 patients, about 30% showed some degree of improvement. Toxicity included retinal damage, seizures, and motor weakness as well as the usual systemic symptoms, but serious toxicity was limited to doses of 75 mg/m^2 or more. The BTCG is now performing a Phase II study with IC cisplatin.

Opening the blood-tumor barrier. Increasing tissue drug concentration in patients by attempting to open the BBB by IC hyperosmolar mannitol has been described by Neuwelt et al[59] who administered MTX. Our animal studies[18] and his[19] predict markedly increased brain concentrations of MTX after IC mannitol. Since previous experience demonstrates CNS toxicity from MTX, there is concern that such patients may ultimately develop brain damage. Neuwelt is also concerned about neurotoxicity from chemotherapeutic agents after BBB modification.[60] He found that adriamycin and cisplatin damaged the dog's brain after BBB disruption. Cisplatin given IC also did so even without BBB disruption. In Neuwelt's clinical studies,[59] MTX was said not to be neurotoxic.

New Drugs and Polychemotherapy

Several new drugs are under investigation for brain tumors. Among the more promising are PCNU, ACNU (a water-soluble nitrosourea produced in Japan),[61] spirohydantoin mustard,[62] dianhydrogalactitol[63] and its parent dibomodulcitol,[64] and aziridinyl benzoquinone (AZQ).[65,66] They are being tested both as single agents, some administered IA, and in combination chemotherapy.

The primary rationale for combination chemotherapy is the observation that gliomas are heterogeneous and that different cell populations respond to different drugs. Several groups around the world have treated patients by this technique, but only a few controlled studies have been performed comparing single-drug treatment with polychemotherapy (reviewed elsewhere[41,67]). The problem remains that the drugs that arc chosen are still only marginally effective and when empirically combined have only a small chance of success. Unfortunately, until a better system is developed to test agents against individual tumors, we must rely on such empirical approaches.

ASSAYS FOR BRAIN TUMOR CHEMOTHERAPY

In Vivo Studies

Animal models of brain tumors have been useful in studying a wide variety of problems, eg, BBB and BTB, pharmacokinetics of drug entry, immunology, and immunotherapy, tumor pathogenesis, and tumor metabolism. There have been many efforts to develop animal models that could be used in brain tumor chemotherapy. The ependymoblastoma model and its use for chemotherapy testing as described by Ausman et al[68] was further developed by Geran et al.[69] The 9L gliosarcoma in the rat brain has been used for many years for chemotherapy experiments.[70] Shapiro et al[71] described the nude mouse system to test chemotherapeutic agents in human tumors. They found that different patients' tumors were responsive to different drugs.[72] In a later study they found that only some of the cells in a tumor were selected for growth in the nude mouse, thus making this system unreliable for testing individual patients' tumors.[73] Both Schold et al[74,75] and Houchens et al[76] have used the nude mouse system as a general human glioma screen to examine new single agents and combination chemotherapy. Schold and Bigner have reviewed animal brain tumor models used in chemotherapy research.[77] Recently, a nude rat brain tumor model has been described.[78]

In Vitro Studies

In vitro investigations of human glioma cell lines have been used to study a variety of tumor characteristics, including heterogeneity, immunology, chemotherapy, and tumor cell metabolism. Conclusions from these studies about the original tumor must be drawn cautiously because tumor cells in long-term tissue culture have been found to change genotypically and phenotypically.[79] For chemotherapy assays on individual patients' tumors, it is especially crucial to test fresh material.

An in vitro assay system to evaluate the degree of chemosensitivity of a given patient's tumor to a panel of chemotherapeutic agents would be quite useful. If a patient's tumor could reliably be shown to be sensitive to specific drugs in vitro, his physician would be able to individualize his chemotherapy in a manner analogous to treating bacterial infections after sensitivity testing. If one could reliably predict agents to which the tumor was resistant, patients could avoid many of the unpleasant and dangerous side effects associated with ineffective drugs. The advent of the Hamburger/Salmon soft-agar assay promised to fulfill many of these goals. The assay is now widely used both in research and in the clinic to predict chemotherapy sensitivity for individual patients' tumors. Unfortunately, its applicability is limited because many systemic tumors do not grow well in soft-agar and because it has not always been reproducible in different laboratories. The clinical applicability of this research tool has been questioned by critics who argue with some justification that it was moved too rapidly into predictive testing.[80]

Assaying Individual Patient's Brain Tumors

Three methods have been reported to assay human gliomas for chemotherapy: the microcytotoxicity assay, the radiolabelled precursor uptake assay, and the colony-forming (clonogenic) assay.

In the microcytotoxicity assay, cells grown in a monolayer are exposed to a drug and then reincubated. Twenty-four hours later the cells that remain attached to the dish surface are considered viable and counted. A sensitive cell line is one in which 75% of the cells die and detach. As a rule these assays are not particularly sensitive; drug concentrations are required that well exceed achievable plasma levels in humans.[3] However, Kornblith et al[81] reported human glioma sensitivity to BCNU at 6.6 μg/mL.

In the precursor uptake assay, tumor cells are exposed to drug and the effect is then measured by determining the uptake of ^{3}H-leucine or ^{35}S-methionine, both measures of protein synthesis.[82] The results of testing several drugs demonstrated variable suppression of uptake. Similar assays have been described measuring the effect of drugs on uptake of ^{3}H-uridine and ^{14}C-leucine.[83] These assays measure protein or DNA synthesis and define drugs that modify cellular metabolism but do not necessarily kill the cell.

The colony-forming assay exposes suspended or plated cells to drug for 1 to 2 hours, replates them with or without soft-agar, and then measures the number of colonies that grow. This assay therefore measures the potential of a drug to block the reproductive capacity of a tumor cell, clinically the most important of its characteristics.

As noted above, our laboratory performs chemotherapy testing as part of our drug-resistance studies, to define heterogeneity of chemotherapy response and to correlate chemotherapy response to the tumor's genotypic and phenotypic characteristics.[5] We do not use a soft-agar assay because we have found that freshly resected gliomas cells do not grow in agar. Rather we use an aqueous monolayer colony-forming assay which we find to be reproducible.[3] Rosenblum et al[84] have pioneered in attempts to develop a human glioma "stem" cell assay. They also do not use soft-agar, but grow the tumors on a "feeder" layer of irradiated 9L gliosarcoma cells. They have reported on a series of in vitro/in vivo correlation studies. In a small number of comparisons (13 untreated patients) the in vitro test predicted response in 5/7 and failure in 6/6.

There are several problems that must be considered if in vitro assay systems are to be used to define appropriate chemotherapy for patients[85]: (1) The nature of the assay. The colony-forming assay would appear to be the most sensitive and the most specific for in vitro testing for human gliomas. However, many cells may not form colonies. In our own studies, we find that astrocytes are often highly motile and wander away from the colony before it has achieved the 25 to 50 cells needed to define it. Only cells that form colonies can be counted in such systems, thus introducing selection. (2) Drug concentrations. It has been suggested that unless drugs are used in the assays at concentrations achievable in vivo, results are unlikely to be clinically applicable.[86] Unfortunately, we often know achievable plasma concentrations, but rarely know achievable tumor tissue concentrations. The QAR experiments reviewed above have permitted us to determine regional drug concentrations in animal brain tumors.[18] It is possible that PET scanning techniques will permit similar measurements in humans. Nevertheless, it would appear prudent to determine dose-response curves rather than test tumors against only 1 or 2 doses. (3) Heterogeneity. All drug assays have used mass cultures derived directly from the patient's tumor. Our studies of regional heterogeneity have shown that testing a portion of a patient's tumor does not reliably indicate the sensitivity of any other part.[2] Furthermore, our finding of clonal heterogeneity indicates that mass culture testing might well misinterpret resistance or sensitivity depending on the proportion of the cell populations present in the assay. Correlation between clonal assays and mass culture assays will need to be done. (4) Response criteria. All in vitro assays must be compared to the patient's response.

Determining the response of a patient to chemotherapeutic agents is difficult at best and relating it to in vitro results is even harder. How are we to compare the in vitro response of the tumor from a patient who lives 8 months with one from a patient who lives 20 months? (5) Other problems include the need for longer exposure time for cell cycle–specific agents, the requirement for certain drugs to be metabolized to an active form, and the need to develop techniques to evaluate combination chemotherapy in vitro.

CONCLUSIONS

Data from the laboratory clearly identify two problems important in the therapy of malignant brain tumor. These are regional and clonal heterogeneity of human brain tumor cells within individual patients and the problems of the blood-brain barrier. The heterogeneity of gliomas is responsible, at least in part, for the development of resistance to chemotherapeutic agents. Intrinsic variation in chemosensitivity has been demonstrated for human glioma cells, and low-dose nitrosourea therapy rapidly produces resistant cell populations. Continued laboratory investigation using modern techniques of molecular biology hopefully will yield clues to the mechanism(s) underlying drug resistance. Two obvious clinical approaches to this problem are increasing drug concentrations to reduce the chances for the development of resistance and the use of multiple agent chemotherapy programs.

The blood-brain barrier represents an important but still ill-understood problem in chemotherapy. Whilc it is evident that the blood-tumor barrier is not closed to chemotherapeutic agents, it is also clear from laboratory studies that its breakdown needs to be defined quantitatively. The barrier is partially open, and the degree of opening must be related to drug entry. One method for increasing drug entry into brain tumors is to deliver the chemotherapeutic agents in higher blood concentrations. The most readily applicable method is that of intraarterial drug injection. Both computer models and animal studies have been utilized to examine this question, and intraarterial drug administration has been carried out in humans. Generally, drug concentrations within the brain in experimental animals (and in some experimental brain tumors) are markedly increased by using intracarotid *v* intravenous drug infusion. Such techniques permit not only an increase in drug concentration within the tumor, but also a lower systemic drug dosage so as to reduce peripheral drug toxicity. The most obvious drug candidates for intraarterial treatment of human gliomas are BCNU and cisplatin.

For chemotherapy of brain tumors to advance beyond its current empiric approach, it must be made more specific, both in terms of its role as a cellular poison and in terms of methods to define individual cellular susceptibility. With respect to the former, continued basic work on the mechanism of action of drugs is necessary and especially on biochemically mediated (induced) and genotypically mediated (selected) cell resistance. With respect to the latter, continued work on individual patient tumor sensitivity assays is needed. While we wait for a "breakthrough," we must learn to use the available drugs better.

REFERENCES

1. Shapiro JR, Yung W-KA, Shapiro WR: Isolation, karyotype and clonal growth of heterogeneous subpopulations of human malignant glioma. Cancer Res 51:2349–2359, 1981

2. Shapiro JR, Pu P-Y, Mohamed AN, et al: Regional heterogeneity in high grade gliomas. Proc Am Assoc Cancer Res 25:375, 1984

3. Yung W-KA, Shapiro WR, Shapiro JR: Heterogeneous chemosensitivities of subpopulations of human glioma cells in culture. Cancer Res 42:992–998, 1982

4. Shapiro JR, Pu PY, Shapiro WR: Resistant cell types in human gliomas, in Salmon SE, Trent JM (eds): Human Tumor Cloning. Orlando, Fla, Grune & Stratton, 1984, pp 133–142

5. Pu PY, Shapiro WR, Shapiro JR: Correlation of chromosome number to BCNU sensitivity in freshly resected human gliomas tested by colony forming assays in monolayer culture. Proc Am Assoc Cancer Res 24:284, 1983

6. Houghten P, Houghten J: Personal communication

7. Look AT, Hayes FA, Nitschke R, et al: Cellular DNA content as a predictor of response to chemotherapy in infants with unresectable neuroblastoma. N Engl J Med 311:231–235, 1984

8. Barlogie B, Hittelman W, Spitzer G, et al: Correlation of DNA distribution abnormalities with cytogenetic findings in human adult leukemia and lymphoma. Cancer Res 37:4400–4407, 1977

9. Rall DP, Zubrod CG: Mechanism of drug absorption and excretion. Passage of drugs in and out of the central nervous system. Ann Rev Pharmacol 2:109–128, 1962

10. Vick NA, Khandekar JD, Bigner DD: Chemotherapy

of brain tumors: The "blood-brain barrier" is not a factor. Arch Neurol 34:523–526, 1977

11. Ausman JI, Levin VA, Brown WE, et al: Brain-tumor chemotherapy: Pharmacological principles derived from a monkey brain-tumor model. J Neurosurg 46:155–164, 1977

12. Levin VA, Landahl HD, Freeman-Dove MA: The application of brain capillary permeability coefficient measurements to pathological conditions and the selection of agents which cross the blood-brain barrier. J Pharmacokinet Biopharm 4:499–519, 1976

13. Levin VA, Patlak CS, Landahl HD: Heuristic modeling of drug delivery to malignant brain tumors. J Pharmacokinet Biopharm 8:257–295, 1980

14. Blasberg RG, Groothuis D, Molnar P: Application of quantitative autoradiographic measurements in experimental brain tumor models. Sem Neuro 1:203–221, 1981

15. Ushio Y, Chernik NL, Shapiro WR, et al: Metastatic tumor in the brain. Development of an experimental model. Ann Neurol 2:20–29, 1977

16. Benda P, Someda K, Messer J, et al: Morphological and immunochemical studies of rat glial tumors and clonal strains propagated in culture. J Neurosurg 34:310–323, 1971

17. Hiesiger EM, Voorhies R, Basler GA, et al: Capillary permeability of experimental brain tumor and cortex after intracarotid hyperosmolar mannitol as measured by quantitative autoradiography (QAR). Neurology 33:108, 1983 (suppl)

18. Hiesiger EM, Voorhies R, Basler GA, et al: Comparison of ^{14}C-methotrexate (^{14}C-MTX) delivery by intravenous vs intracarotid (IC) route without or with IC mannitol in experimental rat brain tumors as measured by quantitative autoradiography (QAR). Proc Am Assoc Cancer 25:363, 1984

19. Neuwelt EA, Bigner D, Frenkel EP, et al: The effects of osmotic modification of the blood brain barrier and adrenal steroid administration on methotrexate delivery of gliomas in rats: The blood brain barrier is a factor. Proc Natl Acad Sci USA 79:4420–4423, 1982

20. Nakagawa H, Groothuis D, Blasberg RG: The effect of graded hypertonic intracarotid infusions on drug delivery to experimental RG-2 gliomas. Neurology 34:1571–1581, 1984

21. Barranco SC, Humphrey RM: The effects of BCNU on survival and cell progression in Chinese hamster cells. Cancer Res 31:191–195, 1971

22. Kann HE Jr: Carbamoylation activity of nitrosoureas, in Prestayko AW, et al (eds): Nitrosoureas Current Status and New Developments. Orlando, Fla, Academic, 1981, pp 95–105

23. Kohn KW, Erickson LC, Laurent G, et al: DNA crosslinking and the origin of sensitivity of chloroethylnitrosoureas, in Prestayko AW, et al (eds): Nitrosoureas Current Status and New Developments. Orlando, Fla, Academic, 1981, pp 69–83

24. DeVita VT, Denhan C, Davidson JD, et al: The physiological disposition of carcinostatic 1,3-bis(2-chloroethyl)-1-nitrosourea in man and animals. Clin Pharmacol Ther 8:566–577, 1967

25. Aronin PA, Mahaley MS Jr, Rudnick SA, et al: Prediction of BCNU pulmonary toxicity in patients with malignant gliomas, an assessment of risk factors. New Engl J Med 303:183–188, 1980

26. Schacht RG, Feiner HD, Gallo GR, et al: Nephrotoxicity of nitrosoureas. Cancer 48:1328–1334, 1978

27. Hansch C, Smith N, Engle R, et al: Quantitative structure-activity relationships of antineoplastic drugs: Nitrosoureas and triazenoimidazoles. Cancer Chemother Rep 56:443–456, 1972

28. Levin VA, Kabra PM: Effectiveness of the nitrosoureas as a function of their lipid solubility in the chemotherapy of experimental rat brain tumors. Cancer Chemother Rep 58:787–792, 1974

29. Levin VA, Liu J, Weinkam J: Comparative pharmacokinetics of 1-(2-chloroethyl)-3-(2,6-dioxo-1-piperidyl)-1-nitrosourea in rats and patients and extrapolation to clinical trials. Cancer Res 41:3475–3477, 1981

30. Levin VA, Resser KJ, McGrath L, et al: PCNU treatment for recurrent malignant gliomas. Cancer Treat Rep 68:969–973, 1984

31. Green SB, Byar DB, Strike TA, et al: Randomized phase II comparison of PCNU and AZQ for the treatment of primary brain tumors (study 8120). Proc Amer Soc Clin Oncol (in press)

32. Spivak SD: Drugs 5 years later: Procarbazine. Ann Intern Med 81:795–800, 1974

33. Edwards MS, Levin VA, Wilson CB: Brain tumor chemotherapy: An evaluation of agents in current use for phase II and III trials. Cancer Treat Rep 64:1179–1205, 1980

34. Zwelling IA, Bradley MO, Sharkey NA, et al: Mutagenicity, cytotoxicity, and DNA crosslinking in V79 Chinese hamster cells treated with cis- and trans-Pt(II) diamminedichloride. Mutat Res 67:271–280, 1979

35. Hayes DM, Cvitkovic E, Golbey RE, et al: High dose cis-platinum diamminedichloride: Amelioration of renal toxicity by mannitol diuresis. Cancer 39:1372–1381, 1977

36. Shapiro WR, Young DF: Neurological complications of antineoplastic therapy. Acta Neurol Scand 70:125–132, 1984 (suppl)

37. Allen L: The role of drug disposition kinetics on cellular transport of the antineoplastic agent VM-26. Drug Metab Rev 8:119–135, 1978

38. Bender RA: Vinca alkaloids and epipodophyllotoxins, in Pinedo HM (ed): Cancer Chemotherapy 1979. The EORTC Cancer Chemotherapy Annual 1. Amsterdam-Oxford, Excerpta Medica, 1979, pp 100–106

39. Krishan A, Paika K, Frei E: Cytofluorometric studies on the action of podophyllotoxin and epipodophyllotoxins (VM-26, VP-16-213) on the cell cycle traverse of human lymphoblasts. J Cell Biol 66:521–530, 1975

40. Creaven PJ, Allen LM: PTG, a new antineoplastic epipodophyllotoxin. Clin Pharmacol Ther 18:227–233, 1975

41. Shapiro WR: Brain tumors, in Pinedo HM, Chabner BA (eds): Cancer Chemotherapy 1983. The EORTC Cancer Chemotherapy Annual 5. Amsterdam, Elsevier, 1983, pp 446–459

42. Krakoff IH, Brown NC, Reichard P: Inhibition of ribonucleoside diphosphate reductase by hydroxyurea. Cancer Res 28:1559–1565, 1968

43. Beckloff GL, Lerner HJ, Frost D, et al: Hydroxyurea

(NSC-32065) in biological fluids: dose-concentration relationships. Cancer Chemotherap Rep 48:57–58, 1965

44. Bourke RS, West CR, Chheda G, et al: Kinetics of entry and distribution of 5-fluorouracil in cerebrospinal fluid and brain following intravenous injection in a primate. Cancer Res 33:1735–1746, 1973

45. Gerosa MA, Dougherty DV, Wilson CB, et al: Improved treatment of a brain-tumor model. Part 2: Sequential therapy with BCNU and 5-fluorouracil. J Neurosurg 58:368–373, 1983

46. Shapiro JR, Shapiro WR: Specific karyotypic and tumorigenic changes in cloned subpopulations of human gliomas exposed to sublethal doses of BCNU, in Chabner BA (ed): Rational Basis for Chemotherapy. New York, A.R. Liss, 1983, pp 45–59

47. Hochberg FH, Parker LM, Takvorian T, et al: High-dose BCNU with autologous bone marrow rescue for recurrent glioblastoma multiforme. J Neurosurg 54:455–460, 1981

48. Levin VA, Kabra PM, Freeman-Dove MA: Pharmacokinetics of intracarotid artery ^{14}C-BCNU in the squirrel monkey. J Neurosurg 48:587–593, 1978

49. Fenstermacher JD, Cowles AL: Theoretic limitations of intracarotid infusions in brain tumor chemotherapy. Cancer Treat Rep 61:519–526, 1977

50. Fenstermacher JD, Gazendam J: Intra-arterial infusions of drugs and hyperosmotic solutions as ways of enhancing CNS chemotherapy. Cancer Treat Rep 65:27–37, 1981 (suppl)

51. Madajewicz S, West CR, Park HC, et al: Phase II study—intra-arterial BCNU therapy for metastatic brain tumors. Cancer 47:653–657, 1981

52. Greenberg HS, Ensminger WD, Chandler WF, et al: Intra-arterial BCNU chemotherapy for the treatment of malignant gliomas of the central nervous system. J Neurosurg 61:423–429, 1984

53. Cascino TL, Byrne TN, Deck MDF, et al: Intra-arterial BCNU in the treatment of metastatic brain tumors. J Neuro-Oncol 1:211–218, 1983

54. Hochberg FH, Pruitt AA, Beck D, et al: The rationale and methodology for intra-arterial chemotherapy with BCNU as treatment for glioblastoma, in Howell S (ed): Intra-arterial and Intra-cavitary Chemotherapy. Boston, Martinus Nijhoff, 1984, pp 97–109

55. Ross RL, Kapp JP, Hochberg F, et al: Solvent systems for intracarotid 1,2-bis(2-chloroethyl)-1-nitrosourea (BCNU) infusion. Neurosurgery 12:512–514, 1983

56. Stewart DJ, Wallace S, Feun L, et al: A Phase I study of intracarotid artery infusion of cis-diamminedichloroplatinum (II) in patients with recurrent malignant intracerebral tumors. Cancer Res 42:2059–2062, 1982

57. Stewart DJ, Benjamin RS, Zimmerman W, et al: Clinical pharmacology of intraarterial cis-diamminedichloroplatinum (II). Cancer Res 43:917–920, 1983

58. Lehane DE, Bryan RN, Horowitz B, et al: Intraarterial cisplatin chemotherapy for patients with primary and metastatic brain tumors. Cancer Drug Del 1:69–77, 1983

59. Neuwelt EA, Frankel EP, Diehl JT, et al: Monitoring of methotrexate delivery in patients with malignant brain tumors after osmotic blood-brain barrier disruption. Ann Int Med 94:449–454, 1981

60. Neuwelt EA, Glasberg M, Frenkel E, et al: Neurotoxicity of chemotherapeutic agents after blood-brain barrier modification: Neuropathological studies. Ann Neurol 14:316–324, 1983

61. Yamashita J, Handa J, Tokuriki Y, et al: Intra-arterial ACNU therapy for malignant brain tumors: Experimental studies and preliminary clinical results. J Neurosurg 59:424–430, 1983

62. Suling WJ, Struck RF, Woolley CW, et al: Metabolism of spirohydantoin mustard in the mouse: Isolation of an alkylating, mutagenic metabolite. Biochem Pharm 32:523–527, 1983

63. Eagan RT, Dinapoli RP, Hermann Jr RC, et al: Combination carmustine (BCNU) and dianhydrogalactitol in the treatment of primary brain tumors recurring after irradiation. Cancer Treat Rep 66:1647–1649, 1982

64. Afra D, Kocsis B, Dobay J, et al: Combined radiotherapy and chemotherapy with dibromodulcitol and CCNU in the postoperative treatment of malignant gliomas. J Neurosurg 59:106–110, 1983

65. Savaraj N, Lu K, Feun LH, et al: Intracerebral penetration and tissue distribution of AZQ. J Neuro-Oncol 1:14–19, 1983

66. Schold SC Jr, Friedman HS, Bjornsson TD, et al: Treatment of patients with recurrent primary brain tumors with AZQ. Neurology 34:615–619, 1984

67. Hiesiger EM, Shapiro WR: Brain tumors, in Pinedo HM, Chabner BA (eds): Cancer Chemotherapy/6, The EORTC Cancer Chemotherapy Annual. Amsterdam, Elsevier, 1984, pp 450–466

68. Ausman JI, Shapiro WR, Rall DP: Studies on chemotherapy of experimental brain tumors: Development of an experimental model. Cancer Res 30:2394–2400, 1970

69. Geran RI, Congleton GF, Dudeck LE, et al: A mouse ependymoblastoma as an experimental model for screening potential antineoplastic drugs. Cancer Chemother Rep 4:53–87, 1980

70. Rosenblum ML, Gerosa MA, Doughter DV, et al: Improved treatment of a brain-tumor model. Part 1: Advantages of single- over multiple-dose BCNU schedules. J Neurosurg 58:177–182, 1983

71. Shapiro WR, Basler GA, Chernik NL, et al: Human brain tumor transplantation into nude mice. J Natl Cancer Inst 62:447–453, 1979

72. Basler GA, Shapiro WR: Brain tumor research with nude mice, in Fogh J, Giovanella B (eds): The Nude Mouse in Experimental and Animal Research. Orlando, Fla, Academic, 1982, pp 475–490

73. Horten BC, Basler GA, Shapiro WR: Xenograft of human malignant glial tumors into brains of nude mice. A histopathological study. J Neuropath Exp Neurol 450:493–511, 1981

74. Schold SC, Rawlings CE, Bigner SH, et al: Intracerebral growth of a human glioma tumor line in athymic mice and treatment with procarbazine, 1,3-bis(2-chloroethyl)-1-nitrosourea, aziridinylbenzoquinone, and cis-platinum. Neurosurgery 12:672–677, 1983

75. Schold SC, Bigner DD: Treatment of five subcutaneous human glioma tumor lines in athymic mice with carmustine, procarbazine, and mithramycin. Cancer Treat Rep 67:811–819, 1983

76. Houchens DP, Ovejera AA, Riblet SM, et al: Human brain tumor xenografts in nude mice as a chemotherapy model. Eur J Cancer Clin Oncol 19:799–805, 1983

77. Schold SC, Bigner DD: A review of animal brain tumor models that have been used for therapeutic studies, in Walker MD (ed): Oncology of the Nervous System. Boston, Martinus Nijhoff, 1983, pp 31–63

78. Saris SC, Bigner SH, Bigner DD: Intracerebral transplantation of a human glioma line in immunosuppressed rats. J Neurosurg 60:582–588, 1984

79. Shapiro JR, Shapiro WR: Clonal tumor cell heterogeneity. Prog Exp Tumor Res 27:49–66, 1984

80. Selby P, Buick RN, Tannock I: A critical appraisal of the "human tumor stem-cell assay." N Engl J Med 308:129–134, 1983

81. Kornblith PL, Smith BH, Leonard LA: Response of cultured human brain tumors to nitrosoureas. Cancer 48:255–265, 1981

82. Morgan D, Freshney RI, Darling JL, et al: Assay of anticancer drugs in tissue culture: Cell cultures of biopsies from human astrocytoma. Br J Cancer 47:205–214, 1983

83. Bogdahn U: Chemosensitivity of malignant human brain tumors. Preliminary results. J Neuro-Oncol 1:149–166, 1983

84. Rosenblum ML, Gerosa MA, Wilson CB, et al: Stem cell studies of human malignant brain tumors. Part 1: Development of the stem cell assay and its potential. J Neurosurg 58:170–176, 1983

85. Shapiro WR, Byrne TN: Chemotherapy of brain tumors—Basic concepts, in Walker MD (ed): Oncology of the Nervous System. Boston, Martinus Nijhoff, 1983, pp 65–100

86. Alberts DS, Salmon SE, Moon TE: Human tumor cloning: Drug sensitivity testing clinical correlations, in Ariel IM (ed): Progress in Clinical Cancer (vol VIII). Orlando, Fla, Grune & Stratton, 1982, pp 147–179

Chemotherapy of Brain Tumors: Physiological and Pharmacokinetic Considerations

Ronald G. Blasberg and Dennis R. Groothuis

THE IMPACT of chemotherapy on the treatment of malignant brain tumors has been disappointing, despite 30 years of trials with different drugs, regimens, and routes of administration. Normally, the blood-brain barrier (BBB) regulates the rate that different compounds in the blood cross the capillaries and enter the brain parenchyma.[1] In brain tumors a similar capillary barrier, here called the blood-tumor barrier (BTB), is almost universally recognized as one major factor impeding successful chemotherapy. However, the extent to which the BTB limits chemotherapeutic drugs from reaching brain tumor cells and the overall effect of the BTB on the exposure of tumor cells to specific drugs are still not fully understood. This review outlines the history of the blood-tumor barrier, describes our current yet fragmentary understanding of the BTB, introduces simple pharmacokinetic modeling of brain tumor-drug exposure using data obtainable in individual patients, and discusses some directions for research efforts that seem promising in the next few years.

THE BLOOD-TUMOR BARRIER

Our understanding of the BTB is intimately related to our understanding of the normal BBB. Physiological and anatomic studies of the normal BBB date back to the turn of the century.[1] More recently Rall and Zubrod listed the drug characteristics that most favored passage across the normal BBB in a 1962 review; these included high lipid solubility, low extent of ionization, and lack of protein binding.[2] Also in the 1960s, electron microscopic (EM) studies established firmly that the functional basis of the normal BBB was related to the structure of the capillary endothelial cells and the interendothelial junctions.[3] At the present time the behavior of the normal BBB is fairly well understood[1,4] although much remains to be learned about local variations as well as its behavior in pathological conditions.

Neuropathologists have long recognized that malignant brain tumors, especially glioblastoma multiforme, typically have blood vessels that are abnormal both in appearance and quantity.[5] With the advent of cerebral arteriography, the characteristic "blush" of the abnormal brain tumor vessels was quickly recognized.[6] In 1952 Moore summarized research on the BTB up to that time, including his own experiments in animals and patients with brain tumors using the in vivo uptake of vital dyes, fluorescein, and radiolabeled markers, and he acknowledged that the structural basis of the BBB was not understood.[7] Although early EM studies indicated that the vessels in brain tumors were abnormal, it was not until the work of Long in human brain tumors[8] and that of Brightman, Vick, and Bigner in experimental brain tumors[9,10] that the extent of these abnormalities was realized. In addition to changes in capillary wall thickness, surface projections, and basement membrane, these investigators found increased numbers of pinocytotic vesicles, fensestrations, and endothelial gaps or defects. Long also reported open interendothelial cell junctions.[8] Similar changes have now been described in a wide spectrum of human and experimental brain tumors,[11-13] although the existence of endothelial cell gaps and open interendothelial cell junctions[11,13] and the functional significance of pinocytotic vesicles[14] and fenestrations remain controversial. Few studies have attempted to quantitate the frequency of the endothelial abnormalities or to correlate the structural and functional changes of brain tumor capillaries.[15] At the present time we do not know the prevalence of the endothelial abnormalities, the local distribution of these changes within a tumor, or which of the changes is primarily responsible for the increases in permeability of the BTB.

From the Nuclear Medicine Department, National Institutes of Health, Bethesda, Md, and the Department of Neurology, Northwestern University, Evanston University, Evanston Hospital, Evanston, Ill.

Dr Groothuis is a recipient of an NIH Research Career Development award and NIH Grant NS12745.

Address reprint requests to Ronald G. Blasberg, MD, Nuclear Medicine Department, Clinical Center, Bldg 10, Rm 1C401, National Institutes of Health, Bethesda, MD 20205.

0093-7754/86/1301-0008$00.00/0

Although the advent of cerebral arteriography and radionuclide brain scanning demonstrated that there were qualitative differences between the normal BBB and the BTB, these changes were not expressed in usable quantitative terms that could help the clinician administer water-soluble chemotherapeutic drugs to brain tumor patients on a more rational basis. In fact, the review of Rall and Zubrod[2] was often quoted as a basis to support the widespread use of lipid-soluble chemotherapeutic agents, such as the nitrosoureas, for the treatment of malignant brain tumors during the 1960s and 1970s. This approach largely neglected the qualitative information that blood-to-tissue transport (permeability in the broad sense) was increased in brain tumors.

During the 1970s quantitative investigations of BTB permeability were initiated, particularly by Levin and co-workers.[16,17] These investigators demonstrated that BTB permeability to water-soluble radiolabeled compounds was increased over normal brain, although the increase was modest. They also noted in the region of brain around tumor that the permeability of the capillaries decreased to values similar to those of the normal BBB.[16] In the late 1970s and early 1980s we began using quantitative autoradiographic (QAR) techniques[18] to measure local blood flow and blood-to-tissue transport in a variety of brain tumor models.[19-31] The advantage of QAR as a technique to measure tissue radioactivity is that measurements can be made in very small tissue regions, 50 × 50 × 20 μm, representing the volume of 100 to 200 cells. Double-label techniques can also be used to obtain concurrent measurements of more than one physiological variable.[32] The ability to define and measure the local distribution of isotopically labeled compounds by QAR can be enhanced by the application of modern image processing techniques and this results in even more precise correlation between histologic features and the physiological parameter being measured.[18,32]

A summary of our blood flow and blood-to-tissue transport studies in seven different experimental brain tumors is shown in Table 1. The average of the mean tumor values presented in the table obscures the wide range of values in different tumors. The range of the individual mean tumor values is indicated by the standard deviation of the average value (Table 1), and the range of variation within an individual tumor is illustrated in Fig 1. These studies have demonstrated that (1) the mean blood flow (F) to most intracerebral tumors does not vary much from one tumor model to the next and is slightly higher than that to normal brain white matter; (2) blood flow within individual tumors varies considerably and is frequently lowest within central and necrotic tumor regions of medium and large size tumors; (3) local values of the blood-to-tissue transfer constant (K) of AIB (alpha aminiosobutyric acid, a water-soluble, small neutral amino acid) vary widely over a range of 1 to 100 times normal brain value; (4) values of K for AIB correlated poorly with tumor size, location, histological classification, or the presence or absence

Table 1. The Averaged Mean Values of Blood Flow (± SD), the Transfer Constant K for AIB (± SD), and the Overall Extraction Fraction Calculated From This Data (Eq. 2) for Several Different Brain Tumor Models in the Rat*

Normal Brain (Parietal Cortex)	Blood Flow (mL/g/min) 1.69			Transfer Constant (mL/g/min) 0.002			Extraction Fraction 0.0024
Tumor Model	N	Blood Flow	Multiple of Normal Cortex	N	Transfer Constant	Multiple of Normal Cortex	
ENU[19,20]	32	0.45 ± 0.20	0.27	28	0.003 ± 0.002	1.5	0.013
MSV[21]	16	0.64 ± 0.21	0.38	16	0.012 ± 0.008	6.0	0.038
WL-256[22,23]	23	0.56 ± 0.39	0.33	75	0.014 ± 0.018	7.0	0.050
RT-9[24,25]	18	0.60 ± 0.20	0.36	19	0.015 ± 0.018	7.5	0.050
ASV[26,27]	46	0.60 ± 0.34	0.36	37	0.030 ± 0.039	15.0	0.10
RG-2[28,29]	18	0.84 ± 0.34	0.50	23	0.037 ± 0.010	18.5	0.088
H-54[30]	13	0.52 ± 0.18	0.31	13	0.058 ± 0.026	29.0	0.22

*At the top are shown typical values for blood flow, the transfer constant, and extraction fraction in normal brain. To fascilitate comparisons, the blood flow and transfer constant data for each of the tumor models are expressed as a multiple of that for normal cortex. Note that these averaged values do not convey the regional variation that can be seen within individual tumors (see Fig 1). The reference sources for the blood flow and transfer constant data are shown in parenthesis next to the tumor model.

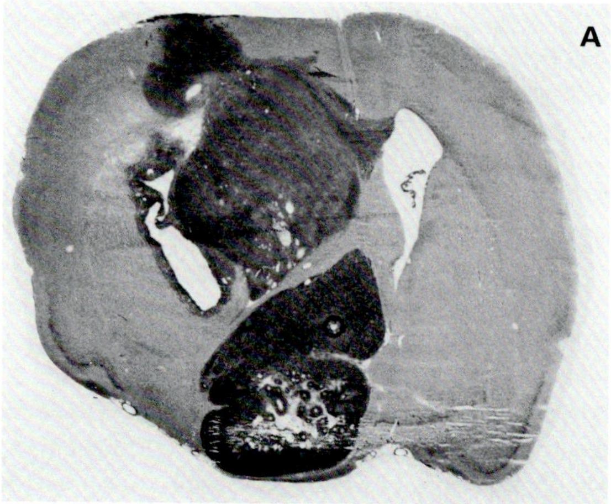
A

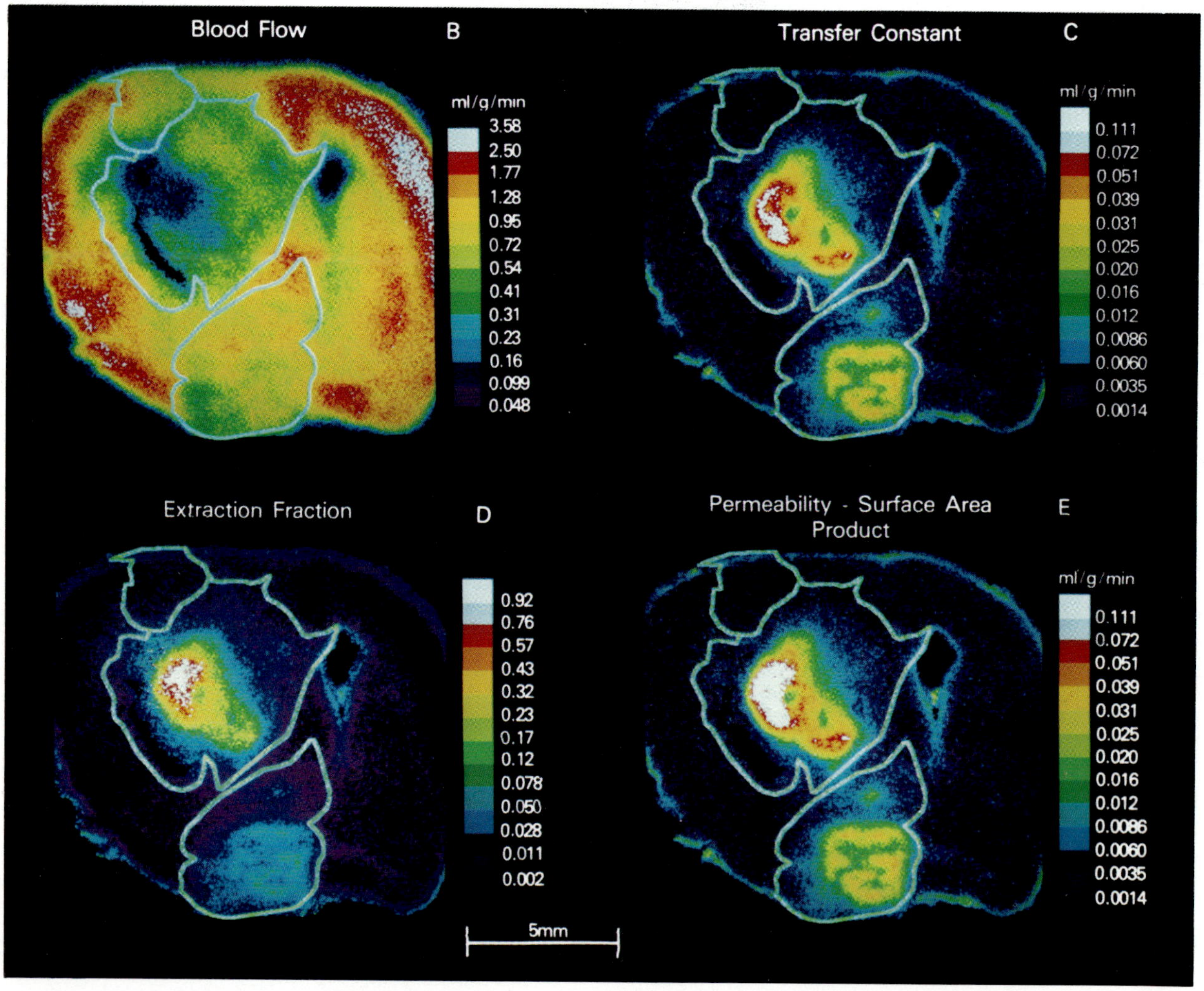
Blood Flow
B
ml/g/min
3.58
2.50
1.77
1.28
0.95
0.72
0.54
0.41
0.31
0.23
0.16
0.099
0.048
Transfer Constant
C
ml/g/min
0.111
0.072
0.051
0.039
0.031
0.025
0.020
0.016
0.012
0.0086
0.0060
0.0035
0.0014
Extraction Fraction
D
0.92
0.76
0.57
0.43
0.32
0.23
0.17
0.12
0.078
0.050
0.028
0.011
0.002
Permeability - Surface Area Product
E
ml/g/min
0.111
0.072
0.051
0.039
0.031
0.025
0.020
0.016
0.012
0.0086
0.0060
0.0035
0.0014
5mm

of necrosis, but do correlate with tumor invasion into choroid plexus and meninges; and (5) despite the comparatively high K and low F values within many of these tumors, an appreciable BTB is present. The latter point is seen more clearly by the mean tumor extraction fractions of AIB estimated from these F and K studies; average values equal to or less than 0.1 were calculated for all but one of the tumor models (Table 1). Thus, the permeability and surface area of tumor capillaries rather than blood flow will determine the rate of delivery of most water-soluble drugs to the cells of the experimental tumors we have studied.

These aforementioned studies were all performed in experimental brain tumors in rats. The question naturally arises about the applicability of these results to human brain tumors. From purely a qualitative point of view, one would expect a similar situation in human brain tumors since the appearance of a tumor on a contrast-enhanced CT scan can vary from one of no visible enhancement to very marked enhancement.[33] Furthermore, even the aggressively malignant glioblastoma multiforme can sometimes lack contrast enhancement on CT.[34] It is only within the past few years that methods have been developed to permit quantitative measurement of physiological parameters in human brain tumors.

Quantitative measurements of blood flow in malignant brain tumors in humans have generally corroborated our observations in experimental brain tumors—mean tumor blood flow values are similar to those in normal tumor free white matter.[35] Quantitative measurements of the rate of blood-to-tissue transport in human brain tumors have been reported in a preliminary fashion only, but they too mirror our earlier observations in the rat brain tumor models.[36–38] Methods have been developed to measure bidirectional capillary transfer constants of water-soluble, iodinated compounds with the CT scanner,[36] and of water-soluble positron-labeled compounds with the PET scanner.[37,38] Our preliminary data suggest that there is marked variability in the values of the transfer constants of water-soluble compounds, both regionally within a tumor and from tumor to tumor, similar to that seen in the experimental brain tumors.

There are several major differences between QAR and PET/CT measurements that must be kept in mind. The first is resolution: QAR is capable of detecting low energy radioisotope emissions with a spatial resolution of 50 to 100 microns; current PET techniques have a resolu-

Fig 1. Histological section of Avian Sarcoma Virus–induced tumors in rat brain (hematoxylin and eosin stain, Panel A) and reconstructed autoradiograhic images of blood flow (Panel B), blood-to-tissue transfer constants of alpha aminoisobutyric acid (AIB) (Panel C), tissue extraction fractions of AIB (Panel D), and permeability-surface area products of the tissue capillaries with respect to AIB (Panel E) of the brain section shown in Panel A.[32] Blood flow and the transport of AIB were measured concurrently using ^{131}I-iodoantipyrine, ^{14}C-AIB and double-label quantitative autoradiography.[32] The images of extraction fraction and permeability-surface area product were derived from the primary images of F and K by a computer using an algorith expressed by equations 2 and 3b, respectively. The images in Panels B–E are color coded to a range of values. Blood flow, the transfer constant, and the permeability-surface area product are expressed in units of mL/g/min; the extraction fraction is without units. The smaller cortical tumor invading meninges is an anaplastic astrocytoma. It is adjacent and contiguous with, but morphologically distinct from, a large polymorphic astrocytoma in putamen that is compressing and obliterating the lateral ventricle medially. A large lateral cyst is present in this polymorphic astrocytoma. The central portion of this tumor contains focal regions of neovascularization that could be associated with remnants of choroid plexus; this area also has several regions containing many small cysts and foci of necrosis. The central portion of this tumor is composed of predominantly anaplastic and gemistocytic tumor cells, whereas the more peripheral dorsomedial region has a uniform cellular appearance with clearly identifiable pilocytic tumor cells and no necrosis or cyst formation. The lower tumor has obliterated the third ventricle; it is also a polymorphic astrocytoma with extensive neovascularization that could be an outgrowth from third ventricular choroid plexus. A large star-shaped area of cyst formation and central necrosis is seen in the ventral portion of this tumor. The cellular morphology of the ventral portion is predominantly anaplastic, whereas clearly identifiable pilocytic tumor cells are seen in the dorsal half of this astrocytoma. Note the following: (A) Blood flow values within the cortical and ventral (3rd ventricular) tumors are similar to that of surrounding brain tissues. The lowest flows were measured in a compact cellular zone of predominantly anaplastic cells adjacent to the large cyst in the central (putamen) tumor; there was little or no evidence of necrosis in this region. (B) The local transfer constants in the cortical tumor are similar to that in normal brain. In contrast, the values of K in the central tumor are variable; the highest values are seen in the same tissue area with the lowest blood flow and are about 100 times that in normal brain. A variable pattern of K is also seen in the ventral tumor; the highest values are associated with areas of neovascularization around areas of necrosis. (C) The permeability-surface area product image is almost a replicate of the transfer constant image except for those regions with relatively high values of K and/or low values of F. In these latter regions the PS products are appreciably greater than the values of K. (D) The extraction fraction image shows variability between the three tumors as well as within the central and ventral polymorphic astrocytomas. The highest extractions are seen in those tumor regions with high K and low F values.

tion of about 0.6 to 1.0 cm and CT techniques have a practical resolution of about 0.1 cm. QAR techniques allow precise correlation of the measured physiological parameter and the corresponding histology. However, the QAR and histological techniques require the sacrifice or sampling of the experimental subject, and the use of many animals to obtain a time course analysis of the isotope distribution. In addition, it is difficult to follow the time course of a pathologic process and its response to therapy using QAR. Since external detectors are used for both PET and CT, studies can be performed in humans and repeated or serial scans can be performed to obtain the distribution-time course of the isotope (or iodinated compound) in the same subject. In addition, sequential studies can be performed over long periods of time in order to follow the course of the disease and/or reponse to therapy in the same subject. In most instances PET or CT techniques do not permit correlation of the measured physiologic parameter with the corresponding pathology.

In view of the respective merits of these imaging techniques, both approaches should be developed and used together. QAR is useful for developing the basic experimental procedures, for studying fundamental biologic processes, and for gaining high spatial resolution and correlation with tissue morphology. PET and CT are useful for investigating and diagnosing human disease and for following the response of an individual patient to therapy. Based on our measurements of F and K in experimental rat brain tumors and our preliminary measurements of K in human brain tumors, we believe that there will be highly individual differences with regard to the degree of BTB alteration in brain tumors. It is likely that there will be over a 200-fold variation in the rate of blood-to-tissue transport of water-soluble compounds and drugs in different brain tumors.

PHARMACOKINETIC CONSIDERATIONS

Our discussion of pharmacokinetics and brain tumor chemotherapy covers two topics. The first relates to the properties of individual drugs and how these affect the rate of drug delivery and the overall exposure of the tumor to the drug. The second is the development of relatively simple pharmacokinetic principles that emphasize an operational approach to estimate the rate of drug delivery and exposure of the tumor, so that quantitative transport and pharmacokinetic data currently measurable in experimental animals and in patients can be used to develop an individualized approach to the chemotherapeutic treatment of brain tumors.

The delivery of systemically administered drugs to brain and brain tissue is influenced by the physiological characteristics of the blood-tissue system and the physiochemical properties of the drugs. For example, the amount of drug that passively diffuses across the BBB is determined by at least four factors[39]: (1) the permeability coefficient (P) of the capillaries with respect to the drug, (2) the luminal surface area (S) of the capillaries, (3) the activity or concentration of unbound drug in the plasma (C_p), and (4) the length of time (t) that the drug circulates through the capillaries. A fifth parameter, blood flow (F), becomes important in situations when the extraction of the drug is high[40] and will be discussed later.

Davson and Danielli first produced an expression that relates the rate at which a compound passively crosses a lipid (or biological) membrane to its physiochemical properties, particularly its lipid solubility and molecular weight.[41] Fenstermacher and Rapoport[42] have discussed this relationship in terms of the octanol/water partition coefficient (o/w):

$$PS = \gamma(o/w)/(\text{molecular weight})^{1/2}$$

Equation 1

where PS is the permeability-surface area product and γ is a proportionality constant. The $(\text{molecular weight})^{1/2}$ term reflects the effect of molecular size, namely diffusivity, on the value of P.

In Table 2 we show four chemotherapeutic drugs of a similar molecular size that are currently used in the treatment of malignant brain tumors, list their respective octanol/water partition cofficients, and estimate the values for the PS product across the BBB using Equation 1. These values indicate the extent to which passive trancapillary diffusion is affected by the physiochemical properties of the drugs.

Before we discuss the impact of individual drug properties on the delivery and the concentration of drug in brain tumors, it is important to

Table 2. Pharmacokinetic Parameters of Four Chemotherapeutic Drugs

Drug	Molecular Weight	log o/w	PS* (mL/g/min)	K* (mL/g/min)	Cl (mL/min/kg)	$T_{1/2}$ (min)	V_D (L/kg)
MTX[53]	454	−2.52	0.00014	0.00014	1.24 ± 0.48	124.8 ± 34.8	0.186 ± 0.062
5-FU[54]	130	−0.95	0.0098	0.0096	16.1 ± 6.5	12.6 ± 3.8	0.310 ± 0.19
AZQ[55]	364	0.50	0.166	0.145	12.2 ± 3.8	43.9 ± 10.2	0.764 ± 0.558
BCNU[56]	214	1.54	2.370	0.588	56.5 ± 56.2	21.5 ± 8.8	3.25 ± 1.60

Abbrev: MTX, methotrexate; 5-FU, 5-fluorouracil; AZQ, aziridinylbenzoquinone; BCNU, 1,3 bis(2-chloroethyl)-1-nitrosourea.

Shown for each drug are the molecular weight (Daltons), $\log_{10}$ of the octanol/water partition coefficient (log o/w), estimated permeability-surface area product (PS*) from the relationship shown in Equation 1 assuming $\gamma = 1$, blood-to-tissue transfer constant (K*) calculated from Equation 3b (see text), and the following pharmacokinetic parameters: Cl, total body clearance; $t_{1/2}$, beta plasma half-life; and V_D, volume of distribution in the steady state. Note that although these four chemotherapeutic drugs are not very different in molecular size, they have markedly different values of log o/w, PS*, K*, Cl, $t_{1/2}$, and V_D. The reference source for the pharmacokinetic data is shown in parentheses next to the drug.

understand the relationships between the above expressions and their influence on blood-to-tissue transport. These expressions have been discussed in detail elsewhere and will be reviewed only briefly here.[39,40] Capillary permeability (P) per se, is a functional characteristic of the capillary membrane(s) with respect to a particular solute and is measured in units of velocity (eg, cm/sec). The amount of blood-borne material that crosses the capillaries from blood into tissue is also dependent on the total surface area of the capillaries available for exchange per unit mass of tissue (S). The functional experession for capillary permeability in tissue where the capillary surface area may not be known is the permeability-surface area product (PS) and is measured in units of volume per unit mass of tissue per unit time (eg, mL/g/min). However, P or PS values cannot be measured directly by in vivo experiments. Experimental results from blood-to-tissue transport experiments are usually expressed in terms of a transfer constant (K) or an extraction fraction (E). The transfer constant is usually calculated from the results of multiple capillary passages of the test substance and can be considered a plasma clearance constant, with units of volume per unit mass per unit time (eg, mL/g/min). E is dimensionless and respresents the fraction of test substance removed from the blood in one capillary passage. Both K and E are expressions of *unidirectional* transfer across tissue capillaries and can be obtained from the appropriate experimental data. These two transfer expressions are related by

$$K = FV_fE \qquad \text{Equation 2}$$

where F is blood flow and V_f is the fractional volume of blood that serves as the source fluid for exchange across the capillaries.[40] Both E and V_f are dimensionless; K and F are defined by the same units. The PS of tissue capillaries can be calculated from E using the relationship derived by Renkin[43] and Crone[44] for a single capillary system:

$$PS = FV_f \ln (1 - E) \qquad \text{(Equation 3A)}$$

or from K[40]:

$$PS = FV_f \ln (1 - K/FV_f) \qquad \text{Equation 3B}$$

providing FV_f, the blood flow–exchangeable fraction product, is known. It is evident that both experimentally obtainable measures of blood-to-tissue transport, K and E, depend on blood flow and capillary permeability and that K will always be less than PS or FV_f. When the ratio of PS/FV_f is less than 0.1, K approaches PS in magnitude, and in this range blood-to-tissue transfer of a drug is mainly dependent on the PS value of the capillaries. When PS/FV_f is greater than 2.3, K approaches FV_f in value and under these conditions blood-to-tissue transfer is mainly dependent on the values of F and V_f. When PS/FV_f is between 0.1 and 2.3, changes in K or E can be caused by changes in any or all of the parameters F, V_f, P, or S.

Examples of these effects are shown in Table 2 where the value of K is calculated for each of the four drugs using the previously estimated PS* values (Table 2) and Equation 3B. For these calculations, a tumor F of 0.6 mL/g/min was assumed (Table 1). V_f was assumed to be 1.0 for the lipid-soluble drugs AZQ and BCNU, and 0.5 (the plasma fraction) for the water-soluble drugs MTX and 5-FU. The ratio of PS^*/FV_f for each drug is MTX, 0.0005; 5-FU, 0.03; AZQ, .28; and BCNU, 3.95. For MTX and 5-FU (where the PS^*/FV_f ratio is <0.1), the values of K^* closely approximate the PS^* values of the capillaries. For BCNU the PS^*/FV_f ratio is >2.3, and the value of K closely approximates blood flow, FV_f. For AZQ the PS^*/FV_f ratio is between 0.1 and 2.3, and blood-to-tissue transport can be expected to depend on any or all of the terms in the ratio.

So far we have limited the discussion to passive, unidirectional flux across the capillaries and the relationships between PS, FV_f, K, and E. The amount of drug available for exchange across the capillaries over time (A_0^T) is dependent on the blood concentration (C_b) and the FV_f product[22]:

$$A_0^T = FV_f \int_0^T C_b(t)dt \quad \text{Equation 4}$$

Similarly, the amount of drug that crosses the capillaries and enters the tumor parenchyma from the blood over time (B_0^T) is dependent on the plasma concentration of free drug (C_p) and the influx constant K[23]:

$$B_0^T = K \int_0^T C_p(t)dt \quad \text{Equation 5}$$

The time course of the blood or plasma concentration, expressed here as a concentration-time integral, is more commonly known as the C × T product or area under the curve (AUC). This term is the "driving force" for blood-to-tissue transport, and with knowledge of the influx constant K it is possible to calculate the amount of drug that enters the tumor parenchyma (Equation 5).

Once a drug enters the extracellular fluid of the tumor it can distribute within the parenchyma and it can be cleared from the system by (1) efflux back into the blood, (2) metabolism to other active or inactive products, or (3) transport (eg, convection or diffusion) into other tissue regions (eg, adjacent brain or CSF). Each of these clearance mechanisms is as important as influx with respect to the time course of drug concentration in the tumor and the overall exposure of the tumor cells to the drug (ie, the C × T product of the tumor).

We are currently using a comparatively simple two-compartment (blood and tissue) pharmacokinetic model to analyze the concentration time course and exposure of the tissue to drug circulating in the blood.[32] This model includes terms to account for drug efflux from tissue into blood (k_2) and for drug metabolism or inactivation in the tissue (k_3). The influx term K_1 is the same as K in the previous equations. The model is purposely kept simple for operational considerations and can be applied to human subjects since it is now possible to obtain measurements of K_1 and k_2 in vivo.[36-38] From standard pharmacokinetic studies it is possible to obtain data from which the rate of clearance of drug from the plasma can be calculated (the so-called beta half-life), and estimate the volume of distribution (V_D) in the steady-state and the rate at which the drug is cleared from the body (Cl). These values have been determined for MTX, 5-FU, AZQ, and BCNU, and they are included in Table 2.

By assuming first order diffusional transport kinetics, first order metabolism and inactivation kinetics and no binding of the drug to plasma constituents or intratissue movement (eg, diffusion), the concentration of parent drug in the tissue (Ci) is given by:

$$\frac{dCi}{dt} = K_1C_p - (k_2 + k_3)Ci \quad \text{Equation 6}$$

where C_p is the concentration of freely exchangeable active drug in plasma and k_3 is a tissue metabolism constant. K_1 has units of mL/g/min and is equivalent to K; k_2 and k_3 have units of reciprocal time.[32] The solution of Equation 6 is:

$$Ci(T) = K_1 \int_0^T C_p(t)e^{-(k_2+k_3)(T-t)}dt \quad \text{Equation 7}$$

This equation can be used to compute the relative drug concentration in tissue over time, and can be used for different values of K_1, k_3, and the equilibrium distribution volume, λ, of the drug in the tissue (where $\lambda = K_1/k_2$ in units of volume per unit mass of tissue), as well as different rates of plasma clearance.[32]

In Figs 2 and 3 we have computed relative changes in the tissue concentrations and tissue exposure that will result from changes in K_1 and k_3. To perform this modeling exercise we have made several assumptions. First, we modeled incremental changes in the PS product of tumor capillaries where ΔPS equals 0.001, 0.01, and 0.1 mL/g/min, respectively. It is assumed that these changes in the PS of tumor capillaries is *not* due

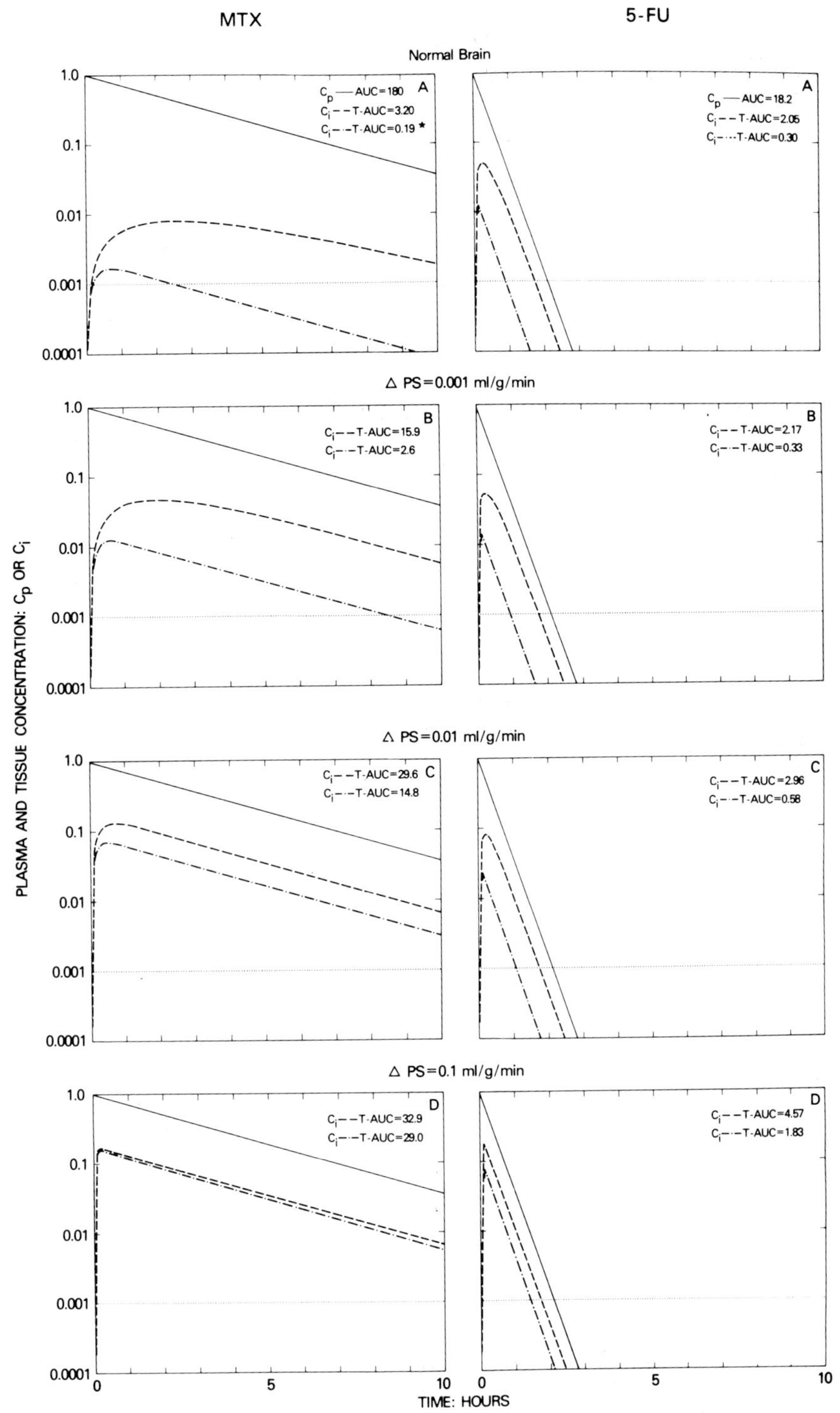

Fig 2. Time courses of MTX and 5-FU concentrations in plasma, C_p, and tissue, C_i, are shown for different increments in the PS of the tissue capillaries (ΔPS; panels A through D) and two different rates of drug metabolism or inactivation in the tissue. The plasma half-lives listed in Table 2 for MTX and 5-FU were used to calculate the time course of relative plasma concentration of the drugs, where $C_p(t) = \alpha \exp(-\beta t)$, α is a unit amount of drug/mL plasma and $\beta = \ln 2/t_{1/2}$, where $t_{1/2}$ = plasma half-life of the drug. This relationship assumes a single exponential plasma clearance of the drug and was used for simplicity; it is also possible to model a more complex plasma clearance using the sum of exponentials. The time course of drug concentration in the tissue was calculated with Equation 7. The influx constant K_1 was calculated from (PS + ΔPS) and the appropriate FV_f value using Equation 3b (see text). The efflux constant k_2 is given by the ratio K_1/λ, where λ is the equilibrium distribution volume of the drug in the tumor. The value of λ was assumed to be the same as the distribution volume V_D (Table 2), except for BCNU (Fig 3) where a value of 0.6 mL/g was used.[56,57] Two rates of drug metabolism in the tumor were estimated from the whole-body distribution and clearance values listed in Table 2, where $k_3 = Cl/V_D$ (dash line) and $K_3 = 10 \cdot Cl/V_D$ (dash-dot-dash line). The tissue-drug exposure or T-AUC is equivalent to the tissue concentration time integral and was calculated for each graph. The units of AUC and T-AUC are amount/mL/min and amount/g/min, respectively. The concept of a "threshold concentration" below which a therapeutic or biological effect is not seen was also included in this exercise. A threshold of 3 log concentrations below the peak plasma concentration is indicated by the horizontal dotted line and was used in all the calculations of T-AUC. The presence of a * (MTX, panel A) indicates that T-AUC was approximately 50% of T-AUC$_\infty$ calculated by Equation 8. In all other cases T-AUC and T-AUC$_\infty$ differed by less than 10%.

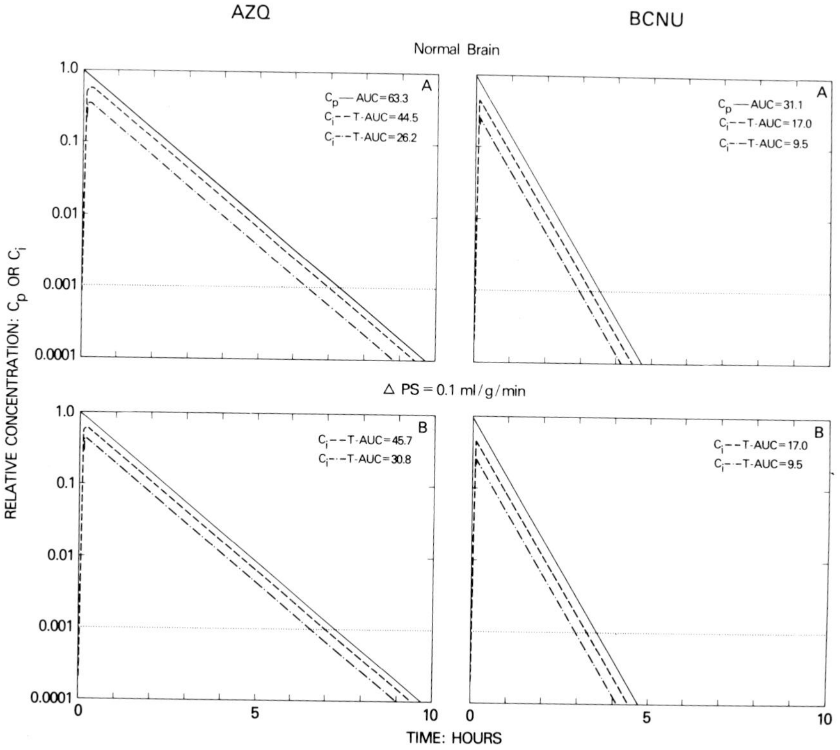

Fig 3. Time courses of AZQ and BCNU concentrations in plasma, C_p, and tissue, C_i, are shown for normal brain and one comparatively large increment in the PS of the tissue capillaries (Panels A and B, respectively). See the legend to Fig 2 for details.

to some general change in the lipid or structural composition of the endothelial cell membranes. Rather we assume that ΔPS of tumor capillaries is due to the presence of aqueous "holes" or "channels" in the BTB that are sufficiently large to avoid steric or sieving limitations due to solute size. Preliminary data comparing aqueous diffusion constants and influx constants of small and large molecules in two experimental tumors support this hypothesis (unpublished observations). In addition, the above increases in the PS product of tumor capillaries (compared to brain capillaries) are reasonable values based on our experimental data in rats (Table 1) and from preliminary studies in humans.[37]

Second, two values were used for k_3; one was equal to the drug concentration clearance constant for the whole body and the other was arbitrarily taken to be 10 times this value. Third, the relative tissue-drug "exposure" or area under the curve, tissue-AUC (T-AUC), was calculated assuming a "threshold concentration" below which a therapeutic or biological effect is not seen. Although this concept is commonly accepted in pharmacology, the modeling results it produces must be viewed with caution since they are specific for the threshold chosen. In the absence of a threshold and for infinite time T-AUC_∞ can be calculated directly from the rate constants by:

$$\text{T-AUC}_\infty = K_1/\beta(k_2 + k_3) \quad \text{Equation 8}$$

where β is the blood or plasma clearance constant with units of reciprocal time. Thus, the differences in both Ci(t) and T-AUC of the four drugs could be due to differences in β, K_1, k_2 (or K_1/λ), k_3 and the threshold concentration or to all of these terms. In the following discussion we will focus on the effects that changes in β, K_1, and k_3 will have on $C_i(t)$ and T-AUC.

The plasma concentration time course of a drug determines the driving force for influx into the tumor. In this modeling exercise the units of plasma concentration are unspecified and C_p has a maximum value of 1.0 U/mL at $t = 0$. A single exponential decline in C_p, based on the drug's plasma half-life, was used in the modeling and β was calculated from this value. The plasma half-lives of the four drugs listed in Table 2 varied from 12 to 124 minutes and AUC varied from 180 to 40 U/mL/min (Figs 2 and 3; Panel A). The value of AUC is directly proportional to the plasma half-life and will always be greater than T-AUC since these drugs are not concentrated in tumor tissue. Thus, the relative driving force for MTX flux across the BTB and BBB is 10-fold higher than that for 5-FU due to the difference in their rate of plasma clearance.

A comparison of MTX and 5-FU in Fig 2 illustrates several additional points. First, the effect of increasing capillary permeability (ΔPS) on Ci(t) and T-AUC is considerably greater for MTX than 5-FU (compare the progression from Panel A through Panel D for both drugs). This difference between MTX and 5-FU is due to the 70-fold difference in PS* on the capillaries of normal brain with respect to the two drugs (Table 2). For example, a small increase in capillary permeability of the tumor in comparison to normal brain (ΔPS of 0.001 mL/g/min) results in an 8-fold increase in the rate of drug delivery (the influx constant times the plasma concentration) for MTX and only a 1.1-fold increase for 5-FU in tumor compared to that in normal brain. For a larger increase in capillary permeability (ΔPS of 0.01 mL/g/min), a 72-fold increase in K_1 is calculated for MTX and only a two-fold increase in K_1 for 5-FU. The same effect is seen for AZQ and BCNU (Fig 3). For an appreciable increase in capillary permeability of the tumor in comparison to normal brain (ΔPS = 0.1 mL/g/min), only a 48% (AZQ) and 0.3% (BCNU) increase in the rate of delivery (at K_1) to the tumor compared to normal brain is obtained, respectively, with each drug. Correspondingly small increases in T-AUC are achieved with AZQ and BCNU under these conditions (Fig 3).

It is intuitively evident that increases in the permeability of tumor capillaries would not substantially increase the rate of flux across the BTB of drugs that cross normal brain capillaries rapidly (eg, $PS/FV_f > 1$). Under these conditions, the rate of flux across the tumor capillaries is determined more by blood flow (FV_f) than the permeability and surface area of the capillaries. This is clearly seen with BCNU (Table 2). Although the estimated PS* value for normal brain capillaries is 2.4 mL/g/min for BCNU, the calculated value of K* is 0.59 mL/g/min and approximates the value for blood flow (FV_f) that was used in the calculation (0.6 mL/g/min; Equation 4). The second point is that tissue metabolism and inactivation have a variable effect on Ci(t) and T-AUC. It can be readily seen from Equation 8 that the effect of metabolism will be large when $k_3 \gg k_2$ and the effect will be small when $k_3 \ll k_2$. Since $k_2 = k_1/\lambda$, it is conceptually simpler to compare k_3 with K_1/λ. This is because the equilibrium distribution volume of a particular drug in the tissue or λ is not likely to vary substantially in different tumors, whereas K_1 can vary widely (Table 1 and Fig 1). Thus, the effect of k_3 on $C_i(t)$ and T-AUC is more likely to be related to changes in K_1 than to changes in λ. This effect is seen in the graphs of Fig. 2. The difference in C_i and T-AUC values for two different rates of metabolism in the tissue (indicated by the dash and dash-dot-dash curves) is largest in Panel A where K_1 is low. In contrast, the same 10-fold difference in tissue metabolism has only a small effect on $C_i(t)$ and T-AUC in Panel D where K_1 is comparatively high. For high PS/FV_f ratios (eg, BCNU) the value of K_1 will approach a maximum value (FV_f) and the values of $C_i(t)$ and T-AUC will depend primarily on the relationship between FV_f and k_3 (Fig 3, BCNU).

A third point not illustrated in the Figures is implicit in Equation 8. For low rates of drug metabolism in the tissue relative to the rate of drug efflux (or K_1/λ), the effects of increasing capillary permeability or blood flow on tumor exposure to the drug is small. Assuming $k_3 \ll k_2$, Equation 8 can be rearranged and reduces to:

$$\text{T-AUC}_\infty = \lambda/\beta \quad \text{Equation 9}$$

Although the maximum value of $C_i(t)$ may differ substantially under these conditions (Equation 7), T-AUC_∞ will be the same for different values of K_1 and, thus, independent of capillary permeability and blood flow.

This condition can be restated in the following manner. For high values of influx, efflux will also be high and in direct proportion to influx since $K_1/k_2 = \lambda$. For lower values of influx, efflux will be correspondingly lower but the tissue exposure will be same (Equation 9). Thus, the BTB and blood flow will have a comparatively small effect on the exposure of the tumor to drugs that are slowly inactivated in the tissue providing $k_3 < K_1/\lambda$. This is an example of the "fast in—fast out" and "slow in—slow out" phenomena.

The corollary to the above discussion is that influx *does* have a direct effect on the tumor exposure to drugs that are rapidly inactivated in the tissue. By assuming $k_3 \gg k_2$, Equation 8 simply reduces to:

$$\text{T-AUC}_\infty = K_1/\beta k_3 \quad \text{Equation 10}$$

Thus, the BTB and/or blood flow can be expected to have an important effect on the exposure of brain tumors to water-soluble drugs that are rapidly inactivated in the tissue (eg, nitrogen-mustardlike alkylating drugs).

This exercise illustrates how several physiological and pharmacokinetic parameters can be combined into a relatively simple operational model that can predict the rate of drug delivery and total exposure of the tumor to the drug. This approach can be used to advantage in patients with brain tumors in the selection and evaluation of specific chemotherapeutic protocols. For example, if K_1 and k_2 of a water-soluble test-marker are known for a particular brain tumor or tumor region and reasonable estimates of β and k_3 of the drug can be made, it may be possible to individualize the selection of patients for treatment with some water-solbule drugs. It should be emphasized that in performing this type of modeling exercise we are talking about relative advantages. Other very important parameters, such as tumor cell chemosensitivity and systemic toxicity, must be considered and included in the selection, dose, and administration schedule of drugs for individualized chemotherapy of brain tumors.

FUTURE DIRECTIONS

In this review we have summarized the history of the BTB and indicated that most recent efforts in the chemotherapy of brain tumors have concentrated on lipid-soluble chemotherapeutic drugs. This has occurred despite qualitative knowledge that the BTB has increased permeability to water-soluble compounds compared to the normal BBB. We have summarized our quantitative autoradiographic data in experimental rat brain tumors. These results indicate that blood flow is generally comparable to that of normal brain white matter, but that the rate of blood-to-tissue transport can vary markedly from one tumor to the next and, in most cases, is the rate-limiting transport step in the delivery of water-soluble drugs to the tumor parenchyma. Preliminary measurements of blood-to-tissue transport indicates that a similar situation probably exists in human brain tumors. We have also shown how pharmacokinetic modeling can be used to identify those situations (ie, patients and drugs) in which the transport of drugs across the BTB is *not* a major limiting condition for tumor exposure and a chemotherapeutic response could be expected from the predicted tumor-drug exposure.

The technology now exists to answer some of the many puzzling questions concerning the role of the BTB in regulating drug delivery to human brain tumors. In the next few years the following topics of investigation will be persued. First, in vivo studies in human brain tumor patients will be necessary to define the magnitude of the variability in the rate of blood-to-tissue transport and blood flow in the tumors, and longitudinal studies can be used to define the effects of therapy (eg, corticosteroids) on these and other physiological and biochemical measurements in individual patients. Second, experimental methods to increase drug delivery, either by increasing blood flow (for lipid soluble drugs) or capillary permeability (for water soluble drugs), should continue to be tested in experimental animals to define those situations where they are most useful.[45,46] Third a continued search for new and more effective drugs must be persued. Pharmacokinetic modeling has indicated that water-soluble drugs with very low rates of tissue inactivation and long plasma half-lives would be advantageous in the systemic treatment of brain tumors,[32] whereas lipid-soluble drugs that cross tumor capillarics readily and are rapidly cleared from the body would be advantageous for intra-arterial chemotherapy of brain tumors.[47,48] Fourth, concomitant with BBB and BTB disruption studies and the development of new drugs, the potential for neurotoxicity must be evaluated.[49] Fifth, new techniques, such as HPLC, can be used in experimental brain tumors to quantitatively define transcapillary transport values and tumor metabolism rate constants of the different drugs that are likely to be used in brain tumor chemotherapy. Sixth, other methods of "drug" delivery, such as monoclonal antibodies, should be carefully explored for both diagnostic and therapeutic potential.[50] Seventh, careful correlative studies can help define which of the ultrastructural abnormalities that have been seen in brain tumors are most responsible for increased capillary permeability. This knowledge could be used to design drug delivery methods that are directed toward a known defect. Lastly, since variability or heterogeneity are likely to remain the catch words in the biologic behavior of malignant brain tumors, continued emphasis should be placed on the development of operational and testable pharmacokinetic models of drug delivery to brain tumors.[51,52]

ACKNOWLEDGMENT

We wish to thank Peter Molnar, Marc Horowitz, and Francine Vriesendorp for their assistance in the experiments summarized in this paper. We also wish to thank Clifford Patlak, Nicholas Vick, and Joseph Fenstermacher for their support and guidance and Mrs Beverly Sisco and Ms Gina Kelsh for excellent secretarial assistance.

REFERENCES

1. Bradbury M: The Concept of a Blood-Brain Barrier. New York, Wiley, 1979

2. Rall DP, Zubrod CG: Mechanisms of drug absorption and excretion: Passage of drugs in and out of the central nervous system. Ann Rev Pharmacol 2:109–128, 1962

3. Reese TS, Karnovsky MJ: Fine structural localization of a blood-brain barrier to exogenous peroxidase. J Cell Biol 37:207–217, 1967

4. Rapoport SI: Blood-brain Barrier in Physiology and Medicine. New York, Raven, 1976

5. Russell DC, Rubenstein LJ: Pathology of Tumors of the Nervous System (4th ed). Baltimore, Williams and Wilkins, 1977

6. Moniz E: L'Angiographie Cerebrale. Paris, Masson and Co, 1934

7. Moore GE: Diagnosis and localization of brain tumors: A clinical and experimental study employing fluorescent and radioactive tracer methods. Springfield, Ill, Charles C Thomas, 1953

8. Long DM: Capillary ultrastructure and the blood brain barrier in human malignant brain tumors. J Neurosurg 32:127–144, 1970

9. Brightman MW, Reese TS, Vick NA, et al: A mechanism underlying the lack of a blood-brain barrier to peroxidase in virally incuded brain tumors. J Neuropath Exp Neurol 30:139, 1971

10. Vick NA, Bigner DD: Microvascular abnormalities in virally induced canine brain tumors: Structural bases for altered blood-brain barrier function. J Neurol Sci 17:29–39, 1972

11. Hirano A, Matsui T: Vascular structures in brain tumors. Hum Path 6:611–621, 1975

12. Waggener JD, Beggs JL: Vasculature of neural neoplasms. Adv Neurology 15:27–49, 1976

13. Vick NA: Brain tumor microvasculature, in Weiss L, Gilbert HA, Posner JB (eds): Brain Metastasis. Boston, GK Hall, 1980, pp 115–133

14. Bundgaard H, Frokjaer-Jensen J, Crone C: Endothelial plasmalemmal vesicles as elements in a system of branching invaginations from the cell surface. Proc Natl Acad Sci 76:6439–6442, 1979

15. Bar-Sella P, Front D, Hardoff R, et al: Ultrastructural basis for different pertechnetate uptake patterns by various human brain tumors. J Neurol Neurosurg Psych 42:924–930, 1979

16. Levin VA, Freeman MA, Landahl HD: The permeability characteristics of brain adjacent to intracerebral rat tumors. Arch Neurol 32:785–791, 1975

17. Levin VA, Landahl HD, Freeman-Dove MA: The application of brain capillary permeability coefficient measurements to pathological conditions and the selection of agents which cross the blood-brain barrier. J Pharmacokin Biopharmaceut 4:499–519, 1976

18. Blasberg RG, Groothuis DR, Molnar P: Application of quantitative autoradiographic measurements in experimental brain tumors. Sem Neurol 1:203–221, 1981

19. Blasberg RG, Kobayashi T, Horowitz M, et al: Regional blood flow in ethylnitrosourea (ENU)-induced brain tumors. Ann Neurol 14:189–201, 1983

20. Blasberg RG, Kobayashi T, Horowitz M, et al: Regional blood-to-tissue transport in ethylnitrosourea (ENU)-induced brain tumors. Ann Neurol 14:202–215, 1983

21. Vriesendorp FJ, Groothuis DR, Vick NA: Murine sarcoma virus induced brain tumors: Concurrent measurements of blood flow and blood-to-tissue transport. J Neuro-Oncol 2:301–314, 1984

22. Blasberg RG, Shapiro WR, Molnar P, et al: Local blood flow in Walker 256 metastatic brain tumors. J Neuro-Oncol 2:195–204, 1984

23. Blasberg RG, Shapiro WR, Molnar P, et al: Local blood-to-tissue transport in Walker 256 metastatic brain tumors. J Neuro-Oncol 2:205–218, 1984

24. Blasberg RG, Molnar P, Horowitz M, et al: Regional blood flow in RT-9 brain tumors. J Neurosurg 58:863–873, 1983

25. Molnar P, Blasberg RG, Horowitz M, et al: Regional blood-to-tissue transport in RT-9 brain tumors. J Neurosurg 58:874–884, 1983

26. Groothuis D, Blasberg RG, Molnar P, et al: Regional blood flow in avian sarcoma virus (ASV)-induced brain tumors. Neurology (Cleveland) 33:686–696, 1983

27. Molnar P, Blasberg RG, Groothuis D, et al: Regional blood-to-tissue transport in avian sarcoma virus (ASV)-induced brain tumors. Neurology (Cleveland) 33:702–711, 1983

28. Groothuis DR, Fisher JM, Pasternak JF, et al: Regional measurement of blood flow in experimental RG-2 rat gliomas. Cancer Res 43:3362–3367, 1983

29. Groothuis DR, Fisher JM, Pasternak JF, et al: Regional measurements of blood-to-tissue transport in experimental RG-2 rat gliomas. Cancer Res 43:3368–3373, 1983

30. Vriesendorp FJ, Peagram C, Bigner DD, et al: Concurrent measurements of blood flow and transcapillary transport in xenotransplanted human gliomas in immune suppressed rats. J Natl Cancer Inst (in press)

31. Groothuis DR, Molnar P, Blasberg RG: Regional blood flow and blood-to-tissue transport in five brain tumor models: Implications for chemotherapy, in Rosenblum M, Wilson C (eds): Progress in Experimental Tumor Research (vol 27): Brain Tumor Biology. Basel, S. Karger, 1984, pp 132–153

32. Blasberg RG, Molnar P, Groothuis DR, et al: Concurrent measurements of blood flow and transcapillary transport in ASV-induced brain tumors: Implication for chemotherapy. J Pharm Exp Ther 231:724–735, 1984

33. Norman D, Stevens EA, Wing SD, et al: Quantitative aspects of contrast enhancement in cranial computed tomography. Radiol 129:683–688, 1978

34. Steinhoff H, Grumme T, Kazner E, et al: Axial transverse computed tomography in 73 glioblastomas. Acta Neurochir 42:45–56, 1978

35. Ito M, Lammertsma AA, Wise RJS, et al: Measurement of regional cerebral blood flow and oxygen utilization in patients with cerebral tumours using ^{15}O and positron emission tomography: Analytical techniques and preliminary results. Neuroradiol 23:63–74, 1982

36. Groothuis DR, Vriesendorp FV: Michael M, et al: Quantitative measurement of brain tumor capillary permeability by CT: Application of canine gliomas and implications for use in patients. Neurology 34:185–186, 1984 (suppl)

37. Hawkins RA, Phelps ME, Huang SC, et al: Simultaneous estimations of blood brain barrier (BBB) permeability and local cerebral blood volume (CBV) in human brain tumors with positron emission tomography and Ga-68 EDTA. J Nucl Med 25:9, 1984 (abstr)

38. Blasberg RG, Wright DC, Patlak CS, et al: Determination of regional blood-tissue transfer constants and initial (plasma) volume in brain and brain tumors using ^{68}Ga-EDTA and dynamic positron emission tomography. J Nucl Med 25:51, 1984 (abstr)

39. Blasberg RG: Pharmacokinetics and metastatic brain tumor chemotherapy, in Weiss L, Gilbert HA, Posner JB, et al (eds): Brain Metastasis. Boston, GK Hall, 1980, pp 146–164

40. Fenstermacher JD, Blasberg RG, Patlak CS: Methods for quantifying the transport of drugs across brain barrier systems. Pharmacol Ther 14:217–248, 1981

41. Davson J, Danielli JF: The Permeability of Natural Membranes. Cambridge, Cambridge University Press, 1943

42. Fenstermacher JD, Rapoport SI: The blood-brain barrier, in Renkin EM, Michel CC (eds): Handbook of Physiology: The Cardiovascular System IV. Bethesda, American Psychological Society, 1984, pp 969–1000

43. Renkin EM: Transport of potassium-42 from blood to tissue in isolated mammalian skeletal muscle. Am J Physiol 197:1205–1210, 1959

44. Crone C: Permeability of capillaries in various organs as determined by use of the indicator diffusion method. Acta Physiol Scand 58:292–305, 1963

45. Neuwelt EA, Barnett PA, Bigner DD, et al: Effects of adrenal cortical steroids and osmotic blood-brain barrier opening on methotrexate delivery to gliomas in the rodent: The factor of the blood-brain barrier. Proc Natl Acad Sci 79:4420–4423, 1982

46. Nakagawa H, Groothuis D, Blasberg RG: The effect of graded hyperosmolal intracarotid infusions on drug delivery to experimental RG-2 rat gliomas. Neurology 34:1571–1581, 1984

47. Eckman WW, Patlak CS, Fenstermacher JD: A critical evaluation of the principals governing the advantaged of intra-arterial infusions. J Pharmacok Biopharm 2:257–285, 1974

48. Collins JM: Pharmacokinetic rational for intra-arterial therapy, in Howell SB, Nijhoff M (eds): Intra-arterial and Intracavity Chemotherapy. Boston, 1985

49. Neuwelt EA, Glasberg M, Frenkel E, et al: Neurotoxicity of chemotherapeutic agents after blood-brain barrier modification: Neuropathological studies. Ann Neurology 14:316–324, 1983

50. Rosen ST, Winter JN, Epstein AL: Application of monoclonal antibodies to tumor diagnosis and therapy. Ann Clin Lab Sc 13:173–184, 1983

51. Levin VA, Patlak CS, Landahl HD: Heuristic modeling of drug delivery to malignant brain tumors. J Pharmacokinet Biopharm 8:257–296, 1980

52. Collins JM, Dedrick RL: Pharmacokinetics of anticancer drugs, in Chabner BA (ed): Pharmacologic Principals of Cancer Treatment. Philadelphia, Saunders, 1982, pp 77–99

53. Breithaupt H, Kuenzlen E: Pharmacokinetics of methotrexate and 7-hydroxy-methotrexate following infusions of high-dose methotrexate. Cancer Treat Rep 66:1733–1741, 1982

54. Collins JM, Dedrick RL, King FG, et al: Nonlinear pharmacokinetic models for 5-fluorouracil in man: Intravenous and intraperitoneal routes. Clin Pharm Ther 28:235–246, 1980

55. Schold SC, Friedman HS, Bjornsson TD, et al: Treatment of patients with recurrent brain tumors with AZQ. Neurology 34:615–619, 1984

56. Levin VA, Hoffman W, Weinkam RJ: Pharmacokinetics of BCNU in man: A preliminary study of 20 patients. Cancer Treat Rep 62:1305–1312, 1978

57. Blasberg RG, Patlak CS, Fenstermacher JD: Intrathecal chemotherapy: Brain tissue profiles after ventriculocisternal perfusion. J Pharmacol Exp Ther 195:73–83, 1975

The Role of Positron Emission Tomography in the Study of Cerebral Tumors

David J. Brooks, Ronald P. Beaney, and David G. T. Thomas

POSITRON Emission Tomography (PET) provides a relatively noninvasive means of regionally determining concentrations of positron-emitting isotopes in tomographic slices of human brain.[1] Suitable positron-emitting isotopes include ^{15}O, ^{11}C, ^{18}F, ^{13}N, and $^{75/76}Br$. Many naturally occurring organic molecules and pharmacological agents can be tagged with these agents and their regional distribution in the brain mapped out. Although PET can be used as a simple imaging device, it has far greater potential as a means of studying regional cerebral blood flow, oxygen, glucose, and amino-acid metabolism, and the transport of substrates across the blood-brain barrier. In addition, it can potentially study brain tumor receptor densities and the binding of monoclonal antibodies to tumours. In practice the application of PET to brain tumor studies has fallen into two main groups—those studies where information about tumor and cerebral physiology has been obtained using tracer kinetic modelling, and those studies where PET has been used primarily as an imaging technique.

Table 1 shows the possible applications of PET to studies of cerebral tumor function and the positron-emitting tracers appropriate for these studies.

THE TECHNIQUE OF POSITRON EMISSION TOMOGRAPHY

In order to carry out a PET scan, a positron-emitting radionuclide tagged to a suitable substrate must be administered to the subject either intravenously—for example, ^{18}F-2-fluro-2-deoxy-glucose (^{18}FDG)—or via inhalation—for example, $^{15}O_2$. The tracer then becomes distributed about the brain and decays, emitting a positron. This positron travels approximately 2 to 3 millimeters before colliding with an electron, resulting in its annihilation. The annihiliation energy is emitted as two 511 keV energy gamma photons at 180° to each other. PET scanners consist of circular or hexagonal arrays of photomultiplier detectors (Fig 1) which detect the paired arrival of these two gamma rays as a "coincident event." Any random noncoincident gamma radiation, or any gamma radiation at an energy other than 511 keV, is ignored by the PET scanner. By counting the number of coincident events in a tomographic slice of brain while the detectors move linearly and rotate angularly, it is possible to reconstruct an image representing the true spatial distribution of radioactivity in the transaxial plane.[2,3] Commercial scanners are now being constructed with a full-width half-maximum (FWHM) resolution of 6 mm and an ability to collect data from seven axial tomographic slices simultaneously. In addition a prototype scanner is under construction with a FWHM resolution of 2 mm.[4] For a review of positron emission tomographic scanners a number of literature reports are available.[3,5–9]

The most important advantage of PET compared to single photon emission tomography (SPECT) is the ability to correct for loss of 511 keV signal due to tissue attenuation. So far the inability to correct for tissue attenuation of γ-radiation has meant that SPECT remains primarily a qualitative imaging technique. Before clinical data derived using PET can be interpreted however, the following factors must also be considered: (1) The resolution of current PET scanners in use is often less than the size of anatomical regions of brain being studied. As a result, adjacent tissue structures may contribute to the signal measured and partial volume effects become a problem.[10] (2) Adequate numbers of coincident events must be detected in a tomographic slice so that the coefficient of variation of the final quantity being measured, for example, oxygen extraction, is acceptably low.[11] (3) The method of correction for tissue attenuation of signal is critical. The most accurate corrections are measured corrections using an external ring

---

From the MRC Cyclotron Unit, Hammersmith Hospital, London, and the Institute of Neurology, National Hospital for Nervous Disease, London.

Address reprint requests to David J. Brooks, MD, MRC Cyclotron Unit, Hammersmith Hospital, Du Cane Rd, London W12 OHS.

0093–7754/86/1301–0009$05.00/0

Table 1. Position-Emitting Tracers and Their Application to the Measurement of Regional Cerebral Function

Application	Radionuclide	$t_{1/2}$	Labelled Tracers
Cerebral blood flow	^{15}O	2.07 min	$C^{15}O_2$, $H_2{}^{15}O$
	^{11}C	22.4 min	^{11}C-alcohols
	^{13}N	10 min	$^{13}NH_3$
Cerebral blood volume	^{15}O	2.07 min	$C^{15}O$
	^{11}C	22.4 min	^{11}CO
	^{68}Ga	68.3 min	^{68}Ga-transferrin, ^{68}Ga-EDTA
Cerebral oxygen utilization	^{15}O	2.07 min	$^{15}O_2$
Cerebral glucose utilization	^{18}F	110 min	(^{18}F)-2-fluoro-2-deoxyglucose
	^{11}C	22.4 min	^{11}C-2-deoxyglucose
			^{11}C-glucose
Amino acid uptake	^{11}C	22.4 min	^{11}C-methionine, leucine, valine
	^{13}N	10 min	^{13}N-aminoacids
Blood-brain-barrier	^{82}Rb	1.25 min	Rb^+Cl^-
function	^{68}Ga	68.3 min	^{68}Ga-EDTA
	^{11}C	22.4 min	^{11}C-3-0-methyl-glucose
			^{11}C-cycloleucine
			^{11}C-methyl-albumin
Cerebral pH	^{11}C	22.4 min	^{11}C-dimethyloxazolidinedione
			$^{11}CO_2$
Drug uptake	^{55}Co	18 h	^{55}Co-bleomycin
	^{11}C	22.4 min	^{11}C-BCNU
	^{13}N	10 min	^{13}N-BCNU
Receptor studies	^{11}C	22.4 min	^{11}C-methyl-spiperone
			^{11}C-bromocryptine
			^{11}C-R05-4864

of a positron emitter such as ^{68}Ge to carry out a 511 keV transmission scan of the subject.[12] Alternative approaches involve calculated attenuation corrections assuming the brain to be an elliptical structure.

TRACER MODELS

In order to derive estimates of tissue function from the distribution of administered tracers, kinetic models are necessary. Such models express tracer uptake in terms of regional cerebral blood flow, transport across the blood-brain barrier (BBB), and either tissue metabolic function or binding affinities of tissue receptors. Such models compare the delivery of tracer to the brain—measured ideally as an arterial plasma input curve, with regional cerebral tracer distribution. Arterial tracer plasma levels can be measured during the course of PET scanning by withdrawing blood samples via an indwelling radial artery cannula and well-counting. Tracer kinetic models broadly fall into two categories—steady state models and dynamic imaging.

Steady-state models are based on the principle that if short-lived positron emitters such as ^{15}O ($t_{1/2}$ 124 secs) or $^{82}Rb^+$ ($t_{1/2}$ 75 secs) are administered continuously at a constant level to a subject, a steady arterial plasma and cerebral level of the tracer results within five half-lives of the isotope concerned. The advantages of the steady-state approach are twofold: first, the equations relating cerebral tracer uptake to blood flow and tracer extraction are relatively simple and so results from different centers are directly comparable. Second, high spatial resolution in theory is possible as one can administer tracer until adequate numbers of coincident events have been obtained and so minimize statistical uncertainties. In practice, however, dosage considerations to the patient limit the amount of tracer that can be administered and hence decide signal-to-noise levels.

Disadvantages of the steady-state approach are, first, the poor temporal resolution and, second, the nonlinearity of the relationship between blood flow and tracer uptake. Dynamic studies, although the spatial resolution is lower, are ideally suited for intervention studies on cerebral function and for accurate measurement of blood flow in high flow regions. In addition, dynamic

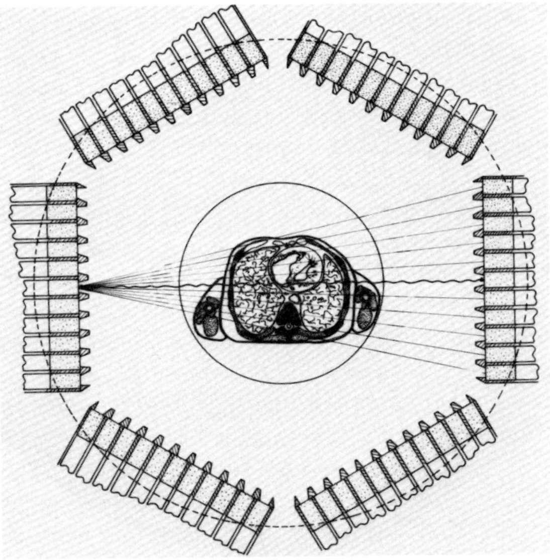

Fig 1. A diagramatic representation of PET scanning at the level of the heart and lungs.

studies can be carried out with all types of positron emitter whereas steady-state models are only useful for short-lived isotopes.

REGIONAL CEREBRAL BLOOD FLOW AND OXYGEN UTILIZATION

The tracer kinetic equations and the method for measuring regional cerebral blood flow (rCBF), oxygen utilization ($rCMRO_2$), and the regional oxygen extraction fraction (rOER) have been extensively documented elsewhere.[12] In this review the results we present are based on steady-state equations using the extended model described by Lammertsma et al[13] to correct for intravascular ^{15}O contributions to the regional cerebral tracer signal. In brief, the method entails sequential inhalation of $C^{15}O_2$ and then $^{15}O_2$, until steady levels of ^{15}O are obtained in arterial plasma and cerebral tissue. When $C^{15}O_2$ is inhaled, carbonic anhydrase in red blood cells rapidly transfers the ^{15}O radionuclide to $H_2{}^{15}O$,[14] and so the cerebral distribution of ^{15}O reflects regional cerebral blood flow. When $^{15}O_2$ is inhaled, the regional cerebral ^{15}O uptake reflects both the regional cerebral blood flow and the fraction of oxygen extracted from the arterial blood supplying the region (rOER). Such regional oxygen extraction is governed by the metabolic requirements of the cerebral tissue. By comparing the ratio of regional ^{15}O uptake during steady-state inhalation of $^{15}O_2$ and then $C^{15}O_2$, rOER values can be computed. Regional oxygen utilisation, $rCMRO_2$, is then derived using the equation:

$$rCMRO_2 = rCBF \times rOER \times \text{arterial oxygen content}$$

Regional cerebral blood volume, rCBV, is obtained by labelling red cells with ^{11}CO as detailed by Phelps et al.[15] The limitations and errors involved in the steady-state approach have been extensively detailed by Lammertsma et al.[11]

Figure 2 shows PET images of regional cerebral blood flow, oxygen extraction fraction, oxygen utilization, and cerebral blood volume, obtained using an E G & G Ortec ECAT II scanner with a FWHM resolution of 1.7 cm^5 for a normal subject. The images are at an axial tomographic level of OM + 6.5 cm (6.5 cm above the orbito-meatal line) and correspond to a peripheral ribbon of cortical grey matter surrounding central white matter in the centrum semiovale. Oxygen utilization by the peripheral cortical grey matter is roughly double that of

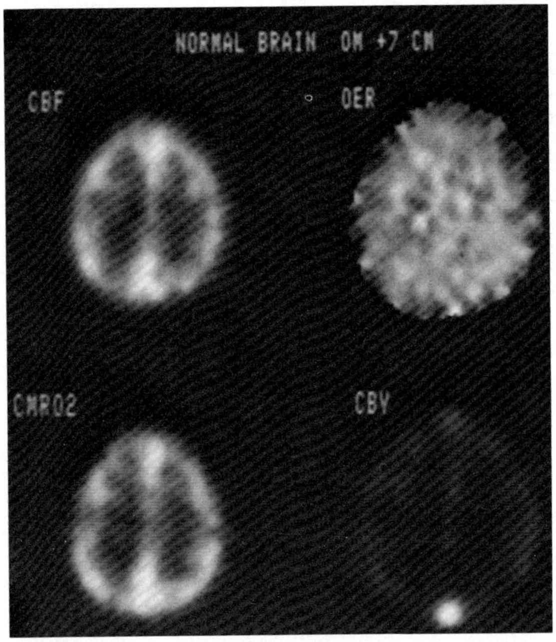

Fig 2. PET images of rCBF, rOER, $rCMRO_2$ and rCBV at OM + 6.5 cm for a normal subject.

Table 2. Mean Values of Regional Cerebral Function for a Group of 13 Normal Subjects*

	Peripheral Cortical Matter (mean ± SD)	Central White Matter (mean ± SD)
rCBF (mL/100 mL/min)	45 ± 10	27 ± 5
rOER	0.40 ± 0.06	0.38 ± 0.06
$rCMRO_2$ (mL O_2/100 mL/min)	3.2 ± 0.3	1.8 ± 0.2
rCBV (mL/100 mL)	4.1 ± 0.6	2.4 ± 0.8
Flow/vol (min^{-1})	11	11

Values apply to tissue at an axial level 6.5 cm above the orbitomeatal line.

central white matter. It can be seen that in normal brain, blood flow is closely coupled to oxygen utilization, grey matter again having double the blood flow of white matter. As a result of this coupling, regional oxygen extraction by normal cerebral tissue is fairly uniform, both grey and white matter extracting roughly 40% of the arterial oxygen supplied. Table 2 summarizes mean rCBF, rOER, $rCMRO_2$, and rCBV values for peripheral cortical grey and central white matter in a group of normal subjects at OM + 6.5 cm. Cerebral blood volume can also be seen to be coupled to blood flow and oxygen utilisation in normal cerebral tissue, the flow:volume (F/V) ratio lying close to 11 min^{-1} for both grey and white matter.

Figure 3A shows an enhanced CT scan image of a patient with a cerebral metastasis from the colon. Figure 3B shows the rCBF, rOER, $rCMRO_2$, and rCBV images at the corresponding axial tomographic level (OM + 8 cm). The tumor corresponds to regions of low rCBF, rOER, and $rCMRO_2$. In practice, blood flow in tumors is found to be highly variable and no longer coupled to blood volume. Low oxygen extraction fractions for tumors, however, are a consistent finding.[16] Table 3 summarizes data on tumor and edema function for a group of patients with cerebral primaries and secondaries. The finding of low rOER values for cerebral tumors is a somewhat surprising finding as tumor necrosis is thought to occur via tissue ischemia and infarction. Such a finding suggests that tumors in fact have a more than adequate oxygen supply for their metabolic needs. It should be pointed out, however, that while on a macroscopic scale tumor hypoxia is never evident in PET studies, one cannot exclude the presence of microscopic regions of tumor hypoxia below the resolution of the scanner.

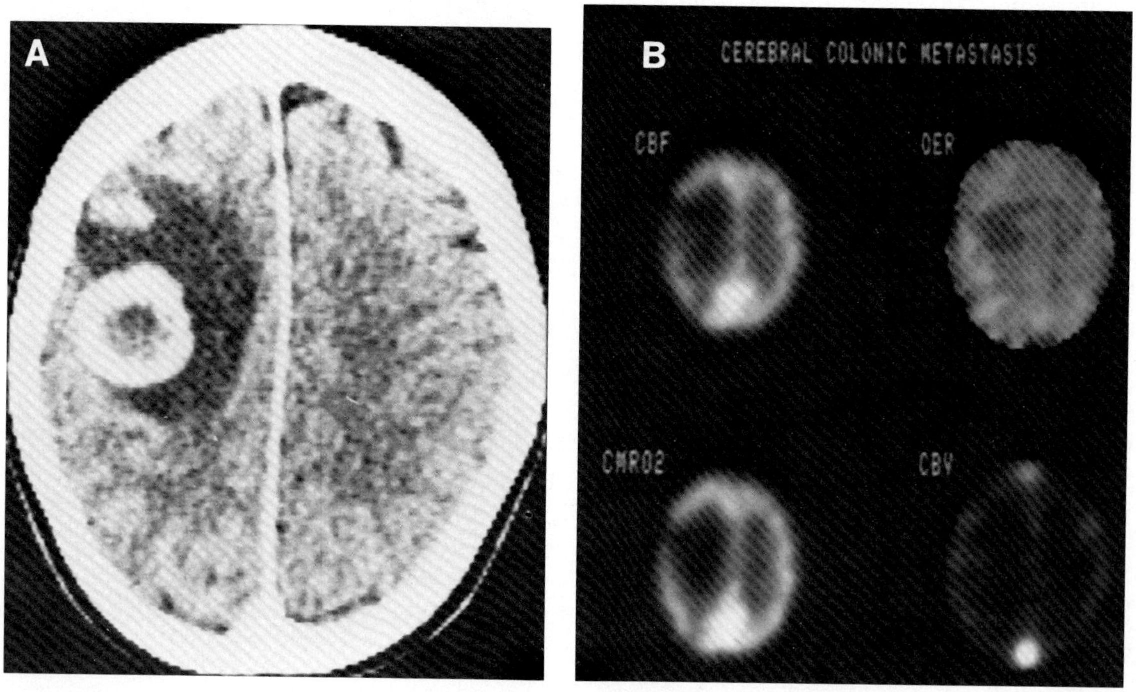

Fig 3. (A) An enhanced CT brain scan of a patient with a cerebral metastasis from the colon. (B) Corresponding PET images at OM + 8 cm of rCBF, rOER, $rCMRO_2$, and rCBV for the patient in Fig 3A.

Table 3. Mean Values of Tumor and Edema Function in Patients With Cerebral Tumors

	Primary Tumors (8) (mean ± SD)	Cerebral Metastases (6) (mean ± SD)	Edema (11) (mean ± SD)
rCBF (mL/100 mL/min)	35 ± 35	18 ± 13	16 ± 6
rOER	0.15 ± 0.10	0.24 ± 0.14	0.44 ± 0.09
$rCMRO_2$ (mL O_2/100 mL/min)	1.0 ± 1.0	0.9 ± 0.6	1.3 ± 0.3
rCBV (mL/100 mL)	4.1 ± 2.3	2.8 ± 2.5	2.2 ± 0.8

Regions of peripheral tumor edema characteristically show a coupled reduction in oxygen utilization and blood flow compared to equivalent regions of contralateral brain tissue. Oxygen extraction fractions in such regions of peripheral edema are generally normal, however, and there is no evidence that tissue ischemia due to locally raised intracranial pressure occurs.

In a study where the oxygen metabolism of the contralateral cortical tissue of tumor patients was studied,[17] it was demonstrated that such cortical tissue had a significantly depressed oxygen utilization and blood flow compared to a group of aged-matched normal control subjects. This depression in cortical function by the tumors was partially reversed following excision biopsy via craniotomy. Patients with acute obstructive hydrocephalus due to posterior fossa tumors have also been studied. Table 4 shows data on cortical function for a group of such patients before and after decompression. Before surgery, compared to age-matched controls, cortical blood flow and oxygen utilization were depressed, probably as a consequence of the raised CSF pressure. Cortical blood volume, however, remained within normal limits, the micro circulation staying dilated in an attempt to maintain normal cortical blood flow. Cortical oxygen extraction was raised in order to try and maintain levels of cortical oxygen utilization in the face of the low blood flow. Two weeks after decompression a significant rise in cortical blood flow occurred but no significant change in cortical oxygen utilization.

Table 4. The Cortical Function of 5 Patients With Acute Obstructive Hydrocephalus Secondary to Cerebral Tumors Before and After Decompression

	Cortical Function	
	Presurgery (mean ± SD)	Postsurgery (mean ± SD)
rCBF (mL/100 mL/min)	27 ± 4	32 ± 4*
rOER	0.53 ± 0.07	0.49 ± 0.02
$rCMRO_2$ (mL O_2/100 mL/min)	2.6 ± 0.1	2.7 ± 0.4
rCBV (mL/100 mL)	4.0 ± 0.7	4.1 ± 0.6
F/V (min^{-1})	7	8

*$P < .01$.

Administration of dexamethasone has been observed acutely to depress both the blood flow and blood volume of contralateral cortical tissue of patients with brain tumors.[18] No consistent effect of dexamethasone on tumor or edema blood flow, or on cerebral metabolism in general was noted by these workers. They postulated that dexamethasone reduces intracranial pressure initially by causing a vasoconstriction, possibly by potentiating the action of catecholamines. This initial vasoconstruction, however, is unlikely to be responsible for the slower resolution of cerebral edema observed after dexamethasone administration.

The effects of radiotherapy on tumor and cerebral oxygen metabolism have also been studied.[19] Following treatment, tumors were found to show a progressive fall in oxygen utilization and blood flow. By contrast blood flow in contralateral brain tissue rose acutely following treatment, suggesting a reactive vasodilation had occurred, and then gradually fell below pretreatment levels. The oxygen utilization of contralateral brain tissue remained relatively unaltered by radiotherapy. Whether the long-term fall in blood flow in the contralateral brain tissue resulted from progressive capillary damage secondary to irradiation, or was due to tumor recurrence which invariably occurred, was not clear.

GLUCOSE UTILIZATION

The glucose analogue ^{18}F-2-fluoro-2-deoxyglucose (FDG) is transported across the blood-brain barrier (BBB) by the same facilitated transport mechanism as glucose.[20] FDG binds more strongly to the carrier than glucose, but is phosphorylated more slowly by hexokinase. FDG-6-phosphate is unable to take part in the glycolytic pathway, or glycogen synthesis, and so once phosphorylated FDG is essentially trapped in the cell, dephosphorylation occurring slowly. Kinetic models have been developed to relate ^{18}F tracer distribution following intravenous FDG administration to regional cerebral glucose utilization, as represented by hexokinase activity.[21–24] There are, however, a number of problems that arise when these models are applied to pathological brain tissue.[25] First, the models rely on the use of a "lumped constant" which relates the relative rates of FDG and glucose transport across the BBB to their relative rates of phosphorylation. The value of the lumped constant in regions of cerebral pathology is uncertain. Second, the models assume that all cerebral neurones and tumors cells are exposed to similar extracellular levels of FDG during tracer accumulation. Where the BBB is disrupted, as in tumors, higher extracellular FDG levels may be present initially leading to artifactual increases in tracer uptake. In spite of these limitations, a number of interesting studies have been carried out on cerebral glucose utilization in tumor patients using FDG.

Brooks and di Chiro[26] showed that FDG uptake by tumors correlated with the clinical grade of the glioma on the Kernohan scale. They also observed a relative depression in glucose utilization by regions of perifocal edematous tissue and adjacent cortical tissue compared to equivalent regions of contralateral brain tissue. Such findings agree well with studies on regional cerebral oxygen utilization in tumor patients.[16]

De la Paz et al[27] noted a similar suppression in glucose utilization in edematous cortical tissue adjacent to tumors compared to contralateral cortical tissue. Those workers also noted suppression of cerebellar glucose utilization in the hemisphere contralateral to the hemisphere containing the tumor—the phenomenen of "crossed cerebellar diaschisis" described by Baron et al[28] in connection with infarcts.

Rhodes and coworkers[25] studied both oxygen and glucose utilization in cerebral tumors using FDG and the oxygen steady-state approach. They used a simplified version of the Sokoloff equation and found a similar glucose extraction fraction for tumors and cortical tissue. Tumor oxygen extraction, however, was characteristically depressed and these workers concluded that tumors have an increased level of nonoxidative metabolism of glucose compared to normal brain tissue in the presence of an adequate oxygen supply. Increased aerobic glycolysis in tumors has been documented by other workers.[29–31] A functional increase in the ability of tumor cells to transport glucose,[32,33] and raised levels of glycolytic enzymes in tumor cells,[34–37] has also been shown. Rhodes et al's observations using PET thus fit in with animal studies on tumor metabolism.

Patronas et al[38] used FDG uptake by tumors as an indicator of prognosis. They showed that length of patient survival correlated with the ratio of glucose utilization (rCMRGlu) for tumors compared to contralateral brain tissue. These workers also studied radiation necrosis following radiotherapy to brain tumors. Using ^{18}FDG they were able to differentiate between regions of tissue necrosis with a low rCMRGlu and recurrent tumor where rCMRGlu was raised.

AMINO ACID METABOLISM

Tracer modeling of amino-acid metabolism is extremely complex as no metabolic analogue of amino-acids which becomes trapped in a similar manner to FDG has been developed. Bustany et al[39] have developed a three-compartment model to quantitate amino-acid metabolism using ^{11}C-methionine. These workers have observed increased ^{11}C-methionine uptake into brain tumors,[40] but whether this represents increased tumor amino-acid metabolism or is an artifact of blood-brain barrier disruption is not clear. Hübner et al[41] have similarly demonstrated increased tumor uptake of ^{11}C-DL-valine and ^{11}C-DL-typtophan.

Bergstrom and coworkers[42] compared tumor imaging with PET using $^{68}Ga^{III}$-EDTA, ^{11}C-glucose, and ^{11}C-methionine as tracers. The first two tracers showed similar tumor extensions to the enhanced CT scan; however, ^{11}C-methionine revealed further tumor extension in tissue judged normal by the other techniques.

TUMOR pH

^{11}C-dimethyl-oxazolidinedione (^{11}C-DMO) and $^{11}CO_2$ are weak organic acids with a pKa of 6.12. When administered intravenously or via inhalation to normal subjects the neutral acid form, but not the anion, crosses the blood-brain barrier. As a consequence, when measured using PET, the relative arterial plasma-to-regional cerebral ^{11}C distributions reflect the pH differences between the plasma and brain compartments. Both the ^{11}C-DMO and $^{11}CO_2$ methods yield a pH of 7.0 for normal brain.[43,59] Rottenberg et al[44] and Brooks et al,[60] have studied the pH of cerebral tumors using ^{11}C-DMO and $^{11}CO_2$ respectively. These workers found that cerebral tumors and normal brain tissue had similar pHs. This result is in agreement with preliminary ^{31}P-nuclear magnetic resonance studies,[46,57] but at variance with microelectrode studies[45] where tumor pH is found to be depressed when compared to surrounding normal tissue. It should be noted, however, that while the PET and ^{31}P-NMA approaches reflect intracellular pH, microelectrode studies to date have all measured extracellular pH.

TRANSPORT ACROSS THE BLOOD-BRAIN-BARRIER

The transport of glucose across the blood-brain barrier in tumors can be specifically studied with ^{11}C-3-O-methyl-glucose, an analogue of glucose that is not metabolised.[47] It has been shown that gliomas have ^{11}C-methylglucose extractine fractions of up to 30% compared to the 15% extractions observed for normal brain tissue.[61] This finding is in agreement with the increased levels of glucose transport previously reported for transformed cells.[32,33] ^{11}C-cycloleucine is a potential transport marker for amino acids being transported via the neutral phenylalanine transport carrier system, but not metabolized.[48,52] So far no kinetic data using this amino acid analogue has been published.

The blood-brain barrier is normally highly impermeable to K^+ cations, permeability values of between 2 to 20 $\times 10^{-7}$ cm sec^{-1} having been measured for this ion in animal studies. Transport of K^+ is thought to be controlled by ATPases situated on the abluminal side of endothelial membranes. $^{82}Rb^+$ is a positron emitter that is chemically similar to K^+ and has a half-life of 75 sec. When infused at a constant rate continuously, a steady level of $^{82}Rb^+$ results after 4 minutes in both arterial plasma and brain tissue. $^{82}Rb^+$ has been used to qualitatively image cerebral tumors.[49] Brooks and coworkers applied a steady-state model to $^{82}Rb^+$ uptake kinetics and have measured quantitative Rb extraction fractions for cerebral tissue.[50]

The $^{82}Rb^+$ steady-state approach requires consecutive measurements of regional cerebral blood flow and blood volume, and yields a BBB permeability of 11 $\times 10^{-7}$ cm sec^{-1} for $^{82}Rb^+$ in normal brain. Figure 4 shows the ^{82}Rb extraction image of the patients whose CT scan and images of cerebral function are shown in Figs 3A and 3B. It can be seen that while the region of blood flow disruption in Fig 3B corresponds to both the tumor and the surrounding area of edema, increased ^{82}Rb extraction is found only in the tumor region. These workers found that increased Rb extraction was only obtained where abnormalities of vascular ultrastructure were present, ie, in cerebral tumors that enhanced on CT scanning, whereas regions of perifocal tumor edema, nonenhancing and contralateral brain tissue tumors had Rb extractions in the normal range (0 to 2.5%).

Table 5 shows the effect of courses of radiotherapy on the permeability of tumors and contralateral brain toward ^{82}Rb, measured as permeability–surface area products. Following a one-week course of 1,000 rad of radiation to a

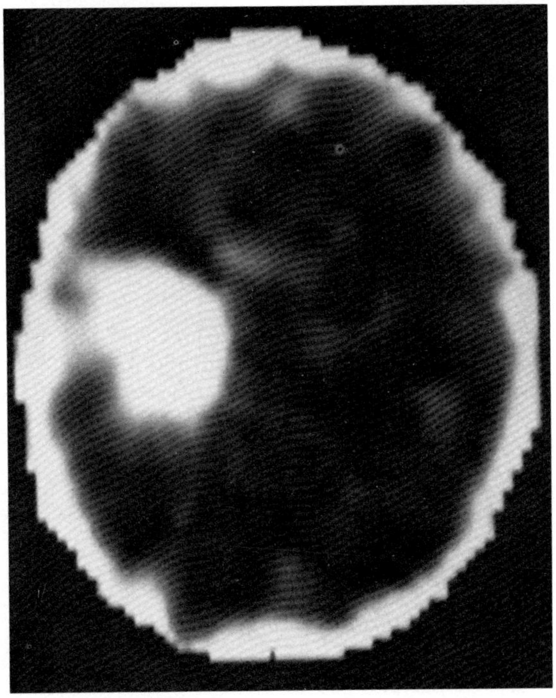

Fig 4. A PET image of ^{82}Rb extraction a OM + 8 cm for the patient in Fig 3A.

Table 5. The Effect of Radiotherapy on Regional Cerebral ^{82}Rb Permeability

Tumor	Dosage	Tumor PS Product (sec^{-1})		Contralateral Brain PS Product (sec^{-1})	
		Pre	Post	Pre	Post
Glioma	1,000 rad over 1 week	184×10^{-5}	225×10^{-5}	10×10^{-5}	25×10^{-5}
Colonic Metastasis	3,000 rad over 2 weeks	93×10^{-5}	222×10^{-5}	9×10^{-5}	10×10^{-5}

glioma, patient 1 showed a 22% rise in tumor and a 250% rise in contralateral brain ^{82}Rb permeability. Patient 2, with a cerebral metastasis from the colon (Fig 3A), showed a 240% rise in tumor ^{82}Rb permeability following a two-week course of 3,000 rads of radiotherapy but here the contralateral brain Rb permeability was hardly affected. The finding of increases in tumor permeability toward Rb following irradiation are not surprising. Rubin et al[51] have shown that an acute dose of 1,000 rads leads to a progressive fragmentation of the microcirculation in Walker cell carcinomas in rats.

Transport of albumin across the blood-brain barrier can be studied with PET using ^{11}C-methyl-albumin. Figure 5A shows the CT scan of a patient with a cerebral metastasis from the breast surrounding by a clearly demarcated region of edema. Figure 5B shows regional cerebral methyl-albumin levels with time for this

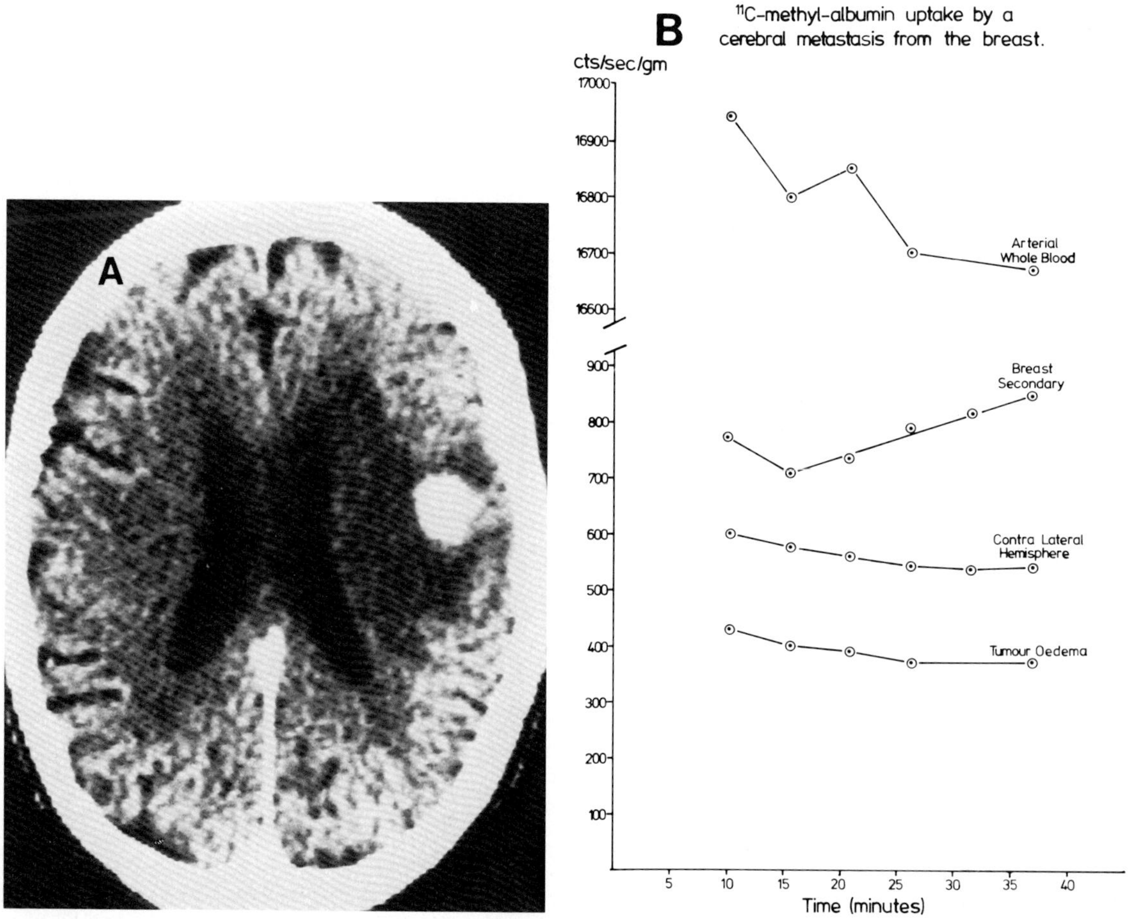

Fig 5. (A) The enhanced CT brain scan of a patient with a cerebral metastasis from the breast. (B) Regional ^{11}C-methyl-albumin cerebral uptake of the patient shown in Fig 5A.

patient after administration of ^{11}C-methyl-albumin. A slow leakage of albumin into the tumor with time is evident, but no uptake by surrounding edematous tissue is seen.

Although no kinetic studies on amino-acid transport using ^{11}C-cyclo-leucine have been carried out, this tracer and ^{11}C-1-aminocyclobutane carboxylic acid have both been shown to be useful for qualitative tumor localization.[52,53] ^{68}Ga-EDTA, a positron-emitting tracer similar to sucrose in size, has been used both qualitatively[42] and quantitatively[62] to detect blood-brain barrier breakdown in tumors.

DISTRIBUTION OF CYTOTOXIC AGENTS

Several studies have been carried out examining qualitatively the distribution of cytotoxic agents labelled with positron emitters. Niewes[54] has demonstrated brain tumor localization using ^{55}Co-Bleomycin. Yamamoto et al[55] have studied the kinetics of uptake of ^{11}C and ^{13}N-labelled BCNU into gliomas. These workers showed that initial uptake of BCNU was dependent on tumor blood flow, and that increased blood-brain barrier disruption, achieved by administering 20% mannitol intravenously, led to an increased glioma BCNU uptake.

FUTURE TRENDS IN TUMOR STUDIES

Tumor Receptor Studies

Gliomas are thought to contain peripheral benzodiazepine receptors which are potentially detectable using the benzodiazepine ^{11}C-R05-4864.[56] With this tracer it should be possible to detect nonenhancing gliomas and to grade them in terms of benzodiazepine receptor status. Prolactinomas contain Type I dopamine receptors,[58] which may be labellable with ^{11}C-methyl-bromocryptine or ^{11}C-methyl-spiperone, a dopamine agonist and antagonist, respectively. Work is also in progress on the use of labeled estrogens using $^{75/76}Br$ to detect prostatic and breast primary and secondary tumors.

Monoclonal antibodies tagged with β-emitters are already in use for treatment of tumor patients. In theory such antibodies, when tagged with positron emitters such as ^{55}Co or ^{68}Ga, could be used for glioma localization.

Manipulation of Tumor Blood Flow

Tumor vasculature is not subject to autoregulation. Vasoactive drugs such as Ca^{II} antagonists and angiotensin could increase tumor blood flow relative to that of normal brain tissue. If this is the case delivery of cytotoxic agents to brain tumors could potentially be improved. PET studies examining the effects of Ca^{II} antagonists on tumor blood flow are currently in progress.

CONCLUSION

PET provides a relatively noninvasive means of studying regional cerebral physiology in patients with brain tumors and of studying the effect of treatment on tumor and cerebral function. At a cruder level PET can be used for tumor localization and has been shown to distinguish tumor recurrence from tissue necrosis following radiotherapy. Nonenhancing tumors which are difficult to visualize on CT scan can often be localized via the region of low oxygen extraction fraction that is their characteristic. It must be remembered, however, that PET is an expensive technique and generally requires an on-line cyclotron for operation. As such it is best suited for studies on regional cerebral physiology and pharmacology in specialized centers and has limited use as a diagnostic tool. Hopefully, the imaging possibilities of PET will become more widely available in the form of single photon emission tomography (SPECT), where an on-line cyclotron is not a prerequisite and a wider range of gamma-emitting tracers can be used. Until, however, a means of measuring the effects of tissue attenuation becomes available, SPECT will be unable to provide absolute values of regional tissue function and this will remain the preserve of positron-emission tomography.

REFERENCES

1. Phelps ME, Mazziotta JC, Huang SC: Study of cerebral function with positron computed tomography. J Cereb Blood Flow Metab 2:113–162, 1982

2. Phelps ME, Hoffman EJ, Mullani NA, et al: Application of annihilation coincident detection by transaxial reconstruction tomography. J Nucl Med 16:210–223, 1975

3. Phelps ME, Hoffman EJ, Huang SC, et al: ECAT: A new computerised tomographic imaging system for positron-emitting radiopharmaceuticals. J Nucl Med 19:635–648, 1978

4. Budinger TF, Derenzo SE, Huesman RH: Instrumen-

tation for positron emission tomography. Ann Neurol 15:535–543, 1984

5. Williams CW, Crabtree MC, Burgiss SG: Design and performance characteristics of a positron emission computed axial tomograph ECAT-II. IEEE Trans Nucl Sci NS-26: 619, 1979

6. Brooks RA, Di Chiro G: Principles of computed assisted tomography (CAT) in radiographic and radioisotopic imaging. Phys Med Biol 21:689–732, 1976

7. Budinger TF, Derenzo SE, Gullberg GT, et al: Emission computed axial tomography with single photon and positron annihilation photon emitters. J Comput Assist Tomogr 1:131–145, 1977

8. Ter-Pergossian MM, Mullani NA, Ficke DC, et al: Photon time-of-flight assistant positron emission tomography. J Comput Assist Tomogr 5:227–229, 1981

9. Di Chiro G, Brooks RA, Sank VJ, et al: The neuro-PET: A new high-resolution 7-slice positron emission tomograph. J Nucl Med 23:59, 1982

10. Hoffman EJ, Huang SC, Phelps ME: Quantitation in positron emission tomography. 1. Effect of object size. J Comput Assist Tomogr 3:299–303, 1979

11. Lammertsma AA, Jones T, Frackowiak RSJ, et al: A theoretical study of the steady-state model for measuring regional cerebral blood flow and oxygen utilisation using oxygen-15. J Comput Assist Tomogr 5:544–550, 1981

12. Frackowiak RSJ, Lenzi GL, Jones T, et al: Quantitative measurements of regional cerebral blood flow and oxygen metabolism in man using ^{15}O and positron emission tomography: theory, procedure and normal values. J Comput Assist Tomogr 4:727–736, 1980

13. Lammertsma AA, Jones T: Correction for the presence of intravascular oxygen-15 in the steady-state technique for measuring regional oxygen extraction ratio in the brain. 1. Description of the method. J Cereb Blood Flow and Metabol 3:416–424, 1983

14. West JB, Dollery CT: Uptake of oxygen-15 labelled CO_2 compared wth carbon-11 labelled CO_2 in the lung. J Appl Physiol 17:9–13, 1962

15. Phelps ME, Huang SC, Hoffman EJ, et al: Validation of tomographic measurement of cerebral blood volume with C-11 labelled carboxyhemoglobin. J Nucl Med 20:328–334, 1979

16. Ito M, Lammertsma AA, Wise RJS, et al: Measurement of regional cerebral blood flow and oxygen utilisation in patients with cerebral tumors using ^{15}O and positron emission tomography: Analytical techniques and preliminary results. Neuroradiology 23:63–74, 1982

17. Beaney RP, Brooks DJ, Leenders KL, et al: Blood flow and oxygen utilisation in the contralateral cortex of patients with untreated intracranial tumors as studied by positron emission tomography with observations on the effect of decompressive surgery. J Neurol Neurosurg Pschiat 48:310–319, 1985

18. Leenders KL, Beaney RP, Brooks DJ, et al: Dexamethanone treatment of brain tumor patients: Effects on regional cerebral blood flow, blood volume, and oxygen utilization. Neurology (in press)

19. Beaney RP: Unpublished observations

20. Sokoloff L, Reivich M, Kennedy C, et al: The (^{14}C) deoxyglucose method for the measurement of local cerebral glucose utilisation: Theory, procedure and normal values in the conscious and anaesthetised albino-rat. J Neurochem 28:879–916, 1977

21. Phelps ME, Huang SC, Hoffman EJ, et al: Tomographic measurement of local cerebral glucose metabolic rate in humans with (F-18)2-fluoro-2-deoxy-D-glucose: Validation of the method. Ann Neurol 6:371–388, 1979

22. Reivich M, Kuhl DE, Wolf A, et al: The ^{18}F-fluorodeoxyglucose method for the measurement of local cerebral glucose utilisation of man. Circ Res 44:127–137, 1979

23. Huang SC, Phelps ME, Hoffman EJ, et al: Non-invasive determination of local cerebral metabolic rate of glucose in man. Am J Physiol 238:E69–E82, 1980

24. Brooks RA: Alternative formula for glucose utilisation using labelled deoxyglucose. J Nucl Med 23:538–539, 1982

25. Rhodes CG, Wise RJS, Gibbs JM, et al: In vivo disturbance of the oxidative metabolism of glucose in human cerebral gliomas. Ann Neurol 14:614–626, 1983

26. Di Chiro G, De La Paz RL, Brooks RA, et al: Glucose utilisation of cerebral gliomas measured by (^{18}F) fluorodeoxyglucose and positron emission tomography. Neurology 32:1323–1329, 1982

27. De La Paz RL, Patronas NJ, Brooks RA, et al: Positron emission tomography study of suppression of grey matter glucose utilisation of brain tumors. AJNR 4:826–829, 1983

28. Baron JC, Bousser MG, Comar D, et al: "Crossed cerebellar diaschisis." A remote functional depression secondary to supratentorial infarction of man. J Cereb Blood Flow Metabol 1:S500–S501, 1981 (suppl)

29. Warburg O: On the origin of cancer cells. Science 123:309–314, 1956

30. Aisenberg AC: The glycolysis and respiration of tumors. Orlando, Fla, Academic Press, 1961

31. Weinhouse S: Changing perceptions of carbohydrate metabolism in tumors, in Arnott MS, Van Eys J, Wang JM (eds): Molecular Interrelations of Nutrition and Cancer. New York, Raven Press, 1982, pp 167–181

32. Hatanaka M, Augl C, Gilden RV: Evidence of functional change in the plasma membrane of murine sarcoma virus-infected mouse embryo cells. Transport and transport-associated phosphorylation of ^{14}C-2-deoxy-D-glucose. J Biol Chem 245:714–717, 1970

33. Hatanaka M: Transport of sugars in tumor cell membranes. Biochem Biophys Acta 355:77–104, 1974

34. Weber G, Cantero A: Glucose-6-phosphatase activity in normal precancerous and neoplastic tissues. Cancer Res 15:105–108, 1955

35. Weber G: Enzymology of cancer cells (Part 1). N Engl J Med 296:486–493, 1977

36. Weber G: Enzymology of cancer cells (Part 2). N Engl J Med 296:541–555, 1977

37. Monakhov NK, Neisfadt EL, Shavlovskii MM, et al: Physiochemical properties and isoenzyme composition of hexokinase from normal and malignant human tissue. J Natl Cancer Inst 61:27–34, 1978

38. Patronas NJ, Di Chiro G, Brooks RA, et al: Work in progress: [^{18}F] Fluorodeoxyglucose and positron emission tomography in the evaluation of radiation necrosis of the brain. Radiology 144:885–889, 1982

39. Bustany P, Sargent T, Saudubray JM, et al: Regional human brain uptake and protein incorporation of ^{11}C-L-methionine studied in vivo with PET. J Cereb Blood Flow Metabol 1:S17–S18, 1981 (suppl)

40. Bustany P: Unpublished results

41. Hübner KF, King P, Gibbs WD, et al: Clinical investigations with carbon-11 labelled amino acids using positron emission computerised tomography in patients with neoplastic diseases. Med Radionuclide Imaging IAEA (Vienna) 515–529, 1981

42. Bergstrom M, Collins P, Ehrin E, et al: Discrepancies in brain tumor extent as shown by computed tomography and positron emission tomography using [^{68}Ga] EDTA, [^{11}C]glucose and [^{11}C]methionine. J Comput Assist Tomogr 7:1062–1066, 1983

43. Syrota A, Castaing M, Rougemont D, et al: Tissue acid-base balance and oxygen metabolism in human cerebral infarction studied with positron emission tomography. Ann Neurol 14:419–428, 1983

44. Rottenberg DA, Gino JZ, Kearfott KJ, et al: In vivo measurement of brain tumor pH using [^{11}C]DMO and positron emission tomography. Ann Neurol 17:70–79, 1985

45. Wike-Hooley JL, Van den Berg AP, Van der Zee J, et al: Human tumour pH and its variation. Eur J Cancer Clin Oncol 21:785–791, 1985

46. Koeze TH, Lantos PL, Iles RA, et al: In vivo nuclear magnetic resonance spectroscopy of a transplanted brain tumor. Br J Cancer 49:357–361, 1984

47. Narahara HT, Özand P: Studies of tissue permeability. IX. The effect of insulin on the penetration of 3-methylglucose-H^3 in frog muscle. J Biol Chem 238:40–49, 1963

48. Berlinquet L, Begin N, Babineau LM: Autoradiographic studies of the distribution of 1-amino-cyclopentane carboxylic acid in normal and cancerous mice. Can J Biochem 40:1111–1114, 1962

49. Yen CK, Yano Y, Budinger TF, et al: Brain tumor evaluation using Rb-82 and positron emission tomography. J Nucl Med 23:532–537, 1982

50. Brooks DJ, Beaney RP, Lammertsma AA, et al: Quantitative measurement of blood-brain-barrier permeability using ^{82}Rb and positron emission tomography. J Cereb Blood Flow Metabol 4:535–545, 1984

51. Rubin P, Casarett G: Microcirculation of tumors. II. The supervascularised state of irradiated regressing tumors. Clin Radiol 17:346, 1966

52. Hayes RL, Washburn LC, Wieland BW, et al: Carboxyl-labelled ^{11}C-1-aminocyclopentane carboxylic acid, a potential agent for cancer detection. J Nucl Med 17:748–751, 1976

53. Washburn LC, Sun TT, Anon JB, et al: Effect of structure on tumor specificity of alicyclic α-amino acids. Canc Res 38:2271–2273, 1978

54. Niewes OE: ^{57}Co-bleomycin scintigraphy and ^{55}Co-bleomycin positron emission tomography (thesis). Groningen, Brukkerij van Deuderen BV, 1983, pp 82–93

55. Yamamoto YL, Diksis M, Sako K, et al: Pharmacokinetic and metabolic studies in human malignant gliomas, in Magistretti PL (ed): Functional Radionuclide Imaging of the Brain. New York, Raven Press, 1983, pp 327–335.

56. Schoemaker H, Morelli M, Deshmukh P, et al: (^{3}H] R05-4864 benzodiazepine binding in the kainate lesioned striatum and Huntingdon's diseased basal ganglia. Brain Res 248:396–401, 1982

57. Ross B, Marshall V, Smith M, et al: Monitoring response to chemotherapy of intact human tumors by ^{31}P nuclear magnetic resonance. Lancet I: 641–646, 1984

58. Creese I: Dopamine receptors explained. TINS 40–43, 1982

59. Brooks DJ, Lammertsma AA, Beaney RP, et al: Measurement of regional cerebral pH in human subjects using continuous inhalation of $^{11}CO_2$ and positron emission tomography. J Cereb Blood Flow Metab 4:458–465, 1984

60. Brooks DJ, Beaney RP, Thomas DGT, et al: Studies on regional cerebral pH on patients with cerebral tumors using continuous inhalation of $^{11}CO_2$ and positron emission tomography. J Cereb Blood Flow Metab (submitted)

61. Brooks DJ, Beane RP, Lammertsma AA, et al: Glucose transport across the blood-brain barrier in normal human subjects and patients with cerebral tumors studied using ^{11}C-3-O-methyl-D-glucose and positron emission tomography. J Cereb Blood Flow Metab (in press)

62. Hawkins RA, Phelps ME, Huang SC, et al: A kinetic evaluation of blood-brain barrier permeability in human brain tumors with [^{68}Ga] EDTA and positron computed tomography. J Cereb Blood Flow Metab 4:507–515, 1984

Immunobiology of Human Gliomas

Dennis E. Bullard, G. Yancey Gillespie, M. Stephen Mahaley, and Darell D. Bigner

MALIGNANT glial neoplasms, which account for almost half of all central nervous system (CNS) tumors,[1,2] remain incurable. The efficacy of standard treatment, surgical resection, and external radiotherapy appears to have reached a plateau, principally because of the intolerable side effects,[3] and adjuvant chemotherapy, as it is currently administered, has met with only marginal success.[1,2] One of the major factors in this poor response to therapy is the biological variability of these tumors. Both phenotypically and genotypically, malignant gliomas are extremely heterogeneous.[4-10] The recognition of this profound heterogeneity and of the limitations of current therapy have stimulated efforts to individualize therapy based upon biologic principles.

The presence of an interaction between malignant gliomas and the immune system has long been known. Ridley and Cavanaugh in 1971 described lymphocytic infiltrates in intracranial tumors and speculated on a possible host-mediated immune response.[11] This and the demonstration of decreased immune functioning in glioma patients suggested the possibility of manipulating the immune system in order to obtain a therapeutic response. However, early attempts at treating malignant gliomas with immunotherapy were not generally successful. Recent scientific progress, most notably the development of monoclonal antibodies (MA), has reopened this area of investigation. In the following review, we outline briefly the normal immune response in man, discuss the data concerning host-tumor interaction, and summarize current data on biologic and immunotherapy agents.

From Duke University Medical Center, Durham, North Carolina.

Supported by Research Grant CA 11898 and CA 32672, from the National Cancer Institute, and PO 1 NS0023, from the National Institute of Neurological and Communication Disorders and Stroke, National Institutes of Health.

Dr Bullard holds Teacher-Investigator Development Award 1 KO7NS00800-01, from the NINCDS.

Address reprint requests to Dennis E. Bullard, MD, Duke University Medical Center, Box 3128, Durham, NC 27710.

0093-7754/86/1301-0010$05.00/0

GENERAL IMMUNE RESPONSE

The human immune system is composed primarily of lymphocytes, macrophages, macrophage-related cells, and specialized epithelial cells including those found in the thymus. When an organism is exposed to an immunogenic foreign molecule, an ordered sequence of physiologic events occurs within this system. Initially, the foreign molecule is recognized as being foreign by a lymphocyte that has been previously committed to responding to specific types of antigens based upon the presence of a specific receptor on the lymphocyte's membrane. Within an expanded clone of lymphocytes, all have the same antigen-specific receptor on their cell surface. Because foreign molecules generally have multiple antigenic determinants, each of which can interact with different populations of lymphocytes, a heterogeneous antibody response usually results.

Lymphocytes have been classically divided into two general classes based upon their functioning; B lymphocytes, which give rise to the antibody-secreting cells, and T lymphocytes, which are thymus-derived and are capable of a wide range of cellular interactions that govern and regulate immune responsiveness. Within the T lymphocyte class, there are several subtypes that have differing and often antagonistic roles, including the activation or suppression of the general immune response. The currently designated groups of T cells include helper (inducer) cells, suppressor cells, killer cells, and those T cells involved in delayed hypersensitivity. In addition, there are also lymphocytes that do not fit into either of these two general categories and appear to mediate certain nonspecific cytotoxic responses. These may be either natural killer (NK) cells that kill other foreign cells directly or K cells that bind and kill antibody-coated target cells by a mechanism known as antibody-dependent cellular cytotoxicity (ADCC).

Normal Cellular Response

Both B and T lymphocytes are derived from stem cells originally located in hematopoietic organs. The T lymphocyte precursors, however, enter the thymus where they mature and differentiate into three general categories: helper T cells, cytotoxic T cells, and suppressor T cells.[12] During this maturation period, cells that are able to recognize autologous antigens are deleted, resulting in T lymphocyte tolerance. Subsequently, the mature T cells leave the thymus and become part of the peripheral T cell population. These T lymphocytes can be characterized on the basis of surface phenotypic antigenic expression.[13,14] The most frequently used designations are the OKT and Leu systems. In the OKT (Leu) designation, human helper cells express OKT4 (Leu3) determinant while both cytotoxic and suppressor cells express OKT8 (Leu2) determinant. While this relationship between functional specialization and antigenic expression appears to hold up in most circumstances, under certain experimental conditions some functional heterogeneity does exist.[15,16] Helper T cells are primarily involved in stimulating B cells into antibody production. As will be discussed later, B cell response to the majority of antigens is dependent upon T cell assistance. Generally, this is by the direct interaction of helper T cells to provide specificity for the antigen to which the response is being generated. Their cell–cell interaction is amplified by production of lymphokines, which are soluble, nonspecific helper factors produced by the T cells. The primary activation of the helper T cells is dependent upon exposure to both an antigen and a compatible major histocompatability complex (MHC) molecule, which are generally on the surface of specialized antigen presenting cells (APC). Although B cells may participate in this, current data suggest macrophages are primarily involved. Conversely, suppressor T cells act through various mechanisms to suppress the immune response. One of these actions is through direct suppression of helper T cells directly or through the release of various factors. The role that suppressor T cells has with B cells or cytotoxic T cells is largely unknown. Cytotoxic T cells corecognize foreign surface antigens and a product of the MHC. The cytotoxic T cells then lyse the target cells. This mechanism is thought to be of particular importance against virus-containing cells and in some forms of tumor rejection. Production of adequate number of T cells appears to be dependent upon stimulation by interleukin-2 (IL-2), which is produced by helper T cells. T cells are also thought to play a role in various other immune responses including delayed hypersensitivity and contact sensitivity by way of their activation of macrophages.[12]

Humoral

Following proper presentation of the antigen to B lymphocytes, the lymphocytes respond by activation, proliferation, differentiation, and antibody production. The sequence of events during activation and proliferation is not totally understood but appears to have two general schemes. Factor-dependent activation, which is limited to a subgroup of B cells, can occur by the interaction of antigen, B cell, and certain helper factors, including B cell growth factor (BCGF) and interleukin-1 (IL-1). Subsequently, differentiating factors, which have sometimes been referred to as T cell replacing factors (TRFs), allow the activated B cells to synthesize and secrete immunoglobulin (Ig). The second pathway for activation of B cells, which appears to be more common, is through direct interaction with T cells. Helper T cells, which are immunologically compatible with the B cell, interact with specific receptors on the surface of the B cell and present the antigen to the B cell in a way that allows it to become activated. The subsequent production of antibody is then influenced by further interaction with the helper T cell and/or soluble factors. During the proliferation phase, the number of B cells increases without actual secretion of antibody. This phase is strongly influenced by BCGF. However, only a small percentage of those cells that proliferate will then go through differentiation and become antibody-secreting cells. The antibodies produced are immunoglobulin (Ig) molecules. These molecules have one or multiple units with each unit formed by two heavy (H) polypeptide chains and two light (L) polypeptide chains. There are five groups of Ig; IgA, IgD, IgE, IgG, and IgM. The type of Ig is determined by the H chain possessed by the molecule. Each unit has two regions, the variable and the constant. In the variable region, which is formed by portions of both the L and H chains, there are two sites for antigen interaction. The binding of antigen at such sites is based on noncovalent interactions that can be expressed as an equilibrium constant or affinity. When binding occurs, biologic responses, such as activation of the complement system or release of mediators of antiphylaxis, occur. Many of these biological responses are determined by the constant region of the molecule.

IMMUNE PARAMETERS IN PATIENTS WITH PRIMARY BRAIN TUMORS

Considerable data exist to document an altered immune status in patients with primary intracranial tumors (Table 1). Unlike patients with cancer elsewhere, patients with gliomas generally do not have disseminated disease nor gross metabolic abnormalities. This circumstance has strongly suggested a direct relationship between immune alteration and glioma presence. At the time of diagnosis, patients with malignant gliomas generally have impaired delayed hypersensitivity responses to common recall antigens, such as tuberculin, Candida, trichophyton, mumps, and streptokinase.[17–19] In addition, there is diminished blastogenic response by peripheral blood leukocytes exposed in vitro to mitogens or in mixed lymphocyte cultures.[18,20,21] Moreover, there is a decrease in the level of circulating lymphocytes, with specific reduction in T cells, which persist through the remainder of the patient's illness.[19,22] Increased monocyte suppressor function has also been reported to occur in patients with glioblastoma multiforme and to be responsible for a portion of the T cell immunodepression.[23,24] These deficits appear to be more pronounced in those patients with the more anaplastic tumors. However, the degree of cellular immune suppression at the time of diagnosis has not proved to be a reliable index of survival time, although further decrease in skin test responsiveness during the course of therapy does appear to correlate with tumor progression.[25]

Table 1. Immune Status of Glioma Patients

Depressed delayed hypersensitivity reactions to recall antigens
Decreased percentage in total number of lymphocytes
Decreased percentage in total number of T cells
Relative decreased T cells and increased suppressor T cells
Impaired mitogen-induced blastogenic response by peripheral mononuclear cells

Recent evidence has suggested that glioblastoma cells may directly interact in cell-mediated immunity. Cultured murine astrocytes and rat C6 glioma cells are known to release an interleukin-1 (IL-1)-like factor that augments the proliferation response of T cells to lectins and the release of IL-2.[26,27] In human glioblastoma cells, however, a different response is seen. Initial IL-1-like factor is released, but the helper factor seen in murine and rat cells is inhibited by another glioblastoma cell-derived factor, which appears to suppress the growth of IL-2–dependent cloned T cell lines and the generation of cytotoxic alloreactive T cells in mixed lymphocyte cultures.[28] This factor has a molecular weight of 97,000 daltons, and has many of the characteristics of the neuroblast growth inhibition factor (NGIF), which has been previously reported to be in the supernate of fetal rat glial cell cultures. If this factor is released by glioblastoma cells in vivo, it may explain at least some of the reported impairment of cell-mediated immunity in glioblastoma patients.[17]

Humoral parameters in patients with glioblastoma are less consistently abnormal. Serum immunoglobulin levels are generally normal, although patients with more anaplastic tumors may have elevated serum IgM levels,[19] but, a similar finding has been reported in patients with benign tumors.[29] While the total number of B cells appears to be normal in these patients, their ability to produce antibodies against tetanus, influenza, or a new foreign antigen (keyhole limpet hemocyanin) appears to be impaired.[19,30] The reason for this is unclear. One hypothesis has been that a soluble blocking factor is present that impairs immune interactions, including in vitro blastogenesis.[18,31] Circulating immune complexes have been reported preoperatively and postoperatively in patients with gliomas.[32,33] Elevated levels appear to correlate with a greater degree of anaplasia and with a shorter survival time among those patients with malignant gliomas. Utilizing panels of immune assays, attempts have been made to predict survival and tumor recurrence based upon serial immune responses. In the hands of some investigators, this has proven worthwhile.[25]

EVIDENCE OF HOST-TUMOR INTERACTION

Cellular Interaction

Since the description of lymphoid cellular infiltrates into brain tumors by Bertrand and Mannen in 1960, the role of mononuclear (MN) cells within CNS tumors has been questioned.[34] Utilizing light microscopy, 30% to 60% of primary human glial tumors have MN cell infiltrates.[11,35–42] This has been speculated to be an example of host response to tumor, but has not been proven. While several studies have reported prolonged survival correlated with the presence of lymphocytic infiltration, this has not been consistently seen, and a wide variation in pathological and histological cell types has been present.[11,35–39,41,42] In the early histopathologic studies utilizing light microscopy, MN cells were seen primarily in the perivascular spaces, as is noted with cell-mediated immune responses to foreign tissue. However, more recent studies utilizing immunohistochemistry and monoclonal antibodies (MA) have demonstrated MN cells diffusely within the parenchyma of gliomas, but not within the surrounding normal tissue.[42] The significance of this, however, is not known. Several attempts have been made to identify the MN cell subpopulations. Both Fc receptor-positive lymphocytes, monocytes, and macrophages, and antigen-antibody complexes have been documented in glial and nonglial CNS tumors.[43,44] It has been postulated that these Fc receptor-positive T cells represent specific suppressor or cytotoxic subsets,[14,39] but these cells have also been documented to be elevated both in situ and in the peripheral blood of patients with non-CNS tumors, and the exact role of these cells has not been confirmed.[45] Recent attempts to define the MN cell infiltrates utilizing MA have shown in a small sampling a predominant suppressor-cytotoxic cell population in glial tumors with a more heterogenous pattern seen in nonglial tumors and no evidence of MN cell infiltrates in normal brain.[42] The significance of these observations has not been determined.

Numerous authors have reported specific cell-mediated antiglioma activity, demonstrated by delayed cutaneous hypersensitivity and in vitro assays, including microcytotoxicity, blastogenic repsonse, and lymphocyte adherence inhibition.[46–53] However, in none of these studies was a true glioma-specific antigenic preparation used and it has been demonstrated that peripheral lymphocytes from glioma patients react as well with cultured adult or fetal glial cells as they do with autologous tumor cells in both cytotoxic and blastogenic assays.[54,55] The possibility that a response is present but masked because of various factors has also been postulated. In vitro studies have suggested that significant cell-mediated cytotoxicity requires an extremely high effector-to-target cell ratio in order to be seen.[31] It has also been reported that the sera from patients with gliomas contain a blocking factor or factors that could prevent the expression of in vitro and in vivo activity by cytotoxic T cells.[17,31,56] Recent work by Fontana et al[26–28] has shown the release of an IL-1-like factor in murine-, rat-, and human-cultured glioma cells. In addition, in cultured human glioblastoma cells, a factor has been identified that inhibits IL-2 with a resultant decrease in the induction of cytotoxic T cells in mixed lymphocyte cultures. Such a factor, if released by glioblastoma cells in vivo, could conceivably be the suppressive or blocking factor previously noted by other authors. It is hoped that further work in this area will shed light on this phenomena.

Humoral Interaction

Preliminary studies in humans appeared to indicate the presence of humoral factors that could interact with autologous and heterologous glioma cells in vitro.[57,58] Subsequently, several authors have reported specific antiglioma antibodies in patient serum utilizing cytotoxicity, antibody-dependent cell-mediated cytotoxicity (ADCC), immunofluorescence, and hemadsorption assays.[31,59–63] The majority of of these studies, however, did not control for tumor-associated versus tumor-specific activity and, in the instances where such controls were employed, positive identification of tumor-specific activity could not be established.[32,43,63] As previously mentioned, immunoglobulin has been found in increased concentrations within malignant gliomas on both glioblastoma cells and bound to Fc-receptor-bearing cells.[44,64] Since immunoglobulin is known to bind to glia in normal human brain, the pertinence of these findings is not known.[65]

EVIDENCE OF SPECIFIC ANTIGENICITY OF GLIOMAS

Implicit in the assumption that the immune system is able to recognize a glioma as being foreign is the presence phenotypically of glioma-specific or glioma-associated antigens. Mahaley and Day immunized rabbits with samples of human glioma and extensively absorbed and fractionated the resulting antisera.[66] Samples of this serum were then conjugated to ^{125}I and injected intraarterially in patients with malignant gliomas 3 to 5 days prior to surgical resection. Samples of normal brain and tumor were then sampled, demonstrating higher levels of ^{125}I-antibody in the tumor in 18 to 20 patients.[67] However, this degree of localization was relatively low and subsequent problems with the polyclonal antisera precluded continuation of this work. In later studies, Coakham et al described rabbit-anti-glioma sera against astrocytomas and glioblastomas.[68–70] Neither of these antisera, however, was demonstrated to be free of cell line contamination by mycoplasma nor HLA-nonreactive. Subsequently, both Miyake and Kitamura and Sato et al produced a rabbit sera against human glioma cells. Unfortunately, the lack of adequate absorption prevented either of these sera from being worthwhile as probes for tumor-specific antigens.[71,72] A more controlled study was done by Kehayov, who immunized rabbits with saline extracts of either normal human brain or human glioblastoma in complete Freund adjuvant followed by multiple boosters without adjuvant.[73] The subsequent serum was extensively absorbed and assayed by immunodiffusion and immunoelectrophoresis. The anti-glioma sera, after absorption with human brain and other organs, reacted with 13/16 glioblastomas and 9/9 astrocytomas with no reaction to normal adult brain or other nonglioma CNS tumors. A lesser degree of reaction was still seen with human fetal brain of 8 to 10 weeks gestation; a general pattern that has also been reported by Trouillas and Wikstrand.[51,74] Despite these separate intriguing findings, a common tumor-associated antigen has not been defined and characterized utilizing polyclonal serologic analysis.

With the development of MA technology, however, much progress in this area has been made. Already, MA have been developed against a wide spectrum of antigens including human neuroectodermal tumor–associated antigens, normal CNS-associated antigens, extracellular matrix proteins, and biochemically defined markers.[75–89] Among these, glial fibrillary acidic protein (GFAP), an intracellular intermediate filament found in normal astroglial cells and astroglial-derived tumors,[75,90–94] has been demonstrated in virtually all types of glial tumors including ependymomas, mixed gliomas, gliosarcomas, angiogliomas, astroblastomas, and glioblastomas.[75,90–92,94–97] Other biochemically defined markers, such as the other intermediate filament proteins, neurofilament (NF), the cytokeratins, desmin and vimentin, S-100, and neuron-specific enolase, have not been as well defined and appear to have less restriction.[75] There has also been demonstrated a pattern of cross-reactivity between nervous system and lymphoid cell markers. Antigens, such as Thy-1 or antigens with similar patterns of reactivity, have been reported on animal and human B and T cells, as well as human brain, glioma, melanoma, endometrial carcinoma, and osteosarcoma tissue.[96–101] Antigens present on both HNT tissue and lymphoid tissue have been demonstrated with MA derived by inoculation either with lymphoid cells or HNT.[87–89,104–108] The identification of these shared antigens poses many questions concerning the interaction between primary intracranial tumors and the human immune system.

Many shared antigens also are present on both CNS and lymphoid tumors and fetal tissue. These shared antigens represent an extremely complex and heterogenous pattern of reactivity. The MA utilized to describe these antigens have most frequently been derived from the immunization of melanoma cell lines, glioma cell lines, or human fetal brain.[87,88,107,109–112] The majority of the MA appeared to identify a shared neuroectodermal-oncofetal antigen with a relatively restricted pattern of reactivity that includes gliomas, neuroblastomas, and melanomas.[107,111] Unfortunately, very few MA have been derived that react only with the type tumor of the immunogen and are operationally specific.[113] In animal work, a MA derived against a nitrosourea-induced rat glioma cell line failed to respond to human or canine gliomas, or to normal rat brain.[114] This pattern of reactivity was similar to that seen by Lee et al,[115] who identified an antigen expressed on virally and chemically induced neurogenic rat tumors, but that was not seen on normal rodent or human cells, despite extensive testing. Whether these antigens represent true tumor or transformation-associated antigens has not been clearly defined, but with the great degree of specificity obtainable from MA, it is hoped that this work can lead to a greater understanding about specificity in human tumors.

IMMUNOTHERAPY

Introduction

A rational approach to the immunotherapy of primary brain tumors is dependent upon the presence of tumor specific antigens and the ability to induce or enhance the host response to these. Immunotherapeutic protocols can be categorized into four general types; restorative or nonspecific, adoptive, passive, and active. *Restorative immunotherapy* is an attempt to stimulate or boost the deficient immune capabilities of the cancer patient in a nonspecific manner. *Adoptive immunotherapy* is the administration of sensitized immune cells, either autologous or allogeneic, in an attempt to transfer specific immunity to the weakly reactive patient. *Passive immunotherapy* operates under the same premise but utilizes the transfer of serum or specifically reactive antibodies rather than cellular components. *Active immunotherapy* employs immunization in a manner that increases the patient's ability to specifically and positively interact with tumor by specific sensitization to tumor-associated or tumor-specific antigens.

Restorative. To date, the use of general immunostimulations in an attempt to restore the immune system in patients with malignant gliomas has not proven successful. In two studies utilizing BCG or *C. parvum,* respectively, no alteration in either immune competence or clinical response was noted in patients with malignant gliomas.[116,117] Since neither of these studies had controlled populations, the adequacy of the immunostimulants used is open to question. However, in a controlled, prospective, randomized study of patients with malignant gliomas following surgical resection and concomitant with adjuvant therapy utilizing radiotherapy and BCNU, the addition of levamisole failed to alter survival times.[118] Currently, there are numerous biologic therapy agents that are being evaluated for their role in augmenting the immune system in patients with malignant gliomas (Table 1).

Adoptive immunotherapy. This form of immunotherapy is an attempt to transfer immune competence to immunosuppressed cancer patients utilizing cellular elements of the immune system. Trouillas and Lapras, in 1970, infused autologous leukocytes directly into the intracranial cavity in three patients with gliomas.[119] Utilizing a similar approach, Takakura et al infused phytohemagglutinin-treated peripheral white blood cells intracranially in patients with recurrent malignant tumors.[120] Seven of the 10 patients had malignant gliomas and had increased survival rates in comparison to historical controls. In a larger but similar study, Young et al injected autologous leukocytes into the tumor bed in patients with recurrent glioblastomas.[121] Prior to infusion, the leukocytes were placed in direct contact with tumor cells. Eight of 17 patients were reported to have significant clinical improvement with survivorship exceeding 17 months. Although each of these studies appears promising, in none were rigid controls maintained in terms of technique, cell population injected, or adequate comparison groups. An alternative form of adoptive immunotherapy has been either allogeneic bone marrow cell transfusions or intrathecal autologous lymphocyte infusions.[122,123] None of these trials, however, has been controlled and the data are virtually impossible to interpret.

Passive immunotherapy. Initial trials of passive immunotherapy utilizing xenogeneic rabbit antiglioma sera indicated some localization within human malignant gliomas, but were not pursued because of the limitations of the polyclonal antisera.[66] With the development of MA technology, however, many of those probelms may be resolved. One of the major potential uses of MA is as a carrier of radiation and drugs for the diagnosis and treatment of brain tumors. MA have been successfully conjugated to a variety of toxins and drugs including the plant toxins, ricin, abrin, and gelonin; the bacterial toxins, diphtheria toxin-A and Pseudomonas aeruginosa; drugs such as chlorambucil, methotrexate, daunomycin, and neocarzinostatin; and multiple enzymes.[76,124] Moreover, MA have been bound to multiple radionuclides including ^{123}I, ^{125}I, ^{131}I, for localization, imaging, and therapeutic purposes.[76,125]

An alternative approach may be based upon new data generated in the field of experimental virology and tumor immunology. It has been noted that spontaneous and chemically induced tumors in animals tend to be poorly antigenic in contrast to virally induced tumors that are strongly antigenic when transplanted in syngeneic animals. The basis for this appears to be that virus-associated tumor systems express a strongly immunogenic and broadly cross-reactive series of viral antigens that are present among all tumors sharing common virion serotypes.[126,127] The majority of work in this area has been performed utilizing C-type retroviruses.[126] Following retrovirus infection in the mouse, viral antigens, most notably gp71, are expressed on the cell surface.[128] Cells expressing this antigen are then susceptible to host cellular and humoral immune response, although normally 100% of animals die within 8 to 12 weeks after infection. However, passive serum therapy with MA anti-gp71 can result in cure of animals infected with friend murine leukemia virus (FLV). In addition to the passive serum response, there is the active development of host antiviral antibodies which appear to play a major role in the survival of the animal.[112,128,129] This form of seroimmunotherapy can also be applied successfully in other species against both leukemias and solid tumors, as long as similar cell surface antigens are present.[130] Once treated, long-term resistance appears to be established and animals are capable of resisting later challenge with either virus or tumor cells. This response appears to specifically require an IgG_{2a} antibody. Kobayashi has demonstrated that chemically induced tumors can be infected with viruses with the development of transplantation resistance to normally fatal tumors.[131] These findings have subsequently been reproduced by other investigators with a variety of murine leukemia viruses.[126,132,133] This has also been successfully done by the administration of live virus to animals bearing tumors in vivo.[134,135] Such an approach could conceivably allow a superinfection of human tumors and subsequent passive serotherapy.

However, with the progress in characterization of human tumor–associated antigens by MA technology, the need for viral antigens may not materialize. It has been shown that murine MA against human cancer–associated antigens have successfully localized in the human tumor tissue following transplantation into athymic mice and rats.[123,136] Moreover, human B cell lymphoma has been treated in man by antiidiotypic MA.[137,138] Theoretically, if tumor-specific antigens can be detected on human tumors, then passive serotherapy with antitumor MA could be successful. From the animal data, it appears that the passive immunization allows a positive adjustment in the interaction between the tumor and the host immune system with the subsequent rejection of the tumor by the host.[106] This exciting new concept, however, awaits much more work in the definition of tumor-specific antigens and biologic mechanisms.

Active immunotherapy. Active immunotherapy is designed to increase a patient's ability to interact specifically with his brain tumor. Generally, this is done by immunization with treated autologous or allogeneic tumor cells or cross-reacting antigen preparations. The initial study in this area was performed by Bloom et al utilizing subcutaneous implantation of autologous tumor cells in a patient with a malignant astrocytoma.[139] Unfortunately, no evidence of an induced response to tumor was noted and the viable tumor cells grew locally. Serologic assays failed to demonstrate any complement-fixing antibodies elicited. In a similar study one year later, Grace utilized the same techniques in six patients.[140] In two of the six patients, the viable tissue grew subcutaneously. In none of the patients was there any serologic evidence for the development of antiglioma antibodies; however, two patients in whom tumor did not grow developed delayed hypersensitivity responses when subsequently tested intradermally with tumor extracts. In a prospective randomized study, Bloom et al treated 27 of 62 patients with malignant gliomas with irradiated autologous tumor cells in addition to radical surgery and postoperative radiation.[141] Only 10 patients had more than one injection and none had more than three. None of the immunized patients demonstrated any response to intradermal test utilizing autologous tumor cell extracts. There was no difference in survival between the immunized and nonimmunized groups. In this study, no attempt was made to select patients preoperatively for immunocompetency, no immune stimulants or adjuvants were utilized, and no patients received more than three immunizations. Trouillas and Lapras randomized 65 patients with malignant gliomas into four treatment groups.[119] In 17 patients, no postoperative treatment was given. In 20 patients, postoperative irradiation was administered. In 18 patients, both postoperative irradiation and immunotherapy with autologous tumor cells emulsified with complete Freund's adjuvant were given. In 10 patients, postoperative immunotherapy alone was given. Unlike the prior studies, Trouillas and Lapras utilized both adjuvant and serial immunizations, with all patients receiving between 4 and 10 injections. Over the two-year course of this study, 25 of 28 patients receiving immunotherapy developed cutaneous hypersensitivity responses to autologous tumor extracts. Survival time for nontreated patients was 5.4 months. For those receiving immunotherapy alone, it was 7.4 months. For those receiving radiation therapy alone, it was 7.5 months, and for those receiving both immunotherapy and radiation therapy, the survival time was 10.1 months. Trouillas later reported immunodiffuse precipitation reactions to autologous glioma extracts in 14 patients receiving similar immunotherapy.[142] The postimmunization sera reacted with autologous glioma extracts and fetal brain extracts, but failed to respond to normal adult brain or meningioma extracts.[50] In 6 of the immunotherapy patients examined at autopsy, lymphocyte infiltration was found in four. During immunotherapy, sera samples were reported to demonstrate cytotoxic antibiotics for glioma cells in complement-mediated in vitro assays. Unfortunately, lack of pathological controls preclude adequate evaluation of the survival times in this study.

Based upon extensive animal investigation, two pilot studies were begun in 1979.[143] Patients with histologically proven anaplastic gliomas underwent immune screening before and/or after surgery. Those found to have normal or slightly less than normal levels of immune competence were given adjunctive immunotherapy as a supplement to radiation and chemotherapy. In the study performed at the National Hospital for Nervous Disease in London, five patients were given viable but HLA-mismatched glioma cell lines mixed with a BCG cell wall preparation in addition to the standard chemotherapeutic regimen which consisted of CCNU, vincristine, and procarbazine. Three of these patients received serial immunization and survived from 383 to 934 days following surgery. Two of the three patients demonstrated evidence of serologic responses to the immunizing cell line. No evidence of allergic encephalitis or untoward systemic reaction was noted clinically or at autopsy in these patients.[144–146] At the University of North Carolina, 20 patients received adjuvant immunotherapy with either of two tissue-cultured glioma cell lines that had been lethally irradiated just prior to inoculation, in addition to the BCG cell wall preparation. The patients were also given levamisole and received chemotherapy bimonthly with BCNU (80 mg/m^2/d IV times 3). The preliminary data from this study demonstrate the production of a significant quantity of serum antibody directed against the immunizing glioma cells, although, as in the other study, approximately 90% of the antibody titer was against nonglioma antigens, which include fetal bovine serum proteins incorporated into the immunizing tumor cells during their tissue culture growth and HLA histocompatability antigens. However, following serial absorption against fetal bovine sera and HLA antigens, there remains in some patients a low, but significant, titer of serum antibody reactive against the original glioma cell preparation. Subsequently, a collaborative phase II trial is now underway comparing the benefit of this adjuvant immunotherapy in a prospective randomized fashion.

BIOLOGICAL RESPONSE MODIFIERS AS THERAPY AGENTS

With the advent of recombinant DNA technology, there has been a strong resurgence of interest in the therapeutic benefit that might be achieved with biologic compounds that have demonstrated antitumor effects. Chief among these substances are the interferons (IFN). There are three major IFN classes (α, β, and γ)

that have been operationally defined on the basis of the combination of cell type source and eliciting stimulus.[147] Various combinations of the 20 allelic forms of IFN-α are produced by human leukocytes in response to exposure to certain viruses. IFN-β is produced by mesenchymal stromal elements (fibroblasts) also in response to virus exposure. IFN-γ is only one of many distinct kinds of "lymphokines and monokines" produced by immune-related cells (lymphocytes and monocytes) as part of their overall responses to antigenic or mitogenic stimulation.

Although all of the IFNs can be quantified on the basis of their antiviral activities, they have all been demonstrated to exert significant antiproliferative activity in vitro and in vivo against various experimental animal tumors and in some human tumors.[148] Possible mechanisms suggested for antitumor activity include direct toxic effects on malignant cells and indirect toxicity mediated through interferon-stimulated lymphocytes (eg, NK cells) or interferon-activated macrophages. Of relevance here is that some human glioma cells cultured in the presence of physiologically attainable levels of IFN exhibit dose-dependent inhibition of growth, while other glioma lines are relatively insensitive. This heterogeneous sensitivity of gliomas to this particular drug should not be that surprising in view of the many other characteristics in which gliomas display heterogeneity.[4-7,9] Nevertheless, the actual role IFNs may eventually play in glioma therapy is just now being explored.

Human IFN-β has been reported to inhibit growth of glioma cell lines when used at concentrations of 30 to 50,000 U/mL.[148-152] Immunocytochemical and other morphologic analyses of IFN-treated glioma cells revealed changes indicative of maturation to more differentiated astrocytic cells that contained increased amounts of GFAP.[151] Human glioma cells have also been found to be sensitive to low concentrations (100 to 1,000 U/mL) of human leukocyte IFN-α in in vitro assays,[148,153,154] although HuIFN-β appears to be more effective in parallel comparisons.[153,154] Nederman and Benedicktsson[153] determined that low-level irradiation (300 rads) of U-251MG glioma cells treated with 100 U of IFN-α/mL produced an additive growth inhibition. In studies involving human glioma biopsy tissue, both IFN-α and IFN-β, in concentrations of 4 to 1,000 U/mL generally caused reduction in RNA and protein synthesis with the latter more effective than the former. In two instances, however, low-dose exposure caused increased synthesis of RNA and protein.[155] Several groups have also studied the effectiveness of human IFNs to retard growth of human gliomas transplanted into nude mice.[154,156,157] In theory, the antiproliferative effect caused by the human interferon on human tumor cells growing in a nude mouse could be separated from an indirect effect (activation of host immune-related cells), since interferons are relatively species restricted in their actions on immune-related cells. Compared with studies done in vitro, however, higher doses are generally required to produce a significant regression of these tumors. Significantly, the degree of inhibition of tumor grwoth mediated by IFN-β was less than that seen with ACNU or vincristine chemotherapy.[157] Bradley et al[154] did not observe any growth inhibition of human tumor implants in nude mice treated with 2,000 U of IFN-α/d for periods of up to 23 days.

There have been several reports in the last few years that describe results of clinical trials in which IFN-α or IFN-β was administered to patients with CNS tumors.[157-167] A number of different routes have been used (intramuscularly, intravenously, intrathecally, intratumorally) and, while the numbers of patients have been small, in some instances transient beneficial responses have been reported. Sano et al[159] have reported the largest such study in which 7/42 patients with recurrent anaplastic gliomas, 3/7 medulloblastoma patients, and 2/5 patients with other gliomas had either complete or partial responses lasting at least four weeks. These patients were given between 1 and 6 $\times$ 10^6 units of IFN-α/d for eight weeks either intravenously or intratumorally.

We have previously reported a phase I trial of HuIFN-α given intravenously to patients beginning within three weeks of surgical resection of an anaplastic glioma.[164] These patients received 10 to 30 μ/m^2 on three consecutive days for three weeks and then began conventional radiation therapy. Survival of this small, but relatively uniform, group of patients has been comparable to that of a larger group of matched, historical patients treated with BCNU chemotherapy and radiotherapy.[166] In a recently completed phase II evaluation of IFN-α as a single agent in the treatment of 15 patients with recurrent gliomas, we have observed tumor reduction (by CT scan) in six patients and stabilization of tumor size in a seventh patient.[167] Here, patients received an intense exposure (up to 900×10^6 U/m^2 over an eight-week period) in a treatment plan utilizing both escalating doses and increasing numbers of treatment days per week. Not surprisingly, patients with smaller tumor volumes were more often responders, further indicating the inherent limitations of therapies based on evoking a biologic antitumor response.

IFN-γ offers the possibility of a substantial improvement in this type of therapy for two reasons: it does not produce the same degree of severe neurotoxicity (somnolence, disorientation, memory loss) observed with IFN-α, thus permitting larger doses to be given for longer treatment intervals. Secondly, IFN-γ may be depressed in brain tumor patients. Elliott et al[169] have recently shown that brain tumor patients' T lymphocytes are defective in the amount of interleukin-2 (T cell growth factor; IL-2) that they can produce. This fact, coupled with the critical role that IL-2 has in regulation of IFN-γ synthesis by human T lymphocytes,[170] would suggest that IFN-γ replacement may serve to circumvent the IL-2 defect. Since IFN-γ specifically triggers activation of mononuclear phagocytes, this treatment may improve the patients' general immune status and, hopefully, their antitumor defenses.

The use of IL-2 as another agent in the Biological Response Modifier armamentarium is gaining support. Although there have been no reports of its therapeutic use in patients with brain tumors, it has been used clinically in patients with other malignancies and in AIDS patients.[171] The theoretical value of IL-2 can be outlined as follows. First, it has been shown that peripheral blood lymphocytes from cancer patients can be stimulated to proliferate in vitro in response to autologous or allogeneic tumor cells or to mitogenic plant lectins (con-A or PHA). If an appropriate amount of IL-2 is present, there is a rapid proliferation of various lymphoid cells, including T lymphocytes, B lymphocytes, and NK cells. T lymphocytes so activated in culture have been shown to have antitumor activity in vitro. At a recent meeting in Bethesda to review the past and future uses of IL-2, a number of anecdotal reports of tumor regression achieved with intralesional or systemic administration of IL-2 that activated patients' lymphocytes was reported.[171] Once the T cells have proliferated, continued growth is highly dependent on IL-2. Starting with 10^5 T lymphocytes, it has been possible to expand these cells to 10^8 cells in a matter of 30 days.[172] The possibility of returning these activated T lymphocytes (or NK cells) back to the patient has been demonstrated.[171] However, without a continued source of IL-2 in vivo, the T lymphocytes quickly revert to their typical quiescent state. This leads to the second proposed use of IL-2 in cancer patients; administering IL-2 systemically in concert with the autoadoptive return of the patients' own in vitro stimulated lymphocytes to maintain their activity for prolonged periods. Alternatively, IL-2 has been given to cancer patients directly in an effort to compensate for a perceived deficit in T lymphocyte activity stemming from an inability to produce sufficient amounts of IL-2 endogenously.[171] This latter treatment may be of special importance to patients with brain tumors in light of the observations of Elliott et al[169] that there appears to be some defect in IL-2 production by lymphocytes from these patients.

FUTURE PROSPECTS FOR IMMUNOTHERAPY

The future of immunotherapy in the management of patients with anaplastic gliomas remains to be defined; however, multimodality approaches combining radiotherapy, chemotherapy, immunotherapy, and biological response modifier therapy have a strong theoretical appeal. Currently much work needs to be done exploring the basic questions involved in this field. It will continue to be important to monitor the immunologic status of glioma patients. Much useful immunological data are now being acquired in current studies that would help to understand the host-tumor interaction and how to optimize this form of therapy.

The rapid evolution of monoclonal antibody technology will soon provide the opportunity for utilization of these antibodies as reagents in neurodiagnostic studies and perhaps as therapeutic agents directly or as carriers of cytotoxic packages in the form of radioactivity or a drug toxic to neoplastic brain cells. Attachment of polyhedral boron to monoclonal antiglioma antibodies may be a means of enhancing radiotherapeutics.[173] With other forms of cancer, tumor cell-specific cytotoxic response has been obtained by the selective uptake of hematoporphyrin derivatives by tumor cells and subsequent activation with selective laser-delivered light.[174] The ability to bind such agents to MA with highly selective delivery and activation is a fertile area for future research.

Autoadoptive immunotherapy using the patient's own peripheral blood mononuclear leukocytes awaits the refinement of techniques to activate, clone, and expand antiglioma effector cells specifically so that they can be safely transferred back to the patient. Systemic versus intratumoral administration of these antitumor cells will need to be compared for risk-benefit ratio.

While there is much yet to be learned and a great deal to be gained in the management of patients with anaplastic gliomas using immunobiological approaches, this arena of clinical and scientific endeavor is evolving quickly. Scientific pursuit of these potentially useful modalities for therapeutic intervention should yield a more thorough understanding of the immunobiology of neoplasia within the CNS.

ACKNOWLEDGMENT

We would like to thank Mrs Rose Hagan and Mrs Karen Vann for their editorial assistance in helping prepare this manuscript.

REFERENCES

1. Walker MD, Green SB, Byar DP, et al: Randomized comparisons of radiotherapy and nitrosoureas for the treatment of malignant glioma after surgery. N Engl J Med 303:1323–1329, 1980

2. Shapiro WR: Treatment of neuroectodermal brain tumors. Ann Neurol 12:231–237, 1982

3. Burger PC, Vogel FS: Surgical Pathology of the Nervous System and Its Coverings (2nd ed). New York, John Wiley, 1982

4. Bigner DD, Bigner SH, Ponten J, et al: Heterogeneity of genotypic and phenotypic characteristics of fifteen permanent cell lines derived from human gliomas. J Neuropath Exp Neurol 40:201–229, 1981

5. Bigner SH, Bullard DE, Pegram CN, et al: Relationship of in vitro morphologic and growth characteristics of established human glioma-derived cell lines to their tumorigenicity in athymic nude mice. J Neuropath Exp Neurol 40:390–409, 1981

6. Bigner DD, Schold C, Bigner SH, et al: How heterogeneous are gliomas? Cancer Treat Reps 65:45–49, 1981

7. Bigner DD: Biology of gliomas: potential clinical implications of glioma cellular heterogeneity. Neurosurgery 9:320–326, 1981

8. Bigner SH, Burger PC, Mark J, et al: Relationship between karotype and histologic parameters of malignant human gliomas (MHG). J Neuropath Exp Neurol 43:335, 1984 (abstr)

9. Bullard DE, Schold SC, Bigner SH, et al: Growth and chemotherapeutic response in athymic mice of tumors arising from human glioma-derived cell lines. J Neuropath Exp Neurol 40:410–427, 1981

10. Shapiro JR, Yung W-KA, Shapiro WR: Isolation, karyotype, and clonal growth of heterogeneous subpopulations of human malignant gliomas. Cancer Res 41:2349–2359, 1981

11. Ridley A, Cavanagh JB: Lymphocytic infiltration in gliomas: Evidence of possible host resistance. Brain 94:117–124, 1971

12. Paul WE: Fundamental Immunology. New York, Raven Press, 1984

13. Evans RL, Wall DW, Platsoucas CD, et al: Thymus-dependent membrane antigens in man: Inhibition of cell-mediated lympholysis by monoclonal antibodies to T_{H2} antigen. Proc Natl Acad Sci USA 78:544–548, 1981

14. Reinherz EL, Schlossman SF: The differentiation and function of human T lymphocytes. Cell 19:821–827, 1980

15. Siegal FP, Rambotti P, Siegal M, et al: Helper cell function of leukemic Leu-2a+, histamine receptor+, $T\gamma$ lymphocytes. J Immunol 129:1775–1781, 1982

16. Thomas Y, Rogozinski L, Irigoyen OH, et al: Functional analysis of human T cell subsets defined by monoclonal antibodies. V. Suppressor cells within the activated OKT4+ population belong to a distinct subset. J Immunol 128:1386–1390, 1982

17. Brooks WH, Netsky MG, Normansell DE, et al: Depressed cell-mediated immunity in patients with primary intracranial tumors. Characterization of a humoral immunosuppressive factor. J Exp Med 136:1631–1647, 1972

18. Brooks WH, Caldwell HD, Mortara RH: Immune responses in patients with gliomas. Surg Neurol 2:419–423, 1974

19. Mahaley MS Jr, Brooks WH, Roszman TL, et al: Immunobiology of primary intracranial tumors. I. Studies of the cellular and humoral general immune competence of brain tumor patients. J Neurosurg 46:467–476, 1977

20. Thomas DGT, Lannigan CB, Behan PO: Impaired cell-mediated immunity in human brain tumours. Lancet 1:1389, 1975

21. Young HF, Sakalas R, Kaplan AM: Inhibition of cell-mediated immunity in patients with brain tumors. Surg Neurol 5:19–23, 1976

22. Brooks WH, Roszman TL, Rogers AS: Impairment of rosette-forming T lymphocytes in patients with primary intracranial tumors. Cancer 37:1869–1873, 1976

23. Braun DP, Penn RD, Flannery AM, et al: Immunoregulatory cell function in peripheral blood leukocytes of patients with intracranial gliomas. Neurosurgery 10:203–209, 1982

24. Braun DP, Penn RD, Harris JE: Regulation of natural killer cell function by glass-adherent cells in patients with

primary intracranial malignancies. Neurosurgery 15:29–33, 1984

25. Brooks WH, Latta RB, Mahaley MS, et al: Immunobiology of primary intracranial tumors. Part 5: Correlation of a lymphocyte index and clinical status. J Neurosurg 54:331–337, 1981

26. Fontana A, Kristensen F, Dubs R, et al: Production of prostaglandin E and an interleukin-1 like factor by cultured astrocytes and C_6 glioma cells. J Immunol 129:2413–2419, 1982

27. Fontana A, McAdam KP, Kristensen F, et al: Biological and biochemical characterization of an interleukein-1 like factor from rat C6 glioma cells. Eur J Immunol 13:685–689, 1983

28. Fontana A, Hengartner H, de Tribolet N, et al: Glioblastoma cells release interleukin 1 and factors inhibiting interleukin 2-mediated effects. J Immunol 132:1837–1844, 1984

29. Weiss JF, Morantz RA, Bradley WP, et al: Serum acute-phase proteins and immunoglobulins in patients with gliomas. Cancer Res 39:542–544, 1979

30. Mahaley MS Jr, Gillespie GY: Immunologic considerations of patients with brian tumors, in Walker MD (ed): Oncology of the Nervous System. Boston, Martinus Nijhoff, 1983, pp 151–165

31. Woosley RE, Mahaley MS Jr, Mahaley JL, et al: Immunobiology of primary intracranial tumors. Part 3. Microcytotoxicity assays of specific immune responses of brain tumor patients. J Neurosurg 47:871–875, 1977

32. de Tribolet N, Martin-Achard A, Louis JA: Circulating immune complexes in patients with gliomas. Acta Neurochir Suppl 28:473–474, 1979

33. Martin-Achard A, de Tribolet N, Louis JA, et al: Immune complexes associated with brain tumors: Correlation with prognosis. Surg Neurol 13:161–163, 1980

34. Bertrand J, Mannen H: Etude des reactions vascularies dans les astrocytomes. Revue Neurologique 102:3–19, 1960

35. Apuzzo MLJ, Mitchell MS: Immunological aspects of intrinsic glial tumors. J Neurosurg 55:1–18, 1981

36. Brooks WH, Markesbery WR, Gupta GD, et al: Relationship of lymphocyte invasion and survival of brain tumor patients. Ann Neurol 4:219–224, 1978

37. Maunoury R, Vedrene C, Constans JP: Infiltrations lymphocytaires dans les gliomes humains. Neuro-Chirurgie 21:213–222, 1975

38. Palma L, DiLorenzo N, Guidetti B: Lymphocytic infiltrates in primary glioblastomas and recidivous gliomas. Incidence, fate, and relevance to prognosis in 228 operated cases. J Neurosurg 49:854–861, 1978

39. Phillips JP, Eremin O, Anderson JR: Lymphoreticular cells in human brain tumours and in normal brain. Br J Cancer 45:61–69, 1982

40. Stavrou D, Anzil AP, Weidenbach W, et al: Immunofluorescence study of lymphocytic infiltration in gliomas. Identification of T-lymphocytes. J Neurol Sci 33:275–282, 1977

41. Takeuchi J, Barnard RO: Perivascular lymphocytic cuffing in astrocytomas. Acta Neuropathol 35:265–271, 1976

42. von Hanwehr RI, Hofman FM, Taylor CT, et al: Mononuclear lymphoid populations infiltrating the microenvironment of primary CNS tumor. Characterization of cell subsets with monoclonal antibodies. J Neurosurg 60:1138–1147, 1984

43. Wood GW, Morantz RA: Immunohistologic evaluation of the lymphoreticular infiltrate of human central nervous system tumors. J Natl Cancer Inst 62:485–491, 1979

44. Wood GW, Morantz RA, Tilzer SA, et al: Immunoglobulin bound in vivo to Fc receptor-positive cells in human central nervous system tumors. J Natl Cancer Int 64:411–418, 1980

45. Kaszubowski PA, Husby G, Tung KSK, et al: T-lymphocyte subpopulations in peripheral blood and tissues of cancer patients. Cancer Res 40:4648–4657, 1980

46. Hitchcock MH, Hollinshead AC, Chretien P, et al: Soluble membrane antigens of brain tumors. I. Controlled testing for cell-mediated immune responses in a long surviving glioblastoma multiforme patient. Cancer 40:660–666, 1977

47. Levy NL: Specificity of lymphocyte-mediated cytotoxicity in patients with primary intracranial tumors. J Immunol 121:903–915, 1978

48. Levy NL: Cell-mediated cytotoxicity and serum-mediated blocking: Evidence that their associated determinants on human tumor cells are different. J Immunol 121:916–922, 1978

49. Sheikh KMA, Apuzzo MLJ, Weiss MH: Specific cellular immune responses in patients with malignant gliomas. Cancer Res 39:1733–1738, 1979

50. Febvre H, Maunoury R, Constans JP, et al: Reactions d'hypersensibilite retardee avec des lignees de cellules tumorales humaines cultivees in vitro chez des marlades porteurs de tumeurs cerebrales malignes. Int J Cancer 10:221–232, 1972

51. Trouillas P: Immunologie des tumeurs cerebrales. L'antigene carcino-foetal glial. Ann Inst Pasteur 122:819–828, 1972

52. Ciembroniewicz J, Oldrich K: Tissue culture study of glioblastoma cells with addition of autologous lymphocytes. Acta Cytol 13:42–47, 1969

53. Eggers AE: Autoradiographic and fluorescence antibody studies of the human host immune response to gliomas. Neurology 22:246–250, 1972

54. Wahlstrom T: Sensitivity to normal brain antigens of blood lymphocytes from patients with gliomas. Acta Path Microbiol Scand 81B:763–767, 1973

55. Wahlstrom T, Saksela E, Troupp H: Cell-bound antiglial immunity in patients with malignant tumors of the brain. Cell Immunol 6:161–170, 1973

56. Kumar S, Taylor G, Steward JK, et al: Cell-mediated immunity and blocking factors in patients with tumours of the central nervous system. Int J Cancer 12:194–205, 1973

57. Kornblith PL, Prieto A Jr, Pollen DA: Alterations in glial and mesenchymal tumor cell membrane resistance with heteroimmune and autologous sera. Ann NY Acad Sci 159:585–590, 1969

58. Mitts MG, Walker AE: Autoimmune response to malignant glial tumors. Preliminary observations. Neurology 15:474–476, 1965

59. Kronblith PL, Dohan FC Jr, Wood W, et al: Human

astocytomas: Serum-mediated immunologic response. Cancer 33:1512–1519, 1974

60. Phillips JP, Sujatanond M, Martuza RL, et al: Cytotoxic antibodies in preoperative glioma patients: A diagnostic assay. Acta Neurochirurg 35:43–52, 1976

61. Quindlen EA, Dohan FC Jr, Kornblith PL: Improved assay for cytotoxic antiglioma antibody. Surg Forum 25:464–466, 1974

62. Pfreundschuh M, Shiku H, Takahashi T, et al: Serological analysis of cell surface antigens of malignant human brain tumors. Proc Natl Acad Sci 75:5122–5126, 1978

63. Martin-Achard A, Diserens A-C, de Tribolet N, et al: Recherche d'anticorps anti-tumeur antibodies dans les serums de malades atteints de gliomes. Schweiz Med Wochenschr 108:959–962, 1978

64. Tabuchi K, Kirsch WM: Detection of IgG on glioblastoma cell surface in vivo. Acta Neurochir 43:93–100, 1978

65. Aarli JA, Aparicio SR, Lumsden CE, et al: Binding of normal human IgG to myelin sheaths, glia and neurons. Immunology 28:171–185, 1975

66. Mahaley MS Jr, Day ED: Immunological studies of human gliomas. J Neurosurg 23:363–370, 1965

67. Mahaley MS Jr: Experiences with antibody production from human glioma tissue. Prog Exp Tumor Res 17:31–39, 1972

68. Coakham H: Surface antigen(s) common to human astrocytoma cells. Nature 250:328–330, 1974

69. Coakham HB, Lakshmi MS: Tumour-associated antigen(s) in human astrocytomas. Oncology 31:233–243, 1975

70. Wahlstrom T, Linder E, Saksela E, et al: Tumor-specific membrane antigens in established cell lines from glioma. Cancer 34:274–279, 1974

71. Miyake E, Kitamura K, Nomoto K, et al: An attempt to detect cell surface antigens in cultured human brain tumors by mixed hemadsorption test. (First Report) Acta Neuropathol (Berl) 37:27–29, 1977

72. Sato K, Raimondi AJ, Dray S, et al: Comparison of tumor-associated surface antigens on cells from medulloblastomas and from other neoplasms of the human nervous system. Childs Brain 4:83–94, 1978

73. Kehayov IR: Tumour-associated water soluble antigen(s) in human glioblastoma demonstrated by immunodiffusion and immunoelectrophoresis. Ann Immunol 127C:703–716, 1976

74. Wikstrand CJ, Bigner DD: Surface antigens of human glioma cells shared with normal adult and fetal brain. Cancer Res 39:3235–3243, 1979

75. Bonnin JM, Rubinstein LJ: Immunohistochemistry of central nervous system tumors. Its contribution to neurosurgical diagnosis. J Neurosurgery 60:1121–1133, 1984

76. Bourdon MA, Coleman RE, Bigner DD: The potential of monoclonal antibodies as carriers of radiation in drugs for immunodetection and therapy of brain tumors. Prog Exp Tumor Res 28:79–101, 1984

77. Carrell S, Schreyer M, deTribolet N, et al: Lymphoid associated differentiation antigens expressed by normal and malignant brain cells. Proc First Monoclonal Antibody to CNS Antigens Workshop, March 31, 1984, Lausanne, Switzerland (in press)

78. deTribolet N, deMuralt B, Diserens AC, et al: Reactivity spectrum of monoclonal antibodies to human gliomas. Proc First Monoclonal Antibody to CNS Antigens Workshop, March 31, 1982, Lausanne, Switzerland (in press)

79. Eisenbarth GS, Jackson RA: Application of monoclonal antibody techniques to endocrinology. Endocrine Reviews 3:26–39, 1982

80. Grahmann FC, Wikstrand CJ, Bigner DD: Human glioma-associated antigens defined by monoclonal antibodies, in Spreafico F (ed): Proc First International Congress Neuroimmunology. New York, Raven Press

81. McComb RD, Wikstrand CJ, Bourdon MA, et al: Antigenic heterogeneity of human malignant gliomas (MGs) demonstrated by reactivity with 10 monoclonal antibodies (MeAs). J Neuropathol Exp Neurol 42:308, 1983 (abstr)

82. McComb RD, Jones TR, Pizzo SV, et al: Localization of Factor VIII/von Willebrand Factor and glial fibrillary acidic protein in the hemangioblastoma: Implications for stromal cell histogenesis. Acta Neuropathol (Berl) 56:207–213, 1982

83. McKay R, Raff MC, Reichardt LF: Proceedings of a Workshop on Monoclonal Antibodies Against Neural Antigens. Cold Spring Harper Reports, Neuroscience 2:1, 1981

84. Schnegg JF, Diserens AC, Carrel S, et al: Human glioma associated antigens detected by monoclonal antibodies. Cancer Res 41:1209–1213, 1981

85. Sears HF, Atkinson B, Mattis J, et al: Phase I clinical trial of monoclonal antibody in treatment of gastrointestinal tumours. Lancet 1:762–765, 1982

86. Sears HF, Herlyn D, Herlyn M, et al: Ex vivo perfusion of human colon with monoclonal anticolorectal cancer antibodies. Cancer 49:1231–1235, 1982

87. Wikstrand CJ, Bigner DD: Expression of human fetal brain antigens by human tumors of neuroectodermal origin as defined by monoclonal antibodies. Cancer Res 42:267–275, 1982

88. Wikstrand CJ, Bourdon MA, Pegram CN, et al: Human fetal brain antigen expression common to tumors of neuroectodermal origin: Gliomas, neuroblastomas, and melanomas. J Immunol 3:43–62, 1982

89. Wikstrand CJ, Bigner SH, Bigner DD: Demonstration of complex antigenic heterogeneity in a human glioma cell line and eight derived clones by specific monoclonal antibodies. Cancer Res 43:3327–3334, 1983

90. DeArmond SJ, Eng LF, Rubinstein LJ: The application of glial fibrillary acidic (GFA) protein immunohistochemistry in neurooncology. A progress report. Pathol Res Pract 168:374–394, 1980

91. Deck JHN, Eng LF, Bigbee J, et al: The role of glial fibrillary acidic protein in the diagnosis of central nervous system tumors. Acta Neuropathol (Berl) 42:183–190, 1978

92. Duffy PE, Huang Y-Y, Rapoport MM: Glial fibrillary acidic protein in giant cell tumors of brain and other gliomas. A possible relationship to malignancy, differentiation, and pleomorphism of glia. Acta Neuropathol (Berl) 52:51–57, 1980

93. Eng LF, Bigbee JW: Immunohistochemistry of the nervous system-specific antigens, in Agranoff BW, Aprison MH (eds): Advances in Neurochemistry. New York, Plenum Press, 1978, pp 43–97

94. Eng LF, Rubinstein LJ: Contribution of immunohistochemistry to diagnostic problems of human cerebral tumors. J Histochem Cytochem 26:513–522, 1978

95. Bonnin JM, Pena CE, Rubinstein LJ: Mixed capillary hemangioblastoma and glioma. A redefinition of the "angioglioma." J Neuropathol Exp Neurol 42:504–516, 1983

96. Deck JHN, Rubinstein LJ: Glial fibrillary acidic protein in stromal cells of some capillary hemangioblastomas: Significance and possible implications of an immunoperoxidase study. Acta Neuropathol (Berl) 54:173–181, 1981

97. Rubinstein LH: Diagnostic applicability of GFA protein immunoperoxidase staining, in Supplement to Tumors of the Central Nervous System, Atlas of Tumor Pathology, Series 2, Fascicle 6. Washington, DC, Armed Forces Institute of Pathology, 1982, pp S21–30

98. Bluestein HG, Zvaifler NJ: Brain-reactive lymphocytotoxic antibodies in the serum of patients with systemic lupus erythematosus. J Clin Invest 57:509–516, 1976

99. Carrel SN, deTribolet N, Gross N: Expression of HLA-DR and common acute lymphoblastic leukemia antigens on glioma cells. Eur J Immunol 12:354–357, 1982

100. Lampson LA: Potential of monoclonal antibodies as tools for the study of human neuroblastoma. Prog Cancer Res Ther 12:221–226, 1980

101. Mitchell KF, Fuhrer JP, Steplewski Z, et al: Structural characterization of the 'melanoma-specific' antigen detected by monoclonal antibody 69115 Nu-4-B. Mol Immunol 18:207–218, 1981

102. Mitchell KF, Fuhrer JP, Steplewski Z, et al: Biochemical characterization of human melanoma cell surfaces: Dissection with monoclonal antibodies. Proc Natl Acad Sci 77:7287–7291, 1980

103. Natali PG, DeMartino C, Quaranta V, et al: Expression of Ia-like antigens in normal human nonlymphoid tissues. Transplantation 31:75–78, 1981

104. Seeger RC, Danon YL, Rayner SA, et al: Definition of a Thy-1 determinant on human neuroblastoma, glioma, sarcoma, and teratoma cells with a monoclonal antibody. J Immunol 128:983–989, 1982

105. Kennett RH, Gilbert F: Hybrid myelomas producing antibodies against a human neuroblastoma antigen present on fetal brain. Science 203:1120–1121, 1979

106. Kirch ME, Hammerling U: Immunotherapy of murine leukemias by monoclonal antibody. I. Effect of passively administered antibody on growth of transplanted tumor cells. J Immunol 127:805–810, 1981

107. Dippold WG, Lloyd KO, Li LTC, et al: Cell surface antigens of human malignant melanoma: Definition of six antigenic systems with mouse monoclonal antibodies. Proc Natl Acad Sci 77:6114–6118, 1980

108. Seeger RC, Siegel SE, Sidell N: Neuroblastoma: Clinical perspectives, monoclonal antibodies, and retinoic acid. Ann Int Med 97:873–884, 1982

109. Brown JP, Nishiyama K, Hellstrom I, et al: Structural characterization of human melanoma-associated antigen p97 with monoclonal antibodies. J Immunol 127:539–546, 1981

110. Liao S-K, Clarke BJ, Kwong PC, et al: Common neuroectodermal antigens on human melanoma, neuroblastoma, retinoblastoma, glioblastoma, and fetal brain revealed by hybridoma antibodies raised against melanoma cells. Eur J Immunol 11:450–454, 1981

111. Saxton RE, Torbett B, Nestor M, et al: Four distinct melanoma cell surface antigens defined by monoclonal antibodies. Proc Amer Assn Cancer Res 24:226, 1983 (abstr)

112. Schafer W, Schwarz H, Thiel H-J, et al: Properties of mouse leukemia viruses. XIII. Serum therapy of virus-induced murine leukemia. Virology 75:401–418, 1976

113. Sikora K, Alderson T, Phillips J, et al: Human hybridomas from malignant gliomas. Lancet 1:11–14, 1982

114. Stavrou D, Suss C, Bilzer T, et al: Monoclonal antibodies reactive with glioma cell lines derived from experimental brain tumors. Eur J Cancer Clin Oncol 19:1439–1449, 1983

115. Lee FH, Hwang KM: Antibodies as specific carriers for chemotherapeutic agents. Cancer Chemother Pharmacol 3:17–24, 1979

116. DeCarvalho S, Kaufman A, Pineda A: Adjuvant chemo-immunotherapy in central nervous system tumors, in Salmon SE, Josen SE (eds): Adjuvant Therapy of Cancer. Amsterdam, Elsevier/North Holland, 1977, pp 495–502

117. Selker RG, Wolmark N, Fisher B, et al: Preliminary observations on the use of corynebacterium parvum in patients with primary intracranial tumors: Effect on intracranial pressure. J Surg Oncol 10:299–303, 1978

118. Mahaley MS Jr, Steinbok P, Aronin P, et al: Immunobiology of primary intracranial tumors. V. Levamisole as an immune stimulant in patients and in the ASV glioma model. J Neurosurg 54:220–227, 1981

119. Trouillas P, Lapras CL: Immunotherapie active des tumeurs cerebrales. A propos de 20 cas. Neuro-Chirurgie 16:143–170, 1970

120. Takakura K, Miki Y, Kubo O, et al: Adjuvant immunotherapy for malignant brain tumors. Jap J Clin Oncol 12:109–120, 1972

121. Young HF, Kaplan AM, Regelson W: Immunotherapy with autologous white cell infusions ('lymphocytes') in the treatment of recurrent glioblastoma multiforme. A preliminary report. Cancer 40:1037–1044, 1977

122. Takakura K, Miki Y, Kubo O: Adjuvant immunotherapy for malignant brain tumors in infants and children. Childs Brain 1:141–147, 1975

123. Neuwelt EA, Clark K, Kirkpatrick JB, et al: Clinical studies of intrathecal autologous lymphocyte infusions in patients with malignant glioma: A toxicity study. Ann Neurol 4:307–312, 1978

124. Shearer WT, Turnbaugh TR, Coleman WE, et al: Cytotoxicity with antibody-glucose oxidase conjugates specific for a human colonic cancer and carcinoembryonic antigen. Int J Cancer 14:539–547, 1974

125. Bullard DE, Bourdon M, Bigner DD: Comparison of various methods for delivering radiolabeled monoclonal antibody to normal rat brain. J Neurosurgery, 1984 (in press)

126. Iglehart JD, Weinhold KJ, Ward EC, et al: Prospects for the immunological management of lethal tumors. Cancer Invest 1:409–421, 1983

127. Kobayashi H, Sendo F: Immunogenecity of viable xenogenized tumor cells, in Kobayashi H (ed): Gann Monograph on Cancer Research No. 23. Immunological Xenogenization of Tumor Cells. Baltimore, University Park Press, 1979, pp 27–39

128. Schafer W, Bolognesi DP: Mammalian C-type oncornaviruses; relationship between viral structure and cell surface antigens and their possible significance, in immuno-

logical defense mechanisms, in Rapp F, Hanna MG (eds): Contemporary Topics in Immunology. New York, Plenum Press, 1977, pp 127–167

129. Hunsmann G, Moenning V, Schafer W: Properties of mouse leukemia viruses. IX. Active and passive immunization of mice against Friend leukemia with isolated viral GP_{71} and its corresponding antiserum. Virol 66:327–329, 1979

130. De Noronha F, Baggs R: Prevention of oncornavirus-induced sarcomas in cats in treatment with antiviral antibodies. Nature 267:54–56, 1977

131. Kobayashi H, Sendo F, Shirai T, et al: Modification in growth of transplantable rat tumors exposed to Friend virus. J Natl Cancer Inst 42:413–419, 1969

132. Kuzumaki N, Klein G: Increased immunogenecity of rat tumors after superinfection with indogenous murine C-type viruses, in Kobayashi H (ed): GANN Monograph on Cancer Research #23. Immunological Xenogenization of Tumor Cells. Tokyo, Japan Scientific Society's Press, 1979, pp 41–45

133. Barbieri D, Belehradek J Jr, Barski G: Decrease in tumor-producing capacity of mouse cell lines following infection with mouse leukemia viruses. Int J Cancer 7:364–371, 1971

134. Greenberger JS, Aaronson SA: In vivo inoculation of RNA C-type viruses inducing regression of experimental solid tumors. J Natl Cancer Inst 51:1935–1938, 1973

135. Kodama T, Kato H, Gotohda E, et al: Regression of established tumors in rats by injection of diethylaminoethyl-dextran and Friend murine leukemia virus. J Natl Cancer Inst 61:403–406, 1978

136. Stuhlmiller GM, Sullivan DC, Vervaert CE, et al: In vivo tumor localization using tumor-specific monkey xenoantibody, alloantibody, and murine monoclonal xenoantibody. Ann Surg 194:592–601, 1981

137. Miller RA, Maloney DG, Warnke R, et al: Treatment of B-cell lymphoma with monoclonal anti-idiotype antibody. New Engl J Med 306:517–522, 1982

138. Nadler LM, Stashenko P, Hardy R, et al: Serotherapy of a patient with a monoclonal antibody directed against a human lymphoma-associated antigen. Cancer Res 40:3147–3154, 1980

139. Bloom WH, Carstaris KC, Crompton MR, et al: Autologous glioma transplantation. Lancet 2:77–78, 1960

140. Grace JT, Jr, Perese DM, Metzgar RS, et al: Tumor autograft responses in patients with glioblastoma multiforme. J Neurosurg 18:159–167, 1961

141. Bloom HJG, Peckham MJ, Richardson AE, et al: Glioblastoma multiforme: A controlled trial to assess the value of specific active immunotherapy in patients treated by radical surgery and radiotherapy. Brit J Cancer 27:253–267, 1973

142. Trouillas P: Immunologie et immunotherapie des tumeurs cerebrales. Revue Neurologique 128:23–38, 1973

143. Mahaley MS Jr, Bigner DD, Dudka LF, et al: Immunobiology of primary intracranial tumors. Part 7: Active immunization of patients with anaplastic human glioma cells: A pilot study. J Neurosurg 59:201–207, 1983

144. Mahaley MS, Gillespie GY, Gillespie RP, et al: Immunobiology of primary intracranial tumors. Part 8: Serological responses to active immunization of patients with anaplastic gliomas. J Neurosurg 59:208–216, 1983

145. Bullard DE, Darling JL, Bigner DD, et al: Specific active immunotherapy with tissue-cultured HLA mismatched human glioma cell in malignant cerebral gliomas. J Neurol Neurosurg Phych 45:946, 1982 (abstr)

146. Bullard DE, Thomas DGT, Darling J, et al: A preliminary study utilizing viable HLA mismatched cultured glioma cells as adjuvant therapy for patients with malignant gliomas. (submitted)

147. Stewart WE: Interferon nomenclature. J Interferon Res 1:6–7, 1980

148. Slimmer S, Masui H, Kaplan NO: Antiproliferative assay for human interferon. Method Enzymol 79:419–422, 1981

149. Lundblad D, Lundblad E: Block of a glioma cell line in S by interferon. Int J Cancer 27:749–754, 1981

150. Wakabayashi T, Yoshida J, Kobayashi T, et al: Effect of interferon on malignant brain tumor. Gan To Kagaku Ryoho 9:1400–1406, 1982

151. Korosue K, Takeshita I, Mannoji H, et al: Interferon effects on multiplication, cytoplasmic protein and GFAP content, and morphology in human glioma cells. J Neuro-Oncol 1:69–76, 1983

152. Cook AW, Carter WA, Nidzgorski F, et al: Human brain tumor-derived cell lines: growth rate reduced by human fibroblast interferon. Science 219:881, 1983

153. Nederman T, Benediktsson G: Effects of interferon on growth rate and radiation sensitivity of cultured, human glioma cells. Acta Radiologica Oncol 21:231–234, 1982

154. Bradley NJ, Darling, JL, Oktar N, et al: The failure of human keukocyte interferon to influence the growth of human glioma cell populations: In vitro and in vivo studies. Brit J Cancer 48:819–825, 1983

155. Bogdahn U: Chemosensitivity of malignant brain tumors. J Neuro-Oncol 1:149–166, 1983

156. Tanaka N, Nagao S, Togho A, et al: Effects of human fibroblast interferon on human gliomas transplanted into nude mice. Gann 74:308–316, 1983

157. Nakamura O, Teramoto A, Yamamoto H, et al: Effect of human fibroblast interferon on malignant brain tumors. No To Shinkei 35:905–911, 1983

158. Salford LG, Stromblad LG, Nordstrom CH, et al: Intratumoral administration of interferon in malignant gliomas. Acta Neurochir 56:30, 1981

159. Sano K, Nagai M, Takakura K, et al: Effects of HUIFN-β on gliomas. Third Annual International Congress for Interferon Research, Miami, Fla, November 1, 1982, abstr

160. Nagai M, Arai T: Interferon therapy for malignant brain tumors: Present and future. No Shinkei Geka 10:463–476, 1982

161. Nagai M, Arai T, Kohno S, et al: Current status of interferon therapy on malignant brain tumor. Gan No Rinsho 29:608–615, 1983

162. Hirakawa K, Ueda S, Nakagawa Y, et al: Effect of human leukocyte interferon on malignant brain tumors. Cancer 51:1976–1981, 1983

163. Nakagawa Y, Hirakawa K, Ueda S, et al: Local administration of interferon for malignant brain tumors. Cancer Treat Rep 67:833–835, 1983

164. Boethius J, Blomgren H, Collins VP, et al: The effect of systemic human interferon-alpha administration to

patients with glioblastoma multiforme. Acta Neurochirurgica 68:239–251, 1983

165. Mahaley MS Jr, Urso MB, Whaley RA, et al: Immunobiology of primary intracranial tumors. IX. Phase I study of human lymphoblastoid interferon. J Biol Resp Mod 3:19–25, 1984

166. Mahaley MS Jr, Urso MB, Whaley RA, et al: Interferon as adjuvant therapy with initial radiotherapy of patients with anaplastic gliomas. J Neurosurg, 1984 (in press)

167. Ueda S, Hirakawa K, Suzuki K, et al: Interferon therapy for brain tumor patients. No Shinkei Geka 10:149–154, 1982

168. Mahaley MS Jr, Urso MB, Whaley RA, et al: Immunobiology of primary intracranial tumors. X. Evaluation of the therapeutic efficacy of interferon in the treatment of recurrent gliomas (in preparation)

169. Elliott LG, Brooks WH, Roszman TL: Cytokinetic basis for the impaired activation of lymphocytes from patients with primary intracranial tumors. J Immunol 132:1208–1215, 1984

170. Reem GH, Yeh NH: Interleukin 2 regulates expression of its receptor and synthesis of gamma interferon by human T lymphocytes. Science 225:429–430, 1984

171. Proceedings of the NIH/Biological Response Modifiers Program Workshop on IL-2, J Biol Resp Mod 3(5), 1984 (in press)

172. Ruscetti FW, Gallo RC: Human T-lymphocyte growth factor: Regulation of growth and function of T lymphocytes. Blood 57:379–394, 1981

173. Barth RF, Johnson CW, Wei WZ, et al: Neutron capture using boronated monoclonal antibody directed against tumor associated antigens. Cancer Detect Prevent 5, 1983 (in press)

174. Hayata Y, Dougherty TJ: Lasers and Hematoprophrin Derivatives in Cancer. New York. Ijaku-Shoin, 1983

Brain Tumors in Children: Current Cooperative and Institutional Chemotherapy Trials in Newly Diagnosed and Recurrent Disease

Jeffrey C. Allen, Julian Bloom, Inta Ertel, Audrey Evans, Denman Hammond, Helen Jones, Victor Levin, Derek Jenkin, Richard Sposto, and William Wara

IN THE PAST 20 years there has been a steady improvement in prognosis in the majority of childhood cancers. This phenomenon is related primarily to the addition of selected chemotherapy regimens to optimum surgical care and radiotherapy. Although survival rates have been slowly increasing due to improved neurosurgical care, radiotherapy, and advances in diagnostic accuracy (CT and MRI), the conventional management and the overall prognosis for children with the majority of primary brain tumors has not improved as dramatically as it has for other childhood cancers. Newer treatment modalities such as chemotherapy have not as yet been incorporated as conventional management.

The reasons for this are complex. Although primary brain tumors collectively are the second most common form of childhood cancer and the most common solid tumors, there are many types of primary malignant childhood brain tumors, each of which is no more common than any particular systemic solid tumor such as neuroblastoma or Ewing's sarcoma. Each requires special management considerations. There are only approximately 250 new cases of medulloblastoma arising in the United States each year and less than half this number of new cases of brainstem glioma and malignant cerebral astrocytoma.[37]

Progress in the field of pediatric neuro-oncology has been delayed in part because large scale disease-specific phase II and III trials have not been conducted until recently. Childhood brain tumors have only recently been the subject of studies of the pediatric cooperative groups, the Children's Cancer Study Group (CSG), the International Society of Pediatric Oncology (SIOP), and the Pediatric Oncology Group (POG).

Nevertheless, over the past 10 years the pace of clinical investigative research has quickened. Summarized below are the results of recent cooperative group phase III trials involving the more common brain tumors such as medulloblastoma, malignant cerebral astrocytoma, and brainstem glioma (Table 1). We are fortunate to have the cooperation and active participation of the leadership of these studies in the preparation of this review. Thereafter, various disease-specific phase II studies in recurrent brain tumors will be reviewed. In addition, some of the new proposals for future institutional and cooperative group trials will be considered.

COOPERATIVE PHASE III TRIALS IN NEWLY DIAGNOSED DISEASE

Medulloblastoma

Medulloblastoma is a type of primitive neuroectodermal tumor usually arising in the roof of the IVth ventricle and the cerebellar vermis. The tumor cells appear uniform with dense carrot-shaped nuclei and scanty cytoplasm. There is usually no particular tissue array, but occasionally Homer-Wright rosettes are evident. In approximately 30% to 40% of cases, there is evidence of differentiation along glial or neuronal lines with focal areas of astrocytoma, ependymoma, or oligodendroglioma.[32] Medulloblastoma is histologically and, in some respects, biologically similar to cerebral hemisphere primitive neuroectodermal tumors and pineoblastoma. These tumors may seed the CNS early in the course of their development and perhaps one in three children, predominantly those under 5 years of age, may have gross metastases in the spinal canal or supratentorial space at diagnosis.[1] Approximately 5% of patients will develop systemic metastases.[22] Contemporary 5-year survival rates for patients of all ages with medullo-

---

From the Children's Cancer Study Group and the International Society of Pediatric Oncology.

Address reprint requests to Jeffrey C. Allen, MD, Memorial Hospital, 1275 York Ave, New York, NY 10021.

0093-7754/86/1301-0011$05.00/0

Table 1. Cooperative Phase III Adjuvant Chemotherapy Trials

Tumor	Cooperative Group	Protocol	Chemotherapy	Dates	Age Limits (yr)	No. of Patients
Medulloblastoma	CSG[18]	942	CCNU, vincristine, prednisone	1975–1981	2–16	232
	POG[12]		MOPP	1979–	1–21	80+
	SIOP[11]		CCNU, vincristine	1975–1979	0–16	276
Cerebral high grade glioma	CSG[17]	943	CCNU, vincristine, prednisone	1976–1981	2–21	63
Brainstem glioma	CSG[21]	944	CCNU, vincristine, prednisone	1977–1980	2–21	69

blastoma who survive operation and who complete radiotherapy approach 50% to 60% with craniospinal radiotherapy alone.[8]

Study Designs

Separate multinstitutional trials for medulloblastoma have been initiated within the past ten years by the Children's Cancer Study Group (CSG),[18] the International Society of Pediatric Oncology (SIOP),[10] and the Pediatric Oncology Group (POG). The CSG has 29 participating institutions; 26 in the USA and 3 in Canada. Its protocols are used to treat over 40% of the 6,000 new cases of childhood cancer diagnosed each year. The POG consists of 38 institutions in the U.S. and Canada. The SIOP group consists of 44 centers from 15 countries primarily in Europe.

As the first series of cooperative studies in childhood primary brain tumors, the main question in the SIOP, CSG, and POG medulloblastoma protocols was whether adjuvant chemotherapy increased disease-free survival (Fig 1). The SIOP and CSG protocols were initiated in 1975 and 1976, and closed for patient accrual after 5 and 6 years, respectively. The data now permit preliminary observations. The POG protocol was opened in 1979 and is still accruing patients.

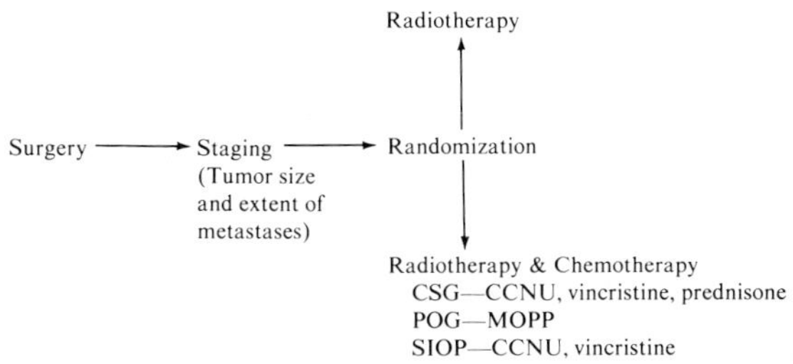

Fig 1. Medulloblastoma cooperative group protocol design.

The CSG and SIOP medulloblastoma protocols had a similar design. This was done intentionally, in hopes of performing intergroup comparisons. However, the two studies also differed in several important respects. The CSG protocol stratified patients at the time of randomization according to a tumor size (T) and metastases (M) staging system designed by Chang.[20] The "T" or tumor stage defined the extent of local growth. There were 4 "T" stages. The "T_1" and "T_2" stages described tumors 3 cm or smaller, which may have invaded adjacent structures but not completely filled the fourth ventricle. The "T_3" and "T_4" stages identified larger tumors that either filled the fourth ventricle, extended up the aqueduct, and/or locally invaded the brainstem, basilar cisterns, or cerebral subarachnoid space.

There were 4 "M" or metastases stages. M_0 was a normal CSF cytology, M_1 represented a CSF cytology containing clumps of medulloblastoma cells, M_2 was widespread supratentorial subarachnoid dissemination now diagnosable by CT scan, M_3 represented gross spinal subarachnoid dissemination as defined by myelography, and M_4 was systemic metastases. The Chang staging system identified a significant correlation between low "T" and "M" stages and a more favorable prognosis.[20]

The CSG 942 protocol committee attempted to reconfirm the importance of the Chang staging system. The CSG neurosurgeons were required to assess the size and invasive nature of the tumor at surgery and designate a T-stage. However, routine postoperative CT scans, myelograms, and bone marrow aspirates were not required, only CSF cytology; therefore, the "T" and "M" stages were not fully evaluated prior to randomization. In the SIOP trial, the medulloblastoma patients were initially stratified by age and sex. The influence of T-stage and brain stem involvement per se were examined later and these patients were not staged with myelograms or CSF cytologies. CSG excluded patients under 2 years, whereas SIOP included all patients under 16.

The nature of the surgical procedure performed in each patient was left to the discretion of the neurosurgeon in both studies. Routine preoperative ventriculo-systemic shunting procedures were discouraged in hopes of reducing the incidence of systemic metastases, and the surgeon was encouraged to remove as much tumor as possible. Following surgery, both the CSG and SIOP surgeons were asked to estimate the extent of resection. This was not confirmed by CT scans since these were not available in the majority of participating institutions when the study was opened.

The treatment regimens were similar but not identical in the CSG and SIOP studies. The control or conventional arm received craniospinal radiotherapy. In both studies the prescribed tumor dose to the posterior fossa was in the range of 5,000 to 5,500 rads administered over 5 to 7 weeks using megavoltage equipment, the cranial dose was 3,500 to 4,000 rads in 5 to 6 weeks, and the spinal dose 3,000 to 3,500 rads in 5 to 6 weeks. Children 3 years and under in the CSG and under 2 years in the SIOP trial had a reduction in radiotherapy dose of approximately 500 rads.

The experimental arm in both protocols included adjuvant chemotherapy (Table 1). Vincristine (1 mg/m^2 during radiation, 1.5 mg/m^2 after radiation—maximum single dose 2 mg) was administered weekly during radiotherapy and then on day 1, 8, and 15 with a 4-week break between cycles for a total of 8 cycles. CCNU (100 mg/m^2) was administered orally every 6 to 7 weeks one month following radiotherapy beginning with the first of the weekly vincristine injections. The CSG but not SIOP added daily prednisone (40 mg/m^2) given daily in 3 divided doses for the first 14 days of each of the postradiation chemotherapy cycles.

The end point of both the CSG and SIOP studies was the time to recurrence or death without recurrence (disease-free survival). In addition to the planned comparison between the chemotherapy and control groups, the CSG and SIOP studies also examined certain other treatment factors such as extent of surgical resection and radiation dose, and disease and host variables such as age, sex, race, pathology, "T" and/or "M" stages, and brain stem involvement.

Results

The complete results of the CSG and SIOP protocols will be published shortly. CSG protocol 942 was opened in 1975 and closed in 1981. There were 233 validated randomized patients in this study. The SIOP study entered 286 fully eligible patients from 1975 to 1979.

All of the survival data are reported as disease-free survival (DFS) or time to first recurrence. This is done because different centers may treat recurrent disease more aggressively than others, possibly obscuring some beneficial effect of the initial treatment regimen if only total survival was to be analyzed.

Pretreatment staging. T-Stage: The T-stage data were grouped into two categories: T_{1+2} and T_{3+4}. In the CSG study there were 78 (34%) patients with T_{1+2} stages and 154 (66%) with T_{3+4} stages. Surprisingly, there was no significant overall difference in DFS between these two groups of "T" stages. For the SIOP study, there were 113 (41%) patients in the T_{1+2} stages and 163 (59%) in the T_{3+4} stages. In this study, the T stage was a very strong prognostic factor with a 28% difference in DFS at 60 months ($P < .001$).

Pretreatment staging. M-Stage: This staging system was only utilized in the CSG study and as stated above, the documentation of the extent of disease at diagnosis was insufficient. For example, myelograms were reported in only 10% of these cases. Since comparisons amongst M_1, M_2, and M_3 stages could not be made because the number of patients in each group was small, the data from these 3 stages were combined (39 patients). The CSG data indicated that the M-stage was a very strong prognostic variable. At 54 months, the DFS was 58.2% for M_0 and 31.8% for M_{1-3} stages ($P < .001$).

Surgery. Total resections were accomplished in 38.5% of CSG patients and 45.5% of SIOP patients. Only 3% of patients in both studies underwent a biopsy only; the remaining patients underwent either a partial or subtotal resection. The extent of resection did not influence DFS in the CSG study but did so in the SIOP study. In the SIOP study, the groups of patients who received either a partial resection or biopsy did significantly less well than patients receiving a total or subtotal resection.

Age and sex. As stated above, CSG restricted entry by age in that patients less than 2 years of age were excluded. SIOP accepted all patients under 16. The age distribution was similar in the two studies. Children aged under 2 years in the SIOP study had a significantly shorter DFS than older patients. Patients in this age group tended to receive a lower dose of radiotherapy in both studies. Both studies showed a greater male incidence; only in the SIOP study was there a difference in survival between the sexes, favoring females.

Treatment regimen. Both the SIOP and CSG studies showed a 10% to 15% advantage in favor of chemotherapy at 54 months. The SIOP data has attained marginal significance at the 5% level, and the CSG data is also marginally significant ($P < .05$) after controlling for the T and M stages. The SIOP and CSG trials achieved a similar standard of DFS in each of the study arms. At 54 months the DFS rates in CCSG were 59% and 49% for test and control groups, respectively, while the corresponding figures for SIOP were 55% and 43%.

The influence of treatment on survival in the various "T" and "M" stage groups was also analyzed. In both studies, patients with locally more extensive tumors (T_{3+4}) benefited from chemotherapy (CSG, $P = .04$; SIOP, $P = .003$). The patients with the smaller primary tumors (T_{1+2}) did not.

Sites of recurrence. The sites of recurrence were compiled in the two studies in those patients who failed therapy. The data are of limited value in that the majority of patients were not completely staged with regard to extent of disease at recurrence. Nevertheless, the data appear to be similar in the two studies. In the CSG study, primary recurrences in the posterior fossa occurred in 55.1% of failed patients whereas 34.6% had initial CNS recurrences outside the posterior fossa. Patients with advanced "M" and "T" stages in the CSG study had a disproportionately higher failure rate in sites outside the posterior fossa.

Radiotherapy. The radiotherapy doses were analyzed in all patients in the two studies, even those who failed to complete the prescribed radiotherapy due to progressive disease. The doses recommended for prophylactic irradiation of brain and spinal cord tended to be lower in the SIOP study compared with CSG. In spite of differences in radiotherapy doses, there were no notable differences in DFS or incidence of disease recurrences outside the posterior fossa between the two studies. These data suggest that a conventional craniospinal dose as great as 3,500 rads may not be necessary in all patients.

Comments on the CSG and SIOP trials

In both studies the overall disease-free survivals at 5 years were in excess of 50%. These data are comparable to those reported in the most optimistic contemporary large institutional experiences[8] and probably represent the upper limit of curability with postoperative megavoltage radiotherapy alone. The chemotherapy of the SIOP study (CCNU and vincristine) added a marginal benefit to DFS at 54 months. This chemotherapy appears to benefit primarily selected groups of high-risk patients—the youngest children, and those with larger or more extensive tumors. Future studies must identify a more effective adjuvant chemotherapy regimen especially for those patients who are less likely to be cured with radiotherapy alone (M_{1-3}) or who are more likely to suffer late effects of radiotherapy (age < 4 years).

Since only T_3 and T_4 cases seemed to benefit to a marginal degree from chemotherapy in both the SIOP and CSG studies, the overall impact of the chemotherapy regimen was limited. It therefore would appear to be premature to offer this type of adjuvant chemotherapy to all newly diagnosed medulloblastoma patients.

In neither the CSG or SIOP studies were patients completely staged prior to therapy. However, patients with some evidence of disseminated disease at diagnosis (M_{1-3}) had a shorter DFS than patients with localized disease (M_0). In a prospective institutional study from Memorial Sloan-Kettering Cancer Center,[1] 30 patients were completely staged prior to therapy. The prognostic significance of an abnormal CSF cytology and/or myelogram was confirmed. All subsequent cooperative medulloblastoma trials should completely stage their patients prior to randomization; the battery of tests should include a CSF cytology, myelogram, post CT scan, and bone marrow aspirate and/or biopsy.

Patients under 4 years appear to have a less favorable prognosis in the CSG study. Other institutional reviews have reported this phenomenon.[1,8] Two factors most likely contribute to this occurrence; the higher incidence of M_{1-3} stages in children under 4 years of age and the planned reduction in radiation dose in children under 3 years.

There appeared to be no correlation between the degree of surgical resection and prognosis in the CSG study. The data were in part flawed by the failure to confirm the surgeon's visual assessment of the degree of surgical resection by a postoperative CT scan. Several other institutional series and the SIOP study have reported a beneficial influence of total resections.[8] Final conclusions must await subsequent studies with CT confirmation. If the surgical management of medulloblastoma is similar to other solid tumors, gross total resections should improve outcome.

The CSG and SIOP cooperative studies have helped to focus the issues for subsequent investigations. Clearly certain host and disease factors have a greater influence on DFS than the chemotherapy. Certain groups of patients (T_{3-4}, M_{1-3}) are more likely to benefit from effective chemotherapy and it is more justifiable to expose these selected high-risk patients to the possible deleterious effects of experimental therapy. Patients with favorable prognostic factors (M_0, T_{1-2}, age > 4) may have a 5-year DFS greater than 60%, and, for these survivors, the greatest concern will be the late effects of treatment.

CSG in conjunction with POG are planning a separate study for the good risk (M_0, T_{1-2}) patients. These patients will be randomized to either the conventional craniospinal dose (3,500 rads in 180 rad daily fractions) or a lower craniospinal dose (2,500 rads) and the posterior fossa dose will be similar in each arm (5,000 rads). The primary area of recurrence in this population is the posterior fossa. Prospective monitoring of psychometric and neuroendocrine function will be performed. Since less than 1/3 of newly diagnosed patients will be eligible for this study by prior CSG data, the combining of CSG and POG patients should allow this study to be completed within six years. SIOP is planning its own study.

For the poor risk (M_{1-3} or T_{3-4}) patients, the CSG proposes to give all patients chemotherapy. The "8 drugs in 1" day[9] protocol will be administered prior to and subsequent to radiotherapy in the experimental arm and the control arm will consist of the chemotherapy arm of the prior CSG study employing CCNU, vincristine, and prednisone. POG will continue with its more recently opened protocol of radiotherapy *v* radiotherapy plus MOPP chemotherapy (mustard, vincristine, prednisone, procarbazine).[12] SIOP is exploring a sandwich chemotherapy protocol including preradiation high-dose intravenous methotrexate with leucovorin rescue, with procarbazine and vincristine for high-risk cases, followed by postradiation CCNU and vincristine.[28]

Given the rarity of medulloblastoma, new treatments can only be validated in a reasonable period of time in multiinstitutional randomized trials. Such protocols must continue to explore the importance of prognostic factors such as age, tumor presentation, and tumor histology or in vitro biology. Single institutions must pilot innovative phase II therapies to identify new treatment alternatives for future phase III cooperative trials.

High Grade Gliomas

Approximately 25% of childhood brain tumors are gliomas of high grade malignancy (malignant astrocytoma and glioblastoma multiforme). These tumors more commonly arise in the cerebral hemispheres (51%), less commonly in the brainstem (37%), and rarely in the cerebellum.[37] Their clinical presentation relates primarily to their size, location, and rapidity of growth. Large infiltrating lesions may cause major shifts in intracranial structures, often with focal deficits and signs of increased intracranial pressure. Focal seizures may be the presenting symptom in over 30% of cerebral glioma cases, especially when the tumor arises in epileptigenic cortical locations in the temporal or frontal lobes.[15] Occasionally, the clinical presentation may mimic that of an intracerebral arterio-venous malformation with a sudden change in sensorium and rapid clinical deterioration as highly malignant tumors may develop spontaneous hemorrhage.[23]

Following conventional radiotherapy, the prognosis for malignant cerebral astrocytomas in children is more hopeful than in adults with about 25% of patients surviving 5 years, but the median survival is less than 20 months.[15] Adjuvant multidrug chemotherapy may improve survival for children[30] as it has for adults with glioblastoma multiforme.

On the basis of this limited survival, the CSG designed a study (CSG 943) for new patients with high grade cerebral astrocytomas to examine the potential benefit of adjuvant chemotherapy in a randomized trial.[17] The drugs and study design were similar to their protocol for medulloblastoma (CSG 942). Although nitrosoureas were known to be active drugs for children with recurrent cerebral astrocytomas,[19] the combination of vincristine, CCNU, and prednisone had not been tried before in any phase II study for this tumor. No other cooperative group has conducted a phase III study with this tumor.

The study was initiated in April 1976, and closed in June 1981, after 63 randomized evaluable patients were accrued with predominantly cerebral malignant astrocytomas—grade 3 (46%) or glioblastomas—grade 4 (42%) were accrued. Maximum surgical debulking was recommended and there was no stratification of patients based on the extent of resection or any other host, disease, or treatment factor. Large focal radiation ports were recommended to a total dose of 5,200 rads in 28 fractions over 5 to 6 weeks for children age 4 to 21 and 4,500 rads in 5 to 6 weeks for children age 2 to 3.

The results of this study indicated that patients receiving adjuvant chemotherapy had a greater DFS than those receiving radiotherapy alone; at 30 months, the DFS was 43.8% for the chemotherapy arm and 21.3% for the radiation therapy only arm. The median DFS for the chemotherapy arm was more than double that of the radiation control (25 *v* 9 months). The treatment differences were still significant when adjustment was made for any imbalance in pathology grade, age, and extent of resection.

The degree of surgical resection also influenced outcome; patients who had a total, subtotal, or partial resection lived longer than those who had a biopsy only. Other variables such as age, sex, conventional pathology grading, and radiation dose and volume did not appear to influence DFS.

The chemotherapy data in this study are very encouraging, especially because of the size of the difference in DFS between the conventional and chemotherapy arms. Previous adult studies in glioblastoma multiforme have also identified a possible treatment advantage to adjuvant chemotherapy with such nitrosoureas as CCNU and BCNU[16] but the results were not nearly so convincing as in the children's study.

Since most children with high grade gliomas are likely to die of recurrent disease, adjuvant chemotherapy may have only postponed the time-to-relapse in the majority of patients. There is still a great need for innovative treatment protocols in this disease. Future CSG protocols for cerebral astrocytoma may include a more aggressive combination chemotherapy regimen such as the "8-in-1"[9] protocol and possibly a combination of external beam and interstitial radiation[7] in selected patients.

Brainstem Glioma

Brainstem gliomas comprise approximately 10% to 15% of primary childhood brain tumors. Although the percentage of patients with histologically verified high grade gliomas in various reported surgical biopsy series is low (16%),[31,26] the majority of patients who die have histologically high grade tumors at autopsy.[27,6] Children with biopsy proven low grade astrocytoma of the brainstem at diagnosis have a better prognosis than those with a high grade histology, but the overall 5-year survival for all patients with this group of tumors is less than 25% and the median survival is less than 1 year.[26] Thus, brainstem glioma appears to be fatal in the majority of children, regardless of the initial histology. Because of its critical location in the brainstem, this tumor is probably the smallest malignant mass to produce such severe morbidity and early demise.

The diagnosis is usually made by clinical criteria only, that is, a history of progressive cranial nerve dysfunction and a gait disorder, a neurologic exam documenting multiple cranial nerve palsies, cerebellar and/or pyramidal tract dysfunction, and a neurodiagnostic study such as a CT or MRI scan identifying an intrinsic brainstem mass. Although mild hydrocephalus is usually present on CT, it is unusual for children to present with symptomatic raised intracranial pressure. Surgical confirmation is usually reserved for those cases with exophytic or cystic lesions or where alternative diagnoses such as an arterio-venous malformation or inflammation are seriously entertained.

Conventional management includes corticosteroids, followed by local, posterior fossa radiation therapy. The child should receive from 5,000 to 5,500 rads in 170 rad daily fractions over 6 to 7 weeks. Although over 50% of children respond to this therapy by clinical and CT criteria, the treatment tends to be palliative. The majority of children develop local recurrences. In one recent study, however, 1/3 of patients had symptoms of meningeal gliomatosis prior to death.[29] Because of the limited efficacy of radiotherapy, adjuvant treatment modalities such as chemotherapy have been investigated.

Before 1977, there was little published experience with single or combination chemotherapy regimens in patients with brainstem gliomas, although it was reported that over 30% of recurrent supratentorial gliomas in adults responded to nitrosoureas.[16]

Over the past 7 years, two multiinstitutional cooperative studies have been conducted by the CSG in patients with brainstem glioma. The first protocol, CSG 944, was a prospective randomized 2 arm study.[21] It was initiated in January 1977, and closed in October 1980, after accruing 69 evaluable patients. Its design was very similar to CSG 942 for medulloblastoma and CSG 944 for malignant glioma. The major study question was to test the potential benefit of adjuvant chemotherapy (CCNU, vincristine, and prednisone) when added to conventional radiotherapy. The eligibility criteria were age 2 to 21 years and a primary tumor arising in the brainstem. Surgical confirmation was not mandatory because of its potential morbidity and the sampling bias provided by the limited amounts of tissue that are usually obtained. Although surgical exploration was performed in 31 patients, tissue sufficient for a histologic diagnosis was available for only 22 patients; 11 patients had astrocytomas and 8 patients had malignant astrocytomas. This study, therefore, included a substantial percentage (42%) of children with high grade tumors than did other reported series.[26,31]

The overall median survival for all patients was 11 months, and there was no significant difference in survival between the two treatment regimens. The 24-month survival rate was 22% for the radiation therapy group and 29% for the radiation therapy and chemotherapy group. The disease-free survival rates were very similar to the total survival rates in that death rapidly followed relapse. The median duration of survival following relapse was 3 months; the retrieval therapies employed, if any, did not significantly prolong life. There was a higher incidence of infectious complications in patients receiving adjuvant chemotherapy (12/35) compared to that with radiotherapy alone (5/33), but there were no fatalities due to infections.

The second multiinstitutional brainstem glioma study conducted by CSG was a single arm pilot study (CSG 904P[24]). Since the historical radiation therapy experience, including the prior CSG protocol 944, was so predictable with a median survival under 12 months, a single arm multiinstitutional study was conducted using historical control data. This pilot study incorporated two new concepts, preradiation chemotherapy and a radiosensitizing agent given concomitantly with radiation therapy. The chemotherapy regimen included preradiation 5-FU and CCNU with hydroxyurea given during radiation therapy. These drugs were selected because of their radiomimetic and possible synergistic effects. In addition, a radiation sensitizing agent, oral misonidazole (0.5 g/m^2), was administered 4 hours prior to each dose of radiation therapy. Misonidazole was added to increase the relative radiosensitivity of hypoxic tumor cells, thought to be a major component of a heterogenous tumor such as a brainstem glioma.

There were 28 evaluable patients in this study. The diagnosis was made clinically in 15 and histologically confirmed in the other 13 patients. One patient had an astrocytoma, 10 had an anaplastic astrocytoma, and 2 had a glioblastoma multiforme. This study had a disproportionately large number of patients with high grade tumors in the surgical group (92%). There were an equal number of males and females, and the median age was 7 years.

The mean dose of radiation therapy was 5,527 ± 280 (SD) given in 5 to 6 weeks. The treatment regimen was well tolerated in 24 patients while 4 developed moderate myelosuppression during radiation therapy that did not require a significant deviation from planned therapy. Two patients had a mild peripheral neuropathy presumably secondary to misonidazole.

The results were disappointing; the median disease-free survival was 32 weeks and the median survival was 44 weeks. These survival figures were similar to those generated from the previous CSG protocol 944. The conclusion was that this multimodality protocol had no significant impact on the quality or length of survival.

Several new treatment alternatives are being considered for future studies. There is an interest in both the CSG and POG groups in hyperfractionation radiation techniques where 2 or 3 treatments of a radiation dose in the range of 80 to 100 rads are given daily instead of the usual single daily fraction.[35] It is anticipated that a cumulative dose in excess of 6,400 rads can be given more safely with this technique. A second line of pursuit is to use new combinations of more aggressive chemotherapy. The present strategy of the CSG is to conduct single arm pilot studies with a variety of new approaches since information can be gathered more quickly and the historical experience is reasonably well documented.

PHASE II STUDIES IN RECURRENT AND NEWLY DIAGNOSED DISEASE

Children with recurrent malignant brain tumors are expected eventually to die from their disease. In these circumstances, new treatment modalities can be ethically studied. All new phase III studies for children with newly diagnosed disease must be firmly based on data derived from carefully executed phase II trials in patients with recurrent disease, for it is difficult to justify untested treatments in newly diagnosed patients unless their prognosis with conventional therapy is unusually poor. In addition, phase III randomized studies are expensive and time consuming and of limited value if promising leads are not available in preliminary studies.

There has been modest experience with single and combination chemotherapy agents for brain tumors in children, the results of which have helped to formulate the recently completed CSG and SIOP studies and the ongoing POG medulloblastoma study. Objective responses in recurrent childhood brain tumors to single agent therapy (eg, vincristine, procarbazine, BCNU, CCNU, and high-dose intravenous methotrexate with leucovorin rescue) have been reported.[16] These studies have usually involved a relatively small number of pediatric patients with a particular histology and some were conducted without the benefit of CT scans. Multidrug regimens such as procarbazine, CCNU, and vincristine (PCV)[13] or mustard, vincristine, procarbazine, and prednisone (MOPP)[12] have also demonstrated activity.

Crafts et al treated 16 patients with recurrent medulloblastoma with several courses of PCV.[13] Improvement was observed in 10 and stabilization in 4 for a median period of 45 weeks. Cangir et al treated 23 children with several cycles of MOPP.[12] Responses were reported in 9/10 patients with astrocytomas and 8/10 patients with medulloblastoma.

A number of treatment regimens for children with recurrent brain tumors are under investigation at the present time. Some are in preliminary phases of development where the risks have yet to be fully evaluated such as with interstitial radiation implants for recurrent gliomas[7] or with new drugs such as carboplatin.[5] However, several chemotherapy studies have recently been completed using single drugs such as cyclophosphamide,[3] AZQ,[34] PCNU,[2] and cisplatin[36] and the multidrug regimen, "8 drugs in 1 day."[9]

There is some controversy about whether to use single or multiagent chemotherapy regimens in phase II studies in children with recurrent brain tumors. Advocates for multidrug studies point out that the desperate nature of the diseases and the heterogeneous nature of the tumors argue strongly for combination chemotherapy. Advocates of single drug studies emphasize the importance of demonstrating that every single drug used against these diseases is effective and of acceptable toxicity. In addition, the water-soluble agents should be used in maximum high doses because of the blood-brain barrier. Multidrug therapy usually requires compromising dosages. At this stage in the development of the field it would appear that single agent studies are desirable at least at the institution level.

The goal of a phase II study is to characterize the frequency and duration of objective responses in a clinically and histologically well-characterized disease while documenting important toxicity. If accurate information can be derived with single agents, then these data can be used in larger cooperative phase II trials involving multiple drugs. Since childhood brain tumors constitute a diverse group of malignancies, it is anticipated that response rates to single agents will vary considerably depending on tumor specificity.

Below is a summary of the results of current phase II single agent studies at Memorial Sloan-Kettering Cancer Center (MSKCC) using cyclophosphamide, PCNU, and cisplatin.

Cyclophosphamide

A total of 18 children with recurrent primary brain tumors (medulloblastoma, 8; glioma, 7; germ cell, 3) received multiple courses of high-dose intravenous cyclophosphamide (80 mg/kg or greater).[3] The overall objective response rate (CR and PR) assessed after 2 courses of chemotherapy was 89% (16 of 18 patients) and the mean response duration was 7 months (2 to 24+ months). Germinomas and medulloblastomas responded most readily. The hematologic toxicity was considerable and frequent hospitalization for fever and neutropenia were required. Nevertheless, cyclophosphamide, perhaps in lower doses, could be included in a multidrug regimen for patients with newly diagnosed brain tumors, especially medulloblastoma and CNS germ cell tumors.

PCNU

PCNU is a relatively new nitrosourea. It is of interest because it has greater lipid solubility than other currently available nitrosoureas such as CCNU and BCNU while retaining cytotoxic activity in various animal studies.[25] A total of 39 children with recurrent primary brain tumors participated in the MSKCC PCNU study.[2] There were 3 categories of tumors: glioma (cerebral, 11; brainstem, 16; and spinal cord, 1); primitive neuroectodermal (medulloblastoma, 5; pineoblastoma, 2; and cerebral hemisphere primitive neuroectodermal, 2); and miscellaneous (ependymoma, 1; meningeal sarcoma, 1; choroid plexus carcinoma, 1). The median age of the study population was 11 years. Only 10 patients had received prior adjuvant chemotherapy (4 with nitrosoureas) in addition to radiation therapy.

All patients had evaluable disease as determined by a neurodiagnostic study such as a CT scan or myelogram. Objective and clinical responses were determined after two doses of PCNU (120 mg/m^2) separated by a 7-week interval. Of 36 evaluable patients, 6 (17%) had objective improvement on a neurodiagnostic test as well as clinical improvement when the steroid therapy was either reduced or eliminated. Partial responses were observed in 5/25 patients with gliomas for 2+, 3, 3+, 6, and 8 months and the single patient with an ependymoma for 5+ months. None of the 9 patients with primitive neuroectodermal tumors responded. Four patients with gliomas had stabilization of their disease for 3, 3+, 3+, and 10 months.

The major toxicity was hematologic, predominantly thrombocytopenia and neutropenia. Of 33 patients evaluable for toxicity, 13 had a nadir platelet count below 50,000 and another 13 had a platelet count below 20,000 requiring platelet transfusions during at least one of their PCNU courses. There were no treatment-related deaths.

We concluded that PCNU has modest activity in children with gliomas with a 20% objective response rate. When the glioma patients with stable disease are included, the overall beneficial outcome approached 36%, a figure similar to those reported for nitrosourea studies in adults and children.[25] Because the toxicity and the response rates with PCNU are similar to that reported in other nitrosourea studies in adults and children,[16] we do not see any particular advantage of replacing such drugs as BCNU or CCNU with PCNU. Our experience indicates that nitrosoureas are useful drugs for glial tumors but not for primitive neuroectodermal tumors.

Cisplatin

A phase II cisplatin study for recurrent childhood primary brain tumors has also been conducted at MSKCC.[36] A total of 31 patients were treated with high-dose intravenous cisplatin (120 mg/m^2) in the following tumor categories: primitive neuroectodermal tumors (medulloblastoma, 12; cerebral primitive neuroectodermal tumor, 6), gliomas (brainstem, 7; cerebral, 2), and miscellaneous (ependymoma, 3; germ cell, 1).

The major side effects of cisplatin are renal and auditory toxicity. Therefore, baseline and follow-up studies of renal and auditory function were performed. Patients were required to have a creatinine clearance greater than 70 cc/min/1.73 m^2 prior to therapy. Cisplatin was administered intravenously with mannitol-enforced diuresis.

Acute drug-related toxicity included seizures secondary to inappropriate ADH secretion and hyponatremia in 3 patients with meningeal disease and moderate to severe nausea and vomiting in the majority of patients. Although transient depression of renal function was common in the first 2 to 3 weeks after treatment, recovery usually occurred by the fourth or fifth week. Only one patient who received 6 courses of cisplatin could not tolerate further therapy because of renal toxicity. High frequency hearing impairment (proportional to the cumulative cisplatin dose) was detectable in all patients and resulted in occasional delays or discontinuation of additional therapy. Only minimal hematologic toxicity was observed.

Objective responses were detected in 9 of 12 patients with medulloblastoma for a median of 8 months (3+ to 18), 1 of 6 patients with cerebral primitive neuroectodermal tumors for 5 months, 1 of 7 brainstem glioma patients for 4 months, 1 of 3 ependymoma patients for 7 months, and 1 of 1 germinoma patient for 3+ months.

The high response rate observed in patients with medulloblastoma (75%) is very encouraging; 4 of the 9 patients who responded had a complete response after 2 courses of cisplatin. The quality of life was generally excellent for the children who responded. We believe that high-dose cisplatin should be included in future studies of patients with recurrent and newly diagnosed patients with "poor risk" (M_{1-3}) primitive neuroectodermal tumors. We encourage the study of other platinum analogues with less auditory and renal toxicity, such as carboplatin.[5]

AZQ

AZQ has been the subject of phase II trials in recurrent primary brain tumors in adults and children in several institutions.[34,14] AZQ appears to induce a response rate similar to that of the nitrosoureas for adults with recurrent malignant astrocytomas, with a combined response and stable disease rate of 50%.[34,14] A response was also observed in one patient with medulloblastoma.[34] The dose and dose schedules have differed in the various clinical trials, ie, 8 mg/m^2 daily for 5 days[34] and 20 mg/m^2 weekly for 2 weeks.[14] Hematologic toxicity was the dose-limiting side effect. There is no published large pediatric brain tumor experience but both the CSG and POG have ongoing phase II studies.

"8 in 1" Protocol

A multidrug regimen has been designed by Dr A. Bleyer and colleagues entitled "8 in 1" or 8 drugs in 1 day.[9] The drugs include methylprednisone, vincristine, BCNU, procarbazine, hydroxyurea, cisplatin, cytosine arabinoside, and cyclophosphamide for primitive neuroectodermal tumors. The doses of several of the drugs are substantially lower than conventional recommendations when they are used individually because of anticipated toxicity from their combination.

The preliminary response and toxicity data are encouraging. Response rates in excess of 70% have been observed for small numbers of patients with medulloblastoma, cerebral primitive neuroectodermal tumors, ependymoma, and cerebral malignant astrocytoma. The regimen is being evaluated in a large cooperative CSG phase II trial and there is interest in employing it as adjuvant therapy for newly diagnosed patients with poor risk medulloblastoma and malignant cerebral astrocytoma in a randomized phase III study for newly diagnosed patients.

Preradiation Phase II Trials in Newly Diagnosed Patients

A relatively new conceptual approach in phase II chemotherapy trials is to administer the study drugs prior to radiotherapy in newly diagnosed patients who have measurable disease. This approach has proved valuable in osteogenic sarcoma patients who received presurgery chemotherapy prior to an en bloc resection.[33] The histologic response to HDMTX helped in the planning of future chemotherapy and made surgery easier in patients who responded.

For brain tumor patients, radiation therapy could be delayed for 6 to 8 weeks while several courses of a single or a multiagent regimen are administered. The benefits of such an approach include (1) determining response rates in untreated disease, (2) treating patients who have no significant limitations of organ tolerance because of previous therapy, (3) anticipating a synergistic or additive effect between radiation therapy and chemotherapy, and (4) using drugs such as MTX before radiation therapy and thereby reduce the likelihood of producing neurotoxicity.

The possible disadvantages of preirradiation chemotherapy include (1) delaying a potentially effective therapy such as radiotherapy while allowing the patient to deteriorate, (2) failing to detect an objective tumor response in such a short period of time (6 to 8 weeks), which might be detectable in a longer trial, and (3) the possible need to compromise the planned course of radiotherapy if bone marrow reserves become impaired.

The feasibility and relative safety of a preradiation chemotherapy phase II trial has been studied at MSKCC in primary brain tumors with several single agents. With respect to the danger of delaying conventional therapy, of a total of 24 newly diagnosed patients with various tumors treated with preradiation chemotherapy, none developed clinical deterioration related to progressive disease. Fourteen children with newly diagnosed brain tumors considered to carry a poor prognosis were treated with two courses of cyclophosphamide (80 mg/kg) over 4 to 6 weeks prior to radiation therapy.[4] Five patients received additional therapy with intrathecal ara-C (50 mg/m^2) and oral hydroxyurea (40 mg/kg) prior to radiation therapy. Objective responses were observed in 8 patients (57%) prior to radiotherapy (medulloblastoma, 3; pineoblastoma, 2; cerebral primitive neuroectodermal, 1; germinoma, 2). Twelve of the 14 children tolerated the subsequent planned dose of craniospinal radiotherapy. Post-radiotherapy chemotherapy was not given. The median survival of this group was only 11 months. Therefore, in spite of the objective responses achieved by chemotherapy in some patients, no survival benefit was observed.

A relatively large multinational pilot study in Europe for patients with medulloblastoma incorporates multiple courses of preradiation HDMTX with vincristine and procarbazine for newly diagnosed patients with medulloblastoma.[28] Preliminary data have not identified serious neurotoxicity.

CONCLUSIONS

The most exciting developments in the field of pediatric neuro-oncology in the past 10 years have not been simply the completion of investigatory clinical trials, although these have been important. More importantly, there now appears to be the "critical mass" of clinical and laboratory personnel who have made a commitment to the emerging interdisciplinary field of pediatric neuro-oncology to understand better and treat more effectively the children afflicted with tumors that in many cases carry a very poor prognosis. There has been a delay in applying old and new knowledge derived from other areas of oncology, primarily due to lack of trained and committed personnel. Hopefully, the next decade will bring rapid developments and significant improvements in the quality and duration of survival for those children. The cancers most likely to yield to multimodal therapy are the primitive neuroectodermal and germ cell tumors.

It is becoming increasingly apparent that the care of such patients is complex and beyond the scope of a single specialist. Teams of physicians must collaborate in the design and implementation of treatment protocols. Closer collaboration with the basic scientists will not only enlighten our understanding of tumor biology and drug pharmacokinetics but also provide leads for new clinical trials. Although certain studies can be accomplished in single institutions, there will always be a need to conduct multiinstitutional studies to corroborate preliminary observations. Only through education of the medical and lay communities can we increase participation in such clinical trials. A necessary corollary to the development of aggressive treatment protocols is the problem of late effects, especially germane to the infant and young child. However, our first obligation is to produce cures with predictable frequency and then to diminish therapy in patients at high risk for late effects and low risk for tumor recurrence.

REFERENCES

1. Allen J, Epstein F: Medulloblastoma and other primary CNS malignant neuroectodermal tumors: The effect of age and extent of disease on prognosis. J Neurosurg 57:446–451, 1982
2. Allen J, Hancock H, Tan C: A phase II trial of PCNU in recurrent primary CNS tumors in children—a negative study. Ann Neurol 12:206, 1982
3. Allen J, Helson L: High dose cyclophosphamide chemotherapy for recurrent CNS tumors in children. J Neurosurg 55:749–756, 1981
4. Allen J, Helson L, Jereb B: Preradiation chemotherapy for newly diagnosed childhood brain tumors—a modified phase II trial. Cancer 52:2001–2006, 1983
5. Bacha D, Caparros B, Allen J, et al: Cis-Diammine [-1,1-cyclobutanedicarboxylate-(2-)-0,0′] platinum II (CBCDA; NSC-241240) in children with cancer. Proc Am Assoc Cancer Res 25:201, 1984
6. Berger M, Edwards M, LaMasters D, et al: Pediatric brainstem tumors: Radiographic, pathologic, and clinical correlation. Neurosurg 12:298–302, 1983
7. Bernstein M, Gutin P: Interstitial irradiation of brain tumors: A review. Neurosurg 9:741–750, 1981
8. Berry M, Jenkin R, Keen C, et al: Radiation therapy for medulloblastoma: A 21-year review. J Neurosurg 55:43–51, 1981
9. Bleyer W, Millstein J, Balias F, et al: 8 drugs in 1 day chemotherapy for brain tumors: a new approach and rationale for preradiation chemotherapy. Med Pediat Oncol 11:213, 1983
10. Bloom H, Thorton-Jones H: Adjuvant chemotherapy for medulloblastoma: The multicentre controlled trial of the International Society of Pediatric Oncology (SIOP) from the Proceedings of the 13th International Congress of Chemotherapy, 1983
11. Bloom HJG: Intracranial tumors: Responses and resistance to therapeutic endeavors, 1970–1980. Int J Pediat Oncol Biol Phys 8:1083–1113, 1982
12. Cangir A, Van Eys J, Berry D: Combination chemotherapy with MOPP in children with recurrent brain tumors. Med Pediat Oncol 4:253–261, 1978
13. Crafts D, Levin V, Edwards M, et al: Chemotherapy of recurrent medulloblastoma with combined procarbazine, CCNU, and vincristine. J Neurosurg 49:589–592, 1978
14. Curt G, Kelley J, Kufta C, et al: Phase II and pharmacokinetic study of Azirinylbenzoquinone [2,5-diaziridenyl-3,6-bis (carboethyoxyamino)-1,4-benzoquinone, diaziquone, NSC182986] in high grade gliomas. Cancer Res 43:6102–6105, 1983
15. Dohrmann G, Farwell I, Flanner J: Glioblastoma multiforme in children. J Neurosurg 44:442–448, 1976
16. Edwards M, Levin V, Wilson C: Brain tumor chemotherapy: An evaluation of agents in current use for phase II and III trials. Cancer Treat Rep 64:1179–1205, 1980
17. Ertel I, Boesal C, Evans A, et al: Adjuvant chemotherapy of high grade astrocytomas in children: Radiation therapy with or without CCNU, vincristine, and Prednisone. Proc ASCO, C-309, 1984
18. Evans A, et al: CSG 942 medulloblastoma study. (submitted)
19. Fewer D, Wilson C, Boldrey E, et al: Phase II study of 1-(2-chlorethyl)-3-cyclohexyl-1-nitrosourea (CCNU:NSU 79037) in the treatment of brain tumors. Cancer Chemotherapy Rep 56:3, 1972
20. Harisiadis L, Chang C: Medulloblastoma in children: A correlation between staging and results of treatment. Int J Radiat Oncol Biol Phys 2:833–841, 1977
21. Jenkin D, Anderson J, Ertel I, et al: Brain stem tumors of childhood: A prospective randomized trial of adjuvant treatment with CCNU, vincristine, and prednisone. (submitted)
22. Kleinman G, Hochberg F, Richardson E: Systemic metastases from medulloblastoma. Cancer 48:2296–2309, 1981
23. Laurent J, Bruce D, Schut L: Hemorrhagic brain tumors in pediatric patients. Child's Brain 8:263–270, 1981
24. Levin V, Edwards M, Wara W, et al: 5-Fluorouracil and 1-(2-chloroethyl)-3-cyclohexyl-1-nitrosourea (CCNU) followed by hydroxyurea, misonidazole, and irradiation for brain stem gliomas: A pilot study of the Brain Tumor Research Center and the Childrens Cancer Group. Neurosurg 14:679–681, 1984
25. Levin V, Resser K, McGrath L, et al: PCNU treatment for recurrent malignant gliomas. Cancer Treat Rep 68:969–973, 1984
26. Littman P, Jarrett P, Bilaniuk L, et al: Pediatric brainstem glioma. Cancer 45:2787–2792, 1980
27. Montravadi R, Phatak R, Bellus S, et al: Brainstem gliomas: An autopsy study of 25 cases. Cancer 49:1294–1296, 1982
28. Neidhart M, Hanefeld F, Henze G, et al: Treatment of medulloblastoma with postoperative combination chemotherapy before neuroaxis irradiation: An interim progress report on the Berlin pilot study and the West German cooperative trial. Proceedings of the XIII meeting of the Int Sec Pediatr Oncol, 1983, p 39
29. Packer R, Allen J, Deck M, et al: Brain stem glioma:

Clinical manifestations of meningeal gliomatosis. Ann Neurol 14:177–182, 1983

30. Phuphanich S, Edwards M, Levin V, et al: Supratentorial malignant gliomas of childhood: Results of treatment with radiation therapy and chemotherapy. J Neurosurg 60:495–499, 1984

31. Reigel D, Scarff T, Woodford J: Biopsy of pediatric brainstem tumors. Child's Brain 5:329–340, 1979

32. Rorke L: The cerebellar medulloblastoma and its relationship to primitive neuroectodermal tumors. J Exp Neuropathol, Exp Neurol 42:1–15, 1983

33. Rosen G, Marcove R, Caparros B, et al: Primary osteogenic sarcoma: The rationale for preoperative chemotherapy and delayed surgery. Cancer 43:2163–2177, 1979

34. Schold S, Friedman H, Bjornsson T, et al: Treatment of patients with recurrent primary brain tumors with AZQ. Neurology 34:615–619, 1984

35. Shin K, Muller P, Geggre P: Superfraction after radiation therapy in the treatment of malignant astrocytoma. Cancer 52:2040–2043, 1983

36. Walker R, Allen J: Treatment of recurrent primary intracranial childhood tumors with Cis-Diamminedichloroplatinum. Ann Neurol 14:371, 1983

37. Young J, Miller R: Incidence of malignant tumors in U.S. children. J Pediatrics 86:254–258, 1975

SUBJECT INDEX

Acquired resistance to chemotherapy, 57, 58–59
Active immunotherapy, 100–101
Adoptive immunotherapy, 99
Adriamycin, clinical trials of, 42
Age
  and anaplastic astrocytoma, 17
  and astrocytoma, 27
  and glioblastoma, 17
  and survival rates, 42, 43
Agents for brain tumor chemotherapy, 61–63. *See also* specific agents
Amino acid metabolism, PET and, 88
Anaplastic astrocytoma, 17, 18(*fs*)
Angiography, cerebral, 29
Antibody-dependent cellular cytotoxicity (ADCC), 94, 97–98
Anticonvulsant therapy, preoperative, 29, 30
Antigenic expression of T cells, 95
Antigen presenting cells (APC), 95
Antigens, glioma-associated, 98–99
Antiglioma activity, cell-mediated, 97
Argon laser and hematoporphyrin, 35–36
Assays for chemotherapy, 64, 66
Astrocytic neoplasms, malignant
  classification of, 16–17
  clinopathologic features of, 17
  therapy for
    complications, 24–25
    recurrence, 20, 23–24
    remission, 20, 22(*fs*)
  topography of, 17, 20
Astrocytomas, non-random karyotypic changes in, 8
Autoadaptive immunotherapy, 104
Avian Sarcoma Virus-induced tumors in rat brain, 72–73(*f*)
Azeridinylbenzoquinone (AZQ)
  for children, 119
  pharmacokinetic parameters of, 75–76
  time courses of, 78(*f*), 79
AZQ. *See* Azeridinylbenzoquinone

B cell growth factor (BCGF), 95
B cell response
  brain tumors and, 96
  normal, 95
BCG, 99, 101
BCNU, 56, 57(*f*), 61(*t*), 62, 99. *See also* Chemotherapy
  clinical trials of, 41
  high-dose intravenous, 63
  intraarterial, 63
  lesions from, 25
  oncogenes and, 11, 12
  pharmacokinetic parameters of, 75–76
  resistance to, 57–59
  time courses of, 78(*f*), 79
Benign brain tumors, lethal, 1
Binding of antigen in immune system, 96
Biological response modifiers as therapy agents, 101–103
Biological variability of human gliomas, 94
Blood-brain barrier (BBB)
  chemotherapy and, 59–61, 66, 74
  normal, 2, 70, 71
  PET and, 89–91
  radiosensitizers and, 46
Blood-to-tissue transport in brain tumor model, 71–73
Blood-tumor barrier (BTB), 59–60, 63–64
  history of, 70–74
  and pharmacokinetic considerations in chemotherapy, 80
Blood types, prognosis and, 42
B-lym family of oncogenes, 6
Brain scan *v* CT scan for malignant gliomas, 29
Broders system for astrocytic neoplasms, 16
BudR, 46
Burkett's lymphoma, specific chromosome alterations in, 4–5
Butterfly gliomas, surgery for, 30

Carbon dioxide laser, 32
CCNU, 61(*t*), 62, 101. *See also* Chemotherapy
  for children, 116
Cell-mediated antiglioma activity, 97
Cellular aspects of chemotherapy, 56–59
Cellular heterogeneity in malignant gliomas, 6–8
Cellular interaction, brain tumors and, 97
Central nervous system (CNS) tolerance and RT, 49–50
C-erb-B-gene, 11
Cerebral edema, 2
Chemotherapy. *See also* specific agents
  agents for, 61–63
  assays for, 64, 66
  blood-brain barrier and, 59–61, 66
  cellular aspects of, 56–59
  for children. *See* Pediatric neurooncology
  clinical trials of. *See* Clinical trials
  discussion of, 56–66
  future directions in, 80–81
  newer methods in, 63–64
  pharmacokinetic considerations and, 74–80
  quality of life and, 43
Children, brain tumors in, 1, 3, 5. *See also* Pediatric neurooncology
Chromosome ploidy as gene amplification, 5
Chromosomes
  gains and losses in gliomas, 8–9
  specific alterations in, 4–5
Cisplatin, 56, 57(*f*), 61(*t*), 62, 63. *See also* Chemotherapy
Classification of malignant astrocytic neoplasms, 16–17
Clinical trials
  cytoreduction and, 39
  discussion of, 38, 44
  nature of, 38–39
  phase II studies in, 38, 41–42
  phase III studies in, 38, 39–41
  prognostic variables in, 42–43
  quality of life and, 43–44
Clinopathologic features of malignant astrocytic neoplasms, 17
Colony-forming assay, 65

Complications of therapy, 24–25, 41
Computerized tomography
glioblastoma and, 17, 18(*fs*)
malignant gliomas and, 28–29
recurrent, 36
stereotactic laser surgery and, 32, 35
surgery and, 30
Cooperative group protocol design for medulloblastoma, 111–112
Cooperative group studies, 38–39, 40(*f*). *See also* Clinical trials
Corpus callosum, surgery for, 30
Corticosteroids
clinical trials and, 39–40
intracranial surgery and, 29
postoperative, 31
Co-transfection of oncogenes, malignancy and, 6
C. *parvum,* 99
C-sis gene and polypeptides of platelet-derived growth factor, 10, 12
CT. *See* Computerized tomography
CUSA surgical instrument, 30
Cyclophosphamide for children, 118
Cytogenetic analysis of tumor cell chromosomal complement, 6–8
Cytoreduction, clinical trials and, 39. *See also* Clinical trials

Deletions and proto-oncogenes, 4–5
Diagnosis and surgery for malignant gliomas, 27–29
Differential diagnosis in malignant gliomas, 28
Digital intravenous angiography (DIVA), 29
Distribution of cytotoxic agents, PET and, 91
DNA in cancer cells, 4
Double minutes (DMs) and duplications of genes, 5
Drug concentrations, increasing, 63–64
Duplications and proto-oncogenes, 4–5
Duration of symptoms, prognosis and, 42

Early draining vein in malignant glioma, 29
Edema, cerebral, 31, 56
Eight in one protocol for children, 119
Electron affinic sensitizers, 47–49
Electron microscope (EM) studies, 70
Enhancing rim of glioblastoma, 20
Epidermal growth factor (EGF) receptors, 10, 11–12
Epipodophyllotoxin, 61(*t*), 62. *See also* Chemotherapy

Factor-dependent activation, 95
Flagyl, 46, 47. *See also* Chemotherapy
5-Fluorouracil, 61(*t*), 62–63. *See also* Chemotherapy
for children, 116
pharmacokinetic parameters of, 75(*t*), 76
time courses of, 77(*f*), 79
Future directions
in chemotherapy, 63–64, 80–81
in immunotherapy, 103–104
in tumor studies, 91

G-banded cells in mammary tumors, 8
Gene dosage hypothesis of oncogenes, 4, 5
Glioblastoma cells, 96
Glioblastoma multiforme, 17, 19(*fs*), 21(*fs*), 42, 56. *See also* Astrocytic neoplasms, malignant
hypoxic cells in, 46
in remission, 22(*fs*)
Gliomas, malignant
antigenicity of, 98–99
chromosome abnormalities and, 9
definition of malignancy in, 16
immune status and, 96(*t*). *See also* Immune system
and oncogenes, 4
surgery for. *See* Intracranial surgery for malignant gliomas
Glucose utilization, PET and, 87–88
Grading of astrocytic neoplasms, 16–17
Growth factors, 10–11
Growth, lethal, in benign and malignant brain tumors, 1

Halogenated pyrimidines, 49
Headache, 28
Heavy particle radiotherapy, 50–52
Hematoporphyrin and argon laser, 35–36
Hemiparesis, 28
Hemostasis after resection, 31
Heterogeneity in malignant gliomas, 6–8, 17, 94
chemotherapy and, 56
Histologic criteria
and classification of fibrillary astrocytic neoplasms, 16–17
prognosis and, 43
HLA antigens and passive immunotherapy, 101
Homogeneous staining regions (HSRs) and duplication of genes, 5
HpD and argon laser surgery, 35–36
Humoral parameters
with brain tumors, 96–98
normal, 96
Hydroxyurea, 61(*t*), 62. *See also* Chemotherapy
Hyperbaric oxygen (HBO) as radiation sensitizer, 46–47
Hyperdiploid cells and chemotherapy, 59
Hyperfractionation and RT, 50
clinical trials of, 40–41
Hyperthermia and brachytherapy, 53–54
Hypervascular gliomas, surgery for, 30
Hypoxia and RT, 46
Hypoxic cell sensitizers, 46
clinical trials of, 40–41

IL-1. *See* Interleukin-1
IL-1-like factor in glioma cells, 97
Immune system. *See also* Immunotherapy
brain tumors and, 96–97
antigenicity of gliomas, 98–99
host-tumor interaction, 97–98
normal cellular response in, 94–96
Immunobiology, monoclonal antibodies and, 3
Immunoglobulin (Ig), 95–96
increased, in malignant gliomas, 97–98
Immunotherapy. *See also* Immune system
active, 100–101
adoptive, 99
discussion of, 99

Immunotherapy *(Continued)*
future prospects for, 103–104
passive, 99–100
restorative, 99
Interferons (IFN), 101–103
Interleukin-1 (IL-1), 95
Interleukin-2 (IL-2)
immunotherapy and, 103
Interstitial brachytherapy, 52–53
Intraarterial chemotherapy, 63
Intracarotid (IC) hyperosmolar mannitol, 60–61
Intracranial surgery for malignant gliomas
diagnosis and, 27–29
discussion of, 27, 36–37
exclusions for, 30
goal of, 30
hematoporphyrin and argon laser, 35–36
and postoperative management, 31
preoperative management of, 29–30
principles for, 30–31
for recurrent gliomas, 36
risk in, 31
stereotactic laser for, 31–35
Intrinsic resistance to chemotherapy, 57–58
Iodine-125 implant, 53
In vitro assays for chemotherapy, 64–65
problems with, 65–66
In vivo assays for chemotherapy, 64
Iridium-192, 53

Karnofsky performance status, 43
Karnofsky Scales, 31, 42
Karyotypic changes, non-random, in astrocytomas, 8
Kernohan system for grading astrocytic neoplasms, 16–17
Keyhole limpet hemocyanin, 96

Lesions from BCNU, 25
Leu system, 95
Level of consciousness, postoperative, prognosis and, 42
Lymphocytes, normal, 94–95

Magnetic Resonance Imaging (MRI) for low grade gliomas, 28–29
Major histocompatibility complex (MHC) and T cells, 95
Malignancy in human glioma, definition of, 16
Memory, difficulties with, 28
Metastasis, cerebral
from breast, 90(*f*)
from colon, 86(*f*)
infrequency of, 2
Methyl-CCNU, 61(*t*), 62. *See also* Chemotherapy
Methylprednisolone, 40
Metronidazole (Flagyl), 46, 47. *See also* Chemotherapy
Microcytotoxicity assay, 65
Misonidazole (MISO), 46, 47–49. *See also* Chemotherapy
for children, 116
clinical trials of, 40–41
Monoclonal antibodies (MA)
and antigenicity in gliomas, 98–99
for drug delivery, 80
and immunobiology, 3

Monoclonal antibodies *(Continued)*
and immunotherapy, 103–104
passive, 99–100
Mononuclear (MN) cells, 97
MTX, 60, 63, 64. *See also* Chemotherapy
pharmacokinetic parameters of, 75–76
time courses of, 77(*f*), 79
Multistep process in malignancy, oncogenes and, 5–6
Mutation hypothesis of oncogenes, 4

Natural killer (NK) cells, 94
Nausea, 28
Near-diploid cells and chemotherapy, 59
Necrosis
and astrocytic neoplasms, 17, 19(*f*)
and RT, 50, 53
Neon ion beam, 52
Neoplasia, recurrent, and radionecrosis, 24(*fs*), 25
Neoplastic cells in systemic cancer, 1
Neuroblastoma, deletions in, 5
Neuroectodermal tumors, blood-brain barrier in, 2
Neurologic deterioration from radiotherapy, 25
New drugs, 64
New methods. *See* Future directions
Nitroimidazoles, 46
Nitrosoureas, 61–62. *See also* Chemotherapy
for children, 118–119
Normal brain, blood-brain barrier in, 2
Numerical abnormalities in amplification of oncogene products, 5

Obtundation, 28
OKT system, 95
Oncogenes
discussion of, 4
and multistep process in malignancy, 5–6
gliomas, 4
potential of, 4
Oncology, history of for brain tumors, 1
Oxygen utilization, PET and, 85–87

Passive immunotherapy, 99–100
PCNU, 61(*t*), 64. *See also* Chemotherapy
for children, 118–119
PDGF-like molecules, 11
Pediatric neurooncology
discussion of, 110, 120
phase II studies in, 117–118
AZQ, 119
cyclophosphamide, 118
eight drugs in one day, 114, 119
PCNU, 118–119
preradiation chemotherapy, 120
phase III trials in
brain stem glioma, 115–117
high-grade gliomas, 114–115
medulloblastoma, 110–111
study design, 111–114
Personality changes, 28
PET. *See* Position Emission Tomography

Pharmacokinetic considerations and chemotherapy, 74–80
blood-brain barrier and, 59–61, 66
Phase II studies, 38, 41–42. *See also* Clinical trials
Phase III studies, 38, 39–41. *See also* Clinical trials
Phenotypes of cancer cells, 4
Photoradiation therapy (PRT), 35–36
pH, tumor, and PET, 88–89
Platelet-derived growth factor (PDGF) and c-sis gene, 10, 12
Point mutation and alterations in DNA, 5
Polychemotherapy, 64
Polypeptide chains in immune system, 95–96
Position Emission Tomography (PET)
amino acid metabolism and, 88
applications of, 84(*t*)
blood-brain barrier and, 89–91
blood flow and, 85–87
discussion of, 83
distribution of cytotoxic agents and, 91
future trends in, 91
glucose utilization and, 87–88
and pH, tumor, 88–89
v QAR, 73–74
regional cerebral, 85–87
technique of, 83–84
tracer models and, 84–85
Postoperative management of malignant gliomas, 31
Precursor uptake assay, 65
Preoperative management for malignant gliomas, 29–30
Preradiation chemotherapy for children, 120
Procarbazine, 42, 61(*t*), 62, 101. *See also* Chemotherapy
Prognosis. *See also* Survival rates
for children with brain tumors, 110
variables in, 42–43
Progress in last 20 years, 3
Proto-oncogenes, 4
Pyrimidine analogues, 46

Quality of life, 43–44
QAR. *See* Quantitative autoradiography
Quantitative autoradiography (QAR), 59
to measure blood flow, 71, 73–74

Radiation therapy (RT)
clinical trials and, 39–41. *See also* Clinical trials
heavy particle, 50–52
interstitial brachytherapy as, 52–53
hyperthermia, 53–54
lesions from, 25
neurologic deterioration from, 25
radiation sensitizers and
electron affinic sensitizers, 47–49
general considerations, 46
halogenated pyrimidines, 49
hyperbaric oxygen (HBO), 46–47
radiation tolerance and, 49–50
radionecrosis from, 24–25
Radiocrenosis, cerebral, 24–25
Rapidly growing cells, chemotherapy and, 57
Ras gene family
cellular transformation and, 5
in malignancies, 5
Rats, brain tumors in, 71–73
Reciprocal translocations and proto-oncogenes, 4–5
Recurrence of glioblastoma, 20, 23–24
Recurrent brain tumors
in children, 117–120
surgery for, 36
Regional cerebral blood flow, PET and, 85–87
Regional heterogeneity in malignant gliomas, 9–10
Resistance to chemotherapy, 57–59
Restorative immunotherapy, 99
Retinoblastoma, deletions in, 5
Ring enhancement on contrast CT scan, in malignant glioma, 28
RT. *See* Radiation therapy

Secondary surgery, 36
Serioimmunotherapy, 100
Sex chromosome in malignant glioma cells, 8–9
Sex differences in malignant astrocytoma, 27
Single photon emission tomography (SPECT) *v* PET, 83
Speech impairment, 28, 43
Stereotactic biopsy
CT guided, 27
for glioblastoma, 20
Streptozotocin, clinical trials of, 41
Surgery. *See also* Intracranial surgery for malignant gliomas
for brain tumor, 2
for medulloblastoma, phase II trials for, 112–113
quality of life and, 43
Survival rates
astrocytic neoplasms, malignant, 16
with brachytherapy, 53
with brainstem glioma, 115
with electron affinic sensitizers, 47–49
with heavy particle radiotherapy, 52
with high-grade gliomas, 115
with hyperbaric oxygen (HBO), 46
with medulloblastoma, 110–112
Symptoms
preoperative
in anaplastic astrocytoma, 17
in glioblastoma multiforme, 17
and prognosis, 42
Systemic cancer, 1

T cell replacing factors (TRFs), 95
T cells
brain tumors and, 96
normal, 94–95
Therapy. *See also* Chemotherapy; Immunotherapy; Surgery
for astrocytic neoplasms. *See* Astrocytic neoplasms, malignant, therapy for
complications of, 24–25
quality of life and, 43–44

Thermal enhancement of radiation, 53–54
Three- *v* four-tiered system for grading astrocytic neoplasms, 16–17
Topography of astrocytic neoplasms, malignant, 17, 20
Transfer constant in brain tumor models, 71–73
α- and β-transforming growth factor (TGF), 12
Tumor blood flow and PET, 91
Tumor receptor studies and PET, 91

Vascular proliferation in astrocytic neoplasms, 17
Vincristine, 101
Viral counterparts of proto-oncogenes, 4
Visual disturbance, 43
Visual field defect, 28
Vomiting, 28

Wilms' tumor, deletions in, 5

POINT OF VIEW

Hospice: The Game Is Not Over

In the mid-1970s, a new wave of social consciousness swept through this country concerning the once taboo subject of death. Indeed, death came out of the closet and into the spotlight. Part of this new cultural awareness was the expectation that as much dignity as possible should accompany death and that everyone's final moments should be surrounded by love and comfort. It was on this point, that is, death with maximal comfort, that the public perceived the medical community had failed to meet its commitment. It was in this background that hospice was discovered. Hospice care, in a simple definition, is the use of modern medical technology to provide supportive care to dying patients and emotional support and counseling to both patients and family members on a 24-hour basis.[1] Hospice was certainly not a new concept. It had been practiced in England for some time thanks to the pioneering work of Dame Cicely Saunders. It was this elaboration of hospice that was imported and popularized in this country. The different health care system in England caused some early problems when we shifted to home- rather than hospital-related emphasis. These problems were resolved and soon hospice was the flag carrier for our new social emphasis on death and dying.

In 1978, there were only 59 identifiable operational hospice programs and by July 1981, this number had increased to 440. As of September 1985, there were 1,700 hospice programs nationally. Hand-in-hand with this phenomenal hospice growth was the development of hospice trade organizations. Some hospice leaders and advocates envisioned hospice care as an alternative to, not a part of, the conventional health care delivery system. They stressed autonomy and separation from this traditional system with emphasis on the discrete unit for providing inpatient care. Debates raged concerning eligibility criteria for admission, prediction of survival, and so on. Somewhere during this process, the medical community, especially the physician, was lost in the shuffle. To some, hospice represented nothing more than a fancy nursing home with a new name while to others, hospice and its nonmedical advocates were a clear intrusion and threat to physicians' practices. Some physicians felt hospice violated their patient-physician relationship.

In the early 1980s, significant light was cast on this new industry as part of the Hospice Project of the Joint Commission on Accreditation of Hospitals (JCAH). Hospice provider models were identified as predominantly independent, hospital based, or home health agency based.[1] Only four of the independent hospices were free-standing inpatient buildings with supplemental home care services. The great majority of the independent programs were community based organizations that provided hospice care in the patient's home with provisions for inpatient care made through formal or informal agreements primarily with hospitals. Hospital-based hospices most often offered both inpatient and home care services. Home health agency hospices provided care either as a service of all agency staff or by a specific hospice team identified within the agency, and rarely had formal arrangements for inpatient care. In addition to identifying hospice structure, the JCAH Hospice Project, perhaps more importantly, clarified five major functions unique to hospice care. The first was the designation of the patient and family or other primary careperson as the unit of care. The second was the delivery of care by a specific interdisciplinary team. These team services included physician, both attending and medical director, nursing, psychosocial, spiritual, volunteer, and bereavement services. The third was the 24-hour availability of team services in both the home care and inpatient setting. The fourth was the importance of continuity of care across the inpatient and home care settings. The final was the recognition of palliation with emphasis on pain and symptom control as the primary goal.[1]

Congress, with a good push from lobbying trade organizations, introduced reimbursement legislation in early 1982. Despite the lack of significant science and information on hospice care, and ignoring testimony from many sources urging that these data were critical for sound legislation, the hospice

Seminars in Oncology, Vol 13, No 1 (March), 1986: pp 128–129

Medicare benefit was enacted on September 3, 1982, as part of the Tax Equity and Fiscal Responsibility Act (TEFRA). The final regulations for this benefit were published in December 1983 and made effective retroactive to November 1, 1983. But, as of July 1985, only 12% (200) of hospices were participating in the Medicare hospice program. Since most hospice programs are losing money, this lack of support for the Medicare program underscores the serious flaws in the TEFRA legislation. Simply stated, the Medicare benefit dictates a restricted model of hospice. This model is not consistent with hospice care as it is currently being delivered in the real world. If a patient lives more than the total 210 day election period (two 90-day and one 30-day periods), the program absorbs the costs for further care. Indeed, the Medicare benefit requires an unheard of level of accurate prognostication. Each patient's reimbursement is capped at $6,500 and if a patient exceeds this amount, the program must continue hospice care despite subsequent financial losses. A hospital-based program must supply, not contract for, the home care services although many of these services may be readily available, leading to duplication of services. On the other hand, home health agency based or community based independent programs can contract for inpatient services. These are just a few examples of the many inequities in the Medicare hospice benefit.

Of critical importance in hospice is that the same level and quality of care be administered both to those patients who are participating in the Medicare hospice benefit and to those who are not. Many programs, because of this restrictive legislation, have opted not to participate in this Medicare benefit. Out of fear of retribution by government regulators, the names of these programs have been changed from hospice to palliative care units. Patients admitted to these "hospice-like" programs are then under the same rules and regulations, including utilization and PRO review, as acute care Medicare patients. As a consequence of this, many hospital-based hospices no longer have clearly defineable inpatient units due largely to retroactive PRO denials.[2] Indeed, hospice appears to be changing rather dramatically with many organizations offering hospice service as merely one of an array of services. This question of uniformity of level and quality of care based on Medicare hospice reimbursement has surfaced as a result of these changes. For example, a patient participating in the Medicare hospice benefit can be admitted to an inpatient unit for respite care, however, the same admission for a patient not participating in the benefit would surely be denied by PRO. In fact, this disparity of care based on Medicare reimbursement status can exist between two patients in a single program. It is on these issues that physicians must take an active role and get back into the game to assure that the same level and quality of care is delivered to each hospice patient regardless of reimbursement status. Physicians must be more involved in hospice care to bring back the sensitized not legislated care to the patient-physician relationship. If physicians do not take a leadership role in these issues, no one else will.

REFERENCES

1. McCann BA, Enck RE: Standards for hospice care: A JCAH hospice project overview, in Engstrom PF, Anderson PN, Mortenson LE (eds): Advances in Cancer Control: Epidemiology and Research. New York, Alan R. Liss, 1984, pp 431–440

2. McCann BA: personal communication

Robert E. Enck, MD
Director of Oncology
Regional Cancer Center at Lourdes Hospital
Binghamton, NY
Member, Hospice Professional and Technical
Advisory Committee, Joint Commission on
Accreditation of Hospitals

ERRATUM

In the article by Zbylut J. Twardowski "Intraperitoneal Therapy in Renal Failure" (*Seminars in Oncology* 12:81–89, 1985 [suppl 4]), an omission was made from Table 1, page 87. The completed table appears below.

Table 1. Differential Diagnosis of Turbid Dialysate

	White Blood Cells (per μg)	% Neutrophils	% Eosinophils	% Mononuclear Cells
Normal	< 100	< 50	< 3	> 50
Bacterial or fungal peritonitis	> 100	> 50	< 3	< 50
Tuberculous peritonitis	> 100	< 50	< 3	> 50
Peritoneal eosinophilia	> 100	< 50	> 20	< 50
Chyloperitoneum	< 100	< 50	< 3	> 50

Data from Nolph with permission.[8]

Pancreatic Cancer Response Rates Are More Than Chance

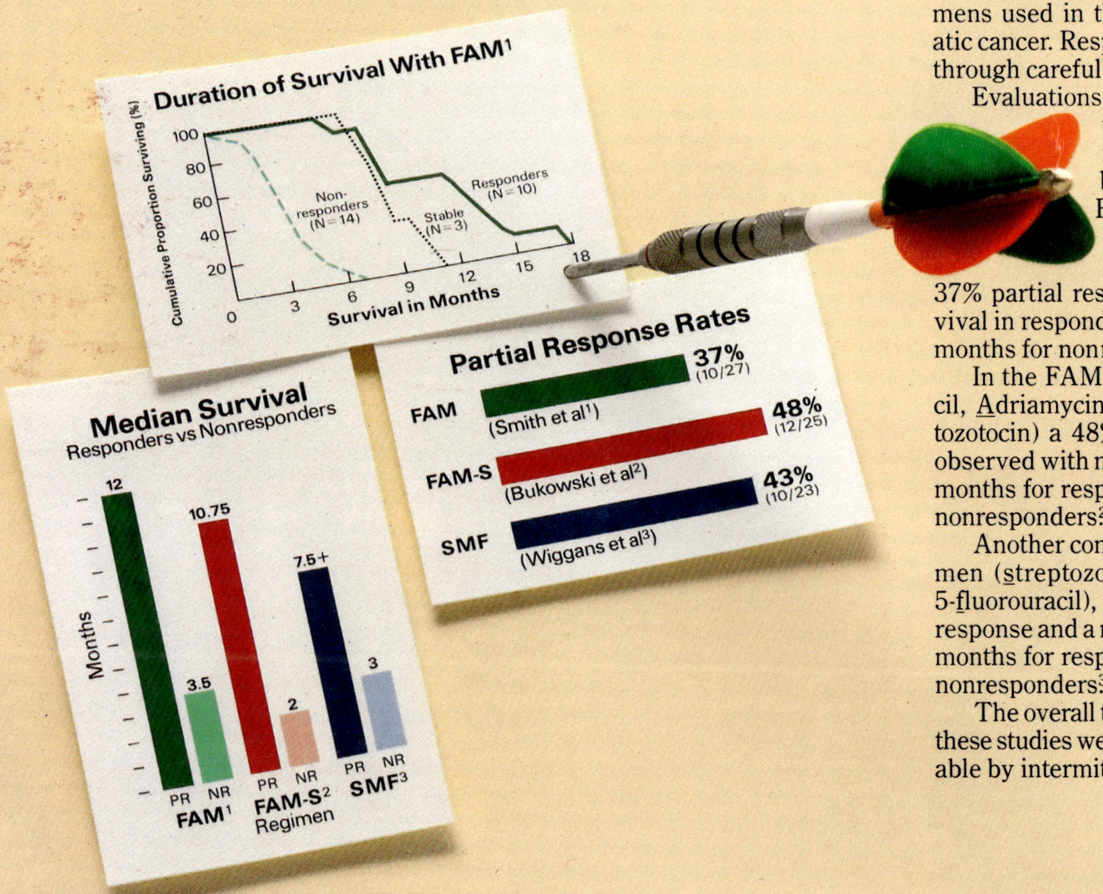

Mutamycin® (mitomycin for injection) is a key component of combination regimens used in the treatment of pancreatic cancer. Response may be enhanced through careful patient profiling.

Evaluations of combination chemotherapy regimens that include Mutamycin have been encouraging. The FAM regimen (5-fluorouracil, Adriamycin and Mutamycin) achieved a 37% partial response and median survival in responders of 12 months vs 3.5 months for nonresponders.[1]

In the FAM-S regimen (5-fluorouracil, Adriamycin, Mutamycin and streptozotocin) a 48% partial response was observed with median survival of 10.75 months for responders vs 2 months for nonresponders.[2]

Another combination, the SMF regimen (streptozotocin, Mutamycin and 5-fluorouracil), produced a 43% partial response and a median survival of 7.5+ months for responders vs 3 months for nonresponders.[3]

The overall toxicity characteristics in these studies were moderate and manageable by intermittent dosage schedules.

Widening the Hope for Cancer Remission

MUTAMYCIN®
mitomycin for injection

Please see full prescribing information on following page.

VOL XIII, NO 2 JUNE 1986

Seminars in Oncology

Biological Response Modifiers

Carl M. Pinsky, *Guest Editor*

Contributors

Carl M. Pinsky
Michael J. Hawkins • Daniel F. Hoth
Robert E. Wittes • Ernest C. Borden • Ralph A. Reisfeld
Alan N. Houghton • David A. Scheinberg • Donald L. Morton
M.J. Mastrangelo • D. Berd • H. Maguire, Jr • Ronald B. Herberman
Steven A. Rosenberg • Susan E. Krown • Steven Gillis
Paul J. Conlon • David Cosman • Thomas P. Hopp
Steven K. Dower • Virginia Price • Diane Y. Mochizuki
David L. Urdal • Janice L. Gabrilove
E. Mihich

GRUNE & STRATTON
Harcourt Brace Jovanovich, Inc.

References:

1. Loehrer PJ, Einhorn LH: Cisplatin. *Ann Intern Med* 100:704-713, 1984.
2. Hainsworth JD, Greco FA, Williams SD, Einhorn LH: VP-16 in the treatment of refractory germinal neoplasms, in Issell BF, Muggia FM, Carter SK (eds): *Etoposide (VP-16): Current Status and New Developments*, pp 243-252. Copyright © 1984 by Academic Press, Inc.

Seminars in Oncology

Vol XIII, No 2 **June 1986**

INTRODUCTION

Biological Response Modifiers

THIS ISSUE is an attempt to present the current status of treatment with Biological Response Modifiers (BRMs) to medical oncologists. It is a comprehensive review of the results available in late 1985 and early 1986, and as such should be looked at as a snapshot in time. Clearly, by the time of publication, much in this rapidly evolving field will have changed. As only one example, when the article assignments were made, recombinant human tumor necrosis factor was not available. By the time of this writing, over 100 patients have been treated. Before publication of this issue, the results in these early patients will be known. However, most of the articles have "future perspectives" sections and some imminent results are described. Also, the main subject addressed by Mihich in his concluding article is prediction of future directions, and expected results, with BRMs.

The articles are arranged in a somewhat arbitrary way. After an introduction by three medical oncologists, the articles are grouped into general topics relating to immunomodulators, human tumor serology, cell-mediated immunity and cytokines before the concluding article on future perspectives. The authors have addressed concepts, and experimental results, as they relate to the practice of oncology. As only one BRM, interferon, has been approved in this country, the purpose of this issue should be viewed more as a preparation for the future and an attempt to put the current literature into perspective than as a prescription for the current practice of oncology.

Another potential use of this volume will be to indicate ongoing clinical trials to which practicing oncologists can refer eligible patients. Finally, it is clear that BRM approaches to cancer therapy will have to be integrated into standard regimens for many common cancers. The results reported in this issue will provide the foundation for rational design of such combination protocols.

Carl M. Pinsky
Frederick, Md
Guest Editor

Clinical Development of Biological Response Modifiers: Comparison With Cytotoxic Drugs

Michael J. Hawkins, Daniel F. Hoth, and Robert E. Wittes

IDENTIFICATION of immunobiologically active cytokines and advances in DNA technology have increased the number of biological response modifiers (BRMs) that are potential candidates for cancer therapy in man. The methods used to screen new agents and to design optimal therapeutic regimens for BRMs take on considerable importance as the number of potential agents increase.

For the purposes of this article, BRMs will be considered as agents that exert their antitumor effects only through mediation of host responses and not by a direct effect on the cancer cell. In general, this effect has been measured on immunocompetent effector cells thought to be capable of mediating tumor killing. Most cytotoxics are selected on the basis of their direct activity against tumor cells. In the clinic, cytotoxics are tested at the maximum tolerated dose (MTD) because the dose response curves are steep and do not show a peak below the MTD. In contrast, potential BRMs must be screened for activity on host effector cells and cannot necessarily be assumed to be optimally therapeutic at the MTD. This article will review the clinical development of BRMs with emphasis on the differences from cytotoxics, the limitations imposed by an incomplete understanding of the mechanisms of immunologically mediated tumor killing, and the lessons learned from clinical trials designed to evaluate interferon (IFN) alpha as a BRM.

PRECLINICAL SCREENING

At the present time, approximately 10,000 potential cytotoxic agents are screened by the National Cancer Institute (NCI) each year using the P388 in vivo murine leukemia model.[1] Agents that prolong survival beyond 125% of controls are selected for further testing. This system permits evaluation of an agent's antitumor effect in the context of toxicity to the host. However, NCI is shifting emphasis in its screening programs for cytotoxic agents from murine tumor systems to human cells to increase the specificity against human tumors.[2] Agents with in vitro activity will be tested further against the same tumor in nude mice to determine if antitumor activity is still present at a dose that can be tolerated by the animal.

Screening of BRMs is operationally more difficult. By definition, the target cell of BRMs is not the malignant cell, but rather a host effector cell that then mediates the antitumor effect (Table 1). More than one class of effector cells can mediate antitumor responses. Lymphokine activated killer (LAK) cells lyse fresh tumor cells in vitro,[3] cause regressions of established tumors in irradiated mice,[4] and have resulted in objective antitumor responses in patients with advanced malignancies.[5] Natural killer (NK) cells are capable of lysing some tumor cell lines following removal from the systemic circulation without a requirement for prior activation, sensitization to the tumor cell line or the presence of antibody on the surface of the tumor cell.[6] The rejection of tumor by animals previously immunized against the same tumor cell line is mediated by cytotoxic T lymphocytes.[7] Macrophages activated to a tumoricidal state have been demonstrated to be the effector cell responsible for eradication of pulmonary metastases in a murine model.[8]

To evaluate potential BRMs rigorously, each agent must be tested in vitro and in vivo for biologic activity on each effector cell and for antitumor activity in standard tumor models. The complexity associated with the evaluation of each agent prevents screening large numbers of potential BRMs as has been done with cytotoxics. The Biologic Response Modifiers Program (BRMP) Preclinical Screening Laboratory (PSL) has evaluated the effects of ten to 20 compounds per year on macrophage, NK cell, the lymphocyte function in tumor-free mice and

---

From the Cancer Therapy Evaluation Program, Division of Cancer Treatment, National Cancer Institute, Bethesda, Md.

Address reprint requests to Michael J. Hawkins, MD, IDB, CTEP, DCT, NCI, 4C19 Landow Building, Bethesda, MD 20892.

0093–7754/86/1302–0002$0.00/0

Table 1. Comparison of the Clinical Development of Cytotoxics and Biological Response Modifiers

Phase of Development	Cytotoxics	Biological Response Modifiers
Preclinical screening	Assess effect on tumor cell	Assess effect on host cell and effect of treated host cell on tumor cell
Phase I	Determine toxicity of agent	Determine toxicity of agent
	Determine dose, route, and schedule that results in maximum drug administration with acceptable toxicity	Determine dose, route, and schedule that produces the maximum biological effect on the host cell
Phase II	Identify malignancies in which the agent has reproducible antitumor activity	Identify malignancies in which the agent has reproducible antitumor activity
Phase III	Determine the role of the agent in treatment of the malignancy	Determine the role of the agent in treatment of the malignancy
Metastatic	Use agents with antitumor activity in phase II	Use agents with antitumor activity in phase II
Adjuvant	Use agents with antitumor activity in phase II	Agents may enhance immunologic responses in the absence of phase II antitumor activity

on tumor growth in metastatic transplant and autochtonous murine tumor models.[9,10] The effect of each agent was assessed at multiple doses and graded for activity relative to positive and negative controls. Most active agents have had effects in multiple assays, and it is not yet clear whether multiple cells are activated by the BRM or if assays thought to be specific actually measure the activity of multiple effector cells. Selective depletion of specific effector cells has been difficult to achieve in in vivo models but must be pursued to fully understand the mechanism of action for each agent.

Following the evaluation of the BRM on effector cell function, the PSL then, in nontumor-bearing mice, determines the optimal immunomodulatory protocol (OIP), defined as the dose and schedule producing maximal enhancement of the effector cell function of interest without compromise of other immunologic responses.[11] Subsequent evaluation of survival in mice bearing sensitive tumors treated with different doses and schedules of the BRM then yields the optimal therapeutic protocol (OTP). For example, Poly IC had a high degree of activity in all assays of effector function and also caused antitumor response in the MBL-2 ascites tumor model. The cumulative dose of the OTP (100 μg twice weekly) was less than the highest nonlethal dose (50 μg daily) but also differed from the OIP (10 μg daily) as measured in nontumor-bearing animals.[12] Because the OIP may differ for tumor-bearing and nontumor-bearing animals, further studies are necessary to determine the effect of tumor burden on immune function and response to selected BRMs.

In other studies conducted by the PSL, the antitumor activity of recombinant IFN gamma in two B16-BL6 metastatic tumor models in C57Bl/6 mice was highly dose and schedule dependent.[13] IFN gamma 50,000 units three times per week significantly reduced the median number of metastases following intravenous or foot pad injection of tumor cells when compared to saline treated controls ($P = .008$ and .0047, respectively). Following 10,000 or 100,000 units of IFN gamma three times weekly the median number of pulmonary lesions in either model did not differ significantly from saline-treated controls ($P > .10$). Studies to identify an effector cell mediating this antitumor effect are currently in progress. However, it is clear that the apparent antitumor effect of IFN gamma is not a simple increasing function of dose. Data such as these have profound implications for clinical developmental strategies.

PHASE I CLINICAL TRIALS

The purposes of phase I trials are to define the toxicities of the investigational agent and to develop a treatment regimen that will be adequately tolerated in subsequent efficacy trials. Patients with normal or near normal organ function are selected for study so that the chance of irreversible organ damage is minimized and drug-related toxicities can clearly be identified. Pharmacokinetic parameters determined during phase I trials can be useful in the design of optimal treatment regimens and for the establishment of dose modification guidelines in patients with compromised organ function.[14] Because the full expression and recovery from toxicity for many cytotoxics does not occur until 2 to 3 weeks after administration, intermittent treatment schedules have frequently been used.

Many phase I trials with BRMs have attempted to obtain preliminary pharmacokinetic, toxicity, and BRM data by escalating the dose of the BRM within each patient after a short observation period (usually three to seven days) following each injection. Because delayed toxicity could result in life-threatening or fatal complications, trials that permit escalation within patients must allow an adequate time interval between injections to permit full recovery from any acute or subacute adverse effects. Although further pharmacokinetic and BRM data may be obtained at the escalated dose levels, prior exposure to the BRM may have altered the responsiveness of effector cells to subsequent doses,[15] and apparent dose-dependent changes in pharmacokinetics cannot be distinguished from altered metabolism due to subclinical organ dysfunction induced by the BRM. In addition, tachyphylaxis to the BRM or cumulative toxicity from prior injections may result in an overestimate or underestimate, respectively, of the single-dose MTD.

The most reliable method, therefore, of establishing the dose of a BRM suitable for prolonged administration is by a classical phase I trial design in which groups of patients are treated at progressively higher dose levels until the MTD is determined.[16] Dose escalation should not generally be performed within patients because evaluation of chronic administration on toxicity, metabolism of the BRM, and effector cell function is a primary objective of these studies. While cytotoxic agents are almost always used at the MTD, the biological response modifying activity of the agent should ideally be evaluated at all dose levels to determine the optimal dose for enhancement of immunologic responses.

In the PSL, the definition of the OIP has been useful because of the high degree of assay reproducibility and the ability to grade all agents relative to positive and negative controls. In the clinic, however, it is frequently not practical to evaluate the BRM for biological activity in all effector cell assays. In addition, the patient population may exhibit considerable heterogeneity. Thus, the OIP becomes much more difficult to determine. Based on preclinical data, a decision can be made to focus on one particular effector system. Variability between patients may remain considerable, however, even if entry onto the study was well controlled for stage of disease, tumor type, prior therapy, organ function, and performance status.[17]

The problems associated with determination of the OIP in man can be demonstrated by a review of the initial phase I BRM trials with IFN alpha. While it was recognized that a number of mechanisms could account for IFN alpha-induced tumor regressions,[18] NK cells were thought to be a likely target for IFN alpha effect since a large preclinical experience demonstrated consistent enhancement of NK cell cytotoxicity following in vitro or in vivo exposure of leukocytes to IFN or IFN inducers.[19–21] It was, therefore, of great interest to determine if treatment regimens that optimized NK cell function in phase I trials resulted in maximum antitumor activity. An assay that used peripheral blood mononuclear cells as effector cells to lyse K562 tumor cell targets was used to assess NK cell function in man.[22] Considerable intra- and interpatient variability in the NK cell assay was demonstrated.[23] Although cryopreserved effector cells from normal donors could be used to help control for day-to-day assay variability, freezing resulted in too much loss of activity to assay all samples together.[24] Given these problems with the clinical NK assay, it is not surprising that many experienced investigators obtained conflicting results (Table 2). The limits of a normal range, as defined by the mean ± 2 standard deviations for a population of cancer patients or normal volunteers, were so large that many investigators resorted to alternative methods of statistical analysis. These included: (1) subset analysis that classified patients based upon pretreatment levels of NK cell cytotoxicity[30]; (2) establishment of a normal range for each patient before IFN administration by analysis of multiple baseline determinations[27]; and (3) comparison of pre- and post-treatment values for each patient with analysis of changes for the group.[31] The use of multiple effector to target cell (E:T) ratios in the conduct of the NK assay further confounded interpretation of the data; some investigators reported results based on a single

Table 2. Initial Biological Response Modification Trials Using IFN Alpha

Institution	Dose Range	Route/Schedule	Kinetics of NK Cell Cytotoxicity	Analysis	NK Assay	Reference
Duke	.1-4.0 MU/m²	IM × 1	Decreased at 12 h with recovery at 24 and 48 h	Percent change from baseline for all patients at E:T ratio 10:1	2 h ^{51}C release, K562 targets, E:T ratio 20, 10, 5, 2.5:1	25
	.5-15 MU/m²	IM 3 times/wk	Maximum after 1 wk, decline during wks 4 and 5 with high doses	Cryopreserved effector cells used as controls	Cells centrifuged to increase contact	
UCLA	1.5-100 MU	IM twice/d × 7 days; Repeat every 28th day	Increased at 2 h from baseline Decreased by day 7	All time points averaged regardless of dose at E:T ratio 25:1	3 h ^{51}Cr release, K562 targets, E:T ratio 25, 10, 5:1	26
BRMP	.1-50 MU	6 hr IV infusion, 5 d/wk	No change in approximately 70% of patients Tendency for decrease at higher doses	Cryopreserved effector cells used as correction factor	4 h ^{51}Cr release, K562 targets, E:T ratio 60, 20, 7:1	27
	.1-50 MU	IM 5 d/wk	No difference by routes of administration	Significant change was considered as ± 15.3% from baseline as determined in each patient		
Wisconsin	.1-30 MU dose levels given in random sequence	IM every week × 6	Maximum enhancement after 3 MU; less enhancement after .1, 1, 10, or 30 MU No carryover effect from week to week	Percent change in lytic units over mean baseline for each patient	6 h ^{51}Cr release, K562 targets, E:T ratio 100, 50, 25, 12.5, 6.25, 3.125:1 Effector cells incubated overnight in media before assay	28
Georgetown	15 MU/m²	IM 3 times/wk × 2 wks; Repeat every 21st day	Increased in 7 patients Decreased or no change in 6 patients	Multiple baselines Comparison of peak pre- and post-treatment values	4 h ^{51}Cr release, K562 targets, E:T ratio 40, 20, 10, 5, 2.5:1 Adherent cells depleted from effector cells	29
	5 MU/m²	IM each wk	Increased in 6 patients, decreased or no change in 4 patients	Lytic unit calculations		

Abbreviation: IM, intramuscularly; IV, intravenously.

E:T ratio,[25,26] while others attempted to use all the data obtained by performing lytic unit calculations.[27-29] Thus the variability of the NK assay in man has become a significant obstacle to determining the effect of IFN alpha administration of NK cell function and correlating changes with antitumor response.

PHASE II CLINICAL TRIALS

After the dose of a cytotoxic has been determined for a treatment schedule in phase I, a series of trials are usually initiated to determine if the agent is active or inactive in each malignancy.[16] Each study limits accrual to a specified number of patients (usually 30 to 40) with a given histologic diagnosis who have disease that can be objectively evaluated so that the rate of response can be determined. Cytotoxic trials have also placed limits on the amount of prior chemotherapy patients may have received, since heavily pretreated patients may have developed resistance to multiple cytotoxic agents and may not tolerate full doses of the new agent. Because no agent yet developed has significant antitumor activity against all types of malignancies, an adequate number of patients with each malignancy must be studied to evaluate adequately the antitumor potential of each agent.

The objectives of phase II trials with BRMs are similar to those of cytotoxics.[32] Empirically derived regimens have shown that certain malignancies are quite sensitive. IFNs alpha have been shown to be highly active against hairy cell leukemia, even in the presence of extensive disease.[33-35] Antitumor responses have also occurred in patients with chronic granulocytic leukemia,[36] cutaneous T cell lymphomas,[37] multiple myeloma,[38] and favorable histology of non-Hodgkin's lymphoma.[39] As always, the clinical significance of these responses ultimately must be determined in phase III trials. In contrast to the hematologic malignancies, IFN alpha has had relatively little activity against most solid tumors.[40,41] Antitumor activity has been reported in malignant melanoma,[42] renal cell carcinoma,[43] and Kaposi's sarcoma.[44,45] In the majority of patients with solid tumors, however, responses have been infrequent or of short duration; it seems unlikely, therefore, that single agent therapy with IFN alpha will have a significant impact on overall survival in these malignancies.

Selection of a dose suitable for phase II testing of a BRM may be difficult for reasons previously outlined here and by others.[46] For example, as a result of the difficulty in establishing an OIP for IFN alpha, a number of doses and schedules have been explored during phase II trials, the dose for a given study depending in part on the malignancy being treated. Highly sensitive malignancies, such as hairy cell leukemia, have responded well to low doses of IFN alpha (2 MU/m^2 daily or three times per week).[33-35] Since this dose has been effective and well tolerated even in patients with poor bone marrow reserve, the effect of higher doses on the time to response and the frequency of complete remissions has not been studied. In less sensitive tumors, higher doses have been associated with greater antitumor activity. In a randomized trial in renal cell carcinoma, for example, 20 MU/m^2 yielded 12 of 41 responses, compared to 0 of 15 at 2 MU/m^2.[43] Similar results have also been observed in a nonrandomized trial in Kaposi's sarcoma[45] and a smaller randomized trial of partially purified leukocyte IFN in renal cell carcinoma.[47] However, in malignant melanoma the response rate was not appreciably higher at 50 MU/m^2 than at 20 MU/m^2 (23% and 20% respectively) in two consecutive phase II studies conducted by the same investigator.[42,48]

Differing sensitivities of malignant cells to the antiproliferative activity of IFN alpha with a plateau of the dose-response curve at high doses could explain the results of these phase II trials, since the antiproliferative effects of IFNs alpha have been well documented in vitro.[49] It is also possible, however, that these results reflect differing mechanisms of antitumor activity and that NK cells, which have been postulated to control normal hematopoietic function in man,[50] are only capable of effectively inhibiting malignant cells of hematologic origin. In one study designed to assess the effect of dose on NK activation, IFN alpha-induced enhancement of human NK cell cytotoxicity was optimal following a single IM dose of 3 MU and was significantly less following .1, 1, 10 or 30 MU.[28] For no malignancy thus far, however, has IFN alpha demonstrated less antitumor activity at the MTD than at lower doses. Thus in the absence of laboratory data suggesting an antitumor role for an effector cell for which the dose of OIP is less than the MTD, it is difficult to develop enthusiasm for further studies of IFN alpha at doses lower than the MTD.

For other BRMs currently in clinical trial, more extensive evaluation of the effect of dose on antitumor activity may be required. From the PSL data mentioned earlier, one might expect the antitumor activity of IFN gamma to show significant dependence on dose and to be optimal at a dose less than the MTD.[13] If an effector cell is identified and an assay that accurately reflects its activity can be developed for clinical trials, treatment regimens can seek to maximize effector cell function and optimize antitumor activity. In the absence of an identified effector cell or a reliable clinical assay, it may be necessary to pursue these preclinical observations empirically by conducting a series of phase II trials using different doses of IFN gamma administered at a fixed schedule.

PHASE III CLINICAL TRIALS

The objective of phase III trials is to determine the role of a new agent in increasing survival or improving the quality of life for patients with a given stage of a malignant disease. The new agent is usually compared to or combined with standard therapy, depending on the single agent activity documented in phase II and the activity of the standard therapy. Phase III trials with cytotoxics follow the same general principles regardless of whether treatment is given for advanced metastatic disease or as an adjuvant to primary therapy. The new cytotoxic is combined with or compared to existing therapy for the disease in a fashion that permits administration of the greatest amount of agent that can be tolerated.[32] Regimens that are highly active in the metastatic setting are also given to patients following primary therapy to treat subclinical metastatic disease and prevent subsequent clinical relapse.

Although cytotoxic chemotherapy should be administered at full doses to achieve maximal antitumor activity, agents must often be used at less than the single agent MTD when combined with other drugs having similar toxicities. Because cytotoxics are generally given in a cyclic fashion to permit recovery from toxicity, new agents may be added at the time of drug administration or during the recovery period. The possibility of unexpected interactions between agents used in combination means that new regimens usually must be tested in pilot studies to document safety before initiation of large-scale trials.

Because many cytotoxic agents may be toxic to effector cells, the addition of BRMs to existing chemotherapy regimens is conceptually complex. At present, there is no model that can be used to combine BRMs with cytotoxic chemotherapy in an optimal manner. Because IFN alpha has activity as a single agent in a number of malignancies, it has been combined with cytotoxic agents in preparation for randomized phase III advanced disease trials that evaluate the contribution of IFN alpha to existing therapy. Combination regimens have been designed to give IFN alpha at the time of chemotherapy administration, between cycles of chemotherapy, and after chemotherapy induced complete remissions (Table 3). The dose of IFN alpha used in each combination was the highest that could be given without compromising administration of cytotoxic agents known to be effective in the disease. IFN alpha is also being tested as a surgical adjuvant in patients with malignant melanoma at high risk for recurrence (Table 3). In this case, the treatment regimen was based on a dose and schedule of IFN alpha with antitumor activity in phase II trials.

In each of these examples, the decision to add IFN alpha to established therapy was based on the single agent activity of IFN alpha against advanced disease. Admittedly there is no way of knowing if the dose of IFN alpha in each case is optimal; however, each regimen was constructed such that administration of known effective therapy was not compromised. In these randomized trials, significant improvement in survival due to the addition of IFN alpha should be detectable, since both groups of patients receive optimal standard therapy. However, rational design of treatment regimens to optimize the activity of IFN alpha in combination with existing therapies will not be possible until a relevant model that correlates with the antitumor activity of IFN alpha is identified.

Design of adjuvant trials in malignancies for which the BRM does not have antitumor activity in advanced disease is much more problematic. It has been proposed that BRMs should be tested in the adjuvant setting because only patients with a small tumor burden might be expected to respond to immunotherapy.[32] Data from the PSL suggesting that the antitumor activity of poly IC is greatest in animals with a low tumor burden supports this approach.[54] It is reasoned that BRMs without activity in metastatic disease could still be of value in phase III trials to enhance or restore immunocompetence that has been compromised by surgery or chemotherapy. However, large scale phase III trials entail the commitment of substantial clinical resources and previous studies using agents without single agent activity in metastatic disease, such as Bacillus Calmette-Guerin (BCG) or *Corynebacterium parvum,* have not convincingly improved survival in the adjuvant setting.[55] In such a setting, the dose and schedule of the BRM and the timing of administration with respect to the cytotoxic or surgery could be critical. Until it is possible to prospectively develop regimens that

Table 3. Schedules of IFN Alpha Used in Combination With Standard Therapy

Tumor Type	Standard Therapy	IFN Alpha Dose/m²	IFN Alpha Schedule	Reference
Multiple myeloma	Melphalan days 8, 10, 12, 15 Prednisone days 8–15 every 28 days	5 MU	days 1, 3, 5, 8, 10, 12, 15	51
Non-Hodgkin's lymphoma	COPA days 1–5 every 28 days	6 MU	days 22–26	52
	CVP every 4 weeks until complete remission	8 MU	After CVP completed: each day × 30 days, every 4 months × 4	53
Malignant melanoma	Surgical resection	20 MU 10 MU	days 1–5 every week × 4 weeks 3 times/wk × 1 year	53

Abbreviations: COPA, cyclophosphamide, vincristine, prednisone, doxorubicin; CVP, cyclophosphamide, vincristine, prednisone.

are likely to use the BRM in an optimal manner, treatment schedules used in phase III adjuvant trials should probably be based on those that produce antitumor responses in advanced disease.

CONCLUSIONS

As oncologists are aware, the development of cytotoxics has been an arduous process. The lack of screening systems that are highly predictive of antitumor activity in the common human solid tumors has been a major roadblock. In addition, despite impressive advances in characterizing the action of many active cytotoxic agents, we still do not have a comprehensive understanding of the biochemical basis of selective tumor cell killing for any drug. Although this lack has seriously hindered the rational development of combination chemotherapy and combined modality approaches, it has not been an insuperable obstacle to progress in treatment, chiefly because oncologists have been able to assume that antitumor effect is roughly proportional to dose. This very fundamental assumption has permitted intelligent empiricism to operate with very gratifying results in at least some tumor types.

BRMs, however, present an additional level of complexity. A truly rational approach to their clinical testing requires that the interaction of the BRM and the host be understood, or at least be formulated in terms of testable hypotheses. If one supposes that an agent kills tumor by activating a certain class of host effector cells, then it is certainly reasonable to administer the agent in a manner that maximizes activation of this class. To do this properly, whether in mice or men, one obviously needs both a tenable hypothesis and laboratory techniques reliable and reproducible enough to measure the BRM effect(s) and correlate it(them) with antitumor effects.

Because we understand only in a rather rudimentary way how the host goes about controlling tumor growth and because our methods of monitoring the effects we have identified leave much to be desired, the goals of rational BRM development are much easier to articulate theoretically than to realize in actual clinical investigation. As outlined previously, a number of very significant conceptual and practical barriers have frustrated our early attempts to approach BRM development in this manner.

Given these serious limitations, how can we approach the development of BRMs in a reasonably efficient manner? The question is an important and timely one, since the number of cytokines that are candidates for clinical trial will increase dramatically over the next few years. In developing a reasonable approach, the lessons learned from years of cytotoxic drug development may provide a useful perspective.

From the preclinical laboratory, we can hope to learn whether the candidate BRM has significant antitumor effects and, if so, what the shape of the dose-response curve is. From experiments in immune-competent animals, we can develop data concerning activation of effector mechanisms that are postulated to mediate the antitumor effect. If preclinical experiments can present clinicians with a coherent body of information concerning the form of dose-response relationships for both antitumor and BRM effects, the implementation of a rational clinical strategy will be greatly expedited. In phase I, one then determines the MTD in the usual manner; in addition, as Herberman has proposed,[32] if patients with minimal prior treatment, excellent performance status, and relatively limited tumor burden can be entered upon such studies, it may be possible to determine the relation of dose to BRM activity using selected effector functions as endpoints. Once this is done, phase II studies can proceed at the MTD and the OIP, if this can be satisfactorily defined in phase I.[46] Randomized trials may ultimately be required to determine the optimally therapeutic regimen.

In situations where a probable effector cell cannot be identified from preclinical studies, an alternative procedure might involve performing the initial phase II evaluation at the MTD only. If antitumor activity is observed, the function of multiple effector cells can be compared in responding and nonresponding patients. Changes in effector cell function that correlated with tumor responses, although not establishing a cause and effect relationship, would provide a rationale for evaluating the antitumor activity of an OIP designed to optimize the effect of the BRM on the putative effector cell.

Obviously successful implementation of either approach requires reproducible assays for the effector functions of interest. In the absence of meaningful clinical monitoring, we do not think that the purely empirical study of a range of doses in phase II is likely to be useful. If, however, the preclinical evaluation suggests a complex dose-antitumor effect relationship in which the effect rises and then falls with continued dose escalation, one might reasonably consider phase II trials at doses other than MTD. Such doses and schedules would have to be selected rather arbitrarily and the possibility of missing the OIP would be very real.

ACKNOWLEDGMENT

The authors thank Edith Altemus for the preparation of this manuscript.

REFERENCES

1. DeVita VT Jr: Principles of chemotherapy, in DeVita VT Jr, Hellman S, Rosenberg SA (eds): Cancer: Principles and Practice of Oncology. Philadelphia, J.B. Lippincott, 1982, pp 144–145

2. Shoemaker RH, Wolpert-DeFilippes MK, Kern DH, et al: Application of a human tumor colony-forming assay to new drug screening. Cancer Res 45:2145–2153, 1985

3. Rosenstein M, Yron I, Kaufman Y, et al: Lymphokine activated killer cells: Lysis of fresh syngeneic NK-resistant murine tumor cells by lymphocytes cultured in interleukin-2. Cancer Res 44:1946–1953, 1984

4. Mule JJ, Shu S, Rosenberg SA: The antitumor efficacy of lymphokine-activated killer cells and recombinant interleukin 2 in vivo. J Immunol 135:646–652, 1985

5. Rosenberg SA, Lotze MT, Muul LM, et al: Observations on the systemic administration of autologous lymphokine-activated killer cells and recombinant interleukin-2 to patients with metastatic cancer. N Engl J Med 313:1485–1492, 1985

6. Herberman RB, Holden HT: Natural cell mediated immunity. Adv Cancer Res 27:305–377, 1978

7. Greenberg PD, Cheever MA, Fefer A: Therapy of established tumors by adoptive transfer of T lymphocytes, in Herberman, RB (ed): Basic and Clinical Tumor Immunology. Boston, Martinus Nijhoff, 1983, pp 301–35

8. Fidler IJ, Barnes Z, Folger WE, et al: Involvement of macrophages in the eradication of established metastases following intravenous injection of liposomes containing macrophage activators. Cancer Res 42:496–501, 1982

9. Fidler IJ, Berendt M, Oldham RK: Rationale for and design of a screening procedure for the assessment of biological response modifiers for cancer treatment. J Biol Response Mod 1:15–26, 1982

10. Talmadge JE, Herberman RB: The preclinical screening laboratory: Evaluation of immunomodulatory and therapeutic properties of biological response modifiers. Cancer Treat Rep 70:171–182, 1986

11. Talmadge JE, Hartmann D: Optimization of an immunotherapeutic protocol with poly (I,C)-LC. J Biol Response Mod 4:484–489, 1985

12. Hartmann D, Adams JS, Meeker AK, et al: Dissociation between therapeutic and toxic effects of polyinosinic-polycytidylic acid solubilized with poly-L-lysine in carboxymethylcellulose [poly (IC)-LC] in tumor-bearing mice. Cancer Res, 1985 (in press)

13. Talmadge JE, Tribble HR, Pennington RW, et al: Immunomodulatory and immunotherapeutic properties of recombinant gamma interferon and recombinant tumor necrosis factor in mice. (submitted for publication)

14. Collins JM, Dedrick RL: Pharmacokinetics of anticancer drugs, in Chabner BA (ed): Pharmacologic Principles of Cancer Treatment. Philadelphia, Saunders, 1982, pp 77–99

15. Maluish AE, Ortaldo JR, Conlon JC, et al: Depression of natural killer cytotoxicity after in vivo administration of recombinant leukocyte interferon. J Immunol 131:503–507, 1983

16. Simon RM: Design and conduct of clinical trials, in DeVita VT Jr, Hellman S, Rosenberg SA (eds): Cancer: Principles and Practice of Oncology. Philadelphia, J.B. Lippincott, pp 198–225, 1982

17. Pross HF, Baines MG: Studies of human natural killer cells. I. In vivo parameters affecting normal cytotoxic function. Int J Cancer 29:383–390, 1982

18. Borden EC: Interferons: Rationale for clinical trials in neoplastic disease. Ann Internal Med 91:472–479, 1979

19. Gidlund M, Orn A, Wigzell H, et al: Enhanced NK cell activity in mice injected with interferon and interferon inducers. Nature 273:759–761, 1978

20. Herberman RB, Ortaldo JR, Bonnard GD: Augmentation by interferon of human natural and antibody-dependent cell-mediated cytotoxicity. Nature 277:221–223, 1979

21. Herberman RB, Djeu JY, Ortaldo JR, et al: Role of interferon in augmentation of natural and antibody-dependent cell-mediated cytotoxicity. Cancer Treat Rep 62:1893–1896, 1978

22. Ortaldo JR, Bonnard GD, Herberman RB: Cytotoxic reactivity of human lymphocytes cultured in vitro. J Immunol 119:1351–1357, 1977

23. Pross HF, Baines MG, Rubin P, et al: Spontaneous human lymphocyte-mediated cytotoxocity against tumor target cells. IX. The quantitation of natural killer cell activity. J Clin Immunol 1:51–63, 1981

24. Strong DM, Ortaldo JR, Pandolfi F, et al: Cryopreservation of human mononuclear cells for quality control in clinical immunology. I. Correlations in recovery of K and NK cell functions, surface markers, and morphology. J Clin Immunol 2:214–21, 1982

25. Koren HS, Brandt CP, Tso CY, et al: Modulation of natural killing activity by lymphoblastoid interferon in cancer patients. J Biol Response Mod 2:151–165, 1983

26. Spina CA, Fahey JL, Durkos-Smith D, et al: Suppression of natural killer cell cytotoxicity of the peripheral blood of patients receiving interferon therapy. J Biol Response Mod 2:458–469, 1983

27. Maluish AE, Ortaldo JR, Sherwin SA, et al: Changes in immune function in patients receiving natural leukocyte interferon. J Biol Response Mod 2:418–427, 1983

28. Edwards BS, Merritt JA, Fuhlbrigge RC, et al: Low doses of interferon alpha result in more effective clinical

natural killer cell activation. J Clin Invest 75:1908–1913, 1985
29. Neefe JR, Sullivan JE, Silgals R: Preliminary observations of immunomodulatory activity of lymphoblastoid interferon-alpha administered every other day or weekly. J Biol Response Mod 2:441–449, 1983
30. Lotzova E, Savary CA, Quesada Jr, et al: Analysis of natural killer cell cytotoxicity of cancer patients treated with recombinant interferon. J Natl Cancer Inst 71:903–910, 1983
31. Edwards BS, Hawkins MJ, Borden EC: Correlation between in vitro and systemic effects of native and recombinant interferons-alpha upon NK cell cytotoxicity. J Biol Response Mod 2:409–417, 1983
32. Herberman RB: Design of clinical trials with biological response modifiers. Cancer Treat Rep 69:1161–1164, 1985
33. Quesada JR, Reuben J, Manning JT, et al: Alpha interferon for induction of remission in hairy cell leukemia. N Engl J Med 310:15–18, 1984
34. Golomb H, Fefer A, Ratain M, et al: Intron A, recombinant alpha-2 interferon (IFN), for the treatment of hairy cell leukemia (HCL). Proc Am Soc Clin Oncol 4:225, 1985 (abstr)
35. Foon KA, Maluish AE, Abrams PG, et al: A phase II trial of recombinant leukocyte A interferon (rIFN-alpha A) for advanced hairy cell leukemia. Proc Am Soc Clin Oncol 4:221, 1985 (abstr)
36. Talpaz M, McCredie KB, Mavligit GM, et al: Leukocyte interferon-induced myeloid cytoreduction in chronic myelogenous leukemia. Blood 62:689–692, 1983
37. Bunn PA Jr, Foon KA, Ihde DC, et al: Recombinant leukocyte A interferon: An active agent in advanced cutaneous T-cell lymphomas. Ann Intern Med 101:484–487, 1984
38. Quesada JR, Alexanian R, Hawkins M, et al: Treatment of multiple myeloma with recombinant alpha-interferon. Blood 67:275–278, 1986
39. Foon KA, Sherwin SA, Abrams PG, et al: Treatment of advanced non-Hodgkin's lymphoma with recombinant leukocyte A interferon. N Engl J Med 311:1148–1152, 1984
40. Kirkwood JM, Ernstoff MS: Interferons in the treatment of cancer. J Clin Oncol 2:336–352, 1984
41. Bonnem EM, Spiegel RJ: Interferon alpha. Current status and future promise. J Biol Response Mod 3:580–598, 1984
42. Creagan ET, Ahmann DL, Green SJ, et al: Phase II study of recombinant leukocyte A interferon (rIFN alpha A) in disseminated malignant melanoma. Cancer 54:2844–2849, 1984
43. Quesada JR, Rios A, Swanson D, et al: Antitumor activity or recombinant-derived interferon alpha in metastatic renal cell carcinoma. J Clin Oncol 3:1522–1528, 1985
44. Krown SE, Real FX, Cunningham-Rundles S, et al: Preliminary observations on the effect of leukocyte A interferon in homosexual men with kaposi's sarcoma. N Engl J Med 308:1071–1076, 1983
45. Groopman JE, Gottlieb MS, Goodman J, et al: Recombinant alpha-2 interferon therapy for Kaposi's sarcoma associated with the acquired immunodeficiency syndrome. Ann Internal Med 100:671–676, 1984
46. Pinsky CM: Applicability of phase I trial results in the design of phase II and III biological response modifier trials. Cancer Treat Rep 69:1171–1173, 1985
47. Kirkwood JM, Harris JE, Vera R, et al: A randomized study of low and high doses of leukocyte A interferon in metastatic renal cell carcinoma: The American Cancer Society collaborative trial. Cancer Res 45:863–871, 1985
48. Creagan ET, Ahmann DL, Green SJ, et al: Phase II study of low-dose recombinant leukocyte A interferon in disseminated malignant melanoma. J Clin Oncol 2:1002–1005, 1984
49. Salmon SE, Durie BG, Young L, et al: Effects of cloned human leukocyte interferons in the human tumor stem cell assay. J Clin Oncol 1:217–225, 1983
50. Wigzell H, Cudkowicz G, Elkins WL, et al: NK cell systems as effectors of resistance to normal and malignant hemopoietic cells, in Jenner CA, Cudkowicz G, Landy M, et al (eds): Natural Resistance Systems Against Foreign Cells, Tumors and Microbes. Proceedings of an International Conference held October 18 to 22, 1976. Orlando, Fla, Academic, 1978 p 29
51. Cooper MR, Fefer A, Thompson J, et al: Alpha-2 interferon (IFN), melphalan (M), and prednisone (P) in the treatment of newly diagnosed multiple myeloma. Proc Am Soc Clin Oncol 4:216, 1985 (abstr)
52. Hawkins MJ, O'Connell MJ, Schiller JH, et al: Phase I evaluation of recombinant A interferon alpha in combination with COPA chemotherapy. Proc Am Soc Clin Oncol 4:229, 1985
53. Hawkins MJ: Evaluation of recombinant alpha interferons in phase III cooperative group trials. The Interferon Letter, II:3, 1985
54. Talmadge JE, Adams J, Phillips H, et al: Immunotherapeutic potential in murine tumor models of polyinosinic-polycytidylic acid and poly-L-lysine solubilized by carboxymethylcellulose. Cancer Res 45:1066–1072, 1985
55. Borden EC, Hawkins MJ: Biological response modifiers as adjuncts to other therapeutic modalities. Semin Oncol 13:144–152, 1986

IMMUNOMODULATORS

Local Administration of Immunomodulators

Carl M. Pinsky

THERE ARE NUMEROUS experimental animal models suggesting that destruction of tumor by local administration of biological response modifiers (BRMs) results in long-lasting tumor immunity. In fact, there are suggestions that such immunity is better induced by destruction in situ than by surgical resection. On the other hand, the clinical data on local administration of BRMs do not permit the conclusion that immunologic mechanisms have been brought into play. Rather, the clinical information is consistent with a bystander effect, namely, local destruction of tumor cells by inflammatory/immunologic reactions that result from the BRM injection. These observations do not minimize the potential utility of the approach, however, because tumor cell necrosis is a useful effect, whatever the mechanism.

There are several clinical situations in which clear-cut antitumor effects appear to result from local administration of BRMs. The most consistent and long-lasting responses have been observed following administration of immunomodulators, a class of BRMs that includes microbial extracts and chemical compounds with pleiotropic and profound effects on the immune system.

INTRALESIONAL ADMINISTRATION

The largest body of data relating to the clinical use of a BRM intralesionally relates to Bacillus Calmette-Guerin (BCG). The first evaluable report concerning the use of BCG by intralesional injection came from Morton et al.[1] In that study, eight patients with 184 lesions of metastatic melanoma were treated, and regression was observed in 90% of the injected lesions. It appeared that an intact cellular immune system was required for this antitumor effect.[1] A number of trials confirmed and extended these observations. Studies that were carried out at Memorial Sloan-Kettering Cancer Center eventually included over 70 patients with diffuse cutaneous melanoma lesions.[2] Conclusions from our work[2] and the work of many other investigators[1,3–7] included the following observations: (1) Large volumes of tumor could be destroyed with sufficient doses of BCG; (2) regression of injected lesions was common; (3) regression of noninjected, distal cutaneous lesions, or organ metastases, was extremely rare; (4) clinically-useful antitumor responses were common; (5) regrowth of lesions that had regressed was rare, but the appearance of new lesions was common; (6) the histologic appearance of lesions suggested a local granulomatous reaction; (7) no proof that systemic immunity appeared could be documented, but responders survived over four times as long as nonresponders; and (8) these responses were achieved at the expense of considerable systemic toxicity.[1–7]

In order to avoid toxicity, a whole series of nonviable microbial or chemical compounds were then evaluated.[8–14] While none were proven better than BCG in direct head-to-head comparisons, a reduction in toxicity was generally seen. Currently, the use of a nonviable compound first is probably indicated. Most recently, we[14] have found that 2,4-dinitrochlorobenezene works quite well in destroying even large numbers of metastatic melanoma skin nodules. Nonresponding lesions can then be treated with BCG. Recently, one other type of nonviable, BRM that has been used intralesionally is monoclonal antibody-directed against melanoma cell-surface antigens. Response rates are not yet reported. Diseases, other than melanoma, in which clinical responses after intralesional injection of BCG have been seen include breast cancer,[15] and lung cancer.[16]

From the Biological Resources Branch, Biological Response Modifiers Program, Division of Cancer Treatment, National Cancer Institute, Frederick Cancer Research Facility, Frederick, Md.

Address reprint requests to Carl M. Pinsky, MD, Chief, Biological Resources Branch, Biological Response Modifiers Program, Division of Cancer Treatment, National Cancer Institute, Frederick Cancer Research Facility, Frederick, MD 21701-1013.

The contents of this publication do not necessarily reflect the view or policies of the Department of Health and Human Resources, nor does mention of trade names, commercial products, or organizations imply endorsement by the US government.

0093–7754/86/1302–0003$0.00/0

The mechanism by which these compounds cause tumor regression is not known. A particularly useful experimental animal model in this regard, is the line 10 transplanted, chemically-induced hepatoma, of strain-2 guinea pigs.[17–19] Predictions from this model that are consistent with the clinical observations include the following: (1) About 0.5 to 1.0 $\times$ 10^7 viable BCG organisms are required to destroy about 1 cm of tumor; (2) granulomatous reactions indicating the presence of activated macrophages, are present in regressing lesions[20]; and (3) relatively large numbers of tumor cells can be destroyed. One prediction from the model that has never been tested adequately in the clinic is that injection of a primary tumor, followed in 1 or 2 weeks by surgical excision of the tumor and draining lymph nodes is most likely to cause long-lasting effects. The only clinical trials to test this prediction, using either BCG[21] or vaccinia virus,[22] are flawed by methodologic problems that render the results uninterpretable. A well-designed clinical trial to evaluate this approach is badly needed.

POST-SURGICAL INTRACAVITARY ADMINISTRATION

The clinical successes seen after local intralesional administration of BCG prompted several trials in which BCG was administered locally as surgical-adjuvant therapy. The first of these was carried out by McNeally et al.[23] After surgical excision of primary lung cancers, BCG was instilled into the pleural cavity. This was a prospective, randomized trial, indicating that the group treated with surgery and intrapleural BCG had a superior postoperative course when compared to the group treated with surgery, alone. Two similarly designed trials, in patients with recurrent, superficial cancer of the urinary bladder, also showed a clear-cut benefit in the group randomized to receive fulguration and BCG as compared to the group who were treated with fulguration alone.[24,25] The intravesical BCG trials are particularly noteworthy because the observations have been reproduced by several independent investigators.[24–26] In fact, many urologists currently consider intravesical BCG to be the treatment of choice in these patients.[24–26]

Pilot studies have been carried out with other microbial BRMs by the intracavitary route. For example, *Corynebacterium parvum* appears to have clinical utility when used by intrapleural or intraperitoneal instillation in patients with otherwise unmanageable effusions from breast[27] or ovarian[28] cancer.

Again, as with intralesional injections, situations in which tumors can be destroyed by intracavitary instillation of a BRM may be a unique opportunity to study mechanisms of action. In particular, in the case of intravesical BCG instillation, one can evaluate the cells[29,30] or cytokines released into the urine. It is also possible to examine the histologic response in the bladder wall sequentially. Although there are some technical difficulties to be overcome, such a systematic study of the mechanism(s) by which local BRM administration results in tumor regression would likely be quite fruitful.

SUMMARY

This summary of results with local BRM administration has been brief because the number of clinical situations in which this approach is applicable is quite limited. On the other hand, when applied in an appropriate patient population, clinical responses are frequent. In addition, detailed study of the effector cells and cytokines that appear in responding patients may yield information concerning the mechanism of action when BRM therapy is effective. Finally, comparison of the results from clinical trials with the results in experimental animals may help to further elucidate the mechanism by which BRMs exert antitumor effects.

REFERENCES

1. Morton DL, Eilber FR, Malmgren RA, et al: Immunological factors which influence response to immunotherapy in malignant melanoma. Surgery 68:158–164, 1970

2. Pinsky CM, Hirshaut Y, Oettgen HF: Treatment of malignant melanoma by intratumoral injection of BCG. Natl Cancer Inst Monogr 39:225–228, 1973 (and unpublished observations)

3. Nathanson L: Regression of intradermal malignant melanoma after intralesional injection of Mycobacterium bovis strain BCG. Cancer Chemother Rep 56:659–665, 1972

4. Mastrangelo MJ, Sulit HL, Prehn LM, et al: Intralesional BCG in the treatment of metastatic malignant melanoma. Cancer 37:684–692, 1976

5. McKhann CF, Hendrickson CG, Spitler LE, et al: Immunotherapy of melanoma with BCG: Two fatalities following intralesional injection. Cancer 35:514–520, 1975

6. Sparks FC, Silverstein MJ, Hunt JS, et al: Complica-

tions of BCG immunotherapy in patients with cancer. N Engl J Med 289:827–830, 1973

7. Rosenberg, EB, Kanner SP, Schwartzman RJ, et al: Systemic infection following BCG therapy. Arch Intern Med 134:769–770, 1974

8. Malek-Mansour S: Remission of melanoma with D.N.C.B. treatment. Lancet 2:503–504, 1973

9. Yamamura, Y, Yoshizaki K, Azuma I, et al: Immunotherapy of human malignant melanoma with oil-attached BCG cell-wall skeleton. Gann 66:355–363, 1975

10. Richman SP, Mavligit GM, Wolk R, et al: Epilesional scarification: Preliminary report of a new approach to local immunotherapy with BCG. JAMA 234:1233–1235, 1975

11. Cohen MH, Jessup JM, Felix EL, et al: Intralesional treatment of recurrent metastatic cutaneous malignant melanoma: A randomized prospective study of intralesional Bacillus Calmette-Guerin versus intralesional dinitrochlorobenzene. Cancer 41:2456–2463, 1978

12. Krown SE, Hilal EY, Pinsky CM, et al: Intralesional injection of the methanol extraction residue of Bacillus Calmette-Guerin (MER) into cutaneous metastases of malignant melanoma. Cancer 42:2648–2660, 1978.

13. Ishihara K, Hayasaka K: Immunotherapy of malignant melanoma. Gann 21:231–235, 1978

14. Kerr D, Krown SE, Livingston PO, et al: Treatment of melanoma skin metastases with intralesional DNCB. Proc Am Soc Clin Oncol 22:528, 1981 (abstr)

15. Pardridge DH, Sparks FC, Goodnight JE Jr, et al: Intratumor Bacillus Calmette-Guerin therapy for chest wall recurrence of carcinoma of the breast. Surg Gynecol Obstet 148:867–870, 1979

16. Holmes EC, Ramming KP, Bein ME, et al: Intralesional BCG immunotherapy of pulmonary tumors. J Thorac Cardiovasc Surg 77:362–368, 1979

17. Zbar B, Tanaka T: Immunotherapy of cancer: Regression of tumors after intralesional injection of living Mycobacterium bovis. Science 172:271–273, 1971

18. Zbar B, Bernstein ID, Rapp HJ: Suppression of tumor growth at the site of infection with living Bacillus Calmette-Guerin. J Natl Cancer Inst 46:831–839, 1971

19. Zbar B, Canti G, Ashley M, et al: Eradication by immunization with mycobacterial vaccines and tumor cells of microscopic metastases remaining after surgery. Cancer Res 39:1597–1603, 1979

20. Hanna MG, Zbar B, Rapp HJ: Histopathology of tumor regression after intralesional injection of Mycobacterium bovis. I. Tumor growth and metastasis. J Natl Cancer Inst 48:1441–1455, 1972

21. Rosenberg SA, Rapp H, Terry W, et al: Intralesional BCG therapy of patients with primary Stage I melanoma, in Terry WD, Rosenberg SA (eds): Immunotherapy of Human Cancer. Amsterdam, Elsevier North Holland, 1982, pp 239–244

22. Everall JD, Ward J, O'Doherty CJ, et al: Treatment of primary melanoma by intralesional vaccinia before excision. Lancet 2:583–586, 1975

23. McKneally MF, Maver C, Kausel HW: Regional immunotherapy of lung cancer with intrapeural B.C.G. Lancet 1:377–386, 1976

24. Pinsky CM, Camacho FJ, Kerr D, et al: Intravesical administration of Bacillus Calmette-Guerin in patients with recurrent superficial carcinoma of the urinary bladder: Report of a prospective, randomized trial. Cancer Treat Rep 69:47–53, 1985

25. Lamm DL, Thor DE, Winters WD, et al: BCG immunotherapy of bladder cancer: Inhibition of tumor recurrence and associated immune responses. Cancer 48:82–88, 1981

26. Brosman SA: Experience with BCG in patients with superficial bladder carcinoma. J Urol 128:27–30, 1982

27. Pinsky CM, Oettgen HF: Unpublished observations

28. Bast RC, Jr, Berek JS, Obrist R, et al: Intraperitoneal immunotherapy of human ovarian carcinoma with Corynebacterium parvum. Cancer Res 43:1395–1401, 1983

29. Staiano-Coico L, Huffman J, Wolf R, et al: Monitoring intravesical Bacillus Calmette-Guerin treatment of bladder carcinoma with flow cytometry. J Urol 133:786–788, 1985

30. Huffman JF, Fradet Y, Cordon-Cardo C, et al: Effect of intravesical Bacillus Calmette-Guerin on detection of a urothelial differentiation antigen in exfoliated cells of carcinoma in situ of the human urinary bladder. Cancer Res 45:5201–5204, 1985

Biologic Response Modifiers as Adjuncts to Other Therapeutic Modalities

Ernest C. Borden and Michael J. Hawkins

DESPITE SIGNIFICANT advances in cancer treatment, no single modality or drug has yet resulted in optimal therapy for any common cancer. It seems unlikely that biological response modifiers will be exceptional in this regard. Rather, effective application will most probably occur in conjunction with the other therapeutic modalities. If immunomodulation is an important component of their mechanism of action, use of biological response modifiers could occur at doses less than those defined as maximally tolerated in the phase I single agent trials.

Our review will focus on three types of biological response modifiers (Table 1): (1) Bacillus Calmette-Guerin (BCG) is an example of a complex biologic from which lessons in clinical development of a biologic are learned; (2) polyribonucleotides and levamisole are examples of chemically-defined immunomodulators that may have a clinical role; and (3) interferons (IFNs) as the biological response modifiers that show the greatest promise for successful therapeutic application in conjunction with other modalities in the near future. In addition to a clinical review, we will also highlight selected model studies to illustrate potential principles for human application.

Substantial preclinical rationale exists for clinical use of other biologics in conjunction with other treatment approaches. These include the use of interleukin 2 (IL-2) and cyclophosphamide, in vitro expanded immune effector cells adoptively transferred for administration with IL-2, and monoclonal antibodies linked to toxic molecules for selective targeting to the neoplastic cell. These approaches are, however, discussed in other articles in this issue.

COMPLEX BIOLOGICALS

The first biological response modifier to enter large-scale clinical trial was the attenuated live mycobacterium, BCG. Its use was based upon its effects in augmenting immune effector cell function, antitumor activity in animal models, and its ability to induce partial or complete regressions when inoculated into cutaneous metastases of patients with malignant melanoma.[1-5] Methanol-extracted residue (MER), as an active component of BCG,[6-8] subsequently entered trials.

Other preclinical and clinical studies have explored effects of *Corynebacterium parvum.* Although some results suggest possible merit,[9,10] only limited active studies continue. Thus, findings with it will not be further detailed. For those interested, preclinical and clinical work with *C parvum* has been reviewed.[11] Other complex microbials, such as *Brucella abortus,* mixed bacterial vaccines, and *Nocardia rubra,* are from a clinical perspective, mostly of historic interest. They did, however, provide impetus for clinical and mechanistic studies of immunomodulators.

Intradermal administration of BCG to patients with stage II malignant melanoma appeared to prolong remission duration and possibly survival in nonrandomized pilot studies using historic or contemporaneous control groups.[12,13] Based on these results, eight prospectively randomized controlled trials have collectively studied almost 2,000 patients with stage I or II malignant melanoma. None of these studies have demonstrated an increase in disease-free survival or a decrease in the frequency of disease recurrence for patients treated with adjuvant BCG compared to patients receiving surgery alone.[14-17] Deviations from the initial treatment regimen and the bias of historic control groups have been cited as possible explanations for the discrepancies between the initial pilot studies and the subsequent randomized trials.[18]

Increased disease-free interval and overall survival have been reported in 30 patients who

From the Departments of Human Oncology and Medicine, University of Wisconsin Clinical Cancer Center, Madison, and the Cancer Therapy Evaluation Program, Division of Cancer Treatment, National Cancer Institute, Bethesda, Md.

Supported in part through the National Institutes of Health by the Eastern Cooperative Oncology Group (CA 21076) and by the Biological Response Modifiers Program, the American Cancer Society and by Triton Biosciences.

Address reprint requests to Ernest C. Bordon, MD, University of Wisconsin Clinical Cancer Center, Madison, WI 53792.

0093–7754/86/1302–0004$05.00/0

Table 1. Biological Response Modifiers Evaluated in Man in Combination With Other Modalities

BCG (MER)	Interleukin-2
Polyribonucleotides	Interferons $\alpha\beta\gamma$
Levamisole	Monoclonal antibodies
Pyrimidinones	

received intrapleural BCG following resection of stage I cancer of the lung.[19] To follow-up these results, over 400 patients were entered into a randomized trial conducted by the National Lung Cancer Study Group to determine the activity of locally administered BCG following surgery for stage I non–small-cell bronchogenic carcinoma.[20] While the overall survival of all patients was unexpectedly good, no differences in overall or disease-free survival were observed between the control and BCG treated groups. Although a large number of patients with metastatic breast cancer have been treated with BCG as an adjunct to chemotherapy,[21,22] large scale, prospectively randomized trials have not been performed. In a prospectively randomized trial of FAC chemotherapy (5-fluorouracil, doxorubicin, cyclophosphamide) in patients with stage II breast carcinoma, there was no difference in relapse rate following adjuvant chemotherapy alone compared to chemotherapy plus BCG.[23]

Following an initial report indicating a significant prolongation of survival over historic controls in patients with acute myelogenous leukemia (AML) treated with BCG, a number of small randomized clinical trials[17,24] were conducted in an attempt to confirm the activity of BCG in AML. In two larger randomized studies of BCG given intradermally to patients with AML in complete remission following chemotherapy, the median duration of survival was not increased.[25,26] When BCG is mixed with irradiated or viable allogeneic blast cells, the median survival of some patients with AML may be improved.[17] However, the increase in survival that occurred in these studies generally could not be explained by the relatively small increase in the median duration of response.

A large number of controlled clinical studies have failed to demonstrate activity of BCG given alone or with cytotoxic chemotherapy as adjuvant therapy in colon carcinoma.[17] However, based on a treatment regimen in which active specific immunotherapy (intradermal administration of tumor cells mixed with BCG) protected guinea pigs from experimental metastasis,[27] a small prospectively-randomized study was initiated in patients with adenocarcinoma of the colon. After a mean follow-up period of 28 months, three of 20 treated patients have had a tumor recurrence compared to nine of 20 control patients.[28] There were no deaths in the immunotherapy plus surgery group while four patients treated with surgery alone have died. Two thirds of the patients who received active specific immunotherapy developed delayed-type cutaneous hypersensitivity to their autologous tumor cells.[29] These cells are currently being evaluated further in an Eastern Cooperative Oncology Group trial in which participating institutions prepare the vaccine using tumor cells removed at the time of primary surgery for Dukes' C carcinoma of the colon.

Experience with BCG in other malignancies has been less extensive. Patients with large-cell non-Hodgkin's lymphoma treated by the Southwest Oncology Group (SWOG) with intradermal BCG as an adjunct to cytotoxic chemotherapy CHOP, cyclophosphamide, doxorubicin, vincristine, and prednisone) had a higher complete response rate (68% *v* 48%, $P = .02$) and overall survival ($P = .02$) than patients treated with CHOP plus bleomycin.[30] As follow-up to this study, the SWOG randomized 716 patients to one of three induction regimens: CHOP, CHOP plus levamisole, or CHOP plus levamisole plus BCG.[31] There was no difference between the complete response rates or median survivals in patients with favorable histology non-Hodgkin's lymphoma after a median follow-up of 37 months. In patients with unfavorable histology, survival following CHOP plus levamisole plus BCG was equal to CHOP alone ($P = .02$) and better than CHOP plus levamisole ($P < .02$).

While BCG may have significant antitumor activity when administered locally (reviewed by Pinsky, this issue), it has not had confirmed clinical systemic effectiveness. Until better measures of immunologic function in man are available to correlate with antitumor responses, it will be difficult to scientifically design alternative schedules for systemic treatment with BCG. Based on a guinea pig model for control of metastatic disease, a series of small clinical trials in AML, the local effects in bladder carcinoma, and the results of a randomized pilot study in colorectal carcinoma, BCG may still have an eventual role in stimulation of immune responses to autologous tumor cells.

PHARMACEUTICALS

Chemically-defined immunomodulators offer several potential advantages to complex microbials. They can be produced by chemical methodologies, purified to homogeneity, and studied by conventional pharmacologic approaches. Such compounds include derivatives of acridines, aziridines, tilorone, cimetidine, prostaglandin inhibitors, polymeric malic anhydrides, pyrimidinones, and imidazoles. In addition, naturally-occurring molecules and their synthetic analogues such as muramyl dipeptide, tuftsin, thymic peptides, microbial polysaccharides, and polyribonucleotides can be considered in this category.

We will focus on two compounds, a low molecular weight pharmaceutical, levamisole, and the synthetic analogue of a naturally-occurring compound, polyriboadenylic-polyribouridylic acid. These compounds exemplify the potential for combination of biological response modifiers with other therapeutic modalities.

Levamisole

Levamisole is an orally active synthetic phenylimidazole that is a potent inhibitor of tumor tissue alkaline phosphatases.[32] It is an immunomodulator that alters T cell and macrophage function in vitro.[33–38] When used as a single agent against murine transplantable neoplasms, antitumor effects have been seen in some models. However, greater antitumor activity in experimental animals has frequently been observed when used in conjunction with chemotherapy.[39–42] Enhanced effectiveness of nitrosoureas and alkylating agents has been demonstrated. In at least some models, timing of levamisole in relation to the cytotoxic drug has been critical.[39,40]

Three large trials have analyzed the effect of levamisole as an adjunct to surgery in lung cancer. In the first of these, levamisole was given preoperatively and continued for three days every 2 weeks.[43] Considering all 211 patients, those receiving levamisole survived somewhat longer ($P \sim .1$). A second trial of identical design in 217 patients given levamisole on a weight-related basis, failed to confirm this effect.[44] Indeed, a higher mortality occurred in the postoperative period among those patients receiving levamisole when compared to controls. This resulted in a significantly shorter ($P < .03$) survival in those patients receiving levamisole. In a randomized trial of 134 patients, use of levamisole at 2.5 mg/kg in conjunction with BCG intrapleurally at surgery did not result in a significant improvement in recurrence-free or overall survival when compared to a control group.[45] Levamisole has also been evaluated in combination with radiotherapy and chemotherapy in inoperable patients who had not received prior therapy.[46] A dose of 2.5 mg/kg was used in 20 patients. Levamisole did not significantly influence time to relapse or survival.[46]

In colorectal cancer, results of two trials have been published, one of levamisole and surgery and one of levamisole in conjunction with 5-fluorouracil (5-FU). In conjunction with surgery, levamisole (150 mg) three days every 2 weeks, was given to a matched group of patients operated on by the same surgeon over the same time interval.[47] In both the overall group and the 40 patients with Dukes B_2 and Dukes C colorectal carcinoma, survival was prolonged by levamisole.[47] In 82 patients with metastatic colorectal carcinoma, levamisole was administered two days weekly (2.5 mg/kg) between 6-week cycles of 5-FU.[48] Survival of patients receiving 5-FU and levamisole was significantly ($P < .05$) greater (15.5 months) than those patients randomized to receive 5-FU alone (9.7 months).

In malignant melanoma, levamisole has been evaluated as an adjunct to surgery.[49] In a prospective study, 104 patients were randomized to receive levamisole (150 mg/day) for three days every 2 weeks and 99 patients were randomized to receive placebo. No beneficial effect on time to first recurrence or survival resulted from levamisole.[49]

In hematologic malignancies, levamisole has been used as maintenance therapy after chemotherapy.[31,50,51] In acute lymphoblastic leukemia (ALL), 393 patients in complete remission were randomized to maintenance therapy with or without levamisole at 100 mg/m^2 daily.[50] In patients considered to be at low risk for recurrence (WBC count at diagnosis $< 50{,}000/\mu L$), the frequency of relapse was significantly less

($P < .001$) in those patients receiving levamisole.[50] In patients with a WBC count at diagnosis of $> 50{,}000/\mu L$, the differences were not significant, although a greater proportion of the levamisole group remained relapse-free (43% *v* 23%, 36 months after diagnosis). In multiple myeloma, after a partial or complete response to combination chemotherapy, 84 patients were randomized to maintenance chemotherapy alone or with levamisole.[51] Levamisole, which was administered at a dose of 100 mg/m^2 for two days each week following the 3-week chemotherapy cycles, resulted in 75% of patients alive at 27 months after initiation of maintenance therapy. In contrast, in the control group of 38, comparable survival was only 14 months, a significant difference favoring levamisole ($P < .02$).

What is one to conclude about application of levamisole to human neoplasia? First, in concert with the animal models, clinical effectiveness has occurred primarily in conjunction with chemotherapy for advanced disease. Prolonged survival has been observed in conjunction with chemotherapy in randomized trials in ALL, multiple myeloma, colorectal carcinoma, and, in data not reviewed above, breast carcinoma.[48,50–53] As an adjunct to surgery in primary breast carcinoma and melanoma, levamisole has not resulted in any increase in overall or relapse-free survival.[54,55] Studies with levamisole as an adjunct to surgery in colorectal carcinoma are ongoing. Second, considering the essentially empiric nature of the dose and schedule chosen for trials to date, it is remarkable that any effect has been observed. Only one phase I trial examining optimal dose and schedule has been published.[56] This found that single doses four times higher than those currently used could be tolerated. Third, it would be rational to pursue additional phase III studies in combination with chemotherapy in breast carcinoma, colorectal carcinoma, and hematologic malignancies. However, before this, phase I studies should be initiated to define either a maximally-tolerated or biologically optimum dose and schedule for use with the planned chemotherapy program.

Poly A:Poly U

Polyadenylic-polyuridylic acid (poly A:poly U) is, like the more potent interferon inducer polyinosinic-polycytidylic acid (poly I:poly C), a double-stranded complex of synthetic polyribonucleotides. Poly I:poly C has been studied more both clinically and in experimental systems. However, with a few exceptions,[57,58] the primary emphasis in poly I:poly C studies has been defining elements of activity of the single agent. In contrast, a major component of the poly A:poly U studies has been its use in combination with other modalities.

Poly A:poly U stimulates antibody production and cell-mediated immune responses.[59–62] The interferon-induced enzyme, 2-5A synthetase and protein kinase, has increased in mice and patients treated with poly A:poly U.[63,64] Studies have demonstrated a reduced incidence of spontaneous leukemias and mammary carcinomas in mice after treatment with poly A:poly U.[65,66] Additionally, in mice bearing mammary carcinomas, treatment reduced the rate of tumor growth and increased mean survival time significantly.[67] C3H/He mice bearing established mammary tumors who received cytoxan and poly A:poly U showed greater tumor inhibition, lower mortality and a higher rate of complete tumor regression than mice treated with either agent alone.[68] NK cell cytotoxicity against YAC-1 target cells in mice treated with a combination of cyclophosphamide and poly A:poly U was significantly greater than in mice treated with either agent alone.[68]

Poly A:poly U has been tested in conjunction with surgery in a randomized trial of 300 patients with breast cancer.[69] All patients had surgery with or without regional radiotherapy. One hundred fifty-five patients were treated with poly A:poly U 30 mg intravenously (IV) weekly for 6 weeks and 145 patients received normal saline IV on the same schedule. After a follow-up period (mean) of 7.25 years, patients treated with poly A:poly U had a significant ($P < .05$) increase in overall survival (75% of treatment group died compared to 65% of control group). This increase in survival was more marked for patients ($P < .02$) with positive lymph nodes (at 7 years, 60% of the treatment group were alive compared to 19% of controls). These results are consistent with the hypothesis that an appropriate immunologic stimulus can improve the success of local treatment. When compared to the trial from Milan, which used combination chemotherapy as an adjunct to surgery for breast carcinoma, the therapeutic results are closely comparable.[70]

INTERFERONS

It seems probable that the most effective uses of IFN in cancer will come in combination with other treatment modalities. Intelligent clinical design can only result from additional studies in preclinical models. A limited number of such studies suggest that IFN will augment antitumor effects of other modalities.[71] These studies have however, only begun to probe the critical variables of dose, timing, and underlying mechanisms.

Human IFNβ has sensitized bronchogenic carcinoma cells in vitro to radiation cytotoxicity.[72] Similar radiation sensitization of mouse 3T3 cells resulted from mouse IFN.[73] In both mouse and human cells, the shoulder of the radiation survival curve was decreased without alteration of the slope of the exponential portion.[72,73] This result suggests interferons may interfere with enzymes important in radiation repair or induce more effective radiation damage with less sublethal cumulative damage. In the limited number of cells tested to date, this effect has been interferon specific, induced by human IFNβ and not IFNα.[72,74]

When combined with cytotoxic chemotherapy in animal tumor models, interferons and interferon inducers have augmented effectiveness of the cytotoxic agents. Leukemias,[75–79] breast carcinoma,[68,80] bladder carcinoma,[58] and neuroblastomas[81] have all been more effectively treated by the combination. These studies have used diverse models: transplantable tumors,[58,68,75–78] established but spontaneous murine leukemia,[76,79] and xenogeneic human tumors in the immunodeficient nude mouse.[80] Prolongation in survival and reduction in tumor size with combined therapy have been at least additive[76–78] and in most instances synergistic.[58,68,75,80,81]

In these studies, interferons have been combined with alkylating agents, antimetabolites, and agents that intercalate DNA. Whether the mechanism of action of the cytotoxic agent influences optimal schedule for a therapeutic effect, has not been explored. However, appropriate scheduling of poly I:poly C and interferon ameliorated significantly systemic and hematopoietic toxicity from 5-fluorouracil in mice.[57] Poly I:poly C may have resulted in a cell cycle delay that allowed time for repair when administered with 5-fluorouracil but not two days before or after.[57] Consistent with this postulate, IFN inhibited cell killing by a derivative of Adriamycin (Adria Laboratories, Columbus, Ohio) for rapidly proliferating but not slow growing clones of human colorectal carcinoma cells.[82]

Phase I and/or phase II clinical trials of IFN and cytotoxic drugs are now being initiated. When given concomitantly with IFNα, vinblastine has not added to the effectiveness of IFN alone. It did, however, add significantly to myelosuppression of IFNα. (J. Whisnant, Burroughs-Wellcome, personal communication, 1985). This suggests, as our in vitro studies with this drug have,[83] that timing may be critical. We have conducted a phase I study of IFNαA with a combination of cytotoxic drugs (vincristine, Adriamycin, cyclophosphamide and prednisone). IFNαA was administered before the cytotoxic drugs; no added WBC count suppression resulted and several tumor responses resulted from the combination.[84]

In vitro and in vivo studies in murine models and human cells have documented substantial synergy between murine gamma interferon and alpha/beta interferon.[85–87] Such combinations have been shown to enhance antiviral activity, antiproliferative activity, antitumor activity, and natural killer cell activation. This synergy appears to be unique to gamma interferon because combinations of alpha and beta have generally only shown additive effects. Synergy between one or more of the interferons and other lymphokines/cytokines, between human IFNα or IFN γ and human lymphotoxin (LT) and tumor necrosis factor (TNF) have also been demonstrated in vitro.[88–90] Based upon these results, phase I clinical trials have been initiated using interferon αA or interferonβ_{ser} and interferon γ; combinations of other lymphokines will undoubtedly soon enter clinical trial.

CONCLUSION

Biologic response modifiers, when used in combination with other treatments, may prove to have a substantially different immunomodulatory profile than when used alone. Side effects of biological response modifiers in combination with other modalities may be very different than those of either agent when used alone. Thus, as soon as specific therapeutic targets and rational doses can be identified, phase I studies of the combination should be initiated. Little is gained by completely defining maximally-tolerated dose of each single agent.

Combinations of antimicrobials have become common approaches to treatment of infections. Enhanced effectiveness may result from either decreased emergence of resistance or synergistic mechanisms of action. Infections as diverse as pulmonary tuberculosis and urinary tract infections with *Escherichia coli* are now treated in this manner. Randomized trials have also validated this approach in neoplastic diseases.

For optimum therapeutic application of biologic response modifiers, innovative preclinical and clinical approaches will continue to be required. Means are at hand to specifically design biological and chemical molecules to a desired end, quantify alterations in host responses, and formulate clinical hypotheses for phase I and II trials. The idea that immunomodulators may only be effective against minimal tumor burdens is changing.[91] Biologics such as interferons and monoclonal antibodies can alone induce regressions in clinically manifest disease. However, complementary and synergistic approaches will clearly provide more potent antitumor effects. Biologicals will augment effectiveness of other modalities by overcoming resistance of tumors to therapeutic attack, whether resulting from genetic resistance, limitations in drug delivery, or disease dissemination. As with surgery, radiation, or chemotherapy, biological response modifiers should not be used alone for optimum effectiveness in cancer treatment.

ACKNOWLEDGMENT

Our studies would not be possible without the continued interest and collaboration of our colleagues in the Division of Clinical Oncology. We are also indebted to the data managers and technical personnel who have contributed to the research programs at the University of Wisconsin Clinical Cancer Center. Preparation of the manuscript resulted from the energies of Ms Mary Pankratz.

REFERENCES

1. Bast RC Jr, Zbar B, Borsos T, et al: BCG and cancer. N Engl J Med 290:1413–1420, 1458–1569, 1974

2. Hanna MG Jr: Immunological aspects of BCG mediated regression of the established tumors and metastases in guinea pigs. Semin Oncl 1:319–335, 1974

3. Baldwin RW, Pimm MV: BCG in tumor immunotherapy. Adv Cancer Res 28:91–147, 1978

4. Nathanson L: Use of BCG in the treatment of human neoplasms: A review. Semin Oncol 1:337–350, 1974

5. Morton DL, Eilber FR, Holmes EC, et al: BCG immunotherapy of malignant melanoma. Ann Surg 180:635–643, 1974

6. Weiss DW: Nonspecific stimulation and modulation of the immune response and the status of resistance by the MER fraction of tubercule bacilli. J Natl Cancer Inst 35:157–171, 1972

7. Weiss DW: MER and other mycobacterial fractions in the immunotherapy of cancer. Med Clin North Am 60:473–497, 1976

8. Hersh EM, Quesada J, Murphy SG, et al: Evaluation of therapy with methanol extraction residue of BCG. Cancer Immunol Immunother 14:4–9, 1982

9. Gall SA, Creasman WT, Blessing JA, et al: Chemoimmunotherapy in primary stage III ovarian epithelial cancer, *in* Terry WD, Rosenberg SA (eds): Immunotherapy of Human Cancer. New York, Exerpta Medica, 1982, pp 337–341

10. Israel L, Edelstein R, Depierre A, et al: Daily intravenous infusions of *Corynebacterium parvum* in twenty patients with disseminated cancer: A preliminary report of clinical and biological findings. J Natl Cancer Inst 55:29–33, 1975

11. Milas L, Scott MT: Antitumor activity of *Corynebacterium parvum.* Adv Cancer Res 26:257–306, 1978

12. Gutterman JU, Mavligit GM, McBride CM, et al: Active immunotherapy with BCG for recurrent malignant melanoma. Lancet 1:1208–1212, 1973

13. Morton DL, Holmes EC, Eilber FR, et al: Adjuvant immunotherapy of malignant melanoma: Preliminary results of a randomized trial in patients with lymph node metastases, in Terry WD, Windhorst D (eds): Immunotherapy of Cancer: Present Status of Trials in Man. Progress in Cancer Research and Therapy, vol 6. New York, Raven, 1978, p 696

14. Veronesi U, Adamus J, Aubert C, et al: A randomized trial of adjuvant chemotherapy and immunotherapy in cutaneous melanoma. N Engl J Med 307:913–916, 1982

15. Quirt I, Shelley W, Bodurtha A, et al. A controlled trial of adjuvant immunotherapy for malignant melanoma. Proc Am Soc Clin Oncol 3:48, 1984 (abstr)

16. Paterson AH, Willans DJ, Jerry LM, et al: Adjuvant BCG immunotherapy for malignant melanoma. Can Med Assoc J 131:744–748, 1984

17. Terry WD, Hodes RJ: Newer methods of cancer treatment, section 1. Immunotherapy, in DeVita VT, Hellman S, Rosenberg SA (eds): Cancer—Principles and Practice of Oncology. Philadelphia, Lippincott, pp 1794–1810, 1982

18. Pinsky CM: Experience with historical control studies in cancer immunotherapy. Stat Med 3:325–329, 1984

19. McKneally MF, Maver C, Lininger L, et al: Four-year follow-up on the Albany experience with intrapleural BCG in lung cancer. J Thorac Cardiovasc Surg 81:485–492, 1981

20. Mountain CF, Gail MH: Surgical adjuvant intrapleu-

ral BCG treatment for stage I non-small cell lung cancer. J Thorac Cardiovasc Surg 82:649–657, 1981

21. Hortobagyi GN, Gutterman JU, Blumenschein GR, et al: Combination chemoimmunotherapy of metastatic breast cancer with 5-fluorouracil, Adriamycin, cyclophosphamide, and BCG. Cancer 43:1225–1233, 1979

22. Blumenschein GR, Buzdar AU, Hortobagyi GN. FAC + BCG as adjuvant therapy in breast cancer: An 8-year update. Recent Results Cancer Res 96:129–132, 1984

23. Buzdar AU, Blumenschein GR, Smith TL, et al: Adjuvant chemotherapy with fluorouracil, doxorubicin, and cyclophosphamide, with or without Bacillus Calmette-Guerin and with or without irradiation in operable breast cancer. A prospective randomized trial. Cancer 53:384–389, 1984

24. Foon KA, Smalley RV, Riggs CW, et al: The role of immunotherapy in acute myelogenous leukemia. Arch Intern Med 143:1726–1731, 1983

25. Vogler WR, Winton EF, Gordon DS, et al: A randomized comparison of postremission therapy in acute myelogenous leukemia: A Southeastern Cancer Study Group trial. Blood 63:1039–1045, 1984

26. Hewlett JS, Chen T, Balcerzak SP, et al: High rate of long-term survival in adult acute leukemia following ten-day chemotherapy (OAP) induction. Arch Intern Med 145:1006–1012, 1985

27. Hoover HC, Peters LC, Brandhorst JS, et al: Therapy of spontaneous metastases with an autologous tumor vaccine in a guinea pig model. J Surg Res 30:409–415, 1981

28. Hoover HC, Surdyke MG, Dangel RB, et al: Prospectively randomized trial of adjuvant active-specific immunotherapy for human colorectal cancer. Cancer 55:1236–1243, 1985

29. Hoover HC, Surdyke M, Dangel RB, et al: Delayed cutaneous hypersensitivity to autologous tumor cells in colorectal cancer patients immunized with an autologous tumor cell: Bacillus Calmette-Guerin vaccine. Cancer Res 44:1671–1676, 1984

30. Jones SE, Grozea PN, Metz EN, et al. Improved complete remission rates and survival for patients with large cell lymphoma treated with chemoimmunotherapy. A Southwest Oncology Group Study. Cancer 51:1083–1090, 1983

31. Jones SE, Grozea P, O'Bryan R, et al: Chemotherapy with cyclophosphamide, Adriamycin, vincristine, and prednisone (CHOP) alone or with levamisole plus BCG for non-Hodgkin's lymphoma (NHL): A Southwest Oncology Group Study. Proc Am Soc Clin Oncol 3:237, 1984 (abstr)

32. Wolberg WH: Binding of colonic tissue membrane to mononuclear peripheral blood leukocytes. Cancer Res 37:3711–3719, 1977

33. Ramot B, Biniaminor M, Shoham CH, et al: The effect of levamisole on E-rosette-forming cells in vivo and in vitro in Hodgkin's disease patients. N Engl J Med 294:809–811, 1976

34. Pike MC, Snyderman R: Augmentation of human monocyte chemotactic response by levamisole. Nature 261:136–137, 1976

35. Wybran J, Govaerts A: Levamisole and human lymphocyte surface markers. Clin Exp Immunol 27:319–321, 1977

36. Nathanson SD, Zamfirescu PL, Portaro JK, et al: Acute effects of orally administered levamisole on random monocyte motility and chemotaxis in man. J Natl Cancer Inst 61:301–306, 1978

37. Groveman DS, Borden EC: In vitro and in vivo effects of levamisole on monocyte chemotaxis in normal donors and patients with colorectal carcinoma. J Biol Response Mod 2:167–174, 1983

38. Schmidt ME, Douglas SD: Effects of levamisole on human monocyte function and immunoprotein receptors. Clin Immunol Immunopathol 6:299–305, 1976

39. Chirigos MA, Fuhrman F, Pryor J: Prolongation of chemotherapeutically-induced remission of a syngeneic murine leukemia by L-2, 3, 5, 6 tetrahydro-6-phenylimidazo(2,1-β)thiazole hydrochloride. Cancer Res 35:927–931, 1975

40. Chirigos MA, Pearson JW, Pryor J: Augmentation of a chemotherapeutically-induced remission of a murine leukemia by a chemical immunoadjuvant. Cancer Res 33:2615–2618, 1973

41. Padarathsingh ML, Dean JH, McCoy JL, et al: Restorative effects of levamisole on cell mediated immune response following chemotherapy with aniline mustard in mice bearing ADJ-PC5 plasmacytoma. Cancer Treat Rep 62:1627–1640, 1978

42. Gordon DS, Hall LS, McDongal JS: Levamisole and cytoxan in a murine tumor model: in vivo and in vitro studies, in Chirigos MA (ed): Control of Neoplasia by Modulation of the Immune System. New York, Raven, 1977, pp 121–133

43. Amery WK, Cosemans J, Gooszen HC, et al: Four year results from double-blind study of adjuvant levamisole treatment in resectable lung cancer, in Terry WD, Rosenberg SA (eds): Immunotherapy of Human Cancer. New York, Excerpta Medica, 1982, pp 123–133

44. Anthony HM, Mearns AJ, Mason MK, et al: Levamisole and surgery in bronchial carcinoma patients: Increase in deaths from cardiorespiratory failure. Thorax 34:4–12, 1979

45. Wright PW, Hill LD, Peterson AV Jr, et al: Preliminary results of combined surgery and adjuvant bacillus Calmette-Guerin plus levamisole treatment of resectable lung cancer. Cancer Treat Rep 62:1671–1675, 1978

46. Liberati AM, Voelkel JG, Borden EC, et al: Influence of non-specific immunologic factors on prognosis in advanced bronchogenic carcinoma. Cancer Immunol Immunother 13:140–144, 1982

47. Verhaegen H, DeCree J, DeCock W, et al: Levamisole therapy in patients with colorectal cancer, in Terry WD, Rosenberg SA (eds): Immunotherapy of Human Cancer. New York, Excerpta Medica, 1982, pp 225–229

48. Borden EC, Davis TE, Crowley JJ, et al: Interim analysis of a trial of levamisole and 5-fluorouracil in metastatic colorectal carcinoma, in Terry WD, Rosenberg SA (eds): Immunotherapy of Human Cancer. New York, Elsevier North Holland, 1982, pp 231–235

49. Spitler LE, Sagebiel R, Allen R, et al: Levamisole in the treatment of melanoma, in Terry WD, Rosenberg SA (eds): Immunotherapy of Human Cancer. New York, Excerpta Medica, 1982, pp 289–297

50. Pavlovsky S, Garay G, Muriel FS, et al: Levamisole therapy during maintenance of remission in patients with acute lymphoblastic leukemia, in Terry WD, Rosenberg SA (eds): Immunotherapy of Human Cancer. New York, Excerpta Medica, 1982, pp 47–54

51. Salmon SE, Haut A, Bonnet JD, et al: Alternating

combination chemotherapy and levamisole improves survival in multiple myeloma: A Southwest Oncology Group Study. J Clin Oncol 1:453–461, 1983

52. Klefström P, Holsti P, Gröhn P, et al: Combination of levamisole immunotherapy with conventional treatments in breast cancer, in Terry WD, Rosenberg SA (eds): Immunotherapy of Human Cancer. New York, Excerpta Medica, 1982, pp 187–194

53. Stephens EJW, Wood HF, Mason B: The influence of levamisole on the survival of patients with disseminated mammary carcinoma treated with chemotherapy, in Terry WD, Rosenberg SA (eds), Immunotherapy of Human Cancer. New York, Exerpta Medica, 1982, pp 199–204

54. Kay RG, Mason BH, Stephens EJ, et al: Levamisole in primary breast cancer. A controlled study in conjunction with L-phenylalanine mustard. Cancer 51:1992–1997, 1983

55. Hakes TB, Currie VE, Kaufman RJ, et al: CMF ± levamisole breast adjuvant chemotherapy: 5 year analysis. Proc Am Soc Clin Oncol 1:83, 1982 (abstr)

56. Lewinski UH, Mavligit GM, Hersh EM: Cellular immune modulation after a single high dose of levamisole in patients with carcinoma. Cancer 46:2185–2194, 1980

57. Stolfi RL, Martin DS, Sawyer RC, et al: Modulation of 5-fluorouracil-induced toxicity in mice with interferon or with the interferon inducer, polyinosinic-polycytidylic acid. Cancer Res 43:561–566, 1983

58. Borden EC, Sidky YA, Groveman DS, et al: Antitumor effects of polyribonucleotides for mouse transitional cell carcinoma enhanced by cyclophosphamide. Cancer Res 45:45–50, 1985

59. Braun W, Nakano M: Antibody formation: Stimulation by polyadenylic and polycytidylic acids. Science 157:819–821, 1967

60. Braun W, Ishizuka M, Yajima Y, et al: Spectrum and mode of action of poly A:poly U in the stimulation of immune responses, in Beers RF, Braun W (eds): Biological Effects of Polynucleotides. New York, Springer Verlag, 1971, pp 139–156

61. Cone ER, Johnson AG: Regulation of the immune system by synthetic polynucleotides. III. Action on antigen reactive cells of thymic origin. J Expl Med 133:665–676, 1971

62. Wanebo HY, Kemeny M, Pinsky CM, et al: Influence of poly A:poly U on immune response in cancer patients. Ann NY Acad Sci 277:288–298, 1976

63. Hovanessian AG, Youn JK, Buffet-Janvresse L, et al: Enhancement of natural killer cell activity and 2-5A synthetase in operable breast cancer patients treated with polyadenylic-polyuridylic acid. Cancer 55:357–362, 1985

64. Hovanessian AG, Riviere Y, Montgnier L, et al: Enhancement of interferon-mediated protein kinase in mouse and human plasma in response to treatment with polyadenylic-polyuridylic acid (poly A:poly U). J Interferon Res 2:209–215, 1982

65. Drake WP, Cimino EF, Mardiney MR, et al: Prophylactic therapy of spontaneous leukemia in AKR mice by polyadenylic-polyuridylic acid. J Natl Cancer Inst 52:941–944, 1974

66. Lacour F, Delage G, Chianale C: Reduced incidence of spontaneous mammary tumours in C3H/He mice following treatment with poly A:poly U. Science 187:256–257, 1975

67. Lacour F, Delage G, Fenster E, et al: Inhibitory action of poly A:poly U on tumor growth. Enhancement of host immune response? in Gottlieb AA, Plescia O, Bishop HL (eds): Fundamental Aspects of Neoplasia. New York, Springer Verlag, 1975, pp 123–138

68. Youn JK, Lacour F, Hue G: Inhibition of C3H/He mouse mammary tumor growth by combined treatment with cyclophosphamide and polyadenylic-polyuridic acid. Cancer Res 42:4706–4711, 1982

69. Lacour J, Lacour F, Spira A, et al: Adjuvant treatment with polyadenylic-polyuridylic acid in operable breast cancer: Updated results of a randomized trial. Br Med J 288:589–592, 1984

70. Borden EC, Verma AK, Wolberg WH: Potential role of polyribonucleotides in human neoplastic disease. J Biol Resp Mod 4:676–769, 1985

71. Borden EC: Interferons and cancer: How the promise is being kept, in Gresser I (ed): Interferons, vol 5. Orlando, Fla, Academic, 1984, pp 43–83

72. Gould MN, Kakria RC, Olson S, et al: Radiosensitization of human bronchogenic carcinoma cells by interferon β. J Interferon Res 4:123–128, 1984

73. Dritschilo A, Mossman K, Gray M, et al: Potentiation of radiation injury by interferon. Am J Clin Oncol 5:79–82, 1982

74. Nederman T, Benediktsson G: Effects of interferon on growth rate and radiation sensitivity of cultured, human glioma cells. Acta Radiol (Oncol) 21:231–234, 1982

75. Chirigos MA, Pearson JW: Cure of murine leukemia with drug and interferon treatment. J Natl Cancer Inst 51:1367–1368, 1973

76. Gresser I, Maury C, Tovey M: Efficacy of combined interferon and cyclophosphamide therapy after diagnosis of lymphoma in AKR mice. Eur J Cancer Clin Oncol 11:97–99, 1978

77. Slater LM, Wetzel MW, Cesario T: Combined interferon-antimetabolite therapy of murine L1210 leukemia. Cancer 48:5–9, 1981

78. Moshowitz SL, Chin-Bow ST, Smith GD: Interferon and cis-DDP: Combination chemotherapy for P388 leukemia in CDF1 mice. J Interferon Res 2:587–591, 1982

79. Bekesi JG, Roboz JP: Prophylactic and therapeutic application of interferon in spontaneous AKR leukemia. Tex Rep Biol Med 41:614–620, 1982

80. Balkwill FR, Moodie EM, Freedman V, et al: An animal model system for investigating the antitumor effects of human interferon. J Res 3:319–326, 1983

81. Tozawa M, Kidowaki T, Tanaka T, et al: Effects of interferon on C1300 mouse neuroblastoma. Cancer Chemother Rep 66:1575–1577, 1982

82. Van der Bosch J, Zirvi JA: Growth state-specific responsiveness of primary cultures of a nude mouse-xenograft human colon carcinoma to 4′-deoxydoxorubicin and a crude human leukocyte α-interferon preparation. Cancer Res 42:3789–3792, 1982

83. Schmid SM, Borden EC, Cummings KB: Recombinant IFN beta antiproliferative interaction with vinblastine for ACHN renal carcinoma cells: Synergistic inhibition with IFN pretreatment. J Urol 133:250A, 1985

84. Hawkins MJ, O'Connell MJ, Schiller JH, et al: Phase I evaluation of recombinant A interferon alpha (rIFN-αA) in

combination with COPA chemotherapy (I-COPA). Proc Am Soc Clin Oncol 4:229, 1985 (abstr)

85. Fleishmann WR, Kleyn KM, Baron S: Potentiation of antitumor effect of virus-induced interferon by mouse immune interferon preparations. J Natl Cancer Inst 65:963–966, 1980

86. Czarniecki CW, Fennie CW, Powers DB, et al: Synergistic antiviral and antiproliferative activities of *Escherichia coli*-derived human alpha, beta, and gamma interferons. J Virol 49:490–496, 1984

87. Schiller JH, Groveman DS, Schmid SM, et al: Synergistic antiproliferative effects of human recombinant α54, β_{ser}, and γ interferons on human cell lines of various histogenesis. Cancer Res 46:483–488, 1986

88. Lee SH, Aggarwal BB, Rinderknecht E, et al: The synergistic anti-proliferative effect of γ-interferon and human lymphotoxin. J Immunol 133:1083–1986, 1984

89. Williamson BD, Carswell EA, Rubin BY, et al: Human tumor necrosis factor produced by human B-cell lines: synergistic cytotoxic interaction with human interferon. Proc Natl Acad Sci 80:5397–5401, 1983

90. Shalaby MR, Aggarwal BB, Rinderknecht E, et al: Activation of human polymorphonuclear neutrophil functions by interferon-gamma and tumor necrosis factors. J Immunol 135:2069–2073, 1985

91. Oldham RK, Smalley RV: Immunotherapy: The old and the new. J Biol Response Mod 2:1–37, 1983

SEROLOGY

Immunochemical Characterization of Human Tumor Antigens

Ralph A. Reisfeld

DEVELOPMENTS of new technologies often pave the way for key advances and new concepts in science. Cancer research, and particularly tumor biology, is no exception to this rule as one can trace its progress by the development and application of new techniques. Technologies that have had the most recent impact on progress in cancer research are those of molecular biology and monoclonal antibodies. The genetic engineering technologies have made the oncogene concept most topical; however, without taking anything away from this exciting new concept, it appears that the most decisive impact of the oncogene concept on cancer research is yet to come. Monoclonal antibodies, on the other hand, have already had a most decisive influence on the progress of cancer research during the last decade, within a few years after Kohler and Milstein pioneered the development of this exciting technology.[1]

Although it is quite likely that monoclonal antibodies will be seminal for further advances in cancer research, it is already quite evident at this time that the hybridoma technique has literally revolutionized the serologic analysis of human tumor-associated antigens and has facilitated a far more precise immunochemical and molecular analysis that now paves the way for exciting new approaches utilizing chemically defined antigens as targets for monoclonal antibody-mediated therapy of human cancer. This includes approaches designed to mediate tumor cell killing by immune effector cells suitably directed by monoclonal antibodies to their tumor target sites[2] and the use of these uniquely specific reagents to target chemotherapeutic drugs, radionuclides, and toxins to human tumor targets.[3,4]

This brief article will make no attempt to review the voluminous literature on human tumor antigens because this has already been done in a number of recent reviews.[3-8] Rather an attempt is made here to describe and review three human melanoma-associated antigens produced and extensively characterized in the author's laboratory. These antigens were selected because they were among the very few monoclonal antibody-defined targets whose structural and functional properties have been thoroughly delineated. The antigens to be discussed are all preferentially expressed on human melanoma cells and are exemplified by a melanoma-associated chondroitin sulfate proteoglycan (MPG), disialoganglioside GD_3 and 9-0-acetylated disialoganglioside GD_3.

Immunochemical Characterization of MPG

Tissue distribution. Table 1 summarizes the tissue distribution of MPG recognized by monoclonal antibody (Mab) 9.2.27 on fresh frozen tissue sections subjected to the immunoperoxidase assay. It is apparent from these data that Mab 9.2.27 recognizes all melanoma tissues and cell lines analyzed thus far and reacts otherwise only with adult and fetal skin and very weakly with fetal aorta.

Molecular profile. The molecular structure of MPG is that of a noncartilagenous type chondroitin sulfate proteoglycan (CSP) as determined by biochemical and immunochemical analyses using Mab 9.2.27.[9,10] This antibody, as well as Mab 155.8, distinguishes distinct epitopes on both a >400 kDa CSP and its 250 kDa core protein containing both N- and O-linked oligosaccharides as demonstrated by several lines of evidence.[9,10,11]

First, the molecular profile of the molecules reacting with both monoclonal antibodies is clearly indicated from sodium dodecylsulfate polyacrylamide gel electrophoresis (SDS-PAGE) analysis of indirect immunoprecipitates obtained by reacting either Mab 9.2.27 or 155.8 with detergent lysates of M21 melanoma cells that were intrinsically labeled with ^{3}H-leucine. Characteristic patterns obtained after digestion of the ^{3}H-leucine–labeled lysate with chondroitinase ABC showed only the 250 kDa component. In contrast, SDS-PAGE profiles obtained from

---

From the Department of Immunology, Scripps Clinic and Research Foundation, La Jolla, Calif.

Supported by NIH Grants No. CA 28420 and AI 10180.

Address reprint requests to Ralph A. Reisfeld, PhD, Department of Immunology, Scripps Clinic and Research Foundation, La Jolla, CA 92037.

0093–7754/86/1302–0005$05.00/0

Table 1. Tissue Reactivity of Mab 9.2.27

Tissues	Reactivity
Fetal	
Colon	—
Liver	—
Small Intestines	—
Thyroid	—
Skin	+ melanocytes
Lung	—
Aorta	± smooth muscle
Tumor	
Lung adenocarcinoma	—
Colon adenocarcinoma	—
Breast adenocarcinoma	—
Prostate adenocarcinoma	—
Pancreas adenocarcinoma	—
Bladder adenocarcinoma	—
Melanoma	+*
Adult	
Lung	—
Stomach	—
Kidney	—
Breast	—
Colon	—
Thyroid	—
Cerebellum	—
Brain cortex	—
Synovium	±
Cartilage	—
Benign Nevus	+
Lymph Node	—
Skin	+ melanocytes

*Reactivity with > 20 melanoma cell lines and all melanoma tissues tested.

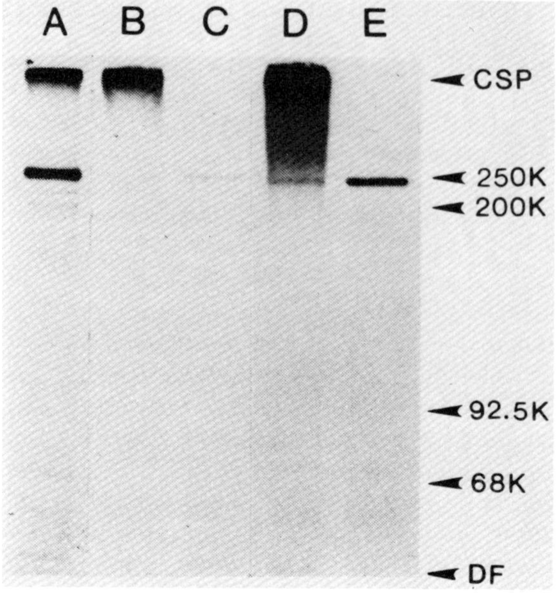

Fig 1. Analysis of indirect immunoprecipitates by SDS-PAGE. Fluorautography of dried 5% gells containing (A) Mab 155.8 immunoprecipitate of a detergent extract from [^{3}H]-leucine-labeled UCLA M21 melanoma cells; (B) $^{35}SO_4{}^{-2}$-labeled UCLA M21 cells; and (C) $^{35}SO_4{}^{-2}$-labeled UCLA M21 cells after chondroitinase ABC digestion. Immunoprecipitates of Mab 9.2.27 with detergent extracts of $^{35}SO_4{}^{-2}$-labeled UCLA M21 cells (D) before and (E) after digestion with chondroitinase ABC shown as controls. (Reprinted with permission[11]).

immunoprecipitates of detergent lysates from $^{35}SO_4{}^{-2}$-labeled M21 cells revealed only a component of >400 kDa, suggesting that the two antibodies each react with one sulfated and one non-sulfated component (Fig 1).[11]

Second, the identity of the glycosaminoglycans (GAG) associated with the CSP recognized by the two monoclonal antibodies is established by alkaline-borohydride treatment of $^{35}SO_4{}^{-2}$-labeled immunoprecipitates and subsequent cellulose acetate electrophoresis. Using appropriate standards as controls, ie, heparin, chondroitin sulfate A/C, chondroitin sulfate B, heparin sulfate, and hyaluronic acid, it is evident that the 0-linked GAG liberated by β-elimination is exclusively of the chondroitin sulfate A and/or C type.[10,11]

Immunochemical identification of two antigenic determinants on MPG. Two lines of evidence indicate that Mabs 9.22.7 and 155.8 recognize separate and distinct epitopes. First, sequential immunodepletion analysis of 155.8 and 9.2.27 reveals that 155.8 partially depletes those molecules recognized by 9.2.27; however, in the opposite direction, initial depletion with 9.22.7 removes all molecules that can be recognized by 155.8. These results combined with data obtained from a series of binding studies with melanoma cells and tissues that show Mab 155.8 binds to a more limited extent than 9.2.27, suggest that either 155.8 recognizes a determinant expressed in smaller numbers on the cell surface or that there is a difference in affinity constants of the two antibodies.[9] Second, use of a competitive binding enzyme linked immunosorbent assay (ELISA) to assess whether Mab 155.8 binds the same epitope or one vicinal to the determinant defined by 9.2.27 indicates that Mab 155.8 is unable to competitively inhibit peroxidase-conjugated 9.2.27 IgG from binding to its determinant on M14 melanoma cells. Taken together, the data from these experiments suggest that the 155.8 determinant is both distinct from and not immediately proximal to that recognized by Mab 9.2.27.[11]

Biosynthesis of MPG

It is quite evidenct from results of the studies described thus far that human malignant melanoma cells synthesize a chondroitin sulfate-rich proteoglycan (CSP) whose core glycoprotein is 250 kDa and contains both N- and O-linked oligosaccharides, as well as O-glycosidically–linked chondroitin sulfate chains. Other investigators have also reported monoclonal antibodies that react preferentially with melanoma type CSP.[12,13] Even though core protein structure varies across tissues of origin studied thus far, the posttranslational modification of such molecules resulting in the formation of a fully matured proteoglycan may be quite similar. For example, the addition of N-linked oligosaccharides likely takes place cotranslationally, most probably within the rough endoplasmic reticulum (RER), as has been suggesting for cartilage proteoglycans.[14] The first core glycoprotein precursor clearly detectable by immunoprecipitation with Mab 9.2.27 from melanoma cells, pulse-labeled with ^{35}S-methionine, is a molecule of 250 kDa that is sensitive to digestion with endo-β-N-acetylglycosaminidase H (Endo H).[9,10] After 15 to 20 minutes of chase in the presence of unlabeled methionine, this precursor increases to 250 kDa and becomes resistant to endo H digestion, including the conversion of high mannose type to complex-type, N-linked oligosaccharides.[15] Also included in this increase in molecular weight is the addition of O-linked, fucose-containing oligosaccharides.[16] Once the core glycoprotein of 250 kDa is thus formed, synthesis of chrondrotin Δ-di-4 and Δ-di-6 sulfated chains is initiated and these chains are elongated essentially as described for cartilage type proteoglycans.[16]

Intracellular transport and cell surface expression of MPG. Several approaches were used to elucidate mechanism(s) by which proteoglycan core protein is transported and segregated into the precise intra-Golgi compartments that serve as sites for glycosaminoglycan addition. One such approach made use of the cationic ionophore monensin because it inhibits the formation of mature proteoglycans in other systems and we found it to arrest core glycoprotein maturation of CSP at a molecular weight of 245 kDa that is Endo-H resistant.[17] NH_4Cl was also used in these experiments because this agent shares many effects of monensin but is really more restricted to the disruption of intracellular pH gradients. Specifically, in the presence of 10 to 15 mmol/L NH_4Cl, the early events of core glycoprotein synthesis appear to be unaffected. The Endo H-sensitive 240 kDa precursor is formed and converted with normal kinetics to a 250 kDa Endo-H-resistant core glycoprotein. The most striking effect of NH_4Cl is the inhibition of proteoglycan synthesis. At equilibrium, M21 melanoma cells synthesized some proteoglycan; however, compared to untreated cells, the amount of proteoglycan produced is significantly reduced and there is a concomitant increase in the amount of core protein present in immunoprecipitates. These findings suggest that glycosaminoglycan addition but not core glycoprotein synthesis is affected by NH_4Cl. The topographical localization of the core glycoprotein accumulation was determined by performing cell surface immunoprecipitation in presence of NH_4Cl. Such an approach revealed that at two hours, the core glycoprotein could be observed on the cell surface, although there was no detectable proteoglycan in whole cell lysates or on the cell surface. At five hours, a small amount of proteoglycan appeared in cell surface immunoprecipitates, but significantly less than in untreated controls. There was, however, a substantial accumulation of core glycoprotein on the cell surface. The interpretation of this result is that chondroitin surface addition to the core protein is not a prerequisite for its cell surface expression. Moreover, it appears from the NH_4Cl inhibition of glycosaminoglycan addition, that following core glycoprotein completion, there is a low-pH mechanism mediating the final processing of core protein to proteoglycan.[17] Taken together, these data imply the existence of two pathways for transporting core glycoprotein to the cell surface, (1) directly to the cell surface devoid of glycosaminoglycan chains following terminal processing of the N-linked oligosaccharides and completion of O-glycosylation, or (2) via an intra-Golgi compartment that serves as the site of chondroitin sulfate synthesis and then to the surface. Implicit in this interpretation is that glycosaminoglycan addition is itself neither a prerequisite nor a signal for cell surface expression of the proteoglycan core glycoprotein.[17]

Evaluation of MPG as a Target for Tumor Cell Destruction

Animal model studies. A previous observation from the author's laboratory indicated that the growth of human melanoma tumors in nude BALB/c mice could be partially suppressed by the simultaneous injection of Mab 9.2.27 and splenocytes from BALB/c mice at the time of tumor cell inoculation.[18] It was assumed that this antibody-dependent suppression of tumor growth was caused by a cell-mediated mechanism and that at least some of the effector cells involved were those with natural killer cell (NK) activity because such cells evoke antibody-dependent cellular cytotoxicity (ADCC).

Here are summarized some of the highlights of a study described in detail elsewhere[18] that examines this hypothesis. Several experiments indicate that simultaneous injection of Mab 9.2.27 and cell populations with NK activity can cause the eradication of established melanoma tumors (mean tumor volume 90 μL) in nude mice. Thus, BALB/c nude mice with 2-week-old melanoma tumors received one of the following as a single intravenous injection: 400 μg 9.2.27 IgG; mononuclear BALB/c splenocytes (2×10^7); 2×10^7 mononuclear splenocytes and 400 μg 9.2.27 IgG. A group of tumor-bearing control mice received no injections. Seven of ten animals injected simultaneously with splenocytes and Mab 9.2.27 were tumor-free 4 weeks after injection. All other animals treated with either antibody or splenocytes alone exhibited large tumors with the exception of one animal in the group that received only spelenocytes. Mice that received only Mab 9.2.27 showed a mean tumor volume that was almost the same as that of control animals whereas tumors of mice that received only effector cells were 50% smaller. Most interestingly, the mean tumor volume of mice that received 9.2.27 IgG together with effector cells was less than 10% of that of control tumors.[19]

Although mature T cells apparently did not play a major role in the type of tumor cell destruction observed in this experiment, several observations strongly suggested that cells with NK activity are the effector cells involved in this process. In this regard, splenocytes obtained from NK-deficient beige C57BL/6 mice were incapable of inducing tumor regression. Specifically, C57BL/6 nude mice with established human melanoma tumors were injected with 9.2.27 IgG, alone or together with splenocytes from NK-deficient C57BL/6 mice that carried the homozygous beige mutation. Results obtained in these experiments illustrated by Fig 2, clearly indicated that none of ten mice that received normal C57BL/6 splenocytes and 9.2.27 IgG showed any tumor growth 4 weeks after injection. In contrast, eight of nine mice that received splenocytes from C57BL/6 bg/bg mice showed large tumors. Because beige mice have low NK activity, these data strongly suggest that NK cells play a key role in the eradication of established human melanoma tumors in the nude mouse model system.[19] These data are illustrated by Fig 2.

Clinical trials. Mab 9.2.27 has been tested in limited phase I clinical trials by Oldham and colleagues.[20] Each patient received single doses of Mab 9.2.27 twice weekly on an escalating

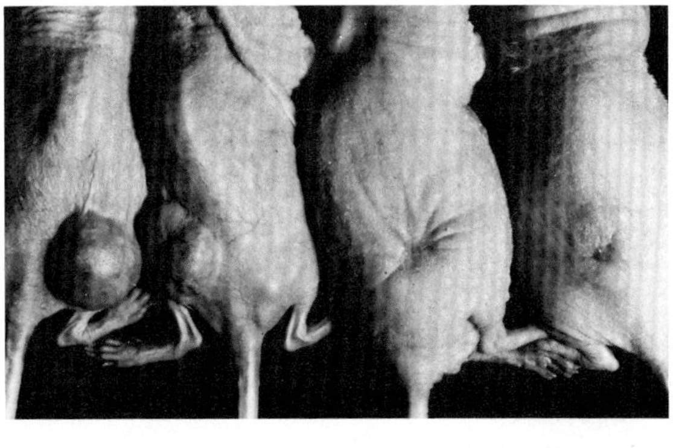

Fig 2. Human melanoma tumor growth in nude mice: effect of Mab 9.2.27 and murine effector cells simultaneously injected into tumor-bearing nude mice. The two mice on the left are representatives of the first group of C57BL/6 nude mice injected once intravenously with Mab 9.2.27 (400 μg) and mononuclear splenocytes (2×10^7) obtained from C57BL/6 beige mice, deficient in NK cells, 14 days after 2×10^7 M21 melanoma cells were injected subcutaneously into these animals. The two mice on the right, apparently devoid of tumor, are representatives of a second group of C57BL/6 nude mice treated in all respects identical to those animals of the first group, except that the effector splenocytes injected into them together with Mab 9.2.27 were obtained from normal C57BL/6 mice. Size of tumors at start of treatment was the same for both groups, ie, 90 to 100 μL. Photographs were taken 28 days after antibody and effector cell injection, ie, 42 days after tumor cell inoculation.

scale, at does of 1, 10, 50, 100, and 200 mg, ie, a total of only 361 mg. When the antibody per se was administered intravenously to eight patients with metastatic malignant melanoma, biopsies of metastatic nodules clearly demonstrated specific tumor localization of the antibody. There was a clear dose relationshp in this localization as 200 mg of antibody was required to show staining of most of the skin nodules; however, the viable tumor cells examined by flow cytometry were clearly not saturated by antibody, suggesting that this highest does injected was still suboptimal. Interestingly enough, none of the patients demonstrated major toxicity to Mab 9.2.27. This is in contrast to results obtained in trials of T101 monoclonal antibody in patients with cutaneous T cell lymphoma and chronic lymphocytic leukemia.[21] In this case, patients treated with 50 mg of T101 during a two hour infusion period developed chest tightness and shortness of breath. Although these symptoms disappeared when the rate of infusion was only one to two mg/hr, a number of patients still developed urticaria after antibody treatment. Mab T101 apparently causes pulmonary toxicity as it binds to some circulating cells leading to microaggregates in the pulmonary microvasculature.[21] This is not the case for Mab 9.2.27 as it does not bind to leukocytes. Only one patient developed serum sickness that responded, however, to steroid treatment and circulating 9.2.27 antiglobulin complexes were not demonstrable. It is also of interest that only 50% of the patients showed even a demonstrable antiglobulin response. This was nevertheless only transient and regulated by higher antibody doses. There was apparent feedback inhibition of the antiglobulin response since no reappearance of antiglobulin levels occurred after the 200 mg dose. Also, pharmacokinetic studies indicated that the clearance rate of murine immunoglobulin was not affected by the transient antiglobulin responses. The data indicate that carefully prepared murine monoclonal antibody can be given to immunologically responsive patients with solid tumors, without eliciting a therapeutically limiting antiglobulin response. Although there was no demonstrable tumor regression, Mab 9.2.27 clearly localized to the tumor, caused no toxic response, and most importantly, flow cytometric and other studies indicated that the treatment did not cause antigenic modulation on the surface of melanoma cells.[20]

In view of the encouraging results in nude mice where Mab 9.2.27 combined with immunological effector cells clearly destroyed established metastatic human melanoma cells, one wonders what this type of regimen could accomplish in patients. Finally, very recent pilot studies in nude mice bearing human melanoma xenografts have shown Mab 9.2.27 to be excellent for targeting of vinblastine and thereby greatly suppressing tumor growth.[22] Thus, it is possible that this antibody may have an excellent potential as a targeting device for chemotherapeutic drug. Also, there is experimental evidence by Hwang et al[23] indicating that Mab 9.2.27 may be applicable for tumor imaging because it showed excellent radiolocalization to human melanoma xenografts in nude mice. When Mab 9.2.27, chelated to 5 mCi ^{111}-Indium with diethylene triamine-pentaacetic acid (DTPA), was injected into melanoma patients either alone or together with the addition of 50 mg unconjugated Mab 9.2.27, serum half-life of both labeled and unlabeled antibody was 30 hours. The labeled antibody was superior for imaging tumors, detecting masses as small as 5 × 5 mm and occult metastases. However, there was substantial uptake of the radioactive tracer by the RES and in vitro incubation at 37 °C revealed gradual loss of the ^{111}-Indium from the chelate. This radionuclide thus may not be optimal for imaging purposes and others such as 99m-technetium may possibly be a better candidate.[24]

Immunochemical Characterization of Disialoganglioside Antigens Expressed on Human Melanoma Cells

Tissue distribution. Human melanoma cells can create a unique antigenic determinant by O-acetylating disialoganglioside GD_3. In this regard, gangliosides represent interesting molecules that may become most useful to mark differentiation events and thus provide markers for tumor metastasis. In this regard, it is well known that the sialic acids of gangliosides have a considerable diversity, largely created by different types of O-substitutions, usually O-acetyl esters at the 4, 7, 8, and 9 positions of the parent molecule, neuraminic acid. Some of the highlights of studies described in detail elsewhere[25,26] are outlined here delineating a highly unique and specific antigenic determinant on human melanoma cells that is comprised by the alkali-labile, 9-O-acetylated product of the neuroectoderm-associated disialoganglioside GD_3. In this regard, Table 2 illustrates that Mab D1.1 directed to this very same antigen epitope is highly restricted in its reactivity with freshly frozen human melanoma tissues and fails to react with a wide variety of normal adult tissues, fetal tissues, and tissues of other neoplasms when tested by the immunoperoxidase assay. In contrast, it is well known that GD_3 per se is associated with various tissues of the neuroectoderm.[25] As illustrated by Table 2, the GD_3 in its nonacetylated form as defined by Mab MB3.6 is indeed present in tissues of human melanoma and adult brain, whereas the 9-O-acetylated GD_3, defined by Mab D1.1, appears only in melanoma tissues and may represent the only truly melanoma-specific antigen detected thus far.

Molecular profiles of disialoganglioside antigens. As shown in initial studies, the 9-O-acetylated GD_3 antigen is highly restricted to human melanoma and is specifically recognized by Mab D1.1[25] an antibody that was originally described by Levine et al[27] to recognize a fetal rat neuroectoderm-associated ganglioside. The first indication that Mab D1.1 recognized an O-acetylated ganglioside came from initial studies that indicated that base treatment of this melanoma-associated ganglioside caused a decrease in its migration on thin layer chromatography (TLC).[25] The purified, alkali-labile ganglioside migrated on TLC between the monosialylated ganglioside standards, GM_1 and GM_2. Thus, increasing periods of alkali treatment first partially and then completely converted this ganglioside to a new doublet, migrating in the same position as GD_3. This observation suggested a structural relationship of this yet undefined ganglioside with GD_3, and the single downward shift in migration on TLC implied the removal of a single, base-labile O-acyl group.

Table 2. Reactivities of Mabs D1.1 and MB3.6 by Immunoperoxidase Assay With Frozen Tissues

Tissues	D1.1	MB3.6
Melanotic		
Melanoma	+	+
Intradermal nevus	—	+
Normal melanocytes	—	+
Normal Adult		
Brain	—	+
Spleen	—	—
Liver	—	—
Lung	—	—
Colon	—	—
Kidney	—	—
Fetal		
Brain	—	+
Spleen	—	—
Liver	—	—
Malignancies		
Oat cell carcinoma	—	—
Astrocytoma	—	—
Glioblastoma	—	—
Neuroblastoma	—	—
Lung adenocarcinoma	—	—
Colon adenocarcinoma	—	—
Breast adenocarcinoma	—	—

Biochemical and immunochemical techniques rather than direct-probe mass spectrometry were used to confirm the structure of this ganglioside because it is relatively unstable and comprises at best only 5% of total melanoma ganglioside. In determining the antigenic characteristics of the de-O-acetylated GD_3, D1.1 was used together with two other monoclonal antibodies, ie, Mab R24[28] and Mab 3.6[29] that recognize only native GD_3 and fail to cross-react with any other gangliosides. Base-induced de-O-acetylation of purified melanoma ganglioside was found to completely destroy their reactivity with Mab D1.1 while causing at the same time a reciprocal increase in the reactivity of Mab R24.[25]

Direct evidence was obtained that Mab D1.1 recognizes an alkali-labile, acetylated form of GD_3 by parallel TLC analysis of both total melanoma ganglioside and the purified ganglioside recognized by Mab D1.1, either with or without prior base treatment followed by direct immunostaining with monoclonal antibodies. Base treatment, ie, overnight incubation at room temperature in an airtight chamber saturated with ammonia, had three effects: First, it caused loss of reactivity with Mab D1.1; second, it resulted in a decrease of mobility on TLC, causing comigration with purified GD_3; and third, the base-treated purified ganglioside now reacted exclusively with Mabs R24 and MB3.6 that are specific for nonacetylated GD_3. It was also corroborated that base treatment of total melanoma gangliosides causes de-O-acetylation of O-acetylated gangliosides with a subsequent decrease in mobility resulting in comigration with their parent gangliosides. Figure 3A depicts the two-dimensional TLC profile of total melanoma ganglioside without alkali treatment. The arrows indicate the position of O-acetylated GD_3 and of a putative O-acetylated GD_2 that under these conditions cannot be distinguished as it is covered, in part, by GD_3. Base treatment produces de-O-acetylation and the resultant decrease in mobility that now clearly shows the two de-O-acetylated ganglioside to comigrate with their parent gangliosides, GD_3 and GD_2, respectively. Coincidentally, these data provide the first evidence for the presence of O-acetylated GD_2 in a human melanoma cell extract (Fig 3B).

Direct evidence was also obtained indicating that the O-acetyl group of acetylated GD_3 was located on the 9-position of its terminal sialic acid residue. To this end, periodate oxidation was done on gangliosides isolated from melanoma cells under conditions that were such that oxidation would occur only between the exocyclic (7, -8, -9) hydroxyl positions of terminal, unsubstituted sialic acid residues. Controlled periodate oxidation of total melanoma gangliosides com-

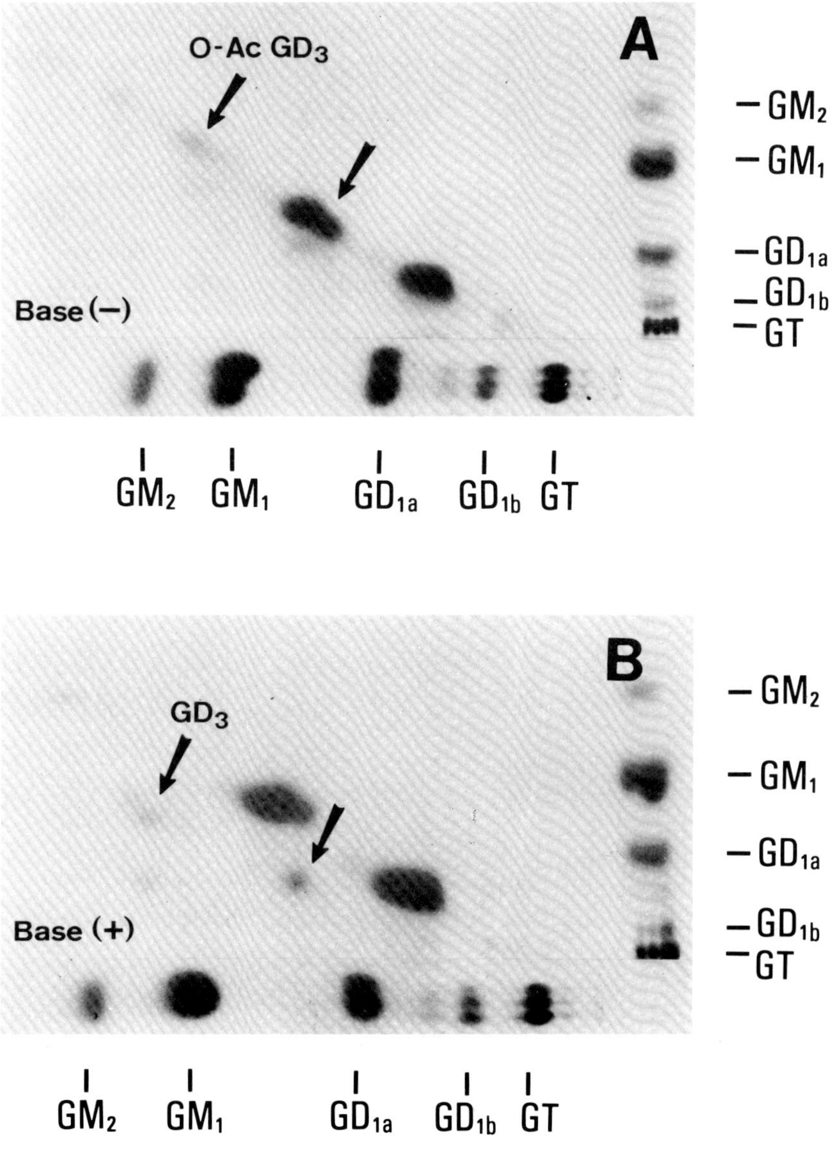

Fig 3. Two-dimensional TLC for identification of alkali-labile gangliosides. Purified gangliosides from M21 melanoma cells were subjected to two-dimensional TLC without intermediate base hydrolysis (A) and with base hydrolysis (B). Gangliosides were visualized with resorcinol reagent. The first dimension was run from right to left. The designated arrows refer to O-acetylated GD_3 and the unmarked arrows indicate the position of putative O-acetylated GD_2.

pletely eliminated their antigenic reactivity with Mabs R24 and MB3.6 that specifically recognize nonacetylated GD_3 as well as reactivity with Mab 126 that reacts specifically with GD_2.[30] However, antigenic reactivity with Mab D1.1 remained unchanged even at the highest periodate concentration used (4 mmol/L), strongly suggesting that the O-acetyl group is indeed located at the 9-position of the terminal sialic acid of GD_3. This finding was also confirmed by chemical means, using the mild acetylating agent N-acetyl-imidazole that is known to selectively O-acetylate the 9-position of the methyl ester/methyl glycoside of sialic acid under appropriate conditions of molar excess. The compound created by this procedure now migrated in the appropriate position on TLC between GM_1 and GM_2 and also specifically reacted with Mab D1.1.

Evaluation of GD_3 as a Target Antigen for Tumor Cell Destruction

The initial hypothesis was that GD_3, which is heavily expressed on most human melanoma cells and like other gangliosides is integrally embedded in the lipid bilayer of these cells, may be an effective target antigen for Mab-mediated cytotoxicity of human melanoma cells. Thus, Cheresh et al[31] tested Mab MB3.6 for its ability to specifically mediate the lysis of ^{51}Cr-labeled human melanoma target cells. In the presence of human serum as a complement source, this antibody effectively lyses within thirty minutes 80% to 100% of four human melanoma cell lines expressing significant levels of GD_3, whereas a melanoma cell line (A375) lacking GD_3 could not by lysed within two hours. Melanoma cells expressing GD_3 were challenged with Mab MB3.6 in the presence of normal human peripheral blood mononuclear leukocytes as effector cells to determine whether this antigen could serve as an effective target for antibody-dependent cellular cytotoxicity (ADCC). Indeed, Mab MB3.6 in the presence of human effector cells could also mediate significant ADCC ranging from 58% to 80% with the four melanoma cell lines expressing GD_3, whereas as expected, no lysis could be detected with the GD_3-negative melanoma cell line A375. In the absence of Mab MB3.6, these same human effector cells could mediate natural killer cell lysis ranging only from 5% to 25% regardless of the GD_3 content of any of the target cell lines.[28]

The finding that Mab MB3.6 could induce the lysis of human melanoma cells served as a rationale to test the effects of this antibody on the ability of cultured human melanoma cells to establish tumors in the athymic nude (nu/nu) mice. Thus, purified Mab MB3.6 was resuspended in phosphate-buffered saline (PBS) pH 7.2, and injected intraperitoneally into animals that had previously (one day earlier) received a subcutaneous injection of 10^7 M14 melanoma cells. In the control group, six of six animals developed sizable tumors between 30 and 40 days after inoculation [mean [$\pm$SE] volume = 370 $\pm$ 65 μL] whereas only one of six animals treated with 70 μg/mL purified Mab MB3.6 in nine separate intraperitoneal injections beginning on day 2 after tumor inoculum developed a small tumor of approximately 150 μL. Further results of additional experiments suggest that Mab MB3.6 can temporarily suppress the growth of human melanoma tumors that before treatment were allowed to grow for seven days to a size of approximately 50 μL in these animals (Fig 4).[31] However, it should be pointed out that when Mab MB3.6 is used in this manner, some

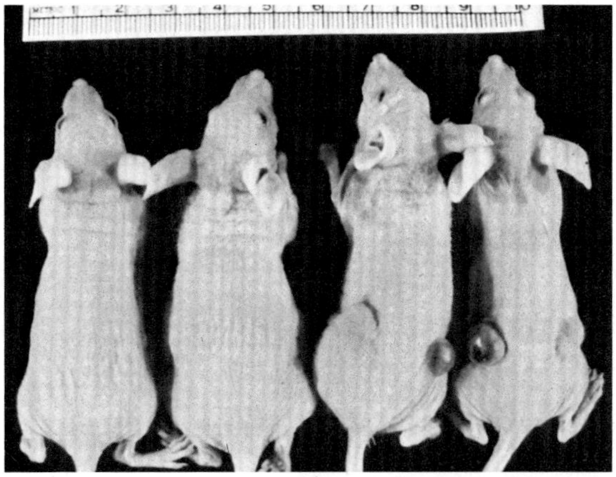

Fig 4. Effects of Mab MB3.6 on human melanoma tumor formation in the athymic nude mouse. FM9m human melanoma cells (10^7) were injected into the right and left flank of 12 nude mice. Tumor formation was allowed to occur for seven days after which six animals received four injections (days 7, 9, 11, and 13) of either Mab MB3.6 (70 μg in 100 μL PBS) or PBS alone. The two animals on the right were in the control (PBS) group and the two animals on the left received Mab MB3.6 treatment. These photographs were taken after the tumors were allowed to develop for 23 days.

tumors will eventually reappear and grow again, especially after antibody injection is stopped for several weeks. In this regard, it is most encouraging that in a very recent experiment this limitation could be overcome when using the armed effector cell approach. Specifically, when established 30 to 50 μL human melanoma tumors are treated at each injection with either anti-GD_3 Mabs MB3.6 or 11C64 together with at least 2×10^6 effector cells, ie, mouse splenocytes, then melanoma tumor growth in most animals is completely suppressed, even several months after the last injection of antibody and effector cells.[32] The results from these experiments suggest that the two monoclonal anti-GD_3 antibodies of IgG3 isotype that can effectively fix human complement and evoke ADCC are also quite effective in suppressing the growth of established melanoma tumors.

In this regard, the report of Houghton et al,[33] is most interesting, as these investigators were able to achieve significant tumor regression in three of 12 melanoma patients treated in phase I clinical trial with R24, another monoclonal anti-GD_3 antibody of IgG3 isotype. Specifically, Mab R24 was injected at dose levels of 8 mg/m^2 over a period of 2 weeks. Inflammatory reactions, consisting of urticaria, pruritus, erythema, and subcutaneous ecchymoses were observed around tumor sites in patients treated with 80 mg/m^2. As was observed in earlier clinical trials with murine monoclonal antibodies, human antimouse antibody appeared in the serum of the patients.[20,21] In this case, peak antibody levels in serum were found to be dose-related and ranged from 0.1 μg/mL to 62 μg/mL. These antibodies were detected in all patients who could be evaluated between 15 and 40 days after the start of therapy. Interestingly, as observed in clinical trials with another murine antimelanoma antibody, 9.2.27,[20] there was again no evidence of antigenic modulation caused by treatment of patients with Mab R24, as continued cell surface expression of GD_3 was observed in the face of substantial levels of circulating and tumor-bound Mab R24.

The data obtained by Houghton and colleagues[33] are, of course, most interesting and one can express cautious optimism regarding the potential usefulness of such treatment. Houghton et al[33] were most cautious in interpreting their data, clearly indicating that some distant tumor metastases were not affected by the antibody, although they later revealed considerable GD_3 expression. The involvement of immunological effector mechanisms(s) is certainly suggested by the 4 to 12-week time intervals required before an approximately 50% decrease in the size of some lesions could be observed. As Houghton et al[33] point out, a variety of mechanisms may be involved, ranging from antibody-directed complement-mediated cytotoxicity and cell-mediated cytotoxicity to tumor cell injury secondary to the inflammatory reaction elicited in the tumor bed by Mab R24. This observation, plus the infiltration of T cells and mast cells, mast cell degranulation, and the depositions of complement components C3, C5, and C9 in the tumor bed certainly supports this hypothesis.

Another observation made by Houghton et al[33] is intriguing, namely that responses to R24 treatment of melanoma tumor-bearing nude rats and mice were actually enhanced by intermittent chemotherapy with Adriamycin (Adria Laboratories, Columbus, Ohio). As pointed out, such treatment may alter tumor cell susceptibility to drugs. Obviously, one may also conclude that antibody-drug conjugates, especially if they involve anti-GD_3 antibodies, may turn out to be a useful modality for immunotherapy of malignant melanoma. Taken together, these results indicate for the first time that a mouse monoclonal antibody recognizing an appropriate target antigen, ie, disialoganglioside GD_3, offers a potentially novel and effective form of immunotherapy for human malignant melanoma.

PERSPECTIVES

It is now increasingly apparent that monoclonal antibodies directed to antigens on human tumor cells not only are excellent probes to delineate the structure and function of these cell surface markers but also offer potentially interesting new approaches for cancer therapy. The experimental data summarized in this brief and obviously incomplete review certainly document this point of view. It should also be obvious from this review that monoclonal antibody-mediated immunotherapy of human cancer is still very much in its infancy and that the handful of clinical trials conducted thus far are not sufficient to make a truly critical evaluation. Data obtained thus far can lead one to be at best cautiously optimistic that new treatment modalities involving monoclonal antibodies can constructively add to existing therapy regimens.

The information available at this time already indicates that monoclonal antibodies per se are not magic bullets that by themselves can cure cancer or have a major impact on cancer therapy. It is far more likely that two major treatment strategies will evolve that will make good use of these unique immunological reagents. The first of these strategies is based on the prediction made by Paul Ehrlich some 80 years ago that antibodies will eventually be the "magic bullets" that target drugs and toxins to tumor cells and thereby assure their ultimate destruction. Although this review simply could not cover a number of attempts made to accomplish this in pre-clinical trials, there is, nevertheless, a fairly massive effort in progress worldwide that makes use of monoclonal antibodies to target chemotherapeutic drugs, radionuclides, plant toxins that interfere with the tumor cell DNA synthesis and differentiation agents to reach and destroy a variety of tumor cells. Results from such studies again warrant some cautious optimism that such attempts to selectively kill tumors cells may ultimately succeed in the clinic and add another modality to cancer therapy. The scattered clinical trials ongoing in this area are two few and as yet too inconclusive to warrant any critical evaluation at this time.

The second of these basic strategies is aimed at improving the tumor host's immunological defense system by arming suitable host cells in such a fashion that they effectively aid in tumor cell destruction. One such approach used in the author's laboratory has been described in this review, ie, arming effector cells with monoclonal antibody that then effectively destroy established human melanoma tumors in athymic (nu/nu) mice. Actually, such approaches are currently being tested clinically in Europe with a murine monoclonal antibody (17–1A) directed to colorectal cancer. The results of such trials presented very recently at the Second Hybridoma Congress[34] provide cause for some optimism, although it is quite clear that this potentially useful treatment modality will have to be tested far more extensively before a critical evaluation can be made. Other approaches that are pioneered and explored by Rosenberg et al[35] are those of treating patients' peripheral lymphocytes with such potent effector molecules as recombinant IL-2 to produce a population of lymphokine-activated killer (LAK) cells that in some instances produced tumor regression, notably in melanoma patients. However, as clearly pointed out by Rosenberg and colleagues[35] these approaches have to be considerably refined to overcome some rather severe clinical problems evoked by this treatment. One such approach is being attempted in the author's laboratory in pre-clinical experiments and consists of arming, ie, targeting LAK cells with monoclonal antibodies directed to GD_3 and other specific cell surface markers of melanoma cells. This is done in the hope that such a maneuver may overcome in part the excessive homing of LAK cells to the lungs. Another interesting and novel approach is being tested in a number of laboratories including that of the author. This strategy is based on the work of Milstein and Cuello[36] who developed the technology of hybrid-hybridomas. The approach presently being tested in the author's laboratory is to produce hybrid monoclonal antibodies, eg, between mouse hybridomas of IgG2a isotype directed to a melanoma-associated chondroitin sulfate proteoglycan and to a mouse or human T cell receptors, respectively. Such antibody constructs proved useful for melanoma tumor cell destruction in vitro and will now be tested for their effectiveness in vivo in nude mouse model systems, especially those bearing spontaneous melanoma metastases.

It is quite clear at this time that a number of new and potentially useful cancer therapy modalities will have to be optimized, first in preclinical animal model systems and then in clinical trials. Once this is accomplished, it seems apparent that the really critical task will be to combine several such optimal treatment modalities is a synergistic fashion to achieve the maximal therapeutic effect on human tumors.

It is obvious that a great deal remains to be done by many research investigators and clinicians in preclinical and clinical trials before some solid achievements in tumor therapy can be recorded and that time is of the very essence to attain some modicum of success in such attempts in the near future.

There is, however, no doubt that murine monoclonal antibodies directed to human tumor-associated antigens have already made a most decisive impact on basic cancer research. As some of the examples cited in this review illustrate, these antibodies have indeed served as exquisitively sensitive and specific molecular and functional probes and have shed considerable light on many areas of work that were most difficult to approach in the past. In this regard, rapid progress is being made in gaining new knowledge in biosynthesis, intracellular transport, regulation of cell surface expression and cell surface receptors of a variety of tumor and differentiation antigens. It is certainly realistic to expect that the knowledge gained in such areas of research coupled with the new and exciting techniques of molecular biology will have the most decisive impact on cancer research in this century. It is also most likely that this type of knowledge will be required ultimately to design approaches that are most effective for the destruction of human tumor cells. In this regard, it is not too much to expect if one postulates that these powerful technologies will have a decisive impact on delineating mechanisms of metastasis and then to develop effective approaches to gain the type of control over metastatic events that will ultimately facilitate a cancer cure.

To be sure, there are still a large number of problems to be solved. To mention just a few, these include a way to cope with massive tumor burden that somehow cannot be debulked by existing treatment modalities, including surgery. Another is to find a way to penetrate and attack the many necrotic tumors with poor blood flow. Both of these problems remain quite formidable at this time. In this regard, there have already been a few attempts made to attain better blood flow at tumor sites, in some cases by making use of complement-induced inflammatory responses and in others by attempting to use monoclonal antibody-directed tumor targeting of molecules such as tumor necrosis factor to induce inflammation, at the tumor site(s) and thereby improve vascularization and blood flow. Needless to say, this is just a beginning and it seems obvious that such approaches can become far more sophisticated with the increasing availability of genetically cloned lymphokines and other potent effector molecules that can impact strongly on the immunological system of the tumor host. Certainly, the key advances made in the molecular delineation of T cell receptors and a variety of T and B cell markers will ultimately have an even more decisive effect on cancer research than it has had thus far.

There is little doubt, at least in the mind of the author, that the combined strategies of hybridoma technology and molecular biology are one of the most powerful experimental tools devised by modern science and that their use will ultimately lead to a marked and sustained progress in cancer research that will hopefully lead to the ultimate conquest of cancer.

ACKNOWLEDGMENT

The author wishes to thank his colleagues, Drs D.A. Cheresh, C.J. Honsik, and R.C. Spiro for contributing their experimental data. The excellent assistance of Ms Bonnie Pratt Filiault in typing this manuscript is gratefully acknowledged. This is Scripps Publication No. 4288-Imm.

REFERENCES

1. Kohler G, Milstein C: Continuous cultures of fused cells secreting antibody of predefined specificity. Nature 256:495–497, 1975

2. Reisfeld RA, Cheresh DA: Human tumor-associated antigens: Targets for monoclonal antibody-mediated therapy. Cancer Surv 4:271–290, 1985

3. Reisfeld RA: Monoclonal antibodies as probes for the molecular structure and biological function of melanoma-associated antigens, in Sell S, Reisfeld RA (eds): Monoclonal Antibodies in Cancer. Clifton, NJ, Humana, 1985, p 205

4. Reisfeld RA, Sell S (eds): Drug Antibody Conjugates, in Monoclonal Antibodies and Cancer Therapy, New York, Alan R. Liss, 1985, p 207

5. Feizi T: Carbohydrate antigens in human cancer. Cancer Surv 4:245–269, 1985

6. Hakamori S: Tumor-associated carbohydate antigens. Ann Rev Immunol 2:103–126, 1984

7. Teh JG, Stacker SA, Thompson CH, et al: The diagnosis of human tumors with monoclonal antibodies. Cancer Surv 4:149–184, 1985

8. Albino AP, Houghton AN: Cell surface antigens of melanocytes and melanoma. Cancer Surv 4:185–211, 1985

9. Bumol TF, Reisfeld RA: Unique glycoprotein proteoglycan complex defined by monoclonal antibody on human melanoma cells. Proc Natl Acad Sci USA 89:1245–1249, 1982

10. Bumol TF, Walker LE, Reisfeld RA: Biosynthetic studies of proteoglycans in human melanoma cells with a monoclonal antibody to a core glycoprotein of chondroitin sulfare proteoglycans. J Biol Chem 259:12733–12741, 1984

11. Harper JR, Bumol TF, Reisfeld RA: Characterization of monoclonal antibody 155.8 and partial characterization of its proteoglycan antigen on human melanoma cells. J Immunol 132:2096–2104, 1984

12. Hellstrom I, Garrigues J, Cabasco L, et al: Studies of a high molecular weight human melanoma antigen. J Immunol 130:1467–1472, 1983

13. Ross AH, Cossu G, Herlyn M, et al: Isolation and characterization of a melanoma-associated proteoglycan antigen. Arch Biochem Biophys 222:370–383, 1983

14. Fellini SA, Hascall UC, Kimura H: Localization or proteoglycan core protein in subcellular fractions isolated from rat chondrosarcoma chondrocytes. J Biol Chem 259:4634–4641, 1984

15. Bumol TF, Walker LE, Reisfeld RA: Biosynthetic studies of proteoglycans in human melanoma cells with a monoclonal antibody to a core glycoprotein of chondroitin sulfate proteoglycans. J Biol Chem 259:12733–12741, 1984

16. Hascall VC, Haskall GK: Proteoglycans, in Hay ED (ed): Cell Biology of Extracellular Matrix. New York, Plenum, 1981, p 39

17. Harper JR, Quaranta V, Reisfeld RA: Biosynthesis and intracellular transport of proteoglycan core protein by human melanoma cells: Involvement of low pH mechanisms, in Reddi AH (ed): Extracellular Matrix Structure and Function, New York, Alan R. Liss, 1985, p 367

18. Schultz G, Staffileno LK, Reisfeld RA, et al: Monoclonal antibody directed effector cells selectively lyse human melanoma cells in vitro and in vivo. Proc Natl Acad Sci USA 80:5407–5411, 1983

19. Schulz G, Staffileno LK, Reisfeld RA, et al: Eradication of established human melanoma tumors in nude mice by antibody-directed effector cells. J Exp Med 161:1315–1325, 1985

20. Oldham RK, Foon KA, Morgan AC, et al: Monoclonal antibody therapy of malignant melanoma: In vivo localization in cutaneous metastasis after intravenous administration. J Clin Oncol 2:1235–1244, 1984

21. Foon KA, Bunn PA, Schroff RW, et al: Monoclonal antibody therapy of chronic lymphocyte leukemic and cutaneous T cell lymphoma: Preliminary observations, in Boss BE, Langman RE, Trowbridge IS, et al (eds): Monoclonal Antibodies and Cancer, Orlando, Fla, Academic, 1983, p 39

22. Bumol TF, Personal communication, April 1985

23. Hwang KM, Morgan AC, Fodstad O, et al: Radiolocalization of xenografted human malignant melanoma by a monoclonal antibody (9.2.27) to a melanoma-associated antigen in nude mice. Cancer Res 45:4150–4155, 1985

24. Abrams PG, Morgan AC, Schroff RW, et al: Localization and biodistribution studies of a monoclonal antibody in patients with melanoma, in Reisfeld RA, Sell S (eds): Monoclonal Antibodies and Cancer Therapy, New York, Alan Liss, 1985, p 233

25. Cheresh DA, Varki AP, Varki NM, et al: A monoclonal antibody recognizes an O-acetylated sialic acid in a human melanoma-associated ganglioside. J Biol Chem 259:7453–7459, 1984

26. Cheresh DA, Reisfeld RA, Varki AP: O-acetylation of disialoganglioside GD_3 by human melanoma cells creates a unique antigenic determinant. Science 225:844–846, 1984

27. Levine JM, Beasley L, Stallcup WB: The D1.1 antigen: A cell surface marker for germinal cells of the central nervous system. J Neurochem 4:820–831, 1984

28. Pukel CS, Lloyd KO, Trabassos LR, et al: GD_3, a prominent ganglioside antigen of human melanoma, detection and characterization of mouse monoclonal antibody. J Exp Med 155:1133–1147, 1982

29. Cheresh DA, Harper JR, Schultz G, et al: Localization of the gangliosides GD_2 and GD_3 in adhesion plaques and on the surface of human melanoma cells. Proc Natl Acad Sci USA 81:5767–6771, 1984

30. Schulz G, Cheresh DA, Varki NM: Detection of ganglioside GD_2 in tumor tissues and neuroblastoma patients. Cancer Res 44:5914–5920, 1984

31. Cheresh DA, Honsik CJ, Staffileno LK, et al: Disialoganglioside GD_3 on human melanoma cells serves as a relevant target antigen for monoclonal antibody-mediated tumor cytolysis. Proc Natl Acad Sci USA 82:5155–5159, 1985

32. Honsik CJ, Reisfeld RA: Model systems for monoclonal antibody-mediated cancer therapy, in Bonavida B, Collier JR (eds): Membrane-Mediated Cytotoxicity, New York, Alan Liss, 1986 (in press)

33. Houghton AN, Mintzer D, Cordon-Cardo L, et al: Mouse monoclonal IgG3 antibody detecting GD_3 ganglioside. A phase I trial in patients with malignant melanoma. Proc Natl Acad Sci USA 82:1242–1246, 1985

34. Steplewski Z, Reisfeld RA: Summary of working group reports, 2nd Hybridoma Congress. Hybridoma, 1986 (in press)

35. Rosenberg SA, Lotze MT, Muul LM, et al: Observations on the systemic administration of autologous lymphokine-activated killer cells and recombinant interleukin-2 to patients with metastatic cancer. N Engl J Med 313:1485–1492, 1985

36. Milstein C, Cuello AC: Hybrid hybridomas and their use in immunochemistry. Nature 305:537–540, 1983

Monoclonal Antibodies: Potential Applications to the Treatment of Cancer

Alan N. Houghton and David A. Scheinberg

THE STUDY of cancer cells by serological probes has a long history that began in the last century and has continued in an uninterrupted fashion to the present.[1] It is the extraordinary resolving power of antibodies that permits molecules on cancer cells to be finely distinguished. The primary concern of the serologist studying cancer has been to define the specificity of the serological reactions in order to identify and characterize the antigenic determinants recognized. A drawback to conventional serological analysis was the reliance on antisera that might contain antibodies of unrelated specificity in addition to the desired antibody. The situation changed dramatically in 1975, when Kohler and Milstein first described a general procedure for the production of monoclonal antibodies (mAb) of defined specificity.[2,3] The power of mAbs was immediately recognized, and has subsequently revolutionized the serological and biochemical analysis of human cancer. MAbs can recognize a single antigenic determinant in a complex mixture of antigens. Potentially, mAbs can be produced in great quantities and in reproducible lots, permitting large scale production for practical applications. The technique introduced by Kohler and Milstein became known as the hybridoma methodology.[4] Briefly, mice are immunized with a source of antigen. Splenocytes from the immunized animals, which include a rich supply of immune B lymphocytes, are fused with an established mouse myeloma cell line. Hybrid cells grow out under selective conditions that kill off nonhybridized mouse myeloma cells (the normal nonhybridized splenocytes die off because they do not usually survive in tissue culture). Hybrid cells combine two critical phenotypes from the original starting cell populations—the ability to produce a specific antibody (from the immune B lymphocytes) and the property of immortality from the cancer cell (the myeloma cell). Immortalized hybrid cells can be isolated by cell cloning procedures that allow identification of hybrid clones secreting individual antibodies of requisite specificity. The hybridoma technology is one of a series of major developments in biotechnology that have occurred in the last decade. Perhaps the most important implication of this rapidly moving area is that discoveries in the laboratory can be quickly translated into clinical applications. Potentially interesting mAbs can be identified and brought into patient studies within several years. A thorough discussion of the characteristics of human tumor antigens detected by mAbs is provided in recent reviews.[5–9] The characterization and potential applications of mAbs are briefly described below.

An initial step in the characterization of a mAb is establishing the pattern of reactivity of the antibody against a panel of cell types. This analysis, called a specificity analysis, defines the reactivity of a mAb against a broad number of normal and malignant cell types. Historically, the serological study of cancer has in major part been a search for antigens that are unique to cancer cells, the tumor-specific antigens, in the hope that such antigens would truly and completely distinguish cancer cells from normal cells. Although tumor-specific antigens have proven to be elusive, the serological scrutiny of cancer cells with mAb has identified a wide range of antigens. Of particular interest is the group of antigens known as differentiation antigens. Differentiation antigens, first noted on T cell leukemias in the mouse,[10,11] can be defined as antigens that identify cells in distinct differentiation pathways or cells at different stages of differentiation within the same pathway.[12] Although differentiation antigens of malignant cells are by definition present on normal cells, a number of differentiation antigens have been shown to have very restricted distribution in normal tissues, and are being intensively studied as targets for diagnosis

From the Division of Medical Oncology, Memorial Sloan-Kettering Cancer Center, New York.

Supported by grants NCI CA 33049 from the National Cancer Institute, and by the Louis and Anne Abrons Foundation, the Alcoa Foundation and the JM Foundation.

Address reprint requests to Alan N. Houghton, MD, 1275 York Ave, Memorial Sloan-Kettering Cancer Center, New York, NY 10021.

0093–7754/86/1302–0006$05.00/0

and therapy of cancer. While mAbs with absolute specificity for cancer cells have been difficult to develop, it has been possible to produce antibodies that identify antigens with higher expression on malignant cells when compared to their normal cell counterpart. These quantitative differences in antigen expression between normal (eg, low expression) and malignant cells (eg, high expression) may prove to be critical in seeking strategies for clinical applications of mAbs. The analysis of antibody specificity remains a cornerstone of the characterization of mAbs—the reactivity of a mAb with normal tissues should be known before any clinical applications are attempted.

Other properties of the antibody molecule may determine their potential applications. The affinity and avidity of an antibody is a measurement of how strongly the antibody binds to a target antigenic determinant and of the stability of the binding. These properties may be very important factors for how effectively and efficiently a mAb localizes to a tumor. The class and subclass of mouse mAbs have been reported to be related to the ability of an antibody to lyse target tumor cells, either by the effect of complement or by immune effector cells. Antibody class may also affect the biodistribution of an antibody in vivo, eg, half-life in the blood and tissue distribution.

The target antigen may determine many of the biological properties of mAbs. Is the antigen secreted/shed or is it on the cell surface or inside the cell? What is the structure of the antigen? Is the antigenic determinant on a glycoprotein, glycolipid, or some other moiety? Is the antigen expressed on all malignant cells in a tumor, or only on a subset of cells? What is the biological function of the antigen for the cell? Biochemical analysis of antigenic structures has important implications for a wide variety of applications of mAbs. Detailed knowledge of the structure and behavior of antigen molecules can facilitate studies of the function of these molecules for the cell, the development of assays for antigen in body fluids, the biodistribution of mAb in patients with cancer, and mechanisms by which mAbs may kill target tumor cells and ways that tumor cells may escape from mAb-mediated destruction of tumors.

MAbs are being applied to broad areas of cancer research. (1) Genes coding for antigens identified by mAbs can be assigned to individual chromosomes through the techniques of somatic cell genetics, or isolated using the method of DNA transfection, or cloned by recombinant DNA technology. (2) In the area of tissue diagnosis, mAbs can finely distinguish different cell types within a tissue, and may be of value in studying embryogenesis and development of normal tissues and of organ malformations. As differentiation markers, panels of mAbs are powerful tools for the histopathological diagnosis of tumors. For instance, it is possible to use antibodies to establish the histogenic origin of undifferentiated metastatic tumors; for example, mAbs are available that distinguish between carcinomas, lymphoma, and malignant melanoma.[13] Cancers can also be subsetted according to the expression of tissue markers. Although the best examples are subsets of T lymphocytes defined by mAbs,[9] a wide variety of cell types have been subsetted according to cell markers.[12,14,15] Classification of cancer subsets according to antigenic phenotypes will depend on careful investigations relating antigen expression to tumor cell biology, morphology, and clinical observations. Antigens secreted or shed by cancer cells can be detected in body fluids (eg, blood, urine, effusions). Numerous attempts have been made to develop assays for tumor antigens to screen for early diagnosis, to moniter therapy, and to detect tumor recurrence after therapy. These tests have generally met with only limited success. This is most frequently due to inadequate sensitivity, detecting patients with only substantial tumor burdens, or to problems of specificity, giving positive reactions in non-cancer conditions. The mAb technology has produced an explosion of activity in this area, as the number of well-characterized tumor markers has increased dramatically. Examples include a novel carbohydrate structure related to the Lewis blood group antigen that is detected in the serum of patients with gastrointestinal cancers,[16,17] and the CA125 antigen that is detected in the serum of patients with ovarian carcinoma.[18] The general role of these new markers awaits extensive investigations and must be regarded cautiously, but their potential utility has been demonstrated in specific patients.

The remaining discussion will focus on the potential application of mAbs in vivo for tumor diagnosis and therapy. This involves the use of labeled antibodies for localization of specific tumor sites and the therapy of patients with cancer using either unmodified mAbs or mAbs conjugated to anticancer agents. The areas of tumor localization and treatment are closely intertwined—the therapeutic efficacy of a mAb may depend on how well the mAb localizes to tumor sites as compared to normal tissues. Thus, information gained from studies of the biodistribution of labeled mAbs, eg, dosimetry of radiolabeled mAbs, can guide approaches for therapy.

STRATEGIES FOR THERAPEUTIC APPLICATION OF MONOCLONAL ANTIBODIES

A number of distinct approaches to cancer therapy with mAb are being explored. At this point, no single strategy has proven to be superior. As more experience has been gained, it has become apparent that mAbs cannot be thought of simply as magic bullets or guided missiles that seek out and destroy the tumor. To be effective, mAbs have to reach tumor sites, but not target most normal tissue. Once an appropriate site has been reached, mechanisms are needed to destroy tumor cells without risking the host. Each approach requires certain prerequisite information about the individual antibody/antigen system being explored. For instance, knowledge about antibody specificity, antibody class and subclass, antibody avidity, or structure and function of the antigen may be critical to the success of a particular scheme. A series of preclinical studies are necessary to fully characterize the effects of mAbs on target tumor cells. Does the mAb kill target cells, either when used alone or in the presence of other components of the immune system? How effective is the antibody when conjugated to a potentially cytotoxic/cytostatic agent? Assays in vitro could include the following: (1) the ability of mAb to mediate destruction of target tumor cells in the presence of human complement (complement-mediated cytotoxicity); (2) the ability of mAb to mediate killing of target tumor cells in the presence of human immune effector cells (antibody-dependent cellular cytotoxicity); (3) the direct biological effects of mAb on target cells, eg, block cell proliferation; and (4) cytotoxic/cytostatic effects of mAb conjugated to anticancer agents. Studies in vitro can be complemented by studies in vivo, the usual model being human tumors xenografted into nude mice. This model is useful in some respects, for instance investigating the ability of a mAb to localize to appropriate tumors. However, the nude mouse model is limited. In most cases one is studying a mouse antibody in a mouse host, which of course does not predict how a mouse antibody will behave in a human host. In addition, the nude mouse accepts xenografted tumor tissue because it does not have an intact immune system. Therefore, antitumor effects that rely on immunological mechanisms in many circumstances cannot be assessed in this model. Preclinical studies both in vitro and in vivo can guide the strategies that should be used for human trials. Three basic strategies are discussed below.

Immune-Mediated Destruction of Tumor Cells

Experimental studies in animals have revealed that passive administration of unmodified antibodies can have antitumor activity.[19] In general, effects have been more substantial against small tumors, and lymphoid tumors have been more susceptible than solid tumors. Monoclonal antibodies directed against differentiation antigens of mouse lymphocytes have been shown to prevent or reduce the growth of tumors and abrogate the development of metastases.[19] Several immune mechanisms may mediate these antitumor effects. The majority of mouse mAbs analyzed to date do not seem to be potent mediators of tumor cell destruction in the presence of human complement or human effector cells. However, a number of mAbs have been identified that are candidates for therapeutic application without further modification.[20-26] Some mouse monoclonal antibodies can activate complement, and complement components can lead to effects on leukocytes, coagulation factors, and other mediators of inflammation. The membrane attack complex produced by the terminal complement components can produce lysis and destruction of target cells. Studies using mouse serum as a source of complement demonstrated that IgM antibodies were powerful activators of complement, while IgG2a and IgG2b subclass antibodies were of medium or low potency.[27] Only an occasional IgG1 subclass antibody activates complement-mediated cytolysis. Complement activation has been suggested to mediate antitumor effects of IgG3, IgG2a, and IgM mouse mAbs against human tumors: (1) IgM and IgG2a, but not IgG1, mAbs against hepatitis B virus surface antigen prevented or suppressed formation of human hepatoma tumors growing in nude mice[28]; (2) Regression of established human breast tumors growing in nude mice was seen after administration of IgG2a and IgG3 complement-fixing mAbs[29]; and (3) Inflammation, complement deposition at tumor sites, and tumor regression were observed after therapy of patients with metastatic malignant melanoma with a complement-fixing IgG3 mAb to G_{D3} ganglioside.[30] One factor that determines whether or not a tumor responds to complement-fixing mAbs may be the density of antigen present on target tumor cells.[31] The number of antigenic sites on a target cell can be increased by combining two or more mAbs. Experiments have suggested that a combination of two antibodies directed against two distinct determinants present on a single antigenic molecule acts synergistically in complement-mediated lysis of target melanoma cells.[32]

Another pathway to the lysis of tumor cells by mAb is by antibody-directed effector cells, called antibody-dependent cell-mediated cytotoxicity (ADCC). A range of cell types have been shown to be active in ADCC, including killer(K) cells, macrophages, natural killer (NK) cells, neutrophils, and even nonimmune cell types such as platelets. Preliminary observation in animal models had revealed that antitumor effects could be detected when noncomplement-fixing antibodies were used for treatment.[20] Because nude mice lack functional T and killer lymphocytes, it was presumed that T cell cytotoxicity and K cell-directed ADCC were not responsible. The antitumor activity of the ADCC mechanism was demonstrated by observing tumor cell lysis when mAbs were incubated with effector cells, eg, splenocytes from nude mice,[33] and subsequent experiments supported antitumor effects in vivo.[20] Further experiments in animal models have substantiated that ADCC mediated by macrophages[34] or NK cells[22,23] can cause rejection of tumors. In the nude mouse model, inhibition of tumor growth by a mAb correlates with its ability to react in ADCC.[35] Mouse mAbs of the IgG2a and IgG3 subclasses have been most effective to date in ADCC assays.[20,25,30] The importance of antibody subclass has been highlighted by experiments that switch an IgG1 mAb to IgG2a and IgG2b subclass while retaining the same antibody specificity, idiotype and avidity.[36] IgG2a mAb had the greatest activity in ADCC assays, and separate observations have shown IgG2a to have tumor inhibiting effects.[35] As with complement-mediated cytotoxicity, the number of antibody binding sites may be important in determining mAbs that are active versus inactive in ADCC.[35] It may be possible to augment the effects of ADCC-reactive antibodies. In one model system, while neither mAb or effector cells alone produced tumor regression, established human melanoma tumors could be eradicated by simultaneously injecting tumor-bearing mice with both mAb and splenocytes with NK activity.[22] One possible explanation for this effect is that mAbs bind to, and arm, cytolytic effector cells, facilitating the ability of the mAbs plus effector cell to eradicate the tumor.[22,23] However, it is likely that binding of mAb to effector cells is more efficient when the mAb is already bound to the target tumor cell.[36]

It is likely that the immunological destruction of established tumors in humans will require multiple arms of the immune system, including soluble components (eg, complement, coagulation factors) and immune cells (eg, NK cells, T cells, B cells, macrophages, neutrophils). The immune response is complex, but inflammation may be a potent way to amplify the antitumor effects of mAbs reaching tumor sites. Thus, mAbs that activate complement, even weakly, may better attract effector cells for ADCC- or T cell-mediated cytolysis. Inflammation can provide several mechanisms for destruction of tumor cells, and fields of inflammation at tumor sites may allow killing of tumor cells that might otherwise escape from mAb binding. New agents are being purified and produced by recombinant DNA technology that might augment immune-mediated tumor destruction. For instance, interferons, interleukin-2, tumor necrosis factor and other lymphokines could enhance the activity of effector cells directed to the tumor by mAbs. Alternatively, effector cells could be stimulated and manipulated ex vivo and then be used for treatment in combination with mAb.

While these approaches to passive immunotherapy with mAbs are being investigated, an interesting and novel strategy is to use mAbs to induce active immunization.[37] In 1974, Jerne proposed the network theory of the immune response, which suggested that antibodies may produce active immunization (or immunosuppression).[38] A critical feature of this theory is that the region of the antibody that binds to antigen (the idiotypic determinant of the antibody)[39,40] can elicit the production of antiidiotypic antibodies, and these antiidiotypic antibodies can exert control over immune responses. In some cases antiidiotypic antibodies may be internal images of the original antigen, and could antigenically mimic the antigen. It has been predicted that immunization with antiidiotypes could be possible, mimicking vaccination with an antigen. Some experimental evidence suggests that antiidiotypes can elicit delayed-type hypersensitivity[41] and protection against microorganisms[42] and tumors.[43,44] It is clear that some patients treated with mAbs develop antiidiotypic antibodies,[45,46] but there is no evidence yet that specific active immunization results from the presence of antiidiotypes.

Monoclonal Antibodies to Growth Factors and Their Receptors

Rapid developments in the arena of cell biology have produced an explosion of information about the biology of tumor cells, including the discovery of oncogenes and of factors that regulate the growth of cancer cells. A fundamental difference between cancer cells and normal cells is the ability of the transformed cell to grow forever without senescence (the property of immortality) and to have reduced requirements for serum (ie, for exogenous growth factors). In 1978, DeLarco and Todaro[47] reported that cells transformed by RNA tumor viruses produced transforming growth factors (TGFs) that bound to growth factor receptors on the cell surface and induced a malignant phenotype in target normal cells. Subsequently, Sporn and Todaro[48] postulated that a cancer cell could produce growth factors that promoted proliferation of the same cell (the autocrine hypothesis). Just in the last several years, the study of oncogenes and growth factors converged with the discovery that the product of the oncogene v-sis was homologous to platelet-derived growth factor (PDGF),[49,50] and the product of another oncogene v-erb-B was homologous to the receptor for epidermal growth factor (EGF).[51] The relationship of growth factors to malignant transformation suggests strategies for interrupting the stimulation of cancer cells by autocrine growth factors. In mouse cells transformed by v-sis, proliferation of the transformed cells can be prevented by adding antibodies to PDGF.[52] Growth of a variety of different cells has been interrupted by incubation of cells with antibodies to growth factors or to receptors for growth factors.[53–59]

Given the intimate relationship between oncogenes, growth factors and proliferation of tumor cells, mAbs to growth factors or their receptors are being explored for therapeutic potential. Two interesting observations in animal models are (1) the inhibition of the growth of epidermal carcinomas observed after treatment with mAbs directed against the receptor for epidermal growth factor[60]; and (2) the inhibition of growth of human small cell lung cancers by treatment with mAbs directed against bombesin, an autocrine growth factor for these tumor cells.[61] It is likely that the flurry of developments in the field of growth factors will provide new pharmacologic approaches to the treatment of cancer.

Radiolabeled Monoclonal Antibodies: Studies of Tumor Targeting

One of the most appealing strategies for the application of mAbs to the diagnosis and treatment of cancer is to conjugate the mAb to a radiolabel or to a cytotoxic, cytostatic, or biological agent. The presumption is that mAbs that have restricted reactivity with tumor cells would bypass most normal tissues in the body and deliver radioactivity, a chemotherapeutic agent, a toxin, or other agents directly to the tumor.

The greatest information concerning this approach comes from studies with radiolabeled antibodies. This area of investigation is presented in more depth in several recent reviews.[62–64] In some respects, studies of radiolabeled mAbs can be considered a necessary step for treatment with mAb-conjugates. The biodistribution of the labeled mAb provides valuable information about tumor versus normal tissue doses, and may allow new strategies for therapy to be developed. Initial studies utilizing radiolabeled rabbit polyclonal antibodies raised against undefined tumor antigens were pioneered by Pressman[65,66] and

Bales.[67] An initial attempt to localize human choriocarcinoma implanted into hamster cheek pouches using I-131-labeled anti-HCG polyclonal antibodies was not very successful,[68] but by 1974 both Goldenberg et al[69] and Mach et al[70] reported images of human xenografted tumors. The coincidence of the development of the hybridoma technology around this time subsequently produce a sharp increase in studies of radiolabeled antibodies.

Animal model systems have provided a way to evaluate factors that may influence the biodistribution and localization of injected antibodies. The study by Ballou et al[71] was the first to show that iodine-125-labeled mAb could localize appropriately to a target tumor (a mouse teratocarcinoma) but not a control tumor in the same animal. Scheinberg et al[72] attached radioactive metal chelates to mAbs, allowing labeling of mAbs with more versatile radiometals such as In-111. Along with iodine radioisotopes, In-111 has become the other standard radiolabel for most mAb studies performed to date.[73] A large number of studies have reported imaging tumors in animal models, including mouse and guinea pig tumors[74–76] and human colon and breast carcinomas, melanoma, sarcoma, and other tumor types growing in athymic mice.[77–86] These studies show that a number of factors can influence the ability of mAb to bind to tumor tissues. Optimally, antibodies of high avidity for tumor cells are required.[87] A critical issue is the specificity of the antibody, particularly in order to evaluate appropriate versus inappropriate localization. The reactivity of mAb with tissues will not always predict the mAb's distribution in vivo, and in some cases mAbs have been shown to localize to tumors preferentially over apparently equally reactive normal tissues.[88] Blood flow, vascular permeability, the site of the tumor, and the state of endothelial cells within the tumor may all impact greatly on the ability of mAbs to access tumor tissue after intravenous administration.[79,83,88] Lymphatic administration of mAbs bypasses the intravenous route, and may provide a more sensitive way to detect tumor in lymph nodes.[89]

Radiolabeled mouse mAbs injected into host animals predictably behave like immunoglobulins and circulate in the vascular system with half-lives of many hours to days, producing considerable background from blood pool. The biodistribution can be affected by the presence or absence of target tissues[74,90] and by the antibody class/subclass. Although it has been the impression that IgM mAbs will not be useful for targeting tumors, no general rules are yet available, and in at least one instance a radiolabeled IgM mAb has been shown to localize to tumor in an animal model system.[91] The better penetration into tumor and more rapid clearance of fragments from blood is an advantage for targeting radioisotopes,[79,92–94] but fragments of mAbs can be hard to generate and the resulting mAb fragment may have a reduced avidity for target tumors.[94] Alternatively, injection of a second antibody directed against the radiolabeled mAb can rapidly clear blood pool background.[95–97] Although labeled mAb in the blood may be cleared, there is evidence that mAb and/or radiolabel is retained at tumor sites for long periods in some systems. In specific cases, radiolabel can be detected at tumor sites weeks after administration and the corresponding tumor to normal tissue ratios of radioactivity have increased over time.[98]

The experience with the injection of radiolabeled antibodies into patients with cancer is more limited, and much of the earlier investigations utilized heterologous and purified polyclonal antisera. In 1978, Goldenberg first reported the detection of cancer in patients using I-131-labeled polyclonal antibodies directed against carcinoembryonic antigen (CEA).[99] Mach et al confirmed that anti-CEA antibodies could be used to image tumors, and found that tumor to normal tissue ratios were generally between 4 and 5 but that only 0.1% of the injected radioactivity was detected in tumors by 6 to 8 days after injection.[100] Subsequent follow-up studies confirmed that tumor sites could be imaged with anti-CEA antibodies, but the percentage of tumor sites detected ranged from 40% to 90%. The great variability in results suggested that more work was needed to establish reproducible methods for imaging. In this regard, one controversial issue is the potential use of computerized subtraction techniques to distinguish blood pool activity from more specific localization. Mach et al reported the first successful localization of tumor in patients with a monoclonal antibody.[63] A number of studies followed, evaluating radiolabeled mAbs in patients with colon[101–111] and breast carcinoma,[106,112] and melanoma.[113–118] These studies demonstrated that (1) In-111 could be used to detect tumors outside of the liver,[107,112,113,117] (2) Single positron emission computerized tomography could be used to obtain dosimetry and tomographic images of tumors,[119] (3) mAb fragments were useful for imaging, sometimes imaging within six to 24 hours, and might be superior to whole immunoglobulin molecules,[103,111,120] and (4) pharmacokinetic data in patients with melanoma of an In-111-labeled mAb directed against the p97 melanoma antigen suggested that the mAb remains primarily in the circulation with a half-life of more than 30 hours.[118] It is clear from these data that mAbs are not simple missiles that seek out tumors; in fact, only a small proportion of injected mAb remains at the tumor site, while most radiolabeled mAb is cleared from the blood pool. However, the ratios of radiolabeled mAb tumor to normal tissues have been favorable, and newer approaches (eg, the use of mAb fragments) will likely improve mAb localization to tumor.

Table 1. Cytotoxic Agents for Conjugation to Monoclonal Antibodies

Therapeutic Agents	References
Isotopes	
Beta Particle Emitters	
Iodine-131	121, 122
Scandium-47	123
Yttrium-90	124
Alpha Particle Emitters	
Bismuth-212	72, 125
Astatine-211	124, 126, 127
Auger Electron Generators	
Iodine-125	125, 128
Bromine-77	129
Fissionable Nuclides	
Boron-10	130
Actinides	131
Protein Toxins and Cytotoxins	
Ricin	55, 132–136
Diphtheria	132
Hematoporphyrin	137
Purothionine	138
Pseudomonas exotoxin	139
Alpha amanitin	140
Chemotherapeutic Drugs	
Vindesine	141
Methotrexate	141
Daunorubicin	142, 143
Doxorubicin	144
Cytosine Arabinoside	145
5-Fluorouridine	145
Biologic Agents	
Interferon	146
Cobra venom factor	147
Liposomes	148–151

RADIOLABELED ANTIBODY AND ANTIBODY CONJUGATES FOR THERAPY

Great effort has been directed towards the use of monoclonal antibodies to target potent cytotoxic or biologically active agents. The success of such a strategy requires that the attachment of the agent alters neither the efficacy or specificity of the mAb nor the function of the agent itself. Moreover, the conjugate must be stable in vivo and, if possible, nontoxic or inactive until it reaches its target. The generation of a local field effect to kill nearby tumor cells that have evaded targeting would be optimal. Numerous agents are being studied to achieve these goals (Table 1).

Of the isotopes, the β particle emitting iodine 131 has been most widely used. Other versatile nuclides are under investigation, including scandium-47 and yttrium-90, both β emitters; bismuth-212 and astatine-211, which emit much shorter ranged and vastly more energetic alpha particles; iodine-125 and bromine-77, which generate short ranged auger electrons; and actinides and boron-10, which are potentially fissionable.

The protein toxins, ricin and diphtheria, have also been the subject of wide interest because of the extreme potency of the active A-chain fragments. The toxic A-chain normally requires a second peptide (the B-chain) in order to bind to target cells. When the A-chain alone is attached to a mAb, the toxic fragment is theoretically inactive unless delivered to a tumor cell by the mAb. Similarly, chemotherapeutic agents, other cell cytotoxins, biologically active molecules, and liposomes are being studied for development of effective mAb conjugates.

Despite this varied array of potential conjugates, a number of technical problems in stability, biological activity, and specificity remain, limiting the success of these cytotoxic mAbs in vivo and delaying their use in humans. Many of these problems will undoubtedly be overcome with new techniques for conjugation under development.

BONE MARROW PURGING WITH MONOCLONAL ANTIBODIES

Rapid progress has been made in the application of mAb to purge tumor cells from human bone marrow in vitro where problems of host response and adverse reactions are less relevant and where conditions can be manipulated more precisely.[152–155] Encouraging clinical trials of mAb purging of malignant lymphoid cells followed by autologous bone marrow reinfusion have recently been summarized.[156] Treatments for small cell lung carcinoma, neuroblastoma, and other cancers are also being approached by this method.[157–159] In addition, the use of mAb to selectively remove T cells from allogeneic bone marrow to abrogate graft versus host disease is being actively investigated.[160]

CLINICAL TRIALS OF MONOCLONAL ANTIBODIES

Despite many unanswered questions about mechanisms of mAb therapy in animal models, a small number of clinical trials in humans have been reported with encouraging results. This use of mAb in patients has raised new issues, but has also answered the questions as to the feasibility of mouse mAb in heterologous human hosts. Because these studies were largely phase 1 and pilot trials, they were aimed primarily at elucidating adverse reactions, host responses to mouse protein, technical problems with mAb administration, and mAb localization to tumor sites, rather than at achieving tumor responses. All of these therapeutic trials have used unmodified, native mAb (Table 2).

The early trials have focused on patients with leukemias and lymphomas because of readily available mAbs and the technical ease of obtaining malignant cells in these patients. The largest body of data has been obtained in trials that used the T65 (Leu-1, T101) antigen as a target. T65 is present on normal T cells, T cell leukemias and lymphomas, chronic lymphocytic leukemia (CLL), and cutaneous T cell lymphoma (CTCL) cells.[46,162–166,172–176] Individual doses ranged from 1 mg to 500 mg and toxicity was minimal with low doses or with slow infusion of high doses. However, dyspnea and chest tightness occurred

Table 2. Trials With Unmodified Mouse Monoclonal Antibody in Patients With Cancer

	Tumor Type	mAb/Antigen	Evaluable Patients	Antigenic Modulation Present*	Human Anti-Mouse Ig†	Tumor Regression‡	Reference
1	ALL	J5/CALLA	4	+	NR	0/4	161
2	ALL (T cell)	Leu-1/T65, and others	6	+	1/3	1/6	162
3	CLL	T101/T65	6	+	0/6	2/6	163
4	CLL	T101/T65	4	+	0/4	0/4	164
5	CLL	T101/T65	13	+	0/13	0/13	165
6	CTCL	Leu-1/T65	7	+	4/8	6/7	162
7	CTCL	T101/T65	10	+	5/10	4/10	168
8	CTCL	T101/T65	4	+	2/4	0/4	164
9	CTCL	T101/T65	7	+	4/4	4/7	166
10	B Cell Lymphoma	Anti idiotype	10	+	5/10	6/10	167
11	Gastrointestinal	17-1A	20	—	9/18	3/20	168
12	Colorectal	17-1A	20	—	10/20	2/20	169
13	Melanoma	96.5/p97 48.7/gp240	5	—	4/5	0/5	170
14	Melanoma	9.2.27/gp240	8	NR	3/8	0/8	171
15	Melanoma	R24/GD3	12	—	12/12	5/12	30

Abbreviations: ALL, acute lymphoblastic leukemia; CLL, chronic lymphocytic leukemia; CTCL, cutaneous T cell lymphoma; NR, not reported.

*Modulation = Disappearance of antigen from the target cell after exposure to mAb.

†Human antibody response to mouse Ig.

‡Tumor regressions include minor, partial, complete and mixed regressions as defined by reference.

transiently in patients given infusions at rates faster than about 0.5 mg per minute, possibly secondary to leukoagglutination of target cells. Fever, rigors, rash, headache, nausea and vomiting, diarrhea, arthralgias, and myalgias were occasionally observed and frequently corresponded to rapid infusion rates, high doses, or the presence of large amounts of circulating target antigen. Tumor regressions occurred in about half of the patients with CTCL—but virtually all were transient. Although target cell binding was demonstrated and leukocyte counts dropped in many CLL patients, no significant sustained responses were reported. Most interestingly, two phenomena were identified that abrogated mAb activity. First, antigen modulation (the disappearance of antigen from the surface of the targeted cells) was observed in the majority of treated patients. This effect appeared rapidly and was dose related. Second, human antimouse Ig developed in the majority of CTCL patients, but surprisingly, in none of the patients with CLL. The human antimouse Ig response was both anti-allotype and antiidiotype; this response may pose a problem for patients receiving multiple mAb infusions.

Therapy of B cell nodular lymphomas using antiidiotype[167,177–179] or other mAb[180] has also provided some new insights as well as one sustained complete remission (now for greater than four years). Single doses of 1 mg to 1,500 mg and total doses of nearly 6,000 mg were used with generally minimal toxicity as described above, although rarely, brief thrombocytopenia, neutropenia, hypotension, and renal dysfunction were observed. Objective responses were common using this approach, but, with the one exception noted, were not durable, lasting 1 to 6 months. In addition, problems in this patient population were identified. The presence of blocking antigen (idiotype) had to be overcome before adequate cell targeting occurred. Second, lymphoma cells escaped targeting via phenotypic alterations of the idiotype, genotypic heterogeneity, as well as antigen modulation. It is unlikely that escape of tumor cells by phenotypic alteration is peculiar to this class of target antigen.

The use of mAbs against the CALLA antigen in mAb therapy of acute lymphoblastic leukemia[161] and myeloid differentiation antigens in mAb treatment of acute myelogenous leukemia[181] have similarly shown minimal toxicity and incomplete, transient responses.

Among the solid tumors, colorectal carcinoma and melanoma have been studied in clinical settings. In gastrointestinal cancer, Sears et al[168,169,182] evaluated 20 patients each in phase 1 and phase 2 studies, using mAb 17-1A. Again, toxicity was minimal, even at single doses of 1,000 mg. As before, human antimouse Ig appeared. Eighty percent of the antimouse Ig studied also contained reactivity directed at the idiotypic determinants on the mAb. Clinical responses were reported in five of 40 patients and did not appear to be related to the dose of mAb.

Three groups studied melanoma using different target antigens.[30,170,171] These studies confirmed the previous reports that higher doses produced higher serum concentrations and allowed more mAb to reach tumor sites. The toxicity of mAb infusions was low and there was a high prevalence of human antimouse Ig responses. Two trials showed no responses, but in the trial evaluating an IgG3 mAb that activates complement and mediates ADCC, three partial responses and two mixed responses were observed in a group of twelve patients.[30] This evidence suggests that careful selection of both the antigen target and the mAb will be critical to the success of mAb mediated therapy.

Overall, preliminary clinical trials have shown that treatment with mouse mAb is generally well tolerated and that tumor targeting obeys dose-response relationships. The problems of antigenic modulation, tumor heterogeneity and tumor escape, and the human antimouse Ig responses were raised by these initial trials. Future trials will begin to evaluate the efficacy of mAb treatment in phase 2 studies and to investigate mechanisms for antitumor effects. The exploration of the clinical application of mAb conjugates is just now starting and little information is available regarding their stability in vivo, biodistribution, and adverse effects or efficacy.

FUTURE DIRECTIONS

The explosion of research that followed the development of methods for producing specific and highly purified mAbs has rapidly led to studies on clinical applications of mAb. MAbs can be used to activate or manipulate the patient's immune system, to interfere with biologic processes crucial to malignant cells, and to deliver lethal agents to cancer cells. Areas of active research interest are: (1) Methods to decrease the human antimouse Ig responses (such as technology to produce human mAb); (2) Genetic and chemical manipulations of the mAb to increase potency or alter biological function; (3) Development of new strategies for therapeutic applications (such as the use of mAb "cocktails" or multimodality treatments of mAb in combination with chemotherapy, lymphokines, or other biological response modifiers).

REFERENCES

1. Old LJ: Cancer immunology: The search for specificity-GHA Clowes Memorial Lecture. Cancer Res 41:361–375, 1981

2. Kohler G, Milstein C: Continuous culture of fused cells secreting antibody of predefined specificity. Nature 256:495–496, 1975

3. Yelton DE, Scharff M: Monoclonal antibodies. A powerful tool in biology and medicine. Annu Rev Biochem 50:657–680, 1981

4. Milstein C, Kohler G: Cell fusion and the derivation of cell lines producing specific antibody, in Haber E, Krause RM (eds): Antibodies in Human Diagnosis and Therapy, New York, Raven, 1977, pp 271–296

5. Hakomori S: Tumor associated carbohydrate antigens. Annu Rev Immunol 2:103–126, 1984

6. Sell S, Reisfeld R (eds): Monoclonal Antibodies in Cancer. Contemporary Biomedicine. Clifton, NJ, Humana, 1985, pp 1–485

7. Mitchell M, Oettgen HF (eds): Hybridomas in Cancer Diagnosis and Treatment. New York, Raven, 1982, pp 1–264

8. Lloyd KO: Human tumor antigens. Detection and characterization with mouse monoclonal antibodies, in Herberman RB (ed): Basic and Clinical Tumor Immunology. Boston, Martinus Nijhoff, 1983, pp 159–214

9. Bernard A, Boumsell L, Dausset J, et al (eds): Leucocyte Typing. Berlin, Springer-Verlag, 1984, pp 1–814

10. Reif AE, Allen JMV: The AKR thymic antigen and its distribution in leukemias and nervous tissues. J Exp Med 120:413–433, 1964

11. Boyse TA, Old LJ: Some aspects of normal and abnormal cell surface genetics. Annu Rev Genet 3:269–291, 1969

12. Houghton AN, Cordon-Cardo C, Eisinger M: Differentiation antigens of melanoma and melanocytes. Int Rev Exp Pathol 28:217–246, 1986

13. Gatter KC, Alcock C, Heryet A, et al: Clinical importance of analysing malignant tumours of uncertain origin with immunohistochemical techniques. Lancet (1):1302–1305, 1985

14. Cairncross JG, Mattes J, Beresford HR, et al: Cell surface antigens of human astrocytoma defined by mouse monoclonal antibodies: Identification of astrocytoma subsets. Proc Natl Acad Sci USA 79:5641–5645, 1982

15. Finstad CL, Cordon-Cardo C, Bander NH, et al: Specificity analysis of mouse monoclonal antibodies defining cell surface antigens of human renal cancer. Proc Natl Acad Sci USA 82:2955–2959, 1985

16. Koprowski H, Herlyn M, Steplewski Z, et al: Specific antigen in serum of patients with colon carcinoma. Science 212:53–55, 1981

17. Magnani J, Steplewski Z, Koprowski H, et al: Identification of the gastrointestinal and pancreatic cancer-associated antigen detected by monoclonal antibody 19-9 in the serum of patients as mucin. Cancer Res 43:5489–5492, 1983

18. Bast RC Jr, Klug T, St John E, et al: A radioimmunoassay using a monoclonal antibody to moniter the course of epithelial ovarian cancer. N Engl J Med 309:883–887, 1983

19. Bernstein ID, Tam MR, Nowinski RC: Mouse leukemia: Therapy with monoclonal antibodies against a thymus differentiation antigen. Science 207:68–71, 1980

20. Herlyn D, Koprowski H: IgG2a monoclonal antibodies inhibit human tumor growth through interaction with effector cells. Proc Natl Acad Sci USA 79:4761, 1982

21. Herlyn D, Steplewski Z, Herlyn M, et al: Inhibition of growth of colorectal carcinoma in nude mice by monoclonal antibody. Cancer Res 40:717–721, 1984

22. Schulz G, Staffileno LK, Reisfeld RA, et al: Eradication of established human melanoma tumors in nude mice by antibody-directed effector cells. J Exp Med 161:1315–1325, 1985

23. Schulz G, Bumol TF, Reisfeld RA: Monoclonal antibody directed effector cells selectively lyse human melanoma cells in vitro and in vivo. Proc Natl Acad Sci USA 80:5407–5411, 1983

24. Imai K, Ng A-K, Glassy M, et al: ADCC of cultured human melanoma cells: Analysis with monoclonal antibodies to human melanoma-associated antigens. Scand J Immunol 14:369–377, 1981

25. Hellstrom I, Brankovan V, Hellstrom KE: Strong antitumor activities of IgG3 antibodies to a human melanoma-associated ganglioside. Proc Natl Acad Sci USA 82:1499–1502, 1985

26. Vogel C-W, Welt SW, Carswell EA, et al: A murine IgG3 monoclonal antibody to a melanoma antigen that activates human complement in vitro and in vivo. Immunobiology 164:309–313, 1983

27. Neuberger MS, Rajewsky K: Activation of mouse complement by monoclonal mouse antibodies. Eur J Immunol 11:1012–1016, 1981

28. Shouval D, Shafritz DA, Zurawski VR Jr, et al: Immunotherapy in nude mice of human hepatoma using monoclonal antibodies against hepatitis B virus. Nature 298:567–569, 1982

29. Capone PM, Papsidero LD, Croghan GA, et al: Experimental tumoricidal effects of monoclonal antibody against solid breast tumors. Proc Natl Acad Sci USA 80:7328–7332, 1983

30. Houghton AN, Mintzer D, Cordon-Cardo C, et al: Mouse monoclonal antibody detecting G_{D3} ganglioside: A phase I trial in patients with malignant melanoma. Proc Natl Acad Sci USA 82:1242–1246, 1985

31. Capone PM, Papsidero LD, Chu TM: Relationship between antigen density and immunotherapeutic response

elicited by monoclonal antibodies against solid tumors. J Natl Cancer Inst 72:673–677, 1984

32. Hellstrom I, Brown J, Hellstrom KE: Monoclonal antibodies to two determinants of melanoma-antigen p97 act synergistically in complement-dependent cytotoxicity. J Immunol 127:157–160, 1983

33. Herlyn D, Herlyn M, Steplewski Z, et al: Monoclonal antibodies in cell-mediated cytotoxicity against human melanoma and colorectal carcinoma. Eur J Immunol 9:657–659, 1979

34. Adams DO, Hall T, Steplewski Z, et al: Tumor undergoing rejection induced by monoclonal antibodies of the IgG2a isotype contain increased numbers of macrophages activated for a distinctive form of antibody-dependent cytostasis. Proc Natl Acad Sci USA 81:3506–3510, 1984

35. Herlyn D, Powe J, Ross A, et al: Inhibition of human tumor growth by IgG2a monoclonal antibodies correlates with antibody density of tumor cells. J Immunol 134:1300–1304, 1985

36. Kipps TJ, Parham P, Punt J, et al: Importance of immunoglobulin isotype in human antibody-dependent, cell-mediated cytotoxicity directed by mouse monoclonal antibodies. J Exp Med 161:1–17, 1985

37. Livingston PL, Oettgen HF, Old LJ: Specific active immunotherapy in cancer treatment, in E Mihich (ed): Immunological Approaches to Cancer Therapeutics. New York, Wiley, 1982, pp 363–404

38. Jerne NK: Towards a network theory of the immune system. Ann Immunol (Paris) 125C:373, 1974

39. Kunkel HG, Mannik M, Williams RC: Individual antigenic specificity of isolated antibodies. Science 140:1218–1220, 1963

40. Oudin J, Michel M: A new allotype form of rabbit serum alpha-globulins apparently associated with antibody function and specificity. Cr Acad Sci 257:805–808, 1963

41. Nepom GT, Nelson KA, Holbeck SL, et al: Induction of immunity to a human tumor marker by in vivo administration of antiidiotypic antibodies in mice. Proc Natl Acad Sci USA 81:2864–2868, 1984

42. Sacks DL, Kelsoe GH, Sacks DH: Induction of immune responses with antiidiotypic antibodies: Implications for the induction of protective immunity. Springer Semin Immunopathol 6:79–85, 1983

43. Kennedy RC, Dreesman GR, Butel JS, et al: Suppression of in vivo tumor formation induced by simian virus 40-transformed cells in mice receiving antiidiotypic antibodies. J Exp Med 161:1432–1449, 1985

44. Gorczynski RM, Kennedy M, Polidoulis I, et al: Altered tumor growth in vivo after immunization of mice with anti-tumor antibodies. Cancer Res 44:3291–3298, 1984

45. Koprowski H, Herlyn D, Lubeck M, et al: Human anti-idiotypic antibodies in cancer patients. Is the modulation of the immune response beneficial for the patients? Proc Natl Acad Sci USA 81:216–219, 1984

46. Shawler DL, Bartholomew RM, Smith LM, et al: Human immune response to multiple injections of murine monoclonal IgG. J Immunol 135:1–6, 1985

47. DeLarco JE, Todaro GJ: Growth factors from murine sarcoma virus-transformed cells. Proc Natl Acad Sci USA 75:4001–4005, 1978

48. Sporn M, Todaro GJ: Autocrine secretion and malignant transformation of cells. N Engl J Med 303:878–883, 1980

49. Waterfield MD, Scarce T, Whittle N, et al: Platelet-derived growth factor is structurally related to the putative transforming protein p28sis of simian sarcoma virus. Nature 304:35–41, 1983

50. Doolittle RF, Hunkapillar MW, Hood LE, et al: Simian sarcoma virus onc gene, v-sis, is derived from the gene (or genes) encoding a platelet-derived growth factor. Science 221:275–281, 1983

51. Downward J, Yarden Y, Mayes E, et al: Close similarity of epidermal growth factor receptor and v-erb B oncogene protein sequences. Nature 307:521–526, 1984

52. Deuel TF, Tong BD, Huang, JS: Autocrine regulation of SSV-transformed cell growth by PDGF-like activity, in Feramisco J, Ozanne B, Stiles C (eds): Cancer Cells. 3. Growth Factors and Transformation. New York, Cold Springs Harbor Laboratory, 1985, pp 87–94

53. Johnsson A, Betsholte C, Heldin C-H, et al: Antibodies against platelet-derived growth factor inhibit acute transformation by simian sarcoma virus. Nature 317:438–440, 1985

54. Trowbridge I, Lopez F: Monoclonal antibody to transferrin receptor blocks transferrin binding and inhibits human tumor cell growth in vitro. Proc Natl Acad Sci USA 79:1175–1179, 1982

55. Trowbridge I, Domingo DL: Anti-transferrin receptor monoclonal antibody and toxin-antibody conjugates affect growth of human tumor cells. Nature 294:171–173, 1981

56. McGrath MS, Pillemer E, Weissman IL: Murine leukemogenesis: Monoclonal antibodies to T cell determinants arrest T lymphoma cell proliferation. Nature 285:259–262, 1980

57. Adkins B, Leutz A, Graff T: Viral oncogenes of the src family induce growth factor production and stimulate transformed chicken myeloblasts to proliferate in an autocrine fashion, in Feramisco J, Ozanne B, Stiles C (eds): Cancer Cells. 3. Growth Factors and Transformation. New York, Cold Springs Harbor Laboratory, 1985, pp 87–94

58. Waldmann TA, Leonard WJ, Depper JM, et al: Structure, function and expression of the receptor for interleukin-2 on normal and malignant lymphocytes, in Feramisco J, Ozanne B, Stiles C (eds): Cancer Cells. 3. Growth Factors and Transformation. New York, Cold Spring Harbor Laboratory, 1985, pp 221–226

59. Mendelsohn J, Trowbridge I, Castagnola J: Inhibition of human lymphocyte proliferation by monoclonal antibody to transferrin receptor. Blood 62:821–826, 1983

60. Masui H, Kawamoto T, Sato JD, et al: Growth inhibition of human tumor cells in athymic nude mice by anti-epidermal growth factor receptor monoclonal antibodies. Cancer Res 44:1002–1007, 1984

61. Cuttitta F, Mulshine J, Moody TW, et al: Bombesin-like peptides can function as autocrine growth factors in human small cell lung cancer. Nature 316:823–826, 1985

62. Larson SM: Radiolabeled monoclonal antitumor antibodies in diagnosis and therapy. J Nucl Med 26:538–545, 1985

63. Mach J-P, Buchegger F, Forni M, et al: Use of radiolabelled monoclonal anti-CEA antibodies for the detection of human carcinomas by external photoscanning and tomoscintigraphy. Immunol Today 2:239–249, 1981

64. Goldenberg DM, DeLand FH: History and status of tumor imaging with radiolabeled antibodies. J Biol Response Mod 1:121–136, 1982

65. Bale WF, Spar IL, Goodland RL, et al: In vivo and in vitro studies of labeled antibodies against rat kidney and Walker carcinoma. Proc Soc Exp Biol Med 89:564–568, 1955

66. Pressman D, Korngold L: The in vivo localization of anti-Wagner osteogenic sarcoma antibodies. Cancer 6:619–623, 1953

67. Pressman D, Day ED, Blau M: The use of paired labeling in the determination of tumor localizing antibodies. Cancer Res 17:845–850, 1957

68. Quninones J, Mizejewski G, Beierwaltes WH: Choriocarcinoma scanning using radiolabeled antibody to chorionic gonadotropin. J Nucl Med 12;69–75, 1971

69. Goldenberg DN, Preston DF, Primus FJ, et al: Photoscan localization of GW-39 tumors in hamsters using radiolabeled anticarcinoembryonic antigen immunoglobulin G. Cancer Res 34:1–9, 1974

70. Mach J-P, Carrel S, Merenda C, et al: In vivo localization of radiolabeled antibodies to carcinoembryonic antigen in human colon carcinoma grafted into nude mice. Nature 248:704–706, 1974

71. Ballou B, Levine G, Hakala TR, et al: Tumor location detected with radioactively labeled monoclonal antibody and external scintigraphy. Science 206:844–846, 1979

72. Scheinberg DA, Strand M, Gansow OA: Tumor imaging with radioactive metal chelates conjugated to monoclonal antibodies. Science 215:1511–1513, 1982

73. Rainsbury R, Westwood J: Tumour localization with monoclonal antibody radioactively labeled with metal chelate rather than iodine. Lancet 2:1347–1438, 1982

74. Colcher D, Zalutsky M, Kaplan W, et al: Radiolocalization of human mammary tumors in athymic mice by monoclonal antibody. Cancer Res 43:736–742, 1983

75. Houston LL, Nowinski RC, Bernstein, ID. Specific in vivo localization of monoclonal antibodies directed against the Thy 1.1 antigen. J Immunol 125:837–843, 1980

76. Bernhard MI, Hwang KM, Foon KA, et al: Localization of In-111- and I-125-labeled monoclonal antibody in guinea pigs bearing line 10 hepatocarcinoma tumors. Cancer Res 43:4429–4433, 1983

77. Buchegger F, Haskell CM, Schreyer M, et al: Radiolabeled fragments of monoclonal antibodies against CEA for localization of human colon carcinoma grafted into nude mice. J Exp Med 158:413–427, 1983

78. Epenetos AA, Nimmon CC, Arklie J: Detection of human cancer in an animal model using radiolabelled tumour-associated monoclonal antibodies. Br J Cancer 46:1–8, 1982

79. Gallagher BM, Sands H, Neacy W, et al: Monoclonal antibody localization and imaging of human mammary carcinoma grown at various sites in the nude mouse. J Nucl Med 25:112, 1984

80. Ghose T, Novel S, Aquino J, et al: Localization of I-131-labeled antibodies in human renal cell carcinomas and in mouse hepatoma and correlation with tumor detection by photoscanning. Cancer Res 40:3018–3031, 1980

81. Herlyn D, Powe J, Alavi A, et al: Radioimmunodetection of human tumor xenografts by monoclonal antibodies. Cancer Res 43:2731–2735, 1983

82. Hwang KM, Fodstad O, Oldham RK, et al: Radiolocalization of xenografted human malignant melanoma by a monoclonal antibody (9.2.27) to a melanoma-associated antigen in nude mice. Cancer Res 45:4150–4155, 1985

83. Mann BD, Cohen MB, Saxton RE, et al: Imaging of human tumor xenografts in nude mice with radiolabeled antibody: limitations of specificity due to nonspecific uptake of antibody. Cancer 54:1318–1327, 1984

84. Moshakis V, McIlhinney RA, Raghaven D, et al: Localization of human tumor xenografts after intravenous administration of radiolabeled monoclonal antibody. Br J Cancer 44:91–99, 1981

85. Pimm MV, Embleton MJ, Perkins AC, et al: In vivo localization of anti-osteogenic sarcoma xenografts. Int J Cancer 30:75–85, 1982

86. Stuhlmiller GM, Sullivan DC, Vervaert CE, et al: In vivo tumor localization using tumor specific monkey xenoantibody, alloantibody, and murine monoclonal antibody. Ann Surg 194:592–601, 1981

87. Haskell CM, Buchegger F, Schreyer M, et al: Monoclonal antibodies to carcinoembryonic antigen: Ionic strength as a factor in the selection of antibodies for immunoscintigraphy. Cancer Res 43:3857–3864, 1983

88. Ballou B, Jaffe R, Taylor RJ, et al: Tumor radioimmunolocation: Differential antibody retention by antigenic normal tissue and tumor. J Immunol 132:2111–2116, 1984

89. Weinstein JN, Parker RJ, Keenan AM, et al: Monoclonal antibodies in the lymphatics: Toward the diagnosis and therapy of tumor metastases. Science 218:1334–1337, 1982

90. East IJ, Keenan AM, Larson SM, et al: Scintigraphy of normal mouse ovaries with monoclonal antibodies to ZP-2, the major zona pellucida protein. Science 225:938–941, 1984

91. Zimmer AM, Rosen ST, Spies SM, et al: Radioimmunoimaging of human small cell lung carcinoma with I-131 tumor specific monoclonal antibody. Hybridoma 4:1–11, 1985

92. Halpern SE, Buchegger F, Schreyer M, et al: Effect of size of radiolabeled antibody and fragments on tumor uptake and distribution in nephrectomized mice. J Nucl Med 25:112, 1984

93. Wahl RL, Parker CW, Philpott GW: Improved radioimaging and tumor localization with monoclonal $F(ab')_2$. J Nucl Med 24:316–325, 1983

94. Ballou B, Reiland J, Levine G, et al: Tumor location using $F(ab')_2$ from a monoclonal IgM antibody: Pharmacokinetics. J Nucl Med 26:283–292, 1985

95. Krizan Z, Murray JL, Hersh EM, et al: Increased labeling of human melanoma cells in vitro using combinations of monoclonal antibodies recognizing separate cell surface antigenic determinants. Cancer Res 45:4904–4909, 1985

96. Goodwin D, Meares C, Diamanti C, et al: Use of specific antibody for rapid clearance of circulating blood background from radiolabeled tumor imaging proteins. Eur J Nucl Med 9:209–215, 1984

97. Sharkey RM, Primus EJ, Goldberg DM: Second antibody clearance of radiolabeled antibody in cancer radioimmunodetection. Proc Natl Acad Sci USA 81:2843–2846, 1984

98. Colcher D, Keenan AM, Larson SM, et al: Prolonged

binding of a radiolabeled monoclonal antibody (B72.3) used for the in situ radioimmunodetection of human colon carcinoma xenografts. Cancer Res 44:5744–5751, 1984

99. Goldenberg DM, DeLand FH, Kimm EE, et al: Use of radiolabeled antibodies to carcinoembryonic antigen for the detection and localization of diverse tumors by external photoscanning. N Engl J Med 298:1384–1388, 1978

100. Mach J-P, Carrel S, Forni J, et al: Tumor localization of radiolabeled antibodies against carcinoembryonic antigen in patients with carcinoma. N Engl J Med 303:5–10, 1980

101. Dykes PW, Hine KR, Bradwell JC, et al: Localization of tumor deposits by external scanning after injection of radiolabeled anti-carcinoembryonic antigen. Br Med J 280:220–222, 1980

102. Chatal J-F, Saccavini J-C, Fumoleau P, et al: Immunoscintigraphy of colon carcinoma. J Nucl Med 25:307–314, 1984

103. Delaloye B, Bischof-Delaloye A, Buchegger F, et al: Detection of colorectal carcinoma by emission-computerized tomography after injection of iodine-123-labeled F(ab) or $F(Ab')_2$ fragments from monoclonal antibodies. J Clin Invest 77:301–311, 1986

104. Delaloye BA, Bischof-Delaloye A, Volant J-C, et al: First approach to therapy of liver metastases in colorectal carcinoma by intrahepatically infused iodine-131 labeled monoclonal anti-CEA antibodies. Eur J Nucl Med 11:37, 1985 (abstr)

105. Dillman RO, Beauregard JC, Sobol RE, et al: Lack of radioimmunodetection and complications associated with monoclonal anti-carcinoembryonic antigen: Antibody cross-reactivity with an antigen on circulating cells. Cancer Res 44:2213–2218, 1984

106. Epenetos AA, Mather S, Granowska M, et al: Targeting of iodine-123-labelled tumour-associated monoclonal antibodies to ovarian, breast and gastrointestinal tumours. Lancet 2:999–1005, 1982

107. Fairweather DS, Bradwell AR, Dykes PW, et al: Improved tumour localization using indium-111 labelled antibodies. Br Med J 287:167–170, 1983

108. Farrands PA, Pimm MV, Embleton MJ, et al: Radioimmunodetection of human colorectal cancers by an antitumour monoclonal antibody. Lancet 2:8295–8298, 1982

109. Moldofsky PJ, Sears HF, Mulhern CB Jr, et al: Detection of metastatic tumor in normal sized retroperitoneal lymph nodes by monoclonal antibody imaging. N Engl J Med 311:106–107, 1984

110. Moldofsky PJ, Powe J, Mulhern CB, et al: Metastatic colon carcinoma detected with radiolabeled $F(ab')_2$ monoclonal antibody fragments. Radiology 149:549–555, 1983

111. Mach J-P, Chatal J-F, Lumbroso J-D, et al: Tumor localization in patients by radiolabeled monoclonal antibody against colon carcinoma. Cancer Res 43:5593–5600, 1983

112. Rainsbury RM, Westwood JH, Coombes RC, et al: Location of metastatic breast carcinoma by a monoclonal antibody chelate labelled with Indium-111. Lancet 2:934–938, 1983

113. Halpern SE, Dillman RO, Witztum KF, et al: Radioimmunodetection of melanoma using In-111 96.5 monoclonal antibody: A preliminary report. Radiology 155:493–499, 1985

114. Larson SM, Carrasquillo JA, Krohn KA, et al: Diagnostic imaging of malignant melanoma with radiolabeled antitumour antibodies. JAMA 249:811–812, 1983

115. Larson SM, Brown JP, Wright P, et al: Imaging of melanoma with 131I-labeled monoclonal antibodies. J Nucl Med 24:123–129, 1983

116. Larson SM, Carrasquillo JA, Krohn KA, et al: Localization of 131I-labeled p97-specific Fab fragments in human melanoma as a basis for radiotherapy. J Clin Invest 72:2101–2114, 1983

117. Murray JL: Rosenblum MG, Sobol RE, et al: Radioimmunoimaging in malignant melanoma with 111-In-labeled monoclonal antibody 96.5. Cancer Res 45:2376–2381, 1985

118. Rosenblum MG, Murray JL, Haynie TP, et al: Pharmacokinetics of In-111-labeled anti-p97 monoclonal antibody in patients with metastatic malignant melanoma. Cancer Res 45:2382–2386, 1985

119. Berche C, Mach J-P, Lumbroso J-D, et al: Tomoscintigraphy for detecting gastrointestinal and medullary thyroid cancers: First clinical results using radiolabelled monoclonal antibodies against carcinoembryonic antigen. Br Med J 285:1447–1451, 1982

120. Buraggi GL, Callegaro L, Mariani G, et al: Imaging with I-131-labeled monoclonal antibodies to a high molecular weight melanoma-associated antigen in patients with melanoma: Efficiency of whole immunoglobulin and its $F(ab')_2$ fragments. Cancer Res 45:3378–3387, 1985

121. Redwood WR, Tom TD, Strand M: Specificity, efficacy, and toxicity of radioimmunotherapy in erythroleukemic mice. Cancer Res 44:5681–5687, 1984

122. Ferens JM, Krohn KA, Beaumier PL: High level iodination of monoclonal antibody fragments for radiotherapy. J Nucl Med 25:367–370, 1984

123. Anderson WT, Strand M: Stability, targeting, and biodistribution of scandium-46- and gallium-67-labeled monoclonal antibody in erythroleukemic mice. Cancer Res 45:2154–2158, 1985

124. Bloomer WD, McLaughlin WH, Lambercht RM: ^{211}At radiocolloid therapy: Further observations and comparison with radiocolloids of ^{32}P, ^{165}Dy, and ^{90}Y. Int J Radiat Oncol Biol Phys 10:341–348, 1984

125. Strand M, Scheinberg DA, Dansow OA, et al: Monoclonal antibody conjugates for diagnostic imaging and therapy in Boss BD, Langman R, Trowbridge I, et al (eds): Monoclonal Antibodies and Cancer. Orlando, Fla, Academic, 1983, pp 125–131

126. Friedman AM, Zalutsky MR, Wung W, et al: Preparation of a biologically stable and immunogenically competent astatinated protein. Int J Nucl Med Biol 4:219–224, 1977

127. Vaughan ATLM, Bateman WJ, Fisher DR: The in vivo fate of a ^{211}At labelled monoclonal antibody with known specificity in a murine system. Int J Radiat Oncol Biol Phys 8:1943–1946, 1982

128. Bloomer WD, Adelstein SJ: 5-^{125}I-iododeoxyuridine as prototype for radionuclide therapy with Auger emitters. Nature 265:620–621, 1977

129. Scheinberg DA: Proteins associated with retroviral tumors and monoclonal antibody diagnosis and therapy.

Baltimore, The Johns Hopkins University 1982, pp 217–218 (thesis)

130. Hawthorne F, Weirsema RJ, Takasugi M: Preparation of tumor-specific boron compounds. 1. In vitro studies using boron-labeled antibodies and elemental boron as neutron targets. J Med Chem 15:449–452, 1972

131. Gansow OA, Atcher RW, Link DC, et al: Generator produced Bi-212: Chelated to chemically modified monoclonal antibody for use in radiotherapy, in Knapp FF, Butler TA (Eds): Radionuclide Generators New Systems for Nuclear Medicine Applications. Washington DC Am Chem Soc 1984, pp 215–227

132. Gilliland DG, Steplewski Z, Collier J, et al: Antibody-directed cytotoxic agents: Use of monoclonal antibody to direct the action of toxin A chains to colorectal carcinoma cells. Proc Natl Acad Sci USA 77:4539–4543, 1980

133. Houston LL, Nowinski RC: Cell-specific cytotoxicity expressed by a conjugate of ricin and murine monoclonal antibody directed against thy 1.1 antigen. Cancer Res 41:3913–3917, 1981

134. Blythman HE, Casellas P, Gros O, et al: Immunotoxins: Hybrid molecules of monoclonal antibodies and a toxin subunit specifically kill tumour cells. Nature 290:145–146, 1981

135. Vitetta ES, Krolick KA, Uhr JW: Neoplastic B cells as targets for antibody-ricin A chain immunotoxins. Immunol Rev 62:159–183, 1982

136. Thorpe PE, Ross WCJ: The preparation and cytotoxic properties of antibody-toxin conjugates. Immunol Rev 62:119–158, 1982

137. Mew D, Wat C, Towers GHN, et al: Photoimmunotherapy: Treatment of animal tumors with tumor-specific monoclonal antibody-hematoporphyrin conjugates. J Immunol 130:1473–1477, 1983

138. Imai K, Nakanishi T, Noguchi T, et al: Selective in vitro toxicity of purothionin conjugated to the monoclonal antibody 225.28S to a human high-molecular-weight melanoma-associated antigen. Cancer Immunol Immunother 15:206–209, 1983

139. Pirker R, FitzGerald DJP, Hamilton TC, et al: Anti-transferrin receptor antibody linked to Pseudomonas exotoxin as a model immunotoxin in human ovarian carcinoma cell lines. Cancer Res 45:751–757, 1985

140. David MB, Preston JF, III: A conjugate of alpha-amanitin and monoclonal Immunoglobulin G to Thy 1.2 antigen is selectively toxic to T lymphoma cells. Science 213:1385–1388, 1981

141. Baldwin RW, Embleton MJ, Pimm MV: Application of tumor-localizing 791T/36 monoclonal antibody in radioimmunodetection of experimental and human tumors and targeting cytotoxic drugs such as vindesine and methotrexate, in Boss BD, Langman R, Trowbridge I, et al: (eds): Monoclonal Antibodies and Cancer. Orlando, Fla, Academic, 1983, pp 265–274

142. Diener E, Diner UE, Sinha A, et al: Specific immunosuppression by immunotoxins containing daunomycin. Science 231:148–150, 1986

143. Tsukado Y, Hurwitz E, Kashi R, et al: Chemotherapy by intravenous administration of conjugates of daunomycin with monoclonal and conventional anti-rat alpha-fetoprotein antibodies. Proc Natl Acad Sci USA 79:7896–7899, 1982

144. Pimm MV, Jones JA, Price MR, et al: Tumour localization of monoclonal antibody against a rat mammary carcinoma and suppression of tumour growth with adriamycin-antibody conjugates. Cancer Immunol Immunother 12:125–134, 1982

145. Hurwitz E, Kashi R, Arnon R, et al: The covalent linking of two nucleotide analogues to antibodies. J Med Chem 28:127–140, 1985

146. Pelham JM, Gray JD, Flannery GR, et al: Interferon-alpha conjugation to human osteogenic sarcoma monoclonal antibody 781T/36. Cancer Immunol Immunother 15:210–216, 1983

147. Vogel CW, Muller-Eberhard HJ: Induction of immune cytolysis: Tumor-cell killing by complement is initiated by covalent complex of monoclonal antibody and stable C3/C5 convertase. Proc Natl Acad Sci USA 78:7707–7711, 1981

148. Huang A, Huang L, Kennel SJ: Monoclonal antibody covalently coupled with fatty acid: A reagent for in vitro liposome targeting. J Biol Chem 255:8015–8018, 1980

149. Leserman LD, Barbet J, Kourilsky F, et al: Targeting to cells of fluorescent liposomes covalently coupled with monoclonal antibody or protein A. Nature 288:602–604, 1980

150. Bragman KS, Heath TD, Papahadjopoulos D: Simultaneous interaction of monoclonal antibody-targeted liposomes with two receptors in K562 cells. Biochim Biophys Acta 730:187–195, 1983

151. Hashimoto Y, Sugawara M, Masuko T, et al: Antitumor effect of actinomycin D entrapped in liposomes bearing subunits of tumor-specific monoclonal Immunoglobulin M antibody. Cancer Res 43:5328–5334, 1983

152. Krolick KA, Uhr JW, Vitetta ES: Selective killing of leukemia cells by antibody-toxin conjugates: Implications for autologous bone marrow transplantation. Nature 295:604–605, 1982

153. Thorpe PE, Mason DW, Brown ANF, et al: Selective killing of malignant cells in a leukaemic rat bone marrow using an antibody-ricin conjugate. Nature 297:594–596, 1982

154. Ritz J, Sallan SE, Bast RC, et al: Autologous bone marrow transplantation in CALLA positive acute lymphoblastic leukemia after in vitro treatment with J5 monoclonal antibody and complement. Lancet 2:60–63, 1982

155. Jansen J, Falkenburg JHF, Stepan DE, et al: Removal of neoplastic cells from autologous bone marrow grafts with monoclonal antibodies. Semin Hematol 21:164–181, 1984

156. Lowder JN, Meeker TC, Levy R: Monoclonal antibody therapy of lymphoid malignancy, in Hoppe R (ed): Cancer Surveys: Advances and Prospects in Clinical, Epidemiological and Laboratory Oncology. Vol 4. Recent advances in the treatment and research in lymphoma and Hodgkin's disease. Oxford, Oxford University Press, 1985, pp 359–375

157. Okabe T, Kaizu T, Ozawa K, et al: Elimination of small cell lung cancer cells in vitro from human bone marrow by a monoclonal antibody. Cancer Res 45:1930–1933, 1985

158. Saarinen UM, Coccia PF, Gerson SL, Eradication of neuroblastoma cells in vitro by monoclonal antibody and human complement: method for purging autologous bone marrow. Cancer Research 45:5969–5975, 1985

159. Bast RC Jr, DeFabritiis P, Lipton J, et al: Elimination of malignant clonogenic cells from human bone marrow using multiple monoclonal antibodies and complement. Cancer Res 45:499–503, 1985

160. Filipovich AH, Youle, RJ, Neville DM, et al: Ex-vivo treatment of donor bone marrow with anti-T-cell immunotoxins for prevention of graft-versus-host disease. Lancet 3:469–476, 1984

161. Ritz J, Pesando JM, Sallan SE, et al: Serotherapy of acute lymphoblastic leukemia with monoclonal antibody. Blood 58:141–152, 1981

162. Levy R, Miller RA, Stratte PT, et al: Therapeutic trials of monoclonal antibody in leukemia and lymphoma: Biologic considerations, in Boss BD, Langman R, Trowbridge I, et al (eds): Monoclonal Antibodies and Cancer. Orlando, Fla, Academic, 1983, pp 5–16

163. Dillman RO, Shawler DL, Dillman JB, et al: Monoclonal antibody in patients with chronic lymphocytic leukemia and cutaneous T cell lymphoma. J Cell Biochem 9A:108,1985 (suppl)

164. Dillman RO, Shawler DL, Dillman JB, et al: Therapy of chronic lymphocytic leukemia and cutaneous T cell lymphoma with T101 monoclonal antibody. J Clin Oncol 2:881–891, 1984

165. Foon KA, Schroff RW, Bunn PA, et al: Effects of monoclonal antibody therapy in patients with chronic lymphocytic leukemia. Blood 64:1085–1093, 1984

166. Foon KA, Schroff RW, Mayer D, et al: Monoclonal antibody therapy of chronic lymphocytic leukemia and cutaneous T-cell lymphoma: Preliminary observations, in Boss BD, Langman R, Trowbridge I (eds): Monoclonal Antibodies and Cancer. Orlando, Fla, Academic, 1983, pp 39–52

167. Meeker TC, Lowder J, Maloney DG, et al: A clinical trial of anti-idiotype therapy for B cell malignancy. Blood 65:1349–1363, 1985

168. Sears HF, Herlyn D, Steplewski Z, et al: Effects of monoclonal antibody immunotherapy on patients with gastrointestinal adenocarcinoma. J Biol Resp Modif 3:138–150, 1984

169. Sears HF, Herlyn D, Steplewski Z, et al: Phase II clinical trial of a murine monoclonal antibody cytotoxic for gastrointestinal adenocarcinoma. Cancer Res 45:5910–5913, 1985

170. Goodman GE, Beaumier P, Hellstrom I, et al: Pilot trial of murine monoclonal antibodies in patients with advanced melanoma. J Clin Oncol 3:340–352, 1985

171. Oldham RK, Foon KA, Morgan C, et al: Monoclonal antibody therapy of malignant melanoma: In vivo localization in cutaneous metastasis after intravenous administration. J Clin Oncol 2:1235–1244, 1984

172. Miller RA, Levy R: Response of cutaneous T cell lymphoma to therapy with hybridoma monoclonal antibody. Lancet 2:226–230, 1981

173. Miller RA, Maloney DG, McKillop J, et al: In vivo effects of murine hybridoma monoclonal antibody in a patient with T-cell leukemia. Blood 58:78–86, 1981

174. Dillman RO, Shawler DL, Sobol RE, et al: Murine monoclonal antibody therapy in two patients with chronic lymphocytic leukemia. Blood 59:1036–1045, 1982

175. Schroff RW, Foon KA, Beatty SM, et al: Human anti-murine immunoglobulin responses in patients receiving monoclonal antibody therapy. Cancer Res 45:879–885, 1985

176. Shawler DL, Miceli MC, Wormsley SB, et al: Induction of in vitro and in vivo antigenic modulation by the anti-human T-cell monoclonal antibody T101. Cancer Res 44:5921–5927, 1984

177. Miller RA, Maloney DG, Warnke R, et al: Treatment of B-cell lymphoma with monoclonal anti-idiotype antibody. N Engl J Med 306:517–522, 1982

178. Raffeld M, Neckers L, Longo DL, et al: Spontaneous alteration of idiotype in a monoclonal B-cell lymphoma: Escape from detection by anti-idiotype. N Engl J Med 312:1653–1658, 1985

179. Meeker T, Lowder J, Cleary ML, et al: Emergence of idiotype variants during treatment of B-cell lymphoma with anti-idiotype antibodies. N Engl J Med 312:1658–1665, 1985

180. Nadler LM, Stashenko P, Hardy R, et al: Serotherapy of a patient with a monoclonal antibody directed against a human lymphoma-associated antigen. Cancer Res 40:3147–3154, 1980

181. Ball ED, Bernier GM, Cornwell GG: Monoclonal antibodies to myeloid differentiation antigens: In vivo studies of three patients with acute myelogenous leukemia. Blood 62:1203–1210, 1983

182. Shen JW, Atkinson B, Koprowski H, et al: Binding of immunoglobulin to human tissues after immunotherapy with anticolorectal carcinoma monoclonal antibody. Int J Cancer 33:465–468, 1984

Active Immunotherapy Against Cancer: Present Status

Donald L. Morton

THE CONCEPT of producing active, specific immunotherapy against cancer is not new. The success of vaccines in inducing active immunity against infectious disease captured the imagination of early oncologists. Consequently, since the turn of the century, many attempts have been made to induce specific immunity in cancer patients by immunization with their own tumors or with those from other patients.[1] Unfortunately, most of these studies were unsuccessful in that few patients exhibited evidence of response to such vaccines, or the absence of suitable controls made the immunotherapy trials impossible to evaluate. Furthermore, rarely were immunologic studies carried out in the immunized patients to determine whether, in fact, the patient had been successfully immunized. Thus, at the present time, there is minimal evidence that this approach to immunotherapy of cancer in man has been successful. As a result, this summary will concentrate on certain of the theoretical aspects of tumor vaccines and review of some of the active, specific immunotherapy trials that included adequate controls to be evaluable.

Although the concept of producing a vaccine against cancer that is similar to the vaccines against infectious disease is theoretically appealing, with few exceptions, cancer vaccines as presently contemplated, are used in a different manner. The vaccines against infectious disease are typically made up of killed, whole microorganisms, nonpathogenic strains of living organisms, or specific microbial antigens. Such vaccines are administered before the development of the infectious disease in an attempt to prevent the disease. There are few examples of the successful use of vaccines where the immunization process is begun after the animal has contracted the infectious disease. The most striking parallel, perhaps, is rabies, in which it has been demonstrated that immunization with the rabies viral antigens after the rabies virus has already been innoculated will prevent the development of the disease. In this case, however, the success of the immunotherapy is due to the long, latency period between infection with the rabies virus and the development of the overt disease. In the case of malignancy, the disease is already present and is inducing, in most cases, an active immune response against the tumor antigens. The purpose, therefore, of active, specific immunotherapy against human cancer is directed at attempts to increase the level of antitumor immunity beyond that which is naturally induced by the growing neoplasm.

Obviously, the rationale for this approach is based upon the assumption that a growing neoplasm does not induce a maximum immune response in the host to the tumor specific antigens it contains. Efforts are made to increase the patient's immunity by altering the tumor antigens in such a way that they become more antigenic or by the use of immunomodulators, such as Bacillus Calmette-Guerin (BCG), which have the ability to enhance the immune response to tumor antigens.

Thus, at the present time, there are well-documented instances from animal tumor models and some serologic evidence in man to suggest that immunity against a growing neoplasm can be enhanced by active immunization.

Some of the approaches to active specific immunotherapy used with human and animal neoplasms are summarized in Table 1.

Most immunotherapy attempts have involved vaccines prepared from whole tumor cells, because progress has been slow in the isolation and purification of human tumor-associated antigens. Furthermore, living tumor cells, when administered intradermally in numbers that are insufficient to cause a progressive tumor growth, generally are the most effective immunogens in animal models. The possibility that living autologous tumor cells could result in tumor growth at the inoculation site has inhibited the use of such vaccines in man. However, theoretically, in certain tumors that share common tumor-associated

---

From the Division of Surgical Oncology, University of California, Los Angeles, Center for Health Sciences.

Address reprint requests to Donald L. Morton, MD, Division of Surgical Oncology, UCLA School of Medicine, Louis Factor Building, Room 9-260, Los Angeles, CA 90024.

0093–7754/86/1302–0007$05.00/0

Table 1. Active Specific Immunotherapy

Whole Tumor Cell Vaccine
Living tumor cells
Autologous
Allogeneic
Inactivated tumor cells
Irradiation
Mitomycin C
Freezing and thawing
Heat
Modification of tumor cells to increase antigenicity
Addition of carrier proteins—eg, rabbit gamma globulin
Viral oncolysates
Chemical modification—eg, iodoacetate
Neuraminidase
Vaccines Composed of Subcellular Components
Crude cell extracts
Isolated cell membranes
Purified solubilized cell surface tumor antigens
Immune Adjuvants
Freund's adjuvant
Bacterial
BCG
Methanol extraction residue of BCG
C parvum
Cyclophosphamide

antigens, such as melanomas, one patient could be immunized with an allogeneic vaccine of living tumor cells from another patient.[2,3] An immune response would be induced against the foreign HLA transplantation antigens on the tumor cells, thereby causing their rejection. In addition, this immunization should induce a strong immune response against the common cross-reacting tumor-associated antigen to which the human leukocyte antigens (HLA) may serve as a helper function.

Most attempts at immunotherapy in man were with vaccines composed of inactivated tumor cells. A variety of different methods render the tumor cells incapable of proliferation, including irradiation, mitomycin C, freezing and thawing or heat treatment. Undoubtedly, all are effective in eliminating progressive tumor growth, but the physical-chemical nature of the tumor antigens of particular neoplasms may be adversely altered by such treatments and the effectiveness of the vaccine diminished.

Repeated efforts have been made to increase the antigenicity of tumor vaccines by modifying the tumor cells in a variety of ways. One method, based upon experiments with other weakly antigenic substances, involved the addition of a highly antigenic carrier protein. Frequently, an immune response could be elicited from a normally nonantigenic substance. The antibodies formed against this complex were specifically directed against the previously nonantigenic substance, as well as against the foreign protein portion of the complex. Early reports using rabbit gamma globulin as a carrier protein attached to autologous tumor cells suggested some therapeutic benefit, but the effectiveness of this type of therapy has not been confirmed.

The finding that the immunogenicity of tumor antigens appears to be augmented following infection of tumor cells by certain viruses has evolved through many attempts to use this approach for active immunization. Despite good evidence for activity in animal models,[4] preliminary evidence of activity in man has not yet been confirmed in randomized clinical trials. Nevertheless, the theoretical basis for this approach is sound and deserves further investigation.

There are many possible ways to modify the tumor-associated antigens in tumor cells by chemicals, such as iodoacetate and other reagents, that will increase the antigenicity of animal neoplasms. Certain substances, such as neuraminidase, were reported to enhance the immune response to animal neoplasms remarkably. Although the mechanism of neuraminidase action has not been completely elucidated, it significantly can enhance the immune response in mice and cause regression of established animal neoplasms by active immunotherapy.[5] The ideal tumor vaccine in many respects would be one composed of the isolated and purified tumor-associated transplantation antigens from the cell surface. Such preparations would have the advantage of safety, stability, and ease of administration. However appealing this concept, most evidence from animal tumor host systems suggests that the whole tumor cell is more immunogenic than the highly purified tumor transplantation antigens. Nevertheless, some work with partially purified preparations has already been carried out in man.[6] Most of the vaccines used today are crude cell extracts or preparations from isolated cell membranes. As stated above, there is always the great danger of inactivating the tumor-associated antigens during preparation of the vaccine, unless immunologic techniques are available for systematically following the isolation-purification procedure. Active investigations are going on, though, in many laboratories and no doubt much progress can be expected in this field soon.

Model experiments with animal neoplasms show that immunologic adjuvants, such as BCG vaccine, *Corynebacterium parvum,* MER (methanol extractable residue of tubercule bacillus), and Freund's adjuvant, are potent stimulants of the immune system that can enhance considerably the humoral and cellular immune response to a variety of different types of antigens. In fact, autoimmune diseases, such as thyroiditis or encephalomyelitis, can be induced in animals following inoculation with normal tissues suspended in complete Freund's adjuvant. Such adjuvants, then, are potentially useful in enhancing the specific immune response to tumor antigens, but there has been little success except in a few instances.

The most convincing data from animal models that active immunization using immune adjuvants might be successful comes from work with syngeneic guinea pigs using BCG. We found, utilizing a methylcholanthrene-induced liposarcoma, that active immunization with BCG and whole tumor cells would cause regressions of previously implanted and growing liposarcoma cells.[7] The experiments of Zbar[8] and Hanna[9] with the L-10 hepatocarcinoma in guinea pigs subsequently demonstrated that intratumoral injection of BCG resulted in regression not only of the established tumor of the skin, but also of regional lymph node metastasis. Subsequently, it was demonstrated that vaccines of BCG mixed with viable, irradiated L-10 cells were effective in eliminating established micrometastasis in the lung even when active immunotherapy was administered up to ten days after intravenous (IV) injection of the L-10 cells. Hanna subsequently demonstrated that there was a crucial interrelationship between the dose of BCG and the viability and number of tumor cells used in the vaccine preparation in order to have optimum activity. Furthermore, it was demonstrated that intratumoral injection of a vaccine composed of BCG cell walls into spontaneous squamous carcinomas of the eyelid in cows frequently resulted in control of the directly injected tumor, as well as of regional lymph node metastasis similar to the guinea pig model.[10] The success of these experiments with active specific immunotherapy in the guinea pig model subsequently led to our studies on active immunization in melanoma and those of Hoover and Hanna in human colonic cancer.

The most convincing evidence that active, specific immunotherapy may be effective in human cancer comes from studies with BCG being used as an adjuvant by injecting it into neoplasms growing in the skin of patients with malignant melanoma. In immunocompetent patients, cutaneous metastasis of malignant melanoma will consistently undergo complete regression following intralesional injection with BCG. This observation, originally reported by Morton and his colleagues,[11] has been confirmed by numerous investigators[1] (also reviewed by Pinsky in this issue). Serial biopsies of injected lesions show an intense lymphocytic and mononuclear cell infiltrate and destruction of melanoma cells. Approximately 90% of the melanoma nodules directly injected with BCG were observed to regress in patients who were immunocompentent as judged by their ability to be sensitized to tuberculin. Thus, it appeared that a large portion of the tumor regression was a result of the induction of a delayed hypersensitivity reaction in the tumor nodule. However, in 15% to 20% of patients receiving intralesional BCG, there is concomitant regression of uninjected nodules and approximately 20% of patients responding in this way remained free of disease over a long period, with some patients having disease remission for as long as 10 years. In these patients, there was evidence of a systemic response to the active immunization to the melanoma-associated antigens because a rising titer of antimelanoma antibodies was observed in some patients and biopsy of uninjected melanoma nodules showing clinical regression were found to contain intense lymphocytic infiltrates. Thus, it appears that active immunization using autologous tumor growing intradermally, when injected with BCG, provides one of the most impressive evidences for the potential success of active, specific immunotherapy in clinical trials. For many years, it appeared that these observations with melanoma metastatic to the skin were a unique instance of the effectiveness of this therapy. However, it has subsequently been found that such treatment is also effective in superficial bladder cancer for which BCG immunotherapy has now become the treatment of choice. The results of administration of immunomodulators is reviewed by Pinsky, this issue.

The above studies that clearly indicate that BCG can act as an effective adjuvant when it is placed in contact with autologous, living tumor cells to induce active, specific immunotherapy have provided the theoretical basis for a number of clinical trials in which this principle is used for adjuvant therapy in an attempt to prevent recurrence of cancer in patients whose primary tumors have been removed by surgery. These studies have involved the use of BCG mixed with allogeneic tissue culture grown melanoma cells administered to melanoma patients or autologous, irradiated tumor cells administered to colon carcinoma patients.

The preliminary results of our earlier trial begun in 1974 have been previously published.[2] Patients with lymph node metastasis of malignant melanoma were randomized following surgical lymphadenectomy into one of three treatment groups: (1) Operation only; (2) operation and adjuvant BCG; and (3) operation, BCG, and immunization with an allogeneic melanoma cell vaccine. Patients were stratified on the basis of age, sex, site of the primary tumor, and whether or not regional lymph nodes appeared to be affected by disease on clinical examination. A total of 140 evaluable stage II patients were admitted to this study and randomized to one of the three arms. Unfortunately, the group of patients receiving the tissue culture grown melanoma cells were injected with tumor cells inadvertently contaminated with hepatitis B virus, presumably, from the human serum supplement in the tissue culture medium. Although all patients subsequently recovered completely as evidenced by normal liver function tests and the disappearance of hepatitis B antigen from their sera, the effect of this occurrence upon the effectiveness of active, specific immunotherapy is unknown at the present time. The results indicate that a higher proportion (52%) of those patients receiving tumor cell vaccine survive 5 years when compared to those patients treated by surgery alone (41%), but the results were not significant ($P = .21$). However, we found that only 37% of those patients immunized with the vaccine developed elevated titers of antibodies specifically reactive with membrane antigens of cultured melanoma cells. Thus, the results would therefore indicate that the active immunization procedure was ineffective in the majority of the patients in this trial. Similar findings have been reported by Livingston.[3] It is of considerable interest, however, that those patients who did respond to the vaccine by the formation of IgM antibody responses to membrane-associated antigens in melanomas had a highly significant, more favorable clinical course than those patients who did not form such a high antibody response to melanoma-associated antigens.[12]

The explanation for the failure to achieve effective immunization to melanoma-associated antigens in these patients remains unknown at the present time. It is possible that inadvertent infection with the hepatitis virus inhibited the response to immunization in our patients. However, it is also well known that many cancer patients are immunosuppressed as judged by tests of their general immunocompetence and this immunodeficiency would be expected to extend to cancer-specific antigens. However, many of our patients who failed to respond to the tumor cell vaccine-associated antigens did, in fact, respond to other antigens such as HLA antigens found in the vaccine. Another likely explanation relates to the possible presence of suppressor cells, which have been demonstrated in animal models to be capable of inhibiting the immune response to tumor antigens and thereby causing accelerated tumor growth. Such suppressor mechanisms appeared to involve both T suppressor cells and macrophages. Consequently, we are presently investigating the possibility of increasing the effectiveness of such vaccines by the use of suppressor cell modification with modulators.

One of the most interesting and well designed clinical studies of active, specific immunotherapy is that of Hoover and Hanna in colorectal cancer.[13] This study involved adoption of principles of active, specific immunotherapy worked out in the guinea pig model using intradermal immunization with BCG and irradiated autologous tumor cells. In this study, patients with high risk colorectal cancer undergoing standard surgical resection were randomized to receive postoperative follow-up alone as the control group or resection plus immunization with active, specific immunotherapy using 10^7 irradiated, autologous tumor cells mixed with 10^7 BCG organisms at weekly intervals for 3 weeks. The results indicated that 67% of the patients so immunized developed delayed hypersensitivity responses to the autologous tumor cells following immunization whereas none were positive before immunization.[14] Furthermore, a recent report of the clinical results of this study after follow-up of 2 to 3 years revealed that patients receiving active, specific immunotherapy had fewer recurrences and death than patients in the control group.[13] These differences are statistically significant, but because of the small number of patients admitted to the trial to the present time, further confirmatory studies in larger series are needed.

CONCLUSIONS

Obviously, the rational application of active specific immunotherapy to human cancer will depend, to a large extent, upon a better knowledge of the nature of tumor-associated antigens in human neoplasms and methods for increasing the immune response against these antigens. Considerable progress has already been made using such immunotherapy in the treatment of selected neoplasms, such as superficial bladder cancer and malignant melanomas, with BCG. These results indicate that active specific immunotherapy has potential as a new treatment modality. Its specificity for cancer cells cannot be achieved by any other known therapeutic modality, but, at the present time, its potency is limited. Therefore, it is unlikely that immunotherapy alone can bolster host defenses sufficiently to reverse this process in advanced disease due to the generalized immunosuppression present in the patient with advanced cancer. In contrast, immunotherapy is a logical adjunct for the treatment of minimal residual disease following definitive cancer surgery, radiation therapy, or chemotherapy. This rationale can be summarized as follows: (1) Patients who have only a small foci of cancer cells remaining after destruction of the major tumor bulk by other types of therapy are the most likely beneficiaries of immunotherapy because the tumor mass that must be destroyed by host defenses is smallest at that point. (2) The specificity of the immune response to cancer cells provides a possible therapeutic tool that has selectivity for small foci of cancer cells not possible with other modalities. (3) Patients with earlier disease are more likely to respond to any immunotherapeutic maneuvers, since the cancer patient's general immune competence is greatest when his disease is localized and is often impaired after metastasis.

Active immunotherapy may prove useful as primary treatment in selected clinical situations, such as superficial bladder carcinomas and metastatic malignant melanoma to the skin. The observation that organ transplant patients with disseminated neoplasms, inadvertently transplanted at the time of kidney transplantation, have regressions of their tumors after cessation of immunosuppressive drugs suggests that the immune response can cause regression of disseminated cancer if the tumor-associated antigens are sufficiently strong.

Thus, it is likely that active specific immunotherapy will play an increasingly important role in the treatment of cancer. The results should improve as our knowledge increases. It should be emphasized, however, that the toxicity, dosage, indications, and results of active immunotherapy are largely unknown at the present time. Furthermore, progress in this field requires a complete integration of laboratory and clinical efforts in order to develop rational approaches. These developmental studies will take considerable time and effort and should precede the clinical application of active specific immunotherapy to significant numbers of cancer patients.

The tumor immunotherapist is faced with a paradox in the clinical application of immunotherapy. Ideally, the patients who are most likely to respond to this therapeutic modality are those who are early in their disease and have minimal residual tumor burden following treatment with other therapeutic modalities. However, many of these patients may have been cured of their cancer by the primary treatment, so the results of such therapy can only be evaluated by controlled clinical trials containing large numbers of patients. Such trials take a long time to complete and are impaired, at the present time, by the inability to induce an enhanced immune response in most of the patients receiving active specific immunotherapy.

We believe that such studies are essential, since it has been demonstrated that enhancement of tumor growth can occur when immunotherapy is applied inappropriately in animal experiments. In order to avoid this, it is necessary to define, by laboratory study, those immune responses that best correlate with clinical course and then develop active immunotherapy programs to stimulate these immune responses in the cancer patient. Until these conditions are better known, the use of this therapeutic modality should be limited to those centers having research teams who monitor the patient's immune response concomitantly with the immunotherapeutic trials. Only when these phase I studies are completed, and we are better informed about the administration of active specific immunotherapy, can we embark upon controlled clinical trials on a large scale basis.

REFERENCES

1. Goodnight JE, Morton DL: Immunotherapy for malignant disease. Annu Rev Med 29:231–283, 1978
2. Morton DL, Holmes EC, Eilber FR, et al: Adjuvant immunotherapy of malignant melanoma: Results of a randomized trial in patients with lymph node metastases, in Terry WD, Rosenberg SA (eds): Immunotherapy of Human Cancer. New York, Elsevier North Holland, 1982, pp 245–249
3. Livingston PO, Takeyama H, Pollack MS, et al: Serological response of melanoma patients to vaccine derived from allogeneic cultured melanoma cells. Int J Cancer 31:567–575, 1983
4. Kobayashi H: Immunological xenogenation of tumor cells. Tokyo, Japan Scientific Societies, 1979
5. Simmons RL, Rios A, Ray PR, et al: Effect of neuraminidase on growth of a 3-methylcholanthrene-induced fibrosarcoma in normal and immunosuppressed syngeneic mice. JNCI 47:1087–1094, 1971
6. Hollingshead A, Arlen M, Yonemoto R, et al: Pilot studies using melanoma tumor associated antigens (TAA) in specific active immunochemotherapy of malignant melanoma. Cancer 49:1387, 1982
7. Eilber FR, Holmes EC, Morton DL: Immunotherapy experiments with a methylcholanthrene-induced guinea pig liposarcoma. JNCI 46:803, 1971
8. Zbar I, Bernstein GL, Bartlett, et al: Immunotherapy of cancer regression of intradermal tumors and prevention of growth of lymph node metastases after intralesional injection of living Mycobacterium bovis (BCG). JNCI 49:119, 1972
9. Hanna MG, Brandhorst JS, Peters LC: Active-specific immunotherapy of residual micrometastasis: An evaluation of sources, doses and ratios of BCG with tumor cells. Cancer Immunol Immunother 7:165–173, 1979
10. Kleinschuster SJ, Rapp HJ, Lueker DC, et al: Regression of bovine ocular carcinoma by treatment with mycobacterial vaccine. JNCI 58:1805, 1977
11. Morton DL, Eilber FR, Malmgren RA, et al: Immunological factors which influence response to immunotherapy in malignant melanoma. Surgery 68:158–164, 1970
12. Jones PC, Sze LL, Liu PY, et al: Prolonged survival for melanoma patients with elevated IgM antibody to oncofetal antigen. JNCI 66:249–254, 1981
13. Hoover HC Jr, Surdyke MG, Dangel RB, et al: Prospectively randomized trial of adjuvant active specific immunotherapy for human colorectal cancer. Cancer 55:1236, 1985
14. Hoover HC Jr, Surdyke M, Dangel R, et al: Delayed cutaneous hypersensitivity to autologous tumor cells in colorectal cancer patients immunized with an autologous tumor cell:Bacillus Calmette-Guerin vaccine. Cancer Res 44:1671–1676, 1984

The Immunoaugmenting Effects of Cancer Chemotherapeutic Agents

M.J. Mastrangelo, D. Berd, and H. Maguire, Jr

SHORTLY AFTER the introduction of cancer chemotherapeutic agents into clinical trials it became apparent that these drugs could suppress host defense mechanisms. This suppression of immunity was felt to be the consequence of a more general inhibition of cell proliferation. The immunopotentiating capacity of certain cancer chemotherapeutic agents was demonstrated inadvertently during studies of immunosuppression. These well-documented but unexplained examples of immune augmentation were not pursued until more recently. Increased knowledge about the complex regulatory network involved in the immune response and a renewed emphasis on active specific tumor immunotherapy have rekindled interest in this area. The immunoaugmenting capacity of chemotherapeutic agents and the application of this phenomenon to tumor therapy will serve as the focus for this review.

Virtually every chemotherapeutic agent has been studied to some extent for its effects on the immune system. Available data for individual drugs are often fragmentary. Frequently studies are not updated as technology advances. Not uncommonly, older work lacks appropriate controls. Adriamycin (Adria Laboratories, Columbus, Ohio) has been systematically evaluated by Mihich[1] in animal models. This presentation will focus on cyclophosphamide (CY) as it has been evaluated both in animals and in man. Those interested in the immunomodulating effects of other chemotherapeutic agents are referred to the reviews by Braun and Harris[2] and Ozer.[3]

From the Division of Medical Oncology, Department of Medicine, The Jefferson Medical College, 1025 Walnut St, Philadelphia.

Supported in part by grants from the National Institutes of Health (R01-CA39248) and the W.W. Smith Charitable Trust.

Address reprint requests to M.J. Mastrangelo, Department of Medicine, The Jefferson Medical College, 1025 Walnut St, Philadelphia, PA 19107.

0093-7754/86/1302-0008$05.00/0

POTENTIATION OF ANTIBODY PRODUCTION IN ANIMALS

Historically the first well-documented demonstration of enhancement of immune responsiveness by a cytotoxic drug was reported by Chanmougan and Schwartz in 1966.[4] These investigators administered 6-mercaptopurine (10 mg/kg/dx7d) to rabbits. One, 5, or 20 days following drug therapy, a subimmunogenic dose (20 μg IV) of bovine gamma globulin was administered. Control animals produced no antibody. All drug pretreated groups produced antibody with the greatest response being noted in the day 1 population.

Similarly, CY has augmented antibody production in several animal models. Results from selected studies are presented in Table 1. Taniguchi and Tada[5] studied the effect of schedule on outcome. When CY was administered one day before antigen, a marked increase in mean antibody titer was noted (passive cutaneous anaphylaxis assay; 348.0 *v* 88.6 for control). Virtually no antibody was produced (0.8 titer) when CY was administered 2 days after antigen. The dose dependence of the phenomenon was shown by Kerckhaert.[6] A dose of 100 mg/kg significantly enhanced antibody production whereas significant suppression was noted at higher doses. Further CY can have a differential effect on the various classes of antibody.[7]

Melphalan[8] and cis-diamine dichloroplatinum[9] can also augment antibody production.

POTENTIATION OF DELAYED-TYPE HYPERSENSITIVITY (DTH) IN ANIMALS

Maguire and Ettore[10] were the first to demonstrate that CY could augment the induction and expression of allergic contact dermatitis. Guinea pigs treated with CY and then contact-sensitized developed much more intense and prolonged allergic contact dermatitis reactions than did control guinea pigs that had received sensitizer alone. This was not due to the induction by CY of a nonspecific increase in skin reactivity, because

Table 1. Modulation of Antibody Production by Cyclophosphamide

Investigators	CY Dose and Schedule	Antigen	Animal	Results
Taniguchi	150 mg/kg	DNP-As	Rat	
and Tada[5]	d − 1			Augmentation
1971	d + 2			Suppression
Kerckhaert	d − 0	SRBC/FCA	Mouse	PFC/10^5 Spl
et al[6]	Control			62
1977	50 mg/kg			70
	100 mg/kg			100
	200 mg/kg			20
Chiorazzi	175 mg/kg	DNP-KLH	Mouse	d14: IgE ↓, IgG ↓
et al[7]	d − 2	primed		d21: IgE ↑ 8x, IgG ↓
1976				d50: IgE ↑, IgG ↓

Abbreviations: DNP-As, dinitrophenylated Ascaris extract; SRBC, sheep red blood cells; FCA, Freund's complete adjuvant; PFC, plaque forming cell; spl, splenocyte; KLH, keyhole limpet hemocyanin.

the reactions to croton oil, a primary irritant, were not affected by CY. A digest of the data taken from the original report is shown in Fig 1. Although rapidly confirmed,[11] this phenomenon did not attract much attention until the early 1970s. The last decade has seen a flourish of activity. Selected studies are presented in Table 2. The ability of CY to augment DTH is clearly dependent on schedule of administration, with d-1 to d-3 being most effective.[12-16] CY administration after immunization is usually immunosuppressive.[12,14,16] Potentiation is not B cell dependent[15] and is seen consistently at (higher) doses that suppress antibody production.[6,7] The augmentation of cellular immunity in animals is more dependent on the schedule of CY administration than it is on dose.

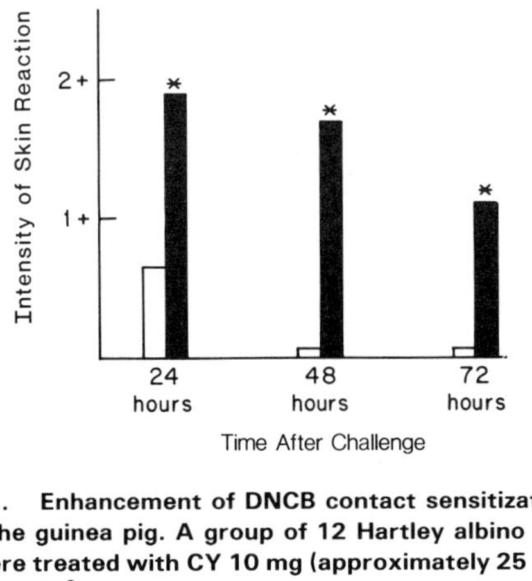

Fig 1. Enhancement of DNCB contact sensitization by CY in the guinea pig. A group of 12 Hartley albino guinea pigs were treated with CY 10 mg (approximately 25 mg/kg or 175 mg/m²) IP daily for five days. On day 5, these guinea pigs, as well as a control group of equal number, were putatively sensitized by the application of 0.5 mg DNCB (1-chloro,2,4-dinitrobenzene) to the skin. Ten days later both groups were challenged by topical application of 0.1% DNCB. The mean intensity of the challenge reaction of each group is shown (open bars = controls, solid bars = CY pretreatment). *, solid *v* open bars, $P < .0001$. Reprinted with permission,[35] by courtesy of Marcel Dekker, Inc.

Local introduction of 4-hydroperoxycyclophosphamide (4-HPCY) (a synthetic derivative of CY that spontaneously hydrolyzes to an active metabolite) into skin drained by antigenically stimulated lymph nodes is as effective as systemically administered CY in facilitating cell-mediated immune reactions.[17]

Turk and Parker[18] have studied the effects of a variety of cytotoxic drugs on contact sensitivity to DNFB in guinea pigs. The data are summarized in Table 3. An effort was made to normalize dosage on the basis of the lethal dose. Several drugs significantly augmented contact sensitivity although not to the degree achieved by CY. Interpretations of these data are limited because only a single dose of each agent was tested. Goto, et al[19] have also demonstrated enhancement of delayed hypersensitivity with a variety of anticancer drugs.

ABROGATION OF TOLERANCE IN ANIMALS

In addition to enhancing the acquisition/expression of immunity to new antigens, CY can also breech natural and acquired tolerance. Yoshida et al[20] were able to provoke significant delayed-type footpad reactions against syngeneic or autologous testicular cells in mice only when immunization was preceded by treatment with CY. A state of specific partial unresponsiveness

Table 2. Modulation of Delayed-Type Hypersensitivity by Cyclophosphamide in Animal Models

Investigator	Animal/Antigen	CY Schedule	CY Dose*	Results
Turk et al[12] 1972	Guinea pig/DNFB	d − 2	300	250% ↑ DTH
		d 0	300	300% ↑ DTH
		d + 4	300	100% ↓ DTH
Askenase et al[13] 1975	Mouse/SRBC	d − 1	0	4 ± 3†
		d − 2	20	10 ± 3
			200	15 ± 2
Mitsuoka et al[14] 1976	Mouse/MHSA	d − 1	0	5.3 ± 1.8‡
		d − 1	15	7.5 ± 1.5
		d − 4	150	16.4 ± 1.2
		d + 4	0	15.2 ± 2.9
		d + 4	150	2.8 ± 0.9
Burrows et al[15] 1976	Mouse§/SRBC	d − 1	200	500% ↑ DTH
Dwyer et al[15] 1981	Guinea pig/H37 Ra	d − 3	0	7.8 mm PPD
		d + 1	300	11.6 mm PPD
			300	3.8 mm PPD

Abbreviations: DNFB, 2,4-dinitrofluorobenzene; SRBC, sheep red blood cells; MHSA, methylated human serum albumin; H37 Ra, strain of mycobacterium tuberculosis.

*mg/kg.

†Percent of increase in footpad thickness at 24 hours ± standard error.

‡Increase in footpad thickness on day 12 with each value representing mean ± standard error (0.1 mm).

§B cell depleted.

to DNCB can be acquired by chronic feeding of DNCB. The intravenous injection of dinitrobenzene-sulfonic acid also induces complete tolerance. Polak and co-workers[21,22] (Table 4) have demonstrated that these states of acquired tolerance can be reversed by a single treatment with cyclophosphamide followed by allergen. This is paralleled by a return of the ability of T cells to proliferate in the draining lymph node following sensitization.

Table 3. Effect of Cytotoxic Drugs on Contact Sensitivity to DNFB in Guinea Pigs

Drug	Dose*	LD	Skin Tests†
None	—	—	1.2 ± 0.12
Cy	300	10	2.9 ± 0.07
Melphalan	5	20	2.2 ± 0.16
Azathioprine	450	0	2.0 ± 0.16
Methotrexate	100	0	1.9 ± 0.29
Chlorambucil‡	10	0	1.3 ± 0.20
Busulphan§	20	0	1.4 ± 0.24
Procarbazine	300	10	1.0 ± 0.16

Abbreviations: DNFB, 2,4-dinitroflurobenzene; LD, lethal dose.

*mg/kg as a single dose 3 days before sensitization.

†Results expressed as the mean intensity (± SE) of the reaction given to an epicutaneous test with 0.25% DNFB 48 hours previously in animals sensitized 7 days before skin test. Reaction intensity was graded on an arbitrary scale of 0 (none) to 3 (confluent redness and swelling).

‡LD80 = 25 mg/kg.

§LD20 = 50 mg/kg.

Reprinted with permission.[18]

EFFECTS OF CY ON TUMOR IMMUNITY IN ANIMAL MODELS

There is an extensive literature documenting the ability of CY to augment anti-tumor immunity in animal systems. The studies cited in this brief review have been selected to highlight the aspects of this phenomenon deemed of most clinical significance.

Early immunoprophylaxis experiments clearly demonstrated the presence of unique antigens on chemically induced murine tumors. The production of antibodies against these antigens has not been successful using conventional approaches. However, pretreatment (d-3) with CY (25 mg/kg) before immunization resulted in antibody production in nine of nine mice.[23] The administration of cyclophosphamide before immunization also facilitated the development of cytotoxic T cells.[24]

Normal mice have been shown to develop concomitant immunity in response to the presence of an antigenic chemically- or virally-induced tumor. This immune response can slow tumor growth and in some systems result in tumor rejection. The development and expression

Table 4. Effect of Cyclophosphamide on Acquired Immunological Tolerance in Guinea Pigs[21,22]

	CY		Results	
Tolerizing Procedure	Dose*	Schedule	MSTR	LN Blasts
$DNBSO_3$, IV				
d − 31, −17	250	d − 3	1.25	108 ± 48
	0	—	0	24.5 ± 9.9
d − 42, −28	250	d − 14	0	64.5 ± 29
DNCB, PO	250	d − 3	3.7 ± 1.15	137 ± 62
3 mg/d × 6d on each of 3 alternate weeks	0	—	1.05 ± 0.94	36 ± 21

Abbreviations: $DNBSO_3$, dinitrobenzene-sulfonic acid sodium salt; DNCB, 2,4-dinitrochlorobenzene; MSTR, mean skin test reactivity based on an arbitrary grading system ranging from 0 (no reaction) to 2 (confluent swelling and redness) and summed for the three challenge doses; LN, lymph node.

*mg/kg.

of concomitant immunity can be augmented by administering CY one to three days before tumor implant.[25–27] Results of representative studies are presented in Table 5. A positive effect was noted over a wide range of doses (25 to 300 mg/kg). Further Baldwin et al,[28] working with the rat hepatoma model, demonstrated that administration of CY three days before initiating a series of immunizations with a 3 mol/L KCl tumor extract generated substantial protection against subsequent challenge with the same tumor whereas CY or tumor extract alone were ineffective (Table 5).

CY has also been used to facilitate immunologically mediated regression of an established MOPC-315 tumor in mice.[29,30] Interestingly CY (15 mg/kg) will cure 92% of animals with large (25 mm in diameter) mature (15 day growth period) tumors but only 10% of animals with small (nonpalpable) immature (four day growth period) tumors. This observation suggested that the therapeutic outcome was dependent at least in part on the generation and expression of concomitant immunity. To test this hypothesis, animals were inoculated with varying doses of tumor cells. After 12 to 13 days of growth, tumor sizes ranged from nonpalpable to large (Table 6). CY was effective in curing animals of these mature tumors, regardless of size, but was ineffective against the nonpalpable immature tumor. That tumor regression was immunologically mediated was suggested by the observations that cured animals could reject a lethal challenge of MOPC-315 tumor cells and that CY was ineffective in immunosuppressed hosts.

CY has also been used to facilitate tumor regression mediated by adoptively transferred immune lymphocytes.[31]

In summary, CY augments the generation of humoral and cellular immune responses against

Table 5. The Effect of Pretreatment With Cyclophosphamide on the Growth of a Subsequent Tumor Inoculum

	CY					
Study	Dose	Schedule	Immunization	Implant (No. Cells)	Additional Comments	
A. Turk et al[25]:	300*	d − 2	—	5 × 10^4	Median Survival:	21.3 ± 0.8†
Meth A Sarcoma in Balb/c Mice	0	—	—	5 × 10^4	(mo ± SD)	15.0 ± 2.0†
B. Ray and Raychandhuri[26]:	25	d − 2	—	2 × 10^6	Tumor Incidence:	3/10‡
MC2 Sarcoma in C3h mice	0	—	—	2 × 10^6	(D13)	9/9‡
C. Maguire[27]: TA3Ha in A	100	d − 3	—	1 × 10^5	Footpad Thickness:	6.7
strain mice	0	—	—	1 × 10^5	(mm)(D14)	8.1
				Challenge: (D13; No. Cells)		
D. Baldwin et al[28]:	40	d 0	d 3–9	1 × 10^3	Tumor Incidence:	3/11
D23 hepatoma in rats	0	—	d 3–9	1 × 10^3		10/10
	40	d 0	—	1 × 10^3		5/5

*mg/kg.
†$P < .001$.
‡$P < .01$.

Table 6. Cyclophosphamide Therapy of MOPC-315 Tumor-Bearing Mice

No. Tumor Cells Innoculated	Day CY Administered	Tumor Size (mm ± SE)	Cured (%)
1×10^5	12–13	nonpalpable	87
5×10^5	12–13	10.8 ± 0.5	87
1×10^6	12–13	17.1 ± 0.5	87
3.5×10^6	12–13	23.9 ± 0.4	100
3.5×10^6	4	nonpalpable	7

NOTE. CY dose = 15 mg/kg.
Reprinted with permission.[29]

tumor associated antigens and facilitates the expression of actively or passively acquired antitumor immunity in tumor-bearing hosts.

IMMUNOPOTENTIATION IN MAN

Study of CY-induced immunopotentiation in man has been limited. Berd et al[32,33] evaluated the effect of two doses (1,000 mg and 300 mg/m^2) of cyclophosphamide administered on day −3 on the acquisition and expression of immunity to KLH (keyhole limpet hemocyanin) by patients with advanced cancer (melanoma and colorectal cancer). The results of these studies are summarized in Table 7. At both doses, the acquisition of DTH was augmented. However antibody was generated only by patients receiving the lower dose of CY, suggesting a greater sensitivity of B lymphocytes to the toxic effects of this agent. These investigators next measured the acquisition of DTH to autologous tumor cells in 19 patients with metastatic melanoma.[34] The patients were treated with an autologous melanoma cell vaccine, either given alone, or given three days after the administration of CY, 300 mg/m^2 IV. The DTH responses of CY-pretreated patients were significantly greater than those of control (vaccine only) patients. Thus, after two vaccine treatments, the median DTH responses (mm induration) were as follows: controls = 4 mm; CY-pretreated = 11 mm; P = .034, Mann-Whitney U test, 2-tailed. Whereas seven of eight CY-pretreated patients developed DTH to autologous melanoma cells of at least 5 mm, only two of seven controls did so (P = .034, Fisher's exact test). Two patients had significant antitumor responses to treatment with CY plus the vaccine, consisting of complete disappearance of skin metastases and a pulmonary nodule in one, and of subcutaneous and liver metastases in the other. Both patients remain free of melanoma after 33 and 24 months, respectively.

MECHANISMS OF IMMUNOPOTENTIATION BY CYLOPHOSPHAMIDE

The data pertaining to the mechanisms of immunopotentiation have been previously reviewed.[35] The first hypothesis proposed to explain CY-induced augmentation of cell-mediated immunity was inhibition of suppressor B cells[36] or their products.[37] Subsequently, Burrows et al[15] and Maguire et al[38] showed that mice lacking detectable B cells and B cell products could be immunopotentiated with CY as effectively as normal mice. Thus the B cell depletion hypothesis does not appear to be valid.

Currently the leading hypothesis is that CY augments immunity by selective toxicity for suppressor T cells and their precursors. There are animal model data that support this hypothesis. Several investigators[24,39] have shown that adoptive transfer of normal T cells abrogates immunopotentiation by CY. Diamantstein et al[40] demonstrated that spleen cells from mice treated

Table 7. Effect of Pretreatment With Cyclophosphamide on the Acquisition of Immunity to KLH by Patients With Advanced Cancer[32,33]

	DTH		Antibody	
Dose* CY	Proportion Positive	Median Response (mm)	Proportion Positive	Titer†
1,000	11/11	18	4/11	—
0	4/11	0	2/11	—
		(P = .025)	(P = .24)	
300	9/9	27	9/9	3
0	7/9	10	4/9	< 1
		(P = < .01)		(P < .01)

Abbreviation: KLH, keyhole limpet hemocyanin.
*Dose in mg/m^2 administered on d − 3.
†Median total antibody titer (Log 2 of the reciprocal of the dilution).

with CY showed an increased (fourfold) mitogenic response to dextran sulfate and that this could be reversed by the addition of normal thymocytes, but not by thymocytes treated with 4-HPCY. The response to dextran sulfate could also be augmented by treatment of spleen cells with 4-HPCY in vitro, but not if the spleen cells had first been depleted of T cells.

Kaufmann et al[41] compared the sensitivity to 4-HPCY of two populations of splenic T cells: (1) those capable of adoptively transferring specific DTH, and (2) those capable of specifically suppressing DTH. The former were resistant to concentrations of 4-HPCY of 3 μg/mL, while the latter were inactivated by 1 μg/mL. Moreover, spleen cells from mice injected with supraoptimal doses of antigen were incapable of adoptively transferring DTH, but regained that capability after exposure to 3 μg/mL of 4-HPCY. Finally, these investigators showed that pretreatment with CY enabled mice to make a DTH response after a supraoptimal dose of antigen. This could be reversed by adoptively transferring normal spleen cells but not by spleen cells that had been exposed to 4-HPCY, even to concentration of 4-HPCY as low as 0.3 μg/mL. These results suggested that antigen-primed suppressor T cells were more sensitive to activated CY than the antigen-primed T cells transferring DTH and that precursors of the antigen-primed suppressor cells were most sensitive of all. B cells, as measured by the mitogenic response to lipopolysaccharide, were about as sensitive to 4-HPCY as T suppressor cells.

Most of the investigation of the mechanism of augmentation of human immunity by CY has involved attempts at showing that CY is selectively cytotoxic for suppressor T cells in vitro.

Ozer et al[42] tested the effect on human lymphocytes of 4-HPCY. These investigators found that one-hour treatment with 4-HPCY did not kill lymphocytes, but did result in marked inhibition of their response to lectins when the concentration exceeded 30 nmol/mL. However, when purified T cells were treated with 4-HPCY and then mixed with untreated B cells, the production of immunoglobulin after stimulation with PWM was increased. This occurred when the concentration of 4-HPCY was 20 nmol/mL or less, and even when it was as low as 10^{-3} nmol/mL. Thus, these authors had circumstantial evidence that activated CY was selectively toxic to suppressor T cells or their precursors.

Ozer et al[42] also studied the effect of in vitro treatment with 4-HPCY on concanavalin A (Con A) inducible suppressor T cells. A one-hour incubation with 4-HPCY in concentrations ranging from 20 nmol/mL to 10^{-2} nmol/mL completely prevented the development of T cells that could suppress pokeweed mitogen-driven immunoglobulin production. On the other hand, treatment of T cells with 4-HPCY after they had been activated by Con A to become suppressors had no effect on their ability to suppress immunoglobulin production. Thus, 4-HPCY appeared to be working by preventing the development of mature suppressor cells, possibly by selective toxicity for a "presuppressor" cell. Ozer et al and others have presented evidence that the presuppressor might have a helper-inducer phenotype (Leu-3 or OKT-4+), rather than the expected suppressor-cytotoxic phenotype (Leu-2 or OKT-8+).

Although these data are interesting, they must be interpreted with caution, because in vivo conditions may be quite different from the in vitro environment. In the experiments of Ozer et al, lymphocytes were exposed to a single active metabolite of CY. Yet the plasma of animals and humans who have received a dose of CY also contains phosphoramide mustard, acrolein, and possibly other as yet unidentified cytotoxic compounds. Moreover in the in vitro experiments, cells were exposed to the one metabolite for an arbitrary length of time, generally one hour. However, cytotoxic compounds are found in the plasma of CY-treated patients for up to 24 hours after administration and may persist even longer in some tissues.

Berd and co-workers have studied the effect of exposure to two doses of CY (1,000 and 300 mg/M^2) in vivo on human lymphocyte composition and function.[43,44] All patients had advanced cancer: High dose, 18 (8, melanoma; 8, colorectal cancer; 2 other); low dose, 25 (16, melanoma; 7, colorectal cancer; 2, other). CY was administered as an intravenous bolus. The results are summarized in Table 8. High dose CY causes a marked depletion of circulating lymphocytes whereas low dose CY does not. Both high and low dose CY impair the generation of nonspecific suppressor T cells without impairing the prolifer-

Table 8. Effect of In Vivo Exposure to Cyclophosphamide on Human Lymphocyte Composition and Function

	Percent Change Compared to Pretreatment					
Day	3		7		20	
Dose	High	Low	High	Low	High	Low
Total B cells	−25	+7	−40	+11	−22	+22
Total T cells	−32	+8	−30	+5	−25	+8
Leu 2 positive	−28	+4	−31	+5	−16	+7
Leu 3 positive	−32	+10	−34	+5	−22	+7
PHA proliferation	−6	−4	−1	−10	−12	−4
Con A suppression*	−32	−23	−21	−32	−32	−58

NOTE. High, 1,000 mg/m^2, d0 IV; Low, 300 mg/m^2, d0 IV; Leu 2, suppressor/cytotoxic T cell subset; Leu 3 helper/inducer T cell subset.

*Con A-inducible suppression: Lymphocytes were incubated with Con A (25 μg/ml) for 48 hours. Suppression was measured by adding these cells to an autologous lymphocyte proliferation reaction to suboptimal (1.0 μg/ml) concentrations of PHA.

ative response to PHA. This preferential impairment of suppressor function is most apparent between three and seven days after CY administration. However, it is premature to conclude that the impairment of this type of T-suppressor activity constitutes the explanation for the augmentation of immunity previously described. There could be other varieties of T-suppressor cells (eg, those inducible by tolerogenic concentrations of antigens) that are even more CY sensitive. Also the possibility that CY diminishes monocyte-mediated suppression must be considered.[45]

IMMUNOPOTENTIATION BY OTHER CYTOTOXIC DRUGS

For a detailed analysis of this subject the reader is referred to the reviews by Braun and Harris,[2] Erke and Mihich,[1] and Berd et al.[35] Only a brief summary will be provided here.

It is clear that CY is not the only cytotoxic drug capable of augmenting immune response. Indeed, Goto et al[19] showed that in mice not only CY but also Thio-TEPA, mitomycin, Adriamycin, fluorouracil, vincristine, and methotrexate could augment the development of DTH to an antigen given four days later. These authors also showed that augmentation was observed if antigen was given after a single dose of drug, but not after the same dose of drug had been given by daily administration over a 2 week period.

There have been no studies showing that the administration of cytotoxic drugs other than CY can augment human immune responses. Several investigators have studied the effect of administration of various combinations of cytotoxic drugs to cancer patients on in vitro lymphocyte function. In general, lymphoproliferative responses to lectins, soluble antigens, and allogeneic lymphocytes are markedly depressed during the period of administration of drugs, but recover to pretreatment levels by three to four days after drug administration is stopped.[46–48] Thus, the kinetics of recovery of lymphoproliferative responses after combinations of drugs is similar to what is observed after CY alone. Frequently, an increase in proliferative responses nine to 14 days after combination chemotherapy has been observed, a phenomenon that has been referred to as "rebound overshoot".[47] Although it is tempting to attribute rebound overshoot to selective elimination of suppressor cells, there are not sufficient data to warrant such a conclusion. Overshoot could just as likely be due to regeneration of functionally efficient lymphocytes from precursor pools, in the same manner as circulating neutrophils recover and rebound after initial depression. Moreover, rebound overshoot of lymphoproliferation has been observed mostly in patients in whom chemotherapy causes tumor regression[48,49] and, therefore, could be a consequence of the decreased tumor burden, rather than a result of the drugs themselves. Braun and Harris[45] reported that 14 of 20 cancer patients developed rebound overshoot of PHA proliferation at at least one point between seven and 28 days after chemotherapy. In each case, rebound overshoot was temporally associated with a decrease in the augmentation of proliferation obtained by adding indomethacin or depleting adherent cells. The authors concluded that rebound overshoot was caused by drug-induced elimination or reduced function of suppressor monocytes. However, they did not directly demonstrate suppression by showing that proliferation could be resuppressed by the addition of the putative suppressor monocytes. Thus, the significance of rebound overshoot remains uncertain.

It seems highly likely that properly controlled studies would demonstrate that a number of cytotoxic drugs can augment human immune response given the proper dose and timing in regard to administration of antigen. As with CY, selective toxicity for some type of suppressor mechanism is likely to be the basis of the immunopotentiation.

SUMMARY AND CONCLUSION

This article has attempted to show that killing of, or damage to, lymphocytes by cancer chemotherapeutic agents does not necessarily lead to immunosuppression, but can just as readily result in immunopotentiation. Although this concept is widely accepted by experimental immunologists, it is not yet fully appreciated by clinical immunologists and clinicians who study cytotoxic agents.

The data accumulated so far suggest that for the most extensively studied drug, CY, the most important variable determining whether one observes immunosuppression or immunopotentiation is the timing of the administration of CY and antigen. In animal system, immunopotentiation is produced by administering CY one to four days before antigens, while administration of CY after antigen generally results in immunosuppression. Although in our own studies immunopotentiation was achieved in patients by giving CY three days before antigen, we did not determine whether this interval was optimal, and further clinical study of this variable is needed. The dose of CY is probably less important than the timing.

It is premature to speculate on the potential usefulness of CY and other cytotoxic drugs in augmenting immunity to clinically important antigens in patients with cancer or other disease states associated with immunosuppression. However, it is clear that the realization that cytotoxic drugs can be immunopotentiating has given a new perspective on immunoregulation. At the very least, these drugs will be valuable tools in the study of human immune responsiveness and the factors that modulate it.

REFERENCES

1. Ehrke MJ, Mihich E: Immunoregulation of cancer chemotherapeutic agents, in Hadden JW, Battisto JR (eds): The Reticuloendothelial System: A Comprehensive Treatise, vol V: The Pharmacology of the Reticuloendoethalial System. New York, Plenum (in press)

2. Braun DP, Harris JE: Modulation of the immune response by chemotherapy. Pharmacol Ther 14:89–122, 1981

3. Ozer H: Effects of alkylating agents on immunoregulatory mechanisms, in Mihich E, Sakurai Y (eds): Biological Responses in Cancer. New York, Plenum, 1985, pp 95–130

4. Chanmougan D, Schwartz RS: Enhancement of antibody synthesis by 6-mercaptopurine. J Exp Med 124:363–379, 1966

5. Taniguchi M, Tada T: Regulation of homocytotropic antibody formation in the rat. IV Effects of various immunosuppressive drugs. J Immunol 107:579–585, 1971

6. Kerckhaert JA, Hofhuis FM, Willers JM: Effects of variation in time and dose of cyclophosphamide injection on delayed hypersensitivity and antibody formation. Cell Immunol 29:232–237, 1977

7. Chiorazzi N, Fox DA, Katz DH: Hapten-specific IgE antibody responses in mice. VI. Selective enhancement of IgE antibody production by low doses of X-irradiation and by cyclophosphamide. J Immunol 117:1629–1637, 1976

8. Baral E, Blomgren H, Wasserman J, et al: Melphalan treatment of human peripheral T cells promotes Ig production by B cells in vitro. Eur J Cancer Clin Oncol 21:81–84, 1985

9. Rihova B, Drobnik J, Riha I: Immunostimulatory effect of cis-diamine-dichloroplatinum. Immunol Lett 8:57–60, 1984

10. Maguire HC Jr, Ettore VL: Enhancement of dinitrochlorobenzene (DNCB) contact sensitization by cyclophosphamide in the guinea pig. J Invest Dermatol 48:39–43, 1967

11. Hunziger N: Effects of cyclophosphamide on the contact eczema in guinea pigs. Dermatologica 136:187–191, 1968

12. Turk JL, Parker D, Poulter LW: Function aspects of the selective depletion of lymphoid tissue by cyclophosphamide. Immunology 23:493–501, 1972

13. Askenase PW, Hayden BJ, Gershon RK: Augmentation of delayed-type hypersensitivity by doses of cyclophosphamide which do not affect antibody responses. J Exp Med 141:697–702, 1975

14. Mitsuoka A, Baba M, Morikawa S: Enhancement of delayed hypersensitivity by depletion of suppressor T cells with cyclophosphamide in mice. Nature 262:77–78, 1976

15. Burrows PD, Gershon RK, Lawton AR, et al: Regulation of delayed hypersensitivity (DTH) in B-cell deprived mice. Fed Proc 35:861, 1976

16. Dwyer JM, Parker D, Turk JL: Suppression of delayed hypersensitivity to tuberculin by antigenic competition. A positive immunoregulatory mechanism sensitive to cyclophosphamide. Immunology 42:549–559, 1981

17. Boerrigter GH, Scheper RJ: Local administration of the cytostatic drug 4-hydroperoxy-cyclophosphamide (4-HPCY) facilitates cell mediated immune reactions. Clin Exp Immunol 58:161–166, 1984

18. Turk JL, Parker D: Effect of cyclophosphamide on immunological control mechanisms. Immunol Rev 65:99–113, 1982

19. Goto M. Mitsuoka A, Sugiyama M, et al: Enhancement of delayed hypersensitivity reaction with varieties of anti-cancer drugs. J Exp Med 154:204–209, 1981

20. Yoshida S, Nomoto, K, Himeno K, et al: Immune response to syngeneic or autologous testicular cells in mice. I. Augmented delayed footpad reaction in cyclophosphamide-treated mice. Clin Exp Immunol 38:211–217, 1979

21. Polak L, Turk JL: Reversal of immunolgical tolerance by cyclophosphamide through inhibition of suppressor cell activity. Nature 249:654–656, 1974

22. Polak L, Geleick H, Turk JL: Reversal by cyclophosphamide of tolerance to contact sensitization. Immunology 28:939–942, 1975

23. Livingston PO, DeLeo AB, Jones M, et al: Comparison of approaches for augmenting the serologic response to the individually specific methylcholanthrene-induced sarcoma-Metha A: Pretreatment with cyclophosphamide is most effective. J Immunol 131:2601–2605, 1983

24. Glaser M: Augmentation of specific immune response against a syngeneic SV40-induced sarcoma in mice depleted of suppressor T cells with cyclophosphamide. Cell Immunol 48:339–345, 1979

25. Turk JL, Parker D, Cameron AEP: The effect of cyclophosphamide on immunological control mechanisms. Int J Tissue React VI:205–211, 1984

26. Ray PK, Ragchaudhuri S: Low-dose cyclophosphamide inhibition of transplantable fibrosarcoma growth by augmentation of the host immune response. JNCI 67:1341–1345, 1981

27. Maguire H: Increased tumor immunity with cyclophosphamide. Proc Am Assoc Cancer Res 18:185, 1977

28. Baldwin RW, Byers VS, Hannant D, et al: Cellular interactions modulating host resistance to tumors. Recent Results Cancer Res 80:338 345, 1982

29. Hengst JCD, Mokyr MB, Dray S: Importance of timing in cyclophosphamide therapy of MOPC-315 tumor-bearing mice. Cancer Res 40:2135–2141, 1980

30. Hengst JCD, Mokyr MB, Dary S: Cooperation between cyclophosphamide tumoricidal activity and host anti-tumor immunity in the cure of mice bearing large MOPC-315 tumors. Cancer Res 41:2163–2167, 1981

31. North RJ, Dye ES, Mills CD, et al: Modulation of anti-tumor immunity—Immunobiologic approaches. Springer Semin Immunopathol 5:193–220, 1982

32. Berd M, Mastrangelo MJ, Engstrom PF, et al: Augmentation of the human immune response by cyclophosphamide. Cancer Res 42:4862–4866, 1982

33. Berd D, Maguire HC Jr, Mastrangelo MJ: Potentiation of human cell mediated immunity by low dose cyclophosphamide. Cancer Res 44:5439–5443, 1984

34. Berd D, Maguire HC Jr, Mastrangelo MJ: Induction of cell-mediated immunity to autologous melanoma cells and regression of metastases after treatment with a melanoma cell vaccine preceded by cyclophosphamide. Cancer Res, 1986 (in press)

35. Berd D, Maguire HC Jr, Mastrangelo MJ: Immunopotentiation by cyclophosphamide and other cytotoxic agents, in Fenichel R, Chirigos M (eds): Immune Modulating Agents and Their Mechanisms. New York, Marcel Dekker, 1984, pp 39–61

36. Katz SI, Parker D, Turk JL: B-cell suppression of delayed hypersensitivity reactions. Nature 251:550–551, 1974

37. Lagrange PH, Mackaness GB, Miller TE: Potentiation of T cell mediated immunity by selective suppression of antibody formation with cyclophosphamide. J Exp Med 139:1529–1539, 1974

38. Maguire HC Jr, Faris LW: Cyclophosphamide intensifies the acquisition of allergic contact dermatitis in mice rendered B-cell deficient by heterologous anti-IgM antisera. Immunology 37:367–372, 1979

39. Rollinghoff M, Starzinski-Powitz A, Pfizenmaier K, et al: Cyclophosphamide-sensitive T-lymphocytes suppress the in vitro generation of antigen-specific cytotoxic T lymphocytes. J Exp Med 145:455–459, 1977

40. Diamantstein T, Willinger W, Reiman J: T-suppressor cells sensitive to cyclophosphamide and to its in vitro active derivative 4-hydro-peroxycyclophosphamide control the mitogenic response of murine splenic B cells to dextran sulfate. J Exp Med 150:1571–1576, 1979

41. Kaufmann SHE, Hah H, Diamantstein T: Relative susceptibilities of T cell subsets involved in delayed-type hypersensitivity to sheep red blood cells to the in vitro action of 4-hydroperoxycyclophosphamide. J Immunol 125:1104–1108, 1980

42. Ozer H, Cowens JW, Colvin M, et al: In vitro effects of 4-hydroperoxycyclophosphamide on human immunoregulatory T subset function. J Exp Med 155:276–290, 1982

43. Berd D, Maguire HC Jr, Mastrangelo MJ: Impairment of concanavalin A-inducible suppressor activity following administration of cyclophosphamide to patients with advanced cancer. Cancer Res 44:1275–1280, 1984

44. Berd D, Golden M, Maguire H, et al: Comparison of the effects of low dose vs. high dose cyclophosphamide (Cy) on peripheral blood lymphocyte (PBL) composition and function. Proc Am Assoc Cancer Res 26:271, 1985

45. Braun DP, Harris JE: Effects of combination chemotherapy on immunoregulatory cells in peripheral blood of solid tumor patients: Correlation with rebound overshoot immune function recovery. Clin Immunol Immunopathol 20:193–214, 1981

46. Hersh EM, Oppenheim JJ: Inhibition of in vitro lymphocyte transformation during chemotherapy in man. Cancer Res 27:98–105, 1967

47. Harris JE, Bagai RC, Steward THM: Serial monitoring of immune reactivity in cancer patients receiving chemotherapy as a means of predicting anti-tumor response, in Daguillard F (ed): Proc 7th Leukocyte Culture Conference, Orlando, Fla, Academic, 1973, pp 443–457

48. Harris JE, Stewart THM: Recovery of mixed lymphocyte reactivity (MLR) following cancer chemotherapy in man, in Schwarz MR (ed): Proc 6th Leukocyte Culture Conference, Orlando, Fla, Academic, 1972, pp 555–579

49. Cheema AR, Hersh EM: Patient survival after chemotherapy and its relationship to in vitro lymphocyte blastogenesis. Cancer 28:851–855, 1971

Effects of Biological Response Modifiers on Effector Cells With Cytotoxic Activity Against Tumors

Ronald B. Herberman

A MAJOR PROBLEM is that most Biological Response Modifiers (BRMs) are very pleiotropic in their actions. It was hoped for some time that as we went from relatively crude microbial agents, for example, Bacillus Calmette-Guerin (BCG) or *Corynebacterium parvum*, to chemically defined, purified, even homogeneous substances, and particularly those with low molecular weight, only one function or action in the host would be observed. However, it has usually been found that low molecular weight homogeneous chemicals tend to be pleiotropic in their effects on the immune system or on other host functions.

What are the biological effects of a BRM that should be focused on? In considering the use of agents for therapeutic efficacy, it seems reasonable to place a strong emphasis on effector cells that can have cytotoxic effects on tumor cells. In classical immunologic terms, cytotoxic T lymphocytes (CTL) would be considered the main candidate for mediation of specific and potent resistance against tumor growth and progression. However, CTL would only be relevant for tumors with immunogenic, tumor associated transplantation antigens. It remains unclear what proportion of human tumors fall in this category. Although CTL with apparent specificity, with restriction to autologous and not allogeneic tumors, have been generated from lymphocytes from some cancer patients,[1,2] it has been technically difficult to extend such approaches to large numbers of patients with a wide variety of tumor types. In addition, studies with spontaneous tumors in rodents have often failed to detect tumor-associated transplantation antigens, in contrast with earlier positive results with tumors induced by oncogenic viruses or chemical carcinogens. Because almost all human tumors are, in the absence of a clearly defined etiology, considered to be spontaneous, the negative results with spontaneous rodent tumors have often been considered to be more clinically relevant.[3] There has also been considerable evidence against a central role for immune T cells in protection against a variety of tumors. For example, the incidence of spontaneous or chemical carcinogen-induced tumors has generally been the same in nude or neonatally thymectomized mice as in euthymic mice.[4] Because thymic-dependent immunity was frequently postulated to be most important for immunosurveillance and for general host resistance against tumors, this has raised questions about the overall role of the immune system in antineoplastic defenses. Similarly, there has been increasing evidence that what had previously been thought to be specific cytolytic T cells reactive against human tumors were actually natural effector cells, especially natural killer (NK) cells.[5]

There is a large amount of data to indicate that NK cells may be quite important for resistance against metastases from tumors.[6,7] If NK activity of mice or rats is depressed by various treatments, including nonspecifically with drugs such as cyclophosphamide, or more selectively with antibodies such as anti-asialo GM_1, or by use of beige mice that have a selective immunologic deficit on NK activity, one sees considerably more metastases than in control animals with normal levels of NK activity. More direct evidence that NK cells are required for resistance against metastases from some tumors has come from experiments with a rat mammary adenocarcinoma.[8] Rats pretreated with anti-asialo GM_1 developed a large increase in the number of lung metastases as compared to controls treated with normal serum. However, when NK activity was selectively restored by adoptive transfer of a purified population of large granular lymphocytes (LGLs), the small subpopulation of lymphocytes that account for virtually all NK activity, there was a concomitant restoration of resistance to the development of metastases.

Another issue that was raised by studies in experimental animals is whether monitoring of

From the Pittsburgh Cancer Institute.
Address reprint requests to Ronald B. Herberman, MD, Director, Pittsburgh Cancer Institute, 230 Lothrop St, Pittsburgh, PA 15213.

0093-7754/86/1302-0009$05.00/0

NK and other immunologic parameters only in the central and convenient sources of lymphocytes, ie, blood or spleen, is sufficient. Most metastases occur in the major organs such as the lungs or liver. Important questions then are: What is the effector activity in these organs, and is that affected in the same way by a BRM as effector cells in the blood or spleen? Procedures have been developed to isolate LGL from the lungs and liver of mice and after administration of a variety of BRMs, including MVE-2, a pyran copolymer, or *C parvum* or interferon. There was a large increase in the number of LGLs accumulating in these organs, accompanied by a marked increase in NK activity.[9] This is encouraging because it shows that the type of effector cells can be increased in the organs where metastases might be present. It also seems important to consider effector cell activity in such sites, because repeated doses of a BRM such as MVE-2 may cease to stimulate augmented NK activity in the spleen but still continues to stimulate high levels of NK activity in the liver or lungs.[10] This has potentially quite important implications for clinical studies, where one generally wants to give the agent repeatedly over a prolonged period of time. Monitoring of NK activity in the peripheral blood of patients receiving repeated high doses of interferon alpha has indicated a hyporesponsiveness to augmentation of NK activity. It would be quite helpful to develop the ability to also sample effector cells from tissue sites to determine the degree of correlation with blood levels.

For each BRM, it would be very desirable to ascertain which effector mechanism is actually responsible for the agent's antitumor effects. This would allow a focus of monitoring effects on that parameter. However, this is difficult to answer, even in experimental tumor systems. This question, however, has been approached with MVE-2, which as noted above can augment NK activity but also can strongly augment macrophage-mediated cytotoxic activity. Experiments have been performed with mice treated with anti-asialo GM_1 in addition to the BRM. When sufficient antiserum was given to ablate NK activity in the liver or lungs, MVE-2 lost its ability to protect against the development of metastases.[11] This supports the conclusion that the NK activity was, in fact, quite important in the protection afforded by the MVE-2 against this tumor. It will be important to extend such an approach to other BRMs and other tumor systems, to determine to what extent augmented NK activity is responsible for therapeutic efficacy.

Ideally, one would like to have all promising BRMs evaluated in depth for their in vivo immunologic and antitumor effects in rodents, and to determine the effector cells required for their therapeutic efficacy. However, a variety of potentially useful BRMs do not cross the species barrier. They might have potent effects, either directly on human tumor cells or indirectly on patients' effector mechanisms, but be entirely ineffective in rodents. For such BRMs, eg, most human interferons and monoclonal antibodies against human tumors, it has been necessary to rely on in vitro preclinical assessments and on studies of human tumor xenografts in nude mice.

As an example of some of the issues to be faced in studies with BRMs, it is worthwhile to consider some of the lessons learned from studies with the interferons. These represent the BRMs that have been most extensively evaluated over the last few years. The interferons represent a family of proteins that induce antiviral resistance in cells. With the advent of recombinant DNA technology, it has been possible to produce large, essentially unlimited quantities of homogeneous materials to work with. However, it has become very clear that each of the interferons that have been examined has quite pleiotropic effects. On one hand, they can directly inhibit the growth of certain tumor cells, and this could be an important mechanism by which they might be useful therapeutically. On the other hand, the interferons are very potent immunomodulators. They can augment NK cell activity and activate macrophages for antitumor cytotoxic activity. They can modulate specific T cell immunity, and change various cell surface structures, eg, tumor-associated antigens and antigens of the major histocompatibility complex, that can be quite important in immune responses against tumors. Any one of these possible effects might account for therapeutic efficacy in some circumstances. For the last several years, the interferons have been in phase I and II clinical trials, and, by now, hundreds of patients have been treated. It has become reasonably clear that certain types of tumors, particularly lymphomas and hairy cell leukemia, are highly responsive to interferon.[12,13] It is quite possible that the high degree of responsiveness that has been seen in these tumors may be related to a direct antitumor effect of interferon. There are at least some hints that higher doses are more effective than lower doses, but some excellent clinical responses have been observed with low doses. In other tumor types in which clinical responses have been seen only infrequently, it seems possible that interferons have little direct antitumor effect but might be effective if they induced potent immunomodulation. The current clinical protocols that are being used with interferon have not been shown to have optimal or even good immunomodulatory effects on parameters that would be expected to be strongly affected, based on either in vitro studies with human peripheral blood mononuclear cells or on studies in animal model systems.[14] A major concern is that one might draw a premature negative conclusion about the lack of efficacy of a BRM such as interferon when it has not been adequately tested under the appropriate circumstances. For evaluation of the potential of interferon to have a therapeutic benefit through some of its immunomodulatory effects, it would seem essential to develop protocols and schedules of administration that produce the desired alterations in the patients' immune functions. Until that has been achieved, there will not be an adequate test of the hypothesis that interferons can have therapeutic efficacy by their ability to augment immunologic effector mechanisms.

Another example of some current problems in the evaluation of BRMs has come from studies with another cytokine, interleukin 2 (IL-2). This is a product of T cells and LGLs that can stimulate the growth and function of T cells and NK cells, and by either one of these effects it might be quite useful therapeutically. In addition, most IL-2 preparations, including the recombinant materials, have recently been found to have macrophage or monocyte-activating properties. This indicates an additional functional effect of IL-2 that might have therapeutic implications and will need to be monitored during clinical trials with IL-2. Preclinical evaluation of IL-2 has been easier than that of interferons, because human IL-2 is active in mice and rats as well as in humans, so that it can be extensively tested both in vitro and in vivo in rodents as well as in humans. Recombinant IL-2 alone was found to have substantial efficacy against pulmonary metastases from B16 melanoma in mice. Significant effects were observed with modest doses of IL-2, as well as with very high doses. This indicates that phase I clinical trials should cover a wide dose range and not be restricted to very high and toxic dose levels.

The combination of IL-2 administration with the adoptive transfer of large numbers of lymphokine-activated killer (LAK) cells has recently been reported to have therapeutic efficacy in some patients with advanced, metastatic disease.[15] These encouraging preliminary results raise many important questions; eg, what is the nature of the LAK cells responsible for the in vivo antitumor effects? What is the optimal way to generate high levels of activity and maximal proliferation in vitro and in vivo of the effector cells? What doses and schedules for administration of IL-2 and LAK cells are optimal for therapy, and can one develop a protocol that will be effective and yet avoid the serious toxicity associated with the initial trial? Will systemically administered LAK cells circulate sufficiently well and reach all of the sites of tumor involvement, or could administration of effector cells directly into the area of the tumor be required instead of, or in addition to, systemic administration, in order to achieve long-lasting therapeutic benefits?

In regard to the nature of LAK cells, it was initially thought that these effector cells must be distinct from NK cells because fresh solid tumor cells are rather resistant to NK activity of unfractionated lymphoid cells.[16] However, studies in several laboratories have indicated that isolated human or mouse LGL have substantial NK activity against autologous or syngeneic, as well as allogeneic fresh tumor cells.[17,18] In addition, recent studies have indicated that the cytotoxic activity of NK cells is strongly augmented by IL-2,[19] and at least a large proportion of LAK activity is derived from lymphocytes with NK associated markers.[20]

To give insight into some of the other issues raised above, experiments have been performed in a mouse tumor model, involving the inoculation of a transplantable renal cell carcinoma under the kidney capsule.[21] This tumor follows a course of growth that is very similar to that seen clinically. After initial growth in the kidney, there is invasion through the capsule into the perinephric fat, and then regional lymph node and venous metastases followed by distant metastases. When therapy was initiated at 1 week after tumor inoculation, nephrectomy was not curative, indicating the early presence of occult metastases. Treatment with IL-2 plus IL-2-stimulated spleen cells also failed to result in long-term survival. Chemotherapy also was not particularly effective, with only a small percentage of the animals showing long-term survival.[22] In contrast, when combined therapy was performed, with Adriamycin (Adria Laboratories, Columbus, Ohio) for cytoreduction, along with IL-2 plus IL-2-stimulated spleen cells, the majority of the mice showed a long-term survival and, in fact, could be shown to be cured of their disease. When treatment was delayed until visible metastases were present,[23] more extensive combination therapy was required. A high percentage of long-term survivors could only be obtained in mice treated by surgical removal of the primary tumor, and by intraperitoneal as well as intravenous administration of chemotherapy plus adoptive immunotherapy with IL-2-stimulated cells together with IL-2. These results emphasize several points: (1) Immunotherapy is likely to only be very effective when there is a low tumor burden, and may have no detectable benefits when given alone to individuals with extensive, advanced disease. Thus, immunotherapeutic efforts should be directed toward the treatment of residual disease, after reduction of tumor burden by surgery, chemotherapy or radiotherapy. (2) Treatment directed at tumor involvement in each of several compartments may be needed for curative effects, presumably due to problems of access of the administered cells or other agents to all of the tumor cells when only systemic administration is used. (3) Dramatic therapeutic results with this approach can be achieved with relatively modest and nontoxic doses of IL-2 and cells. (4) It is also of note that recent evidence indicates that most or all of the effector cells in this experimental model have markers of NK cells and not of CTL (Salup R, personal communication, 1985).

BRMs appear to have considerable promise for therapy of malignant disease. This conclusion is based mainly on many positive therapeutic results with a wide variety of BRMs in experimental animal tumor systems.[4] The major challenge appears to be how to translate such therapeutic efficacy into a clinically applicable setting. It seems that empirically designed clinical studies, even with highly promising BRMs, will be unlikely to produce even close to optimal therapeutic efficacy. Rather, it will probably be essential to systematically evaluate the range of biological effects of each agent, particularly on anti-tumor effector cells, determine the optimal BRM dose in well-designed phase I studies, and only then perform the appropriate phase II and III therapeutic trials.

REFERENCES

1. Vanky F, Argov S: Human tumor-lymphocyte interaction in vitro VII. Blastogenesis and generation of cytotoxicity against autologous tumor biopsy cells are inhibited by interferon. Int J Cancer 26:405–411, 1980

2. Vose BM, Bonnard GD: Antigens of human tumours defined by cytotoxicity and proliferative responses of cultured lymphoid cells. Nature 296:359–361, 1982

3. Hewitt HB: Animal tumor models and their relevance to human tumor immunology. J Biol Response Mod 1:1:107–119, 1982

4. Stutman O: Chemical carcinogenesis in nude mice. Comparison between nude mice from homozygous matings and heterozygous matings and effects of age and carcinogen dose. J Natl Cancer Inst 62:353–358, 1979

5. Herberman RB (ed): Natural Cell-Mediated Immunity Against Tumors. Orlando, Fla, Academic, 1980

6. Herberman RB: Antimetastasis and immunoregulatory functions of NK cells. Fed Proc (in press)

7. Hanna N: Review of evidence for the role of NK cells in immunoprophylaxis of metastasis, in Herberman RB, Wiltrout RH, Gorelik E (eds): Immune Responses to Metastases. Boca Raton, Fla, CRC (in press)

8. Barlozzari T, Leonhardt J, Wiltrout R, et al: Direct evidence for the role of LGL in the inhibition of experimental tumor metastases. J Immunol 134:2783–2789, 1985

9. Wiltrout RH, Mathieson BJ, Talmadge JE, et al: Augmentation of organ-associated natural killer activity by biological response modifiers: Isolation and characterization of large granular lymphocytes from the liver. J Exp Med 160:1431–1449, 1984

10. Talmadge JE, Herberman RB, Chirigos MA, et al: Augmentation of induction of hyporesponsiveness of murine natural killer cell activity in different anatomical compartments by various immunomodulators including recombinant interferons and interleukin 2. J Immunol 135:2483–2491, 1985

11. Wiltrout RH, Herberman RB, Zhang S-R, et al: Role of organ-associated NK cells in decreased formation of

experimental metastases in lung and liver. J Immunol 134:4267–4275, 1985

12. Foon KA, Sherwin SA, Abrams PG, et al: Recombinant leukocyte A interferon: An effective agent in the treatment of advanced non-Hodgkin's lymphoma. N Engl J Med (in press)

13. Quesada JR, Reuben J, Manning JR, et al: Alpha interferon for induction of remission in hairy cell leukemia. N Engl J Med 310:15–18, 1984

14. Maluish AE, Leavitt R, Sherwin SA, et al: Effects of recombinant interferon-alpha on immune function in cancer patients. J Biol Response Mod 2:470–481, 1983

15. Rosenberg S, Lotze MT, Muul LM, et al: Observations on the systemic administration of autologous lymphokine activated killer cells and recombinant IL-2 to patients with metastatic cancer. N Engl J Med 313:1485–1492, 1985

16. Grimm EA, Ramsey KM, Mazumder A, et al: Lymphokinin activated killer cell phenomenon. II. Precursor phenotype is serologically distinct from peripheral T lymphocytes, memory cytotoxic thymus-derived lymphocytes, and natural killer cells. J Exp Med 157:884–897, 1983

17. Serrate SA, Vose BM, Timonen T, et al: Association of human natural killer cell activity against human primary tumors with large granular lymphocytes, in Herberman RB (ed): NK Cells and Other Natural Effector Cells. Orlando, Fla, Academic, 1982, pp 1055–1060

18. Uchida A, Yanagawa E: Natural killer cell activity and autologous tumor killing activity in cancer patients: Overlapping involvement of effector cells as determine in two-target conjugate cytotoxicity assay. J Natl Cancer Inst 73:1093–1100, 1984

19. Ortaldo JR, Mason L, Gerard JP, et al: Effects of natural and recombinant IL-2 on regulation of IFN production and natural killer activity: Lack of involvement of the TAC antigen for these immunoregulatory effects. J Immunol 133:779–783, 1984

20. Itoh K, Tilden AB, Kumagai K, et al: Leu 11^+ lymphocytes with natural killer (NK) activity are precursors of recombinant interleukin 2 (or IL-2)-induced activated killer (AK) cells. J Immunol 134:802–807, 1985

21. Salup R, Herberman RB, Wiltrout R: Role of NK activity in development of spontaneous metastases in murine renal cell cancer. J Urol 134:1236–1241, 1985

22. Salup R, Wiltrout R: Adjuvant immunotherapy of established murine cancer by interleukin 2-stimulated cytotoxic lymphocytes. Cancer Res (in press)

23. Salup R, Wiltrout R: Chemoimmunotherapy of advanced murine renal carcinoma, in Oppenheim JJ, Jacobs B (eds): The Role of Leukocytes in Host Defense. New York, Alan R. Liss, (in press)

The Adoptive Immunotherapy of Cancer Using the Transfer of Activated Lymphoid Cells and Interleukin-2

Steven A. Rosenberg

CELLULAR IMMUNE responses play an important role in the rejection of experimental allografts and tumors in murine model systems. Because of the central role played by lymphocytes in the rejection of tissue, sporadic attempts were made to interfere with the growth of established cancer in experimental models by the adoptive transfer to tumor-bearing hosts of lymphoid cells with antitumor reactivity.[1-4] The major obstacle to the development of this approach in murine tumor models was the inability to easily generate large numbers of syngeneic lymphoid cells with antitumor reactivity. In selected immunogenic tumor model systems, the repeated immunization of normal mice with irradiated tumor cells sometimes gave rise to immune lymphocytes, which when adoptively transferred, could mediate the regression of established growing murine malignancies. This technique was successful in only a limited number of murine models and was not applicable to the treatment of human malignancy. The application of this approach to the treatment of humans with cancer awaited the development of a technique for generating autologous lymphoid cells in large numbers with selective antitumor reactivity.

In 1980, we first described a phenomenon we subsequently called the lymphokine activated killer (LAK) cell phenomenon.[5-9] The incubation of normal murine splenocytes or human peripheral blood lymphocytes in the lymphokine interleukin-2 (IL-2) resulted in the generation of lymphoid cells with the ability to lyse fresh, non-cultured, natural killer (NK)–resistant cancer cells in short-term chromium release assays. These LAK cells appeared to have specificity for cancer cells and were not lytic to fresh normal lymphocytes or liver or lung cells. An example of the lymphokine activated killer cell phenomenon is shown in Table 1.[10]

The in vitro selectivity of LAK cells for malignant target cells led us to explore the possible use of these cells in the adoptive immunotherapy of a variety of murine malignancies. Conclusions drawn from extensive studies of the use of this approach in the treatment of pulmonary and hepatic metastases from a variety of animal tumor models are summarized in Table 2.[9,11-13] The central feature of successful adoptive immunotherapy using this approach involved the adoptive transfer of both LAK cells as well as IL-2. Extensive studies of the mechanisms of these effects revealed that transferred LAK cells proliferated in the tumor-bearing host with retention of specific antitumor reactivity.[14,15] It appeared that these LAK cells, expanding in vivo under the influence of IL-2, were responsible for tumor destruction. These cells are exquisitely sensitive to the continued presence of IL-2 and when IL-2 administration ceases, these lytic cellular infiltrates resorb.

We also demonstrated that the administration to mice of very high doses of IL-2 alone was capable of generating LAK cells in vivo and also mediated antitumor effects.[16,17] The study of a wide variety of animal tumor models revealed, however, that optimal therapeutic effects against established pulmonary and hepatic metastases were obtained when the combination of LAK cells and IL-2 was given. A direct relationship existed between the number of LAK cells transferred, the amoung of IL-2 given, and the therapeutic effect achieved in murine models[18]; this point is especially relevant to the application of this approach to the treatment of human malignancy.

THE USE OF LAK CELLS AND IL-2 IN THE IMMUNOTHERAPY OF HUMAN CANCER

The success of this adoptive immunotherapy approach in animal models depended on the administration of relatively large doses of IL-2 in conjunction with LAK cells. The availability of only very small amounts of IL-2 produced by stimulated lymphocytes limited the potential

From the Surgery Branch, Division of Cancer Treatment, National Cancer Institute, Bethesda, Md.

Address reprint requests to Steven A. Rosenberg, MD, PhD, Chief of Surgery, National Cancer Institute, Bldg 10, Rm 2B42, Bethesda, MD 20892.

0093–7754/86/1302–0010$0.00/0

Table 1. Generation of Human LAK Cells

	Effector Cell (% lysis ± 1 SEM)			
	LAK		Fresh PBL	
Target Cell	40:1*	10:1	60:1	15:1
Autologous sarcoma	76 ± 6	73 ± 1	−4 ± 10	−9 ± 1
Allogeneic sarcoma	88 ± 3	78 ± 2	7 ± 2	−1 ± 1
Colon cancer	62 ± 1	41 ± 3	−16 ± 1	−14 ± 1
Esophageal cancer	78 ± 5	62 ± 2	0 ± 4	−1 ± 1
Adrenal cancer	68 ± 2	41 ± 3	−16 ± 1	−20 ± 2
K562 Cultured cell line	105 ± 6	89 ± 2	46 ± 3	15 ± 1

*Effector to target ratio in four-hour ^{51}Cr release assay.

application of this approach to the human. The use of recombinant DNA technology to clone the gene for IL-2 and express it to high concentrations in *Escherichia coli* and the purification of this recombinant IL-2 to homogeneity provided a means for the production of large quantities of IL-2, thus facilitating the use of this treatment approach in humans.[19,20] In all of our studies, the biologic activity of recombinant IL-2 appeared identical to that of naturally derived IL-2.[20]

Table 2. Characteristics of the Immunotherapy of Established Murine Lung and Liver Metastases With LAK Cells and IL-2

1. Established lung and liver metastases can be inhibited by treatment with LAK cells and IL-2. Both LAK cells and IL-2 are required and either alone is less effective.
2. A direct relationship exists between the number of LAK cells administered and the therapeutic effect.
3. A direct relationship exists between the amount of IL-2 administered and the therapeutic effect.
4. Three day incubation of splenocytes appears optimal for the generation of LAK cells effective in vivo.
5. Immunotherapy with LAK cells and IL-2 is effective in hosts suppressed by total body irradiation or treatment with cyclophosphamide. Therapy is also effective in "B" mice (thymectomized, lethally irradiated, reconstituted with T cell depleted bone marrow).
6. Allogeneic LAK cells are effective in conjunction with IL-2.
7. Irradiated LAK cells (3,000 rads) are less effective than non-irradiated cells.
8. LAK cells effective in immunotherapy can be generated from the splenocytes of tumor bearing mice.
9. Successful therapy of immunogenic and nonimmunogenic sarcomas, melanoma, and a colon adenocarcinoma has been demonstrated.
10. The precursor of the LAK cells effective in vivo is a non-T cell (Thy 1^-).
11. Metastases that persist after in vivo therapy with LAK cells plus IL-2 are sensitive to LAK cell lysis both in vitro and in subsequent in vivo experiments.
12. Administration of IL-2 leads to in vivo proliferation of transferred LAK cells.

To apply this treatment approach to humans it was necessary to demonstrate that large numbers of activated lymphocytes could be administered to cancer patients with safety. It was also necessary to demonstrate that IL-2 could be administered systemically to humans and to establish the maximium tolerated doses of IL-2 by a variety of routes of administration. We, therefore, undertook a series of studies to evaluate the tolerance of humans to the infusion of large numbers of activated killer cells as well as the separate infusion of natural and recombinant IL-2 before attempting to combine these treatments in humans.[21–24] The clinical trials that led to the development of our current treatment approach using the combination of activated killer cells and IL-2 is presented in Table 3.

Before the availability of large amounts of recombinant IL-2, we had described other techniques for generating activated killer cells such as the use of incubation with lectin (phytohemagglutinin or concanavalin-A) or by pooled allosensitization.[25–29] In early trials, we demonstrated that the cells obtained from repeated leukaphereses could be activated to become killer cells by incubation in phytohemagglutinin (PAK cells) and could be reinfused into cancer patients with safety.[21,22] Up to 1.7×10^{11} activated cells from up to 15 successive leukaphereses were administered to patients. The major toxicities of this treatment included fever and chills that lasted several hours and a small decrease in the pulmonary diffusion capacity that also rapidly returned to normal. These PAK cells were administered either alone or in conjunction with cyclophosphamide or in conjunction with activated macrophages. When recombinant IL-2 became available, we performed a study of LAK cell administration in six patients with advanced

Table 3. Clinical Studies Leading to the Development of our Current Treatment Approach

Clinical Study	No. of Patients	Findings
1. Adoptive transfer of phytohemagglutinin activated killer (PAK) cells	10	Large numbers (up to 1.7×10^{11}) of activated killer cells, obtained from up to 15 successive leukaphereses, could be infused safely into humans
2. Adoptive transfer of PAK cells plus cyclophosphamide	6	Activated killer cells could be safely infused in conjunction with high-dose cyclophosphamide (50 mg/kg)
3. Adoptive transfer of PAK cells plus activated macrophages	5	Activated killer cells plus activated macrophages could be safely infused
4. Adoptive transfer of lymphokine-activated killer (LAK) cells	6	LAK cells (activated with recombinant IL-2) could be safely infused into humans
5. Administration of natural (Jurkat-derived) IL-2	16	Natural (Jurkat-derived) IL-2 could be safely infused into humans at doses up to 2 mg
6. Administration of recombinant IL-2	23	Recombinant IL-2 (from *E coli*) could be safely administered though significant toxicity was seen at high doses

NOTE. No tumor responses were seen in any of the above patients.[21-24]

cancer and observed similar toxicity to that using PAK cells.[22] Although no clinically positive effects were seen in any patient treated with activated killer cells, we did demonstrate that safe administration of these large numbers of activated killer cells could be performed.

Concomitant with the administration of activated killer cells alone, we began clinical trials utilizing the administration of IL-2 alone to patients. Sixteen patients received natural IL-2 that was purified from the Jurkat cells line.[23] In these 16 patients, we explored a variety of dose regimens and determined that IL-2 could be safely infused into humans in individual bolus doses up to 2 mg. The difficulty in obtaining large amounts of IL-2 from this natural cell line precluded the use of higher doses of IL-2. At these lower doses of IL-2, only minor toxicity was seen.

When recombinant IL-2 became available, we were able to administer much higher doses to patients.[24] In trials evaluating a variety of doses and dose schedules, up to 1 million U/kg were administered as individual intravenous bolus doses (specific activity of IL-2 is about 3 million U/mg). Using continuous infusions up to 10,000

Table 4. Summary of LAK Cell–IL-2 Treatment Plan

Week	Day	Day of Week	Treatment
1	1	Monday	IL-2 (q8h)
	2	Tuesday	IL-2 (q8h)
	3	Wednesday	IL-2 (q8h)
	4	Thursday	IL-2 (q8h)
	5	Friday	IL-2 (q8h)
	6	Saturday	
	7	Sunday	
2	8	Monday	Leukapheresis-1
	9	Tuesday	Leukapheresis-2
	10	Wednesday	Leukapheresis-3
	11	Thursday	Leukapheresis-4
	12	Friday	Leukapheresis-5/IL-2/LAK cells (1 + 2)
	13	Saturday	IL-2 (every 8 hours) + LAK (3)
	14	Sunday	IL-2 (every 8 hours)
3	15	Monday	IL-2 (every 8 hours) + LAK (4 + 5)
	16	Tuesday	IL-2 (every 8 hours)
4 and 8	Assess for antitumor response. Responding patients re-treated when progressive disease occurs.		

U/kg/h were infused. At these doses of IL-2, dose-limiting toxicity was reached. One of the primary toxicities of high dose intravenous IL-2 is a capillary permeability leak syndrome resulting in major fluid retention and fluid accumulation in visceral organs. A variety of other toxicities have been observed and have been described by us elsewhere.[22,23,30] It should be emphasized that no antitumor responses were seen in any of the 39 patients treated in these phase I trials of the administration of IL-2 to patients with advanced cancer.

In November 1984, we received permission from the Food and Drug Administration to begin clinical trials using the adoptive transfer of LAK cells in conjunction with recombinant IL-2 to patients with advanced cancer. All patients had advanced malignancy and had failed all standard therapies when available. In addition, no patient received any other form of therapy for the 30 days before entrance into this protocol or during the course of treatment in this protocol and the immediate 2-month follow-up.[31]

Though the protocol varied as we gained more experience with the combined administration of LAK cells and IL-2, the basic outline of this treatment plan is shown in Table 4. Patients received IL-2 for several days before discontinuing IL-2 and beginning five daily ieukaphereses. Following a short period of IL-2 administration, we have observed a substantial rebound in the number of LAK cell precursors in the circulation when IL-2 administration is stopped. Cells obtained from leukapheresis are put into culture using techniques we have described in detail[31] and after three to four days these cells were harvested and reinfused into the autologous patient along with the administration of IL-2. LAK cells were given intravenously (IV), generally through central venous catheters and IL-2 was also given IV at doses between 10,000 U/kg and 100,000 U/kg every eight hours. All patients had measurable cancer and were followed for at least 2 months to determine whether any antitumor responses were seen.

Table 5. Results of LAK–IL-2 Treatment Protocol as of 1/20/86*

	No. of Patients	No. of Responses
Colorectal	14	3
Melanoma	10	5
Renal	5	5
Sarcoma	5	0
Lung adenocarcinoma	4	1
Esophageal adenocarcinoma	1	0
Lymphoma	1	0
Gastrinoma	1	0
Total	41	14 (34%)

*Results of first treatment; plus eight patients awaiting 2-month follow-up; plus one patient who died during treatment and one patient lost to follow-up (received chemotherapy before posttreatment evaluation).

Results of treatment in the first 41 patients are shown in Table 5.[31,32] Detailed information concerning the exact number of doses of IL-2, the total number of units, the number of LAK infusions and the total number of LAK cells infused in each patient are shown in Table 6. Significant toxicity was seen in this trial consistent with our early experience using IL-2 alone. These toxicities are summarized in Table 7. Responses have been seen in patients with colorectal cancer, malignant melanoma, renal cell cancer, and in one patient with an unresectable lung adenocarcinoma. Regression of metastases have been observed in the lung, liver, and subcutaneous tissue. One complete response was seen and the remainder were partial regressions lasting from several months to a maximum of 16 months but follow-up is still short.

DISCUSSION

The adoptive transfer of LAK cells in conjunction with IL-2 represents a new approach to the immunotherapy of cancer that is capable of causing at least partial regressions in selected patients with advanced cancer who have failed all other available treatments. The treatment is extremely cumbersome and is associated with substantial toxicity. At the present time the majority of patients that respond experience partial remissions but not complete regressions when a single course of therapy is given.

Improvements are required in the performance of this therapy before it can be more widely applied. The procedure must be simplified, its potency increased, and its toxicity decreased. In our future efforts we will be exploring the use of multiple courses of therapy as opposed to the single therapeutic course listed above. Other approaches to be explored will be the use of allogeneic LAK cells, the direct arte-

Table 6. Immunotherapy With LAK Cells and IL-2 First Treatment With Autologous LAK Cells and IL-2

Patient	Diagnosis	No. of IL-2 Doses	Units IL-2 ($\times 10^{-3}$)	No. of LAK Infusions	Total No. of Cells Infused ($\times 10^{-10}$)	Comments
1	Melanoma	47	790	9	4.2	Complete regression of subcutaneous metastases
2	Colorectal cancer	35	510	9	4.3	Partial regression of pulmonary metastases
3	Melanoma	40	800	13	12.6	No response
4	Osteosarcoma	90	1,340	14	7.4	No response
5	Melanoma	70	700	13	11.6	No response
6	Sarcoma	76	760	9	6.6	No response
7	Melanoma	68	680	10	5.9	Partial regression of pulmonary metastases
8	Colorectal cancer	42	280	10	6.4	Partial regression of liver metastases
9	Melanoma	65	1,490	10	7.8	No response
10	Colorectal cancer	51	510	5	2.8	Treatment discontinued: IL-2 toxicity—no response
11	Colorectal cancer	76	760	10	18.4	No response
12	Colorectal cancer	71	1,830	10	9.7	No response, disease stable
13	Colorectal cancer	48	1,180	10	7.9	No response, disease stable
14	Sarcoma	66	940	10	12.6	No response
15	Esophageal cancer	68	1,200	9	10.1	No response
16	Renal cell cancer	27	2,280	5	9.9	Partial regression of pulmonary metastases
17	Colorectal	14	1,400	4	1.8	Treatment discontinued: IL-2 toxicity (hepatic), no response
18	Colorectal	36	2,200	5	5.0	No response
19	Lung adenocarcinoma	12	1,200	5	6.6	Partial regression of primary lung adenocarcinoma
20	Sarcoma	37	2,670	9	11.7	No response
21	Renal cell cancer	35	2,500	9	8.4	Partial regression of pulmonary metastases
22	Melanoma	22	1,840	5	4.4	Partial regression of pulmonary metastases
23	Colorectal cancer	39	3,180	10	17.1	No response
24	Melanoma	40	3,280	10	13.4	No response
25	Lung adenocarcinoma	36	2,880	10	9.2	No response
26	Colorectal cancer	39	3,180	10	3.6	No response
27	Melanoma	46	3,520	10	9.8	Partial regression of pulmonary and subcutaneous metastases
28	Lung adenocarcinoma	20	2,000	5	3.9	No response
29	Rhabdomyosarcoma	18	1,800	5	3.7	No response
30	Colorectal cancer	24	1,950	5	3.1	Partial regression of pulmonary metastases
31	Renal cell cancer	18	1,440	5	7.3	Partial regression of pulmonary metastases
32	Renal cell cancer	21	1,470	5	3.1	Partial regression of pulmonary metastases
33	Colorectal cancer	19	1,270	5	4.2	No response
34	Melanoma	17	1,700	10	21.2	No response
35	Lung adenocarcinoma	19	1,900	10	6.6	No response
36	Colorectal cancer	10	1,000	4	2.5	No response
37	Colorectal cancer	11	1,100	5	2.2	No response
38	Gastrinoma	15	1,500	9	4.3	No response
39	Lymphoma	18	1,800	10	27.9	No response
40	Renal cell cancer	25	2,500	5	12.3	Partial regression of lung metastases
41	Melanoma	20	2,000	8	5.3	Partial regression of subcutaneous, lung and liver metastases

rial infusion of LAK cells into organs bearing metastases and use of expanded LAK cells. The use of LAK cells expanded in vitro may provide the larger number of cells that animal models predict will have greater antitumor effects. Attempts to abrogate the toxicity of this treatment approach by the administration of steroids are under way. The combination of LAK cells and IL-2 therapy with chemotherapy or radiation therapy are also areas that deserve exploration as does the intraperitoneal instillation of LAK cells and IL-2 in patients with intraperitoneal carcinomatosis from diseases like ovarian and colorectal cancer. Finally, animal models

Table 7. Toxicity of Therapy With LAK Cells and IL-2 in 41 Patients

	No. of Patients* (Total 41)
Fever	34
Nausea or vomiting	28
Diarrhea	28
Confusion	14
Weight gain (>10% body weight)	22
Dyspnea	34
Serum creatinine >2 mg%	25
Serum bilirubin >2 mg%	32
Eosinophilia >5%	39
Anemia requiring transfusion	40
Thrombocytopenia (<50,000/μL)	18

*One additional patient died three days after completion of therapy related to complications of therapy.

predict that smaller amounts of disease will be more responsive to therapy and plans are underway to begin studies of the use of this treatment approach in patients with stage II melanoma following surgical removal of involved lymph nodes.

REFERENCES

1. Rosenberg SA, Terry W: Passive immunotherapy of cancer in animals and man. Adv Cancer Res 25:323–388, 1977
2. Rosenberg SA: The adoptive immunotherapy of cancer: Accomplishments and prospects. Cancer Treat Rep 68:233–255, 1984
3. Fefer A, Cheever MA, Greenberg PD: Lymphocyte transfer as potential cancer immunotherapy, in Mihich E (ed): Immunological Approaches to Cancer Therapies. New York, John Wiley & Sons, 1982, p 333
4. Kedar E, Weiss DW: The in vitro generation of effector lymphocytes and their employment in tunor immunotherapy. Adv Cancer Res 38:171–287, 1983
5. Yron I, Wood TA, Spiess P, et al: In vitro growth of murine T cells, V. The isolation and growth of lymphoid cells infiltrating syngeneic solid tumors. J Immunol 125:238–245, 1980
6. Lotze MT, Grimm E, Mazumder A et al: In vitro growth of cytotoxic human lymphocytes, IV. Lysis of fresh and cultured autologous tumor by lymphocytes cultured in T cell growth factor (TCGF). Cancer Res 41:4420–4425, 1981
7. Grimm EA, Mazumder A, Zhang HZ, et al: The lymphokine activated killer cell phenomenon: Lysis of NK resistant fresh solid tumor cells by IL-2 activated autologous human peripheral blood lymphocytes. J Exp Med 155:1823–1841, 1982
8. Rosenstein M, Yron I, Kaufmann Y, et al: Lymphokine activated killer cells: Lysis of fresh syngeneic NK resistant murine tumor cells by lymphocytes cultured in interleukin-2. Cancer Res 44:1946–1953, 1984
9. Rosenberg SA: Lymphokine activated killer cells: A new approach to the immunotherapy of cancer. JNCI 75:595–603, 1985
10. Rayner AA, Grimm EA, Lotze MT, et al: Lymphokine-activated killer (LAK) cells. Analysis of factors relevant to the immunotherapy of human cancer. Cancer 55:1327–1333, 1985
11. Rosenberg SA: Adoptive immunotherapy of cancer using lymphokine activated killer cells and recombinant interleukin-2, in DeVita VT, Hellman S, Rosenberg SA (eds): Important Advances in Oncology, 1986. New York, J.B. Lippincott, 1986, pp 55–91
12. Mule JJ, Shu S, Schwarz SL, et al: Adoptive immunotherapy of established pulmonary metastases with LAK cells and recombinant interleukin-2. Science 225:1487–1489, 1984
13. Lafreniere R, Rosenberg SA: Successful immunotherapy of murine experimental hepatic metastases with lymphokine-activated killer cells and recombinant interleukin-2. Cancer Res 45:3735–3741, 1985
14. Ettinghausen SE, Lipford EH, Mule JJ, et al: Systemic administration of recombinant interleukin-2 stimulates in vivo lymphoid cell proliferation in tissues. J Immunol 135:1488–1497, 1985
15. Ettinghausen SE, Lipford EH, Mule JJ, et al: Recombinant interleukin-2 stimulates in vivo proliferation of adoptively transferred lymphokine activated killer (LAK) cells. J Immunol 135:3623–3635, 1985
16. Chang AE, Hyatt CL, Rosenberg SA: Systemic administration of recombinant human interleukin-2 in mice. J Biol Response Mod 3:561–572, 1984
17. Rosenberg SA, Mule JJ, Spiess PJ, et al: Regression of established pulmonary metastases and subcutaneous tumor mediated by the systemic administration of high dose recombinant IL-2. J Exp Med 161:1169–1188, 1985
18. Mule JJ, Shu S, Rosenberg SA: The anti-tumor efficacy of lymphokine-activated killer cells and recombinant interleukin-2 in vivo. J Immunol 135:646–652, 1985
19. Tanaguchi T, Matsui H, Fujita T, et al: Structure and expression of a cloned cDNA for human interleukin-2. Nature 302:305–310, 1983
20. Rosenberg SA, Grimm EA, McGrogan M, et al: Biological activity of recombinant human interleukin-2 produced in E. coli. Science 223:1412–1415, 1984
21. Mazumder A, Eberleing TJ, Grimm EA, et al: Phase I study of the adoptive immunotherapy of human cancer with lectin activated autologous mononuclear cells. Cancer 53:896–905, 1984
22. Rosenberg SA: Immunotherapy of cancer by the systemic administration of lymphoid cells plus interleukin-2. J Biol Response mod 3:501–511, 1984
23. Lotze MT, Frana LW, Sharrow SO, et al: In vivo administration of purified human interleukin-2, I. Half life and immunologic effects of the Jurkat cell line derived IL-2. J Immunol 134:157–166, 1985
24. Lotze MT, Matory YL, Ettinghausen SE, et al: In vivo administration of purified human interleukin-2, II. Half life, immunologic effects and expansion of peripheral lymphoid cells in vivo with recombinant IL-2. J Immunol 135:2863–2875, 1985

25. Strausser JL, Mazumder A, Grimm EA, et al: Lysis of human solid tumors by autologous cells sensitized in vitro to alloantigens. J Immunol 127:266–271, 1981

26. Mazumder A, Grimm EA, Rosenberg SA: Lysis of fresh human solid tumor cells by autologous lymphocytes activated in vitro by allosensitization. Cancer Immunol Immunother 15:1–10, 1983

27. Mazumder A, Rosenstein M, Rosenberg SA: Lysis of fresh NK-resistant tumor cells by lectin activated syngeneic and allogeneic murine splenocytes. Cancer Res 43:5729–5734, 1983

28. Mazumder AM, Grimm EA, Zhang HZ, et al: Lysis of fresh human solid tumors by autologous lymphocytes activated in vitro with lectins. Cancer Res 42:913–918, 1982

29. Mazumder A, Grimm EA, Rosenberg SA: Characterization of the lysis of fresh human solid tumors by autologous lymphocytes activated in vitro with phytohemagglutinin. J Immunol 130:958–964, 1983

30. Lotze MT, Matory YL, Rayner AA, et al: Toxicity of interleukin-2 in patients with cancer. Cancer Res (in press)

31. Rosenberg SA, Lotze MT, Muul LM, et al: Observations on the systemic administration of autologous lymphokine-activated killer cells and recombinant interleukin-2 to patients with metastatic cancer. N Engl J Med 313:1485–1492, 1985

32. Rosenberg SA, Lotze MT, Muul LM, et al: A new approach to the therapy of cancer based on the systemic administration of autologous lymphokine activated killer cells and recombinant interleukin-2. Surgery (in press).

CYTOKINES

Interferons and Interferon Inducers in Cancer Treatment

Susan E. Krown

INTERFERONS (IFNs) have been referred to as prototypic biological response modifiers, second only to corticosteroids in the diversity of physiologic changes they induce.[1] Originally described as antiviral proteins in 1957,[2] it was not until more than 20 years later that sufficient supplies of partially purified human IFNs were available for evaluation in a variety of human tumors, although crude preparations had been administered to cancer patients as early as 1966.[3] Furthermore, it was not until 1981 that supplies of human IFNs produced in bacteria using recombinant DNA techniques and purified to homogeneity became available, permitting evaluation of the effects of single IFN species in the absence of contaminating proteins. It is now possible to summarize the accomplishments made thus far in the clinical application of IFNs in cancer and, more importantly, to formulate a series of questions concerning the optimal use of IFNs and to suggest approaches to answering them.

IFNs have also been referred to as "inducible inducers," ie, their production can be induced in cells by a wide variety of agents (eg, viruses, synthetic polyribonucleotides, certain fungal extracts, bacteria and bacterial products, mitogens, and specific antigens, to name a few), and their application to cells induces, in turn, the production of a wide range of substances (eg, various proteins, enzymes, prostaglandins, histocompatibility antigens) that may mediate many of IFN's effects. As part of a more general consideration of the therapeutic activity of IFNs, it appears logical to include a brief discussion of the effects of IFN inducers in cancer patients. However, as Stewart[4] has pointed out, what "interferonologists" refer to as interferon inducers are called other types of inducers by those whose interest lies in evaluating the effects of other cytokines (eg, tumor necrosis factor, colony stimulating factor, lymphotoxin, etc). Thus, in evaluating the effects of crude or partially purified IFN preparations, and particularly when evaluating the effects of so-called "IFN inducers" as potential therapeutic agents, the possible contribution of biologically active substances other than IFNs needs to be considered.

INTERFERON SPECIES—CHARACTERIZATION AND NOMENCLATURE

Interferons are a group of proteins and glycoproteins, subdivided according to differences in antigenic, biologic, and chemical properties. The three distinct antigenic types of IFNs are designed α, β and γ. IFNs α and β are stable at low pH, whereas treatment of IFN-γ at pH2 neutralizes its activity. IFNs α and β can be induced in cells of diverse origin, although those used in clinical trials have been induced, respectively, in leukocytes or lymphoblastoid cell lines and fibroblasts by viruses or synthetic polyribonucleotides. IFN-γ is an exclusive product of T lymphocytes induced by stimulation with T cell mitogens or antigens. Only single genes have been found coding for human IFNs β or γ. In contrast, at least a dozen different genes coding for IFN-α subtypes have been defined, and variations in biological activity between these subtypes have been described. Recombinant alpha IFN preparations contain products of single IFN-α genes, whereas those induced in human cells contain multiple IFN-α gene products. Although differences exist, all classes of IFN possess antiviral, immunomodulatory, and antiproliferative activities that may play a part in tumor control.

Recognizing a need for clear and consistent terminology for the many IFN species, an international committee met in 1980 to formulate recommendations for a standardized IFN nomenclature.[5] The recommendations included the abbreviation IFN for interferon, followed by the designation α, β or γ to indicate the antigenic

From the Clinical Immunology Service, Department of Medicine, Memorial Sloan-Kettering Cancer Center, New York.

Supported by grants from Hoffmann-La Roche Inc, Merck Sharp and Dohme, the American Cancer Society, and the National Institutes of Health (CA-08748 and CA-33049), and by a contract from the National Institutes of Health (CM-07435).

Address reprint requests to Susan E. Krown, MD, Memorial Sloan-Kettering Cancer Center, 1275 York Ave, New York, NY 10021.

0093-7754/86/1302-0011$05.00/0

type of IFN. When a particular IFN subtype is referred to, the antigenic type is followed by a numeric or letter designation (eg, IFN-α_2, IFN-αA), and IFNs from particular cellular sources are similarly identified (eg, IFN from leukocytes, IFN-α [Le]; IFN from lymphoblastoid cell lines, IFN-α [Ly]). Recognizing that IFNs from cells of different species have a restricted and characteristic range of cells on which they show activity, a prefix (eg, Hu for human, Mu for murine) is used to designate the species of origin; recombinant DNA-derived IFNs generally are preceded by the prefix *r* (eg, rIFN-α_2).*

Until the introduction of recombinant alpha IFNs into clinical trials in 1981, alpha IFNs prepared from human leukocytes (HuIFN-α [Le]) stimulated with Sendal virus and purified by acid precipitation techniques were those most frequently investigated in clinical trials. Although such preparations can be purified to homogeneity, the products available for clinical trials have generally not exceeded approximately 1% purity, and have had specific activities in the range of 1 to 3 $\times$ 10^6 units per milligram of protein. HuIFN-β has generally been induced in cultured foreskin fibroblasts by synthetic polyribonucleotides. Although the specific activity of the IFN-β preparations used in clinical trials reported thus far has been of the order of 10^7 U/mg of protein, the introduction of polyacrylamide-gel electrophoresis has recently permitted purification to > 1.5 $\times$ 10^8 U/mg. Production and purification of HuIFN-γ has been difficult, and supplies for clinical trials have been scarce. In the only clinical investigation reported in detail thus far,[6] the IFN-γ tested was induced in buffy coat mononuclear cells using two T cell mitogens, and was purified by a four-step chromatographic technique to a specific activity of 5.2 $\times$ 10^7 U/mg of protein (approximately 40% pure). Although this material apparently did not contain interleukin 2 or lymphotoxin, other HuIFN-γ preparations in use in preliminary clinical trials have reportedly contained variable quantities of these lymphokines. Although they have shown substantial antitumor activity, the natural IFNs described above are not likely to be developed as commercial pharmaceuticals for a variety of reasons, including high cost, relative impurity, and the variability in terms of protein heterogeneity, pyrogenicity, endotoxin content, etc, that is probably inherent in the production of any biological by natural means.

HuIFN-α (Ly) is induced in cultured Namalwa cells derived from a patient with Burkitt's lymphoma. Like HuIFN-α (Le), it contains a mixture of various IFN species, of which approximately 90% are alpha IFNs and the remaining 10% are IFN-β. Although some preparations used in early clinical trials had specific activities of only about 10^7 U/mg protein, current production and purification methods yield a product of at least 90% purity, with a specific activity of 1 to 2 $\times$ 10^8 U/mg.

The molecular cloning of human IFNs in *Escherichia coli* has permitted the large-scale production of highly purified single molecular species of various alpha IFNs, as well as IFNs-β and γ. The two most intensively studied rIFN-α preparations, rIFN-α_2 (Schering-Plough, Kenilworth, NJ) and rIFN-αA (Hoffmann-La Roche, Nutley, NJ), have been purified, respectively by affinity chromatography and monoclonal antibody columns. Both preparations are greater than 98% pure, with specific activities of at least 2 $\times$ 10^8 U/mg of protein. IFNs β and γ induced in eukaryotic human cells are glycosylated, whereas the recombinant DNA produced molecules are not. Nevertheless, the recombinant molecules recently introduced into clinical trials apparently show biological effects in vitro similar to those of the native products. Whether the lack of glycosylation will affect the absorption, distribution, and fate of these IFNs in vivo remains to be determined.

CLINICAL DEVELOPMENT OF INTERFERONS

Because of the limited supplies of IFN available when clinical trials were initiated in cancer patients, it was often difficult to determine maximally tolerated doses, treat patients for extended

*Since submission of this manuscript, new recommendations have been made for naming particular subspecies of alpha interferons (See Lancet 1: 644–645, 1985). The following designations have been proposed: Interferon alfa-2a (IFN-α2a) for rIFN-αA (Roferon-A, Hoffmann-LaRoche, Nutley, NJ); interferon alfa-2b (IFN-α2b) for rIFN-α_2 (Intron-A, Schering-Plough, Kenilworth, NJ); interferon alfa-Nl (IFN-αNl) for HuIFN-α(Ly) (Wellferon, Burroughs-Wellcome). Further modifications in standardized nomenclature are expected from the Interferon Nomenclature Committee and the World Health Organization.

periods, or conduct trials with large numbers of patients. The limited supplies also meant that most of the early studies with IFNs (particularly HuIFN-α [Le]) used empirically derived doses and treatment schedules. With the more recent development of improved methods for large scale production and purification of IFNs, and, in particular, the development of recombinant DNA technology, it has now become possible to design trials to determine the optimal conditions for the use of IFNs in terms of tumor regression and modulation of a variety of biological functions. For the most part, naturally produced IFNs have had only limited phase I trials, somewhat more extensive phase II trials, and few phase III trials have yet been reported. Alpha IFNs produced by recombinant DNA techniques and HuIFN-α (Ly) have had somewhat more phase I testing, are now being studied intensively in phase II trials, and phase III trials are just beginning. Recombinant IFNs β and γ have only begun to be tested in phase I trials, and only very preliminary results of these studies are available.

PHASE I TRIALS OF INTERFERONS

In addition to defining the toxicity and maximally tolerated dose of an agent, more recent phase I trials of IFNs are attempting to define drug doses and/or treatment schedules that induce maximal (optimal) changes in biologic responses thought to be of relevance to tumor control. This represents a novel approach to the study of a potential anticancer agent, and recognizes that a maximal dose in terms of subjective and/or objective side effects may far exceed the amount required to influence a particular cell function. It also recognizes that such cell functions (usually immune effector cell functions have been measured) may actually be impaired if too low or too high a dose is administered, while it is assumed for an agent that acts by its direct cytotoxicity to tumor cells, that the largest safely tolerated dose will also be the dose most likely to result in the greatest tumor cell destruction. Unfortunately, it is not clear which, if any, of the many effector cell functions that can be measured are directly related to tumor control, nor is it at all clear by what mechanism(s) IFN's antitumor effects are achieved in vivo in any particular tumor type. The usual patient composition of a phase I study, including patients with different tumor types, at different stages of disease, and having had different prior treatments, makes the determination of an optimal treatment regimen for an IFN, or an understanding of its mechanism of action, particularly difficult.

A number of studies have been conducted to define the toxicity and maximal tolerated dose (MTD) of alpha IFNs given by various routes and schedules. In general, the MTD has been highest for recombinant DNA produced IFNs, somewhat lower for HuIFN-α (Ly), and still lower when HuIFN-α (Le) was tested. These differences in MTD may be related to the presence of multiple IFN-α subtypes in HuIFN-α (Ly) and (Le), or to the presence of non-IFN proteins, particularly in preparations of HuIFN-α (Le). Differences in MTD have also been seen for different routes of administration (IV bolus, IV infusion, IM, or SC), for different treatment schedules (eg, daily *v* intermittent treatment), and when different criteria for dose-limiting toxicity were used (ie, objective laboratory evidence of toxicity *v* subjective symptoms). Differences in the patient populations studied may also have contributed to differences in the apparent MTD. It is noteworthy that despite differences in IFN subtypes, doses, schedules, routes of administration, and patient composition, therapeutic effects have been observed in every phase I trial of IFN-α reported thus far.

The effects of treatment with IFN alpha on immune function are even more complex and difficult to interpret, and only a few of these studies (primarily of NK cell cytotoxicity) will be cited as examples. Maluish et al[7] reported that rIFN-αA administered either as twice daily or three times weekly doses, produced no consistent augmentation of NK cell cytotoxicity and, in fact, resulted in decreased cytotoxicity in many patients, particularly those treated at higher doses. Cunningham-Rundles, at Memorial Sloan-Kettering Cancer Center, has observed an increase in NK cell cytotoxicity in approximately one third of the patients treated with once daily doses of rIFN-αA in our phase I trial, with a decrease in only about 15%. No dose-response was noted over a range of 1 million units (MU) to 54 MU. A study comparing single IM doses of two purified recombinant subspecies of IFN-α (rIFN-αA and rIFN-αD), showed that both subspecies enhanced NK cell cytotoxicity equally well at 24 hours, but that a 15 μg dose (3 MU) resulted in significantly greater NK cell stimulation than a 45 μg dose.[8]

Golub et al[9] evaluated the effects of daily treatment with partially purified HuIFN-α (Le) in patients with malignant melanoma, and found that doses of 3 or 9 MU/day for 42 days generally induced a decline in NK activity on day 1, followed by increasing cytotoxicity with a peak at day 7, and a gradual decline to pretreatment levels thereafter. Patients treated at a lower dose (1 MU) tended to lack the decline at day 1 and maintained the elevated NK activity past day 7. No correlation was noted by these investigators between the initial NK level and the subsequent response to IFN treatment. Ernstoff et al[10] monitored NK cell function in another group of melanoma patients treated as part of the same therapeutic trial, and also found a peak increase in NK activity at day 8, but only in those patients who showed subnormal NK activity before treatment. In none of the trials of which we are aware was a relationship observed between therapeutic response and the effects of treatment on NK cell cytotoxicity. It should be evident from these few examples that consistent and reproducible changes in NK cell function (and in other in vitro tests) have not been observed. It is thus impossible, at this time, to define an optimal biologic response modifying dose or schedule for a given type of IFN-α.

IFN-α is well absorbed after IM or SC injection, whereas the available evidence indicates that after IM injection of HuIFNs β and γ, serum IFN levels are not detected. In a phase I trial of HuIFN-γ, comparing the effects of IM injection, IV bolus injection, and prolonged infusion, only the latter schedule induced sustained serum IFN levels and reproducible biologic effects (neutropenia and increased serum β_2-microglobulin levels).[6] However, in a trial of HuIFN-β in which the same routes of administration were compared, systemic toxicity, white blood cell count depression and enhanced NK cell cytotoxicity were observed after IM injection even in the absence of detectable serum antiviral activity.[11] Thus, the level of IFN-β in the serum may have limited value as a predictor of in vivo activity. In vitro evidence suggests that IFN-γ activates cells more slowly than either IFNs α or β, and the prolonged in vivo exposure achieved by IV infusion may be of greater importance for HuIFN-γ than for other IFN species.

Phase I and II trials have defined a wide spectrum of side effects associated with IFN treatment (Table 1). Although best described for alpha IFNs, preliminary evidence indicates that qualitatively similar toxicities are observed with IFN-β and IFN-γ. It was initially hoped that IFNs, as natural human proteins, might lack significant toxicity, and the side effects observed in early trials were often ascribed to contaminants in the impure IFN preparations. Although such contaminants may have contributed to the observed adverse reactions, it is now apparent that IFN species purified to homogeneity have a range of characteristic toxicities similar to those of the impure material. This should not come as a surprise because, despite IFNs' natural origins, the conditions under which they are normally induced in vivo (eg, acute virus infections) are themselves associated with a range of toxic reactions.

Detailed descriptions of IFN-induced toxicity have been dealt with in several recent reviews[12,13]

Table 1. Interferon Toxicity

Constitutional	Hematologic
Fever*	Neutropenia†
Chills*	Thrombocytopenia*
Myalgias*	Anemia
Arthralgias	Coagulation Abnormalities
Anorexia*	Hepatic
Fatigue, Weakness†	Elevated transaminases†
Altered Taste	Altered drug metabolism (suppression of cytochrome p-450 activity)
Weight Loss*	
Cardiovascular	
Hypertension	
Hypotension (orthostatic)	Nervous System
Arrhythmias (atrial, ventricular)	Headache
	Lethargy*
Myocardial infarction	Confusion
Gastrointestinal	Decreased concentration*
Nausea	Mood alterations (especially depression)
Vomiting	
Diarrhea	EEG abnormalities
Altered Taste	Seizures
Renal/Metabolic	Peripheral neuropathy
Hypocalcemia	Other
Hyperkalemia	Oral Herpes simplex
Azotemia	Hair loss
Proteinuria	Antibodies to IFN
Interstitial nephritis	

*Common side effects.

†Usual dose-limiting toxicity in phase I trials.

and will not be discussed in detail here, although a few comments are in order. Although the acute side effects associated with the institution of IFN treatment may be marked (fever, chills, malaise, flu-like symptoms), these signs generally abate with continued treatment and rarely necessitate dosage attenuation. The primary dose-limiting side effects of IFN treatment, which occur with repetitive doses, are constitutional symptoms (severe fatigue, weakness, and lowered performance status), leukopenia and elevated serum hepatic transaminases. The other side effects listed in Table 1, although observed relatively infrequently, may be severe, particularly those relating to the central nervous system and the cardiovascular system. It is particularly important to exclude patients who have a history of heart disease from IFN trials, particularly trials in which high IFN doses are administered, because such patients appear most likely to experience serious arrhythmias and myocardial infarction during the course of treatment. Although IFN-induced depression of hepatic cytochrome P-450 activity has not been of major clinical importance thus far, the ability of this enzyme system to detoxify (or activate) other drugs may prove more important as combinations of IFN with other agents are investigated more intensively.

Some patients, particularly those with renal cell carcinoma, have developed neutralizing antibodies after treatment with rIFN-αA. The development of such antibodies has not been associated with other sequelae, ie, evidence of allergic reactions, or an increased incidence of viral infections. The development of neutralizing antibodies has often been accompanied by a decrease in the toxic reactions associated with IFN administration but has not invariably led to decreased therapeutic effects. The antibodies produced generally do not neutralize the multispecies HuIFN-α (Le), but neutralize a restricted range of recombinant DNA-produced IFN-α species. Neutralizing antibodies to HuIFN-α (Le) have also been reported both in patients treated with this IFN, and in some patients without prior IFN treatment, most notably those with certain autoimmune diseases. Neutralizing antibody to IFN-β has also been reported in individuals treated for nasopharyngeal carcinoma with HuIFN-β. Serine-substituted rIFN-β also induces antibodies in a high proportion of patients, but these antibodies apparently do not neutralize IFN-β activity.

PHASE II TRIALS OF INTERFERONS

The results of therapeutic trials with various alpha IFNs in a wide range of tumors are summarized in Table 2. The specific treatments used have been reviewed[1,12,13] and will not be discussed in detail, except to point out major differences in activity between different IFN-α preparations or treatment regimens. Included as tumors in which IFN-α can be considered clearly active are those in which multiple studies have confirmed antitumor activity and those like chronic myelocytic leukemia where extremely high response rates in single studies indicate substantial activity. In another group of tumors, considerable preliminary evidence also suggests antitumor activity for alpha IFNs, but confirmatory evidence of activity, or longer patient follow-up, is probably required before their clinical usefulness can be conclusively demonstrated. The third group is comprised of tumors in which there are at least some reports of antitumor activity, but in which the results of different studies have varied considerably (ie, breast cancer, malignant melanoma, multiple myeloma), or where low response rates or small patient numbers do not permit firm conclusions. The final group comprises tumor types in which several studies have failed to demonstrate antitumor activity for IFN-α.

In several tumors, differences in response rates have been observed when different IFN doses were used. In Kaposi's sarcoma, for example, low doses of rIFN-α induced negligible antitumor effects whereas high doses induced major responses in 30% to 40% of patients.[14] A similar dose response was seen in a randomized study comparing high and low doses of rIFN-αA in patients with renal cancer.[15] In patients with mycosis fungoides, reduction of the dose of rIFN-αA because of severe constitutional toxicity was associated with worsening of lesions. Upon re-escalation of the IFN dose, several patients again showed regression of skin lesions.[16]

Possible differences in the activity of various IFN-α preparations have also been observed. In patients with metastatic breast cancer, several initial trials with relatively low and well tolerated doses of HuIFN-α (Le) induced responses in over

Table 2. Summary of IFN-α Activity in Published Phase II and Phase I/II Trials

	IFN Type		
	HuIFN-α(Le)	HuIFN-α(Ly)	rIFN-α
Active			
Chronic myelocytic leukemia	+	NT	NT
Hairy cell leukemia	+	NT	+
Favorable histology NHL	+	+	+
Renal cell carcinoma	+	+	+
Kaposi's sarcoma	NT	+	+
Juvenile laryngeal papillomatosis	+	+	NT
Initial Studies Positive-Confirmation Required			
Mycosis fungoides	NT	NT	+
Superficial bladder carcinoma	+	NT	+
Unfavorable histology NHL	±	+	+
Nasopharyngeal carcinoma	+	NT	NT
Malignant gliomas	NT	+	NT
Equivocal or Conflicting Results, or Small Patient Numbers Further Study Required			
Breast cancer	+	±	±
Malignant melanoma	—	—	+
Osteosarcoma (adjuvant)	+	NT	NT
Midgut carcinoid tumors	±*	NT	NT
Multiple myeloma	+	—	+
Acute leukemias	±	±	NT
Chronic lymphocytic leukemia	±	±	NT
Hodgkin's disease	±	NT	NT
Ovarian cancer	±	±	NT
Prostate cancer	±	NT	NT
Cervical cancer	+	NT	NT
Inactive			
Non-small cell lung cancer	—	NT	—
Small cell lung cancer	NT	—	NT
Colorectal carcinoma	—	—	—
Osteosarcoma (metastatic)	—	NT	NT

Abbreviations and symbols: +, activity demonstrated; ±, minimal activity and/or inconsistent results in different trials; —, no demonstrable activity; NT, not tested or not yet reported; NHL, non-Hodgkin's lymphoma.

*Subjective improvement and decrease in excretion of tumor products, but no objective tumor regression.

20% of patients. However, subsequent trials with HuIFN-α (Ly) and rIFN-α, given in substantially higher doses, induced responses only rarely. In renal cell carcinoma, although all types of IFN-α tested have induced responses, relatively low doses of HuIFN-α (Le) were as effective as substantially higher doses of HuIFN-α (Ly) and rIFN-α. Low doses of the latter preparations were generally ineffective in this tumor. In malignant melanoma, minimal activity has been observed with HuIFN-α (Le) and HuIFN-α (Ly), whereas high doses of rIFN-αA and rIFN-α_2 have induced responses in a substantial proportion of patients. Differences in activity have also been reported when different IFNs were used to treat patients with unfavorable prognosis histologic subtypes of non-Hodgkin's lymphoma and those with multiple myeloma. These differences in apparent antitumor activity may reflect differences in the sensitivity of tumors of diverse origin to different IFN-α subtypes. However, the possibility exists that differences in the characteristics of the patients treated in different studies may account, at least in part, for the variation in observed response rates.

INTERFERON INDUCERS

One is tempted to say that, compared to IFN, relatively few trials of IFN inducers have been conducted. However, when one considers the large number of agents shown to be capable of inducing IFN production in animals[4] (including—in addition to the obvious viruses and synthetic polyribonucleotides, fungi, fungal extracts and products, whole bacteria and bacterial products, chlamydia, rickettsiae, mycoplasmas, protozoa, mitogens, and a variety of synthetic inducers including anionic polymers and low molecular weight inducers such as tilorone, cationic dyes including quinacrine, and various substituted pyrimidines), it must be admitted that many such agents have been used in clinical trials for years, but were not specifically studied for their IFN-inducing capabilities. One may speculate that IFN inducers have been used in cancer therapy since the time of William Coley, who began to administer mixed bacterial toxins to cancer patients close to a century ago.

Although many agents are capable of inducing IFN under appropriate experimental circumstances, only polyriboinosinic-polyribocytidylic acid (poly IC) and poly IC complexes have been shown to consistently induce IFN in humans. Several phase I trials of poly IC were performed in the late 1960s and early 1970s in advanced cancer patients.[17,18] The side effects were, in some cases, similar to those observed with exogenously administered IFNs, ie, fever and flu-like symptoms. In addition, abnormalities in liver enzymes, coagulation abnormalities and acute hypersensitivity reactions were occasionally observed, although no antibodies to poly IC were detected. In general, low and inconsistent serum levels of IFN were observed, and there was no clear relationship between the dose of poly IC and the amount of IFN induced. Refractoriness to IFN induction was observed after one or more doses, but the optimal interval between doses was not determined.

The modest and inconsistent ability of poly IC to induce IFN was believed to be the result of serum nucleases that could rapidly hydrolyze and inactivate the compound. This led to efforts to develop stabilized complexes of poly IC that were more resistant to hydrolysis. Two such complexes, poly ICLC and poly ICL, were developed. Poly ICLC consists of poly IC complexed with poly-L-lysine and stabilized with carboxymethylcellulose; poly ICL lacks the carboxymethylcellulose. Both compounds induced a wide range of side effects including fever, severe chills, hypotension, malaise, dyspnea, nausea, vomiting, headache, myalgias, and arthralgias.[19–21] A serum sickness-like reaction with erythema overlying tender joints was noted in some patients treated with poly ICLC. Two of five patients treated with poly ICL showed acute hypersensitivity reactions during treatment. Antibodies to poly IC, poly-L-lysine, poly I, and the poly ICL complex were detected in the serum of these patients in an ELISA assay, and were also detected in the posttreatment serum of some patients treated with poly ICL, or poly ICLC, who had shown no hypersensitivity reactions.[21] Although poly IC complexes proved to be better inducers of IFN than poly IC, there was tremendous individual variation in serum IFN titers after a given dose, and maximum tolerated doses for given individuals also varied over a wide range. The IFN induced by poly ICLC and poly ICL has been characterized as IFN-α by antigenic and biologic criteria.

There is limited evidence of therapeutic activity for poly IC and its complexes. Early reports suggested a possible increase in remission duration in patients with acute myelocytic leukemia given poly IC during maintenance chemotherapy, but this was not confirmed in a randomized trial. Although poly IC treatment had no effect on recurrence rates or the development of invasive disease in patients with superficial bladder cancer, a significant prolongation in survival has been reported for patients treated with poly IC compared to those treated with local tumor fulguration alone.[22] In phase I trials of poly ICLC, partial regression of metastatic renal cell cancer and remission of acute lymphocytic leukemia have been observed in single patients. However, a subsequent phase II trial of poly ICLC in childhood leukemia showed no antitumor effects. Preliminary reports have also suggested possible therapeutic activity in small numbers of patients with multiple myeloma and juvenile laryngeal papillomatosis.

FUTURE PROSPECTS

The results of the clinical trials conducted thus far strongly suggest that IFNs will prove to be useful additions to currently available cancer treatments. For diseases like renal cell cancer and hairy cell leukemia, IFNs have induced responses in a significantly higher proportion of patients than conventional therapies. In such tumors, a continuing role for IFN treatment seems likely, although it still remains to be determined whether such treatment modifies their natural history. For other tumors in which IFNs have shown activity but for which effective treatments already exist (eg, lymphomas, breast cancer), a role for IFN will be more difficult to define. Such a role might be determined through studies of IFN in combination with cytotoxic drugs or radiation therapy, or in trials in which IFN is used in patients with minimal tumor burden in an attempt to prevent or delay tumor recurrence.

A number of critical questions must be addressed before the role of IFNs in cancer therapy can be precisely defined and before recommendations can be made for wide-scale application.

What Is an Optimal Dose and Schedule?

In some tumors this question has been partially answered (eg, in renal cell cancer and Kaposi's sarcoma, in which high doses proved superior to low doses of rIFN-αA). For the most part, however, the answer to this question has been elusive whether the endpoint measured was tumor regression or modification of a particular biological response, for example, natural killer cell cytotoxicity. It may be that optimal doses and schedules may vary for different tumors, for different IFNs, and even for different patients. Definition of an optimal treatment regimen will undoubtedly depend, at least in part, upon answers to another question.

What Are the Mechanisms of Interferons' Antitumor Effects?

Again, this may differ for different tumors and for different types of IFNs. In some tumors, IFNs may serve primarily as antiproliferative agents. In others, they may modify immune effector cell mechanisms. In some cases, IFNs may affect the differentiation of tumor cells, while in others (eg, laryngeal papillomas) one may speculate that IFN's antiviral effects play a role in tumor control. It is also possible to speculate that IFNs may modify the expression of cell surface antigens on tumor cells, rendering them more susceptible to control by existing immune effector mechanisms. Although it is not the purpose of this discussion to elaborate on all these possibilities, it is clear that better definition of these potential mechanisms could result in improvements in clinical trial design. Such definitions will require the development of in vitro and animal models, as well as the development and application of better tests to monitor patients treated with IFNs. Such tests may prove to be useful probes for understanding IFNs' mechanism(s) of action by defining functional changes induced by IFNs that are associated with antitumor response, or by predicting which patients are most likely to respond to IFN treatment. If modification of a particular biological response could be shown to be associated with antitumor activity, protocols aimed at finding an IFN dose and schedule inducing an optimal change in that response should be devised.

As an increasing number of highly purified IFNs become available, a third question becomes important.

Which Is the Best Interferon for a Particular Tumor?

Differences in biological activities exist between the three broad antigenic types of IFNs, and between the various IFN-α subspecies. Although there is, as yet, insufficient clinical experience to determine whether these differences will prove to be of major therapeutic significance, at least some case reports exist of patients in whom treatment with HuIFN-α (Le) was successful after a trial of HuIFN-β failed.[23] Furthermore, the observation that the multispecies HuIFN-α (Le) given at relatively low doses was as effective as high doses of a single IFN-α species (rIFN-αA) in inducing regression of renal cell cancer, whereas low doses of rIFN-αA were ineffective, suggests an important contribution of other IFN-α subtypes to the observed tumor responses. More substantial evidence suggesting possible therapeutic differences between IFNs has been obtained in in vitro studies. Although the growth of almost all normal and transformed cell lines can be inhibited by IFNs, differences in relative potencies exist between IFNs α, β, and γ for cells of diverse origin.[24,25] Furthermore, a unique role for IFN-γ in the treatment of certain lymphohematopoietic tumors has been suggested by the results of in vitro studies that indicate that this IFN, but not IFN-α or IFN-β, can induce terminal differentiation of leukemic cells of B cell, monocytic, and myeloid origin.[26–28] These types of observations merit formal study in carefully designed clinical trials.

Although most IFN trials in humans have concentrated on evaluating its activity as a single agent, it is clear that no single drug or treatment modality has resulted in the optimal treatment for any common cancer. Now that the activity and toxicity of at least some IFN species have been evaluated for some years, another important question arises.

How Can Interferons Be Best Combined With Existing Approaches to Cancer Treatment?

Addressing this question will pose a particular challenge because the results of in vitro and animal studies and some clinical trials have already suggested a large number of possible combinations of IFNs with other therapeutic modalities that have the potential for increasing the efficacy of treatment. Among the possibilities suggested by the results of in vitro and animal studies are combinations of IFNs with chemotherapeutic agents, other immunomodulators, other IFN species, radiation therapy, hyperthermia, and hormones.

Combinations of murine IFN-α/β and various chemotherapeutic agents have shown additive or synergistic antitumor activity against a variety of murine leukemias. Synergistic inhibition of tumor growth has also been observed for human IFN-α/chemotherapy combinations in certain human tumors growing in nude mice or cell cultures, eg, cyclophosphamide and IFN-α in breast cancer, doxorubicin and IFN-α in ovarian cancer, vinblastine and IFN-α in renal cancer and difluoromethylornithine (DFMO) and IFN-α in malignant melanoma.[1,13] Few reports of IFN/chemotherapy combinations in cancer patients have been published thus far. In the single published trial using fixed doses of HuIFN-α (Le) and vinblastine in renal cell cancer, increased toxicity, but no increase in antitumor activity over that seen with IFN alone, was observed.[29] A phase I trial of the combination of HuIFN-α (Le) and orally administered DFMO demonstrated increased gastrointestinal toxicity for the combination over that seen at similar doses of DFMO alone.[30] The observation of two partial and one minor response among seven patients with malignant melanoma treated as part of this trial is noteworthy, and suggests that further investigation of this combination is warranted. The unexpectedly severe toxicity of such combinations in some cases suggests that phase I trials, to define toxicity, optimal doses, and schedules of such combinations, should routinely precede efficacy trials. Another area in which IFN/chemotherapy combinations warrant investigation has been suggested by the results of studies in mice, in which the ability of IFN to slow cell cycling, with accumulation of cells in G_0/G_1, has been used to protect mice from toxic doses of a cell-cycle specific drug, 5-fluorouracil.[31] The possibility has been suggested that, depending upon the relative sensitivities of normal and tumor cells to the antiproliferative effects of IFN, that variations in the timing of IFN and an S-phase specific drug might be used to increase the therapeutic index.

Various immunomodulators, when combined with murine IFN or IFN inducers, have been reported to increase antitumor activity or to increase in vivo IFN induction. Synergistic cytotoxic effects of human IFNs α and γ in combination with tumor necrosis factor (TNF) against a panel of human tumor cell lines has also been reported.[32] Considerable evidence suggests that the combination of IFN-γ with either IFN-α or IFN-β induces synergistic antiviral and antitumor effects.[33] Synergistic antitumor activity has been described both in vitro for murine and human tumor cell lines, and in intact mice bearing transplanted or radiation-induced tumors. The synergistic effects may be explained by the existence of separate cell surface receptors for IFNα/β and IFN-γ,[34] and by the induction by IFN-α/β and IFN-γ of distinct groups of polypeptides[35] that may mediate the anticellular effects of IFN.

Under most experimental conditions, IFN has been shown to act as a radiation sensitizer,[13] possibly by altering the distribution of cells through the phases of the cell cycle. Certain clinical observations also support a potential role for human IFN-α as a radiation sensitizer. In patients with small cell lung cancer treated with a combination of radiation therapy, chemotherapy, and HuIFN-α (Le), an increased incidence of severe radiation pneumonitis has been observed. Anecdotal reports have also appeared of regression or stabilization of pulmonary osteosarcoma metastases after treatment with low dose radiation and HuIFN-α (Le). Severe oral mucositis has also been reported in two patients with Kaposi's sarcoma receiving concomitant radiation and rIFN-αA therapy.[36] Under certain experimental conditions, however, both IFN and poly ICLC have been reported to act as radioprotective agents in mice, and it has been suggested that this effect may be mediated through stimulation of NK cell activity.[37] These experimental and clinical data suggest that additional studies to investigate the nature of the interactions between radiation and IFN should be undertaken to define the conditions under which these treatment modalities can be safely and successfully combined.

A number of other observations also suggest potential clinical applications. Hyperthermia has been reported to increase the antiproliferative effects of IFN in tumor-bearing mice and in human transitional cell carcinoma cell lines.[38] In the latter case, the increased antiproliferative effects were associated with a marked increase in the production of an IFN-induced enzyme, 2-5A synthetase. The increased expression of estrogen receptors observed in cultured human breast cancer cells treated with IFN-α[39] has also suggested the possibility of combining IFN with anti-estrogens in patients with breast cancer. Many other examples exist, offering numerous possibilities and challenges.

CONCLUSIONS

Over the next few years we can anticipate that answers to many of the questions regarding the optimal use of IFNs posed in the previous section will be forthcoming. Trials are already underway, or planned, to intensively evaluate IFNs other than IFN-α, to investigate the effects of IFN-α in combination with cytotoxic drugs, radiation therapy and IFN-γ, and to evaluate the potential of IFN-α as adjuvant therapy following conventional surgical or chemotherapeutic treatments in tumors such as malignant melanoma or nodular lymphomas. As biological differences between different IFN-α subtypes are better defined, and structure-activity analysis of these molecules proceeds, it is likely that IFN-α hybrids, prepared by gene splicing techniques, will be engineered to maximize specific antiviral, antiproliferative, or immunomodulatory effects. Preliminary, in vitro studies also suggest that different IFN species and IFN-α subtypes may differ in their tissue specificities,[1] and continued studies along these lines may permit the selection of the most appropriate IFN type for a given tumor.

The future for IFN inducers is more difficult to forsee. With the increasing availability of exogenous IFNs, many have expressed doubts regarding a continued role for these compounds, particularly in view of their toxicity, the variable levels of IFN induced and the refractoriness to IFN induction that invariably develops during the course of treatment. However, there are at least theoretical advantages to this approach, including differences in tissue distribution of IFNs induced in vivo. The induction of biologically active substances other than IFNs by such agents certainly deserves further study, as does the development of less toxic inducers that show less variability in their IFN-inducing capabilities. Using the methods currently available to monitor the effects of such compounds on lymphokine production, it should soon be possible to determine whether continued investigation of these agents is warranted.

REFERENCES

1. Borden EC: Interferons and cancer: How the promise is being kept, in Gresser I (ed): Interferon V, Orlando, Fla, Academic, 1984, p 43

2. Isaacs A, Lindenmann J: Virus interference. I. The interferon. Proc R Soc Lond (Biol) 147:258–267, 1957

3. Falcoff E, Falcoff R, Fournier F, et al: Production en masse, purification partielle et characterization d'un interferon destive a des essais therapeutiques humans. Ann Inst Pasteur 111:562–569, 1972

4. Stewart WE II: The Interferon System. Vienna, Springer-Verlag, 1979, p 27

5. Stewart WE II, Blalock JE, Burke DC, et al: Interferon nomenclature. J Immunol 125:2353, 1980

6. Gutterman JU, Rosenblum MG, Rios A, et al: Pharmacokinetic study of partially pure γ-interferon in cancer patients. Cancer Res 44:4164–4171, 1984

7. Maluish AE, Ortaldo JR, Sherwin S, et al: Immunological monitoring of patients receiving recombinant leukocyte A interferon. Proc Am Soc Clin Oncol 1:39, 1982

8. Edwards BS, Hawkins MJ, Borden EC: Comparative in vivo and in vitro activation of human NK cells by two

recombinant interferons alpha differing in antiviral activity. Cancer Res 44:3135–3139, 1984

9. Golub SH, Dorey F, Hara F, et al: Systemic administration of human leukocyte interferon to melanoma patients. I. Effects on natural killer function and cell populations. J Natl Cancer Inst 68:703–710, 1982

10. Ernstoff MS, Hebert GZ, Kirkwood JM: Parameters of interferon action. Natural killer (NK) activation during a phase II trial. Proc Am Assoc Cancer Res 23:247, 1982

11. Hawkins MJ, Krown SE, Borden EC, et al: American Cancer Society phase I trial of naturally produced β-interferon. Cancer Res 44:5934–5938, 1984

12. Kirkwood JM, Ernstoff MS: Interferons in the treatment of human cancer. J Clin Oncol 2:336–352, 1984

13. Krown SE: Clinical trials of interferons in human malignancy, in Pfeffer L (ed): Mechanisms of Interferons' Actions. Boca Raton, CRC Press, 1986 (in press)

14. Real FX, Krown SE, Krim M, et al: Treatment of Kaposi's sarcoma with recombinant leukocyte A interferon (rIFN-αA). Proc Am Soc Clin Oncol 3:55, 1984 (abstr)

15. Quesada JR, Gutterman JU, Rios A: Investigational therapy of renal cell carcinoma with recombinant alpha interferon. Proc Am Assoc Cancer Res 24:195, 1983

16. Bunn PA Jr, Foon KA, Ihde DC, et al: Recombinant leukocyte A interferon: An active agent in advanced cutaneous T cell lymphoma. Ann Intern Med 101:484–487, 1984

17. Robinson RA, De Vita VT, Levy HB, et al: A phase I–II trial of multiple-dose polyriboinosinic-polyribocytidylic acid in patients with leukemia or solid tumors. J Natl Cancer Inst 57:599–601, 1976

18. Field AK, Young CW, Krakoff IH, et al: Induction of interferon in human subjects by poly I:C. Proc Soc Exp Biol Med 136:1180–1186, 1971

19. Levine AS, Sivulich M, Wiernik PH, et al: Initial clinical trials in cancer patients of polyriboinosinic-polyribocytidylic acid stabilized with poly-L-lysine, in carboxymethylcellulose (poly ICLC), a highly effective interferon inducer. Cancer Res 39:1645–1650, 1979

20. Krown SE, Kerr D, Stewart WE II, et al: Phase I trial of poly ICLC in patients with advanced cancer, in Hersh EM, Chirigos MA, Mastrangelo MJ (eds): Augmenting Agents in Cancer Therapy. New York, Raven, 1981, p 165

21. Krown SE, Friden GB, Khansur T, et al: Phase I trial with the interferon inducer poly I:C/poly-L-lysine (poly ICL). J Interferon Res 3:281–290, 1983

22. Kemeny N, Yagoda A, Wang Y, et al: Randomized trial of standard therapy with or without poly I:C in patients with superficial bladder cancer. Cancer 48:2154–2157, 1981

23. Gobel V, Arnold W, Wahn V, et al: Comparison of human fibroblast and leukocyte interferon in the treatment of severe laryngeal papillomatosis in children. Eur J Pediatr 137:175–176, 1981

24. Borden EC, Hogan TF, Voelkel JC: The comparative antiproliferative activity in vitro of natural interferons α and β for diploid and transformed human cells. Cancer Res 42:4948–4953, 1982

25. Broxmeyer HE, Lu L, Platzer E, et al: Comparative analysis of the influences of human gamma, alpha and beta interferons on human multipotential (CFU-GEMM), erythroid (BFU-E) and granulocyte-marcophage (CFU-GM) progenitor cells. J Immunol 131:1300–1305, 1983

26. Al-Katib A, Wang CY, Koziner B: γ-interferon (IFN-γ)-induced phenotypic changes of chronic lymphocytic leukemia (CLL) and non-Hodgkin's lymphoma (NHL) cells. Proc Am Assoc Cancer Res 25:235, 1984

27. Kelley VE, Fiers W, Strom TB: Cloned human interferon-γ, but not interferon-α or -β, induces expression of HLA-DR determinants by fetal monocytes and myeloid leukemic cell lines. J Immunol 132:240–245, 1984

28. Ralph P, Harris PE, Punjabi CJ, et al: Lymphokine inducing "terminal differentiation" of the human monoblast leukemia line U937: a role for γ interferon. Blood 62:1169–1175, 1983

29. Figlin RA, de Kernion JB, Maldazys J, et al: Human leukocyte interferon (IFN)/vinblastine (VBL) therapy for metastatic renal cell carcinoma (RCCa). Proc Am Soc Clin Oncol 3:49, 1984

30. Talpaz M, Quesada J, Gutterman JU: Phase I study of difluoromethylornithine (DFMO) and leukocyte interferon (IFNα) in cancer patients (pts.) Proc Am Soc Clin Oncol 3:63, 1984

31. Stolfi RL, Martin DS, Sawyer RC, et al: Modulation of 5-fluorouracil-induced toxicity in mice with interferon or with the interferon inducer, polyinosinic-polycytidylic acid. Cancer Res 43:561–566, 1983

32. Williamson BD, Carswell EA, Rubin BY, et al: Human tumor necrosis factor produced by human B-cell lines: Synergystic cytotoxic interaction with human interferon. Proc Natl Acad Sci USA 80:5397–5401, 1983

33. Czarniecki CW, Fennie CW, Powers DB, et al: Synergistic antiviral and antiproliferative activities of *Escherichia coli*-derived human alpha, beta and gamma interferons. J Virol 49:490, 1984

34. Anderson P, Yip YK, Vilcek J: Specific binding of ^{125}I-human interferon-γ to high affinity receptors on human fibroblasts. J Biol Chem 257:11301–11304, 1982

35. Weil J, Epstein CJ, Epstein LB, et al: A unique set of polypeptides is induced by γ interferon in addition to those induced in common with α and β interferons. Nature 301:437–439, 1983

36. Real FX, Krown SE, Nisce LZ, et al: Unexpected toxicity from radiation therapy in two patients with Kaposi's sarcoma receiving interferon. J Biol Response Mod 4:141–146, 1985

37. Ortaldo JR, McCoy JL: Protective effects of interferon in mice previously exposed to lethal irradiation. Radiat Res 81:262–266, 1980

38. Borden EC, Groveman DS, Merritt JA: Augmented antiproliferative effects of alpha interferons at increased temperature. Proc Assoc Cancer Res 24:195, 1983

39. Dimitrov NV, Meyer C, Einhorn S, et al: Interferon as an estrogen receptor modifier. Proc Am Assoc Cancer Res 22:373, 1981

Lymphokines: From Conjecture to the Clinic

Steven Gillis, Paul J. Conlon, David Cosman, Thomas P. Hopp, Steven K. Dower, Virginia Price, Diane Y. Mochizuki, and David L. Urdal

THROUGHOUT THE DECADE of the 1960s, and for the most part, well into the 1970s, the existence of lymphokines as discrete chemical entities remained, to a certain extent, unproven and unsupported by hard chemical or molecular data. Toward the late 1970s, with the development of discrete, reproducible, and unequivocal assays for lymphokine function, which took advantage of monitoring the response of cloned lympokine-dependent cell lines, lympokines in general entered into a world of new credibility. Molecules that were previously dismissed by several investigators as almost mythical components of culture supernates, began to take on characteristics more akin to proteins with defined size, ion exchange characteristics, as well as enzymatic and proteolytic sensitivities. The later advent of sophisticated biochemical approaches (particularly high pressure liquid chromatography) and molecular biology led to the precise biochemical and molecular characterization of lympokine gene products. In addition, recombinant DNA techniques capable of directing the biosynthesis of lymphokine proteins in heterologous prokaryotic expression systems provided both the commercial and scientific impetus to produce sufficient quantities of homogeneous lymphokine protein for testing in both preclinical and clinical conditions.

The progression from bioassay, to cell line source, to purified protein, to protein sequence, to oligonucleotide screening of cDNA libraries, to isolation of an appropriate lymphokine gene cDNA clone, and finally to large-scale production of lymphokine protein for in vivo testing is now a pathway that has been traveled by several molecules. First by interferon-γ, and then in rapid succession by Interleukin-2 (IL-2), granulocyte-macrophage colony stimulating factor, and Interleukin-1 (IL-1). Several of the abovementioned lymphokines are now as far along as phase II and phase III clinical trials, and important clinical data detailing the therapeutic use of these molecules is now at hand. In the following paragraphs, we will review several of the approaches used in the molecular characterization of lymphokines, and will hopefully illuminate areas of potential therapeutic utility that have been uncovered by preclinical experimentation in animal model systems using purified recombinant lymphokine proteins.

INTERLEUKIN-2

Originally known as T cell growth factor,[1] investigators in the late 1970s became intrigued with IL-2 simply as a component of conditioned medium from mitogen-activated leucocytes that had the capacity to maintain in long-term in vitro culture clones of antigen-specific activated T cells.[2] This in vitro use of the molecule should still not be overlooked, as it provided both clinical and basic immunologists with the ability to grow, for the first time, large numbers of various types of T cells (helper cells, suppressor cells, and, particularly, cytotoxic T lymphocytes and natural killer [NK] cells) that led to several important studies on the role of such cell types in both health and disease situations.[3-5] In addition, IL–2-dependent culture of T cell clones has been instrumental in unlocking the mystery surrounding the molecular nature of the T cell antigen receptor,[6] as well as providing a useful reagent for identification of histocompatibility gene products in clonal mixed lymphocyte cultures.[7] Finally, IL–2-dependent growth of T cells has led to the understanding of an extremely important system controlling the replication of immune cells—a system involving the binding of IL-2 in a hormone-line fashion to a specific receptor that sits on the surface of cells that have the capacity to respond to the lymphokine.[8] As such, IL-2 itself was an instrumental reagent in molecular dissection of the IL-2 receptor,[9] and of the hormone/high affinity receptor interaction that is critical to T cell replication.[10]

It was in vitro experimentation in the late 1970s and early 1980s that provided clues to the potential importance of IL-2 as a regulator of immune responses. Addition of IL-2 to various in

From the Immunex Corporation, Seattle.

Address reprint requests to Steven Gillis, PhD, Immunex Corp, 51 University St, Seattle, WA 98101.

0093–7754/86/1302–0012$05.00/0

vitro immune reactions provided remarkable effects. IL-2 was shown to be able to boost the generation of antigen-specific cytotoxic T cells,[11] to augment NK cell activity,[12] and to reverse immune suppression caused by glucocorticoids.[13] Furthermore, because of its ability to cause replication of T cells that produced yet other lymphokines which, in turn, acted on B lymphocytes, IL-2 was shown to enhance plaque-forming cell responses and antibody secretion in vitro.[14] Finally, tumor-specific cytolytic T cells maintained in culture for long periods of time in IL-2, were shown to have significant therapeutic effect upon adoptive transfer into appropriately challenged mice.[15]

The capacity to demonstrate IL-2's effectiveness in augmenting immune responses in vitro was an important step forward for understanding the power of this lymphokine in controlling T cell-dependent immune reactivity. However, in order to fully test the capacity of this hormone to enhance immune responses in vivo, clearly large amounts of truly homogeneous IL-2 would be required. With the development of an unequivocal assay for IL-2 activity in the late 1970s,[16] it took biochemically-oriented immunologists some 2 to 3 years to develop reproducible schemes for purifying natural IL-2 in large quantity.[17–19] Despite the elegance of these procedures, the ability to produce milligram quantities of IL-2 (amounts required by large-scale in vivo animal model experiments) could not be generated using these techniques. With the publishing of the cloning of the human IL-2 gene in early 1983,[20] molecular biologists devised numerous schemes for both bacterial and yeast-based expression of recombinant human and murine IL-2. Since that time, several individual investigators and competing commercial organizations have produced gram quantities of recombinant IL-2 for investigational purposes.

IL-2 has now entered phase II clinical trials as a treatment for malignancy, either alone or in conjunction with IL–2-activated killer cells. Significant recent attention has focused on the successful preliminary results of therapeutic investigations conducted by Steven Rosenberg.[21] In these investigations, leukophoresed cancer patients were given back their own in vitro IL–2-activated T cells in conjunction with large quantities of IL-2. Such a treatment protocol is in part based on successful animal studies previously reported by both Rosenberg[22] and Cheever et al.[23] A separate chapter in this book will deal with the human clinical utility of human IL-2 plus LAK cells in cancer situations, thus repetition of results of these studies in an additional setting would be inappropriate. In addition, single agent phase II trials of IL-2 in cancer patients are under way, but only preliminary results are currently available.

However, in addition to its potential as an anticancer therapeutic, IL-2 holds considerable promise as an agent that could be used therapeutically to augment immune responses in patients whose immune reactivity had been severely compromised by treatment with various cytoreductive therapies (ie, chemotherapy and transplantation). Specific examples of IL-2's potential effects in these clinical situations have been demonstrated in our laboratories in animal model systems; for example, in a model testing the capacity of C57Bl/6 mouse splenocytes to mount a cytotoxic T cell response following alloantigen (P815 mastocytoma cells) challenge. Using this model system, in vivo IL-2 administration has been shown to overcome immune deficiency caused either by prior in vivo administration of hydrocortisone or cyclophosphamide. Figure 1 details immune responsiveness of immunocompromised animals following in vivo IL-2 therapy. Normal mice given P815 tumor cells intraperitoneally (IP) (10^7 cells on day 0) contain splenocytes that, when harvested ten days after alloantigen challenge, mount an excellent cytotoxic T cell response manifested in vitro by specific lysis of ^{51}chromium-labeled P815 mastocytoma cells. Treatment of animals on days −1 or 0 with hydrocortisone acetate (2.5 mg IP) resulted in the generation of a spleen cell population incapable of responding to P815 tumor cell challenge. Treatment of various cohorts of hydrocortisone pretreated alloantigen-challenged mice with either a carrier solution (saline containing human serum albumen at 1 mg/mL), or various sources of IL-2, revealed that treatment of immunocompromised mice with either natural human or recombinant IL-2 IP daily, 1 μg/mouse for eight days, had the capacity to restore the cytolytic response against alloantigen to either normal or supernormal levels. Moreover, it should be noted that the in vivo

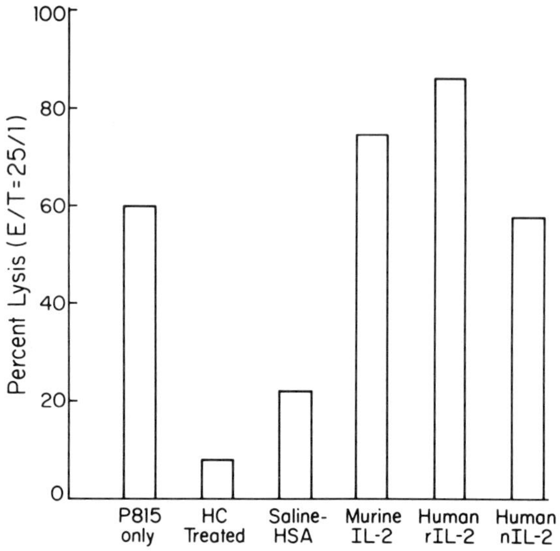

Fig 1. Comparison of various sources of IL-2 to restore the cytolytic response to allogeneic tumor challenge following hydrocortisone acetate-induced suppression. Twenty-four hours after HC and allogeneic tumor cell administration, various groups of mice were treated IP for eight days with PBS-HSA, or 5×10^5 U IL-2 derived from the murine T cell lymphoma, LBRM-33-5A4 (murine IL-2), human recombinant IL-2 (rIL-2), or natural human IL-2 derived from the leukemic cell line, Jurkat (nIL-2). One group received no P815 tumor cell administration following HC pretreatment, but did receive 5×10^5 U/d rIL-2. On day 9, splenic cytolytic activity was measured against ^{51}Cr-labeled P815 cells. Lytic activity is shown at an effector to target cell ratio of 25:1.

administration of recombinant IL-2 in the absence of allogeneic tumor cell challenge did not lead to the generation of cytotoxic T cells having the capacity to kill P815 tumor cells. Thus, both antigenic stimulation and IL-2 were required for the in vivo generation of alloreactive cytolytic T lymphocytes (CTL).

In subsequent experiments, we determined that IL-2 therapy (1 μg IP/dose) could be administered on an every other day schedule without abrogating to any extent the capacity of the treatment to restore immune responsiveness in hydrocortisone-treated animals. Alternatively, steroid-induced immune deficiency, as manifested in the above-detailed model system can be overcome by treatment of animals with recombinant IL-2 via gradual release from an implanted mini-osmotic pump.

We have used an additional model to study the efficacy of IL-2 therapy on immunocompromised mice. In this particular model, the radiomimetic drug, cyclophosphamide, was given to animals intravenously (IV) at a dose of 40 mg/kg body weight six days following allogeneic tumor cell administration. Treatment of C57Bl/6 mice in such a manner significantly reduced the cytolytic activity manifested by murine spleen cells harvested from treated animals on day 10. However, if similarly cyclophosphamide-treated mice were given 2 μg of recombinant IL-2 IP 48 hours after cyclophosphamide treatment, then a significant cytotoxic response to the allogeneic P815 tumor cells was observed.

A comparison of the capacity of natural and recombinant-derived human IL-2 to overcome cyclophosphamide-induced unresponsiveness in the generation of alloreactive cytotoxic T cells is shown in Fig 2. Animals were injected IP with 2×10^7 P815 cells followed six days later by IV treatment with either carrier protein only, or 40 mg/kg body weight cyclophosphamide. Two days later, on day 8, various cohorts of mice received either carrier protein only, natural, pure, human IL-2 (2 μg IP), or pure, recombinant human IL-2.

As suggested above, the normal cytolytic response to allogeneic tumor cells was depressed

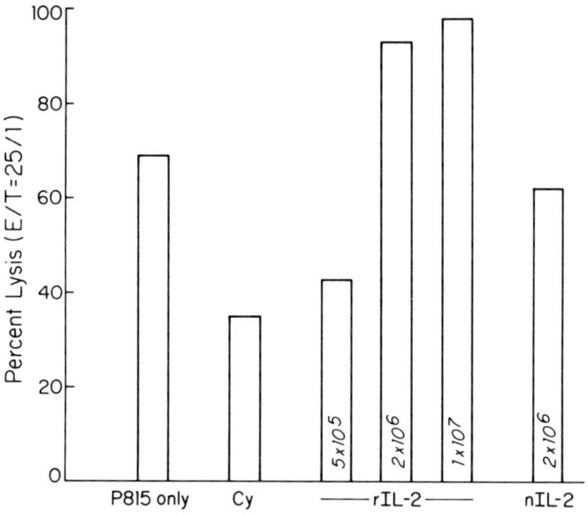

Fig 2. Comparison of natural and recombinant-derived human IL-2 to overcome cyclophosphamide-induced unresponsiveness in the generation of alloreactive cytotoxic T cells. Animals were injected IP with 2×10^7 P815 cells followed six days later by IV treatment with either vehicle only, or 40 mg/kg body weight Cy. Two days later, on day 8, groups received vehicle only, natural human IL-2 (2×10^6 U/animal IP), or recombinant-derived human IL-2 (5×10^5, 2×10^6, or 2×10^7 U/animal IP). On day 9, spleen cells were harvested, pooled, and tested for lytic activity against the tumor cell targets P815. Data depict the lysis at an E to T ratio of 25:1.

by cyclophosphamide treatment on day 6 (from 70% to 35% specific lysis). However, exogenous recombinant IL-2 therapy reconstituted the lytic response in a dose-dependent fashion. Animals receiving one half of a μg of recombinant IL-2 on day 8 did not contain splenocytes that were not remarkably different in their activity from those harvested from animals receiving cytoxan therapy. However, if animals were given either 2 or 10 μg of recombinant IL-2 following cytoxan, a substantial degree of lysis of P815 cells was observed (93% and 98%, respectively). Moreover, natural human IL-2, at 2 μg per animal, was also capable of restoring the cytotoxic T lymphocyte response to levels seen in untreated controls.

Indeed, as seen in the glucocorticoid-induced immune suppression model, on a unit basis, recombinant-derived IL-2 was slightly more efficient in restoring responsiveness than a similar concentration of naturally derived lymphokine. It is also important to note that resulting lytic activity was specific for the immunizing P815 cell, and did not result in any significant lysis of third party target cells. Thus, the in vivo IL–2-activated population in these experiments appears to mediate antigen-specific cytotoxic reactivity, consistent with the notion that the effector cell is of the T cell lineage.

Further investigations in these animal model systems concerning the role of IL-2 in vivo will do much to increase our understanding of the regulation of the immune response. Both models of drug-induced immunosuppression provide systems that could be used to better predict the efficacy of IL-2 in human clinical situations. Nevertheless, on the basis of the data detailed above, it would appear that IL-2 as a therapeutic modality holds promise as a reagent that can overcome immune suppression induced either by steroid hormones or by chemotherapeutic agents such as cyclophosphamide.

INTERLEUKIN-1

IL-1 is a protein product produced by macrophages that has diverse biological functions both within and outside the immune response. Activities that have previously been attributed to IL-1 include its capacity to act as an endogenous pyrogen,[24] its ability to cause lymphoid cell activation and thymocyte proliferation,[25] as well as its ability to induce proliferation of fibroblasts[26] and promote bone resorption and cartilage degradation.[27] Additionally, IL-1 molecules have been thought to be involved in promoting release of collagenase and prostaglandins from synovial cells,[28] and to initiate a broad series of reactions leading to acute phase protein synthesis and release from liver cells.[29] Finally, IL-1 has been implicated in muscle proteolysis and the stimulation of neutrophil secretion.[30]

The capacity of a single macrophage product to function in such diverse systems of biological activity both within and outside of the immune response has, for many years, puzzled cellular immunologists, cell biologists, and clinicians. However, recently it was discovered that two distinct genes are capable of coding for protein products that exhibit IL-1 activities.[31] These two gene products have been subsequently termed IL-1α and IL-1β. Quite interestingly, both genes code for primary translation products that are some 33,000 molecular weight in nature. The biologically active portion of the molecule(s) resides in the 17,500 molecular weight C-terminal portion of each protein.

We have isolated cDNA clones capable of directing the synthesis of both IL-1α and IL-1β gene products in heterologous hosts. Current optimal expression of IL-1 activities has been carried out by directing the synthesis of IL-1 in *Escherichia coli* expression plasmids, as detailed in Fig 3. In both cases, IL-1 gene expression is controlled by the actions of the heat inducible P_L promoter. This directs the synthesis of both C-terminal IL-1α and IL-1β in significant quantities. In fact, using the expression system detailed in Fig 1, we routinely produce approximately 20 to 40 mg of pure recombinant IL-1 product/L fermentation broth. This high yield takes into account whatever losses occurred during extraction and ion exchange column chromatography of *E coli*-directed IL-1 gene product.

Being able to produce large quantities of pure recombinant IL-1α and IL-1β has allowed us to continue to examine which of these gene products is responsible for several of the activities that were previously ascribed to a single IL-1 protein. For example, both IL-1α and IL-1β have the ability to induce in vitro B cell proliferation and antibody synthesis, as measured by plaque-forming cell responses in vitro. However, IL-1α

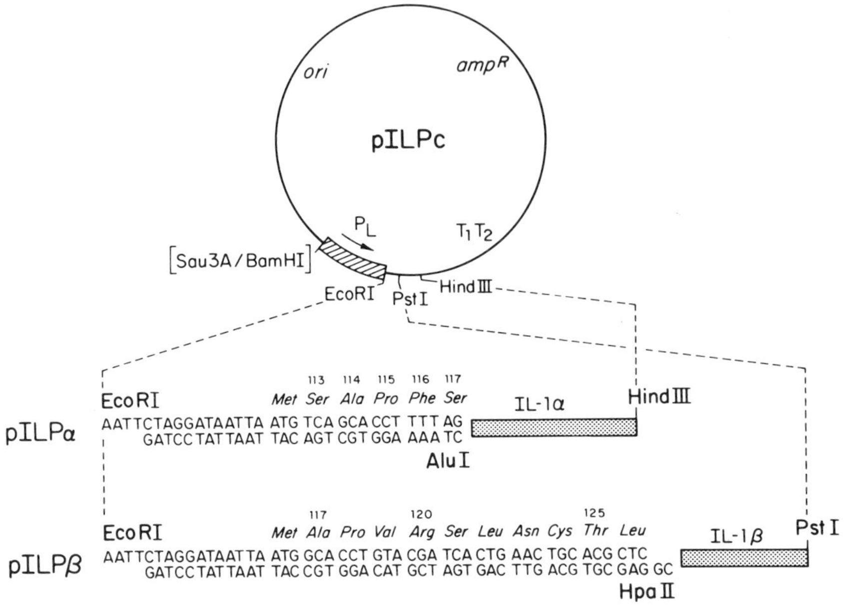

Fig 3. ***E coli*** **expression plasmids capable of directing synthesis of either IL-1α or IL-1β.**

and IL-1β do not equally share in every instance their capacity to mediate certain biological effects. For example, Fig 4 shows the comparative ability of purified recombinant human IL-1α and IL-1β to maintain proliferation of human dermal fibroblasts. As can be seen from these experiments, subconfluent cultures of human dermal fibroblasts are cultured for 120 hours in the presence of fetal calf serum containing medium in the presence or absence of either IL-1α or IL-1β. IL-1α promotes maximal fibroblast proliferation, as assessed by thymidine incorporation, at concentrations well below 2×10^{-11} mol/L, whereas IL-1β only causes half-maximal fibroblast proliferation at a concentration of 2×10^{-10} mol/L. Thus, with respect to proliferation of fibroblastoid cell types, it would appear that IL-1α is a more potent molecule on a weight basis.

Conversely, IL-1β appears to be a far more potent inducer of bone resorption. Figure 5 details the comparative effects of recombinant human IL-1β and human IL-1α on the capacity

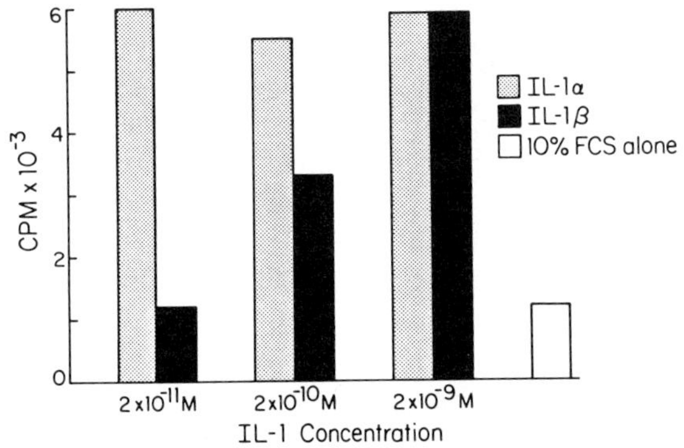

Fig 4. Comparative abilities of IL-1α and IL-1β to induce human dermal fibroblast proliferation. Cells were cultured in replicate 200 μL volumes (2×10^5 cells/mL) for five days, and pulsed for the last 18 hours of culture with 0.5 μCi of ^{3}H-Tdr (80 Ci/mmol/L). ^{3}H-Tdr incorporation was determined by liquid scintillation counting after harvesting the culture on to glass fiber filter strips with the aid of a multiple automated sample harvester. □, IL-1α; ■, IL-1β; □, 10% FCS alone.

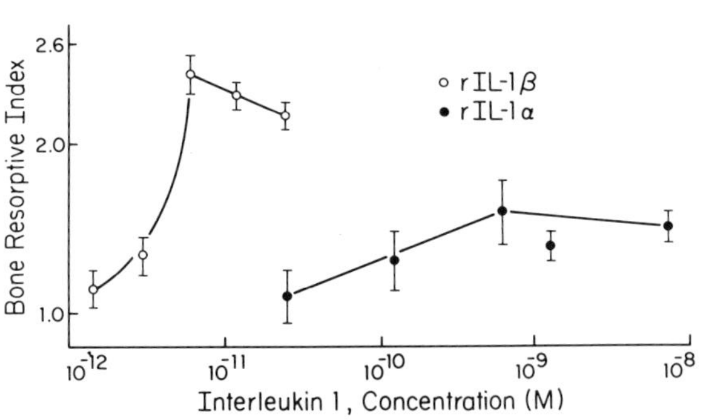

Fig 5. Bone resorptive effect of recombinant β and α human interleukin 1. Rat long bones were labeled with ^{45}Ca and incubated in cultures containing various concentrations of IL-1α and IL-1β. After 24 hours, supernates were harvested and the amount of ^{45}Ca present determined. Bone resorption index equals:

$$\frac{\text{Amount of } ^{45}\text{Ca release in cultures containing IL-1}}{\text{Amount of } ^{45}\text{Ca release in medium only control cultures}}$$

to cause bone demineralization. In these particular experiments, rat long bones are preincubated with ^{45}calcium, then cultured for varying periods of time in the presence or absence of recombinant IL-1 proteins. Bone cultures are then monitored for IL–1-mediated release of calcium over time. The bone resorptive index refers to a value determined by dividing the amount of ^{45}calcium release from cultures containing IL-1 by the level of ^{45}calcium release observed in control cultures. As is evident from the data presented in the figure, IL-1β is a far more potent inducer of ^{45}calcium release from rat long bones than is IL-1α. IL-1α appears to have a half-maximal bone resorption activity of somewhere between 10^{-9} and 10^{-10} mol/L. IL-1β, on the other hand, promotes half-maximal bone resorption at a concentration well below 5×10^{-11} mol/L. Most interestingly, IL-1β as well causes a far greater release of ^{45}calcium from rat long bones than does IL-1α. This more potent ability at an even lower molar concentration is reflected by the higher bone resorption index observed in cultures containing IL-1β.

In the past, therapeutic use of IL-1 has been conjectured due to its capacity to promote dermal fibroblast and gingival fibroblast proliferation. In such settings, it is conceivable that IL-1 might function as a wound healing agent, or as a protective compound to promote gum cell health in cases of plaque-induced oral disease. However, recent new evidence of IL-1 as a radioprotective agent suggests that, in addition to its immune and fibroblast stimulatory activity, IL-1 may be of therapeutic use due to its capacity to protect from radiation-induced bone marrow failure. Figure 6 shows such protective effects.

In these particular experiments, C57Bl/6 mice were exposed to a lethal dose of irradiation (in this particular case, 950 rad). Twenty hours before administration of a lethal irradiation dose, animals were given a single intraperitoneal injection of a control solution, or one containing 100 or 75 ng of human recombinant IL-1α. As is evident from the survival data detailed in Fig 6, IL-1α is extremely radioprotective. In fact, administration of 100 ng of human IL-1α 20 hours before radiation exposure resulted in greater than 75% survival, as compared to a cohort of mice treated with control carrier protein solution. The capacity of IL-1 to function in

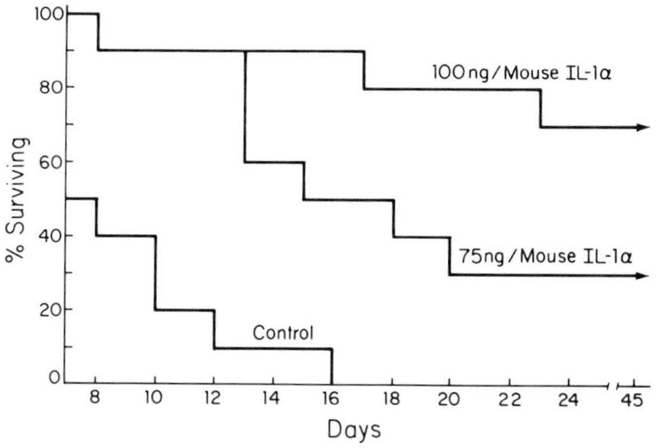

Fig 6. C57Bl/6 mice were exposed to lethal dose (950 r) of irradiation. Twenty hours before exposure, various groups of mice received either 100 or 75 ng of purified recombinant human IL-1α IP. Survival in cohorts of treated and control animals (10 mice/group) is plotted.

such a manner might bode well for its use in bone marrow transplant situations or in allowing cancer patients to receive higher doses of radiation treatment as a cytoreductive therapy.

In addition to being able to probe the biological activities of both IL-1α and IL-1β, the ability to generate large quantities of these recombinant human monokines has enabled us to examine the existence of a class of high affinity receptor sites on the surface of IL-1 responsive cells through which the hormone functions. Indeed, we have recently described the use of radiolabeled binding assays to detail the existence of IL-1 receptors on responsive cell types.[32,33] What has become increasingly interesting of late, and continues to be one of the most exciting aspects of IL-1 research is that, although both IL-1α and IL-1β are only 25% homologous at the amino acid level and thus represent extremely different molecular entities, they appear to bind to cells through a single class of high affinity receptor sites. Data in Fig 7 details the capacity of unlabeled pure recombinant human IL-1α, or natural IL-1β to inhibit the binding of radiolabeled IL-1's, regardless of whether the radiolabeled ligand used was recombinant human IL-1α, recombinant human IL-1β, or natural IL-1β. As is evident from consulting the data in Fig 7, all three species of IL-1 inhibit the binding of each radiolabeled IL-1 species to the same extent, with half-maximal inhibition of binding occurring at a concentration of approximately 5×10^{-9} mol/L. In addition, such binding inhibi-

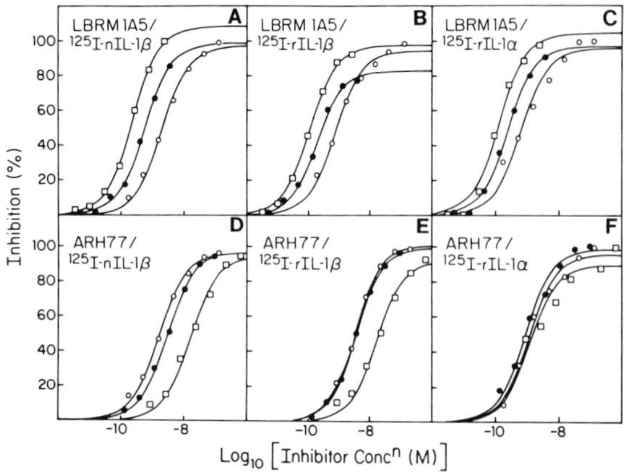

Fig 7. Cross competition between ●, nIL-1β, ○, rIL-1β, and □, rIL-1α for the IL-1 receptor on murine and human cells. Murine LBRM-33-1A5 cells (3.1 × 10^7/mL) or human ARH77 cells (2.1 × 10^7/mL) were incubated with various concentrations of unlabeled nIL-1β, rIL-1β, and rIL-1α at 8 °C for two hours, on a rocker platform. Concentrations of ^{125}I-IL-1's were: (A) nIL-1β, 3.9 × 10^{-10} mol/L; (B) rIL-1β, 1.9 × 10^{-9} mol/L; (C) rIL-1α, 9.2 × 10^{-10} mol/L; with the LBRM-33-1A5 cells; and (D) nIL-1β, 9 × 10^{-10} mol/L; (E) rIL-1β, 1.9 × 10^{-9} mol/L; and (F) rIL-1α, 4.6 × 10^{-9} mol/L for the ARH77 cells. Maximal binding was measured with ^{125}I-IL-1 alone and nonspecific binding was measured with 10 μg/mL of homologous unlabeled IL-1. All data have been corrected for nonspecific binding by subtraction. The cells were greater than 90% viable by trypan blue exclusion at the end of the assay.

tion curves are relatively equivalent, whether the IL-1 response is a T cell represented by the LBRM-33-1A5 cell line (top panel), or the ARH77 B cell line (bottom panel).

Given the fact that the structure of IL-1 genes was only described in June 1985, the rapid progress made with characterization of biological activities of these hormones, as well as the mechanism through which they interact with cells (ie, the existence and activity of a class of high-affinity binding sites) bodes well that additional revelations regarding the mechanism of IL-1 function and its therapeutic ability will continue to emerge in the near future.

GM-CSF

Although the general topic is dealt with in greater detail in a separate section of this treatise, recombinant hematopoietic growth factors (particularly colony stimulating factors) hold great potential as lymphokines with significant therapeutic benefit. One molecule in particular, so-called granulocyte-macrophage colony stimulating factor (GM-CSF), has recently made the transition from being a poorly defined culture supernate activity, to a defined protein produced via recombinant DNA technology. As have other groups,[34] we have isolated a cDNA clone for human GM-CSF[35] and have used this cDNA to direct the synthesis of GM-CSF activity in a variety of heterologous expression systems in both yeast and *E coli*. Figure 8 details SDS polyacrylamide gel electrophoresis of fractions from high pressure liquid chromatography of *E coli*-derived GM-CSF. After being produced in bacteria, this material was extracted with 6 mol/L urea and subjected to replicate rounds of ion exchange chromatography before being chromatographed on a C18 radiopak microbond column (Water's Chemical). Fractions containing pure GM-CSF eluted from this column previously equilibrated in 0.1% trifluoracetic acid with buffer containing 42% to 44% acetonitrile.

Human GM-CSF holds promise for clinical therapeutic benefit in a variety of model systems. First, because colony stimulating factors in general have been shown to cause terminal differentiation of leukemic cells,[36] GM-CSF may be of value in a therapeutic setting as a cytostatic agent in the treatment of leukemia and lymphoma.

In addition, given its capacity to promote the growth and differentiation of granulocytes and macrophages, its use in conjunction with bone marrow transplantation therapy may provide for more effective engraftment of marrow, and

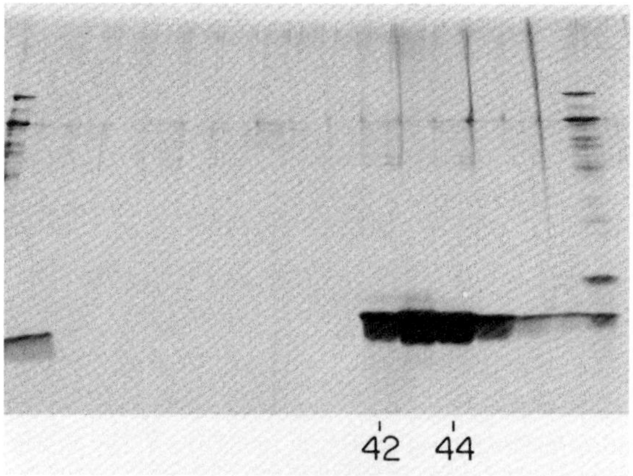

Fig 8. A silver stained SDS polyacrylamide gel shows pure *E coli*-derived recombinant human GM-CSF (fraction 42–45) prepared via ion exchange chromatography and HPLC procedures.

therefore be of value as an adjunct therapy in marrow transplantation therapies aimed at treatment of leukemia and aplastic anemia.

Finally, because GM-CSF has the ability to augment de novo marrow generation of granulocytes and macrophages, its use as an adjunct therapy in cancer patients may be of value in boosting circulating white cell levels following cytoreductive therapy. Such an effect may not only promote recovery of patients from infections occurring during chemotherapy or radiation-induced immunosuppression, but may actually allow for administration of stronger or more frequent dosages of already approved chemotherapeutic agents.

Most interestingly, we have recently shown that GM-CSF can function as a macrophage-activating factor, promoting the activation of macrophages to point where they have the capacity to recognize and destroy human tumor cells. Data detailed in Table 1 confirms the capacity of GM-CSF function in this manner. Human peripheral blood mononuclear cells cultured for 24 hours in a variety of stimuli were assessed for their capacity to mediate destruction of radiolabeled A375 human melanoma tumor cells. As has been detailed in the literature, bacterial endotoxin (lipopolysaccharide) is a potent mediator of macrophage-mediated tumor cell kill, as is interferon-γ, provided that low concentrations of endotoxin are present.[37] Cells incubated in the presence of GM-CSF (500 U/mL) in a solution lacking endotoxin were also capable of mediating potent specific cytotoxicity of the A375 melanoma target.

Table 1. GM-CSF Activates Macrophage-Mediated Tumor Cell Kill

	% Cytotoxicity (A375 Melanoma)				
		LPS (ng/mL)			
Lymphokine	None	10.0	1.0	0.1	0.01
None	0	84	83	0	0
IFN 100 U/mL	0			40	
10 U/mL	0			28	
1 U/mL	0			25	
GM-CSF 500 U/mL	63				

NOTE. Purified peripheral blood monocytes were prepared and cultured in the presence of either lipopolysaccharide (LPS-W, Difco Laboratories, Detroit), purified natural IFN_{γ} (Meloy Laboratories, Springfield, VA) or purified recombinant GM-CSF. After 24 hours, the culture medium was replaced and (^{125}I) iododeoxyuridine-labeled A375 target cells were added. After an additional 72 hours, residual adherent A375 cells were harvested and counted to determine the percentage of cytotoxicity.

On the basis of such experiments, it is hoped that GM-CSF will find an important niche in the therapeutic manipulation of patients with solid tumors. In addition, the capacity of GM-CSF to activate macrophages holds important clinical promise not only in the management of cancer patients, but in patients suffering from parasitic or bacterial infections, as well. For example, recent experiments in our laboratory have confirmed the capacity of GM-CSF to mediate therapeutic benefit in murine parasite models. Figure 9 demonstrates representative experiments. In these studies, C57Bl/6 mice were infected with an inoculation of *Tripanosoma cruzi* on day 0. Animals then received daily administration of either GM-CSF (5 μg IP until day 5), or carrier protein (an identical dosage of mouse serum albumen). Replicate cohorts of mice (5 mice/group) were then monitored every

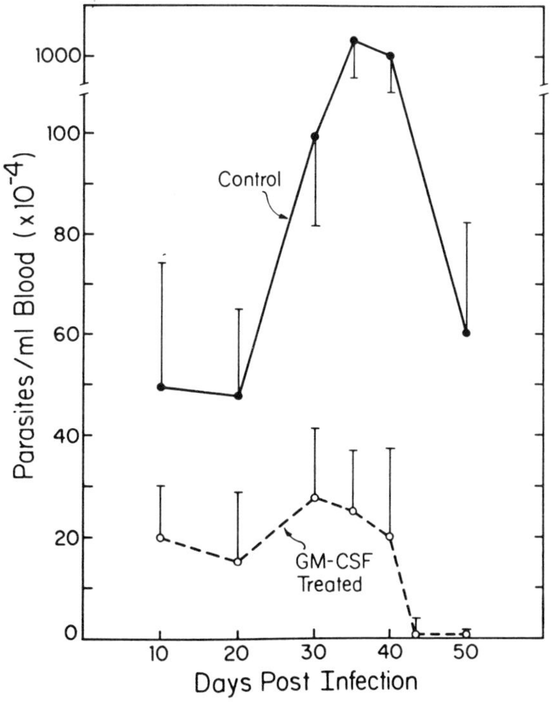

Fig 9. C57Bl/6 mice were inoculated with 2 × 10^4 *T cruzi* IP on day 0. Replicate groups of mice were then treated on days 0–4 with either 5 μg of recombinant murine GM-CSF or mouse serum albumen IP. Parasitemia was determined by visual inspection of blood smears from samples taken over time.

ten days for level of circulating parasites in the blood. As is evident from the data presented in Fig 9, GM-CSF treatment led to a sustained, marked diminution of resultant parasitemia. These experiments, together with data from additional infectious models suggest that the future for use of GM-CSF in therapeutic settings remains bright.

Unfortunately, space prohibits detailing results of experiments with additional lymphokines, like IL-1 and IL-2 together with GM-CSF, that have made the transition from ill-defined serum or supernate factors, to defined molecular entities produced in large quantity by recombinant DNA technology. Many of these additional molecules, including interferon-γ, tumor necrosis factor, lymphotoxin, are close to, or in, human clinical trials. Although some of the lymphokines currently being developed as therapeutic entities may not show reproducible ability to beneficially affect patients suffering from a wide variety of diseases, it remains clear that clinical trial of lymphokines as biological response modifiers continues to show itself as an avenue of great potential promise. Scientific progress in this area has moved exceptionally rapidly in the past 5 years. Molecules, which several years ago carried with them a certain mythical or mystical quality, are now becoming proven molecular entities that may, with continued good fortune and savvy clinical application, become therapeutic realities.

ACKNOWLEDGMENT

Experimentation with IL-2, IL-1, and CSF was conducted in collaboration with Hoffmann-La Roche, Syntex (USA), and Behring Werke A.G., respectively.

REFERENCES

1. Gillis S, Smith KA: Long-term culture of tumor-specific cytotoxic T-cells. Nature 268:154, 1977

2. Gillis S, Baker PE, Ruscetti FW, et al: Long-term culture of human antigen-specific cytotoxic T-cell lines. J Exp Med 148:1093, 1978

3. Flomenberg N, Welte K, Mertelsmann R, et al: Interleukin-2 dependent natural killer (NK) cell lines from patients with primary T-cell immunodeficiencies. J Immunol 130:2635, 1983

4. Merluzzi VJ, Welte K, Savage DM, et al: Expansion of cyclophosphamide resistant cytotoxic precursors in vitro and in vivo by purified human interleukin-2. J Immunol 131:806, 1983

5. Domzig W, Stadler BM, Herberman RB: Interleukin-2 dependence of human natural killer (NK) cell activity. J Immunol 130:1970, 1983

6. Saito H, Kranz DM, Takagaki Y, et al: Complete primary structure of a heterodimeric T-cell receptor deduced from cDNA sequences. Nature 309:757, 1984

7. Palacios R: Mechanism of T-cell activation: Role and functional relationship of HLA-DR antigens and Interleukins. Immunol Rev 63:73, 1982

8. Leonard WJ, Depper M, Uchiyama T, et al: A monoclonal antibody that appears to recognize the receptor for human T-cell growth factor; partial characterization of the receptor. Nature 300:267, 1982

9. Cosman D, Cerretti DP, Larsen A, et al: The human receptor for Interleukin-2: Cloning, sequence and expression. Nature 312:768, 1984

10. Robb RJ, Munck RA, Smith KA: T-cell growth factor receptors. Quantitation, specificity, and biological relevance. J Exp Med, 154:1455, 1981

11. Baker PE, Gillis S, Ferm MM, et al: The effect of T-cell growth factor on the generation of cytolytic T-cells. J Immunol 121:2168, 1978

12. Henney CS, Kuribayashi K, Kern DE, et al: Interleukin-2 augments natural killer cell activity. Nature 291:335, 1981

13. Gillis S, Crabtree GR, Smith KA: Glucocorticoid-induced inhibition of T-cell growth factor production. I. The effect on mitogen-induced lymphocyte proliferation. J Immunol 123:1625, 1979

14. Marrack P, Graham SD, Kushnir E, et al: Nonspecific factors in B-cell responses. Immunol Rev 63:33, 1982

15. Mazumder A, Rosenberg SA: Successful immunotherapy of natural killer-resistant established pulmonary melanoma mestastases by the intravenous adoptive transfer of syngeneic lymphocytes activated in vitro by Interleukin-2. Science 225:1487, 1984

16. Gillis S, Ferm MM, Ou W, et al: T-cell growth factor: Parameters of production and a quantitative microassay for activity. J Immunol 120:2027, 1978

17. Gillis S, Watson J: Biochemical and biological characterization of lymphocyte regulatory molecules. V. Identification of an Interleukin-2 producer human leukemia T-cell line. J Exp Med 152:1709, 1980

18. Frank MB, Watson JD, Mochizuki DY, et al: Biochemical and biological characterization of lymphocyte regulatory molecules. VIII. Purification of interleukin-2 from a human T-cell leukemia. J Immunol 127:2361, 1981

19. Stern AS, Pan YCE, Urdal DL, et al: Purification to homogeneity and partial characterization of interleukin-2 from a human T-cell leukemia. Proc Natl Acad Sci USA 81:871, 1984

20. Taniguchi T, Matsui H, Fujita T, et al: Structure and expression of a cloned cDNA for human interleukin-2. Nature 302:305, 1983

21. Rosenberg SA, Lotze MT, Muul LM, et al: Observations on the systemic administration of autologous lymphokine-activated killer cells and recombinant interleukin-2 to patients with metastatic cancer. N Engl J Med 313:1485–1492, 1985

22. Mule JJ, Shu S, Schwarz SL, et al: Adoptive immunotherapy of established pulmonary metastases with LAK cells and recombinant Interleukin-2. Science 225:1487–1489, 1984

23. Cheever MA, Greenberg PD, Fefer A, et al: Augmentation of anti-tumor efficacy of long-term cultured T-lymphocytes by in vivo administration of purified interleukin-2. J Exp Med 155:969, 1982

24. Dinarello CA, Goldin NP, Wolff SM: Demonstration and characterization of two distinct human leukocytic pyrogens. J Exp Med 139:1369, 1974

25. Oppenheim JJ, Gery I: Interleukin-1 is more than an interleukin. Immunol Today 3:113, 1982

26. Schmidt JA, Mizel SB, Cohen D, et al: Interleukin-1: A potential regulator of fibroblast proliferation. J Immunol 128:2177, 1982

27. Dewhirst FE, Stashenko PP, Mole JE, et al: Purification and partial sequence of human osteoclast activating factor: Identity with interleukin-1β. J Immunol 135:2562, 1985

28. Mizel SB, Dayer JM, Krane SM, et al: Stimulation of rheumatoid synovial cell collagenase and prostaglandin production by partially purified lymphocyte-activating factor (interleukin-1). Proc Natl Acad Sci USA 78:2474, 1981

29. Selinger MJ, McAdam KP, Kaplan MM, et al: Monokine-induced synthesis of serum amyloid: A protein by hepatocytes. Nature 285:498, 1980

30. Kampschmidt RF, Upchurch HF: Neutrophil release after injection of endotoxin or leukocytic endogenous mediator into rats. J Retic Soc 28:191, 1980

31. March CJ, Mosley B, Larsen A, et al: Cloning, sequence and expression of two distinct human interleukin-1 complementary DNAs. Nature 315:641, 1985

32. Gillis S, Urdal DL: Detection and characterization of high affinity plasma membrane receptor for interleukin-1. J Exp Med 162:501, 1985

33. Dower SK, Call SM, Gillis S, et al: Similarity between the interleukin-1 receptors on a murine T-lymphoma cell line and on a murine fibroblast cell line. Proc Natl Acad Sci USA 83:1060, 1986

34. Gough NM, Gough J, Metcalf D, et al: Molecular cloning of cDNA encoding a murine haematopoietic growth regulator, granulocyte-macrophage colony stimulating factor. Nature 309:763, 1984

35. Cantrell MA, Anderson D, Cerretti DP, et al: Cloning, sequence and expression of a human granulocyte-macrophage colony stimulating factor. Proc Natl Acad Sci USA 82:6250, 1985

36. Moore MAS, Kurland J, Broxmeyer HE: Regulatory interactions in normal and leukemic myelopoiesis, in Clarkson B, Marks PA, Till JE (eds): Differentiation of Normal and Neoplastic Hematopoietic Cells. Cold Spring Harbor Conferences on Cell Proliferation, vol 5, p 393, 1978

37. Le J, Prensky W, Yip YK, et al: Activation of human monocyte cytotoxicity by natural and recombinant immune interferon. J Immunol 131:2821, 1983

Differentiation Factors

Janice L. Gabrilove

CANCER CAN BE VIEWED as a disorder resulting from an uncoupling of gene expression that controls cellular proliferation and differentiation. This concept does not necessarily imply that the maturation block is irreversible, and much attention has been paid to neoplastic cell line models, which can be induced to terminal differentiation following exposure in vitro to a variety of chemical or chemotherapeutic agents.[1]

Normal cell development is classically depicted as proceeding from an immature stem cell, which possesses unlimited self-renewal to committed progenitors and terminally, lineage-specific differentiated cells with limited, restricted or no self-renewal capacity. The strategy of the induction of tumor cell differentiation is based upon the idea that by inducing cell maturation, one decreases and eventually extinguishes the self-renewal capacity of the malignant clone.

Deviant cell maturation, resulting in a cellular phenotype exhibiting a relative maturation arrest and the potential to manipulate this phenotype in a therapeutically advantageous fashion, is best illustrated by human hematopoietic tumors. For this reason, we have chosen for the purpose of this review to focus our discussion on the nonphysiologic as well as physiologically important inducers of myeloid leukemic cell differentiation. It is hoped that this will serve as a model for an understanding and appreciation of the potential relevance as well as the already clinically applied therapeutic utility of cell maturation therapy.

From the Department of Medicine, Division of Leukemia/Lymphoma and Clinical Immunology, Memorial Sloan-Kettering Cancer Center, and the Cornell University Medical College, New York.

Supported by the National Cancer Institute, Grants CA 00966, CA 23766, CA 20194. Dr Gabrilove is a recipient of a Junior Faculty Fellowship Award from the American Cancer Society and a Clinical Investigator Award from the NCI.

Address reprint requests to Janice L. Gabrilove, MD, Department of Medicine, Division of Leukemia/Lymphoma and Clinical Immunology, Memorial Sloan-Kettering Cancer Center, 1275 York Ave, New York, NY 10021.

0093-7754/86/1302-0013$05.00/0

The concept of biological modification of myeloid leukemic cell growth and differentiation has been based upon various observations suggesting that transformed leukemic stem cells may be induced to normality with respect to morphology, function, and regulation. This reversal of malignancy in leukemia, while an attractive goal, is one that is rarely attainable in its entirety in clinical or experimental systems. What is more feasible and has proved attainable is removal of the maturation block in the leukemic lineage with resulting development of varying but incomplete functional and phenotypic features of lineage-specific differentiation.

Inducers of myeloid cell differentiation can be divided into the following categories: (1) chemotherapeutic agents, (2) polar compounds, (3) phorbol diesters, (4) vitamin analogs, and (5) physiologically-important cytokines. The initial identification of active agents, and our understanding of myeloid leukemic cell differentiation, has been aided, to a great extent, by the development of both murine and human leukemic cell lines, which represent various stages of myeloid cell maturation. The most frequently used cell lines include the following: (1) The murine myelomonocyclic WEHI-3B(D+) and M1, and (2) the human early myeloblast and/or erythroblast (K562), myeloblast (KG-1), promyelocyte (HL-60), and monocytoid (U937) leukemia cell lines. One can monitor for distinct morphological, antigenic, histochemical, and functional properties that accompany the erythroid, granulocyte, or macrophage differentiation of leukemic cells. In addition, self renewal can be assessed by measuring recloning capacity. We will refer to these cell lines, throughout our discussion in the following pages, because they have served as a foundation, supporting additional investigations concerning the differentiation of leukemic cells from patients with newly diagnosed or relapsed acute nonlymphocytic leukemia (ANLL), both in vitro and in vivo.

CHEMOTHERAPEUTIC AGENTS

Of the variety of chemotherapeutic agents used in cancer chemotherapy, it is becoming apparent that some may be effective because of their capacity to selectively induce tumor cell differentiation, and this property may be more important than their cytotoxic potential.[2] Some of the more standard agents such as mitomycin, Adriamycin (Adria Laboratories, Columbus, Ohio), bleomycin, daunomycin, cytosine arabinoside, methotrexate, 5-azacytidine[2–4] as well as some of the newer investigational agents such as homoharringtonine,[5] have been shown to induce M1 and HL-60 leukemic cell differentiation.

In recloning studies of primary human leukemias cultured in methylcellulose, a decreased self-renewal potential of clonogenic cells (plating efficiency 2 [PE-2]) can be observed with various chemotherapeutic agents that are independent of their chemosuppressive action on primary leukemic cloning efficiency.[6] This action on PE-2 is a likely differentiation index because more primitive leukemic stem cells with extensive proliferative potential are differentiated into a nonself-renewing compartment. Furthermore, this PE-2 parameter has been shown to correlate with clinical response.[6]

The combination of low doses of the above antineoplastic drugs with other differentiation-inducing proteins may prove effective when neither type of agent can induce differentiation directly. In this regard, differentiation-resistant clones of murine myeloid leukemic cells M1 that failed to respond to a protein differentiation factor could be sensitized by the addition of low doses (less than required for cytotoxicity) of actinomycin D, daunomycin, mitomycin C, hydroxyurea, bleomycin, 5-fluorouracil, prednisone, or dexamethasone to terminal differentiation when combined with protein factor.[4,7]

One particular chemotherapeutic agent, cytosine arabinoside (ara-C), has been the subject of extensive investigation.[2,8–10] Cytosine arabinoside is one of the most effective single agents for the treatment of myeloid leukemia and is conventionally considered to act by incorporation in DNA and inhibiting DNA replication. While ara-C is cytotoxic by virtue of its ability to inhibit DNA replication, it is capable at low doses of inducing differentiation of leukemic myeloblasts in vitro.[2,8–10]

One possible mechanism by which ara-C may promote differentiation of leukemic cells was suggested by the finding that ara-C increases the degree of methylation of DNA in cultured murine P815 mastocytoma cells; presumably, ara-CTP incorporated into DNA during synthesis serves as the substrate for postsynthetic enzymatic methylation.[11] Because transcriptional activity in certain regions of the cellular genome varies inversely with the degree of methylation in those regions, Beohm and Drahovsky have hypothesized that ara-C induced DNA hypermethylation may inhibit transcription of genes required for neoplastic cell proliferation.[11]

Complete or partial remissions by treatment with low dose ara-C have already been reported in patients with myelodysplastic syndromes (MDS) or ANLL.[12–18] Where clinical responses have been obtained, the evidence points to a differentiating role for the drug rather than a cell kill effect. The progressive evolution of recovery, the absence of aplasia, the simultaneous presence of normal islets of promyelocytes and leukemic myeloblasts,[14] morphologic[12,14] and bone marrow culture[18] studies of specimens from patients treated with low-dose ara-C, support the hypothesis that the observed therapeutic effectiveness is due at least in part to induction of cell differentiation. In at least one study, leukemic marrow cultures were exposed to low doses of ara-C and a reduction in blast cells and increase in more mature granulocyte and macrophage elements was noted in two out of three patients.[10] Subsequent low dose ara-C treatment in vivo resulted in complete remission in the two patients that showed a strong in vitro response.[10]

POLAR-PLANAR COMPOUNDS

Dimethyl sulfoxide (DMSO) and hexamethylene bisacetamide (HMBA, NSC-95580) are two of the most active polar-planar compounds that trigger cell differentiation.[19] These are low molecular weight (ie, <300 daltons) compounds with a polar hydrophilic moiety and a planar hydrophobic portion. HMBA is one of the most widely studied of these agents, having activity in both solid tumor derived and leukemic cultured cell lines including neuroblastoma, mesenchymal glioblastoma multiforme, teratocarcinoma, melanoma, Friend murine erythroleukemia and the human promyelocytic leukemia, HL-60.[19–21] The precise mechanism of action is unknown. Cellular uptake of HMBA appears to be necessary for differentiation; HMBA linked to glutathione (which cannot penetrate the cell membrane) is inactive. Induction of differentiation is both concentration (1.5–2.0 mmol/L for 50% of cells to differentiate) and time dependent.[19,20] It takes up to eight hours for equilibration of intracellular and extracellular drug concentration, and differentiation is not detected until 18 hours after first drug exposure.[20] The lag time may indicate that there is a need for continuous HMBA presence during a sequence of biochemical changes and/or that induction is cell-cycle dependent. Phase I studies have already begun to evaluate this differentiation agent. A five-day continuous infusion regimen of HMBA, has been recently evaluated over a dose ranging from 4.8 to 42.3 g/m^2/d. At 24 g/m^2/d, a steady-state plasma level of 1–2 mmol/L appears to be achievable. Additional trials are forthcoming and should promise for the efficacy of this agent.

VITAMIN ANALOGS

Retinoids

Retinoic acid, a metabolite of vitamin A, is of critical importance in normal epithelial cell maturation, and in the proliferation and differentiation of normal and malignant hematopoietic cells. A vitamin A analog, 13-cis-retinoic acid at concentrations of 10^{-6} mol/L has been shown to inhibit tumor and leukemic cell growth[22] and also induces differentiation in tumor and leukemic cell lines as well as cells from patients with newly diagnosed promyelocytic leukemia.[23–26] In addition, retinoids (3×10^{-8} mol/L–10^{-7} mol/L) would appear to enhance normal hematopoietic cell proliferation by increasing the responsiveness of cells to the action of CSF and EPO[3]. Several clinical trials have already been conducted utilizing retinoic acid including chronic myelogenous leukemia (CML)[27] and myelodysplastic syndrome[28] and in cases of acute promyelocytic leukemia.[29] Arlin et al[27] found peak blood levels of 2.7 mmol/L 13-cis-retinoic acid (comparable to in vitro levels required for differentiation) in patients with CML, where 13-cis-retinoic acid was added to daunorubicin, cytosine arabinoside and thioguanine to determine if it could increase the incidence and duration of remission induced by cytoxic chemotherapy. No obvious clinical benefit was seen with regards to eradication of the leukemic clone. The role of 13-cis-retinoic acid in delaying the onset of blastic transformation will have to be answered in a separate trial comparing standard chemotherapy with or without the addition of 13-cis-retinoic acid. Although only clinical benefit has been shown in cases of acute promyelocytic leukemia, the understanding of the real role of retinoids in the treatment of these diseases is still unclear and awaits further controlled trials. It would seem that retinoic acid might be a useful agent for purging of bone marrow in the setting of autologous transplantation, given its differential effect on normal versus leukemic progenitors.

Vitamin D

Vitamin D is a major regulator of calcium transport. 1,25 dihydroxyvitamin D_3, (1,25 $(OH)_2D_3$), the most active hormonal form, has been demonstrated to induce the maturation of both normal and leukemic immature myeloid cells, (both from cell lines and patients with newly diagnosed ANLL) along the monocyte/macrophage pathway in vitro and in vivo.[3,30] Its effects are concentration dependent with maximum induction of monocytic differentiation when cells are exposed to concentrations of 10^{-6} mol/L.[3] $1,25(OH)_2D_3$ has been used in patients with malignant osteopetrosis, with correction in their bone bending and resorptive deficiencies in patients monocytes[31] and is presently being evaluated in the treatment of patients with myelodysplastic syndrome.[32] Several analogs of vitamin D with lower toxicity to therapeutic action, should be of interest, with regard to future clinical implementation.

PHORBOL ESTERS AND TELEOCIDINS

Phorbol esters that appear to bind to protein kinase C can induce a full spectrum of macrophage differentiation features in both leukemic cell lines and fresh leukemic cell cultures. The effect of phorbol esters is concentration dependent.[3] In contrast to other differentiation-inducing agents, they are most unlikely to have therapeutic value, not only because of their tumor promoting and strong inflammatory activities, but also because they do not appear to provide a differential kill of leukemic versus normal hematopoietic cells. Interestingly enough, a clinical trial of phorbol myristate acetate (PMA) in patients with myelodysplastic syndrome is presently in progress. The results of this study are not available at this time.

CYTOKINES

More recently, interest in biological response modifiers has focused on the identification and potential clinical use of physiologic hematopoietic protein regulators that might interfere with leukemic cell growth.

Materials of biological origin capable of inducing leukemic cell differentiation were first described in the mouse. Fibach and Sachs reported that serum from mice injected with endotoxin induced granulocyte and macrophage differentiation of the mouse myeloid leukemia cell line M1.[33] The existence of a special type of colony stimulating factor (CSF), with exceptional differentiation activity on leukemic cells, was subsequently further substantiated.[34] Biochemical purification of murine postendotoxin serum, utilizing ammonium sulfate precipitation, gel filtration, and phenyl sepharose column chromatography, demonstrated that a differentiation activity, termed differentiation factor[34] or granulocyte-macrophage differentiation factor,[34] copurified with a subspecies of CSF with predominant neutrophil colony stimulating factor (G-CSF) for normal mouse bone marrow myeloid progenitors.[34] More recently, this differentiation factor has been purified to apparent homogeneity and has been shown to be identical to murine G-CSF.[35] Murine G-CSF has three important properties: (1) It promotes the differentiation of the murine myelomonocytic leukemia cell line WEHI-3B(D+)[35]; (2) the self-renewal capacity of murine myeloid leukemia cells cultured in G-CSF is decreased[36]; and (3) the in vivo leukemogenicity of myeloid leukemia cells is suppressed when cells are cultured continuously in the presence of G-CSF.[37] It would be important to identify and isolate either the human analog or a human protein with similar differentiation-inducing capabilities as murine G-CSF, so that its effectiveness on human myeloid leukemias could be assessed. Several human sources of differentiation activities for human and mouse myeloid leukemic cells have been detected in or partially purified from the following: Human post endotoxin serum,[38] conditioned medium (CM) from a human hepatoma cell line,[39] human placenta,[40] cultures of human T lymphocyte leukemia virus (HTLV-I) infected umbilical cord blood or adult bone marrow T lymphocytes,[41] HTLV-III positive cell lines HUT 102,[42] and day 2 CM from phytohemagglutinin-stimulated leukocytes (PHA-LCM).[43]

Recently we have purified two pluripotent colony-stimulating factors for hematopoietic stem cells, pluripoietin (PPO) and pluripoietin-alpha (PPO-alpha) from the conditioned medium of the bladder carcinoma cell line 5637.[44–46] Both factors have differentiation-inducing activities for the human promyelocytic leukemic cell line HL-60.[45,46] In addition, pluripoietin induces differentiation of the murine myelomonocytic leukemic cell line WEHI-3B(D+).[44,45] Pluripoietin has also recently been molecularly cloned,[47] and has no sequence homology to any of the other molecularly cloned colony stimulating factors. Recombinant pluripoietin has also been shown to bind to specific receptors on leukemic cells, and to induce the differentiation of leukemic cells from patients with newly diagnosed ANLL.[47]

Pluripoietin may represent the human biological counterpart of murine G-CSF. It differs from murine G-CSF in that it promotes the growth of human mixed pluripotential progenitors (CFU-GEMM) and human early erythroid BFU-E, a property not described for murine G-CSF; however, it is biologically similar to mouse G-CSF in that it promotes predominantly the growth of neutrophil colonies and it differentiates WEHI 3B (D+). A direct molecular comparison of PPO and murine G-CSF is not possible because the amino acid sequence of G-CSF is not known.

Other lymphokines and cytokines that have no CSF activity have been shown to be potent inducers of both normal and leukemic myeloid cell maturation. There is increasing evidence to suggest a role for gamma interferon in the regulatory control of cells of the monocyte macrophage lineage. Gamma interferon induces differentiation of immature myeloid cells along the monocytic pathway and induces or enhances expression of class II HLA antigens during this process.[48] In addition, gamma interferon induces (1) phagocytosis, (2) the acquisition of tumorcidal activity, and (3) the expression of new receptors for Fc, and interleukin-2 on mature monocytic cells.[48–50] A 46,000 dalton molecular weight (SDS-PAGE) differentiation factor for HL-60 cells, which is not identical to gamma interferon, has also been purified from a human T lymphocyte, HUT 102 cell line conditioned medium.[42] This factor also works synergistically with retinoic acid to induce differentiation of the human monoblast cell line U937. The relationship of this factor to lymphotoxin (TNF-beta) is unclear.

The data that we have briefly reviewed have significant clinical implications in the area of biological response modification. The therapeutic application of maturation-induced death of malignant cells is only beginning to surface in the clinical arena. Additional support of this novel approach are the recent exciting observations of Reitsma et al,[51] which demonstrate a reduction in C-myc mRNA levels within four hours of HL-60 exposure to $1,25(OH)_2D_3$, preceding by eight hours the onset of other measurable phenotypic changes. These data would suggest that differentiation induction can be associated with a switching off of particular oncogenes thought to be intimately associated with the malignant phenotype and possibly the process of cell transformation. The future availability of new recombinant proteins with specific differentiation inducing activity will certainly add an additional important component to the developing biologic armamentarium.

REFERENCES

1. Bloch A: Induced cell differentiation in cancer therapy. Cancer Treat Rep 68:199–204, 1984
2. Sachs L: Control of normal cell differentiation and the phenotypic reversion of malignancy in myeloid leukemia. Nature 274:535–539, 1978
3. Koeffler HP: Induction of differentiation of human acute myelogenous leukemia cells: Therapeutic implications. Blood 62:709–721, 1983
4. Hozumi M: Fundamentals of chemotherapy of myeloid leukemia by induction of leukemia cell differentiation. Adv Cancer Res 38:121–169, 1983
5. Boyd AW, Sullivan JR: Leukemic cell differentiation in vivo and in vitro: Arrest of proliferation parallels the differentiation induced by the antileukemic drug Harringtonine. Blood 63:384–392, 1984
6. Buick RN, Chang JA, Curtis JE, et al: Self-renewal capacity of leukemic blast progenitors. Cancer Res 4:4849–4852, 1981
7. Hayashi M, Okabe-Kado J, Hozumi M: Sensitization of resistant myeloid leukemia clone cells by anti-cancer drugs to factors stimulating differentiation. Exp Cell Res 139:422–427, 1982
8. Griffin JD, Munroe P, Major D, et al: Induction of differentiation of human myeloid leukemia cells by inhibitors of DNA synthesis. Exp Hematol 10:774–781, 1982
9. Lotem J, Sachs L: Different blocks in the differentiation of myeloid leukemic cells. Proc Natl Acad Sci USA 71:3507–3511, 1974
10. Michalewicz R, Lotem J, Sachs L: Cell differentiation and therapeutic effect of low doses of cytosine arabinoside in human myeloid leukemia, Leuk Res 8:783–790, 1984
11. Boehm TLJ, Drohovsky D: Elevated level of enzymatic DNA methylation in cells treated with I-B-D-arabinofuranosylcytosine. Cancer Res 42:1537–1540, 1982
12. Boccaroni MO, Turo S: Differentiation of myeloid leukemic cells: New possibilities for therapy. Br J Haematol 42:485–487, 1979
13. Castaigne SMT, Daniel H, Tilly P, et al: Does treatment with ara-C in low dosage cause differentiation of leukemic cells? Blood 62:85–86, 1983
14. Housset M, Daniel MT, Degas L: Small doses of ara-C in the treatment of acute myeloid leukaemia: Differentiation of myeloid leukaemic cells? Br J Haematol 51:125–129, 1982
15. Manhoharan A: Low dose cytarabine therapy in hypoplastic acute leukemia. N Engl J Med 309:1652–1653, 1983
16. Mufti GJ, Oscier DG, Hamblin TJ, et al: Low doses of cytarabine in the treatment of myelodysplastic syndrome and acute myeloid leukemia. N Engl J Med 309:1653–1654, 1983
17. Wisch JS, Griffin JD, Kufe DW: Response of preleukemic syndromes to continuous infusion of low-dose cytarabine. N Engl J Med 309:1599–1602, 1983
18. Moloney WC, Rosenthal DS: Treatment of early acute non-lymphatic leukemia with low dose cytosine arabinoside. Haematol Blood Trans 26:59–62, 1981
19. Spremulli EN, Dexter DL: Polar solvents: A novel class of antineoplastic agents. Clin Oncol 2:227–241, 1984
20. Marks PA, Rifkind RA: Erythroleukemic differentiation. Ann Rev Biochem 47:419–498, 1978
21. Reuben RC: Studies on the mechanism of action of hexamethylene bisacetamide, a potent inducer of erythroleukemic differentiation. Biochim Biophys Acta 588:310–321, 1979
22. Lotan R, Giotta G, Nork E, et al: Characterization of the inhibitory effects of retinoids on in vivo growth of murine melanoma. JNCI 60:1035–1041, 1978
23. Strickland S, Mahdavi V: The induction of differentiation in teratocarcinoma stem cells by retinoic acid. Cell 15:393–403, 1978
24. Meyskens FL, Fuller BB: Characterization of the effects of different retinoids on the growth and differentiation of a human melanoma cell line and selected subclones. Cancer Res 40:2194–2196, 1980
25. Breitman TE, Selonick SE, Collins SJ: Induction of differentiation of the human promyelocytic leukemia cell line (HL–60) by retinoic acid. Proc Natl Acad Sci USA 77:2936–2940, 1980
26. Breitman T, Collins S, Keene B: Terminal differentiation of human promyelocytic leukemia cells in primary culture in response to retinoic acid. Blood 57:1000–1004, 1981
27. Arlin Z, Mertelsmann R, Berman E, et al: 13-cis-retinoic acid does not increase the true remission rate and the

duration of true remission (induced by cytotoxic chemotherapy) in patients with chronic phase chronic myelogenous leukemia. J Clin Oncol 3:473–476, 1985

28. Gold EJ, Mertlesmann R, Itri M, et al: Phase 1 clinical trial of 13-cis-retinoic acid in myelodysplastic syndromes. Cancer Treat Rep 67:981–986, 1983

29. Flynn PJ, Miller WJ, Weisdorf DJ, et al: Retinoic acid treatment of acute promyelocytic leukemia: In vitro and in vivo observations. Blood 62:1211–1218, 1983

30. Potter GK, Mohamed AN, Dracopoli NC, et al: The action of $1,25(OH)_2D_3$ in nude mice bearing transplantable human myelogenous leukemic cell lines, Exp Hematol 13:722–732, 1985

31. Bar-Shavit Z, Tietelbaum SL, Reitsma P, et al: Induction of monocyte differentiation and bone resorption by 1,25-Dihydroxyvitamin D_3. Proc Natl Acad Sci USA 80:5907–5911, 1983

32. Koeffler HP, Reichel H, Reinhold M, et al: Interaction of 1,25 dihydroxyvitamin D_3 and the hematopoietic system, in Golde DW, Gale R (eds): Leukemia: Recent Advances in Biology and Treatment, New York, Alan R. Liss, 1985, pp 399–413

33. Fibach E, Sachs L: Control of normal differentiation of myeloid leukemic cells IV. Induction of differentiation by serum from endotoxin treated mice. J Cell Physiol 83:177–185, 1974

34. Metcalf D: Clonal extinction of myelomonocytic leukemic cells by serum from mice injected with endotoxin. Int J Cancer 25:225–233, 1980

35. Lotem J, Sachs L: In vivo inhibition of the development of myeloid leukemia by injection of macrophage–granulocyte-inducing protein. Int J Cancer 28:375–386, 1981

36. Burgess A, Metcalf D: Characterization of a serum factor stimulating the differentiation of myelomonocytic leukemic cells. Int J Cancer 26:647–654, 1980

37. Nicola N, Metcalf D, Matsumoto M, et al: Purification of a factor inducing differentiation in murine myelomonocytic leukemia cells: Identification as granulocyte colony-stimulating factor. J Biol Chem 258:9017–9023, 1983

38. Moore MAS, Gabrilove J, Sheridan AP: Therapeutic implications of serum factors inhibiting proliferation and inducing differentiation of myeloid leukemic cells. Blood Cells 9:125–137, 1985

39. Gabrilove J, Welte K, Lu L, et al: Constitutive production of leukemia differentiation, colony-stimulating erythroid burst-promoting, and pluripoietic factors by a human hepatoma cell line: Characterization of the leukemia differentiation factor. Blood 66:407–416, 1985

40. Nicola NA, Metcalf D, Johnson GR, et al: Separation of functionally distinct human granulocytic-macrophage colony stimulating factors. Blood 54:614–627, 1979

41. Salahuddin S, Markhan PD, Lindner SG, et al: Lymphokine production by cultured human T cells transformed by human T cell leukemic lymphoma virus I. Science 223:703–707, 1984

42. Olsson IL, Sarngadharan MG, Breitman TR, et al: Isolation and characterization of a T lymphocyte-derived differentiation and proliferation of HL-60 leukemic cells in the presence of leukocyte condition medium. Leuk Res 4:301–307, 1980

43. Elias L, Wogenvich F, Wallace J, et al: Altered pattern of differentiation and proliferation of HL-60 leukemic cells in the presence of leukocyte conditioned medium. Leuk Res 4:301, 1980

44. Welte K, Platzer E, Lu I, et al: Purification and biochemical characterization of human pluripotent colony stimulating factor. Proc Natl Acad Sci USA 82:1526–1530, 1985

45. Plitzer EP, Welte K, Gabrilove JL, et al: Biological activities of a human pluripotent hematopoietic colony stimulating factor on normal and leukemic cells. J Exp Med 162:1788–1801, 1985

46. Gabrilove J, Welte K, Harris P, et al: Pluripoietin-alpha; a second human hematopoietic colony stimulating factor produced by the human bladder carcinoma cell line 5637. Proc Natl Acad Sci USA (in press)

47. Souza LM, Boone TC, Gabrilove J, et al: Recombinant pluripotent human granulocyte colony-stimulating factor: Effects on normal and leukemic myeloid cells. Science (in press)

48. Perussia BET, Dayton V, Fanning P, et al: Immune interferon and leukocyte-conditioned medium induce normal and leukemic myeloid cells to differentiate along the monocyte pathway. J Exp Med 158:2058–2080, 1983

49. Pace JL, Russel SW, Torres BA, et al: Recombinant mouse-G-interferon induces the primary step in macrophage activation of tumor cell killing. J Immunol 130:2011–2013, 1983

50. Friedheim H, Cannistra SA, Levine H, et al: Expression of interleukin 2 receptors and binding of interleukin 2 by gamma interferon-induced human leukemic and normal monocytic cells. J Exp Med 162:1111–1116, 1985

51. Reitsma PH, Rothberg PG, Astrin SM, et al: Regulation of myc gene expression in HL-60 leukemia cells by a vitamin D metabolite. Nature 306:492–494, 1983

FUTURE PERSPECTIVES

Future Perspectives for Biological Response Modifiers: A Viewpoint

E. Mihich

BIOLOGICAL RESPONSE Modifiers (BRMs), have been recently identified as a group of diversified agents within a programmatic area of potential therapeutic interest. The definition of BRM includes agents or approaches that alter interactions between tumors and host toward therapeutic advantage, primarily through modification of host response to tumors.[1] While there is little doubt that BRMs as a whole provide approaches toward the development of new types of useful cancer therapies, it is also likely that different types of BRMs have different degrees of potentiality in this respect, whether used alone or in combination with other BRMs or other modalities of treatment. In some cases the information available relates to phenomena observed primarily in vitro, as, for example, in the case of tumor differentiating agents; in such cases predictions can be based only on the assumption that concepts derived from in vitro phenomena have a counterpart in vivo, an expectation not necessarily fulfilled.

In this article, primary attention is given to BRMs that presumably act through a modification of host defenses against a tumor because, as a whole, more information is available about these agents than about other BRMs. The potentiality of interfering with regulation of tumor growth and/or differentiation is also briefly considered, however, as this approach is bound to increase in its therapeutic relevance. Whenever possible, reference is made to review articles to maximize information transferral.

A somewhat coarse critique of cancer immunotherapy might suggest that this modality, as known to date in clinical practice, is of relatively little value, certainly less valuable than established approaches based on cytoreductive combination chemotherapy. As immunotherapy, defined in broad terms, represents a major portion of the BRM modality, there is a tendency in some quarters to generalize the frustrations derived from the experience gained in the past with nonspecific immunotherapy and to apply them a priori to BRM as a whole. This skepticism is also in part the consequence of early over optimistic and premature pronouncements that have elicited greater expectations than warranted and when not realized have placed undeserved discredit on the BRM field in general. Nevertheless it is now evident that some types of immunotherapy have clinical activity under specific conditions. This evidence is consistent with current knowledge of the mechanisms of immune responses and their regulation in experimental systems. This knowledge supports the concept that immunotherapeutic treatments can be effective under conditions present in any one patient perhaps only at certain stages of the evolution of tumor-host interactions. Given the fact that even so-called nonspecific immunoaugmenting agents have shown activity against tumors in humans,[1] it seems reasonable to expect that unique agents with intrinsic specificity and selectivity of action may hold promise towards therapeutic applications. There is little doubt that known BRMs have, in general, limited potency. Also, much more knowledge needs to be acquired on the regulation of biological responses in man before the BRMs can be utilized optimally. The limitations are counterbalanced, however, by the rapid progress being made in obtaining large amounts of biologicals in purified form through modern biotechnology. The opportunity is thus provided to verify in humans the validity of proposals often based on results obtained in vitro or in animal experimentation until recently severely restricted by the limited availability of the agents under study. Moreover, although the toxicity of BRMs is not insignificant,[2] it is not necessarily related

---

From the Grace Cancer Drug Center, Roswell Park Memorial Institute, New York State Department of Health, Buffalo.

Address reprint requests to E. Mihich, MD, Grace Cancer Drug Center, Roswell Park Memorial Institute, New York State Department of Health, 666 Elm St, Buffalo, NY 14263.

0093-7754/86/1302-0014$05.00/0

to mechanisms also involved in their antitumor actions; this suggests novel opportunities in the design of selective treatments.

THE GENERAL BASIS FOR BRM ACTION

It may be reasonably said that a common denominator in the action of most novel BRMs is the presence of a specific receptor or binding structure on the surface of the cells directly affected by the agent. This appears to be the case when the target cell is a tumor cell on which the BRM acts directly as well as when the target cell is a host cell being triggered to exert antitumor action either directly or through a cascade of effects. In terms of agents, this appears to be the case for cytokines, such as lymphokines, interferons (IFNs), lymphotoxins, and tumor necrosis factor (TNF), obviously for antibodies and complement, for transferred antigen-specific cells and for differentiation and growth factors. Exceptions are likely to be found among immunomodulating chemicals and bacterial products. The effects of these agents may be due as much to selective stimulation of target host cells such as macrophages as to selective elimination of a target host cell involved in negative feed-back control mechanisms; both effects may be based on selective action on intracellular metabolism not necessarily requiring the existence of an agent-specific surface receptor moiety.

In most cases, natural BRMs may have a primary cellular basis for their action different from that of cytotoxic anticancer agents, most of which affect the synthesis or function of DNA. Except for differentiation factors, BRMs ultimately cause tumor cell elimination either through direct cytotoxic action on tumor cells or through a cascade of effects resulting in increased antitumor action of host defenses. It remains to be seen whether the presumed basic differences in proximal cellular action between BRMs and cytotoxic drugs noted above might condition a favorable use of these two types of agents in combination. Although at first sight one might expect that this would be the case, too little is known about the ultimate mechanisms of tumor cell death induced by BRMs to exclude the possibility that these mechanisms may be in some cases similar to those of cytotoxic drugs such that synergistic action may be precluded. Clearly this is an area where increased information must be sought through systematic studies that should be emphasized in the future.

Considering BRMs from a different point of view, and focusing on those acting through an augmentation of host defenses against tumor, one may divide them somewhat dogmatically into antigen-dependent and antigen-independent agents. Given the complex interactions existing in the regulation of the various networks of host defense, this separation must always be viewed with caution, but it is useful in formulating reasonable projections in the therapeutic use of the agents considered.

Predominantly antigen-dependent effects are those caused by immunomodulating natural and synthetic drugs, perhaps by the IFNs, by some lymphokines, by certain anti-T cell monoclonal antibodies and by thymic factors restoring T cell functions.[3] The antitumor effects of adoptively transferred T cells, both the classical T cytotoxic effector cells,[3] and possibly the recently discovered lymphokine activated killer (LAK) cells,[4] and those of passively transferred antitumor monoclonal antibodies, both by themselves and as delivery vectors,[3] are also dependent on the presence of tumor-associated antigens (TAAs). Therefore, the action of this type of BRMs will depend not only on TAA expression but also on TAA accessibility as affected by such factors as tumor vascularization and intercellular spaces on the one hand and immunological blocking and neutralizing phenomena on the other.

Predominantly antigen-independent effects are those induced through activation of macrophages or of natural killer (NK) cells. Macrophages may be activated to become cytotoxic to tumor cells and several BRMs seem to have antitumor action through the involvement of activated macrophages.[1,3] Nevertheless, a definitive demonstration that activated macrophages are uniquely active against primary tumor cells has not been obtained in some cases.[5] While cell transfer experiments involving cell subset selection suggested that activated macrophages have indeed antitumor action, in some studies this action was dependent on host immunocompetence and tumor immunogenicity.[1,5] The overall clinical experience with *Bacillus Calmette-Guérin* (BCG) and *Corynebacterium parvum* does not support the proposal that macrophage activation may be, by itself, very effective against human cancer.[6] Nevertheless substantial evidence accumulated in experimental tumor systems strongly suggests that activated macrophages may exert antitumor action through recognition of target tumor cells independent of cell population heterogeneity, particularly in the treatment of metastasis.[7] In the near future powerful muramyl dipeptide (MDP) derivatives with primary macrophage activating action in animals are expected to be tested in cancer patients[7-9]; these clinical trials may show whether or not macrophage activation represents a valid approach to the treatment of metastatic cancer. While most studies are concerned with the action of systemic macrophages, attention should also be given to intratumor resident macrophages as potential modifiers of tumor cell populations.[10,11]

The effectiveness of the NK cell system against human tumor cells in vivo has not yet been verified. In view of the substantial evidence for the cytotoxic activity of these cells in experimental systems and in human systems in vitro,[11,12] there is little doubt that the potential in vivo antitumor activity of NK cells in humans deserves intensive investigations.

The existence and function of TAA conditions the effectiveness of antigen-dependent BRM treatments and also provides the basis for the development of active immunization regimens. With the advent of monoclonal antibody technology, TAAs have been shown on human tumors such as melanomas, renal cell carcinoma, astrocytoma and other solid tumors.[13,14] TAAs have also been demonstrated on acute leukemia cells.[15] In a few cases of melanoma, it was shown that TAAs may be immunogenic in the patient of origin. In most cases, however, antibodies against TAAs are not found in the tumor-bearing patient, possibly due to a variety of mechanisms of tumor escape.[16] The occurrence of tumor escape phenomena points at the need to clarify the mechanisms involved so that treatments may be developed based on an inhibition of such escape. As a whole, the large body of evidence indicating the existence of potentially exploitable tumor immunity offers encouragement toward the possibility of developing antigen-dependent immunotherapies.

FUTURE PROJECTIONS FOR BRM THERAPIES

Projections about future developments in this area of therapeutics should stem from a realization of current achievements and should be cognizant of the fundamental need for further basic knowledge of the mechanisms regulating tumor immunity in humans. Knowledge in this area is essential not only to develop new types of BRM treatments but also to be able to utilize available BRMs optimally. Indeed only after the status of tumor immunity can be measured in a patient and the therapeutically relevant targets of BRM action are identified for each agent, will it be possible to accurately determine the conditions for the appropriate administration of a BRM and to design regimens based on a knowledge of the optimal BRM dose (OBRMD) in that particular patient. Admittedly fulfillment of these requirements represents no small task and may in fact not be completely achievable at the present status of knowledge. Nevertheless, in projecting future opportunities for developing effective anticancer treatment with BRMs, it is of paramount importance to project the need for basic studies in humans that would answer the questions implicit in the requirements noted above.

Immunomodulating Agents

It is becoming apparent that most immunoaugmenting agents ultimately alter regulatory mechanisms through a cascade of effects on components of the system and thus in broad terms may be defined as immunomodulating agents. In a very strict and dogmatic sense, however, only a few of these agents are true immunomodulators such that they have potential for affecting a response in opposite directions through effects on single target cells within a regulatory network. The current clinical status of this type of agent has been considered in a recent critique[3] and will not be reviewed herein. These agents can be divided into products obtained mainly from microorganisms or fungi, synthetic compounds and anticancer drugs.

Among the natural products (Table 1), BCG was the first agent tested in a large number of clinical trials. These trials yielded relatively little progress. In a few controlled studies, it was shown that stimulation of host defenses with BCG could induce measurable effects in

Table 1. Partial List of Immunomodulating Agents

Agents	Cells Primarily Affected in a Selective Manner	References*
Microorganisms or microbial and fungal products		
BCG	MO, NK	1, 17, 18
C Parvum	MO, NK	18, 19
NCWS	MO, T	20
PSK	MO, T	21, 22
OK432	MO, T_c, NK, T_s	23
Lentinan	T, MO, NK	24, 25
Glucan	MO	26
Synthetic Compounds		
Alkyllysophospholipids	MO, T	27
Azimexon	MO, T, NK	28, 29
Levamisol	MO, T	1, 28, 30
Isoprinosine	MO, T, NK	28, 31
Bestatin	MO, NK	32
Muramyldipeptide	MO, T	33, 34
PGE inhibitors	MO, NK	35, 36
Poly ICLC	MO	37
Tufstin	MO	28, 38
Anticancer Drugs		
Cyclophosphamide	T_s	39, 40
Adriamycin	MO, T	41, 42
Vincristine	B	43, 44
Vinblastine	T	43, 44
6-MP	B	43, 45

Abbreviations: NK, natural killer; MO, macrophage; T_s, T suppressor cell.

*Whenever possible, review articles have been cited to maximize information transferral.

humans[3] when the agent was given systemically or better so when it was given regionally or intralesionally. Perhaps equally important was the lesson learned with BCG. In fact those clinical trials clearly showed how slow patient accruals, excessive diversification of aims, differences among preparations used, lack of adequately comparable prospective variables among groups of patients studied, and premature reporting of results can each contribute to misleading conclusions about the potential value of a BRM. In the future, randomized trials are to be considered essential in such investigations. Another aspect of the experience gained with BCG and other immunoaugmenting BRMs is that in most cases where prolongation of median survival of a group of patients is seen, ultimate convergence of treated and control survival curves is also noted. It is not clear whether a reduced effectiveness of continuous BRM treatments in the presence of a growing tumor escaping host control mechanisms provides a sufficient explanation for that rather common observation. It is also not clear whether or not, or to what extent, tumor mass per se may affect the efficacy of host defenses. Undoubtedly the evolution of tumor host relationships during a continuous BRM treatment in humans is an area of investigation deserving high priority in the future, not only in studies of these types of BRMs, but in the field as a whole.

Several extractive natural product shown in Table 1 are being tested clinically, at this time, mainly in Japan. Of these, a protein bound polysaccharide (PSK) seems to have immunoaugmenting activity with predominant effects on infections but, to date, without unequivocal antitumor effects in humans; a *Streptococcal* preparation, OK432, is undergoing intensive clinical trials with reportedly positive responses in a variety of tumors[1,23]; *Nocardia rubra*-cell wall skeleton (N-CWS) in randomized trials appears effective on metastatic lung tumor among others.[20] Lentinan showed activity against advanced gastric cancer in combination with Ftorafur.[46] It is rather difficult to sort out the compound with the highest priority based on the clinical results reported to date, nor is this task facilitated by a knowledge of the mode of action of these agents. Indeed, whereas PSK is primarily a macrophage activator, OK432 is an NK cell stimulator, N-CWS is a macrophage activator, and Lentinan is a T cell stimulator; each of these agents also affects more than one additional immune function. It is therefore impossible to decipher the critical alteration that is relevant to therapeutic action, let alone the possibility of using any of these agents as probes to verify whether any one specific alteration in the immune system may result in a useful antitumor effect. Therefore, while the pursuit of careful clinical studies with such agents is laudable as the results may ultimately provide some benefit to some patients, it is doubtful that these trials will lead to progress in the field beyond the knowledge already basically derived from the studies with BCG. These studies may also be complicated by the essential requirement that reproducible, possibly purified to homogeneity or, even better, synthetic preparations be used. Clinical studies on natural extractive products should optimally be postponed until the active moiety can be prepared synthetically or by genetic engineering procedures.

Among the examples of synthetic immunomodulators listed on Table 1, Levamisol[1,28] and Bestatin[32] have already been tested in man, both showing statistically significant but biologically not outstanding antitumor activity; however, in the future both are expected to be studied further, particularly in the adjuvant setting. A compound of great interest is muramyl tripeptide-phosphatidylethanolamine (MTP-PE), a synthetic analog of MDP, which in mice specifically activates macrophages to become cytotoxic for tumor cells, particularly when given encapsulated in liposomes.[47] Because of its selective activity on macrophages, with a relative minor component of T cell involvement, this agent may provide a very useful tool to assess the validity of macrophage-activating therapies against cancer; it is expected that clinical trials with this agent will start during 1986.

In recent years, the immunomodulating activity of certain anticancer drugs has been well demonstrated in experimental systems and has been thoroughly reviewed.[43,44,48] For example, cyclophosphamide affects precursors of T suppressor cells, both in mice[49] and in humans,[39,40] and is more discriminatory than available monoclonal antibodies directed against T cell phenotype markers. Likewise, in mice Adriamycin (Adria Laboratories, Columbus, Ohio) selectively induces maturation of macrophages and eliminates an adherent T down-regulator cell, along with stimulation of lymphokinc production.[41,42,50] Whether this antibiotic has comparable effects in humans is not yet known. Other anticancer drugs, both antimetabolites and agents reacting directly with intracellular macromolecules, also have been shown to exert selective and in some cases specific effects on the immune systems in mice.[43,48,51] Thus the old concept is no longer tenable that anticancer drugs are primarily immunosuppressive and relatively nonspecific and nonselective in their actions on the immune system.[43,51]

In view of the fact that these agents do have specific immunomodulating activity, it is reasonable to propose that clinical investigations be initiated to verify this activity in humans. Subsequently protocols should be designed to examine the possibility that this activity may have therapeutic value, for instance in remission maintenance regimens when presumably the patient's immune system is somewhat less influenced by the disease experience than it might be in the presence of overt tumor masses. Indeed it may be possible to utilize certain anticancer drugs not only for their cytotoxic action on tumors, but also for their therapeutically favorable immunomodulating action and (see below) for their capacity to favor tumor cell differentiation.

In concluding discussion of this broad group of BRMs, certain considerations are in order with reference to their potential as anticancer therapeutic agents. It is apparent that a relatively large number of agents are already available that have immunomodulating activity in experimental systems in vitro and in vivo. Because of species differences and differences among the models used, some of which are not readily reflecting the situation existing in cancer patients, and the fact that immunomodulating activity is as much dependent on pharmacologic parameters as it is on immunologic parameters,[43,48] it may be difficult to identify the more promising agents among seemingly comparable BRMs. It is therefore important that in the future priority be given to studies aimed at defining appropriate models for the selection of BRMs that deserve to be tested in man. Also, as alluded to above, efforts should be made to clarify relevant parameters of tumor immunity in man, their possible changes as a function of disease type and stage, and the effects of BRMs on thcm. Only thcn an OBRMD may bc determined during phase I trials, this leading to the design of optimal regimens and patient selection for phase II trials.

Admittedly these simply stated needs imply a very large amount of work and the solution of problems that may be beyond total feasibility at the current level of basic knowledge. In the opinion of this author, however, these are important needs for all BRMs, not only for immunomodulating agents, that deserve urgent attention and concerted efforts.

Given progress in the direction just mentioned, it is important that the mode of action of new immunomodulators be clarified in meaningful models. This is critical not only to the design of appropriate regimens in clinical trials but also to the use of any given agent as a probe to verify whether a given specific immunomodulation has therapeutic relevance in man.

A tumor can stimulate the development of

suppressor functions of T[5,16] and non-T[16] cells. There needs to be in vivo clinical verification of the proposal that selective inhibition of T suppressor cells with cyclophosphamide[39,40,49,52] may have therapeutic value, perhaps in combination with other agents. Such an inhibition could also be achieved with monoclonal antibodies (MoAbs)[53] and also through inhibition of suppression mediators.[16] In addition to the implicit potential value of this type of approach, the information acquired through its implementation may elucidate, at least in part, the reason why human tumors are usually not immunogenically effective in eliciting a productive antitumor response.

Another possibility for tumor escape is the formation of blocking TAA-antibody complexes.[16] It is possible that these complexes, other serum blocking factors and suppressor cell activating factors may be removed by extracorporeal passage through columns coated with protein A or other immunoabsorbants[54]; these approaches are currently being verified in clinical trials and should be pursued in conjunction with other means of potentially therapeutic immunomodulations such as mentioned above.

Additional approaches based on drug-induced augmentation of macrophage or NK functions or the modification of T helper to T suppressor cell ratios should be vigorously pursued,[3] also with emphasis on modification of intratumor effectors.

Well-studied specific immunomodulators may be invaluable in assessing the clinical potentiality of such therapies as those based on macrophage activation, NK cell stimulation, T suppressor cells inhibition, and T helper cell or T effector cell stimulation. It is obvious that immunomodulators with specific effects on possibly a single target host cell type are preferable to agents that have effects on multiple target cells, this precluding the possibility of using them as discriminating probes.

The rational use of immunomodulating agents in cancer therapeutics can be optimally implemented only when tumor immunity and its regulation can be reliably measured in cancer patients, this being a formidable task at present. Compromises and approximations may be in some cases acceptable hoping that semi-empirical progress may yield therapeutic advantages and also clarify the central issues at hand. Finally, it seems important that the therapeutic potential of immunomodulation by BRMs be verified and its limitations defined for each of the possible approaches mentioned above (eg, macrophage activation therapies), in more than one disease type, before any one is discarded as nonviable.

Cytokines

In a broad sense, cytokines are cell products with biological activity on another cell or on themselves that are produced in response to a variety of endogenous or exogenous stimuli. Within such a broad definition one might distinguish subgroups defined by function,[55] for example, cell regulators or cytotoxic agents; or by cell origin, for example lymphokines (made by lymphocytes) or other cytokines made by other normal or tumor cells, see below. It is customary to group cytokines according to both criteria, but giving emphasis on their functions. Consequently one may consider cytokines as follows: (1) IFNs are cytokines made in response to viral infection or to other inducers by leukocytes, fibroblasts or lymphocytes. (2) Lymphokines are regulators of components of the immune response made by lymphocytes; regulators made by cells of the monocyte-macrophage type are customarily included in this group. (3) Lymphotoxins (LTs) are cytotoxic factors produced by activated lymphocytes and therefore are also lymphokines. (4) TNF is one of the cytotoxic factors produced by macrophages. (5) Growth factors other than those produced by lymphocytes are biologicals such as epidermal growth factor (EGF), tumor growth factor (TGF), or colony stimulating factors (CSFs). (6) Differentiation factors, each specific for a given target cell, are produced by a variety of cell types. There are many other cytokines[56] that may be classified as helper factors (for example, transferrin or complement components), suppressor factors (for example, soluble immune suppressor factors [SIRs]), factors acting on inflammatory cells (for example, macrophage migration inhibitory factor [MIF]), or factors acting on vascular endothelium (for example, increased vascular permeability factor or the complex sets of interacting factors promoting vascularization of tumors). Although it is estimated that there are more than 100 different cytokines, their precise number can be determined only through structural analysis and the production of individual pure moieties by genetic engineering.[56] Given this large pool of biological factors with unique specificities of action, it is likely that this group of agents will represent a source of potentially valuable new anticancer agents, acting directly on cancer cells or indirectly through a modification of host mechanisms. Therefore, cytokines are bound to be the object of intensive study in the foreseeable future. Such studies are made feasable and realistic by the availability of pure compounds in quantities by genetic engineering procedures.

Given the plethora of factors found even within an apparently similar functional group, it is important in this area of BRMs that preclinical relevant models be developed that would facilitate the selection of those cytokines that have a greater probability to show activity against human cancer. In this article only the future potentiality of IFN, certain lymphokines, TNF, and certain growth and differentiation factors are considered.

Interferons. Natural IFNs are a group of glycoproteins with major, but apparently not absolute, species specificity. Proteins with comparable biological activity have been obtained in recent years through recombinant DNA technology, this demonstrates that the carbohydrates in the natural products are not essential at least for some of the effects of IFN. The main biologic actions of the IFNs include antiviral, antitumor, immunomodulating, and cell differentiating activities. These actions appear to be shared by the three classes of natural IFNs, namely α, β, and γ, but it is not yet precisely known to what extent specific quantitative differences exist among them. Physicochemical heterogeneity occurs within and among IFN types,[57] even more so with the advent of recombinant DNA IFNs molecules and hybrids thereof. With the availability of an increasing number of diversified IFN molecules, the profiles of biologic activity of each is bound to become more diversified too; it is not yet known whether mixtures of molecules may ultimately be required for optimal anticancer activity in general or for specific activity in patients with a given tumor type. The mode of action and pharmacology of the IFNs have been reviewed repeatedly.[58] It is not clear whether the antitumor activity of all or some of the IFNs is due primarily to their direct anticell action or to their immunomodulating effects or even, perhaps, to differentiating effects analogous to those demonstrated in vitro in various cell systems. Direct effects on tumor cells and immunomodulation may both be relevant in humans, perhaps one prevailing over the other depending upon target tumor type, dose, and regimens.[3] Optimal regimens have not yet been defined in humans for any IFN. This uncertainty also pertains to the optimal dose, although in some clinical studies the antitumor effects of high doses were better than those of the lower doses tested.[59] These uncertainties are in part the consequence of the fact, alluded to above, that the mode of antitumor action of the IFNs is not yet known and, therefore, that a parameter of possibly relevant BRM action could not yet be identified on which to base the determination of the OBRMD. Because of this, until now IFNs have been tested clinically essentially according to criteria established for trials of anticancer cytotoxic drugs. In the case of IFN, however, the evaluation of antitumor activity is rendered more difficult by the relatively slow onset of antitumor effects.

In the light of the preceding considerations, it is obvious that any future projection about BRMs must include provisions for a large effort towards the clarification of the relevant mode(s) of antitumor action of each IFN molecule that is tested in man, the determination of optimal regimens, target cell specificities and possible synergisms in combination with other BRMs or cytotoxic drugs. The opportunities for combinations with other BRMs may be particularly propitious for IFNγ,[49] itself a lymphokine, for which synergism has already been proposed in combination with IFNα and IFNβ[3,56] or such agents as macrophage-activating MDP derivatives[60] or TNF.[61] The difficulties to be met in such future investigations are not only those intrinsic to the topic itself but also those related to the fact that well-founded priorities should be established in selecting for detailed study those IFNs, among an increasing number of molecules and their combinations, which hold the greatest promise of therapeutic action in humans.

A systematic investment of efforts in pursuing IFN investigations seems justified by the results obtained to date. Although most of the clinical experience has been obtained thus far with various types of IFNα, phase I and initial phase II trials for IFNβ and IFNγ also suggest therapeutic interest. In fact, IFNγ appears to exert more pronounced immunomodulation and greater antiproliferative activity than IFNα or β.[56] It can be said that IFNα has activity against a few types of human tumors when tested as a single agent. Thus a 10% to 15% objective response rate has been seen in patients with renal cell carcinoma, melanoma, and myeloma, around a 20% response rate among patients with Kaposi's sarcoma, about a 40% response rate in patients with various types of lymphomas and about a 80% to 90% response rate among patients with hairy cell leukemia and mycosis fungoides; a high incidence of responses has also been seen in patients with benign papilloma of the larynx.[3] It may be argued that IFNα has shown activities against certain types of cancer generally comparable to those exhibited by several established cytotoxic anticancer agents at comparable stages of development. There is little doubt that these indications of activity, obtained as they have been under empirical and probably suboptimal conditions, are likely to be confirmed in future investigations hopefully carried out with a greater knowledge of relevant mechanisms of response. Moreover, as is the case with cytotoxic agents, it should be expected that the therapeutic potentality of the IFNs can be fulfilled only when these agents are used in appropriate combination regimens.[3] In conclusion, it may be reasonably predicted that certain IFN molecules will ultimately find some useful application in clinical cancer therapeutics, this justifying the pursuit of further basic and clinical investigations of this group of BRMs.

Lymphokines. The lymphokines are peptide moieties secreted by lymphocytes that regulate immune responses through differentiation, amplification, and inhibition of cell functions; some of them also have a cytotoxic effector function.[62]

Lymphokines as a family of agents have therapeutic potential from different points of view. For instance, a lymphokine like IL-2 may stimulate the differentiation and proliferation of cytotoxic T lymphocytes (CTLs) and thus may be useful in augmenting T effector function in the treated hosts or in facilitating proliferation in culture of clones of CTLs sensitized against authochthonous tumors thus allowing their subsequent adoptive transfer to the patient of origin.[63] These applications have not yet been verified in humans. Recently, however, it was reported that IL-2, when given to patients along with culture generated lymphokine activated killer (LAK) cells, maintained LAK activity in vivo and caused objective responses in treated individuals,[64] in parallel with results obtained in mouse tumor models. The LAK cells have T cell phenotypic characteristics, are generated nonspecifically and kill target tumor cells that are not affected by NK cells.[4] Given the promising initial results obtained with this new type of adoptive cell tranfer therapy, it is likely that treatments based on the utilization of LAK cells plus IL-2 administration will undergo intensive investigation in the foreseeable future. The fact that in vivo administration of high doses of IL-2 alone may elicit the generation of endogenous LAK cells and inhibit pulmonary metastasis in experimental murine models has been recently reported.[65] The requirement for extremely high doses suggests that the regulation of such cells may be a suitable target area for further exploration and a possible site of intervention in development of new therapies. Indeed, in mice it was recently found that PGEs down regulate LAK cells such that indomethacin (IM) causes them to increase in activity; consequently combinations such as those of IL-2 with IM or of IM with Adriamycin, the latter inducing increased IL-2 production (see preceding section), can be reasonably designed for study in experimental systems with possible applications in humans. The cooperative interactions between IL-2 and IFNγ in the generation and replication of LAK cells has also been recently demonstrated in humans,[66] this pointing at the likelihood that combinations of lymphokines may acquire practical therapeutic value in the future based also on a concerted augmentation of cellular defenses.

Stimulation of T cell proliferation by IL-2 in vivo has been demonstrated in mice as well as in humans.[63,64] Of particular interest is the observation that in patients with AIDS, IL-2 administration resulted in some correction of the abnormal Th/Ts ratios observed in these patients and of their T cell defects.[56]

With the advent of recombinant DNA IL-2, it should be expected that the therapeutic potential of this lymphokine will be definitively ascertained in the foreseeable future. Several questions of a pharmacologic nature need to be answered, however, before IL-2 and other lymphokines can be optimally used in humans. In fact the half life of lymphokines in blood is generally rather short and improvements in mode of administration are desirable such as application by continuous infusion or administration of agent incorporated into liposomes. Moreover, relationships seem to exist between lymphokine action and certain hormones, including those of the neuroendocrine system,[67] and these need to be carefully explored. The possibility that tumors of the lymphoid system may respond to lymphokine administration cannot be excluded a priori although in experimental systems such tumors have been generally insensitive to such regulation.[56]

Lymphotoxin is possibly an effector moiety instrumental in the cytotoxic activity of sensitized T cells and deserves to be tested in humans as an antitumor cytotoxic substance. Only recently it has been obtained in purified form and adequate quantities through genetic engineering, and the results of the initial clinical trials have not yet been reported.

Of the more than 100 lymphokines available,[56] factor(s) involving macrophage activation (MAF and/or IFNγ) may also represent a useful moiety based on the assumption that activated macrophages will represent an effective means to attack cancer, a reasonable projection at the present state of knowledge.[7] Macrophages may indeed represent a heterogenous cell population of considerable potential value in cancer therapeutics. When suitably activated, they have been found to kill tumor cells selectively without causing cytotoxicity in normal cells in experimental model systems. Taken as a whole, they represent a factory producing multiple types of substances ranging from cytokines like macrophage cytolytic factor or TNF to pharmacological regulators such as PGE_2 that also affect cells of the host defense system, eg, NK cells. It is reasonable to expect that stimulation or activation of macrophages, their adoptive transfer and/or the exogenous administration of some of their products (produced by genetic engineering) will find useful application in cancer therapeutics. TNF, mentioned below as an example, has already reached the stage of phase I clinical trial.

TNF. Tumor necrosis factor is a glycoprotein produced by macrophages conditioned by BCG or other stimulating agents and triggered by endotoxin; this compound has tumor necrotizing effects similar to those caused by endotoxin but clearly does not contain endotoxin.[1] In contrast to endotoxin, TNF is toxic in vitro for murine or human tumor cells but not for normal cells.[61] Recently TNF polypeptide has been obtained by genetic engineering and its structure identified.[68,69,70] These preparations have been found to exert all the biological effects of natural TNF. It was found that specific binding sites for TNF, presumably a specific receptor, exist on sensitive target tumor cells and that the number of such receptors is correlated with sensitivity; entry of TNF into cell lysosomes, after binding to the receptor, seems to be a prerequisite for cytotoxic action. Indeed injection of TNF by micromanipulator directly into cytoplasm has no cytotoxic effect. Treatment of target cells with pronase, with cytoskeleton disrupting agents or with lysomotropic agents also abolished TNF activity, this suggesting directions of further work aimed at clarifying the mode of action of this potentially important molecule.[71]

Very recently, Cerami and co-workers reported that cachectin, a macrophage-produced factor, has a major role in the cytotoxic effects of LPS[72] and that the cachectin polypeptide is almost identical to TNF.[73] Although the marked similarities between cachectin and TNF are interesting, further work is required. While the mode of action of TNF is being actively investigated in a number of laboratories, the phase I trial of TNF has begun in Japan and elsewhere. Although any assessment of the therapeutic potentiality of TNF for the treatment of human cancer must await the results of at least the phase II trials, the clinical studies of this agent represent the first deliberate attempt to utilize therapeutically a toxic product of a cell capable of killing tumor target cells. Lymphotoxin has an identity of about 30% with TNF[68] and is produced by sensitized cytotoxic T lymphocytes; it is to be expected that this compound will also be tested in man before too long. Other cytotoxic biological products are known or will no doubt be identified in the future and should be developed toward clinical trial provided that their biological effects have a measure of specificity or selectivity for tumor cells. In the case of TNF, this prerequisite has been met. However, it is not yet known whether the cytotoxic activity of TNF can be dissociated from the hemorrhagic necrosis effect nor whether the latter effect may lead to complications that may be difficult to control in the case of certain human tumor types and/or sites. It is reasonable to conclude that intensive preclinical and clinical studies of TNF are warranted at this time, with emphasis on a definition of the clinical effects and the optimal conditions for treatment and, at the same time, on a clarification of the mode of action of the product and of the structure activity relationships involved in cytotoxic and hemorrhagic effects, respectively.

Growth factors (GFs) and Differentiation Factors (DFs). GFs and DFs represent different sets of molecules that are functionally somewhat related and include a large number of individual entities. Both GF and DF require binding to a specific receptor on the surface of cells to exert their function and in most cases an opposing relationship exists between them when tumor cells are the target. GFs are known that are secreted by one cell and act on another cell; certain GFs are secreted by a cell that also has a specific receptor for it such that the GF produced acts on the producer cell itself.[74]

Several GF and DF have been studied extensively. For example, NGF (normal growth factor) has been well characterized as a small basic protein made up of subunits; the linear sequence of one resembling pro-insulin. Using an antibody against NGF it was possible to show in vivo that the maturation of sensory neurons includes an NGF-dependent stage, this providing an example of the possibility to demonstrate a maturation activity in vivo by the use of anti-DF antibodies.[75] Indeed, thus far in most cases the function of differentiation factors has been demonstrated in cell culture systems, this always implying the possibility of noncorrespondence between in vitro model and in vivo situation.

In several neuronal tumors, differentiation can be functionally demonstrated in the presence of NGF,[76,77] this supporting the important concept that, at least in certain situations, neoplastic cells are still capable of responding to normal regulatory factors in analogy to the sensitivity to hormones of certain tumors at certain stages of their progression. Similarly human leukemic cell lines, particularly of the myeloid type, retain their sensitivity to DF or, for that matter, also to retinoic acid, certain drugs, corticosteroids, and PGEs.[78] Moreover, murine embryonal cancer cells have been shown to respond with differentiation to retinoic acid[1] possibly through an effect on GF receptors. A number of agents (see below) have been shown to be able to effect differentiation of leukemic cell lines, particularly in the presence of minimally active concentrations of DF.

GF and DF may interact at the cellular level. Competition between certain GFs for receptors has been shown in the sense that tumor growth factors (TGFs) can compete with EGF at the specific receptor thus perhaps conditioning disregulated growth.[74] Inhibition of the synthesis of a GF receptor by a DF has been exemplified by the inhibition of EGF receptor by NGF,[77] this suggesting that regulation of GF receptor synthesis may be a realistic site of therapeutic intervention.

The interplay between regulatory factors in the case of epithelial cells has just begun to be explored and appears to be as complex as the interplay between regulatory factors involved in the function of the immune system or of the hematopoietic system. For instance, PDGF, a platelet derived growth factor of MW 35,000 that is released from the α granules of platelets,[79] is a limiting factor for the growth of fibroblasts in culture; it is known that a relatively brief exposure of fibroblasts to PDGF will make them responsive to proliferating stimuli by the somatomedins, polypeptide hormones with insulin-like activity.[79] Thus a cascade of responses to factors acting in sequence can be realistically visualized in the maintenance of a proliferative state; such a cascade of responses may offer multiple opportunities for sequential therapeutic intervention.

Despite the fact that, with a few notable exceptions such as those just mentioned, information on GFs and DFs has been obtained primarily in culture, it is reasonable to predict that the functions of GF and DF provide potentially useful sites for therapeutic intervention.[78]

Limitations are also to be considered, however, as for instance those related to (1) the extreme specificity of these factors, especially DF, such that they are likely to act only on cells at specific stages of differentiation, or (2) the heterogeneity of tumor cell populations with respect to responsiveness to regulatory factors.

Based on the assumption that tumor growth is dependent on GFs in vivo and that a decrease of GF function may favor DF function and vice versa, it is conceivable that treatments may be found that would limit the synthesis of GF receptors or interrupt the signal from GF-receptor complex to the proliferation program in the cell, whether this signal is mediated by tyrosine-specific protein kinases or by other mechanisms involving intracellular proliferation factors.[78] As mentioned above, the synthesis of GF receptors has been shown to be susceptible to inhibition by other agents, such as NGF. The signal from the GF-receptor complex may be mediated by oncogene products such as tyrosine-specific protein kinase. Although it is not clear whether a decrease of this enzyme activity could bring about decreased proliferation with consequent facilitation of differentiation, it is known that differentiation induced by DF or other agents is preceded by a decrease in oncogene expression.[80] Competition with GFs for their receptor may be affected by synthetic GF analogs; alternatively antibodies may be used as receptor blocking agents. For instance, it was found that EGF has significant sequence homology and shared functional activities with urogastrone, a small polypeptide inhibiting gastric secretion.[1] Bombesin, an analog of gastrin-releasing factor with analogy to a family of peptides stimulates proliferation of 3T3 mouse fibroblasts and other cell types in vitro and in vivo. It was recently found that human small-cell lung cancer cell lines produce bombesin-like peptides and express a high affinity receptor for them.[81] Exogenous peptide also stimulates growth of these lung cancer cells, this suggesting an autocrine function for bombesin-like peptides. A monoclonal antibody to bombesin was found to block the binding of the peptide to the receptor and to inhibit the growth of the lung cancer cells in vitro and that of related xenografts in vivo.[81] The possibility to neutralize the GF per se using anti-GF antibody is contingent upon the accessibility of natural GF to that antibody, accessibility that may be limited in some cases in view of the circumscribed pericellular zone of diffusion that at least some GF are likely to have. The results with bombesin, however, support the concept that antibodies directed against GF, also of the autocrine type, may have therapeutic potential. Certainly this type of approach should be intensely pursued.

The availability of specific receptor for GF may also be reduced through binding of phorbol ester (TPA) to it. Because TPA is a carcinogenesis promoter, potentially useful analogs need to be found that are devoid of this action but retain GF receptor binding capacity.[78]

Administration of exogenous DFs or of functional synthetic analogs, stimulation of endogenous DF production or release by such agents as dexamethasone, LPS or polyIpolyC[78] or stimulation of the synthesis of DF receptors represent the other side of the coin in trying to induce cell differentiation for a therapeutic purpose.

Several compounds are known to have differentiation-inducing effects on certain types of neoplastic cells. For instance, HL60 cells are induced to differentiate upon exposure to such polar compounds as dimethylformamide, hexamethylene bisacetamide (HMBA), or butyric acid,[78,82] although the exact mechanisms involved are not clear at this time. Interferon is also a potent differentiating agent.[83]

The possibility of inducing neoplastic cell differentiation by the concerted action of anticancer drugs inhibiting DNA synthesis and exogenous DF has been extensively explored by Bloch.[78,84–85] In his pioneering studies, he showed that preservation of transcription mechanisms for the essential transferral of differentiation-related information and of protein synthesis are essential for the action of DF to occur in conjunction with the DNA inhibition caused by the drugs. These agents affect the proliferation program in target cells, also as evidenced by decreases of oncogene expression,[86] such that exogenous or endogenous DF may now induce differentiation.

The information briefly alluded to above, taken as a whole, substantiate the important concept that the oncogenic arrest of cell differentiation that appears to be instrumental in effecting neoplastic transformation, is not necessarily an irreversible phenomenon.[78] This offers encouragement to the proposition that induction of differentiation and inhibition of GF effects on neoplastic tumor cells may be a viable and effective approach in the future development of selective nontoxic therapies of cancer.

Monoclonal Antibodies (MoAbs)

The use of MoAbs in the treatment of cancer is dependent on the presence on the target cancer cells of TAA epitopes in larger amounts than on normal cells. This prerequisite is likely to be met in many instances. Given this general feasability, it is reasonable to predict that MoAbs, because of their unique specificity, will find useful applications in cancer therapeutics as effectors against tumor cells, as selective delivery systems of compounds to tumor cells and/or as immunomodulating or growth regulating agents.

Despite the large number of MoAbs that are now available in many laboratories,[56] only a few pilot studies have been conducted thus far in patients with solid tumors, such as pancreas, melanoma, and colorectal carcinoma[6,87] with the majority of the studies being conducted in patients with leukemia and lymphoma.[5,56,88] Antiidiotypic antibodies have been used with success in a patient with B cell lymphoma who was refractory to chemotherapy.[89] In cases of cutaneous T cell lymphomas, transient responses of skin lesions and lymph nodes were noted.[90] In patients with pancreatic tumors, a few cases of complete tumor regression were seen, with about 20% of patients with colorectal carcinoma responding.[91]

Much information has been obtained during early clinical trials that is consistent with knowledge acquired in animals and will be useful in guiding more definitive clinical studies.[3] Antigenic modulation is observed particularly in hematological diseases but is transient in nature. Effective circulating antibody levels can normally be obtained only after circulating TAA has been complexed, this representing a potential problem in those cases where tumors shed substantial amounts of TAA in the circulation. It seems likely that the MoAbs used clinically to date are not cytotoxic to target cells through complement action but mark tumor cells for attack by K cells through an antibody-dependent cellular cytotoxicity (ADCC) response; given this mechanism it would appear that ADCC effector cells are the limiting step. Therefore treatment with other agents aimed at increasing ADCC effector function, for instance IFN in combination with certain MoAbs are in order. The MoAbs studied to date are of mouse origin and consequently they elicit antimouse antibodies in the treated patient; this possibly may limit the institution of prolonged treatments[3] or may actually provide new approaches to the control of cancer.[91]

In humans, it would appear that MoAbs selectively bind to tumor, albeit with different affinity, and can exert antitumor activity in inverse relationship to tumor mass and/or TAA shedding. Because of antigenic diversity within tumor cell populations and the exquisite specificity of MoAbs, it is possible that mixtures of reagents may be required for optimal therapeutic application. Although the results obtained on a few patients with lymphoma using antiidiotypic antibodies have been exciting, in practice the routine development of such antibodies for individual patients is fraught with difficulties, among others the fact that the long time needed to raise such MoAbs requires that the patient survives long enough to be treated.

It would seem that efforts should be placed in different directions in this promising area of BRM development. Selective MoAbs of proven interest should be made in large quantity and rigorously tested in clinical trials that would include determination of such parameters as dose and schedule dependence. The toxicological features of MoAbs may not represent as many difficulties as initially feared and have been discussed recently.[2] It would be useful to develop large amounts of MoAbs in culture rather than continuously depending on i.p. mouse hybridoma growth, thereby simplifying purification and preclinical toxicologic experimentation. The availability of MoAbs of human origin would be desirable even though their advantages may not be as great as anticipated due to the intrinsic genetic heterogeneity of the human population. Of considerable importance and promise could be studies aimed at developing MoAb fragments that would retain the desired biological activity and might be made synthetically or by recombinant DNA technology. In view of the plethora of MoAbs available, it will become soon important to establish a MoAb registry and build a data base for orderly comparisons and systematic development.

The development of MoAbs as selective delivery vectors for anticancer drugs, toxins or radioisotopes (the later for topical irradiation or radioimaging) has been studied using model systems in culture and in animals, but its realistic potentiality for the treatment of human cancer has not yet been thoroughly tested. Intracavitary administration of ^{131}I radiolabeled MoAb had tumor-reducing effects.[92] This type of conjugate has been tested in children with neuroblastoma[93] and in adult patients with melanoma[94] and with hepatoma.[95] MoAbs covalently linked to a toxin appeared to eliminate in vitro tumor cells from bone marrow before transplantation.[53] It is unlikely that MoAbs conjugated with toxins may be safely used systemically[53] until means are devised to avoid the uptake of such conjugates by the reticuloendothelial system (RES), particularly in liver, with consequent local toxicity; progress in this direction is being achieved.[96] MoAbs linked with daunorubicin,[97] vindesine,[98] MTX,[99] or mitomycin C[100] have been primarily tested against various target human tumor cells in vitro, with clinical trials being at a very preliminary stage. The use of MoAbs as modulators of the host response has not yet been explored systematically but may be of interest in instituting specific antisuppressor therapies of cancer, based on the assumption that increased suppressor activities is a significant mechanism of tumor escape.[16] The use of MoAbs to block GF receptors and thus facilitate differentiation has just begun (see preceding section).

Despite the fact that, as a whole, the use of MoAbs as effectors in the treatment of cancer is still at a rather primitive stage, there is little doubt that this approach should be pursued intensely. In fact while much needs to be learned on the determinants and mechanisms of MoAb action, the potential of MoAbs in cancer therapeutics seems real given the demonstrated feasibility of the approach and the unique specificity intrinsic to an antibody interaction with antigen. In this area as it is in some other areas of BRM development, there is an excess of agents available in pilot laboratory quantitates relative to developmental capacities, this calling for the establishment of strict priorities based on comparative evaluations made in relevant preclinical models; human tumor xenografts in nude mice have been widely used to this end. In considering MoAbs as vectors, it would seem that early efforts in development towards systematic clinical trial should be given to MoAb conjugates with drugs or radiolabeled isotopes, with toxin conjugates restricted for the moment to such in vitro uses as bone marrow tumor cell elimination before the transplantation. Drug conjugates seem to be the safest to study first, given the knowledge already acquired on the toxicity of the anticancer agents to be used. Toxicity problems related to accumulation and nonspecific binding at unwanted sites are still to be overcome in connection with the use of isotope conjugates. When toxin conjugates can be prepared devoid of the characteristic causing them to be accumulated in the RES, this application of MoAbs may deserve high priority.

Active Immunization

Many attempts have been made in the past to prepare vaccines based on the use of killed or attenuated autologous or allogeneic tumor cells and/or tumor cells modified through virus infection or haptenic alterations.[1,101–103] The assessment of human cancer vaccines is very difficult, however, in terms of the selection of appropriate antigen type and form, dose, and regimen. Perhaps very important is the timing of vaccination during the evolution of tumor-host relationships in the progression of the disease in any one patient. The actual evaluation of the clinical results obtained also poses major difficulties. Nevertheless, the unequivocal demonstration of immunogenic TAA in certain diseases, for example, melanoma[104] indicates the feasibility of developing specific active immunotherapy and provides encouragement toward its further development. In this area, perhaps even more than in other BRM areas, it is essential that progress be achieved in understanding relevant parameters of immunoregulation in humans and their changes during disease progression in order to be able to measure the modifications induced by a vaccine given at a particular time according to a particular modality. It is only based on such measurements that optimal conditions for vaccine utilization in further trials can be defined. Indeed it is reasonable to project that improper vaccine utilization could actually induce untoward effects such as augmented tumor growth. To mention only an obvious consideration, if shedding of TAA is instrumental in determining untoward immune suppressive or blocking effects,[16] then the administration of TAA in an unsuitable form or by an unfavorable route or regimen could also cause untoward effects. It is conceivable that such problems may be minimized if combined with an antisuppressor treatment, for example with a drug such as cyclophosphamide or a MoAb directed against suppressor cell determinants; this approach should be studied carefully in relevant animal models before it is tested in humans.

Active immunization with PPD conjugated to cells from a MCA-induced mouse sarcoma resulted in augmented immunogenicity of tumor cells in syngeneic hosts with pre-existent delayed hypersensitivity to BCG.[105] Pooled allogeneic cells from patients with AML have been used as vaccines after surface modification with neuraminidase, in sequence with remission induction chemotherapy[106]; in these randomized trials beneficial effects were noted, but it is not yet clear whether specific TAA or nonspecific immunization determined the effects seen.

In syngeneic guinea pigs bearing hepatocarcinoma, the possibility was investigated that vaccines using BCG modified tumor cells, rendered nontumorigenic by irradiation, may be effective in the treatment of metastatic disease when given in sequence with chemotherapy, notably before it.[107] It appears that hypersensitivity reactions occurred at the site of lung metastasis with infiltration of metastatic nodules by lymphocytes and cells of the mononuclear-macrophage type; the ensuing inflammatory reactions disrupted the structure of the metastatic nodules with increased permeability to such molecules as antitumor MoAbs. Thus it appeared that the disruption of anatomic obstacles to the uptake of drugs or biologicals may augment the effects of such treatment given after immunization.[107,108] The reported success of this sequence of treatment suggests that other modalities of immunotherapy causing inflammatory reactions in target tumors may also provide hitherto unsuspected advantages when given before other treatments.

While attempts to develop vaccines using modified tumor cells may eventually lead to useful clinical applications, the demonstration of the existence of TAA in human tumor suggests that active immunization could be achieved with purified TAA preparations. The usage of MoAbs to isolate TAA in sufficient quantity to allow purification and subsequent production of pure TAA by genetic engineering procedures seems realistic at this time. When such preparations become available for clinical trial, many important questions would have to be answered. For instance, it will then be possible to define TAA immunogenicity, whether common TAA from allogeneic origin are effective, whether antitumor effector cells are stimulated selectively in comparison to suppressive mechanisms, how to avoid the formation of unwanted immune complexes, what are the optimal conditions of treatment, and so on.

It is obvious that active specific immunotherapy based on the existence of TAA is an important BRM approach that should be studied intensively. It is also clear, at the present state of knowledge, that the effective utilization of this mode of treatment is somewhat in the future as it must await the acquisition of substantial basic information before it can be optimally developed.

Adoptive Transfer of Cells

The adoptive transfer of cells into tumor bearing hosts as a means to augment cell defenses and inhibit tumor growth has been extensively investigated in mice using T cells for transfer.[63] These cells had been sensitized with target tumor either in vivo or in vitro. By selective elimination with antisera, it was found that the transfer of T helper cells or amplifier cells from immunized mice was sufficient; however, the cooperation of recipient host effector cells was required for the antitumor effect to occur.[109] Cells sensitized in vitro and grown in the presence of IL2 when transferred into mice given exogenous IL2 at relatively low doses can lyse tumor cells without requiring further multiplication, however, these cells are also capable of proliferation.[109,110] These investigations provided much information upon which to design optimal studies in humans. It was found that T cell transfer is most effective following cytoreductive chemotherapy. In continuous long-term cultures in the presence of IL2, methods have been developed for obtaining different functional subsets of antigen-specific T lymphocytes, thus permitting attempts for diversified cell transfers. The potential therapeutic effectiveness of the transferred cells against tumor has been verified as have the complicating factors derived from the interactions of transferred cell functions with immunoregulatory networks in the recipient host.[110]

More recently it has been found that mouse spleen cells or human peripheral blood leukocytes grown in culture for three days in the presence of extremely high concentrations of IL2 are activated to generate cells that, upon intravenous infusions to tumor bearing mice or combined with radiolabeled tumor targets in four hour assays in culture, kill different types of tumor cells without requiring specific sensitization.[4,111] In vivo IL-2 administration is required to sustain the activity of these LAKs. It is of interest that these cells are different from NK cells, have T cell phenotype, but do not require sensitization for development of lytic activity. This new type of functional cell may provide useful means to exploit cell transfers as an effective therapeutic modality, in conjunction with IL2 administration. Indeed pilot clinical trails carried out by S. Rosenberg at the National Cancer Institute, USPHS seem to indicate that significant objective responses can be obtained in cancer patients through adoptive transfer of LAK cells.

As more information is acquired on the regulation of IL2 production and LAK cells function, it will be possible to design improved combination therapies. For instance, combination treatments of LAK cells with IL2 and Adriamycin may exploit the immunomodulating effects of the drug that include augmented IL2 production[50]; combinations with indomethacin may be advantageous in view of the functional inhibition of LAK cells demonstrated for PGE_2.[112]

In addition to the transfer of T cells and LAK cells, bone marrow transplantation should be mentioned as a proven means to exert therapeutic effects in preconditioned leukemic patients.[113] There is some evidence suggesting that the therapeutic effects of the transferred bone marrow cells against leukemia are related to graft-versus-host disease probably mediated by transferred T cells, although final proof must await further study.[113,114]

While the adoptive transfer to T cells and LAK cells, and the clinical therapeutic utilization of bone marrow transplantation in patients with leukemias have received much attention with consequent accumulation of a wealth of significant information, not much is known about the therapeutic potential of adoptive transfer of non-T cells such as NK cells or macrophages. The difficulties in developing these types of adoptive transfer lie in part in the relative paucity of information on how to efficiently develop large populations of these cells in culture. As more information is obtained on cytotoxic factors produced by NK cells[115] and macrophages,[68–73] it is conceivable that the administration of related recombinant DNA cytotoxin may pre-empt the need to develop adoptive transfer therapies with these cells.

CONCLUDING REMARKS

As discussed in the preceding sections of this article, a large number of structural or functional analogs can be expected to become available within diversified groups of BRMs for evaluation and possible development towards clinical trial. Moreover, several priority agents have already been identified and have been tested in humans or are designated for eventual clinical evaluation. While such a wealth of products with diverse mechanisms of antitumor action hold promise for exciting new developments in therapeutics, it also provides warnings that this promise may not be fully and/or speedily realized unless progress is achieved in several areas of knowledge. Relevant and different experimental model systems need to become available to reliably establish priorities in the choice of products to be developed. The mechanism of antitumor action of the selected agents must be clarified such that the relevant OBRMD can be identified. Additional basic information needs to be obtained on the regulatory mechanisms of tumor immunity in humans and on the changes that are likely to occur during the evolution of the neoplastic disease. Means must be developed to measure the status of tumor immunity in humans before, during and after BRM treatments in order to establish the OBRMD in man and to design protocols accordingly. Given fulfillment of these essential needs, a tall order, it can be reasonably projected that substantial progress will be made in the therapeutic exploitation of different types of BRMs. Expectations within each group of BRM, have already been briefly outlined in the preceding sections of this article. Several additional comments need to be made that pertain to the development of most of the BRMs discussed herein.

Whenever possible pure products should be used in the development of BRMs towards clinical trials. The fact that a natural product has been found to be of therapeutic interest in experimental models is promising, but the product should be obtained in pure form by chemical means or by bioengineering for ultimate development towards clinical trials. The availability of pure agents will reduce the possibility that inconsistencies of results are related to batch differences and will also increase the likelihood of defining pertinent BRM activity without possibly complicating interferences or toxicities due to impurities or the action of co-isolated known or new BRM moieties.

In some cases, agents obtained by genetic engineering may not have the total profile of antitumor activities exhibited by the natural product or, conversely, may have more salient specific effects; this might be the case, for instance, with the IFNs where heterogeneity among products within the same type have been described. In such cases it is important that maximally purified natural products be compared with each of their recombinant DNA analogs such that specific differences may be recognized and measured, and appropriate protocols may be designed, in some cases possibly using mixtures of recombinant DNA molecules.

It is conceivable that certain BRMs or groups of BRMs may have greater utility as agents restoring or augmenting host defenses against opportunistic infections in cancer patients than as antitumor agents. This may be the case for certain immunoaugmenting natural products or for certain restorative agents such as the thymic factors. Indeed, although statistically significant prolongation of survival of patients with certain types of cancer have been reported in randomized trials,[1] in general thymic factors have been shown to restore depressed immune activities more readily than to affect human tumors therapeutically.[56] It is conceivable that thymic factors may be particularly effective in correcting certain immunodeficiency syndromes that occur in connection with certain types of cancer.

Major opportunities for exploitation of BRMs with therapeutic advantages are likely to be identified in studies of combination treatments. Such studies should include combinations of BRMs with clinically effective cytotoxic anticancer agents with a view to verify the extent to which these agents might affect the action of the combinant BRM not only in a synergistic manner, possibly consequent to cytoreduction of tumor mass, but also in an antagonistic manner, possibly consequent to depression of a host defense component required for the expression of that BRM's action. Evaluation of doses and sequences of administration would be important, with the possibility that, as mentioned in a preceding section, BRM treatment may usefully precede drug treatment[56,108,116] and not only the converse, as one might predict based on the perceived expectation that BRMs may be more effective in the presence of a small tumor burden. Studies of combination treatments should also include combining different BRMs concurrently or in appropriate sequence. As alluded to in preceding sections, combinations of cytokines already provide promising examples of synergism such as those of IFNγ plus IL2[117] or of IFNγ plus TNF.[61,118] Combinations of cytokines with macrophage stimulating agents also appear promising.[7,60]

Novel approaches in this area should also be identified based on progress made in the understanding of tumor cell biology. For instance, resistance to drugs of certain tumor cells has been found to be associated with increased expression of GF receptors[119] and also, for pleiotropic resistance, to an increase in P170 glycoprotein,[120] while agents with calcium channel blocking activity have been found to overcome pleiotropic resistance through increased retention of active drugs.[121] It is appealing to predict in this case that inhibitors of specific molecular phenomena involved in the expression of GF receptors, or anti-GF receptor MoAbs, may be usefully combined with anti-P170 MoAbs or with agents such as calcium channel blockers in attempts to overcome resistance to drugs. Many such examples could be proposed for study;

efforts based on this type of approach should certainly be intensified. There is little doubt that study of combination treatments will yield fruitful therapeutic results.

While efforts should continue along lines such as those indicated in this article, new approaches should be pursued and new ideas tested in areas of BRM action not traditionally considered until now as being a part of this appraoch. In considering the biology of metastasis, several possibilities of intervention may be offered such as for instance, (1) inhibitors of certain enzymes such as the collagenases that appear to be involved in tumor invasion[122]; (2) fragments or analogs of laminin and/or MoAbs against laminin receptors[123]; (3) cyclooxygenase inhibitors in order to decrease platelets aggregation[124] and thus reduce metastatic seeding. Each of these types of treatments could be combined with each other, with other BRMs affecting the metastatic tumor cell or with cytotoxic anticancer drugs. Studies of cell population sociology have emphasized the importance of cell-to-cell interactions in controlling the patterns of behavior of transformed[125] or neoplastic[126] cells. It is already known that modulation of cAMP levels in normal cells may affect the expression of neoplastic patterns of behavior in transformed cells.[125] Whether selective modulation of intracellular mediators such as cAMP or of intercellular communications and regulatory messenger molecules may affect tumor progression is not yet known, but related questions should provide a fertile terrain for investigation.

The neovascularization of tumors intended as an organic system seems affected through a cascade of actions by heparin and other factors interacting with each other.[122,127] The possibility to interfere with tumor neovascularization would seem particularly appealing in attempts to modify the physiopathology of metastasis. The complex interactions between mechanisms of oncogene expression, the role of oncogene products, the function and regulation of GF receptors, the relationships between GF and DF dependent mechanisms are each likely to provide potentially useful sites for therapeutic exploitation. These different approaches cannot be discussed within the scope of this article but are alluded to because in the future they are likely to provide additional dimensions to the development of BRMs and combinations involving BRMs in therapeutics.

In conclusion, the future of BRMs in cancer therapeutics can be considered with a measure of cautious optimism in the light of progress achieved in the recent past and the reasonable projections that now can be formulated. The fact that to date BRMs have shown only limited activity in patients with cancer may be discouraging to some investigators. Nevertheless it should also be a stimulus towards conducting careful basic and clinical experimentation aimed at verifying the promise derived from animal investigations and at obtaining further fundamental information on BRM mechanisms and the molecular biology of cancer that would provide a basis for the optimal utilization of these types of agents.

REFERENCES

1. Mihich E, Fefer A (eds): Report on the Biological Response Modifiers by the Subcommittee of the DCT Board of Scientific Advisors. J Natl Cancer Inst Monogr No 63, 1983

2. Mihich E, Kanter PM: The toxicology of biological response modifiers. Proceedings of International Seminar on the Immunotoxicological System as a Target for Toxic Damage, Luxembourg, November 1984 (in press)

3. Mihich E: Biological response modifiers: Their potential and limitations in cancer therapeutics. Cancer Invest 3:71–83, 1985

4. Grimm EA, Mazumder A, Zhang HZ, et al: Lymphokine-activated killer cell phenomenon, lysis of natural killer-resistant fresh solid tumor cells by interleukin 2-activated autologous human peripheral blood lymphocytes. J Exp Med 155:1823–1841, 1982

5. Mastrangelo MJ, Berd D, Maguire HC: Current condition and prognosis of tumor immunotherapy: A second opinion. Cancer Treat Rep 68:207–219, 1984.

6. Mastrangelo MJ, Berd D, Bellet RE: Critical review of previous reported clinical cancer immunotherapy with nonspecific immunostimulants. Ann NY Acad Sci 277:94–123, 1976

7. Fidler IJ, Berendt MJ: The biological diversity of malignant neoplasms, in Mihich E (ed): Biological Responses in Cancer: Progress Toward Potential Applications, vol 1. New York, Plenum, 1982, pp 269–299

8. Lederer E, Chedid L: Immunomodulation by synthetic muramyl peptides and trehalose diesters, in Mihich E (ed): Immunological Approaches to Cancer Therapeutics. New York, John Wiley and Sons, 1982, pp 107–135

9. Dukor P, Tarcsay L, Baschang G: Immunostimulants. Annu Rep Med Chem 14:146–167, 1979.

10. Mantovani A: Effect of glucocorticoid hormones on the immune system, in Mihich E, Sakurai Y (eds): Biological

Responses in Cancer: Progress Toward Potential Applications, vol 3. New York, Plenum, 1985, pp 155–180

11. Adams DO, Johnson WJ: Activation of murine mononuclear phagocytes for destroying tumor cells: Analysis of effector mechanisms and development, in Norman SJ, Sorkin E (eds): Macrophages and Natural Killer Cells: Regulation and Function, Advances in Exp Med and Bio, vol 155. New York, Plenum, 1982, pp 707–737

12. Herberman RB, Santoni A: Regulation of natural killer cell activity, in Mihich E (ed): Biological Responses in Cancer: Progress Toward Potential Applications, vol 2. New York, Plenum, 1984, pp 121–144

13. Brown JM, Rosenberg SA: Serologic analysis of human solid tumor antigens, in Mihich E (ed): Immunological Approaches to Cancer Therapeutics. New York, John Wiley and Sons, 1982, pp 1–37

14. Oettgen HF: Host defense against cancer, in Burchenal JH, Oettgen HF (eds): Cancer: Achievements, Challenges and Prospects for the 1980s, vol 2. Orlando, Fla, Grune & Stratton, 1981, pp 309–330

15. Ritz J, Griffin JD: Cell-surface antigens in acute leukemia, in Mihich E (ed): Biological Responses in Cancer: Progress Toward Potential Applications, vol 1. New York, Plenum, 1982, pp 1–21

16. Ozer H: Tumor immunity and escape mechanisms in humans, in Mihich E (ed): Immunological Approaches to Cancer Therapeutics. New York, John Wiley and Sons, 1982, pp 39–73

17. Byers VS, Baldwin RW: Immunoregulation by bacterial organisms and their role in the immunotherapy of cancer, in Chedid L, Miescher PA, Mueller-Eberhard HJ (eds): Immunostimulation. Berlin, Springer-Verlag, 1980, pp 73–94

18. Mastrangelo MJ, Berd D: Immunotherapy with microbial products, in Mihich E (ed): Immunological Approachs to Cancer Therapeutics. New York, Wiley-Interscience, 1982, pp 75–105

19. Tuttle RL, Cantrell J: *C. Parvum*—determinants of biologic activity, in Hersh EM, Chirigos MA, Mastrangelo MJ (eds): Augmenting Agents in Cancer Therapy. New York, Raven, 1981, pp 53–69

20. Yamamura Y, Yasumoto K, Ogura T, et al: Nocardia rubra—cell wall skeleton in the therapy of animal and human cancer, in Hersh EM, Chirigos MA, Mastrangelo MJ (eds): Augmenting Agents in Cancer Therapy. New York, Raven, 1981, pp 71–90

21. Ehrke MJ, Reino JM, Eppolito C, et al: The effect of PS-K, a protein bound polysaccharide on immune responses against allogeneic antigens. Int J Immunopharmacol 5:35–42, 1983

22. Kasamatsu T: Clinical cancer immunotherapy, in Yamamura Y (ed): Immunomodulation by Microbial Products and Related Synthetic Compounds. Tokyo, Exerpta Medica, 1982, pp 463–476

23. Ishida N, Hoshino J: A streptococcal preparation as a potent biological response modifier OK-432. Tokyo, Exerpt Medica, 1985

24. Izawa M-A, Ohno K, Amikura K, et al: Lentinan augments the production of interleukin 3 and colony stimulating factor(s) by T cells, in Aoki J, Tsubura E, Urushizaki I (eds): Manipulation of Host Defence Mechanisms, Tokyo, Excerpta Medica, 1983, pp 59–69

25. Aoki T, Miyakoshi H, Horikawa Y, et al: Staphage lysate and lentinan as immunomodulators and/or immunopotentiators in clinical and experimental systems, in Hersh EM, Chirigos MA, Mastrangelo MJ (eds): Augmenting Agents in Cancer Therapy, New York, Raven, 1981, pp 101–112

26. Chirigos MA (ed): Immune Modulation and Control of Neoplasia by Adjuvant Therapy—Glucan. New York, Raven, 1978 pp 171–280

27. Munder PG, Modolell M, Bausert W, et al: Alkyllysophospholipids in cancer therapy, in Hersh EM, Chirigos MA, Mastrangelo MJ (eds): Augmenting Agents in Cancer Therapy. New York, Raven, 1981, pp 441–458

28. Chirigos MA, Mastrangelo MJ: Immunorestoration by chemicals, in Mihich E (ed): Immunological Approaches to Cancer Therapeutics, New York, Wiley-Interscience, 1982, pp 191–239

29. Bicker U: Aziridine dyes: Preclinical and clinical studies, in Hersh EM, Chirigos MA, Mastrangelo MJ (eds): Augmenting Agents in Cancer Therapy. New York, Raven, 1981, pp 523–537

30. Symoens J, Rosenthal M, DeBrabander M, et al: Immunoregulation with levamisole, in Chedid L, Miescher PA, Mueller-Eberhard HJ (eds): Immunostimulation, Berlin, Springer-Verlag, 1980, pp 195–214

31. Hadden JW, Giner-Sorolla A: Isoprinosine and NPT15392: Modulators of lymphocyte and macrophage development and function, in Hersh EM, Chirigos MA, Mastrangelo MJ (eds): Augmenting Agents in Cancer Therapy, New York, Raven, 1981, pp 497–522

32. Umezawa H (ed): Small Molecular Immunomodifiers of Microbial Origin: Fundamental and Clinical Studies of Bestatin. Oxford, Pergamon, 1981, pp 1–254

33. Lemaire G, Tenu J-P, Petit, J-F, et al: Effects of microbially derived products on mononuclear phagocytes, in Hadden JW, Szentivanyi A (eds): The Reticuloendothelial System, A Comprehensive Treatise, vol 8. Pharmacology, New York, Plenum, 1985, pp 181–246

34. Chedid L, Parant M, Riveau G: Immunopharmacological activities of MDP, in Webb DR (ed): Immunopharmacology and the Regulation of Leukocyte Function. New York, Marcel Dekker, 1982, pp 159–182

35. Goodwin JS: Prostaglandin E and cancer growth: potential for immunotherapy with prostaglandin synthetase inhibitors, in Hersh EM, Chirigos MA, Mastrangelo MJ (eds): Augmenting Agents in Cancer Therapy, New York, Raven, 1981, pp 393–415

36. Leung KH, Ehrke MJ, Mihich E: Modulation of the development of cell-mediated immunity. Possible role of the products of the cyclo-oxygenase and the lipoxygenase pathways of arachidonic acid metabolism. Int J Immunopharmacol 4:195–204, 1982

37. Levy HB, Stephen ES, Harrington D, et al: Polynucleotides in the treatment of disease, in Hersh EM, Chirigos, MA, Mastrangelo MJ (eds): Augmenting Agents in Cancer Therapy. New York, Raven, 1981, pp 135–176

38. Najjar VA, Fridkin M (eds): Antineoplastic immunogeneic and other effects of the tetrapeptide tuftsin: A natural macrophage activator. Ann NY Acad Sci 419:1–273, 1983

39. Hengst JCD, Kempf RA: Immunomodulation by

cyclophosphamide, in Mitchell MS, Fahey JL (eds): Clinics in Immunology and Allergy, vol 4, Immune Suppression and Modulation. London, W.B. Saunders, 1984, pp 199–216

40. Ozer H: Effects of alkylating agents on immunoregulatory mechanisms. in Mihich E, Sakurai Y (eds): Biological Responses in Cancer, vol 3, Immunomodulations by Anticancer Drugs. New York, Plenum, 1985, pp 95–130

41. Ehrke MJ, Mihich E: Adriamycin and other anthracyclines, in Mitchell MS, Fahey JL (eds): Clinics in Immunology and Allergy, vol 4, Immune Suppression and Modulation. London, W.B. Saunders, 1984, pp 259–277

42. Mihich E, Ehrke MJ, Ishizuka M: Immunomodulations by antibiotics, in Mihich E, Sakurai Y (eds): Biological Responses in Cancer, vol 3, Immunomodulation by Anticancer Drugs. New York, Plenum, 1985, pp 71–94

43. Ehrke MJ, Mihich E: Immunoregulation by cancer chemotherapeutic agents, in Hadden JW, Szentivanyi A (eds): The Reticuloendothelial System: A Comprehensive Treatise, vol 8, Pharmacology. New York, Plenum, 1985, pp 309–347

44. Spreafico F, Vecchi A: The immunomodulatory activity of certain cancer chemotherapeutic agents, in Mihich E, Sakurai Y (eds): Biological Responses in Cancer, vol 3, Immunomodulations by Anticancer Drugs. New York, Plenum, 1985, pp 131–154

45. Miller FR, Kataoka T: Interactions of antimetabolites with tumors and the immune system, in Mihich E, Sakurai Y (eds): Biological Responses in Cancer, vol 3, Immunomodulations by Anticancer Drugs. New York, Plenum, 1985, pp 33–70

46. Taguchi T, Furue H, Kimura T, et al: End-point result of randomized controlled study on the treatment of gastrointestinal cancer with a combination of lentinan and chemotherapeutic agents, in Tsubura E, Urushizaki I, Aoki T (eds): Rationale of Biological Response Modifiers in Cancer Treatment, Excerpta Medica, International Congress Series 690. Amsterdam, 1985, pp 151–166

47. Fidler IJ: Optimization and limitations of systemic treatment of murine melanoma metastases with liposomes containing muramyl tripeptide phosphatidyl ethanolamine. Cancer Immunol Immunother, 1986 (in press)

48. Ehrke MJ, Mihich E: Immunological effects of anticancer drugs, in Berkarda B, Karrer K, Mathe G (eds): Clinical Chemotherapy, Vol III, Antineoplastic Chemotherapy. Stuttgart, Germany, Thieme-Stratton, 1984, pp 475–499

49. Cowens JW, Ozer H, Ehrke MJ, et al: Inhibition of the development of suppressor cells in culture by 4-hydroperoxycyclophosphamide. J Immunol 132:95–100, 1983

50. Ehrke MJ, Maccubbin D, Ryoyama K, et al: Correlation between Adriamycin-induced augmentation of interleukin 2 production and of cell mediated cytotoxicity. Cancer Res 46:54–60, 1986

51. Ehrke MJ, Mihich E: Effects of anticancer agents on immune responses. Trends in Pharmacological Sciences 6:412–417, 1985

52. North RJ: The murine antitumor immune response and its therapeutic manipulation, in Kunkel HG, Dixon FJ (eds): Advances in Immunology. Orlando, Fla, Academic, 1984, pp 89–155

53. Vitetta ES, Uhr JW: The potential use of immunotoxins in transplantation, cancer therapy and immunoregulation. Transplantation 37:535–538, 1984

54. Hersh E: Perspectives for immunological and biological therapeutic intervention in human cancer, in Mihich E (ed): Immunological Approaches to Cancer Therapeutics. New York, John Wiley and Sons, 1982, pp 505–540

55. Waksman BH: Overview: Biology of lymphokines, in Cohen S, Pick E, Oppenheim JJ (eds): Biology of the Lymphokines. Orlando, Fla, Academic, 1979, pp 585–616

56. Oldham RK: Biologicals and biological response modifiers: New approaches to cancer treatment. Cancer Invest 3:53–70, 1985

57. Stewart WE: Heterogeneities of human interferons, in Mihich E (ed): Biological Responses in Cancer: Progress Toward Potential Applications, vol 2. New York, Plenum, 1984, pp 19–44

58. Borden EC, Edwards BS, Hawkins MJ, et al: Interferons: Biological response modification and pharmacology, in Mihich E (ed): Biological Response in Cancer: Progress Toward Potential Applications, vol 1. New York, Plenum, 1982, pp 169–218

59. Real FX, Krown SE, Krim M, et al: Treatment of Kaposi's sarcoma with recombinant leukocyte A interferon. Proc Am Soc Clin Oncol 3:55, 1984

60. Fidler IJ, Schroit AJ: Synergism between lymphokines and muramyl dipeptide encapsulated in liposomes: In situ activation of macrophages and therapy of spontaneous cancer metastates. J Immunol 133:515–518, 1984

61. Williamson BD, Carswell EA, Rubin BY, et al: Human tumor necrosis factor produced by human B-cell lines: Synergistic cytotoxic interaction with human interferon. Proc Natl Acad Sci USA 80:5397–5401, 1983

62. Mizel SB: The interleukins: Regulation of lymphocyte differentiation, proliferation, and functional activation, in Mihich E (ed): Biological Responses in Cancer: Progress Toward Potential Applications, vol 1. New York, Plenum, 1982, pp 89–119

63. Cheever MA, Greenberg PD, Fefer A: Lymphocyte transfer for cancer therapy: Prerequisites for efficacy and the use of long-term cultured T lymphocytes, in Mihich E (ed): Biological Responses in Cancer: Progress Toward Potential Applications, vol 2. New York, Plenum, 1984, pp 145–183

64. Rosenberg SA, Lotze MT, Muul LM, et al: Observations on the systemic administration of autologous lymphokine-activated killer cells and recombinant Interleukin-2 to patients with metastatic cancer. N Engl J Med 313:1485–1492, 1985

65. Rosenberg SA, Mule JJ, Spiess PJ, et al: Regression of established pulmonary metastases and subcutaneous tumor mediated by the systemic administration of high-dose recombinant interleukin 2. J Exp Med 161:1169–1188, 1985

66. Shiiba K, Suzuki R, Kawakami K, et al: Interleukin 2-activated killer cells: Generation in collaboration with interferon γ and its suppression in cancer patients. Cancer Immunol Immunother 21:119–128, 1986

67. Dinarello C: Interleukin-1. Rev Infect Dis 6:51–95, 1984

68. Pennica D, Nedwin GE, Hayflick JS, et al: Human tumor necrosis factor: Precursor structure, expression and homology to lymphotoxin. Nature 312:724–729, 1984

69. Shirai T, Yamaguchi H, Ito H, et al: Cloning and

expression in *Escherichia coli* of the gene for human tumor necrosis factor. Nature 313:803–806, 1985

70. Wang AM, Creasey AA, Ladner MB, et al: Molecular cloning of the complementary DNA for human tumor necrosis factor. Science 228:149–154, 1985

71. Niitsu Y, Urushizaki I, Hayashi H: Antitumor effects of TNF. Abstr of 14th International Congress of Chemotherapy, Kyoto, Japan, p 14, 1985

72. Beutler B, Mahoney J, LeTrang N, et al: Purification of cachectin, a lipoprotein lipase-suppressing hormone secreted by endotoxin-induced RAW 264.7 cells. J Exp Med 161:984, 1985

73. Beutler B, Greenwalkd D, Hulmes JD, et al: Identity of tumor necrosis factor and the macrophage-secreted factor cachectin. Nature 316:552, 1985

74. Todaro GJ: Properties of growth factors produced by sarcoma virus-transformed cells, in Moore MAS (ed): Progress in Cancer Research and Therapy, vol 23, Maturation Factors and Cancer. New York, Raven, 1982, pp 115–128

75. Johnson E, Gorin P, Osborne P, et al: Use of an autoimmune approach to study the biological role of nerve growth factor, in Moore MAS (ed): Progress in Cancer Research and Therapy, vol 23, Maturation Factors and Cancer. New York, Raven, 1982, pp 1–8

76. End D, Guroff G: Nerve growth factor and epidermal growth factor responsiveness of pheochromatocytoma cells, in Moore MAS (ed): Progress in Cancer Research and Therapy, vol 23, Maturation Factors and Cancer. New York, Raven, 1982, p 9–28

77. Goodman R, Herschman HR: Pheochromocytoma cells as neuronal models: Effects of EGF and NGF, in Moore MAS (ed): Progress in Cancer Research and Therapy, vol 23, Maturation Factors and Cancer. New York, Raven, 1982, pp 29–40

78. Bloch A: Induced cell differentiation in cancer therapy. Cancer Treat Rep 68:199–205, 1984

79. Scher CD, Locatell KL, Lilliquist T, et al: Control of cell growth by somatomedins and the platelet-derived growth factor, in Moore MAS (ed): Progress in Cancer Research and Therapy, vol 23, Maturation Factors and Cancer. New York, Raven, 1982, pp 57–71

80. Westin EH, Wong-Staal, F. Gemmann EP, et al: Expression of cellular homologues of retroviral onc genes in human hematopoietic cells. Proc Natl Acad Sci USA 79:2490–2494, 1982

81. Cuttitta F, Carney DN, Mulshine J, et al: Bombesin-like peptides can function as autocrine growth factors in human small-cell lung cancer. Nature 316:823–826, 1985

82. Gallo RC, Breitman TR, Ruscetti FW: Proliferation and differentiation of human myeloid leukemia cell lines in vitro, in Moore MAS (ed): Progress in Cancer Research and Therapy, vol 23, Maturation Factors and Cancer. New York, Raven, 1982, pp 255–272

83. Buessow SC, Gillespie GY: Interferon-α and γ promote myeloid differentiation of HL-60, a human acute promyelocytic leukemia cell line. J Biol Resp Med 3:653–662, 1984.

84. Bloch A: Induction of tumor-cell maturation as a target for cancer therapy, in Harraps KR, Davis W, Calvert AH (eds): Cancer Chemotherapy and Selective Drug Development. Boston, Martinus Nijhoff, 1984

85. Craig RW, Sakagami H, Hromchak R et al: Enhancement of ML-1 human myeloblastic leukemia cell differentiation by combinations of anticancer agents and human leukocyte conditioned medium. Proc Am Assoc Cancer Res 26:266, 1985

86. Craig RW, Block A: Early decline in C-Myb oncogene expressions in the differentiation of human myeloblastic leukemia (ML-1) cells induced with 12-O-tetradecanoylphorbol-13-acetate. Cancer Res 44:442–446, 1984

87. Koprowski H: Mouse monoclonal antibodies in vivo, in Boss BO, Langman RE, Trowbridge IS, et al (eds): Monoclonal Antibodies and Cancer. Orlando, Fla, Academic, 1983, pp 17–37

88. Oldham RK: Biologicals and biological response modifiers: Fourth modality of cancer treatment. Cancer Treat Rep 68:207–219, 1984

89. Miller RA, Maloney DG, Warnicki ER, et al: Treatment of B cell lymphoma with monoclonal anti-idiotype antibody. N Eng J Med 306:517–522, 1982

90. Miller RA, Levy R: Response of cutaneous T cell lymphomas to therapy with hybridoma monoclonal antibody. Lancet 2:226–280, 1981

91. Koprowski H, Herlyn D, Lubeck M, et al: Human antiidiotype antibodies in cancer patients: Is the modulation of the immune response beneficial for the patient. Proc Natl Acad Sci USA 81:216–219, 1984

92. Hammersmith Oncology Group and Imperial Cancer Research Fund (Royal Post-graduate Medical School and Hammersmith Hospital, London) Courtenay-Luck KA, Epenetos AA, Hainan KE, et al (eds): Antibody-guided irradiation of malignant lesions: Three cases illustrating a new method of treatment. Lancet 1:1441–1443, 1984

93. Lashford L, Jones D, Pritchard J, et al: Therapeutic application of radiolabelled monoclonal antibody UJ13A in children with disseminated neuroblastoma. Cancer Drug Del 2:233, 1985

94. Rosenblum MD, Murray JL, Lamki L, et al: Comparative clinical pharmacology of two antimelanoma antibodies ZME-018 and 96.5 labeled with [^{111}IN]. Cancer Drug Del 2:234, 1985

95. Order SE, Klein JL, Leichner PK, et al: The treatment of hepatocellular cancer: A clinical model for radiolabeled antibody therapy. Cancer Drug Del 2:235, 1985

96. Vitetta ES: Immunotoxins, in Hadden JW, et al (eds): Advances in Immunopharmacology 3. Oxford, Pergamon, 1986 (in press)

97. Nepo AG, Hindenburg A, Mesa-Tejada R, et al: Toxicity, uptake and intracellular distribution of daunorubicin conjugated to tumor-directed monoclonal antibodies. Proc Am Assoc Cancer Res 26:220, 1985

98. Ford CHJ, Bartlett SE, Casson AG, et al: Vindesine monoclonal anti-CEA conjugate efficacy and specificity with 9 human cancer cell lines. Cancer Drug Del 2:230, 1985

99. Baldwin RW: Tumour inhibitory properties of monoclonal antibody 791T/36-drug conjugates. Cancer Drug Del 2:230, 1985

100. Hara T, Takahashi Y: Conjugates of mitomycin C with antitumor antibody with or without serum albumin as intermediary. Cancer Drug Del 2:231, 1985

101. Livingston PO, Oettgen HF, Old LJ: Specific active immunotherapy in cancer treatment, in Mihich E (ed):

Immunological Approaches to Cancer Therapuetics. New York, John Wiley and Sons, 1982, pp 363–404

102. Kobayashi H: Modification of tumor antigenicity in therapeutics: Increase in immunologic foreignness of tumor cells in experimental model systems, in Mihich E (ed): Immunological Approaches to Cancer Therapuetics. New York, John Wiley and Sons, 1982, pp 405–440

103. Kobayashi H: The biological modification of tumor cells as a means of inducing their spontaneous regression: An over-view. J Biol Response Mod 5:1–11, 1986

104. Carey TE, Takahasi T, Resnick LA, et al: Cell surface antigens of human malignant melanoma. I. Mixed hemadsorption assays for humoral immunity to cultured autologous melanoma cells. Proc Natl Acad Sci USA 73:3278–3283, 1976

105. Lachmann PJ, Sikora K: Coupling PPD to tumor cells enhances their antigenicity of BCG-primed mice. Nature 27:463–464, 1978

106. Bekesi JG, Holland JF, Roboz JP: Immunotherapy trials with neuraminidase-modified tumor cells, in Mihich E (ed): Immunological Approaches to Cancer Therapuetics. New York, John Wiley and Sons, 1982, pp 441–486

107. Hanna MG Jr, Key ME: Immunotherapy of metastases enhances subsequent chemotherapy. Science 217:367–369, 1982

108. Hanna MG Jr, Key ME, Oldham RK: The biology of cancer therapy: Some insights into adjuvant treatment of metastatic solid tumors. J Biol Resp Modif 2:295–309, 1983

109. Cheever MA, Greenberg PD, Fefer A: Potential for specific cancer therapy with immune T lymphocytes. J Biol Resp Modif 3:113–127, 1984

110. Cheever MA, Thompson JA, Kern DE, et al: Interleukin-2 administered in vivo induces the growth and augments the function of cultured T cells in vivo. J Biol Resp Modif 3:462–467, 1984

111. Mule JJ, Shu S, Schwartz SL, et al: Adoptive immunotherapy of established pulmonary metastases with LAK cells and recombinant interleukin-2. Science 225:1487–1489, 1984

112. Ehrke MJ, Maccubbin D, Salazar D, et al: Evaluation of the link between Adriamycin-induced effects on NK or LAK activities and modulation of soluble mediators. Int J Immunopharmacol 7:307, 1985

113. Thomas ED, Fefer A, Storb R: Bone marrow transplantation in the treatment of neoplastic disease, in Mihich E (ed): Immunological approaches to cancer therapeutics. New York, John Wiley and Sons, 1982, pp 299–332

114. Weiden PL, Flournoy N, Sanders JE, et al: Antileukemic effect of graft-versus-host disease contribution to improved survival after allogeneic marrow transplantation. Transplant Proc 13:248–251, 1981

115. Wright SC, Bonavida B: Studies on the mechanism of natural killer cytotoxicity. III. Activation of NK cells by interferon augments the lytic activity of released natural killer cytotoxic factors (NKCF). J Immunol 130:2960–2964, 1983

116. Key ME, Brandhorst JS, Hanna MG Jr: Synergistic effects of active specific immunotherapy and chemotherapy in guinea pigs with disseminated cancer. J Immunol 130:2987–2992, 1983

117. Welte K, Mertelsman R: Human interleukin 2: Biochemistry, physiology and possible pathogenetic role in immunodeficiency syndromes. Cancer Invest 3:35–49, 1985

118. Williams TW, Bellanti JA. In vitro synergism between interferons and human lymphotoxin: Enhancement of lymphotoxin-induced target cell killing. J Immunol 130:518–520, 1983

119. Biedler JL, Myers MB, Spengler BA: Multiple pathways to multidrug-resistance. Proc Am Assoc Cancer Res 26:388–390, 1985

120. Bell DR, Gerlach JH, Kartner N, et al: Detection of P-glycoprotein in ovarian cancer: A molecular marker associated with multidrug resistance. J Clin Oncol 3:311–315, 1985

121. Tsuruo T, Iida H, Tsukagshi S, et al: Cure of mice bearing P388 leukemia by vincristine in combination with a calcium channel blocker. Cancer Treat Rep 69:523–525, 1985

122. Gullino P: Angiogenesis, tumor vascularization and potential interference with tumor growth, in Mihich E (ed): Biological Responses in Cancer: Progress Toward Potential Applications, vol 4. New York, Plenum, 1985, pp 1–20

123. Thorgeirsson UP, Turpeenniemi-Hujanen, Liotta L: Mechanisms of tumor invasion and their potential theapeutic modification, in Mihich E (ed): Biological Responses in Cancer: Progress Toward Potential Applications, vol 4. New York, Plenum, 1985, pp 21–46

124. Menter DG, Onoda JM, Taylor JD, et al: Effect of prostacyclin on tumor cell-induced platelet aggregation. Cancer Res 44:450–456, 1984

125. Bertram JS: Inhibition of the carcinogenic process and of expression of the neoplastic phenotype, in Mihich E (ed): Biological Responses in Cancer: Progress Toward Potential Applications, vol 2. New York, Plenum, 1984, pp 45–120

126. Heppner G: Tumor Heterogeneity. Cancer Res 44:2259–2265, 1984

127. Folkman J: How is blood vessel growth regulated in normal and neoplastic tissue (GHA Clowes Memorial Award Lecture). Proc Am Assoc Cancer Res 26:384–385, 1985

SUBJECT INDEX

Action of BRMs, 235–236
Active immunotherapy
  future directions for, 246–247
  with MoAbs, 169
  present status of, 180–185
Acute lymphoblastic leukemia (ALL), 146–147, 172(*t*)
Acute myelogenous leukemia (AML) and BCG, 145, 146
Acute nonlymphocytic leukemia (ANLL), 228, 229
ADCC, 156, 168, 178, 245
Adjuvant therapy, 137–138
  with BCG, 144–146
  discussion of, 144, 148–149
  future directions in, 235
  with IFNs, 148
  with levamisole, 146–147
  with MoAbs, 168
  with poly A:poly U, 147
Adoptive immunotherapy
  future directions for, 247–248
  LAK cells and IL-2 in, 200–205
ALL, 146–147, 172(*t*)
Allergic contact dermatitis and CY, 186–187, 188(*t*)
AML and BCG, 145, 146
ANLL, 228, 229
Antibody-dependent cellular cytotoxicity (ADCC), 156, 168, 173, 245
Anti-extrogens and IFN, 216
Antigens, human tumor. *See also* Monoclonal antibodies
  discussion of, 153
  disialoganglioside GD3 and, 157–161
Antiidiotypic antibodies, 169, 245
Antimicrobials, combinations of, 149
Ara-C, 229
Arrhythmias from IFNs, 211
Autocrine hypothesis, 169

Bacillus Calmette-Guerin (BCG), 180, 181(*t*), 195, 247
  adjuvant therapy with, 144–145, 183–184
  clinical studies of, 144–145
    phase III, 137
  future projections for, 236–237
  intralesional administration of, 141–142
  postsurgical intracavitary administration of, 142
Bacterial infections, GM-CSF for, 225
B cell depletion and CY, 190, 191(*t*)
BCG. *See* Bacillus Calmette-Guerin
Bestatin, 237(*t*), 238
Biologic Response Modifiers Program, 132–133
Bladder cancer, 142, 146, 148, 182–183
Bombesin, 244
Bone marrow purging with MoAbs, 172
Bone marrow reserve, IFN alpha and, 136
Bone marrow transplantation
  future of, 248
  and GM-CSF, 224–225
Bone resorption and IL-1, 222–223
Breast cancer, 141, 142, 145, 147, 148, 168, 171, 211–212, 214
Brucella abortus, 144

CALLA antigen, 173
Carcinoembryonic antigen (CEA), 170
CEA, 170
Cell lines, murine and human leukemic, 228–232
Chemotherapeutic agents. *See also* Cytotoxic drugs
  differentiation factors and, 228–230
Chondriotin sulfate-rich proteoglycon (CSP), 155
Chronic granulocytic leukemia and IFN alpha, 135
Clinical development of BRMs
  difficulties of, 138
  discussion of, 132, 138–139
  phase I trials in, 133–135
  phase II trials in, 135–136
  phase III trials in, 136–138
  preclinical screening in, 131–132
Colon cancer, 145, 146, 148, 171, 182
Colony stimulating factors (CSFs), 239
Colorectal cancer, 172(*t*), 183–184, 203
Concanavalin A (Con A) and 4-HPCY, 191, 192(*t*)
Conjugation of MoAbs, 169
Contact sensitivity and CY, 186–187, 188(*t*)
COPA and IFN alpha, 137(*t*)
Corynebacterium parvum, 137, 142, 144, 181(*t*), 182, 195
CSFs, 239
CSP, 155
CTL, 195
Cutaneous T cell lymphoma, 135, 157
CVP and IFN alpha, 137(*t*)
CY. *See* Cyclophosphamide
Cyclophosphamide (CY), 144, 238
  antibody production and, 186, 187(*t*)
  discussion of, 186, 193
  DTH and, 186–187, 188(*t*), 190, 191
  pretreatment with, 188–189
  tumor immunity and, 188–190
  mechanisms, 190–192
Cyclophosphamide-induced unresponsiveness, IL-2 for, 220–221
Cytokines, 231–232. *See also* specific types
  future directions for, 239–240
Cytosine arabinoside (ara-C), 229
Cytotoxic drugs
  action of, 235
  and BRMs, 137, 145
  clinical trials of, 132, 133, 134, 135, 136–137, 138
  dose and timing of, 192–193
  and IFNs, 148, 215
  immunodilating effects of, 186, 192–193. *See also* Cyclophosphamide
  and MoAbs, 171
Cytotoxic T lymphocytes (CTL), 195

Delayed-type hypersensitivity (DTH), 192
  and CY, 186–187, 188(*t*), 190, 191
DFMO and IFNs, 215
DFs. *See* Differentiation factors
Differentiation antigens, 165–166

Differentiation factors (DFs)
chemotherapeutic agents and, 228–230
discussion of, 228
future directions for, 243–244
polar-planar compounds and, 229–230
vitamin analogs and, 230–232
Difluoromethylornithine (DFMO) and IFN, 215
Dimethyl sulforide (DMSO), 229
2,4-Dinitrochlorobenzene (DNCB), 141
and CY, 188, 189(*t*)
2,4-Dinitrofluorobenzene (DNFB), contact sensitivity to, 187, 188(*t*)
Disialoganglioside GD3, 157–161
DMSO, 229
DNA, effect of ara-C on, 229
DNA technology, effect of on BRMs, 166, 207, 218, 221, 224
DNCB. *See* 2,4-Dinitrochlorobenzene
DTH. *See* Delayed-type hypersensitivity
Dukes' C carcinoma of the colon, 145, 146

Effector cells with cytotoxic activity, 195–200
EGF, 169, 239
Encephalomyelitis, 182
Epidermal carcinomas and MoAbs, 169
Epidermal growth factor (EGF), 169, 239
Escherichia coli
cloning of human IFNs in, 208
and GM-CSF, 224
and IL-1, 221
and IL-2, 201

FAC chemotherapy and BCG, 145
Freund's adjuvant, 181(*t*), 182
Future directions, 236, 248–250
for active immunization, 246–247
for adoptive transfer cells, 247–248
for cytokines, 239–240
for DFs, 243–244
discussion of, 235–236, 248–250
for GFs, 243–245
for IFN inducers, 216
for IFNs, 240–241, 213–216
for IL-1, 223–224
for immunomodulating agents, 236–239
for lymphokines, 241–242
for MoAbs, 245–246
for TNF, 242–243G

GAG, 154
Genes coding for antigens identified by MoAbs, 166
Glycosaminoglycans (GAG), 154
GM-CSF, 224–226
Granular lymphocytes (LGLs), 195, 196
Granulocyte-macrophage colony stimulating factor (GM-CSF), 224–226
Growth factors (GFs), 239
future directions for, 243–245
and MoAbs, 169

Hairy cell leukemia, 135, 136, 197, 213–214, 241
Hematologic malignancies and levamisole, 146
Hexamethylene bisacetamide, (HMBA), 229–230
Histopathological diagnosis of tumors, MoAbs and, 166
HLA antigens, 181, 183
HMBA, 229–230
Host effector cell as target of BRMs, 132
4-HPCY and splenic T cells, 191
HuIFN-α, 208, 209, 210, 211. *See also* Interferons
Human leukocyte antigens (HLA), 181, 183
Human leukocyte IFN alpha, (HuIFN-α), 208, 209, 210, 211. *See aso* Interferons
Hybridoma methodology, 153, 165, 170
Hydrocortisone, IL-2 for immune deficiency from, 219–220, 221

IFNs. *See* Interferons
IL-1, 221–224. *See also* Interleukin-2
IL-2. *See* Interleukin-2
Immunomodulating activity of traditional agents, 186, 238
Immunosuppression, chemotherapy and radiation-induced,
GM-CSF for, 225
IL-2 for, 219–221
Inactivated tumor cells, vaccine from, 181
Inflammation and MoAbs, 168
Interferon alpha (IFN α), 132, 134–135, 136, 137, 209–210. *See also* Interferons
Interferon gamma (IFN γ), 133, 134, 207, 208, 209, 214, 215, 218. *See also* Interferons
Interferon inducers, 207, 212–213. *See also* Interferons
future of, 216
Interferons (IFNs), 144, 239. *See also* Interferons alpha; interferon gamma; Interferon inducers
action of, 235–236
adjuvant therapy with, 148, 214, 215–216
clinical development of, 208–209
clinical trials of, 196–197, 209–212
discussion of, 207, 216
dose, optimal, for, 209, 214
future prospects for, 213–216, 240–241
hyperthermia and, 216
immunomodulating effects of, 196–197
mechanisms of antitumor effects of, 209, 214
nomenclature of, 207–208
selection of, 214–215
species of, 207–208
subspecies of, 208*n*
therapeutic effects of, 209
toxicity of, 210–211
Interleukin-1 (IL-1), 221–224. *See also* Interleukin-2
Interleukin-2 (IL-2), 144. *See also* Interleukin-1
adoptive immunotherapy with, 200–205, 247–248
clinical development of, 218–219
clinical trials for, 219–220
dose trials for, 202–203
future directions for, 204, 241–248
for immunosuppression induced by cytoreductive therapies, 219–221
and LAK cells, 200–205
preclinical evaluation of, 197
renal cell carcinoma and, 198
Intradermal administration of BCG, 144

Intralesional administration of BRMs, 141–142
Iodine radioisotopes and MoAbs, 170

Juvenile laryngeal papillomatosis and ICLC, 213

Kaposi's sarcoma, 135, 211, 241
Keyhole limpet hemocyanin (KLH) and CY, 190
KLH and CY, 190
Kohler and Milstein, hybridoma methodology and, 153, 165

Lentinan, 237
Leukaphereses, 201, 203
Leukemias, 135, 145, 146–147, 157, 172, 173, 213, 224, 228–229
Levamisole, 144, 146, 237(*t*), 238
  adjuvant therapy with, 145, 146–147
LGLs, 195, 196
Liver metastasis, LAK cells and IL-2 for, 200, 201(*t*)
Living tumor cells, vaccine from, 180–181
Local administration of BRMs, 141–142
LTs. *See* Lymphotoxins
Lung cancer, 142, 145, 146, 172, 200, 201(*t*), 203
Lymph nodes
  BCG for metastasis in, 183
  MoAbs for tumor detection in, 183
Lymphomas, 135, 172, 173, 221, 241
Lymphocytes, immune, adoptive transfer of, 200
Lymphokine activated killer (LAK) cell phenomenon, 200
Lymphokine activated killer (LAK) cells, 132, 200. *See also* Natural killer cells
  adoptive transfer of, 248, 200–205
  future directions for, 203–204
  and IL-2, 197, 200–205, 241
Lymphokines, 239. *See also* Lymphokine activated killer cells; specific types
  action of, 235
  future directions for, 241–242
  molecular characterization of, 218, 226
Lymphotoxins (LTs), 239
  action of, 235–236
  future directions for, 242

Macrophage activation
  and GM-CSF, 225
  and lymphokines, 242
Markers, tumor, 157, 169–172. *See also* Monoclonal antibodies
Maximum tolerated dose (MTD) of BRMs, 132, 134, 138–139, 144, 209
Melanoma-associated antigens and BCG, 183. *See also* Antigens, human tumor
Melanoma-associated chondroitin sulfate progeoglycan (MPG), 153–157
Melanomas, 137, 141, 144, 146, 147, 153–154, 157, 159–161, 168, 171, 172, 182, 183, 203, 212, 241, 246
Melphalan and IFN α, 137(*t*)
MER, 144, 181(*t*), 182
Metastic disease, clinical trials of cytotoxins and BRMs for, 136–138
Methanol-extracted residue (MER), 144, 181(*t*), 182. *See also* BCG

Mixed bacterial vaccines, 144
MoAbs. *See* Monoclonal antibodies
Modification of tumor cells to increase antigenicity, 181
Monoclonal antibodies (MoAbs). *See also* Antigens, human tumor
  bone marrow purging with, 172
  clinical trials of, 172–173
  discussion of, 165–167
  future directions for, 173–174, 245–246
  therapeutic applications of
    discussion, 167
    immune-mediated destruction, 167–169
    growth factors and their receptors, 169
    nude mouse model, 167
    targeting of tumor, 169–172
MOPC-315 tumor in mice, CY and, 189
Mouse MoAbs, 167–168, 170, 172(*t*), 174
MPG, 153–157
MTD, 132, 134, 138–139, 144, 209
MTP-PE, 238
Multiple myeloma, 135, 137(*t*), 212, 213. *See also* Myeloma
Murine tumor models and LAK, 200, 201(*t*)
Muramyl tripeptide-phosphatidylethanol amine (MTP-PE), 238
MVE-2, 196
Mycosis fungoides, IFN for, 211, 241
Myeloma, 241. *See also* Multiple myeloma
Myocardial infarction from IFN, 211

National Cancer Institute screening programs, 132–133
N-CWS, 237
Natural killer (NK) cells, 156, 160, 195–196, 239
  and IFN alpha, 134–135, 136, 209–210
  and IL-2, 197
Neovascularization of tumors, 250
Network theory of the immune response, 169
Neuraminidase, 181
Neuroblastoma, 148, 149
Nocardia rubra, 144
Nocardia rubra-cell wall skeleton (N-CWS), 237
Non-Hodgkin's lymphoma and IFNs, 135, 137(*t*), 145, 212

OIP of BRMs, 133
OK432, 237
Optimal immunomodulatory protocol (OIP) of BRMs, 133
Optimal immunomodulatory therapeutic protocol (OTP) of BRMs, 132
OTP of BRMs, 132
Ovarian cancer and *Corynebacterium parvum,* 142

P388 in vivo murine leukemia model, 132
PAK cells, 201–202
Parasitic infections, GM-CSF for, 225–226
Passive immunotherapy with MoAbs, 167–168
PDGF, 169
PE-2, 229
PHH proliferation, 192
Pharmaceuticals, 146–149
Phase clinical trials of BRMs, 133–138
Phorbol esters and teleocidins, 230–231
Phytohemagglutinin (PAK cells), 201–202

Platelet-derived growth factor (PDGF), 169
Plating efficiency 2 (PE-2), 229
Plaque-induced oral disease, IL-1 for, 223
Polar-planar compounds, 229–230
Polyadenylic-polyuridylic acid (poly A:poly U), 147
Poly A:poly U, 147
Poly IC, 133, 137, 213
Polyribionosinic-polyribocytidylic (poly IC), 133, 137, 213
Polyribonucleotides, 144
Postsurgical intracavity administration of BRMs, 141, 142
Preclinical screening for cytotoxic drugs and BRMs, 132–133
Preclinical Screening Laboratory (PSL), 133–134
Prednisone and IFN, 137(*t*)
Present status of active immunotherapy, 180–185
Protein bound polysaccharide (PSK), 237
Pulmonary osteosarcoma metastasis and IFNs, 215–216

Radiation therapy and IFNs, 215
Radiolabeled MoAbs, 169–172
Radioprotective agent, IL-1 as, 223
Rebound overshoot of PHA proliferalism, 192–193
Recombinant human tumor necrosis factor, 131
Renal cell cancer, 135, 136, 197–198, 203, 211, 213, 241
Resistance to cytotoxic drugs, 135
Retinoids, 230

Solid tumors and IFN α, 135–136
Somatic cell genetics and MoAbs, 166
Specificity analysis of MoAbs, 165
Squamous carcinomas, 182
Steroid-induced immune deficiency and IL-2, 219–220, 221
Subcellular components, vaccine from, 181
2-5A Synthetase and protein kinase, 147
Systemic immunity for intralesional administration of BCG, 141

T202, 157
TAA, 235, 239, 245, 246, 247
T cell dependent immune reactivity, IL-2 and, 218, 219
T cell growth factor. *See* Interleukin-2
T cells, 235
  and CY, 190–192
  IL-2 dependent growth of, 218, 219
TGF, 239
Thymic-dependent immunity, 195
Thyroiditis, 182
Tissue diagnosis and MoAbs, 166
TNF. *See* Tumor—necrosis factor
Transforming growth factors (TGFs), 169
Tumor-associated antigens (TAA), 235, 239, 245, 246, 247
Tumor enhancement with immunotherapy, 185
Tumor necrosis factor (TNF) action of, 235–236, 239
  future directions for, 242–242
  and IFNs, 215

Vaccina virus, 142
Vitamin analogs, 230–232
Vitamin D, 230

Whole tumor cell vaccine, 180–181
Wound healing agent, IL-1 as, 223

XIII, NO 3 SEPTEMBER 1986

Seminars in Oncology

Plasma Cell Myeloma and the Myeloma Proteins

Mehdi Farhangi, *Guest Editor*

Contributors

Steven M. Rosen
Joel N. Buxbaum • Blas Frangione
Mehdi Farhangi • Michael Potter • Daniel R. Jacobson
Susan Zolla-Pazner • Gregory R. Mundy • Donald R. Bertolini
Brian G.M. Durie • Robert A. Kyle • John P. Garton • Jonathan R. Sporn
O. Ross McIntyre • Philip R. Greipp • Morie A. Gertz
M. Robert Cooper • Charles E. Welander • Alan Solomon
Giampaolo Merlini • Elliott F. Osserman

GRUNE & STRATTON
Harcourt Brace Jovanovich, Inc.

Seminars in Oncology

Vol XIII, No 3 **September 1986**

Plasma Cell Myeloma and the Myeloma Proteins Introduction and Dedication

THIRTEEN YEARS have passed since two consecutive issues of *Seminars in Hematology* were devoted to immunoglobulin diseases. Major discoveries have been made in the genetics of immunoglobulin, the B cell differentiation stages, and the DNA rearrangements and other molecular events giving rise to antibody diversity. Recent discoveries have provided better understanding of the structure of monoclonal immunoglobulins and heavy and light chain variants. The cell kinetics and prognostic indicators in plasma cell myeloma are better defined, and a more lucid picture of the circulating monoclonal B cell in this disease is emerging. The induction of plasmacytoma in BALB/c mice has taught valuable lessons in oncogenesis and now serves as a model for the study of the *myc* oncogene in B cell neoplasms. The mechanisms of immune deficiency and the nature of humoral factors causing bone destruction in myeloma have been elucidated.

Monoclonal immunoglobulins with well-defined antibody activity are increasingly being identified. Myeloma proteins have now been recognized as the prime cause of several clinical disorders. Amyloidogenic and nephrotoxic light chains have been sorted out and systemic light chain (or immunoglobulin) deposition disease has been described and increasingly diagnosed.

Since the discovery in the 1960s that the alkylating agents melphalan and cyclophosphamide and the corticosteroids were efficacious for the treatment of myeloma, some other agents have been found to be effective including the nitrosoureas, Adriamycin (Adria Laboratories, Columbus, Ohio), and vincristine. Efforts to define the most efficacious combination of drugs and scheduling are continuing. Interferon *a* has been shown to be effective in a minority of previously-treated myeloma patients, and future studies will no doubt clarify the role of this agent for remission induction and maintenance. Intensive research efforts in this disease have provided us with not only a better understanding of pathogenesis and treatment but with major discoveries in the biology of the immune system. Many distinguished investigators deserve credit for this work but one of them is very special to me.

Nearly 30 years have passed since Elliott F. Osserman began a life-long research in the plasma cell dyscrasias. His pioneering insight into the nature of amyloid tissue deposits is an example of the clear thinking and searching mind that have characterized his work. His continuously productive research laboratory has trained and inspired researchers all over the world. Because of his unceasing quest for new knowledge and a life of devotion to research in cancer, I am dedicating this issue of the *Seminars* to this astute physician and scientist.

Mehdi Farhangi
Guest Editor

The Structure of Immunoglobulins and Their Genes, DNA Rearrangement and B Cell Differentiation, Molecular Anomalies of Some Monoclonal Immunoglobulins

Steven M. Rosen, Joel N. Buxbaum, and Blas Frangione

THE HUMORAL IMMUNE response is characterized by its exquisite specificity and its equally specific memory. These two qualities are the result of a number of complex processes that are regulated at the levels of gene rearrangement, mRNA transcription and cell-cell interaction. Defects in these processes can be seen in a number of pathologic states. Studies of variant immunoglobulin products, which occur in the course of disease, have given us insight into the details of the physiologic events involved in antibody formation. In addition, it now appears that some immunoglobulin molecules, which are structurally variant, can actually cause human disease.

GENERAL FEATURES

There are five classes of immunoglobulins (Igs) in man: IgG, IgA, IgM, IgD, and IgE (Fig 1). They all have the same basic four-chain structure: Two identical heavy and two identical light chains (Fig 2). The heavy (H) chain in each Ig is class specific, with differing lengths, disulfide bridge patterns, numbers of domains, degree of polymerization, amino acid sequences, and number and types of oligosaccharides. IgG and IgA can be further divided into subclasses based on the presence of specific antigenic determinants (representing defined chemical structures) present on the H chains. The subclass designations are gamma 1,2,3, and 4 and alpha 1 and 2, respectively.[1,2]

The light (L) chains exist in two different chemical types, κ and λ, which can also be distinguished immunologically. Both L chain types can combine with any of the heavy chains.

The different classes, subclasses, and types of Ig polypeptide chains are called isotypes. They are present in all individuals and are the products of different structural genes.

Each Ig chain consists of two regions. One is designated the variable(V) region; the other is designated the constant (C) region. The V region is the amino terminal portion of the chain, H or L, and consists of approximately 110 amino acids of varying composition. The C region is the carboxyl portion of the chain and has the same primary structure as all other chains of the same class, subclass and type. The C regions of κ and λ chains contain 110 residues. The C regions of γ, α, and δ are three times larger whereas those of μ and ϵ are four times the size. All these regions are homologous in structure and are related to each other with respect to their evolution from a common precursor. Each homology region folds into a somewhat similar conformation, a compact globular domain.[3]

V regions sharing certain similarities in their amino acid sequence can be classified as belonging to a single subgroup. Four V κ and six V λ subgroups have been identified in this way. The V regions of the H chains can also be divided in a similar fashion. There has been some discrepancy when subgroups defined by amino acid analysis have been compared with those sharing experimentally established DNA homologies, with a larger number of V_H groups seen by the latter technique. Certain positions in the V regions are highly conserved. Other amino acids vary to a much greater extent. These are clustered in three areas of both chains (amino acids 24 to 34, 50 to 56, and 89 to 97 in the L chains and residues 31 to 35, 50 to 65, and 95 to 102 in the H chains). These are called the hypervariable or complementarity determining regions (CDR) and are directly involved in antigen binding. Antibodies, produced by immunization of an animal with a single monoclonal Ig, which react only with the immunizing Ig, are referred to as

From the Departments of Pathology and Medicine, and The Kaplan Cancer Center, New York University Medical Center, New York.

Supported by Veterans Administration research funds and NIH grants AM 01431, and AM 02594.

Address reprint requests to Blas Frangione, MD, PhD, Department of Pathology, New York University Medical Center, 550 First Ave., New York, NY 10010.

0093-7754/86/1303-0002$05.00/0

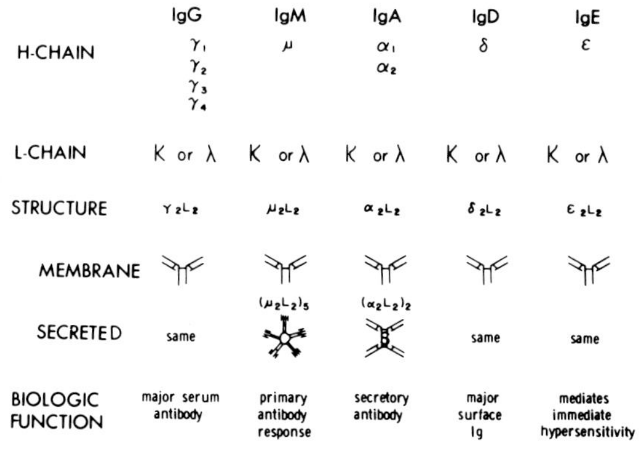

Fig 1. Each of the different classes and subclasses of immunoglobulin is depicted along with its associated basic subunit structures. The membrane and secreted forms of the immunoglobulins are shown schematically for each H chain isotype. The major biological function of each isotype is stated.

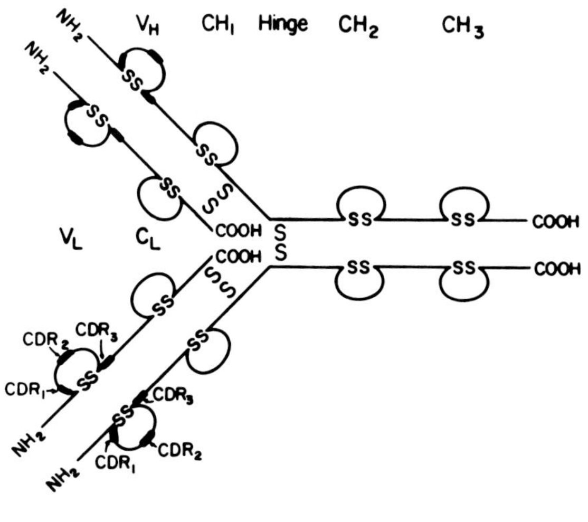

Fig 2. The gross three-dimensional structure of the H_2L_2 IgG heterodimer is dominated by intrachain disulfide loops that create three-dimensional domains (V_H, C_H1, C_{H2}, and C_H3). The carboxy terminal portions of the molecule are responsible for the effector functions specific to the class of the H chain. The amino terminal portion of the molecule, comprised of both H and L chains, serves to bind the antigen. Those major regions (V_H and V_L) that contain the contact points of the antigen binding site have specific clusters of amino acids that determine the specificity of the combination with antigen in a stable fashion, ie, CDRs 1, 2, and 3 of both H and L chains. S-S: disulfide bridges. Hinge contains the inter H-H disulfide bridges (reprinted with permission[25] by courtesy of Marcel Dekker, Inc.)

antiidiotypic and appear to have specificity for the chemical structures related to the binding site.[4,5]

IMMUNOGLOBULIN G

IgG molecules consist of identical pairs of H and L chains (molecular weights of 50,000 and 25,000, respectively) linked by disulfide bridges. Papain splits IgG into three fragments that retain biologic activity, two Fab (antigen binding), containing the entire L chain and the two amino terminal domains of the H chain, and one Fc (fragment crystallizable), composed of the disulfide-linked carboxy-terminal halves of the H chains. The Fc contains the sites responsible for mediating most biologic functions. The demarcation of the H and L polypeptide chains into defined regions associated with specific biologic functions is a striking feature of the Ig system.[6,7]

Normal human IgG contains a mixture of H_2L_2 molecules containing H chains of all four γ subclasses. IgG activates complement by the classic pathway, with the γ_1 and γ_3 subclasses being most effective. IgG_4 does not fix complement in the native state but does so after proteolytic cleavage. IgG is the only Ig class providing passive immunity to the newborn, because μ, δ, ϵ, and α classes do not cross the placenta. IgG proteins also interact with receptors for the Fc fragment on polymorphonuclear leucocytes, monocytes, macrophages, and platelets, a property probably related to the initiation or maintenance of the inflammatory response. Most IgG molecules have a slow catabolic rate, with a half-life of approximately 3 weeks, IgG_3, however, is degraded more rapidly. Immunologic memory, ie, the humoral anamnestic response, is related to the production of antibodies of the IgG class. Some antigens may even elicit preferential production of a specific subclass.

IgG_1 and IgG_4 proteins contain four interchain bridges. Two such bonds join the H chains to each other in the hinge region and two join the H and L chains. IgG_2 molecules are crosslinked by four inter-H chain disulfides and two H-L bonds. IgG_3 has structural and biologic features not shared by the other three subclasses. It does not bind to staphylococcal protein A, which is tightly bound by the others; it has a more rapid turnover, and it is the most potent subclass activating the first component of the complement system. Structurally the γ 3 chain has the highest molecular weight of all the human γ chains because of an extended hinge region that contains a quadruplicated 15 amino acid segment.[8,9]

IMMUNOGLOBULIN M

The IgM molecule is a pentamer composed of five identical H_2L_2 subunits and one nonhomologous chain, the J chain. The J chain facilitates the formation of the polymer. IgM antibodies are the first to appear in the course of most immune responses and represent the major or only Ig class comprising the response to some antigens, eg, aggregated immunoglobulins, I and other red cell antigens. Most antigenic stimuli result in a switch to other Ig classes after the initial IgM burst. IgM is predominantly intravascular; its turnover is rapid; it can initiate complement activation. The pentamer has a valence of 10 for small antigens but may not exceed 5 for larger ligands, presumably as a consequence of steric considerations. The μ chain with a molecular weight of 70,000 contains five domains (V and $C_{mu1\text{-}4}$) rather than the four found in IgG.[10]

An IgM monomer appears to be, together with IgD, the major Ig protein found on the surface of B lymphocytes. When both are found on the same cell, the V regions are identical, hence they have the same antigen binding specificity.[11] The membrane μ molecule differs from the secreted IgM of the same specificity in both size, ie, monomer *v* pentamer, and in the presence of a carboxy-terminal hydrophobic segment on the μ chain that allows it to anchor itself in the plasma membrane. The molecular mechanisms allowing the production of these two forms of the same polypeptide will be discussed below.[12]

IMMUNOGLOBULIN A

IgA is produced in large quantities in areas adjacent to secretory surfaces. Secretory IgA represents a first line of local defense against environmental pathogens.[13,14] IgA-producing cells assemble two H_2L_2 monomers and a J chain into the dimer, which is taken up by secretory component-producing epithelial cells that join the IgA with their own product and secrete the entire complex into the intestinal lumen as secretory IgA (SIgA). It has been noted that there are two classes of IgA. Whereas 90% of serum IgA is IgA_1, external secretions contain equal proportions of both classes. It is interesting to note that regions of the gut populated by large numbers of bacteria contain a protease that specifically cleaves the hinge region of IgA_1.[15] The increased ratio of IgA_2 to IgA_1 seen in secretions may represent an evolutionary adaptation of man to what has become the normal flora of the gut.

The J chain is structurally unrelated to H and L chains. It combines covalently with the H chains of IgA and IgM so that one J chain is present in each polymeric molecule, regardless of the size of the polymer. The linkage is by a disulfide formed between J and the penultimate residue bond (cysteine) of both the μ and α chains. J is a 15,000 dalton polypeptide with a single oligosaccharide moiety. While most serum IgM circulates as the 19S polymer, only 10% of serum IgA is polymeric, the bulk being the H_2L_2 monomer.[16]

IMMUNOGLOBULIN D

The functional role for this class remains uncertain. It is present in normal serum in very low quantities, yet is found on the surface of most B lymphocytes as a membrane Ig, usually in association with IgM, both molecules having the same V_H and V_L regions.[11,17] Intact IgD has a molecular weight of 160,000 and contains about 10% carbohydrate. Serum IgD and IgD myeloma proteins are predominantly of the λ type.[18]

IMMUNOGLOBULIN E

The IgE class contains most of the molecules bearing the biologic and immunochemical characteristics of reaginic antibodies. They have the ability to bind reversibly, but with high affinity, to specific membrane receptors on basophils and mast cells. The combination of specific cell-bound antibody with antigen triggers a series of events that ultimately lead to the release of vasoactive amines and other pharmacologically active substances responsible for the clinical manifestations of immediate hypersensitivity. The serum level of IgE, even in the most severely allergic individual, seldom exceeds 1 μg/mL.

IgE has a molecular weight of 180,000 of which approximately 12% is carbohydrate. A comparison of the size of the ϵ H chain with those of the other H chain classes shows it to be about the same size as the μ chain, 11,000 daltons larger than γ, α, or δ. Thus, both IgE and IgM H chains possess an extra domain. The ability of the IgE molecule to bind to specific cell surface receptors is mediated through sites localized within the Fc region.[19–21]

GENETIC POLYMORPHISMS: ALLOTYPES

Allotypes are genetically determined structural variants of Ig's that are inherited according to Mendelian laws and detected serologically. In humans, each appears to be the product of a single autosomal codominant gene. Three sets of allotypic markers have been recognized in human Ig's, the linked Gm and Am factors and the independently inherited Km system. The Gm specificities are located in the γ constant region. The Am locus is α chain specific, with the A2m(2) allotype dominant in the IgA2 subclass. The Km factors are associated with κ L chains, and so are found in all the Ig classes. There are three allelic forms, $Km^{1,2}$, Km^{1}, and Km^{3}. All serologic allotypic specificities are due to amino acid differences that involve interchanges at one or two contiguous positions that are not critical to the overall function of the antibody molecule.[22]

IDIOTYPES AND THE COMBINING SITE

Idiotypes are antigenic determinants localized within the V region that correspond to the antigen binding site of a given antibody molecule. Antibody specificity results from the molecular complementarity between determinant groups on the antigen molecule and amino acid residues in the active site. Both H and L chains contribute to the combining site. The interaction between antigen and antibody involves weak noncovalent associations, including electrostatic bonding, hydrogen bonding, and van der Waals interactions. Amino acid sequence analysis and affinity labeling of antibody polypeptide chains have suggested that the hypervariable regions of both H and L chains were involved in antigen binding. Definitive evidence was obtained by x-ray crystallographic analysis. The hypervariable regions exhibit insertions, deletions, and amino acid substitutions when antibodies of the same V region subgroup but different specificities are compared with each other. Sequence modifications of this type have a very significant effect on the size and shape of the combining site, hence specificity. Additional diversity can be generated by the combination of different pairs of H and L chains. It has recently become apparent that even monoclonal antibodies can combine with a spectrum of sterically-related molecules (multispecificity). Thus, every antibody will react with the inducing antigen, but each antibody will differ in the family of disparate antigens it can bind (cross reactivity).[4,23,24]

IMMUNOGLOBULIN GENE STRUCTURE

Germline Gene Families

The structure and properties of normal human immunoglobulin genes have been reviewed in depth elsewhere.[25] Immunoglobulin genes consist of three families encoded on three separate chromosomes. Each family consists of variable and constant gene segments that are not contiguous in germline DNA, being separated by thousands of nucleotides (Fig 3).[26]

κ genes. In man, the κ gene family has been localized to chromosome 2.[27] The variable gene segments number between 15 and 30 and are located at the 5′ end of the gene complex. The V_κ gene segments encode a promoter, the site at which RNA polymerase initiates transcription, a leader segment coding for a hydrophobic polypeptide region that is thought to play a role in the binding of polyribosomes synthesizing immunoglobulins to the endoplasmic reticulum, and the first 95 amino acids of the V region of the L chain protein.[28] The remaining residues in the expressed L chain V region are not encoded by the V region gene per se but are derived from one of four J_κ segments, which are contiguous with the DNA coding for the constant region. The constant region gene segment encodes the remaining amino acids (109 to 214), the termination codon, a 3′ untranslated region followed by a polyadenylation signal.

λ genes. The λ L chain locus, on chromosome 22, has a similar general configuration but has some characteristics that are distinct from the κ locus.[29] In humans, there are at least six V subgroups.[30] In contrast with the C_κ locus, which contains only one gene, the $C\lambda$ locus contains at least six nonallelic genes. The number of $C\lambda$ genes seems to be polymorphic in different human populations. Some of these constant region segments have been shown to possess their own J segments, a characteristic likely to be shared by all $C\lambda$ genes. In neither of the light chain chromosomes, nor on the heavy chain

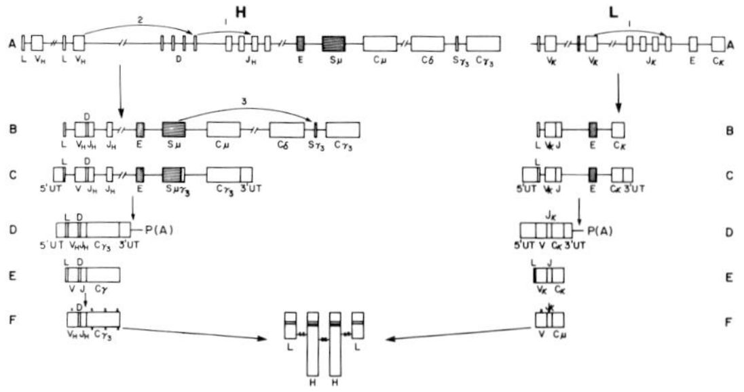

Fig 3. A schematic view of our current understanding of the process of Ig H and L chain gene rearrangement and expression. The protein coding, or exonic, gene segments are shown as open rectangles. The enhancer and μ switch segments are indicated by boxes with chevrons. The H chain locus on line A undergoes D-J joining and then V to D-J joining. With the rearranged gene configuration, the cell can synthesize either cytoplasmic or membrane IgM. In the course of the maturation of the immune response, a specific clone may give rise to antibodies of the same specificity but of different class. These molecules have the same V region but different C regions. In order to accomplish this, the rearranged locus (B) undergoes switch recombination where the same V region is brought adjacent to a new C region with deletion of the DNA 5′ to the new C region gene. The primary transcript (C) is processed with methylation of the 5′ terminus, splicing out of the intronic or noncoding sequences, and addition of polyadenylic residues to the 3′ terminus. The initial translation product (E) contains a leader segment that is later removed to give a processed H chain protein (F). The positions identified by x are the glycosylation sites of the H chain protein. The L chain locus is less complex than the H chain locus and need only undergo a V-J recombination to be expressed (A and B). Its primary transcript (C) is processed and translated in the same manner as the H chain (D and E). The mature L chain (F) is able to combine with the H chain via interchain disulfide bonds to form a stable tetramer containing two identical H and two identical L chains.

chromosome, have the V and C regions been physically linked to each other.

H chain genes. The germline H chain genes possess a configuration that is more complex than those coding for the L chains. The V_H cluster is at the 5′ portion of the locus. On the basis of protein sequence data, the locus has been divided into three major V_H groups.[31] However recent data from analyses of murine V_H regions suggest a larger number of V_H families in both humans and mice. In a normal V_H segment, the first exon codes for the hydrophobic signal sequence, which is separated from a second exon that codes for the last four or five amino acids of the signal sequence and the first 95 amino acids of the V_H region.

The first major organizational departure of the H chain locus from those of the L chain is a region of 2–9 diversity(D) segements that is 3′ to the V region.[32] Each D contains approximately 30 nucleotides. In each complete H chain, one of these contributes to CDR 3. 3′ to the bulk of the D region is the J_H cluster, which consists of six functional J_H segments. 3′ to the J cluster is the switch region, a 3 kb stretch of DNA containing short repeated sequences.[33] It is involved in the process of class switching, by which different C_H region genes can be expressed with the same V gene. Such a mechanism is necessary for a single B cell clone of defined specificity to produce antibodies of different Ig classes with the same antigenic target. 3′ to the switch region is the constant region complex covering an as yet undetermined length of DNA but containing the genes for $C\mu$, $C\delta$, $C\gamma_3$, $C\gamma_1$, $C\psi\epsilon$, $C\alpha_1$, $C\psi\gamma_1$, $C\gamma_2$, $C\gamma_4$, $C\epsilon$, and $C\alpha_2$ in that order. In humans, there appears to be two discrete clusters, each containing two γ constant region genes, an α gene, and an ϵ or pseudo-ϵ gene.[34] These have apparently arisen by duplication after speciation, because the mouse genome does not display a similar configuration.

Ig Gene Expression: Gene Rearrangements

The expression of Ig genes during B cell development is an apparently ordered phenomenon whereby the H chain gene undergoes rearrangement and expression before the L chain genes.[35] The first detectable event appears to be the translocation of one of the D segments to a position in apposition to a J segment. Specific recognition units exist that allow a D_H to join a J_H, and a V_L to join a J_L.[36] A V_H cannot join directly to a J_H, nor can a D or a J_H join to another D or J_H. The recognition sequences on either end of the D segment consist of a nanomer and a heptamer of specific sequences separated by a 12 base pair (bp) spacer. On the 3′ end of each V region and the 5′ end of each J segment are nanomer-heptamer sequences separated by a 22 to 23 bp spacer. It is the length rather than the composition of the spacers that is critical. While both the sequence and length of the nanomers and heptamers are important. A segment bearing a 12 bp spacer can only recombine with a segment having a 23 bp spacer, hence the constraints on specificity of segment recombination.

T cells appear to be able to carry out DJ_H joins but apparently go no further. After a successful

DJ join, any V on the B cell chromosome can translocate and join with the DJ via the 5′ recombination sequence of the D and its 3′ recombination sequence. The site of VDJ joining is reflected in the amino acid sequence of CDR 3.[37] Hence the protein product of the same germline V gene can vary in its CDR 3 depending which D and J are used in its recombination. In addition, it has been noted that additional variability is generated by the insertion of bases at the VD and DJ junctions by terminal deoxynucleotidyl transferase (Tdt).

If VDJ recombination produces a DNA sequence that is in-frame with the rearranging VH, ie, each nucleotide triplet codes for an amino acid, then a functional H chain is produced. If an in-frame rearrangement does not occur, the other H chain allele is free to rearrange one of its V segments. Cells in which both VDJ events are unsuccessful are presumably incapable of expressing any Ig product.

The production of a successful VDJ join signals the κ chromosome that it is free to rearrange one of its V regions. L chain rearrangement requires the translocation of the V segment to one of the J_κ's.[38] If this is successful then the rearrangement process stops, if not, the other κ allele is free to rearrange. If neither of these produces a functional protein then the λ genes rearrange. In both H and L chain gene rearrangements, only one allele is expressed.[39] In the case of the L chain, it is only one allele at one locus. This phenomenon has been termed allelic exclusion and operates at the level of the single cell.

The rearranged H and L chain genes contain both exons, regions carrying the information coding for the amino acids comprising the protein, and introns, regions that do not carry information related to the primary sequence. The H chain exons include those for the bulk of the leader sequence, the V region itself and one for each of the constant region domains, ie, C_H1, C_H2, C_H3 and C_H4 for the μ chain, C_H1-3 for the γ, α, and δ chains. The hinge region has its own nonhomologous exon in the γ, α, and ϵ genes.

The L chain genes have only three exons, one for the leader, one for the V region and a single C region exon.

Each of the Ig loci contains several elements that are related to the regulation of expression. The human and murine H chain and κ loci contain segments in their intervening sequences that have the capacity to increase the rate of transcription of their respective genes.[40]

Transcript processing. When the genes are transcribed into RNA, the entire linear gene is copied as a single molecule including all the exons, the intervening sequences (introns) between them, and approximately 200 bp beyond the identifiable end of the gene. A specific sequence, AAATAAAA, signals where a variable number of adenylic acid residues are added to the end of the transcript.[41] The primary transcript must then be processed to remove the noncoding material and form a functional mRNA containing only the information necessary to specify the amino acid sequence of its H or L chain product. The cellular apparatus carrying out this function is not specific for Ig's. It is used to process the transcripts of virtually all synthesized proteins. So-called splice signals are found at the 5′ and 3′ ends of all introns that tell the splicing enzymes which pieces of RNA are to be removed.

The B cell uses specific types of splicing to carry out two particular lineage specific functions.[42] All H chain classes have a small 3′ exon that codes for a hydrophobic carboxy-terminal extension that allows the insertion of the chain into the cell membrane to serve as a cell surface receptor for antigen. B cells that express IgM on the cell surface splice out the intron between C_4 and the membrane exon. B cells that express cytoplasmic or secreted IgM polyadenylate μ mRNA just beyond C_4. In cells that produce both forms of IgM, two mRNAs are found, differing by the presence or absence of the RNA coding for the membrane exon. When other Ig's are expressed on the cell surface, the same process is used to code for the synthesis of their intramembranous portions.

The second instance in which a specific splicing event occurs is that in which IgM and IgD with the same antigen binding specificity are expressed on the surface of the same cell.[43] In this case, a single long transcript encompassing the single rearranged V region and the two contiguous constant region genes is produced. Different molecules of the transcript are then processed differently with some having the entire C spliced out and the VDJ joined to the delta constant region, while others have the entire δ gene spliced away. These two instances use what has been termed alternative splicing.

Class switching. During the course of the immune response to a given antigen, the antibody response matures so that the initial IgM antibody is supplemented with antibodies of similar or identical specificities but with different H chain classes. The biologic functions of the various classes have been reviewed earlier. In our discussion of the structure of the H chain gene complex, we noted that the genes coding for all the H chain constant regions are found in a linear array on chromosome 14. Mu is closest to the V region and δ is contiguous with μ. The remainder of the genes are in two discrete clusters, an undetermined distance from δ, with an as yet undetermined amount of DNA between them. The order of the genes in each cluster has been defined as have the distances between the members.

We have discussed, vide supra, the mechanism whereby B cells express two membrane molecules with the same specificity but with different H chain constant regions, ie, μ and δ. In that case, differential splicing of a single long transcript is used. Expression of a murine IgA molecule by pre-B cells has also been demonstrated to use a similar mechanism. It has been suggested that pre-B cells may differ from Ig-producing cells that class switch later in the development of the lineage. If plasma cells expressing IgG are examined for the presence of μ genes on the same chromosome, they cannot be found. Based on a series of similar observations in murine plasma cell tumors, it has been hypothesized that class switch occurs by deletion of the heavy chain constant region genes between the utilized V region and the C region to be used.[44] Each C_H gene has a region 5′ to its coding sequence that consists of a long series of short repeats. In the μ gene it occupies about 3000 bp and is called the switch region. It is retained after VDJ recombination because it is located between the J cluster and the first constant region exon. The other H chain genes have similar regions that are homologous to that found in μ but appear to be less homologous the further the c region is from Cμ. Recombination appears to occur using the homologous areas in each C gene with the DNA between the μ switch and that utilized deleted.[45] Hence the V region with its D and J are placed in a position analogous to their original position in the rearranged μ gene with a different C immediately 3′.

IG VARIANTS

The number and complexity of the processes described above suggest that there are many opportunities for error. In fact, the nature of some of the structures and processes we can now explore experimentally were originally suspected or hypothesized on the basis of the analysis of apparent errors in the process. In the course of studying human lymphoproliferative diseases, which are usually associated with the production of an intact monoclonal immunoglobulin, eg, multiple myeloma and macroglobulinemia, unusual Ig products have been identified. The discovery of a variant Ig in the bodily fluids of patients depends upon several features of the protein: It must be stable; it must be present in sufficient quantity to be detectable by the methodology available; it should not be absorbed out of the serum by the tissues during the time of its circulation. Any of these features will make detection technically difficult. Biologically, its presence should not be a selective disadvantage to the cell producing it. The best studied of the variant Ig's reflect these characteristics, however it is not clear that they are the most meaningful of all the possible variations on the Ig theme.

H CHAIN VARIANTS

Human heavy chain disease (HCD) is a lymphoproliferative disorder characterized by cells that synthesize an abnormal H chain and usually fail to produce L chains.[46] The aberrant H chain proteins may be detected in the serum, urine, or both. In the presence of normal renal function, proteins larger than 60,000 dalton will not appear in the urine. Covalently-bound dimers or polymers of an H chain fragment larger than this will not be excreted.

HCDs of the three major Ig classes have been described. Each seems to have a fairly typical clinical picture, although some patients have exhibited the protein abnormality in a somewhat different clinical setting. Alpha chain disease seems to occur most often in the course of abdominal lymphoma of the Mediterranean type with lymphoid hyperplasia of the bowel and enlargement of the mesenteric lymph nodes.[47] Biopsy samples from the affected tissues have been shown to produce the proteins. The μ variant has been described most frequently in the course of atypical chronic lymphocytic leukemia. γ chain disease is the most pleiotypic in its presentation, behaving as a lymphoplasmacytic disorder with involvement of liver, spleen, lymph nodes and bone barrow. Synthesis of the truncated protein has been found in the three latter sites and in lymphoid cells obtained from the peripheral blood.

γ H Chain Disease Proteins

The amino acid sequence of a number of γ HCD proteins has been determined (Fig 4).[48] Some of these contain internal deletions beginning in the V_H region at residues 2 to 100, and extending to the beginning of the hinge region (residue 216). Six of the sequenced proteins fall into this category. Three of them have normal amino termini. The others do not. The original HCD protein (CRA), has 11 amino acids of uncertain origin at its amino terminus. The unusual amino termini may reflect the presence of genomic events that either accompany, or are part of, the process that results in the deleted protein.

An additional group of internally deleted molecules is characterized by resumption of normal sequence at the carboxy-termnus of the hinge, ie, residue 252. One of these (HAL) circulates as a 55 kilodalton noncovalently linked dimer that dissociates to the 25 kilodalton monomer on exposure to 6 mol/L guanidine.[49] Thus it lacks the inter-H S-S bonds. Sequence studies have shown that the monomer contains only four cysteines and that the deletion encompasses the majority of the V region, the C_H1 domain and the entire hinge region.

Three other proteins have been described that exhibit deletions involving only the hinge region, ie, residues 216 to 230.[50] These lack a full complement of cysteines involved in H-H and H-L disulfide bonding so that the chains exist as noncovalently linked dimers and tetramers that dissociate without prior reduction. It is easy to conceive how these types of proteins could arise via small alterations in DNA that alter splicing around the hinge sequence without actually deleting the genetic information coding for the hinge.

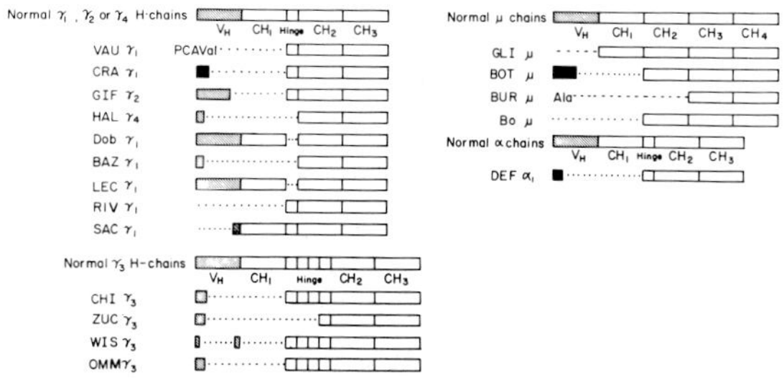

Fig 4. The structures of a number of human H chain variants are depicted. Normal H chain structure is shown for each immunoglobulin class. The variable protein segments are indicated by the shaded areas. The blackened regions show an abnormal amino-acid sequence. The dotted lines depict regions of deletion. The Mcg protein has a deletion identical to that of Dob and is not shown.

An unusual protein, (WIS), appears to have three normal V region residues followed by five unusual amino acids that are homologous with the V-C junction and a normal hinge, CH2 and CH3.[51] Hence the deleted portions of the V region and the deleted CH1 appear to be interrupted by a small stretch of apparently normal amino acid sequence in an abnormal place (vide infra).

Several proteins with apparent N terminal H chain deletions have been reported. These are particularly informative when viewed with respect to the signal hypothesis that states that the N terminal hydrophobic leader sequence is required for synthesis of proteins which are either membrane associated or secreted. According to this hypothesis, which has strong experimental support in a number of systems, the absence of such a sequence will result in a protein product that cannot be secreted. Because all the N terminally deleted HCD proteins have been isolated from serum or urine, it is evident that they must have been secreted by the Ig-producing cell. Therefore it is likely that they all have some sort of functional leader sequence.

One of these proteins is the most extensively studied of any of the HCD molecules. The serum of patient (OMM) contained an 80,000 dalton dimer of a protein that had a reduced size of 39 kilodaltons. Its amino terminal residue was glycine, an amino acid usually found as the seventh amino acid of the hinge. The sequence after the glycine was identical with that of the normal γ_3

hinge region.[52] Amino terminal amino acid analysis of the short γ_3 protein isolated from the cytoplasm and secretions of a lymphoid cell line established from the patient's peripheral blood revealed a blocked amino terminus (PCA-val), a feature characteristic of normal γ_3 H chains, suggesting that the protein was synthesized as an internally, rather than N-terminally, deleted molecule. Further support for the observation was gained by in vitro translation analysis of mRNA isolated from the cells. These studies showed that the mRNA encoded a normal hydrophobic leader segment. cDNA prepared from the mRNA template was sequenced and revealed the normal leader followed by bases coding for 14 normal V region amino acids, a proline codon, not noted in any other human or murine V region in this position, and sequence coding for a normal hinge region, C_H2, C_H3, a chain terminating codon and a normal polyadenylation signal. These observations confirmed the suspicion that the (OMM) protein and others like it were not truly N-terminal deletions, but represented internal deletions followed by postsynthetic degradation.[53] The rearranged γ gene containing the deletion was cloned from the (OMM) cell line and analyzed in detail. As suspected, the DNA coding for the V region beyond normal residue 14 is missing; residue 15, proline, is probably derived from the J region DNA that is present, as is much of the intervening sequence between J and the middle of the switch region. The remainder of the switch region and half of the CH1 exon are missing. Sequence resumes in the middle of the CH1 and is normal through the end of the constant region.

The OMM HCD protein, with its apparent N terminal deletion, is actually generated by two internal DNA deletions and a splice correction followed by postsynthetic proteolysis (unpublished observations). Another HCD molecule, (RIV), appears to have been generated in a similar fashion.[54] The protein (WIS) (vide supra) resembles these two variants except that the DNA events in the latter are visible in the amino acid sequence of the former.[51]

The molecular event that results in the failure of L chain expression in γ and α HCD cells that possess partial V region deletions is not known.

α H Chain Disease Proteins

There is less known about the molecular defects in the α chain proteins. All the reported patients have proteins belonging to the α_1 subclass. This is somewhat surprising because 10% of IgA molecules are of the α_2 subclass and should be proportionately represented among the deleted molecules.[55] This may reflect a propensity for preferential involvement of the α_1 locus. J chain synthesis is unaffected and J has been shown to be associated with the α fragment polymers in some instances. The α HCD protein, (DEF), has a monomeric molecular weight of 29.3 kilodaltons.[56] Its amino terminus is heterogeneous and biosynthetic labeling suggested a certain degree of postsynthetic degradation. As in the internally deleted γ molecules, it contains a segment of normal V sequence contiguous with a normal hinge residue, valine. The remainder of the constant region appears to be normal.

Based on the relatively sparse data, it appears that the α proteins will have defects similar to those identified in the γ molecules and their genes. Similarly, L chains have not been found to be synthesized by cells producing the deleted α chains.

μ H Chain Proteins

Mu HCD proteins are found in the serum and have molecular weights ranging from 180 to 520 kilodaltons.[57] They are usually covalently linked decamers of the short μ chain, indicating that the cysteines involved in normal intersubunit interaction are present. Not all of the polymers analyzed contain J chain, again suggesting that J chain facilitates, but is not required for, polymerization. A major difference between cells producing μ HCD proteins and those associated with α and γ HCD is the retention of L chain synthesis in the former.

The serum protein (BO) is a decamer with a molecular weight of 520 kilodaltons.[58] It appears to be missing the V_H and C_H1 domains. (BUR) contains only the C_H3 and C_H4 domains, while (BOT) has some unusual amino acids at its amino terminus followed by a deletion of the V region and CH1 with normal sequence resuming at the CH_2.[59] The GLI serum protein is lacking the amino-terminal 130 amino acids.[60] Biosynthetic analysis indicated that the small μ chain could not be the product of N terminal proteolysis of a normal chain.[61] Despite the resumption of normal sequence at ala_{131} and the presence of cys_{140} and intracellular L chains, the normal H-L disulfide was not formed. Interheavy chain disulfides were normal. These observations suggested the need for more than ten residues on the amino terminal side of the μ cysteine to allow the formation of the H-L bond.

The protein structure of the serum protein (BW) has not been analyzed, however biosynthetic analysis has show the production of a 58 kilodalton μ protein and an apparently normal κ chain.[62] Northern blot analysis of mRNA isolated from the cells indicated that the membrane, secreted and precursor forms of the message were approximately 300 bases shorter than normal. The gene coding for the aberrant protein was isolated and found to contain four normal constant region exons with proper splice signals. A structurally normal V_H was also present, however the gene appeared to contain an insertion of sequences of unknown origin coupled with a deletion of normal intron material that interfered with normal splicing, leading to a truncated mRNA and an amino-terminally shortened protein.

H Chain Variants Leading to Half Molecule Formation

Serum and urine samples from several patients with either plasma cell leukemia or multiple myeloma have been found to contain molecules in which the H and L chains are bound to each other but no interheavy chain disulfide bonding is present.[63] Examination of most of these has revealed that the L chains are normal but the H chains are short. At least three have been of the IgA class, the remainder have been IgGs. Although detailed amino acid sequence analysis of the proteins has not been performed, there is suggestive evidence that at least one of the variants, the (WAL) protein, displays a C terminal deletion.[64] It is not clear why such a deletion should result in the absence of interheavy chain disulfide formation. One of the other patients had both H_2L_2 and HL half molecules in the serum, suggesting that the interheavy chain S-S bonds could form but that the reaction was not thermodynamically favored because of the aberrant α chain structure. At least two similar cases have been noted in the mouse myeloma system.

HUMAN L CHAIN VARIANTS

The most common of all variations in Ig production seen in human lymphocytes and plasma cells is that of extreme excess L chain production.[65] Twenty percent of patients with myeloma have only monoclonal L chains in their serum or urine. Using biosynthetic analysis, we have found that the plasma cells from 90% of myeloma patients synthesizing IgA proteins and 75% of patients making IgGs or monoclonal IgMs also make substantial amounts of excess L chains.

Some B lymphomas, which make small amounts of secreted Ig's, have been associated with increased excretion of monoclonal L chains in the urine.[66] Biosynthetic analyses of these cells have shown L chain production in excess of H chain synthesis by the same cells. The molecular explanation for the excess has not been determined. It has been proposed that the unbalanced synthesis is a function of cellular immaturity and may be used as a tumor cell marker. Subsequent analysis has indicated that exposure of the tumor cells to phorbol esters stimulates maturation and leads to balanced synthesis.

There have been fewer investigations of pure L chain producers in myeloma. Immunofluorescent studies have indicated that some of these cells are synthesizing proteins bearing H chain determinants. In at least one case, a short γ chain was synthesized, which assembled with a small portion of the synthesized L chains to form a polymer smaller than 150 kilodaltons that was secreted and degraded.[67] Free L chains were found in the urine.

Some murine L chain producers have been analyzed and found to contain H chain mRNA while others did not appear to be producing the message.

Variants Producing High Molecular Weight L Chain Polymers

When light chains are produced in excess, they usually exist as monomers or disulfide linked dimers.[68] λ chains are predisposed to dimerization because of the availability of a penultimate cysteine residue. When cytoplasmic lysates of λ chain producing myelomas are examined it is clear that the dimer is the dominant form intracellularly and in the secretions. κ producing cells tend to have monomers intracellularly and monomers and dimers in their secretions. In vivo excess L chains of both classes are excreted and catabolized by the kidneys. In the presence of renal disease and excess free L chain production by myeloma cells, free L chains become detectable in the serum.[69] In the presence of normal renal function, dimers and monomers are filtered but molecules larger than 60 kilodaltons do not pass across the glomerulus. Several patients have been described in whom substantial amounts of free L chains were detected in the serum in the face of relatively normal renal function.[70] The molecules were isolated and found to be tetramers of a monoclonal L chain, usually, if not always, of the λ class. In one instance, biosynthetic analysis of the cells producing the L chains revealed that the tetramers were assembled intracellularly.[71] The primary structural feature of the molecules that allows tetramerization has not been established. Some investigators have suggested that these polymers occur more frequently than has been reported. The cells producing them do not appear to have any deficit in secretion.[72]

Variant L Chains Found in Serum in Association With Normal or Abnormal H Chains

The SAC L chain is an internally deleted κ L chain.[73] Abnormal sequence starts at residue 17 with 13 amino acids not homologous to any normal κ sequence. Amino acid 31 is homologous to residue 99 of a normal κ chain with the remaining sequence identical to C_κ. This type of anomaly suggests that normal DNA structure resumes within J_κ. It is not possible to discern if the original defect generated a deletion or a new splice donor site without detailed molecular biologic analysis.

The protein (SM) is composed of H and L chains both of which are shorter than normal.[74] The H chain has not yet been fully characterized although preliminary studies suggested that it was internally deleted. The L chain that probably belongs to the λ_2 subgroup has a normal sequence from residues 1 to 30. The constant region is intact from the usual gln_{110} to the carboxy terminus. The protein also belongs to that 15% of human L chains that are glycosylated, bearing a carbohydrate moiety at position 25. Although no nucleic acid analysis was performed on the cells synthesizing (SM), it can be surmised that the defect represents either a pure deletion, the insertion of an abnormal donor splice site by point mutation, or a deletion with a splice correction to yield normal protein sequence beginning at a usual intron-exon border.

NONSECRETORY MYELOMA

Approximately 1% of all patients with multiple myeloma are deemed to be of the nonsecretory variety.[75] In these individuals, the proliferating cell has the morphologic appearance of a plasma cell, but no monoclonal Ig protein or related molecules can be identified in the serum or urine. Cells from a number of these patients have been studied in detail. Immunofluorescent analysis of the bone marrows have revealed no cytoplasmic staining with anti-Ig reagents, strong staining with anti-κ or anti-λ reagents, strong staining with anti-H chain reagents with little or no anti-L chain fluorescence, brilliant staining with anti L chain sera with little or no anti-H chain binding.[76–78] In the plasma cell of one patient, staining for both α and μ determinants was detected, with monoclonal proteins of neither class evident in the serum or urine.[79] It has been noted that, among these patients with nonsecretory disease in whom L chain immunofluorescence is found, κ staining populations have been more frequent than λ.

Electron microscopic examination of the cells in most cases revealed morphologic features consistent with plasma cells, however, there has been significant heterogeneity with respect to the degree of development of the cytoplasmic organelles. Some patients' cells show well-developed endoplasmic reticulum of Golgi apparatus while others contain sparse flattened cisternae.[80,81]

Biosynthetic analyses have also suggested that no one pattern fits all the patients. In some cases, no synthesis was demonstrable. In most, however, a low level of synthesis could be detected. Free L chains were the most readily detected molecular species, but in some cases molecules with H chain antigenic determinants, but sizes much smaller than intact H chains, were seen.

In general, it appears that most nonsecretors are actually hyposecretors when examined by a combination of immunofluorescent, biosynthetic, and immunochemical techniques. The true nonsecretors are a mixed lot, with some cells synthesizing defective molecules that are difficult to analyze, while others produce nothing. The molecular defects in these cells have not yet been elucidated.

VARIANT IG MOLECULES, THE DEPOSITION OF WHICH, APPEAR TO BE ASSOCIATED WITH ORGAN COMPROMISE

AL Amyloidosis

Detailed structural analysis of the fibrils extracted from the amyloid deposits of patients with the primary, or the myeloma-associated, form of the disease has revealed that the amino acid sequence is identical with that of an immunoglobulin L chain.[82] Biosynthetic analysis of bone marrow cells from patients with AL deposition indicate that they all produce free monoclonal L chains of the same class as the deposited protein, even though free L chains cannot be detected in the sera or urines of 10% to 20% of them.

In several patients whose serum or urine contained a monoclonal L chain, the sequences of the tissue fibril and the urine protein were identical. In most patients, the fibrils are composed of fragments of the L chain rather than the entire molecule. In all fibrils analyzed thus far, the fragments start with the amino terminus of the intact chain. It has been suggested that certain L chains, notably those of the V λ_{VI} subgroup,[83] are predisposed to precipitation after relatively limited specific proteolysis. Recent data have suggested an alternate hypothesis based on the observation that bone marrow cells from 20% to 30% of the individuals with AL disease synthesize peptides bearing L chain antigenic determinants that appear to be smaller than the intact chains. Some of the smaller molecules are clearly short L chains. Others may represent unglycosylated forms of glycosylated L chains. These observations suggest that the fragments themselves may be predisposed to tissue deposition or that may be more susceptible to deposition after additional proteolysis. In one patient in particular, reduction and alkylation of biosynthetically labeled anti-λ precipitated molecules yielded a mixture of intact L chains and a fragment of 10 to 12 kilodaltons.[84]

It is not yet clear how frequently aberrant biosynthetic products can be detected in this disease. The nature of the abnormality leading to the production of such proteins has not been investigated in detail. Any of the molecular defects described in the preceding sections could be responsible.

Monoclonal Immunoglobulin Deposition Disease (MIgDD)

A number of patients have now been described who have developed organ dysfunction, most commonly renal but occasionally hepatic or cardiac, secondary to the deposition of monoclonal Ig's in their tissues.[85] Some of these individuals have had multiple myeloma but most appear to have no other underlying disease. In most cases, the deposits have contained monoclonal κ chains by immunofluorescence but in some, monoclonal λ molecules have been detected. Occasionally, monoclonal H chains of the γ or α class have been noted with the L chains. In no case has the material been extracted from the tissue for analysis. Several laboratories have carried out biosynthetic analyses of the Ig's produced by the marrow cells of the patients in question.[85,86] In some cases, short H chains of the deposited class have been synthesized. In other individuals, short or normal L chains of the same class as the deposits have been found. There has been no evidence of degradation of a normal precursor to yield the short molecules, however this has not yet been rigorously excluded. Thus, another class of clinically significant aberrations in monoclonal Ig proteins has emerged and is subject to analysis using the tools of modern molecular biology.

The association between MIgDD and AL amyloidosis is not yet established. The deposits in the former do not bind Congo Red or metachromatic dyes. They do not have the characteristic fibrillar structure of amyloid. They appear to conserve the antigenic determinants of Ig molecules better than those comprising the amyloid deposits because they are usually readily stainable by conventional anti-Ig immunofluorescent reagents. Only recently has it become possible to obtain reasonable immunohistochemical identification of tissue amyloid. Lastly, amyloid deposits have never been found to contain Ig H chain molecules. While H chain related fibrils may ultimately be detected, for the moment it appears to be a distinguishing characteristic between AL and MIgDD. Both conditions present an opportunity for analysis of aberrations in the expression of the Ig loci, which may yield more insight into their structure and regulation of expression under normal circumstances (see also Soloman, this issue).

CONCLUSION

The analysis of departure from normal in biologic processes has been an extremely productive approach in a variety of systems. In the Ig producing cell, it has served to raise a number of questions concerning the normal mechanisms of secretion, the organization of the genes coding for the polypeptides, the relationships between H and L chain synthesis, and the functions of different portions of the Ig molecules. We also believe that the production of Ig polypeptides with certain types of structural defects lead to disease because of the instability of these molecules under normal physiologic conditions. The investigation of the newly recognized variations should give us additional insights into the function of normal Ig-producing cells. These insights in turn, should enable us to deal more effectively with the diseases.

REFERENCES

1. World Health Organization: Review of the notation for allotypic and related markers of human immunoglobulins. Eur J Immunol 6:599–601, 1976

2. Natvig JB, Kunkel HG: Human immunoglobulins: Classes, subclasses, genetic variants and idiotypes. Adv Immunol 16:1–59, 1973

3. Edelman GM, Cunningham WE, Gall PD, et al: The covalent structure of entire IγG immunoglobulin molecule. Proc Natl Acad Sci USA 63:78–85, 1969

4. Kabat EA, Wu TT, Bilofsky H: Variable regions of immunoglobulin chains. Sequences of proteins of immunological interest. Bethesda, Md, National Institutes of Health, 1983

5. Capra JD, Kehoe JM: Hypervariable regions, idiotype and the antibody combining site. Adv Immunol 20:1–40, 1975

6. Porter RR: The combining sites of antibodies. Harvey Lect 65:157–174, 1971

7. Spiegelberg H: Biological activities of immunoglobulins of different classes and subclasses. Adv Immunol 19:259–294, 1974

8. Frangione B, Milstein C, Franklin EC: Chemical typing of immunoglobulins. Nature 221:149–151, 1969

9. Michaelsen TE, Frangione B, Franklin EC: Primary structure of the "hinge" region of human IgG3. J Biol Chem 253:883–889, 1977

10. Putnam F: Immunoglobulins. I. Structure, in Putnam FW (ed): The Plasma Proteins: Structure, Function and Genetic Control. Orlando, Fla, Academic, 1977, pp 2–143

11. Vitetta EA, Uhr JW: Immunoglobulin-receptors revisited. A model for the differentiation of bone marrow-derived lymphocytes is described. Science 189:964–969, 1975

12. Rogers J, Early P, Carter C, et al: Two mRNA's with different 3′ ends encode membrane-bound and secreted forms of immunoglobulin μ-chain. Cell 20:303–312, 1980

13. Tomasi TB Jr: The gamma A globulins. First line of defense, in Good RA Fisher DW (eds): Immunobiology. Stamford, Conn, Sinauer, 1971, pp 76–83

14. Roux ME, McWilliams M, Phillips-Quagliata J, et al: Differentiation pathways of Peyer's patch precursors of IgA plasma cells in the secretory immune system. Cell Immunol 61:141–183, 1981

15. Mulks ME, Plaut AG, Feldman HA, et al: IgA proteases of two distinct specificities are released by Neiseria Meningitidis J Exp Med 152:1442–1447, 1980

16. Cann GM, Zaritsky A, Koshland ME: Primary structure of the immunoglobulin J chain from the mouse. Proc Natl Acad Sci USA 79:6656–6660, 1982

17. Fu SM, Winchester RJ, Kunkel HG: Occurrence of surface IgM, IgD, and free light chains on human lymphocytes. J Exp Med 139:451–456, 1974

18. Takahashi N, Tetaert D Debuire B, et al: Complete amino acid sequence of the delta heavy chain of human immunoglobulin D. Proc Natl Acad Sci USA 79:2850–2854, 1982

19. Ishizaka K, Ishizaka T, Lee EH: Biologic function of the Fc fragments of E myeloma protein. Immunochemistry 7:687–702, 1970

20. Dorrington KJ, Bennich H: Structure-function relationships in human immunoglobulin E, Immunol Rev 41:3–25, 1978

21. Holowka D, Metzger H: Further characterization of the β-component of the receptor for immunoglobulin in E. Mol Immunol 19:219–227, 1982

22. Kunkel HG, Kindt T: Allotypes and idiotypes, in Benaceraff B (ed): Immunogenetics and Immunodeficiency. Lancaster, England, Medical and Technical Publishing, 1975, pp 56–80

23. Poljak RJ, Amzel LM, Avey HP, et al: Three-dimensional structure of the Fab′ fragment of a human immunoglobulin in at 2.8Å resolution. Proc Natl Acad Sci USA 70:3305–3310, 1973

24. Davies DR, Padlan EA, Segal DM: Immunoglobulin structures at high resolution, in Inman FP, Mandy WJ (ed):

Contemporary Topics in Molecular Immunology, vol 4. New York, Plenum, 1975, pp 127–155

25. Alexander A, Rosen S, Buxbaum J: Immunoglobulin genes in health and disease. Clin Immunol Rev, 4:31, 1985

26. Hozumi N, Tonegawa S: Evidence for somatic rearrangement of immunoglobulin genes coding for variable and constant region. Proc Natl Acad Sci USA 73:3628–3632, 1976

27. Malcolm S, Barton P, Murphy Y, et al: Localization of κ light chain variable genes to the short arm of chromosome 2. Proc Natl Acad Sci USA 79:4957–4961, 1982

28. Proudfoot N, Brownlee G: 3′ Non-coding region sequences in eucaryotic messenger RNA. Nature 263:211–213, 1976

29. Erickson J, Martinis J, Croce C: Assignment of the genes for human lambda immunoglobulin genes to chromosome 22. Nature 294:173–177, 1981

30. Kabat W, Wu T, Bilofsky H, et al: Sequences Of Proteins Of Immunological Interest. US Dept of Health and Human Services Public Health Service, Bethesda, Md, National Institutes of Health 1983, p 14

31. Matthyssens G, Rabbits T: Structure and multiplicity of genes for the human immunoglobulin heavy chain variable region. Proc Natl Acad Sci USA 77:6651–6655, 1980

32. Siebenlist U, Ravetch J, Korsemyer S, et al: Human immunoglobulin D-segments encoded in tandem multigenic families. Nature 294:631–636, 1981

33. Rabbitts T, Forster A, Milstein C: Human immunoglobulin heavy chain genes: Evolutionary comparisons of $C\mu$ $C\delta$ and $C\alpha$ genes and associated switch sequences. Nucleic Acids Res 9:4509–4518, 1981

34. Migone N, Oliviero S, Delange G, et al: Proc Natl Acad Sci USA 79:3260–3263, 1982

35. Ravetch J, Siebenlist U, Korsmeyer S, et al: Structure of the human immunoglobulin mu locus: Characteristic of embyonic and rearranged D and J genes. Cell 27:583–590, 1981

36. Early P, Huang H, Davis M, et al: An immunoglobulin heavy chain variable region is generated from three segments of DNA: VH, D, and J. Cell 19:981–988, 1980

37. Desiderio S, Yancopoulos G, Paskind M, et al: Insertion of N regions in H chain genes is corrected with terminal deoxytransferase in B cells. Nature 311:752–756, 1984

38. Sakano H, Huppi K, Heinrich G, et al: Sequences at the somatic recombination sites of immunoglobulin L-chains. Nature 280:288–291, 1979

39. Alt F, Yancopoulos G, Blackwell T, et al: Ordered rearrangement of immunoglobulin H-chain variable region segments. EMBO J 3:1209–1218, 1984

40. Queen C, Baltimore D: Immunoglobulin gene transcription is activated by downstream enhancer elements. Cell 33:741–749, 1983

41. Proudfoot NJ, Brownlee G: 3′ non-coding region sequences in eucaryotic mRNA. Nature 263:211–215, 1976

42. Early P, Rogers J, Davis M, et al: Two mRNAs can be produced from a single immunoglobulin μ gene by alternative RNA processing pathways. Cell 20:313–321, 1980

43. Cheng H, Blattner F., Fitzmaurice L, et al: Structure of genes for membrane and secreted murine IgD H-chains. Nature, 296:410–414, 1982

44. Honjo T, Katoaka T: Organization of immunoglobulin heavy chain genes and allelic deletion model. Proc Natl Acad Sci USA 75:2140–2144, 1978

45. Yaoita Y, Honjo T: Deletion of immunoglobulin heavy chain genes from the expressed allelic chromosome. Nature 286:850–854, 1980

46. Frangione B, Franklin E: Structural Variants of Human and Murine Immunoglobulins. Contemp Top Mole Immunol 4:89–126, 1977

47. Seligman M, Mihaesco E, Hurez D, et al: Immunochemical studies in four cases of alpha chain disease. J Clin Invest 48:2374–2388, 1969

48. Frangione B: Structure of atypical immunoglobulins—relationship to genetic control mechanisms, in Litman GW, Good RA (eds): Immunoglobulins. New York, Plenum, 1972, pp 257–272

49. Frangione B, Lee L, Harber E, et al: Protein hal: partial delection of a " " immunoglobulin gene(s) and Apparent reinitiation at an internal AUG Codon. Proc Natl. Acad Sci USA 70:1073–1077, 1973

50. Fett J, Deutsch H, Smithies O: Hinge region deletion localized in the IgG globulin Mcg. Immunochemistry, 10:115–118, 1973

51. Franklin E, Prelli F, Frangione B: Human Heavy Chain Protein Wis: Implications for the organization of immunoglobulin genes. Proc Natl Acad Sci USA 76:452–456, 1978

52. Adlersberg JB, Franklin EC, Frangione B: Repetative hinge region sequences in human IgG3. Isolation of a 11,000 dalton fragment. Proc Natl Acad Sci USA 72:723–727, 1975

53. Alexander A, Steinmetz M, Barritault D, et al: Gamma heavy chain disease in man: cDNA supports partial gene deletion model. Proc Natl Acad Sci USA 79:3260–3265, 1982

54. Guglielmi P, Bakhshi A, Mihaesco E, et al: DNA deletion in human gamma heavy chain disease. Clin Res 32:348A, 1984 (abstr)

55. Mihaesco E, Seligman M, Frangione B: Studies of alpha chain disease. Ann NY Acad Sci 1971, pp 489–500

56. Wolfenstein-Todel C, Mihaesco E, Frangione B: Alpha chain disease protein def: Internal deletion of a human immunoglobulin alpha heavy chain. Proc Natl Acad Sci USA 71:974–978, 1974

57. Wetter O, Linder K-H, Leene W: Mu chain secretion by peripheral blood lymphocytes in mu chain disease. Eur J Cancer 13:985–992, 1977

58. Mihaesco C, Mihaesco E, Miglierina R, et al: Physicochemical and immunological properties of a mu chain disease protein. Immunochemistry 13:3945–3952, 1976

59. Lebreton J, Ropartz C, Rousseaux J, et al: Immunochemical and biochemical study of a human fc mu like fragment (mu chain disease). Eur J Immunol 3:179–184, 1975

60. Franklin E, Frangione B, Prelli F: The defect in the mu heavy chain disease protein GLI. J Immunol 116:1194–1199, 1976

61. Buxbaum J, Franklin E, Scharff M: Immunoglobulin M heavy chain disease: Intracellular origin of the mu chain fragment. Science 169:770–773, 1970

62. Bakhshi A, Guglielmi P, Siebenlist U, et al: A DNA insertion/deletion necessitates an aberrant RNA splice

accounting for a mu heavy chain disease. Proc Natl Acad Sci USA (in press)

63. Bernier G, Johnson C, Fanger M: Structural and biosynthetic studies of a human half IgA half molecule. J Immunol 119:1260–1265, 1977

64. Spiegelberg H, Heath V, Lang T: Human IgG half molecules, structural and antigenic analysis. Biochemistry 14:2157–2167, 1975

65. Williams R, Brunning R, Wollheim F: Light chain disease: An abortive variant of multiple myeloma. Ann Intern Med 65:471–486, 1966

66. Gordon J: Molecular aspects of immunoglobulin expression by human B cell leukemias and lymphomas. Adv Cancer Res 41:71–154, 1984

67. Preud'homme J, Morel-Maroger L, Brouet J, et al: Synthesis of abnormal immunoglobulins in lymphoblastic disorders with visceral light chain depletion. Am J Med 69:703–710, 1980

68. Milstein C: Interchain disulfide bridge in Bence-Jones proteins and in gamma-globulin B chains. Nature 205:1171–1173, 1965

69. Solomon A, Fahey J: Bence Jones proteinemia. Am J Med 37:206–222, 1964

70. Caggiano V, Dominguez C, Opfell R, et al: IgG myeloma with closed tetrameric Bence-Jones proteinuria. Am J Med 47:978–985, 1969

71. Buxbaum J, Hurley M, Chuba J, et al: Amyloidosis of the AL type. Clinical, morphologic and biochemical aspects of the response to therapy with akylating agents. Am J Med 67:867–868, 1979

72. Stone M, Frenkel E: The clinical spectrum of light chain myeloma: A study of 35 patients with special reference to the occurrence of amyloidosis. Am J Med 58:601–619, 1975

73. Smithies O, Gibson D, Fanning E, et al: Partial sequences of two unusual immunoglobulin light chains, rzf and sac. Biochemistry 10:4912–4919, 1978

74. Garver F, Chang L, Mendicino Jr, et al: Primary structure of a deleted human lambda type immunoglobulin light chain containing carbohydrate: Protein sm. Proc Natl Acad Sci USA 72:4559–4563, 1975

75. Hobbs J: Immunochemical classes of myelomatosis. Br J Haematol 16:599–606, 1969

76. River G, Tewksbury D, Fudenburg H: Non-secretory multiple myeloma. Blood 40:204–206, 1972

77. Hurez D, Preud'homme J-L, Seligman M: Intracellular monoclonal immunoglobulin in non-secretory human myeloma. J Immunol 104:263–264, 1970

78. Preud'homme J-L, Hurez D, Danon F, et al: Intracytoplasmic and surface bound immunoglobulins in non-secretory and Bence Jones myeloma. Clin Exp Immunol 25:428–463, 1976

79. Mancilla R, Davis G: Non-secretory multiple myeloma. Am J Med 63:1015–1022, 1977

80. Azar H, Zaino E, Pham T, et al: Non-secretory plasma cell myeloma. Am J Clin Pathol 42:618–629, 1972

81. Gach J, Simar L, Salmon J: Multiple myeloma without M type proteinemia. Am J Med 50:835–844, 1974

82. Glenner G: Amyloid deposits and amyloidosis: The beta fibrilloses. N Engl J Med 302: 1283–1292, 1980

83. Solomon A, Frangione B, Franklin EC: Bence Jones proteins and light chains of immunoglobulins: Preferential association of the V_{VI} subgroup of human light chains with amyloidosis (AL). J Clin Invest 70:453–460, 1982

84. Picken M, Gallo G, Buxbaum J, et al: Characterization of renal amyloid derived from the variable region of the lambda light chain subgroup II. Am J Pathol (in press)

85. Gallo G, Feiner H, Katz L, et al: Nodular glomerulopathy associated with nonamyloidotic kappa light chain deposits and excess immunoglobulin light chain synthesis. Am J Pathol 99:621–624, 1980

86. Preud'homme H-L, Morel-Maroger L, Brouet J, et al: Synthesis of abnormal heavy and light chains in multiple myeloma with visceral deposition of monoclonal immunoglobulin. Clin Exp Immunol 42:545–533, 1980

Plasmacytomas in Mice

Michael Potter

MANY OF THE DETAILS of plasmacytoma induction in mice have been reviewed[1-6] and this article, therefore, will be only a brief discussion and summary of recent findings. As the review articles contain references to the previous literature, only pertinent and new references will be cited here.

INDUCTION OF PLASMA CELL TUMORS

A number of years ago it was fortuitously discovered that BALB/c mice carrying intraperitoneally implanted Millipore diffusion chambers containing C3H mammary tumor tissue developed plasmacytomas. Thinking that this process was a form of chronic immunization, we sought to find other means to chronically immunize BALB/c mice and this led us to use various immunologic adjuvant mixtures containing antigens. The best known of these was Freund's Adjuvants (FA), a mineral oil in water emulsion. It was shown that adjuvants like FA (Lieberman's Adjuvant containing staphylococcal antigens) also induced plasmacytomas. Later mineral oil alone was shown to be an effective inducing agent and no antigen needed to be added. The chronic immunization hypothesis appeared to be incorrect. Because of the ease of administration, mineral oils or chemically defined components of mineral oils such as pristane (2, 6, 10, 14 tetramethylpentadecane) became commonly used plasmacytoma inducing agents, even though the underlying mechanism of plasma cell tumor development remained obscure. Pristane is now the best studied agent. Although pristane can be found in fossil mineral oils, it is also generated biologically. Marine copepods metabolically convert the alkane phytane (of plant origin) into pristane.[1] These organisms are consumed by filter feeding fishes and mammals. Whale livers consequently contain large amounts of pristane and are a source of the material used today. Pristane, like mineral oils is probably not effectively metabolized by mammals and for this reason it is regarded as an unlikely mutagen or carcinogen. The action of pristane as a plasma cell tumor inducing agent is indirect and appears to be related to its inflammatory properties in the peritoneal cavity. The presence of the oil in the peritoneal space stimulates the influx of large numbers of cells of the monocyte-macrophage series and neutrophils for the purpose of containing the foreign material. This influx is chronic and persists as long as there is free oil in the peritoneum. The mineral oils or pristane in the peritoneal cavity are emulsified into variable sized globules. Some of these are small enough to be phagocytized but other larger globules are surrounded by several cells.[5] The phagocytic cells that have engulfed or adhered to oil droplets in turn adhere to peritoneal surfaces on the mesentery, omentum, abdominal wall, diaphram, and pelvic fat. They provoke an angiogenic reaction from mesenteric blood vessels that leads to vascularization of much of the accumulating oil laden cells. The vascularized tissue is called an oil granuloma (OG).[5] OG formation begins within a few days of the injection of pristane and continues to accumulate. Most of the surfaces of OG are covered by mesothelial cells. The importance of the OG to plasma cell tumor development is demonstrated by the fact that these tumors originate in this tissue, ie, the fully developed plasmacytoma and a series of progressive preneoplastic plasma cell proliferations are found within the OG. To cope with the continuous demand for phagocytic cells both in the peritoneal space and for renewal of cells in the fixed OG, there are probably major changes in hematopoiesis in the bone marrow. However, there have only been a few studies of the increased production of bone marrow precursors. Pietrangeli et al[7] have described increased proliferation of B lymphocytes in the bone marrow after intraperitoneal (IP) mineral oil injection and it is assumed that macrophages and

From the Laboratory of Genetics, National Cancer Institute, National Institutes of Health, Bethesda, Md.

Address reprint requests to Michael Potter, MD, Laboratory of Genetics, National Cancer Institute, NIH, Bethesda, MD 20892.

0093–7754/86/1303–0003$0.00/0

neutrophil precursors are also very active because the bone marrow is the primary source of these cells.

Plasma cell tumors are diagnosed in pristane-injected mice by the appearance of plasma cells in the peritoneal fluid. These cells appear after a minimal latent period between 115 and 120 days.[8] The mean latent period based on detecting tumor cells in ascites in BALB/cAnPt mice is 210 to 220 days after the injection of pristane[8] and is continuous thereafter. The average incidence of plasmacytomas in a group of BALB/c AnPt mice is 60% (range: 50% to 70%) by 300 days.[8] After 200 days, BALB/c mice may succumb to other complications of pristane such as arthritis[9] ascites formation (obstruction of peritoneal lymphatics) and intestinal adhesions.

The induction of plasmacytomas in inbred mice is highly strain dependent. Most of the commonly used inbred strains of mice, A, C3H, CBA, C57BL, DBA/2, SWR, and others are resistant.[2,10] An exception is NZB/B1, which is susceptible.[11,12] Not all BALB/c sublines are susceptible; the BALB/cJ subline in comparison to other sublines is resistant to plasmacytoma induction.[6,9] Some attempt has been made to determine the number of genes that determine susceptibility and resistance by studying induction in F1 and first generation backcross hybrids of BALB/c AnPt and a resistant strain.[3] BALB/c AnPt and DBA/2 appear to differ by at least three resistance genes. As yet, genes determining susceptibility or resistance have not been identified and characterized.

An important feature of the plasmacytomas in BALB/cAnPt mice is the high incidence of tumors that produce IgA myeloma proteins. Over 66% of all the tumors that are established in transplant produce IgA myeloma proteins.[13]

PRENEOPLASTIC PLASMA CELL LESIONS IN THE OIL GRANULOMA

Our laboratory is currently studying the early stages of plasma cell tumor formation and it appears that there are several different patterns of proliferation that may be sequential. First, the OG becomes diffusely populated with plasma cells, the predominant type being an IgA forming cell (unpublished observations with E.B. Mushinski). Second, aggregates of these cells are seen. These contain 25 cells or less. Third, larger aggregates of 50 to several hundred plasma cells are found. These often contain atypical cells and are called foci of proliferating plasma cells, chiefly, because mitotic figures can be seen in the plasma cells. There are several kinds of foci, one is diffusely distributed in a region of the oil granuloma, and often appears to have cells that are migrating into surrounding tissue. The second kind of focus has a metastatic appearance, ie, it is a relatively compact mass of cells often located near a mesothelial surface. The cells in metastatic foci are usually more atypical.

During the minimal latent period (0 to 120 days), more mice develop foci, and more foci are found per mouse. Foci appear to increase progressively in an individual mouse and involve more and more of the OG. These foci ultimately fuse to form confluent masses of cells. Free tumor cells appear in the peritoneal space. Primary plasmacytomas rarely metastasize beyond the peritoneum but they are readily transplantable to syngeneic recipients. Successful peritoneal transplantation however, requires conditioning of the new host by an IP injection of pristane.[4] This suggests that the tumor cells require special factors for growth that are provided by the OG.

The fundamental reason why plasma cells are located and then subsequently proliferate in the OG is not known. Their presence could reflect primary antibody formation in the OG if circulating antigen gains access to the OG and could be presented to circulating B lymphocytes. Also, the omentum is known to contain islands of lymphoid tissue called milk spots, and these are a potential tissue for antibody formation. Alternatively, though, the OG may simply provide a homing environment for memory cells or derivatives of natural immune responses that are generated in lymph nodes, spleen, and Peyer's patches. This homing environment may have the added feature of supplying factors that permit proliferation of plasma cells.

PLASMACYTOMA DEVELOPMENT AND INFLAMMATION

An important feature of peritoneal plasmacytoma development is the close association of plasma cells with phagocytosing macrophages and neutrophils.[14] This occurs both in the peritoneal space and in the fixed OG. The process of phagocytosis is known to generate oxygen radicals (superoxide anion, hydroxyl radical, singlet oxygen, hydrogen peroxide). It is assumed that the plasma cells in the OG are exposed to exogenously generated radicals. In studies reported by others, it has been shown in cultures containing lymphocytes and phagocytes that have been exposed to macrophage activating agents, eg, phorbol esters that chromosome breaks and other types of damage develop in the lymphocytes.[15]

Further evidence that some product of the chronic inflammation is playing an important role in plasmacytoma development in mice is provided by the finding that the continuous administration of the nonsteroidal antiinflammatory drug indomethacin in the drinking water during the latent period strikingly inhibits plasmacytoma development.[14] The mice do develop a characteristic peritoneal OG. However, indomethacin appears to inhibit the formation of multiple plasma cell focal proliferations. Plasma cells are seen in the OG including both aggregates and scattered cells, and even occasional focal proliferations, but the progressive formation of multiple foci appears to be inhibited.[14] The biochemical basis for this striking inhibition in plasmacytoma development is not yet defined. Indomethacin has several known biochemical actions. First, it is a powerful inhibitor of prostaglandin synthetase and therefore blocks the formation of prostaglandins and thromboxanes and also lipid radical by-products. Further, indomethacin has been shown to have other pharmacologic actions and one of these is its ability to inhibit the formation of radicals by neutrophils.[4,14] One possibility that seems relevant is that indomethacin's major inhibitory action is the reduction of potential genotoxic radicals that are generated in the OG, because these could potentially mutagenize proliferating plasma cells. But other explanations are also possible, for example, it might be argued that the reduction in prostaglandin formation alleviates a putative immunosuppressed environment that compromises immunologic surveillance processes that may normally control plasma cell proliferation and tumor development. Preliminary evidence did not support this latter notion[14] but further studies will be required to completely rule it out.

The association of spontaneous plasmacytoma development with chronic inflammation has also been described.[16] Spontaneous plasmacytomas are very rare but do occur late in life in a few strain C3H mice. Dunn noted that these tumors arose in the wall of the ileocecal region in inflammatory tissue that formed under ulcerations of the mucosa. In a special inbred stain of rats called Lou/C, developed in Louvain, Belgium, by Hervé Bazin, 30% to 40% of the rats develop immunocytomas that are morphologically similar to the murine plasmacytomas.[17–19] These tumors arise in the ileocecal lymph node itself. However, these lesions have not been associated with ulcerations in the gut wall,[19] and no direct association with inflammatory tissue has yet been made. A feature of the spontaneous rat immunocytomas, however, is a high incidence of IgE producing tumors.[18] This suggests that cells differentiated to produce IgE are at increased risk of transforming to a neoplastic state. Because IgE immunoglobulins are associated with parasitic infestations, it is possible that a connection to parasitic infestations should be further sought, particularly because the tumors in the terminal ileocecal node drain a specific segment of the gut that often harbors helminthic and protozoan parasites.

NONRANDOM TRANSLOCATIONS INVOLVING CHROMOSOME 15

A salient feature of the induced plasmacytomas in mice is the occurrence of nonrandom chromosomal breaks and recombinations involving the D2/D3 band in chromosome (chr) 15. For details and references of the following discussion see reference no. 4. One of three types of anomalies is found in 98% of these tumors. The most common is a reciprocal translocation involving chr 15 and chr 12, which appears in about 70% of the tumors. The second type is a reciprocal exchange of chr 6 and chr 15. A third type rarely found is a deleted segment of chr 15. The break sites in chrs 6, 12, and 15 occur in the same band regions and the genes located at these break sites have now been identified: Ig κ locus (chr 6), Ig heavy chain locus (chr 12) and the c-*myc* oncogene on chr 15. The break site in chr 12 is associated clearly with immunoglobulin heavy chain switch region sites, and the availability of the chr 12 for the reciprocal exchange with chr 15 may be associated with the process of IgC_H switching. In the mouse heavy chain gene complex, there are seven switch genes, located 5′ of Cμ, Cγ3, Cγ1, Cγ2b, Cγ2a, Cε and Cα. The most commonly involved switch site in rcpt12;15 is Sα. Moreover the chr 12 involved in the reciprocal translocations is not the one that is transcribing heavy chain messenger RNA for Ig biosynthesis, but is in fact, the inactive or nonproductive chromosome. Many of the plasmacytomas with rcpt12;15 synthesize and secrete IgA, using the productively switched chromosome but, interestingly, also show evidence that a switch to Sα has occurred on the translocated chromosome. However, it is difficult to establish the time and site of the reciprocal translocation with existing evidence. It is possible that the translocations represent a mistake that occurs when the cell is normally undergoing the switch from Sμ to Sα, for example. It is also possible that the translocation event is dissociated from the switching step. For example, abortively switched chromosomes may be more vulnerable to subsequent nonspecific chromosome breaks. This notion is speculative and remains to be demonstrated.

C-MYC GENE DEREGULATION IN PLASMACYTOMAS

The significant end result of the nonrandom chromosomal translocations is the activation of the c-*myc* oncogene.[4] The molecular basis of c-*myc* oncogene activation is currently being worked out, there are apparently several different ways in which this takes place and not all of them are clearly understood. In the most common situation, the continuity of the c-*myc* gene is disrupted by the translocation. C-*myc* has three exons, E1, E2, and E3. The latter two code for the c-*myc* protein (a 67 kilodalton DNA binding protein usually found in the nucleus). E1 and its 5′ flanking sequences contain noncoding regulatory sequences that control the transcription of the c-*myc* gene. Many, but not all rcpt 12;15 translocations break c-*myc* in the first intron between E1 and E2, thereby dissociating the coding exons from the regulatory ones. In a second type of reciprocal translocation involving chrs 12 and 15, the breakpoint in c-*myc* occurs 300 to 500 base pair 5′ of E1. In these transcripts of the c-*myc* RNA have a prolonged half life,[20] potentially providing another way to effectively increase the availability of c-*myc* gene products. The break site in the rcpt6;15 translocation occurs at a considerable distance from c-*myc* and at present it is not known how this disturbs the function of the c-*myc* gene.[21]

Abnormal c-*myc* gene expression has been found in a number of other B cell neoplasms (Table 1). In bursal lymphomas in the chicken, which are lymphomas of non-Ig secreting B lymphocytes, the c-*myc* gene is activated by a retroviral insertion into the c-*myc* locus. Many of these inserts actually disrupt the chicken c-*myc* gene 5′ of E2 in much the same way as occurs in the plasmacytomas.[22] The Burkitt's lymphoma in man, another B lymphocytic neoplasm, is associated with a set of translocations (t2;8, t8;14, t8;22) that are homologous to those found in the mouse.[21] The breakpoints in chrs 2, 14, and 22 occur in Igk, Igh and Igλ, respectively, while the common breakpoint in chr 8 occurs in c-*myc*. In Burkitt's lymphomas, the switch mμ (Sμ) site is the one most commonly involved. In rat immuno-

Table 1. Association of the c-*myc* Locus With Various Forms of Neoplasms of the B-Lymphocyte-Plasma Cell Lineage

Tumor	Species	B Cell Stage	Mechanism
Bursal lymphoma[22]	Chicken	B lymphocyte	Insertion of ALV usually into the c-*myc* locus
Burkitt's lymphoma[23]	Man	B lymphocyte	Reciprocal chromosomal translocation with Ig-loci
Induced peritoneal plasmacytomas[1-6]	BALB/c mouse	Plasma cell	Reciprocal chromosomal translocation with Ig-loci
Spontaneous illeocecal l.n. immunocytomas[17-19]	Lou/c rat	Plasma cell	Reciprocal chromosomal translocation with Ig-loci
Pre B B cell lymphomas[25]	$(C57BL \times SJL)_{f1}$ mice	Pre-B and lymphocytes	Transgenic mice carrying *E-c-myc*

cytomas or plasmacytomas, the t6;7 translocation is found in high frequency again involving breakpoints in the c-*myc* and Ig heavy chain loci.[23,24] The specific location within the rat *Igh* is not yet known. Finally, and very recently, transgenic mice carrying c-*myc* loci linked to the Ig enhancer (Eμ) sequences develop pre-B and B cell lymphomas in a very high percentage of the mice by 3 to 4 months of age.[25]

A common feature in many of these tumors of the B lymphocytic lineage is loss of normal control of c-*myc* transcription. For example, in bursal lymphomas the normal cellular controls are replaced by viral promoters,[22] while in the tumors associated with chromosomal translocations, the normal regulatory sequences are displaced[4] and in a few of these, Ig-enhancer sequences are found in close proximity.[26,27] Dramatically in the transgenic mice the regular association of the Eμ and c-*myc* results in a high incidence of spontaneous B lymphocytic tumors.[23]

The physiological function of the c-*myc* gene product is currently not known. The human c-*myc* gene product P62$^{c\text{-}myc}$ binds to a component in interphase nuclei, and is easily extracted from nuclei by mild salt concentrations, conditions that do not affect the nuclear matrix or major chromatin proteins.[28] Evan et al[28] suggest that binding of P62$^{c\text{-}myc}$ to nuclei could be reversibly modulated by physiological changes in salt concentration.

While current evidence indicates the c-*myc* gene is transcribed throughout the cell cycle at constitutive rates,[29–31] transcription is amplified roughly ten-fold when certain cell types are activated into mitosis.[32] This burst of transcription appears in the G_1 phase of the mitotic cycle and is followed by a return to the constitutive state. This kind of result suggests c-*myc* normally functions during G_1. In cells that have deregulated c-*myc* genes, the levels of the c-*myc* gene product would remain high throughout the cell cycle. It is tempting to speculate that deregulation of c-*myc* in an Ig secreting cell or plasma cell could interfere with the process of maturation to a postmitotic state. This kind of effect would have especially important consequences in terminally differentiated cells such as plasma cells where the cessation of mitosis is associated with the process of cellular elimination. In earlier stages of B lymphocytic development, resting cells are activated into the mitotic cycle by exogenously derived growth factors. The presence of a deregulated c-*myc* gene may then facilitate entry into or completion of the mitotic cycle.

COMPARISON OF MULTIPLE MYELOMA AND INDUCED PLASMACYTOMAS

Multiple myeloma (MM) and the induced peritoneal plasmacytomas (PCTs) in mice appear to be different forms of Ig-secreting tumors (Table 2). Typically, MM is a spontaneously arising tumor, appearing predominantly

Table 2. Comparison of Plasma Cell Tumor Formations in Mouse, Man, Rat

	Multiple Myeloma (Man)	Induced Plasmacytomas (BALB/c Mouse[1–6])	Spontaneous Immunocytomas (Lou/c rats[17–19])
Etiology	Unknown	Induced by IP mineral oil, plastics	None known
Genetic background	Heterogeneous	Homogeneous	Homogeneous
Role of specific genes	None known	Implicated but not identified	Implicated but not identified
Male/female incidence	Males > females	No difference	3/1
Nonrandom chromosomal anomalies	No consistent types[33]	rcpt12;15 rcpt6;15	t6;7 in a high proportion
myc gene deregulation	None implicated	Deregulated	Deregulated
Site of development	Bone marrow	Peritoneal connective tissues	Ileocecal lymph node
Role of inflammation	Not demonstrated	Implicated	? parasitic infection suspected
Heavy chain classes	IgG > IgA	IgA ≫ IgG	IgE = IgG ≫ IgA
Progression	MGUS → MM (11%)[34]	Foci → Pct	?

in older individuals, where the PCTs require an inductive process and first appear in relatively younger animals. The neoplastic cells in MM accumulate in the bone marrow, divide slowly, and in general are morphologically mature. In contrast, the cells of the PCTs develop in the peritoneal connective tissues and OG, and at the time they become clinically manifest, they are proliferating relatively rapidly and morphologically exhibit varying degrees of atypia; in general they are less mature than their human counterpart. Further, the PCTs in mice are consistently associated with nonrandom chromosomal translocations and activation of *myc* transcription. Although there have been several cytogenetic studies of MM,[33-35] translocations involving the c-*myc* locus on chr 8 are not characteristic of this disease. In sharp contrast, translocations involving c-*myc* on chr 8 are found in over 95% of Burkitt's lymphomas, a neoplasm of B lymphocytes.[36]

Despite these differences in MM and PCTs, there are similarities that relate to the progression of the tumors. Both kinds of plasma cell tumors appear to progress through stages. MM may develop from a monoclonal gammopathy of undetermined significance (MGUS) after several years of stationary growth,[37] but also may present with osteolytic lesions and still progress slowly. However, late in the course of MM, more aggressive plasma cell types may emerge,[38,39] such as dermal metastases, cells in the peripheral blood or in effusions. Also cytogenetic studies show that abnormal clones appear.[34] In the PCTs, some of the earlier preplasmacytoma stages are associated with the accumulation of large numbers of plasma cells in the OG (M. Potter, unpublished observations). Thus, the two processes may go through similar progressive changes but differ chiefly in the anatomic sites where these accumulations occur and by the rate of progression. The failure, though, to find chr 8 translocations even in the late stages of MM is unexplained. Recently, amplification of c-*myc* has been described in plasma cell leukemia.[40] Both MM and PCTs in mice then may be associated with the accumulation of slowly proliferating, relatively normal appearing plasma cells in tissues before the emergence of malignant clones.

REFERENCES

1. Potter M: Pathogenesis of plasmacytomas in mice, in Becker FF (ed): Cancer. A Comprehensive Treatise, (ed 2) vol 1. New York, Plenum, 1982, pp 135–159

2. Potter M: Genetics of susceptibility to plasmacytoma development in BALB/c mice. Cancer Surv 3:247–264, 1984

3. Potter M, Wax JS: Role of genes in the susceptibility to plasmacytomas, in Skamene E (ed): Genetic Control of Host Resistance to Infection and Malignancy, Progress in Leukocyte Biology, vol 3. New York, Liss, 1985, pp 793–804

4. Potter M: Progression in plasmacytoma development in BALB/c mice, in Klein G (ed): Advances in Viral Oncology, 1986 (in press)

5. Anderson AO, Wax JS, Potter M: Differences in the peritoneal response to pristane in BALB/cAnPt and BALB/cJ mice. Curr Top Microbiol Immunol 122:242–253, 1985

6. Potter M, Wax JS, Blankenhorn E: BALB/c subline differences in susceptibility to plasmacytoma induction. Curr Top Microbiol Immunol 122:234–241, 1985

7. Pietrangeli CE, Osmond DG: Regulation of B-lymphocyte production in the bone marrow. Role of macrophages and the spleen in mediating responses to exogenous agents. Cell Immunol 94:147–158, 1985

8. Potter M, Wax JS: Peritoneal plasmacytomagenesis in mice. A comparison of three pristane dose regimens. JNCI 71:391–395, 1983

9. Potter M, Wax JS: Genetics of susceptibility to pristane-induced plasmacytomas in BALB/cAn: Reduced susceptibility in BALB/cJ with a brief description of pristane-induced arthritis. J Immunol 127:1591–1595, 1981

10. Morse HC III, Hartley JW, Potter M: Genetic considerations in plasmacytomas of BALB/c, NZB, and (BALB/c × NZB)F_1 mice, in Potter M (ed): Progress in Myeloma. New York, Elsevier/North Holland, 1980, pp 263–279

11. Morse HC III, Riblet R, Asofsky R, et al: Plasmacytomas of the NZB mouse. J Immunol 121:1969–1972, 1978

12. Warner NL: Review. Autoimmunity and the pathogenesis of plasma cell tumor induction in NZB and hybrid mice. Immunogenetics 2:1–20, 1975

13. Potter M: Immunoglobulin producing tumors and myeloma proteins of mice. Physiol Rev 52:631–719, 1972

14. Potter M, Wax JS, Anderson AO, et al: Inhibition of plasmacytoma development in BALB/c mice by indomethacin. J Exp Med 161:996–1012, 1985

15. Emerit I, Cerutti P: Icosanoids and chromosome damage, in Thaler-Dao H (ed): Icosanoids and Cancer. New York, Raven, 1984, pp 127–137

16. Dunn TB: Plasma cell neoplasms beginning in the ileocecal area in strain C3H mice. JNCI 19:371–391, 1957

17. Bazin H, Deckers C, Beckers A, et al: Transplantable immunoglobulin secreting tumors in rats. I. General features of Lou/Wsl strain rat immunocytomas and their monoclonal proteins. Int J Cancer 10:568–580, 1972

18. Bazin H, Beckers A, Deckers C, et al: Transplantable immunoglobulin secreting tumors in rats. V. Monoclonal

immunoglobulins secreted by 250 ileocecal immunocytomas in Lou/wsl rats. JNCI 51:1359, 1973

19. Bazin H: Mechanisms of B Cell Neoplasia, Basel, Switzerland, Editiones Roches, 1985, p 208

20. Piechaczyk M, Yang J-Q, Blanchard JM, et al: Posttranscriptional mechanisms are responsible for accumulation of truncated c-*myc* RNAs in murine plasma cell tumors. Cell 42:589–597, 1985

21. Cory S, Graham M, Webb E, et al: Variant (6;15) translocations in murine plasmacytomas involve a chromosome 15 locus at least 72 kb from the c-*myc* oncogene. EMBO J 4:675–681, 1985

22. Shih G-K, Linial M, Goodenow MM, et al: Nucleotide sequence 5′ of the chicken c-*myc* coding region: Localization of a noncoding exon that is absent from myc transcripts in most avian leukosis virus-induced lymphomas. Proc Natl Acad Sci USA 81:4697–4701, 1984

23. Klein G, Klein E: Myc/Ig juxtaposition by chromosomal translocations. Some new insights, puzzles and paradoxes. Immunol Today 6:208–215, 1985

24. Sumegi J: Mechanisms in B Cell Neoplasia, Basel, Switzerland, Editiones Roche, 1985, pp 244–247

25. Adams JM, Harris AW, Pinkert CA, et al: The c-*myc* oncogene driven by immunoglobulin enhancers induces lymphoid malignancy in transgenic mice. Nature 318:533–538, 1985

26. Fahrlander PD, Sumegi J, Yang J-Q, et al: Activation of the c-*myc* oncogene by the immunoglobulin gene enhancer after multiple switch region-mediated chromosomal rearrangements in a murine plasmacytoma. Proc Natl Acad Sci USA 82:3746–3750, 1985

27. Corcoran LM, Cory S, Adams JM: Transposition of the immunoglobulin heavy chain enhancer to the *myc* oncogene in a murine plasmacytoma. Cell 40:71–79, 1985

28. Evan GI, Hancock DC: Studies on the interaction of the human c-*myc* protein with cell nuclei: $P62^{c\text{-}myc}$ as a member of a discrete subset of nuclear proteins. Cell 43:253–261, 1985

29. Hann SR, Thompson CB, Eisenman RN: C-*myc* oncogene protein synthesis is independent of the cell cycle in human and avian cells. Nature 314:366–369, 1985

30. Thompson CB, Challoner PB, Neiman PE, et al: Levels of c-*myc* oncogene mRNA are invariant throughout the cell cycle. Nature 314:363–369, 1985

31. Blanchard JM, Piechaczyk M, Dani C, et al: C-*myc* gene is transcribed at a high rate in Go arrested fibroblasts and is posttranscriptionally regulated in response to growth factors. Nature 317:443–445, 1985

32. Persson H, Gray HE, Godeau F: Growth dependent synthesis of c-*myc* encoded proteins: Early stimulation by serum factors in synchronized mouse 3T3 cells. Mol Cell Biol 5:2903–2912, 1985

33. Ueshima Y, Rowley JD: Chromosome studies in patients with multiple myeloma and related paraproteinemias, in Wiernik PH, Canellos GP, Kyle RA, et al: (eds): Neoplastic Diseases of the Blood, New York, Churchill-Livingstone, 1985, pp 513–528

34. Dewald GW, Kyle RA, Hicks GA, et al: The clinical significance of cytogenetic studies in 100 patients with multiple myeloma, plasma leukemia or amyloidosis. Blood 66:380–390, 1985

35. Philip P: Chromosomes of monoclonal gammopathies. Cancer Genet Cytogenet 2:79–86, 1980

36. Lenoir GM, Preud'homme JL, Bernheim A, et al: Correlation between immunoglobulin light chain expression and variant translocation in Burkitt's lymphoma. Nature 298:474–476, 1982

37. Kyle RA: Monoclonal gammopathy of undetermined significance. Natural history in 241 cases. Am J Med 64:814–825, 1978

38. Greipp RR, Kyle RA: Clinical morphological and cell kinetic differences among mulitple myeloma monoclonal gammopathy of undetermined significance and smoldering multiple myeloma. Blood 62:166–171, 1983

39. Bergsagel DE, Pruzanski W: Some unusual manifestations of plasma cell neoplasia, in Wiernick PH, Canellos GP, Kyle RA, et al (eds): Neoplastic Diseases of the Blood, vol 1. New York, Churchill-Livingstone, 1985, pp 553–573

40. Sumegi J, Hedberg T, Bjorkholm M, et al: Amplification of the c-*myc* oncogene in human plasma cell leukemia. Int J Cancer 36:367–371, 1985

Immunosuppression and Infection in Multiple Myeloma

Daniel R. Jacobson and Susan Zolla-Pazner

BACTERIAL INFECTIONS are major causes of morbidity and mortality in patients with multiple myeloma. A variety of immune deficiencies have been identified in such patients, and are thought to play a role in their high incidence of infection. In vitro and in vivo studies in humans and mice have provided insight into the pathogenic mechanisms underlying the observed immune deficits. In this report, we review the spectrum of infections frequently seen in patients with myeloma. We then examine the nature of immune disorders found in these patients and the mechanism underlying this altered immunity. Finally, we consider strategies for reducing the incidence of infection in these patients.

CLINICAL FINDINGS

Between 1953 and 1963, three studies of patients with multiple myeloma[1–3] and one study of patients with myeloma or Waldenstrom's macroglobulinemia[4] were published that described a high incidence of infection, particularly of the lower respiratory tract. In these studies, 20% to 72% of patients had at least one episode of pneumonia. Half of these patients had multiple episodes. *Streptococcus pneumonia* was by far the most common pathogen isolated, and gram-negative pneumonia was rarely described. The urinary tract was the second most common site of infection, with *Escherichia coli* and other gram-negative rods being the predominant pathogens.[3,4] The incidence of infection was threefold higher among patients with myeloma than among those with macroglobulinemia in one study, though the patterns of infection were similar.[4]

From the Departments of Medicine and Pathology, New York Veterans Administration Medical Center and New York University Medical Center, New York, NY.

Supported by Grant CA-15585 from the National Institutes of Health and research funds from the Veterans Administration.

Address reprint requests to Susan Zolla-Pazner, PhD, Veterans Administration Hospital, 408 First Ave, Room 16028W, New York, NY 10010.

0093–7754/86/1303–0004$05.00/0

In contrast to these early reports, studies since 1972 document an increased frequency of gram-negative rod isolates from infected myeloma patients.[5–9] This difference reflects the fact that pneumonia accounts for a smaller percentage of total infections and that an increased percentage of pneumonias results from gram-negative infection. In all series, the overall incidence of infection ranges from 0.8 to 2.22 infections per patient per year, which is seven- to 15-fold greater than the infection rate in hospitalized control groups without malignancy.[4,9] Infection is the leading cause of death in both early and recent studies of patients with myeloma, accounting for 20% to 50%[9,10] of deaths.

A decreased percentage of infections with gram-positive organisms, combined with a relatively stable incidence of infection per patient-year, led several investigators to conclude that gram-positive infections had become less prevalent than in previous years.[5,7,8] This conclusion was drawn by comparing recent data with historical observations. Caution must be exercised in drawing conclusions about overall trends in incidence of infection by comparing data derived from differing institutions, patient populations, and study durations. Only two single-institutional reports of the incidence of gram-positive infection over sequential time periods have appeared.[9,11] Twomey found the incidence of gram-positive infection in patients with myeloma for the period 1950 to 1963 similar to that for 1964 to 1971.[9] In his study, the decreased percentage of gram-positive organisms isolated during the latter period was entirely the result of a marked increase in the incidence of hospital-acquired gram-negative infection. The total number of infections was higher during the latter time period in this study. In another study, the incidence of pneumococcal bacteremia in patients with neoplastic disease at Memorial Hospital was compared for the time periods 1955 to 1971 and 1972 to 1978. The percentage of patients with multiple myeloma who experienced pneumococcal bacteremia more than doubled during the latter period.[11] No single-institutional study of myeloma patients has reported a decreasing incidence of gram-positive infection.

Thus, one can state only that in recent years gram-negative infections have increased in frequency, while the incidence of gram-positive infection has remained the same or increased.

Several investigators have studied the reasons for the increased incidence of serious gram-negative infections in patients with myeloma. Savage et al found a biphasic pattern of bacterial infection: *S pneumonia* and *Haemophilus influenza* infections tended to occur within 8 months of diagnosis and during response to chemotherapy as determined by a decreasing level of monoclonal protein.[6] Infection with gram-negative bacilli typically occurred in patients with refractory, advancing disease. Previous antibiotic therapy, instrumentation, immobilization, and colonization with hospital flora were all suggested as possible contributing factors to the risk of gram-negative bacillary infection. Azotemia (BUN $>$ 35) was found to be significantly related to infection with gram-negative bacilli, but not with *S. pneumonia* or *H. influenza.* It was uncertain whether azotemia represented an independent risk factor for infection, or whether this association reflected the fact that azotemia identified myeloma patients with a poor prognosis.[12] Most,[7,13] but not all,[5] investigators agree that azotemia correlates with incidence of infection. The risk of potentially fatal urosepsis associated with instrumentation of the urinary tract and with neurogenic bladder caused by vertebral collapse has been emphasized,[7-9] as has the risk of infection from an indwelling intravenous (IV) catheter.[7] In one study, all fatal infections were hospital-acquired[7]; thus, the standard admonition to minimize indwelling foreign bodies is particularly applicable to patients with myeloma.

Savage et al also examined the relationship between bacteremia and chemotherapy-induced neutropenia.[6] Nine of 19 episodes of gram-negative bacillary sepsis, and 12 of 13 episodes of sepsis with *S. pneumonia* and *H. influenza* occurred in the absence of neutropenia. This lack of correlation of infection and neutropenia has been noted by others as well.[5-9] Duration of disease may[5] or may not[7] play a role in the incidence of infection. In another study, Perri et al noted that during the first 2 months after the start of initial chemotherapy, patients were at increased risk for infection, and patients who responded to chemotherapy exhibited a lower risk of infection during the period of response.[13] Infections with fungi, Herpes virus, *Mycobacteria tuberculosis,*[3,9,14] and *Pneumocystis carinii*[15] have been infrequently described in patients with myeloma.

The increased risk of bacterial infection led investigators to study the immune response in patients with multiple myeloma. The first immune abnormality appreciated was an impaired humoral response to immunization. Patients with myeloma mount a weak or no primary antibody response to immunization with a variety of bacterial and viral antigens.[2,4,16,17] In one study, patients responded to 28 of 88 antigens (32%), while controls responded to 75 of 92 (87%).[4] Furthermore, inability to respond to immunization correlated with frequency of infection.[4] Patients with myeloma also have decreased levels of normal immunoglobulins, including antibodies against specific bacterial[18,19] and viral[20] antigens and against lipid A.[21,22] This results from both a decreased synthesis and an increased catabolism of normal immunoglobulins.[23-25] Although one cannot predict which patients will respond to immunization based on the level or pattern of abnormal immunoglobulin,[4,26-28] in one study, patients with higher levels of M protein tended to mount a poorer antibody response.[28] The secondary antibody response to previously encountered antigens is nearly normal in that the antibody titer rises by a normal amount; however, when the preimmunization titer is low, the postimmunization titer is also low.[26-28] The tendency for the primary response to be more profoundly suppressed than the secondary response is consistent with experimental models that have shown the secondary immune response always to be more refractory to suppression.

MECHANISMS OF IMMUNE SUPPRESSION

The mechanisms of humoral immune suppression induced by plasma cell tumors have been studied both in humans and in a mouse model of myeloma. In the mouse model, plasmacytomas (PC) are serially transplanted subcutaneously, intraperitoneally, or IV within inbred strains of mice. As with myeloma patients, PC-bearing mice demonstrate a decreased antibody response to immunization with T dependent and T independent antigens, suggesting that the immune suppression is not primarily T cell mediated.[29–35] As with human myeloma, where patients show a variable tendency toward infection, different PC cause a variable degree of immune suppression. For all PC, as the tumor mass increases, so does the degree of immune suppression.[32] This holds true for nonsecretory PC as well, indicating that the immunosuppression is not mediated directly by the monoclonal immunoglobulin.[32] The secondary immune response is usually, though not always, intact in PC-bearing mice,[32–34] again analogous to the case in patients with myeloma.

The mechanism underlying the immunosuppression in PC-bearing mice has been studied in vivo and in vitro. The primary mechanism responsible for the decreased humoral response to antigens involves suppressor monocyte/macrophages. PC tumor cells secrete a protein termed "PC factor". PC factor has no direct immunosuppressive properties, but it induces a monocyte/macrophage population to secrete a second humoral substance, termed "plasmacytoma-induced macrophage substance" (PIMS), which suppresses antibody production and B cell proliferation.[36–42] Thus, splenic B cells from PC-bearing mice did not proliferate in response to mitogens, unless macrophages were removed before culture. After removal of macrophages, the B cells responded normally, suggesting that B cells of PC-bearing mice are intrinsically normal, but inhibited by the suppressor macrophages.[42] Recent experiments have shown that the affected B cells are arrested in the late G_{-1} phase of the cell cycle, preventing clonal expansion and antibody production (Berman J, and Zolla-Pazner S, submitted for publication.) Normal macrophages become suppressor macrophages and secrete PIMS when cocultured with PC.[38] It has been proposed that this PC-induced immunosuppressive mechanism is not qualitatively different from normal mechanisms that control antibody production, and that the immunosuppression seen in PC-bearing mice represents a quantitatively exaggerated form of naturally occurring feedback inhibition.[37,43]

A second immunoregulatory mechanism described in PC-bearing mice is mediated by T cells. PC-bearing mice have increased numbers of T cells carrying membrane-bound Fc receptors (FcR) specific for the isotype of the paraprotein being secreted by the PC. Most of these FcR^+ cells express a suppressor phenotype and negatively control nonmalignant B cells producing the same immunoglobulin isotype.[44–47] They are also capable of suppressing the growth and secretion of PC producing the isotype for which they are specific.[48] The expansion of this isotype-specific T suppressor population appears to be caused directly by the monoclonal protein. Thus, for example, $T\alpha$ cells do not increase in the presence of nonsecretory PC,[49] but are induced in normal mice injected with IgA.[46] However, at least certain FcR^+ cells can act as helper cells. Thus, IgD-producing tumors in mice induce $T\partial$ cells with helper phenotype and helper function, which enhance the humoral immune response of their hosts.[50,51] $T\alpha$ and $T\epsilon$ cells with helper phenotype and function have also been described.[52,53] Thus, these paraprotein-induced FcR^+ T cells have a complex effect on the immune response of their hosts that varies depending on the isotype of the tumor and the phenotype of the induced FcR^+ T cell. Like the suppressor macrophages in PC-bearing mice, the isotype-specific T cells in PC-bearing mice appear to reflect an exaggerated normal immunoregulatory mechanism.

In vitro studies using human cells suggest similar mechanisms of immunosuppression by macrophages and T cells, although in humans the details have been less completely described. Several groups have described a circulating phagocytic mononuclear cell from myeloma patients that suppresses secretion of mitogen-stimulated normal human B cells in culture.[23,54–56] These cells, present also in the blood of healthy individuals,[54] appear to mediate the immunosuppression of the humoral immune response in patients with myeloma. Again, this suggests exaggeration of a normal control mechanism.

Other human studies have shown that, as with PC-bearing mice, patients with myeloma have increased numbers of T cells with Fc receptors specific for the isotype of the myeloma paraprotein.[57,58] These cells suppress pokeweed mitogen-induced immunoglobulin secretion,[59] and may contribute to the immune dysfunction in patients with myeloma. One group has described similar suppression mediated by a non-B, non-T, nonphagocytic lymphoid cell bearing Fc receptors for IgG.[60,61] A further observation suggests that $T\mu$ cells, which function as helper T cells,[62] are depleted in patients with myeloma.[58] While a dearth of these cells could hypothetically cause immunosuppression, no significant correlation was found between the level of circulating Tμ cells and serum IgM levels.[58] Helper and suppressor cells have also been enumerated using the T4 and T8 cell surface markers. In untreated patients, T4$^+$ cells were reduced in three studies[63–65] and were within normal limits in a fourth,[66] and T8$^+$ cells were normal in three studies[63,64,66] and increased in one study.[65] The helper-to-suppressor ratio (T4/T8) was significantly decreased in only the one study that demonstrated an increased number of T8 cells in untreated patients.[65] These complex and contradictory results regarding the function of the FcR$^+$ T cells and the number of T4 and T8 cells in patients with myeloma leave the role of these T cells undefined in the immunosuppression of multiple myeloma.

A third type of suppression occurs in myeloma in which production of the light chain isotype is suppressed in nonmalignant intestinal plasma cells[67] and in peripheral blood lymphocytes.[68, 69] Thus, in κ-myeloma the nonmalignant B cells show a low κ:λ ratio and vice versa. The mechanism and significance of this suppression is unknown.

Whereas a consistent picture of humoral immunosuppression in multiple myeloma has emerged, studies of cell-mediated immunity (CMI) and T cell function are less clear. Patients with myeloma demonstrate suppressed development of delayed-type hypersensitivity to dinitrofluorobenzene.[16] The response to commonly encountered antigens that stimulate delayed-type hypersensitivity, such as candida, mumps, and tubercle bacillus, is sometimes impaired and sometimes normal.[3] The severe humoral immunosuppression and relative sparing of CMI in patients with myeloma contrasts with that in Hodgkins's disease and sarcoidosis, in which CMI is severely impaired but antibody responsiveness is normal. Mice with PC more consistently retain normal cell-mediated immunity than do patients with myeloma.[43,70,71]

In vitro studies of T cell function in human and murine hosts of plasma cell tumors have yielded conflicting results: Increased, normal, and decreased responses to mitogens have all been reported. The results of such studies may indicate that T cell hyporesponsiveness, when present, results from an altered population of T cells, rather than from active suppression mediated by a suppressor cell. This aspect of myeloma has been reviewed previously.[43]

Studies of circulating lymphocyte populations in myeloma are similarly complex. A few early studies reported an increased number of circulating polyclonal B cells.[72–74] More recent studies indicate, in contrast, that polyclonal B cells are markedly reduced.[68,75–81] Many studies using antiidiotypic antibodies have reported a large circulating monoclonal lymphocyte pool bearing the idiotype of the secreted M protein.[74,79–85] Two recent studies, on the other hand, reported an absence of circulating monoclonal lymphocytes related to the malignant plasma cells.[76,78] These latter investigators provided an explanation for the apparent discrepancy in the literature: they suggested that monoclonal immunoglobulins may be bound to circulating nonmalignant mononuclear cells (probably the increased population of T cells bearing isotype-specific Fc receptors, discussed previously), giving falsely high values for the number of circulating cells derived from the malignant clone. However, evidence does exist for a small but finite subset of circulating cells that are a part of the malignant population: In one study, three of four patients' circulating cells contained the same immunoglobulin gene rearrangements seen in the malignant plasma cell clone.[86]

Nonspecific host defense mechanisms have also been studied in patients with myeloma. The pattern of infection in myeloma patients, with a preponderance of such organism as *S. pneumonia, Staphylococci, H. influenza, Neisseria meningitidis,* and *E. coli,* which require complement activation for maximal host resistance,[87–91] suggested that complement activity may be abnormal in patients with myeloma. Most myeloma patients' sera demonstrate decreased complement activity, even in the absence of a consistent decrease in identified complement components.[92–94] Cheson et al demonstrated that sera from myeloma patients are nearly always deficient in their ability to activate C3, resulting in reduced binding of C3b to strains of pneumococci that activate complement by both the classical and alternative pathways.[94] Using mixing experiments, they showed that the deficiency was not attributable to a lack of specific antipneumococcal antibodies. The defect in C3 binding correlated with the presence of *S. pneumonia* infections. Similar conclusions of defective functional complement activity, using different assays, have been reached by other groups[92,93]; however, they have not found a correlation between defective complement activation and incidence of infection.[92,93] Levels of several complement proteins, including Clq, C2, C3, C4, and factor B were found to be decreased in some infected myeloma patients, but no consistent pattern of deficiency has emerged.[93–96]

Granulocyte function has also been studied in myeloma patients. A heat-labile factor is present in myeloma plasma, but not serum, which inhibits in vitro adherence of granulocytes.[96–99] In vivo granulocyte migration, as measured by the skin window technique, is also defective in patients with myeloma.[97,100] Granulocytes from myeloma patients have been shown to have decreased receptors for IgG and C3b.[101] Abnormalities in neutrophil function have not correlated with incidence of infection,[96] but have correlated with disease progression.[96,99] Monocyte chemotaxis has been reported as decreased[102,103] or normal[103] in myeloma, and monocyte phagocytic function as normal.[103]

The data discussed here all concern the immune system in the presence of untreated disease. A small number of studies address the question of treatment-induced changes in the immune system. In two studies, treatment with melphalan caused a decrease in the previously normal response of lymphocytes from patients with myeloma to pokeweed mitogen.[72,104] In two mouse studies, low doses of melphalan or cyclophosphamide abrograted the suppression of antitumor immunity seen with large tumor burdens,[105,106] while another study showed restoration of depressed mitogen-induced proliferative responses after tumor eradication with melphalan.[71]

PROPHYLAXIS AND THERAPY

Of all therapeutic interventions directed at the immune dysfunction of multiple myeloma, the pneumococcal vaccine has been most extensively studied. This vaccine has been shown to be effective in nonimmunosuppressed "at risk" populations, and is recommended for use in such groups.[107,108] In patients with myeloma, both serologic and clinical studies have been performed. In three studies, pre- and postimmunization levels of antipneumococcal antibodies were compared with control subjects.[26–28] Patients with myeloma had markedly diminished preimmunization antibody titers. Therefore, even though these patients generally exhibited normal (three- to four-fold) rises in antibody titers, they exhibited low postimmunization titers as well. The patients postimmunization titers were considered nonprotective, ie, less than 215 to 300 ng of antibody nitrogen/mL.[26,109]

In regard to clinical recommendation for the use of pneumococcal vaccine, one group of investigators advises not to administer the pneumococcal vaccine to patients with myeloma[28]; most, however, citing the low cost and toxicity and possible benefit in some patients, have recommended its use.[26,27,109]

Two clinical studies have demonstrated little, if any, protection from pneumococcal disease among vaccinated patients.[107,110] It has been pointed out, however, that these studies were not specifically designed to evaluate efficacy of pneumococcal vaccine in immunosuppressed populations, and much larger number of patients would have been needed to prove a small benefit.[107] The Health and Public Policy Committee of the American College of Physicians, therefore suggested that patients with multiple myeloma "may be offered the vaccine but should be informed of their potential inability to respond to it and thus be protected by it."[108]

In support of this recommendation, a single animal study demonstrated that PC-bearing mice are protected from fatal pneumococcal sepsis by immunization, though their degree of protection was less than in a control group.[111]

Since normal secondary antibody responses occur in myeloma patients, the data summarized here suggest that higher antibody levels and increased protection might be attainable via repeated immunization. Although, in the general population, reimmunization has not been recommended because of the risk of severe local and mild systemic reactions,[108,112] reimmunization has not been studied in immunosuppressed groups with low preimmunization antibody levels. Furthermore, even after a response to immunization, myeloma patients frequently show a rapid fall in antibody levels. In one study, 18 months after immunization, the mean antibody concentrations returned to preimmunization levels or lower for 50% of the antigens administered.[28] Currently, it is recommended that nonimmunosuppressed patients should not be reimmunized for at least 3 to 5 years,[109] but the applicability of this recommendation to immunosuppressed populations is uncertain. Whether myeloma patients specifically might benefit from repeated immunizations merits study.

Passive immunization in myeloma patients has been less frequently studied. In a classic study by Salmon et al, intramuscular gamma globulin given in the same dose as used successfully in patients with agammaglobulinemia was unsuccessful in reducing the incidence of infection.[113] These investigators postulated that the increased catabolism of immunoglobulins seen with myeloma may have been responsible for the inefficacy of gamma globulin, and that a higher dose may have been effective. The availability of intravenous gamma globulin, allowing administration of larger doses, has rekindled interest in this therapeutic possibility. In a phase I study, IV gamma globulin was well tolerated by myeloma patients and normal levels of immunoglobulins were attained.[114] No infections occurred in this study group, but the numbers were too small to draw clinical conclusions. Should further studies demonstrate efficacy of IV gamma globulin in infection prophylaxis, it might be expected to protect against both gram-positive and gram-negative infections. It has been suggested that the potential benefit of IV gamma globulin in myeloma patients may derive from not only antibodies against specific bacterial antigens, but also from antibodies against lipid A and/or core polysaccharide.[25] The ultimate role of IV gamma globulin in patients with myeloma has not yet been defined, and requires further study.

It has also been suggested that the use of prophylactic antibiotics be considered in patients with myeloma.[11,115] Others caution against their use because of the risk of developing antibiotic resistance.[14,116] While it may be reasonable to consider prophylactic antibiotic usage in the rare patient who develops repeated infections with the same organism, no data support this approach; given the potential risks, extreme caution is mandated. Finally, one group has shown that oral *Bacillus subtilis* spores[117] and oral lysozyme[118] were able to improve some measures of humoral and cell-mediated immunity and to decrease the frequency of infection in patients with myeloma, but these approaches must be considered experimental at present.

SUMMARY

Patients with multiple myeloma are at increased risk of severe bacterial infection. A variety of immune deficits has been described in such patients, including a decreased primary antibody response and defects in complement and granulocyte function. The depressed humoral response appears to result primarily from the activity of suppressor monocytes. Pneumovax (Merck Sharp & Dohme, West Point, Penn) should be administered to patients with myeloma, although its effectiveness in this population has not been proven. The role of other potential modalities of treatment and prophylaxis, such as IV gamma globulin, requires further study.

REFERENCES

1. Snapper I, Turner LB, Moscovitz HL: Multiple Myeloma. Orlando, Fla, Grune & Stratton, 1953, p 29

2. Zinneman HH, Hall WH: Recurrent pneumonia in multiple myeloma and some observations on immunologic response. Ann Intern Med 41:1152–1163, 1954

3. Glenchur H, Zinnerman HH, Hall WH: A review of fifty-one cases of multiple myeloma. Arch Intern Med 103:173–183, 1959

4. Fahey JL, Scoggins R, Utz JP, et al: Infection, antibody response and gamma globulin components in multiple myeloma and macroglobulinemia. Am J Med 35:698–707, 1963

5. Meyers BR, Hirschman SZ, Axelrod JA: Current patterns of infection in multiple myeloma. Am J Med 52:87–92, 1972

6. Savage DG, Lindenbaum J, Garrett TJ: Biphasic pattern of bacterial infection in multiple myeloma. Ann Intern Med 96:47–50, 1982

7. Espersen F, Birgens HS, Hertz JB, et al: Current patterns of bacterial infection in myelomatosis. Scand J Infect Dis 16:169–173, 1984

8. Shaikh BS, Lombard RM, Appelbaum PC, et al: Changing patterns of infections in patients with multiple myeloma. Oncology 39:78–82, 1982

9. Twomey JT: Infections complicating multiple myeloma and chronic lymphocytic leukemia. Arch Intern Med 132:562–565, 1973

10. Kyle RA: Subject Review: Multiple myeloma—Review of 869 cases. Mayo Clin Proc 50:29–40, 1975

11. Chou M, Brown AE, Blevins A, Et al: Severe pneumoccocal infection in patients with neoplastic disease. Cancer 51:1546–1550, 1983

12. Witts LJ, Blackburn EK, Callender ST, et al: Report on the first myelomatosis trial: Part I. Analysis of presenting features of prognostic importance. Br J Haematol 24:123–139, 1973

13. Perri RT, Hebbel RP, Oken MM: Influence of treatment and response status on infection risk in multiple myeloma. JAMA 71:935–939, 1981

14. Cohen HJ, Rundles RW: Managing the complications of plasma cell myeloma. Arch Intern Med 135:177–184, 1975

15. Gordon H, Bandmann M, Sandbank U: Multiple myeloma associated with progressive multifocal leukoencephalopathy and *Pneumocystis carinii* pneumonia. Isr J Med Sci 7:581–588, 1971

16. Cone L, Uhr JW: Immunological deficiency disorders associated with chronic lymphocytic leukemia and multiple myeloma. J Clin Invest 43:2241–2248, 1964

17. Larson DL, Tomlinson LJ: Quantitative antibody studies in man. II. The relation of the level of serum proteins to antibody production. J Lab Clin Med 39:129–134, 1952

18. Marks J: Antibody formation in myelomatosis. J Clin Pathol 6:62–63, 1953

19. Lawson HA, Stuart CA, Paull AM, et al: Observations on the antibody content of the blood in patients with multiple myeloma. N Engl J Med 252:13–18, 1955

20. Heath RB, Hamilton F, Malpas JS: Production of antibodies against viruses in leukaemia and related diseases. Br J Haematol 10:365–370, 1964

21. Fink PC, Galanos C: Serum anti-lipid A antibodies in multiple myeloma and Waldenstrom's macroglobulinameia. Immunobiology 169:1–10, 1985

22. Stoll C, Schedel I, Peest D, et al: Serum antibodies against common antigens of bacterial lippolysaccharides in healthy adults and patients with multiple myeloma. Infection 13:115–119, 1985

23. Broder S, Humphrey R, Durm M, et al: Impaired synthesis of polyclonal (non-paraprotein) immunoglobulins by circulating lymphocytes from patients with multiple myeloma. N Engl J Med 293:887–892, 1975

24. Waldmann TA, Strober W: Metabolism of immunoglobulins, in Kallos P, Waksman BH (eds): Progress in Allergy. Basel, Karger, 1969, p 87

25. Morell A, Terry WD, Waldmann TA: Metabolic properties of IgG subclasses in man. J Clin Invest 49:673–680, 1970

26. Lazarus HM, Lederman M, Lubin A, et al: Pneumococcal vaccination: The response of patients with multiple myeloma. Am J Med 69:419–423, 1980

27. Shildt RA, Rubin RR, Schiffman G, et al: Polyvalent pneumococcal immunization of patients with plasma cell dyscrasias. Cancer 48:1377–1380, 1981

28. Birgens HS, Espersen F, Hertz JB, et al: Antibody response to pneumococcal vaccination in patients with myelomatosis. Scand J Haematol 30:324–330, 1983

29. Fahey JL, Humphrey JH: Effect of transplantable plasma-cell tumors on antibody response in mice. Immunology, 5:110–115, 1962

30. Havas HF, Schiffman G: The effect of an IgM plasmacytoma (TEPC-183) on the primary immune response of BALB/c mice. Immunology 34:1–8, 1978

31. Smith F, Grenan MM, Owens J: Effect of a transplanted plasma-cell tumor on antibody formation. J Natl Cancer Inst 25:803–812, 1960

32. Zolla S: The effect of plasmacytomas on the immune response of mice. J Immunol 108:1039–1048, 1972

33. Hirano S, Imamura Y, Takaku F, et al: Immune response in mice wtih plasma-cell tumor (X5563) assayed by agar plaque technique. Blood 31:252–257, 1968

34. Zolla S, Naor D, Tanapatchaiyapong P: Cellular basis of immunodepression in mice with plasmacytomas. J Immunol 112:2068–2076, 1974

35. Ullrich S, Zolla-Pazner S: Immunoregulatory circuits in myeloma. Clin Haematol 11:87–111, 1982

36. Tanapatchaiyapong P, Zolla S: Humoral immunosuppressive substance in mice bearing plasmacytomas. Science 186:748–750, 1974

37. Kolb J-P, Arrian S, Zolla-Pazner S: Suppression of the humoral immune response by plasmacytomas: Mediation by adherent mononuclear cells. J Immunol 118:702–709, 1977

38. Kennard J, Zolla-Pazner S: Origin and function of suppressor macrophages in myeloma. J Immunol 124:268–273, 1980

39. Krakauer RS, Strober W, Waldmann TA: Hypogammaglobulinemia in experimental myeloma: The role of suppressor factors from mononuclear phagocytes. J Immunol 118:1385–1390, 1977

40. Katzmann JA: Myeloma-induced immunosuppression: A multistep mechanism. J Immunol 121:1405–1409, 1978

41. Hamburger AW: Inhibition of B-lymphocyte clonal proliferation by spleen cells from plasmacytoma-bearing mice. J Natl Cancer Inst 65:1337–1343, 1980

42. Berman JE, Zolla-Pazner S: Contorl of B cell proliferation: Inhibition of responses to B cell mitogens induced by plasma cell tumors. J Immunol 134:2872–2878, 1985

43. Zolla-Pazner S: Immunodeficiency induced by plasma cell tumors: Comparison of findings in human and murine hosts, in Potter M (ed): Progress in Myeloma. New York, Elsevier, 1980, pp 171–184

44. Hoover RG, Dieckgraefe BK, Lake J, et al: Lymphocyte surface membrane immunoglobulin in myeloma. III. IgA plasmacytomas induce large numbers of circulating, adult-thymectomy-sensitive, $\Theta+$, Lyt-1^{-} 2^{+} lymphocytes with IgA-Fc receptors. J Immunol 129:2329–2331, 1982

45. Hoover RG, Lynch RG: Isotype-specific suppression of IgA: Suppression of IgA responses in BALB/c mice by $T\alpha$ cells. J Immunol 130:521–523, 1983

46. Hoover RG, Dieckgraefe BK, Lynch RG: T cells with Fc receptors for IgA: Induction of T cells in vivo and in vitro by purified IgA. J Immunol 127:1560–1563, 1981

47. Mathur A, Lynch RG: Increased $T\gamma$ and $T\mu$ cells in BALB/c mice with IgG and IgM plasmacytomas and hybridomas. J Immunol 136:521–525, 1986

48. Muller S, Hoover RG: T cells with Fc receptors in myeloma: Suppression of growth and secretion of MOPC-315 by $T\alpha$ cells. J Immunol 134:644–647, 1985

49. Hoover RG, Lynch RG: Lymphocyte surface immunoglobulin in myeloma. II. T cells with IgA-Fc receptors are

markedly increased in mice with IgA plasmacytomas. J Immunol 125:1280–1285, 1980

50. Xue B, Coico R, Wallace D, et al: Physiology of IgD. IV. Enhancement of antibody prodcution in mice bearing IgD-secreting plasmacytomas. J Exp Med 159:103–113, 1984

51. Coico RF, Xue B, Wallace D, et al: Physiology of IgD. VI. Transfer of the immunoaugmenting effect of IgD with Tδ containing helper cell populations. J Exp Med 162:1852–1861, 1985

52. Kiyono H, McGhee JR, Mosteller LM, et al: Murine Peyer's Patch T cell clones. Characterization of antigen-specific helper T cells for immunoglobulin A responses. J Exp Med 156:1115–1130, 1982

53. Ishizaka K: Regulation of IgE synthesis. Annu Rev Immunol 2:159–182, 1984

54. Twomey JJ, Laughter AH, Rice L, et al: Suppression of lymphocyte responses by monocytes with untreated and treated multiple myeloma. Blood 60:316–322, 1982

55. Knapp W, Baumgartner G: Monocyte-mediated suppression of human B lymphocyte differentiation in vitro. J Immunol 121:1177–1183, 1978

56. Peest D, Brunkhorst U, Schedel I, et al: In vitro immunoglobulin production by peripheral blood mononuclear cells from multiple myeloma patients and patients with benign monoclonal gammopathy. Scand J immunol 19:149–157, 1984

57. Hoover RG, Hickman S, Gebel HM, et al: Expansion of Fc receptor-bearing T lymphocytes in patients with immunoglobulin G and Immunoglobulin A myeloma. J Clin Invest 67:308–311, 1981

58. Oken MM, Kay NE: T-cell subpopulations in multiple myeloma: Correlation with clinical disease status. Br J Haematol 49:629–634, 1981

59. Moretta L, Mingari MC, Moretta A, et al: Human T lymphocyte subpopulations: Studies of the mechanism by which T cells bearing Fc receptors for IgG suppress T-dependent B cell differentiation induced by pokeweed mitogen. J Immunol 122:984–990, 1979

60. Paglieroni T, MacKenzie MR: Studies on the pathogenesis of an immune defect in multiple myeloma. J Clin Invest 59:1120–1133, 1977

61. Paglieroni T, MacKenzie MR: Multiple myeloma: An immunologic profile. III. Cytotoxic and suppressive effects of the EA rosette-forming cell. J Immunol 124:2563–2570, 1980

62. Moretta L, Webb SR, Grossi CE, et al: Functional analysis of two human T-cell subpopulations: Help and and suppression of B-cell responses by T cells bearing receptors for IgM or IgG. J Exp Med 146:184–200, 1977

63. Bergman L, Mitrou PS, Kelker W, et al: T-cell subsets in malignant lymphomas and monoclonal gammopathies. Scand J Haematol 34:170–176, 1985

64. Mellstedt H, Holm G, Pettersson D, et al: Idiotype-bearing lymphoid cells in plasma cell neoplasia. Clin Haematol 11:65–86, 1982

65. Mills KHG, Cawley JC: Abnormal monoclonal antibody-defined helper/suppressor T-cell subpopulations in multiple myeloma: Relationship to treatment and clinical stage. Br J Haematol 53:271–275, 1983

66. Wahlin A, Roos G, Holm J: T-cell subsets in multiple myeloma. Blut 51:291–295, 1985

67. Leonard RCF, MacLennan CM, Smart Y, et al: Light chain isotype-associated suppression of normal plasma cell number in patients with multiple myeloma. Int J Cancer 24:385–393, 1979

68. Van Camp B, Reynaert PH, Broodtaerts L: Studies on the origin of the precursor cells in multiple myeloma, Waldenstrom's macroglobulinaemia and benign monoclonal gammopathy. I. Cytoplasmic isotype and idiotype distribution in peripheral blood and bone marrow. Clin Exp Immunol 44:82–89, 1981

69. Werne A, Joshua DE, Kronenberg H: Light chain isotype associated suppression of surface immunoglobulin expression on peripheral blood lymphocytes in myeloma during plateau phase. Br J Haematol 58:483–489, 1984

70. Zolla-Pazner S, Sullivan B, Richardson D: Cellular specificity of plasmacytoma-induced immunosuppression. J Immunol 117:563–568, 1976

71. Padarathsingh ML, McCoy JL, Dean JH, et al: Examination of general and tumor-specific cell-mediated immune responses in mice bearing progressively growing plasmacytomas. J Natl Cancer Inst 58:1701–1707, 1977

72. Mellstedt H, Holm G: In vitro studies of lymphocytes from patients with plasma cell myeloma. I. Stimulation by mitogens and cytotoxic activities. Clin Exp Immunol 15:309–320, 1973

73. Mellstedt H, Jondal M, Holm G: In vitro studies of lymphocytes from patients with plasma cell myeloma. II. Characterization of cell surface markets. Clin Exp Immunol 15:321–329, 1973

74. Jones SV, McFarlane H: T and B cells in myelomatosis. Br J Haematol 31:545–552, 1975

75. Dillman RO, Royston I, Meserve BL, et al: Alterations of peripheral blood B-lymphocyte populations in plasma cell disorders. Cancer 48:2211–2217, 1981

76. King MA, Wells JV: Cell-bound immunoglobulin on peripheral blood mononuclear cells of patients with myeloma. Clin Exp Immunol 45:522–556, 1981

77. Bast EJEG, Van Camp B, Reynaert P, et al: Idiotypic peripheral blood lymphocytes in monoclonal gammopathy. Clin Exp Immunol 47:677–682, 1982

78. Pilarksi LM, Mant MJ, Ruether BA, et al: Severe deficiency of B lymphocytes in peripheral blood from multiple myeloma patients. J Clin Invest 74:1301–1306, 1984

79. Lindstrom FD, Hardy WR, Eberle BJ, et al: Multiple myeloma and benign monoclonal gammopathy: Differentiation by immunofluorescence of lymphocytes. Ann Intern Med 78:837–844, 1973

80. Abdou NI, Abdou NL: The monoclonal nature of lymphocytes in multiple myeloma. Ann Intern Med 83:42–45, 1975

81. Chen Y, Bhoopalam N, Yakulis BS, et al: Changes in lymphocyte surface immunoglobulins in myeloma and the effect of an RNA-containing plasma factor. Ann Intern Med 83:625–631, 1975

82. Sato I, Abo T, Onodera S, et al: Detection of monoclonal B lymphocytes in multiple myeloma by immunofluorescence tests of surface immunoglobulins. Scand J Haematol 21:433–444, 1978

83. Kubagawa H, Vogler LB, Capra JD, et al: Studies on the clonal origin of multiple myeloma—Use of individually specific (idiotype) antibodies to trace the oncogenic event to

its earliest point of expression in B-cell differentiation. J Exp Med 150:792–807, 1979

84. Schedel I, Peest D, Stunkel K, et al: Idiotype-bearing peripheral blood lymphocytes in human multiple myeloma and Waldenstrom's macroglobulinaemia. Scand J Immunol 11:437–444, 1980

85. Carmagnola AL, Boccadoro M, Massaia M, et al: The idiotypic specificities of lymphocytes in human monclonal gammopathies: Analysis with the fluorescence activated cell sorter. Clin Exp Immunol 51:173–177, 1983

86. Berenson K, Wong R, Kim K, et al: Clonal antibody gene rearrangements of peripheral blood lymphocytes in multiple myeloma patients. Blood 66:232a, 1985 (suppl)

87. Winkelstein JA, Abramovitz AS, Tomasz A: Activation of C3 via the alternative complement pathway results in fixation of C3b to the pneumococcal cell wall. J Immunol 124:2502–2506, 1980

88. Verhoef J, Peterson PK, Kim Y, et al: Opsonic requirements for staphylococcal phagocytosis. Immunology 33:191–197, 1977

89. Corrall CJ, Winkelstein JA, Moxon ER: Participation of complement in host defense against encapsulated *Haemophilus influenzae* types a, c, and d. Infect Immun 35:759–763, 1982

90. Petersen BH, Lee TJ, Synderman R, et al: *Neisseria meningitidis* and *Neisseria gonorrhoeae* bacteremia associated with C6, C7, or C8 deficiency. Ann Intern Med 90:917–920, 1979

91. Van Dijk WC, Verbrugh HA, van der Tol ME, et al: Role of *Escherichia coli* K capsular antigens during complement activation, C3 fixation, and opsonization. Infect Immun 25:603–609, 1979

92. Cheson BD, Plas PR, Rothstein G: Defective opsonization in multiple myeloma. Blood 55:602–606, 1980

93. Kraut EH, Sagone AL: Alternative pathway of complement in multiple myeloma. Am J Hematol 11:335–345, 1981

94. Cheson BD, Walker HS, Heath ME, et al: Defective binding of the third component of complement (C3) to *Streptococcus pneumoniae* in multiple myeloma. Blood 63:949–957, 1984

95. Schifferli JA, Pascual M, Deleamont P, et al: Meningococcemia in a patient with acquired complement deficiency and myeloma. N Engl J Med 311:1381–1382, 1984

96. MacGregor RR, Negendank WG, Schreiber AD: Impaired granulocyte adherence in multiple myeloma: Relationship to complement system, granulocyte delivery, and infection. Blood 51:591–599, 1978

97. Spitler LE, Spath P, Petz L, et al: Phagocytes and C4 in paraproteinaemia. Br J Haematol 29:279–292, 1975

98. Penny R, Galton DAG: Studies on neutrophil function. II. Pathological aspects. Br J Haematol 12:633–645, 1966

99. Hopen G, Glette J, Halstensen A, et al: Granulocyte function in malignant monoclonal gammopathy. Scand J Haematol 31:133–143, 1983

100. Ziegler JB, Hansen PJ, Penny R: Leucocyte function in paraproteinaemia. Aust NZ J Med 5:39–43, 1975

101. Naess A, Hopen G, Solberg CO: Decrease of Fcγ and C3b receptor-bearing granulocytes and of T lymphocytes in myelomatosis. Scand J Haematol 33:83–90, 1984

102. Dammacco F, Miglietta A, Ventura MT, et al: Defective monocyte chemotactic responsiveness in patients with multiple myeloma and benign monoclonal gammapathy. Clin Exp Immunol 47:481–486, 1982

103. Blom J, Nielsen H, Larsen SO, et al: A study of certain functional parameters of monocytes from patients with multiple myeloma: Comparison with monocytes from healthy individuals. Scand J Haematol 33:425–431, 1984

104. MacKenzie MR, and Paglieroni T: Multiple myeloma: An immunologic profile. I. Peripheral blood studies. J Immunol 118:1864–1870, 1977

105. Bocian RC, Ben-Efraim S, Dray S, et al: Melphalan-mediated protentiation of antitumor immune responsiveness of immunosuppressed spleen cells from mice bearing a large MOPC-315 tumor. Cancer Immunol Immunother 18:41–48, 1984

106. Mokyr MB, Dray S: Some advantages of curing mice bearing a large subcutaneous MOPC-315 tumor with a low dose rather than a high dose of cyclophosphamide. Cancer Res 43:3112–3119, 1983

107. Bolan G, Broome CV, Fracklam RR, et al: Pneumococcal vaccine efficacy in selected populations in the United States. Ann Intern Med 104:1–6, 1986

108. Health and Public Policy Committee: Position Papers: Pneumococcal Vaccine. Ann Intern Med 104:118–120, 1986

109. Landesman SH, Schiffman G: Assessment of the antibody response to pneumococcal vaccine in high-risk populations. Rev Infect Dis 3:S184–S197, 1981 (suppl)

110. Shapiro ED, Clemens JD: A controlled evaluation of the protective efficacy of pneumococcal vaccine for patients at high risk of serious pneumococcal infections. Ann Intern Med 101:325–330, 1984

111. Havas HF, Schiffman G, Schmitz J: Effect of TEPC-183 plasmacytoma on resistance of passively or actively immunized BALB/c mice to infection with *Streptococcus pneumoniae*. Cancer Res 44:3299–3302, 1984

112. Borgono JM, McClean AA, Vella PP, et al: Vaccination and revaccination with polyvalet pneumococcal polysaccharide vaccines in adults and infants (40010). Proc Soc Exp Biol Med 157:148–154, 1978

113. Salmon SE, Samal BA, Hayes DM, et al: Role of gamma globulin for immunoprophylaxis in multiple myeloma. N Engl J Med 277:1336–1340, 1967

114. Gordon DS, Hearn EB, Spira TJ, et al: Phase I study of intravenous gamma globulin in multiple myeloma. Am J Med 76:111–116, 1984 (suppl)

115. Bergsagel DE: Plasma cell myeloma, in Williams WJ, Beutler E, Erslev AJ (eds): Hematology. New York, McGraw-Hill, 1983, pp 1078–1104

116. Scharff MD, Uhr JW: Immunologic deficiency disorders associated with lymphoproliferative diseases. Semin Hematol 2:47–67, 1965

117. Vacca A, Pantaleo G, Ronco M, et al: Chemoimmunotherapy for multiple myeloma using an intermittent combination drug schedule (melphalan + prednisone) and alternating courses of bacillus subtilis spores. Chemioterapia 2:300–306, 1983

118. Vacca A, Campobasso N, Iodice G, et al: Cyclic lysozyme administration as a tool for immunopotentiation in patients with multiple myeloma. Chemotherapy 4:147–155, 1985

Bone Destruction and Hypercalcemia in Plasma Cell Myeloma

Gregory R. Mundy and Donald R. Bertolini

PATHOGENESIS OF THE BONE LESIONS

Cellular Mechanisms

MYELOMA is almost always associated with a marked increase in destructive osteolytic bone lesions. Bone destruction in myeloma is responsible for the most distressing clinical features of this disease, including intractable bone pain, fractures occurring either spontaneously or following trivial injury, and hypercalcemia with its attendant symptoms and signs. Eighty percent of patients present with bone pain as a predominant symptom.[1] The bone lesions occur in several patterns. Occasionally, patients develop single osteolytic lesions that are associated with solitary plasmacytomas. Some patients have diffuse osteopenia, which mimics the appearance of osteoporosis, and is due to the myeloma cells being spread diffusely throughout the axial skeleton. In most patients there are multiple discrete lytic lesions occurring at the site of deposits or nests of myeloma cells.

Bone scans in myeloma show very little abnormality. Isotopic bone scans are performed with labeled bisphosphonates that are taken up at sites of mineral deposition and reflect increased activity of bone forming cells. Myeloma is characterized by discrete lytic lesions with little increase in formation and this is probably the explanation for the difference in appearance between the bone scan in myeloma and the bone scan in breast cancer, where osteoblast activity is frequently increased. Similarly, serum alkaline phosphatase, which also reflects osteoblast activity, is usually not increased in patients with myeloma, unless they have coexistent pathological fractures.

Most available evidence suggests that the mechanism of bone destruction in myeloma is primarily osteoclastic. This was first suggested in a study in which morphologic examination was performed on autopsy and biopsy samples of bone from a series of 37 patients with myeloma.[2] In this series, active osteoclastic bone resorption was found predominantly in specimens that contained more than 20% marrow myeloma cell infiltration. In specimens of bone from myeloma patients that contained few or no myeloma cells, little osteoclast activity or evidence of active bone resorption was observed. This suggested that the myeloma cells caused the osteoclast activity that led to increased bone resorption. The association between increased osteoclasts on bone resorbing surfaces and areas of heavy myeloma cell infiltration was confirmed in a later study using the technique of quantitative bone histomorphometry on undecalcified transiliac bone biopsies from 118 patients with myeloma.[3] Surprisingly, no decrease in mean trabecular bone volume was observed, but abnormalities were observed in bone formation. Bone forming surfaces were increased away from the areas of heavy myeloma cell infiltration but the osteoid seams were reduced in thickness and had a lowered calcification rate. The authors suggested that the activity of individual osteoblasts may be reduced in many patients with myeloma, accounting for these latter findings.

Further evidence that the mechanism of bone resorption in myeloma is primarily osteoclastic is provided by data that show drugs that are specific inhibitors of osteoclast activity such as the bisphosphonates, mithramycin, and corticosteroids are usually very effective in lowering the serum calcium in patients with myeloma.[4,5,6]

Not all workers have found increased osteoclastic resorption in myeloma. Schechter et al[7] saw little evidence of osteoclastic activity in the patients they studied. MacDonald et al[8] suggested that murine myeloma cells had the capacity to destroy bone directly in vitro independent of osteoclasts, in a similar manner described earlier for human breast cancer cells.[9] Whether this phenomenon has an in vivo significance is not currently known.

In some patients with myeloma, osteosclerosis

From the University of Texas Health Science Center, San Antonio.

Supported in part by grants AM28149, CA29537, RR0136, and AM07464 from the National Institutes of Health.

Address reprint requests to Gregory R. Mundy, MD, Medicine/Endocrinology, University of Texas Health Science Center, 7703 Floyd Curl Dr, San Antonio, TX 78284.

0093–7754/86/1303–0005$05.00/0

rather than osteolytic bone destruction is the major radiologic finding. This feature probably occurs in less than 1% of all patients.[10] These patients frequently have peripheral neuropathy and they may or may not have other multisystem features that have been referred to as the polyneuropathy, organomegaly, endocrinopathy, M protein, skin changes (POEMS) syndrome (see article by Farhangi et al, this issue). Hypercalcemia has not been reported in this condition to our knowledge. In the study of Valentin-Opran et al,[3] which reported histomorphometric data on bone biopsies from 118 patients, three had considerable increase in trabecular bone volume, suggesting that these biopsies represented the osteosclerotic variant. The molecular mechanism for the increase in osteoblast activity in this small subset of patients with myeloma is unknown and has not been investigated to our knowledge.

Pathogenetic Factors

The increase in osteoclast activity in myeloma is likely to be due to production of a local factor by the myeloma cells that increases osteoclast activity. The supporting evidence comes from in vitro studies in which it has been shown that lymphoid cell lines derived from patients with myeloma,[11] marrow myeloma cells,[2,12] and explants of bone containing myeloma cells[13] produce a factor or factors that stimulate osteoclast activity in organ cultures of fetal rat bones. The first observation was made using lymphoid cell lines.[11] Culture media harvested from lymphoid cell lines derived from patients with myeloma, Burkitt's lymphoma, and other lymphomas contained bone resorbing activity with similar chemical and biological characteristics to the bone resorbing activity present in phytohemagglutinin-stimulated peripheral blood leukocyte cultures, which is known as osteoclast activating factor or OAF.[14] One of these lymphoid cell lines, 8226, produced λ light chains with the same antigenic determinants as the Bence Jones protein in the urine of the patient from whom this cell line was derived, suggesting that this lymphoid cell line was in fact derived from the myeloma cells. The bone resorbing activity was distinguished from other bone resorbing factors such as parathyroid hormone, prostaglandins of the E series and the vitamin D metabolites by dose-response curves, gel filtration chromatography, heat lability, extraction in lipid solvents, and immunoassay. In a further study, Mundy et al[2] examined short-term cultures of marrow cells aspirated from patients with myeloma. Six of the seven marrow cultures contained similar bone resorbing activity. Again the bone resorbing activity had similar dose-response curves to the osteoclast activating factor found in normal activated peripheral blood leukocyte cultures and was distinguished from well-characterized bone resorbing factors such as parathyroid hormone and prostaglandins of the E series. Similar bone resorbing activity was not present in a series of patients with other types of hematologic disorders not usually associated with bone lesions or hypercalcemia. These findings were confirmed by Josse et al,[12] who also showed that the bone resorbing factor produced by marrow myeloma cell cultures had no effect on cyclic AMP accumulation in bone and the production of the factor was inhibited by indomethacin, suggesting that it was dependent on prostaglandin synthesis. These workers showed that the effects of the factor on bone were independent of inhibition of prostaglandin synthesis. Similar results had been previously shown for the OAF produced by activated peripheral blood leukocytes.[15–17]

Thus, from these studies, it is apparent that myeloma cells in culture produce a local osteoclast stimulating factor (or factors) that is macromolecular and is clearly distinguished from parathyroid hormone, prostaglandins of the E series and the vitamin D metabolites, but has similar biological and chemical characteristics to the bone resorbing activity present in normal activated leukocyte culture supernatants.

Similar bone resorbing activity has been found in other hematologic neoplasms. In patients with various forms of lymphoma, macromolecular bone resorbing activity similar to that present in lymphoid cell lines derived from patients with lymphoma, normal activated peripheral blood leukocytes, and myeloma cell cultures has been identified.[11] In one patient with lymphosarcoma cell leukemia, the bone resorbing activity was characterized in some detail.[18] In this patient, the cultured tumor cells produced a bone resorbing factor that was chromatographically and pharmacologically similar to osteoclast activating factor produced by normal peripheral blood leukocytes. Recently, it has been shown that many of these patients have a T cell lymphoma that is associated with the HTLV type I virus.[19] HTLV type I infected cells produce a range of lymphokines including macromolecular bone resorbing activity.[20] Moreover, many of these patients have increased circulating concentrations of 1,25 dihydroxyvitamin D.[21-24] It appears likely that in addition to producing macromolecular bone resorbing activity, these tumor cells also have the capacity to metabolize 25 hydroxyvitamin D to its most biologically active metabolite, 1,25 dihydroxyvitamin D, and this may be playing a part in the pathogenesis of hypercalcemia by increasing calcium absorption from the gut as well as increasing bone resorption.[25] The circulating concentrations of 1,25 dihydroxyvitamin D are usually low or low-normal in patients with myeloma.

Potential Factors Involved in the Bone Destruction in Myeloma

The pathogenesis of the bone lesions in myeloma is related to increased production of a local bone resorbing factor by the myeloma cells. This bone resorbing activity has similar characteristics to the bone resorbing activity produced by activated peripheral blood leukocytes that was formerly called osteoclast activating factor or OAF. It is now clear that OAF represents a family of bone resorbing factors that are produced by lymphocytes and monocytes following exposure to an antigen to which they have previously been exposed or a nonspecific mitogen such as phytohemagglutinin.

OAF was first identified in the supernatant media harvested from cultures of peripheral blood leukocytes activated by the mitogen phytohemagglutinin and by dental plaque.[14] Knowledge in this area has advanced considerably by recent observations that several purified and recombinant lymphokines and monokines resorb bone in vitro. The implications of this new knowledge on the entity that we previously called OAF is obvious. For many years, all of the lymphokines and monokines (including OAF) remained poorly characterized biological activities that resisted attempts at purification using traditional techniques. This was so because of their high potency and the cumbersome assays required for monitoring biological activity. However, with the advent of the biotechnology companies into this field over the last 2 or 3 years, a number of lymphokines have been purified to homogeneity using industrial team efforts and large facilities for mass purification. Several of these have now been molecularly cloned and engineered for expression in bacteria or mammalian cells. In general, those cytokines that have been purified, cloned, and expressed are those with potential commercial value. They have included proteins such as lymphotoxin, tumor necrosis factor, the interferons (all of which may have value as anticancer agents), and interleukin (IL) 1. Lymphotoxin is a multifunctional lymphokine that has cytolytic and cytostatic effects on neoplastic tumor cells.[26] Recently, human lymphotoxin has been purified to homogeneity, a complementary DNA sequence isolated, the gene cloned and sequenced, and recombinant human lymphotoxin has been expressed in *Escherichia coli.*[27] Tumor necrosis factor is a monocyte product that has identical biological activity and partial sequence homology at the amino acid level to lymphotoxin, but is encoded by a separate single copy gene and has a different receptor to human lymphotoxin. Tumor necrosis factor has also recently been purified, cloned and expressed in *E coli.*[28] Lymphotoxin is produced primarily by T lymphocytes as well as B lymphocytes and tumor necrosis factor by monocytes.

We have tested purified recombinant human preparations of these cytokines on bone resorption in vitro, and found that they stimulate osteoclastic bone resorption in vitro in concentrations between 10^{-7} and 10^{-9} mol/L. They have similar dose-response curves and time course of action to parathyroid hormone (PTH) and to the bone resorbing activity in crude activated leukocyte cultures.[29]

IL 1 is a monocyte product that recently has also attracted the attention of the biotechnology industry. Like the other cytokines, it is also produced in such small amounts that the purification of quantities sufficient for biochemical characterization has proved difficult without the resources of an industrial biotechnology. In the case of IL 1, this was also more difficult because a wide range of biological activities has been attributed to this factor, including stimulation of thymocyte proliferation by the induction of IL 2 release, stimulation of B lymphocyte maturation and proliferation, fibroblast growth factor activity, and the induction of acute phase protein synthesis by hepatocytes. It has also been reported to stimulate prostaglandin and collagenase release from synovial cells and gingival fibroblasts, and to be identical to endogenous pyrogen. Recently it has become apparent that the IL 1 activities reside in two distinct proteins that show only distant homology to each other. These proteins are encoded by two separate genes. The complementary DNAs for these proteins have now been cloned and the clones engineered for expression so that these forms of IL 1 are now becoming available for in vitro testing.[30,31] Gowen et al[32] showed that highly purified IL 1 resorbs bone in vitro, and this has now been confirmed with homogenous pure preparations[33] and with recombinant IL 1.[34] Dewhirst et al[35] have used a bone resorption assay to purify the OAF in short-term activated leukocyte cultures, and found that IL 1 accounts for most of the biological activity in these cultures. Thus, it appears likely that OAF may be comprised of IL 1, lymphotoxin and tumor necrosis factor and possibly other molecules as well. At the present time, there is no information about the relative importance of these molecules in supernatant media of neoplastic lymphoid cells, the timecourse of their production by activated leukocyte cultures or how they interact one with another.

Recently, we have studied the effects of another lymphokine, γ interferon, on osteoclastic bone resorption. The rationale for these studies is based on two observations of others. First, Nedwin et al[36] showed that γ interferon enhanced both the production and cytotoxic effects of lymphotoxin and tumor necrosis factor, and so we reasoned it may also interact with these cytokines on bone. Second, Jilka et al,[37] suggested that α interferon (which has many similar biological effects to γ interferon), may inhibit osteoclastic bone resorption when used in large concentrations. To our surprise, our observations indicate that γ interferon (unlike α interferon), has little effect on osteoclastic bone resorption stimulated by parathyroid hormone or by 1,25 dihydroxyvitamin D, but inhibits osteoclastic bone resorption stimulated by the osteoclast activating factors (by IL 1, lymphotoxin and tumor necrosis factor).[34]

Thus, the OAFs represent a family of bone resorbing factors in supernatant media harvested from activated peripheral blood leukocytes. The relationship of these factors to each other is unknown at the present time. However, one or several of these factors acting in concert may be responsible for regulation of normal bone turnover and formation of the bone marrow cavity by activation of endosteal osteoclasts. These factors may be important in all of the lymphoproliferative disorders associated with bone destruction and hypercalcemia such as myeloma, adult T cell lymphoma, and Burkitt's lymphoma, as well as in the less frequent monocytic malignancies associated with hypercalcemia. The OAFs also may be important in the localized bone destruction that occurs around accumulations of chronic inflammatory cells in conditions such as periodontal disease, rheumatoid arthritis, and cholesteatoma. Understanding the relationship of these factors to each other and the control of their production and effects should prove of major importance in understanding the process of normal bone turnover and bone remodeling.

PATHOGENESIS OF THE HYPERCALCEMIA

Hypercalcemia in myeloma is due primarily to increased bone resorption. However, the pathogenesis is more complex than just a simple increase in bone resorption. First, only about 20% to 40% of patients with myeloma develop hypercalcemia.[1] Moreover, although hypercalcemia occurs in those patients who have the largest tumor volume, not all patients with the largest tumor burdens develop hypercalcemia. In addition, we have found that measurements of total body myeloma cell number and production of bone resorbing activity by bone marrow myeloma cells in vitro do not correlate closely with the production of hypercalcemia.[38] In contrast, there is a highly significant correlation ($P < .001$) between the amounts of bone resorbing activity produced by cultured marrow myeloma cells and the extent of bone destruction. Thus, other factors in addition to production of bone resorbing activity must be involved in the pathogenesis of the hypercalcemia. Because hypercalcemia occurs almost always in patients with impairment of renal function, we suggest that the increased bone resorption in myeloma leads to increased entry of calcium into the extracellular fluid. Patients with normal homeostatic control mechanisms (particularly patients with normal renal function) are able to compensate for this increase in extracellular fluid calcium and maintain the serum calcium in the normal range by increasing urine calcium excretion. However, in patients with impaired renal function, this increase in bone resorption overwhelms the normal homeostatic mechanisms and the patients develop hypercalcemia. This is more likely to occur in patients who produce Bence Jones protein or are predisposed for other reasons such as myeloma kidney, chronic infection, or uric acid nephropathy to impaired renal function.[1] In many cases, impairment of renal function may also be due to the direct effects of hypercalcemia on the kidney.

TREATMENT

Treatment of bone destruction and hypercalcemia in myeloma will be considered under two categories, first, the treatment of osteolytic bone lesions and second, the treatment of hypercalcemia.

Indications for Treatment

We consider that all patients with hypercalcemia require specific treatment to inhibit bone resorption. As in other malignant diseases, hypercalcemia due to increased bone resorption is likely to worsen very rapidly. This is particularly true in myeloma, where hypercalcemia can impair renal function in a situation where there are a number of other factors that are also deleterious to the kidney such as Bence Jones proteinuria, hyperuricemia, urinary tract infection, and, in a few patients, amyloid.

Principles of Treatment

Underlying Disease

Hypercalcemia and increased bone resorption can be improved in many patients with myeloma by treatment with cytotoxic drug therapy. In many situations, this will lead to a decrease in bone pain and a lowering of the serum calcium. This is particularly likely to occur if corticosteroids, which also inhibit bone resorption in myeloma, are part of the treatment regimen. Even in patients with myeloma who respond to cytotoxic drug therapy, bone lesions are unlikely to recalcify,[1] possibly because there is usually only about a one log reduction in myeloma cell mass.

Inhibition of the bone resorption

The primary goal of therapy for the hypercalcemia of myeloma should be the inhibition of osteoclastic bone resorption. A number of therapeutic agents that inhibit osteoclastic bone resorption are available. These include corticosteroids, calcitonin, mithramycin, and the bisphosphonates.

Corticosteroids. Corticosteroids are frequently effective in controlling osteoclastic bone resorption in myeloma.[39] As already indicated, they are often part of the initial therapeutic regimen. The inhibitory effects of corticosteroids on bone resorption are dependent on the stimulus. They are much less effective against PTH than they are against other factors. Corticosteroids inhibit the bone resorbing activity produced by activated peripheral blood leukocytes in low concentrations,[18,40] and this is possibly why they are very effective in lowering the serum calcium in many patients with myeloma and related diseases. The mechanism by which they exert their effect may be due to impairment of formation of new osteoclasts, as has been shown in a feline marrow cell culture system for generation of cells with osteoclast characteristics.[41] Although most patients with myeloma and hypercalcemia respond to corticosteroid therapy, some do not,[5] particularly those late in the course of their disease.

Plicamycin (mithramycin). Plicamycin is an agent that is a powerful inhibitor of bone resorption, possibly by exerting a cytotoxic effect on bone resorbing cells.[42,43] It is frequently used as a form of treatment of hypercalcemia and is usually effective.[6,44] However, we do not advocate its use as a primary agent in this situation because it is directly nephrotoxic and its side effects are more frequent in patients with impaired renal function.[4] Because many patients with myeloma and hypercalcemia have impaired renal function before treatment, we think it should be used as a third line drug for therapy.

Calcitonin and corticosteroids. Calcitonin and corticosteroids used in conjunction are almost always effective in patients with hypercalcemia due to myeloma.[5] These patients may be extremely difficult to treat because they frequently do have impaired renal function, which makes the use of other agents that lower the serum calcium such as oral phosphate or plicamycin difficult or impossible to use. There are no contraindications for use of combined corticosteroid/calcitonin therapy in patients with impaired renal function. Although the effects may be relatively short-lived, we find that withdrawal of calcitonin for several days followed by its reintroduction almost always results in return of the serum calcium into the normal range or into a range that is not associated with symptoms due to hypercalcemia. We have treated several patients for a number of months with this form of therapy in situations where no other agent was suitable.[4] Moreover, the effects of combined therapy are very rapid with lowering of serum calcium usually occurring within 12 hours. The combination is more effective than either agent used alone and seems to be more effective in myeloma than in patients with solid tumors and hypercalcemia.[5]

Calcitonin and glucocorticoids are also very effective inhibitors of bone resorption in vitro.[45] Calcitonin treatment alone leads to the escape phenomenon, characterized by loss of effectiveness despite the continued presence of calcitonin.[46] Glucocorticoids prevent the escape phenomenon both in vitro and in vivo.[4,5,47] Whether the effects of the combination on bone, as suggested by these data, or on the kidney, as suggested by recent clinical studies of Ralston et al,[48] are more important will require further study.

Bisphosphonates. Recently the bisophosphonates have been used to lower the serum calcium in patients with hypercalcemia and myeloma. The bisphosphonates are very effective inhibitors of osteoclastic bone resorption. These drugs are pyrophosphate analogues that suppress bone resorption by mechanisms that are still not clearly defined but probably involve binding of the drug to the bone surface as well as direct inhibition of osteoclast activity.[4] The agent 3-amino-1-hydroxypropane-1, 1-diphosphonate (APD) has been shown to be particularly effective in patients with secondary osteolytic lesions due to breast cancer and myeloma and has also been extremely effective in lowering the serum calcium.[49] More recently, Siris et al[50] showed that another bisphosphonate (Cl_2MDP) was also very effective in lowering the serum calcium, relieving bone pain, and reducing bone turnover in patients with myeloma. Neither of these two bisphosphonates are available for use in the United States. However, the older bisphosphonate, ethane-1-hydroxy-1, 1-diphosphonate (EHDP) or etidronate, has been used intravenously in the treatment of hypercalcemia.[51] Its effects are possibly slower and less reliable than the newer bisphosphonates. Cl_2MDP was withdrawn from testing in the United States because of potential toxicity.

Fluoride. A number of years ago, it was suggested that fluoride may be useful in the treatment of myeloma because fluoride therapy results in positive calcium balance and improved radiologic and morphologic appearances.[52–54] In a large double blind cooperative study of 150 patients with myeloma treated with fluoride, there was no apparent beneficial effect either on the patient's symptomatology, on the clinical course of the disease, or on survival over a period of 53 to 70 months.[55] A later study[56] suggested that the addition of supplemental calcium to the fluoride regimen improves the morphologic and radiographic abnormalities in myeloma. However, it is well known that fluoride will produce similar changes in normal bone and this study did not provide convincing evidence that the bone lesions in myeloma were in any way altered by fluoride therapy. We feel the use of fluoride in the treatment of the bone lesions in myeloma is not warranted by the existing evidence.

Other agents. Recently, other cytotoxic drugs such as gallium nitrate[57] and cisplatinum[58] have been used in the therapy of hypercalcemia associated with malignant disease. Both of these agents appear to be effective in preliminary studies, although their effects to impair renal function make it unlikely that they will turn out to be useful agents in myeloma.

Promotion of Renal Calcium Excretion

As in other forms of hypercalcemia, promotion of a saline diuresis in myeloma may transiently lower the serum calcium and improve renal function because sodium and calcium handling by the renal tubules are linked. This can be achieved with the use of saline infusions. Some workers also use furosemide, although that produces marginal additional benefits to saline infusion.[4,59] Great care must be used in the use of large volumes of intravenous fluids in myeloma, since frequently the impairment of renal function is fixed and large volumes of fluids will lead to the rapid onset of congestive cardiac failure. For this reason, administration of large volumes of fluids to patients with myeloma should be accompanied by central venous pressure monitoring.

Practical Guide to Treatment

Our own approach to the treatment of hypercalcemia in myeloma is (1) institution of cytotoxic drugs for treatment of myeloma; (2) the cautious use of intravenous saline to promote a saline diuresis with careful observation for the development of cardiac failure; and (3) the institution of calcitonin and corticosteroids, which in our experience is almost universally effective. We use salmon calcitonin in doses of 200 to 400 Medical Research Council (MRC) units intramuscularly (IM) or subcutaneously each 12 hours, and prednisone 40 to 60 mg daily or equivalent doses of hydrocortisone parenterally. In those patients who fail to respond to calcitonin and corticosteroids, we may use mithramycin (10 to 25 g/kg body weight by slow intravenous (IV) infusion, the absolute dose depending on renal function), although in practice this is usually hazardous because many of these patients have preexisting impairment of glomerular filtration.

Treatment of Painful Bone Lesions Without Hypercalcemia

For a number of years, clinicians have attempted to devise therapeutic approaches in myeloma that would relieve disabling symptoms due to skeletal destruction. This was first attempted with the use of fluoride and later calcium and fluoride, although this combination was ineffective and, in fact, detrimental because of the associated side effects. More recently, several groups have shown that the newer generation bisphosphonates will relieve bone pain, and produce a rapid, sustained, and significant decrease in the urinary excretion of calcium and hydroxyproline indicating decreased bone turnover.[49,50] This was shown first with APD[49] and then with Cl_2MDP.[50] Unfortunately, neither of these drugs are currently available for use in the United States. However, active research in this area is likely soon to lead to the introduction of other suitable and nontoxic agents of this class that will be useful as oral forms of therapy to relieve the symptoms caused by bone destruction and its complications in patients with myeloma.

ACKNOWLEDGMENT

The authors are grateful to Nancy Garrett for her help in the preparation of this manuscript.

REFERENCES

1. Snapper I, Kahn A: Myelomatosis. Basel, Switzerland, Karger, 1971
2. Mundy GR, Raisz LG, Cooper RA, et al: Evidence for the secretion of an osteoclast stimulating factor in myeloma. N Engl J Med 291:1041–1046, 1974
3. Valentin-Opran A, Charhon SA, Meunier PJ, et al: Quantitative histology of myeloma induced bone changes. Br J Haematol 52:601–610, 1982
4. Mundy GR, Martin TJ: The hypercalcemia of malignancy: Pathogenesis and management. Metabolism 31:1247–1277, 1982
5. Binstock ML, Mundy GR: Effects of calcitonin and glucocorticoids in combination in hypercalcemia of malignancy. Ann Intern Med 93:269–272, 1980
6. Mundy GR, Wilkinson R, Heath DA: Comparative study of available medical therapy for hypercalcemia of malignancy. Am J Med 74:421–432, 1983
7. Schechter GP, Wahl LM, Horton JE: In vitro bone resorption by human myeloma cells, in Potter M (ed): Progress in Myeloma. New York, Elsevier North Holland, 1980, pp 67–80
8. McDonald DF, Schofield BH, Prezioso EM, et al: Direct bone resorbing activity of murine myeloma cells. Cancer Lett 19:119–124, 1983
9. Eilon G, Mundy GR: Direct resorption of bone by human breast cancer cells in vitro. Nature 276:726–728, 1978
10. Bardwick PA, Zvaifler NJ, Gill GN, et al: Plasma cell dyscrasia with polyneuropathy, organomegaly, endocrinopathy, M protein, and skin changes: The POEMS syndrome. Medicine 59:311–322, 1980
11. Mundy GR, Luben RA, Raisz LG, et al: Bone resorbing activity in supernatants from lymphoid cell lines. N Engl J Med 290:867–871, 1974
12. Josse RG, Murray TM, Mundy GR, et al: Observations on the mechanism of bone resorption induced by multiple myeloma marrow culture fluids and partially purified osteoclast-activating factor. J Clin Invest 67:1472–1481, 1981
13. Gailani S, McLimans WF, Mundy GR, et al: Controlled environment culture of bone marrow explants from human myeloma. Cancer Res 36:1299–1304, 1976

14. Horton JE, Raisz LG, Simmons HA, et al: Bone resorbing activity in supernatant fluid from cultured human peripheral blood leukocytes. Science 177:793–795, 1972

15. Raisz LG, Luben RA, Mundy GR: Effects of osteoclast activating factor from human leukocytes on bone metabolism. J Clin Invest 56:408–413, 1975

16. Yoneda, T, Mundy GR: Prostaglandins are necessary for osteoclast activating factor (OAF) production by activated peripheral blood leukocytes. J Exp Med 149:279–283, 1979

17. Yoneda T, Mundy GR: Monocytes regulate osteoclast activating factor production by releasing prostaglandins. J Exp Med 150:338–350, 1979

18. Mundy GR, Rick ME, Turcotte R, et al: Pathogenesis of hypercalcemia in lymphosarcoma cell leukemia—Role of an osteoclast activating factor like substance and mechanism of action for glucocorticoid therapy. Am J Med 654:600–606, 1978

19. Bunn PA, Schechter GP, Jaffe E, et al: Clinical course of retrovirus associated adult T cell lymphoma in the United States. N Engl J Med 309:257–264, 1983

20. Bertolini DR, Sarin P, Mundy GR: Production of macromolecular bone resorbing activity by human T-cell leukemia virus (HTLV) transformed cell lines. Calcif Tissue Int 36:284A, 1984 (abstr)

21. Breslau NA, McGuire JL, Zerwekh JE, et al: Hypercalcemia associated with increased serum calcitriol levels in three patients with lymphoma. Ann Intern Med 100:1–7, 1984

22. Rosenthal N, Insogna KL, Godsall JW, et al: Elevations in circulating 1,25 dihydroxyvitamin D in three patients with lymphoma-associated hypercalcemia. J Clin Endocrinol Metab 60:29–33, 1985

23. Zaloga GP, Eil C, Medbery CA: Humoral hypercalcemia in Hodgkin's disease. Arch Intern Med 145:155–157, 1985

24. Davies M, Hayes ME, Mawer EB, et al: Abnormal vitamin D metabolism in Hodgkin's lymphoma. Lancet 1:1186–1188, 1985

25. Fetchick DA, Bertolini DR, Sarin P, et al: Metabolism of 25 hydroxyvitamin D by human T cell lymphotropic virus-transformed cord blood lymphocytes. J Clin Invest, 1986 (in press)

26. Evans CH: Lymphotoxin—an immunologic hormone with anticarcinogenic and antitumor activity. Cancer Immunol Immunother 12:181–190, 1982

27. Gray PW, Aggarwal BB, Benton CV, et al: Cloning and expression of cDNA for human lymphotoxin, a lymphokine with tumour necrosis activity. Nature 312:721–724, 1984

28. Pennica D, Nedwin GE, Hayflick JS, et al: Human tumour necrosis factor: Precursor structure, expression and homology to lymphotoxin. Nature 312:724–729, 1984

29. Bertolini DR, Nedwin G, Bringman T, et al: Stimulation of bone resorption and inhibition of bone formation in vitro by human tumour necrosis factors. Nature 319:516–518, 1986

30. March CJ, Mosley B, Larsen A, et al: Cloning, sequence and expression of two distinct human interleukin-1 complementary DNAs. Nature 315:641–647, 1985

31. Marx JL: Interleukin-1 genes are cloned. Science 228:1076–1077, 1985

32. Gowen M, Wood OD, Ihrie EJ, et al: An interleukin 1 like factor stimulates bone resorption in vitro. Nature 306:378–380, 1983

33. Heath JK, Saklatvala J, Meikle MC, et al: Pig interleukin 1 (catabolin) is a potent stimulator of bone resorption in vitro. Calcif Tissue Int 37:95–97, 1985

34. Gowen M, Nedwin G, Mundy GR: Preferential inhibition of cytokine-stimulated bone resorption by recombinant interferon gamma. J Bone Min Res 1:75, 1986 (abstr 67)

35. Dewhirst FE, Stashenko PP, Mole JE, et al: Purification of partial sequences of human osteoclast activating factor: Identity with interleukin 1 beta. J Immunol 135:2562–2568, 1985

36. Nedwin GE, Svedersky LP, Bringman TS, et al: Effect of interleukin-2, interferon-gamma, and mitogens on the production of tumor necrosis factors alpha and beta. J Immunol 135:2492–2497, 1985

37. Jilka RL, Hamilton JW: Inhibition of parathormone stimulated bone resorption by type 1 interferon. Biochem Biophys Res Commun 120:553–558, 1984

38. Durie BGM, Salmon SE, Mundy GR: Relation of osteoclast activating factor production to the extent of bone disease in multiple myeloma. Br J Haematol 47:21–30, 1981

39. Lazor MZ, Rosenberg LE: Mechanisms of adrenal-steroid reversal of hypercalcemia in multiple myeloma. N Engl J Med 270:749, 1964

40. Strumpf M, Kowalski MA, Mundy GR: Effects of glucocorticoids on osteoclast-activating factor. J Lab Clin Med 92:772–778, 1978

41. Suda T, Testa NG, Allen TD: Effects of hydrocortisone on osteoclasts generated in cat bone marrow cultures. Calcif Tissue Int 35:82–86, 1983

42. Minkin C: Inhibition of parathyroid hormone stimulated bone resorption in vitro by the antibiotic mithramycin. Calcif Tissue Res 13:249–257, 1973

43. Raisz LG, Trummel CL, Wener JA, et al: Effect of glucocorticoids on bone resorption in tissue culture. Endocrinology 90:961–967, 1972

44. Stamp TCB, Child JA, Walker PG: Treatment of osteolytic myelomatosis with mithramycin. Lancet 1:719–722, 1975

45. Raisz LG, Trummel CL, Simmons H: Induction of bone resorption in tissue culture: Prolonged response after brief exposure to parathyroid hormone or 25-hydroxycholecalciferol. Endocrinology 90:744–751, 1972a

46. Wener JA, Gorton SJ, Raisz LG: Escape from inhibition of resorption in cultures of fetal bone treated with calcitonin and parathyroid hormone. Endocrinology 90:752–759, 1972

47. Au WYW: Calcitonin treatment of hypercalcemia due to parathyroid carcinoma-synergistic effect of prednisone on long-term treatment of hypercalcemia. Arch Intern Med 135:1594–1597, 1975

48. Ralston SH, Gardner MD, Dryburgh TJ, et al: Comparison of aminohydroxpropylidene diphosphonate, mithramycin and corticosteroids/calcitonin in treatment of cancer-associated hypercalcemia. Lancet 2:907–910, 1985

49. Van Breukelen FJM, Bijvoet OLM, Van Oosterom

AT: Inhibition of osteolytic bone lesions by (3-amino-l-hydroxypropylidene)-l,l-bisophosphonate (A.P.D.) Lancet 1:803–805, 1979

50. Siris ES, Sherman WH, Baquiran DC, et al: Effects of dichloromethylene diphosphonate on skeletal mobilization of calcium in multiple myeloma. N Engl J Med 302:310–315, 1980

51. Ryzen E, Rude RK, Elbaum N, et al: Use of intravenous etidronate disodium in the treatment of hypercalcemia, in Garattini S (ed): Bone Resorption, Metastasis, and Diphosphonates: New York, Raven, 1983, p 99–108

52. Cohen P: Fluoride and calcium therapy for myeloma bone lesions. JAMA 198:583–586, 1966

53. Carbone PP, Zipkin I, Sokoloff L, et al: Fluoride effect on bone in plasma cell myeloma. Arch Intern Med 121:130–140, 1968

54. Cohen P, Gardner FH: Induction of subacute skeletal fluorosis in a case of multiple myeloma. N Engl J Med 271:1129–1133, 1964

55. Harly JB, Schilling A, Glidewell O: Ineffectiveness of fluoride therapy in multiple myeloma. N Engl J Med 286:1283–1288, 1972

56. Kyle RA, Jowsey J, Phil D, et al: Multiple myeloma bone disease. The comparative effect of sodium fluoride and calcium carbonate or placebo. N Engl J Med 293:1334–1338, 1975

57. Warrell RP, Bockman RS, Coonley CJ, et al: Gallium nitrate inhibits calcium resorption from bone and is effective treatment for cancer-related hypercalcemia. J Clin Invest 73:1487–1490, 1984

58. Kukla LJ, Abramson EC, McGuire WP, et al: Cis-platinum treatment for malignancy-associated humoral hypercalcemia in an athymic mouse model. Calcif Tissue Int 36:559–562, 1984

59. Suki WN, Yium JJ, Von Minden M, et al: Acute treatment of hypercalcemia with furosemide. N Engl J Med 283: 836–840, 1970

Staging and Kinetics of Multiple Myeloma

Brian G.M. Durie

MULTIPLE MYELOMA (MM) is the major malignancy of plasma cells.[1] Osteolytic lesions in bones or diffuse osteoporosis with or without fractures are features that distinguish myeloma from related lymphoid malignancies. The malignant plasma cells are usually present in bone marrow material and monoclonal immunoglobulin is present in the serum and/or urine in 99% of cases. Anemia, hypercalcemia, and/or renal insufficiency are frequent accompaniments of stage III multiple myeloma.[2] However, patients with MM can present with a variable spectrum of features and at different stages of disease development. In addition, there is a variable rate of progression from early to later stages of the disease. For example, patients with monoclonal gammopathy of undetermined significance (MGUS) can remain clinically stable for many years.[3] Conversely, there can be rapid progression from stage I to stage III disease with development of advanced symptomatic myeloma. It is therefore clinically important to carefully classify patients in terms of both tumor burden and rate of disease progression. The staging and kinetics of MM will be critically reviewed emphasizing aspects that have proven to be important both for understanding of the biology of the disease, as well as for clinical decision making and patient counseling.

MGUS, SMOLDERING, AND INDOLENT MYELOMA

It is essential to identify patients who have some features of multiple myeloma, however, remain clinically stable without therapy for many years.[4-7] The diagnostic features of MGUS, smoldering, and indolent myeloma are detailed in Table 1. It is often difficult to distinguish between these entities on the one hand and patients with more active MM in the early stages on the other. Using routinely available clinical and laboratory parameters, the only way to definitively diagnose active myeloma (versus MGUS) is to have clear evidence of disease progression.[3] This has spurred additional investigations to allow prediction of stable disease that does not require treatment without waiting for possible disease progression. The tritiated thymidine labeling index of bone marrow plasma cells has proven to be a useful parameter.[2,8] Patients with MGUS and smoldering myeloma invariably have extremely low labeling indices (LIs) of bone marrow plasma cells. Although 10% to 20% of early stage myeloma patients can also have a LI of <1%, such patients usually have obvious, overt myeloma.[2,5,8] Serial follow-up of the LI can be extremely helpful in documenting a transition from low values to higher values at the time of (or even preceding by several months) the development of clinically overt disease.[9]

A number of parameters in addition to the LI have been evaluated in patients with MGUS as compared to more active myeloma. Although suppression of the normal serum immunoglobulins increases progressively with the stage of disease in patients with MM, 10% to 15% of patients with MGUS can also have significant suppression of the normal serum immunoglobulins (Table 2).[10] Likewise, although the number of circulating monoclonal B lymphocytes increases progressively with the stage of disease, again patients with MGUS can also have a small percentage of circulating monoclonal B lymphocytes.[11] Plasma cell cytochemistry has been felt by some investigators to provide additional useful information.[12,13] For example, the plasma cell acid phosphatase (AP) tends to be strongly positive in plasma cells of patients with active MM while remaining extremely low in patients with MGUS.[13] Thus far, no large study has been carried out to evaluate the utility of plasma cell AP in distinguishing between MGUS and active MM in a prospective fashion. Another stain that appears to provide similar information is the plasma cell β-glucuronidase.[14] Again, patients with MGUS have a very low β-glucuronidase

From the Department of Internal Medicine, Section of Hematology/Oncology, College of Medicine, University of Arizona Medical Center, Tucson.

Address reprint requests to Brian G.M. Durie, MD, Department of Internal Medicine, Section of Hematology/Oncology, College of Medicine, University of Arizona Medical Center, Tucson, AZ 85724.

0093-7754/86/1303-0006$05.00/0

Table 4. Effect of Prognostic Factors on Survival

Prognostic Factor	Observed Deaths/Expected Deaths: All Groups	Treatment Group: A	B	C
Stage				
I	0.55	0.79	0.22	0.57
II	0.95 $P \leq 0.001$*	0.84	1.21	0.83
III	1.31	1.22	1.26	1.44
BUN†				
<30 mg/dL	0.84	0.80	0.91	0.80
	$P \leq 0.001$			
>30 mg/dL	1.84	1.84	1.47	2.27

*The significance of stage and BUN as prognostic variables was tested with the log rank test for trend. The *P* values for stage and BUN indicate that these factors have a strong prognostic value. Similar trends are seen within the three treatment groups.

†Blood urea nitrogen, 30 mg/dL = 10.7 mmol/L.

Reprinted by permission of The New England Journal of Medicine 301:746, 1979.[33]

Table 5. Stratification of Myeloma Patients According to Two Simple Variables Sβ2M and Serum Albumin Level

Stratification (Stage)	No. of Patients*	Number Alive (%)	Median Survival† (months)
I Low risk			
Sβ2M <6 μg/mL, and SA >3.0 g/dL	81	63 (78)	55
II Intermediate			
Sβ2M ≥6 μg/mL, but SA >3.0 g/dL	46	19 (41)	19
III Poor risk			
SA ≤3.0 g/dL	18	6 (33)	4

*Two patients had missing serum albumin values: The total number of patients in this correlation is 145.

†I *v* II, $P < .001$; II *v* III, $P < .05$.

Reprinted with permission.[20]

(MWJ), plus two new variables related to disease activity, (the $S\beta_2M$ level and the instantaneous rate of bone resorption), were included. The study confirmed the validity of the three MSS in the prediction of survival duration, with a slight but significant advantage for the DS-MSS. Among single variables, $S\beta_2M$ was the most powerful indicator of prognosis ($P < .0001$), serum albumin level being the only variable adding to this significantly ($P = .02$). Of major interest, $S\beta_2M$ alone was a better indicator than the MRC and MWJ MSS. Finally, $S\beta_2M$ and the serum albumin level, (variables not included in the three MSS), were better indicators than the classical DS MSS and could be combined simply to give a very powerful system of stratification. The derived staging system using $S\beta_2M$ and serum albumin is summarized in Table 5.

Pretreatment Tumor Mass, Cell Kinetics, and Prognosis

Although clinical staging is prognostically important, other factors such as the intrinsic drug sensitivity of the predominant myeloma cell clone and cell kinetics must be taken into consideration.[39] The majority of patients with MM at the time of diagnosis are in a stage of indolent growth. However, a subgroup with more rapid doubling as determined from changes in M component level and measurements of tritiated thymidine turnover and incorporation has been identified.[2,40,41] The kinetics of the predominant clone in this subgroup of patients have proved to be very important. The total number of DNA-synthesizing myeloma cells (S cells) in the body can be calculated by multiplying the LI (the percentage of myeloma cells incorporating tritiated thymidine during a one-hour flash label) and the total myeloma cell mass. The subgroup of patients with both a high cell mass and a high labeling index (>3%) have a median survival of only 5.3 months.[2] Of interest, while rare in the general population of myeloma patients, involvement of the central nervous system is a special feature of the high tumor burden, high labeling subgroup.[2]

It is also important to appreciate how tumor burden and pretreatment kinetics influence response to induction therapy and survival. The pretreatment labeling index does not influence the likelihood of response to induction chemotherapy.[2] However, a preponderance of stage II or III patients with a high pretreatment labeling index (>3%) have a short median duration of remission and short overall survival.

It must be emphasized that the tritiated thymidine labeling index of myeloma cells is only a reflection of the biologically important subcompartment of proliferating tumor cells. What is happening to the underlying myeloma stem cell pool has to be evaluated by more direct approaches, such as a myeloma clonogenic assay system. Using such an assay, it is possible to measure the tritiated thymidine suicide of myeloma colonies.[39] Initial studies have indicated that the suicide index or growth fraction of the stem cell pool is usually very high, although some patients appear to have a predominant G_0 population of clonogenic myeloma cells. There is also a wide range of inherent drug sensitivity of the myeloma clones.[39] In a detailed study of 97 patients, both pretreatment drug resistance and selective sensitivity at the time of relapse were accurately detected. Although LI and in vitro sensitivity were clearly independent variables, a high LI (>3%) plus in vitro resistance were associated with a subsequent survival duration of <6 months. The studies allowed preliminary dissection of the complex interrelationship between cell kinetics and drug sensitivity.

Kinetics of Tumor Regression With Chemotherapy

For patients with MM, there is a characteristic mode of tumor regression with induction chemotherapy. In responsive patients, tumor regression occurs rapidly at first, and then slows as the tumor reaches a plateau stage.[42] Plateau has been defined as a stable state with minimal change in the serum/urine M component level or measured myeloma cell mass for a minimum of 4 to 6 months. This state can persist in spite of ongoing treatment for a period of several months to a number of years. With good responses to treatment, the plateau tumor load is one to two logs smaller than the pretreatment tumor burden. Responses of this magnitude occur in about half of patients treated with standard approaches and are associated with the relief of symptoms and substantial prolongation of survival. The retardation of the regression as it slows toward the plateau phase appears analogous to the plateau effect that occurs during the reverse process of advancing tumor growth at the time of clinical diagnosis.[26] The mechanisms responsible for this plateau phenomenon are currently unclear, but remain crucial for the understanding of apparent resistance to ongoing therapy. It is likely that there are several factors involved, including heterogeneity in the myeloma stem cell compartment, modulation by host factors, and clonal competition/inhibition.[43]

In a recent analysis of 127 patients who had serial measurements of myeloma cell mass, the incidence and significance of the plateau phase were investigated.[42] A stable plateau phase occurred in 44% of patients receiving induction chemotherapy and during the plateau phase the tumor cells were cytokinetically stable. Another group of patients (38%) had an unstable course, with significant ongoing cell turnover in spite of therapy. Another 9% had steady regression continuing beyond 1 year of therapy. This study was based on findings after the first 6 months of initiation of treatment. Reports concerning the initial 6 months have indicated that many more patients have high tritiated thymidine labelling indices and evidence of possible cell recruitment.[41,44] Data on the first 6 months of treatment, as well as in early relapse, weighed heavily in a prior pilot study that suggested that an expansion of the growth fraction was associated with induction of a remission.[45] It now seems that although early expansion of the growth fraction may be an important part of successful induction, the dominant kinetic feature of stable remission (once accomplished) is reversion to a kinetically quiescent state. Studies with idiotypic antibodies have shown that the myeloma cells with very low thymidine incorporation have idiotypic markers and are therefore part of the predominant myeloma clone.[46]

There are many implications of these findings. Because the plateau phase is generally an indolent state when cells resistant to initial induction are dormant (functional G_0 state), one would predict that intensive therapy during this period would not be especially useful. However, it is worth considering other approaches such as immunomodulation. Although a small population of cycling tumor stem cells may persist during plateau, as reflected by a low overall LI despite high tritiated thymidine suicide index of clonogenic myeloma cells,[39] this is not an ideal situation for therapy with currently available cytotoxic agents. A more reasonable approach is the introduction of additional drugs, including those with some cycle specificity, such as vincristine, during the kinetically active initial 6-month induction period or during early relapse.

Conversely, patients in whom >75% tumor regression has been achieved and who are apparently in a plateau phase can be followed carefully without any therapy, since little benefit can be expected from indefinite treatment without cell-kill in these patients. However, patients in the unstable group could be expected to relapse quickly when treatment is withdrawn. Because of the potential leukemogenic effect of prolonged treatment with alkylating agents,[47] and other complications of treatment, it has become increasingly important to be able to identify and treat only those patients who need such therapy—for example, those in the unstable group.

Immunology and Disease Activity or Stage in Myeloma

Research is ongoing in many areas of myeloma immunology and has been extensively reviewed.[48] The roles of T lymphocytes, B and pre-B lymphocytes, macrophages, and the effects of a variety of humoral mediators have all been examined.[48] T lymphocyte subpopulations in myeloma have been studied by a number of techniques, including determination of Fc receptor type, sheep red blood cell binding, reactivity with idiotypic antisera, and using monoclonal antibodies to evaluate helper or suppressor subpopulation phenotypes. A number of types of T lymphocyte imbalances have been noted. Although from animal studies there is now strong evidence for an important regulatory function for idiotypic T lymphocytes, with respect to the malignant plasma cell clone, in humans the findings are much more preliminary.[9] In a recent study by Mellstedt et al,[49] the ratio between OKT4 and OKT8 lymphocytes (helper to suppressor ratio) was extremely low in patients with treated myeloma or Waldenstrom's macroglobulinemia compared to controls ($P < .001$).[49] In addition, the ratio was low in 27% of patients with MGUS and 38% of untreated patients with myeloma, especially those with high cell mass.[49] The latter finding suggested that the increase in the OKT8 suppressor population was in some way a response to the increasing tumor burden. Additional similar findings have recently been reported.[9] T lymphocyte subpopulations were investigated with respect to myeloma disease activity. The treated patients who were in stable plateau had a very low OKT4/OKT8 ratio, which in this instance was associated with an absolute increase in the OKT8 population. Again, this suggested a regulatory or functional role for these suppressor lymphocytes in response to the residual tumor burden. This hypothesis has been tested by coincubation of separated OKT8 lymphocytes with the myeloma cell line 8226.[9] A striking inhibition of myeloma clonogenic growth was demonstrated with increasing concentrations of these separated OKT8 lymphocytes. Because no idiotypic studies were carried out, the true specificity of this type of suppressor lymphocyte subpopulation is currently unknown. Further studies are clearly warranted. The understanding of myeloma immunology has recently been expanding by studies of bone marrow immunotyping of both myeloma cells and accessory cells.[50-52] CALLA-positive myeloma has been identified as an aggressive subtype of myeloma and can be added to the list of important prognostic factors.

Circulating B Lymphocytes in Myeloma

The major question with respect to circulating B lymphocytes is the identification and quantitation of the number of circulating B lymphocytes that are part of the myeloma clone.[53] Various authors using antiidiotypic sera have demonstrated the presence of a significant number of circulating B lymphocytes sharing the same idiotypic specificity as the M component. There has been a question that the M component on these lymphocytes was a result of passive absorption. Despite this, a preponderance of evidence now supports the presence of a subpopulation of lymphocytes representing myeloma precursors in the circulation. The following are the most critical points in favor of this conclusion[54]: (1) The capacity of these idiotypic lymphocytes to reexpress their surface immunoglobulin; (2) the non–self-renewal characteristics of truly mature myeloma cells; (3) the aneuploid pattern of peripheral lymphocytes in some patients with myeloma; (4) the data from the murine plamacytoma model in which maturation in vivo from lymphocytic cells to myeloma cells was clearly demonstrated. In a study by Pettersson et al[55] a clear relationship was established between the number of circulating monoclonal B lymphocytes and disease stage using the Durie/Salmon method.

Evaluation of Bone Involvement

In the initial evaluation of patients with MM, the extent and type of bone involvement is an important question. A number of investigators have recently evaluated the role of radionuclide bone scanning in comparison with routine skeletal roentgenograms for initial staging evaluation and subsequent follow-up of MM. Using 99mTc polyphosphate, methylene diphosphonate, or other phosphonates, there is general agreement as to the conclusions.[18,56–58] First, the extent of lytic lesions is seriously underestimated by bone scanning. Large lytic lesions frequently do not show up at all on technetium phosphate scans. For the skull, spine, pelvis, proximal femura, and shoulder girdle regions, routine radiography is clearly the preferable method of evaluation. At the time of initial evaluation, it is extremely unusual for a patient to have a positive bone scan at any site in the presence of entirely normal roentgenograms. However, about 10% to 20% of patients will have lesions in addition to those evident on x-ray evaluation, which show up on bone scan only. The commonest sites for these additional bone scan positive regions are the ribs, cervical spine, and shoulder girdle regions. The ribs are a particular site of bone scan positivity commented on by several authors. Obviously, ribs are frequently not well seen on routine chest roentgenogram. With special rib films, lesions found on bone scanning, however, can usually also be demonstrated on roentgenograms. There are two possible situations in which bone scanning may be clinically useful.[59] In patients with severe localized bone pain, the bone scan may be positive before the appearance of demonstrable lesions on roentgenograms. This also appears to be true in patients who have refractory myeloma and progressive disease in whom new areas of positive uptake (hot spots) may be of poor prognostic import. Using gallium scanning, Waxman et al have noted similar findings, that is, high gallium uptake identifying a subgroup of patients (five of 18) with rapidly progressive disease.[60] Further studies will be necessary to evaluate the clinical importance of these findings.

Flow Microfluorometry in MM

Flow microfluorometry has added a new dimension to the evaluation of myeloma cells from the bone marrow of patients with MM and related disorders. The current and potential applications have recently been extensively reviewed.[4] The major advantage of flow cytometry is that a very large number of cells can be evaluated for the presence or absence of specific properties. The critical aspect is the specificity. To obtain specific information, one needs to have specific stains or antibodies that will allow quantitation of the property of interest. Because bone marrow specimens from patients with MM normally contain a large mixture of cells, there is an urgent need for specific antibodies for myeloma cells that can be used to discriminate that population and then allow evaluation in detail of the myeloma clones. The primary method of evaluation thus far has been to look at DNA content. However, RNA, protein, and other substances can be quantitated.

To the present time, DNA content has been most extensively evaluated. Several investigators have reported a very high frequency of aneuploidy in MM samples.[61–65] Approximately 75% of patients do have abnormal DNA content of the myeloma cells (aneuploidy). In most instances, this represents the presence of excess DNA. The DNA content is expressed as an index relative to the DNA content of normal granulocytes. The exact basis for the aneuploidy remains uncertain at the present time. Cytogenetic studies have indicated presence of hypodiploidy in samples containing excess DNA. This suggests that different populations are being evaluated by the different techniques. The most interesting finding using the flow cytometry method has been the documentation of discrete populations of myeloma cells with excess DNA. This has suggested the presence of multiple clones in the bone marrow specimens from some patients. In analyses of DNA content of peripheral blood cells, a very important observation has been the finding of a 13% frequency of aneuploidy in the peripheral blood. This confirms as discussed above that myeloma cells are frequently present in the circulation of myeloma patients.

Cytoplasmic RNA is increased in approximately 90% of patients with myeloma, although it is not specific for myeloma cells. Nonetheless, the RNA index (ratio of mean RNA content of $G_{1/0}$ myeloma cells to that of lymphocyte controls) has been shown to be inversely related to degree of bone marrow infiltrate with myeloma cells.[61] In addition, the RNA index is predictive of response, with high levels being associated with good response to treatment and low RNA index levels correlating with more aggressive myeloma behavior.[61] Because of the difficulties in distinguishing myeloma cells from other types of marrow cells, cell cycle analyses have thus far been rather limited. Perhaps with other techniques, such as evaluating the kinetics of clonogenic cells in soft agar or methyl cellulose, more direct evaluation of myeloma growth kinetics will be possible.[39] However, with the introduction of many new monoclonal antibodies, it is hoped that flow cytometry can be expanded to allow more detailed analyses of a whole range of myeloma cell properties. With continued improvement in the technology of cell sorters themselves, this promises to be an area of expanding research.

The Role of Staging and Kinetics in Myeloma

As can be seen from the above review, the staging and kinetics of MM and related gammopathies have many facets. There is ever expanding knowledge of the basic biology of the various disease categories and particularly, recently some indication that induction and relapse treatment can be tailored more precisely to the needs of the individual patient. For example, patients with low tumor burden and minimal growth, as reflected by low thymidine incorporation, can be classified as having MGUS, indolent myeloma or smoldering myeloma, all of which can be safely followed without treatment. Conversely, as recent studies suggest,[59] patients with advanced aggressive myeloma can be identified and can be seen to benefit from more aggressive combination induction therapy. Following induction chemotherapy, patients in stable plateau phase can now be considered for careful follow-up off maintenance therapy, thus possibly reducing the potential risk of a secondary leukemia associated with ongoing alkylating agent maintenance therapy. This type of approach is obviously still investigational and should continue to be practiced only in a study setting until it has been clearly established which patients can safely be followed without maintenance therapy as opposed to those requiring some form of maintenance to prevent early relapse. In the relapse phase of the disease, both kinetic information and results of in vitro drug sensitivity testing can be made available to direct the selection of treatment. Hopefully, the more detailed application of some of these concepts can lead to improved overall survival of patients with MM and related gammopathies.

REFERENCES

1. Durie BGM, Salmon SE: Multiple myeloma, macroglobulinaemia and monoclonal gammopathies, in Hoffbrand AV, Brain MC, Hirsh J (eds): Recent Advances in Haematology. Edinburgh, Churchill Livingstone, 1977, pp 243–261

2. Durie GBM, Salmon SE, Moon TE: Pretreatment tumor mass, cell kinetics, and prognosis in multiple myeloma. Blood 55:364–372, 1980

3. Kyle RA: Monoclonal gammopathy of undetermined significance (MGUS): review, in Salmon SE (ed): Clinics in Haematology. London, Saunders, 1982, pp 123–150

4. Alexanian R: Localized and indolent myeloma. Blood 56:521–525, 1980

5. Boccadoro M, Gavarotti P, Fassati G, et al: Low plasma cell ^{3}[H] thymidine incorporation in MGUS, smoldering myeloma and remission phase myeloma: A reliable indicator of patients not requiring therapy. Br J Haematol 58:689–696, 1984

6. Kyle RA, Greipp PR: Smoldering multiple myeloma. N Engl J Med 302:1347–1349, 1980

7. Kyle RA, Greipp PR: "Idiopathic" Bence Jones proteinuria. Long term follow up in seven patients. N Engl J Med 306:564, 1982

7a. Dollinger MR, Golbey RB, Kamofsky DA: Cancer Chemotherapy. DM 1969, p 11

7b. Durie BGM, Salmon SE: Staging kinetics, and flow cytometry of multiple myeloma, in Wiernik P, et al (eds): Neoplastic Diseases of the Blood. New York, Churchill Livingstone, 1985

8. Greipp PR, Kyle RA: Clinical, morphological, and cell kinetic differences among multiple myeloma, monoclonal gammopathy of undetermined significance, and smoldering multiple myeloma. Blood 62:166–171, 1983

9. Durie BGM, Ludwig CU: Smoldering myeloma: An analysis of patients developing overt disease. Blood 60:143a, 1982 (suppl 1) (abstr)

10. Pruzanski W, Gidon MS, Roy A: Suppression of polyclonal immunoglobulins in multiple myeloma: Relationship to the staging and other manifestations at diagnosis. Clin Immunol Immunopathol 17:280–286, 1980

11. Mellstedt H, Holm G, Pettersson D, et al: Idiotype-bearing lymphoid cells in plasma cell neoplasia, in Salmon SE (ed): Clinics in Haematology. London, Saunders, 1982, p 65

12. Bataille R, Durie BGM, Sany J, et al: Myeloma bone marrow acid phosphatase staining: A correlative study of 38 patients. Blood 55:802–805, 1980

13. Cassuto JP, Hammou JC, Pastorelli E, et al: Plasma cell acid phosphatase, a discriminative test for benign and malignant monoclonal gammopathies. Biomedicine 27:197–199, 1977

14. Seigneurin D, David J, Sotto JJ, et al: β-Glucuronidases plasmocytaires dans les dysglobulinemies. Interet diag-

nostique de leur mise en evidence. Pathol Biol (Paris) 27:467, 1979
15. Miliani A, Anichini P, di Guglielmo R, et al: Etude cyto-enzymologique des plasmocytes medullaries des dysglobulinemies monoclonales myelomateuses et non myelomateuses. Nouv Rev Fr Hematol 24:27–33, 1982
16. Norfolk D, Child JA, Cooper EH, et al: Serum β_2 microglobulin in myelomatosis: Potential value in stratification and monitoring. Br J Cancer 39:510–515, 1979
17. Karlsson FA, Wibell L, Ervin PE: β-$_2$ microglobulin in clinical medicine. Scand J Clin Lab Invest 40:27–37, 1980 (suppl 154)
18. Bataille R, Durie BGM, Grenier J: Serum β-$_2$ microglobulin and survival duration in multiple myeloma: A simple, reliable marker for staging. Br J Hematol 55:439–447, 1983
19. Garewal H, Durie BGM, Kyle RA, et al: Serum β_2 microglobulin in the initial staging and subsequent monitoring of monoclonal plasma cell disorders. J Clin Oncol 2:51–57, 1984
20. Bataille R, Durie BGM, Grenier J, et al: Prognostic factors and staging in multiple myeloma: A reappraisal. J Clin Oncol 4:80–87, 1986
21. Boccadoro M, Durie BGM, Frutiger Y, et al: Independent utility of plasma cell thymidine labelling index and serum β-$_2$-microglobulin as prognostic factors in monoclonal gammopathies. 1986 (submitted for publication)
22. Durie BGM, Ludwig CU: Smoldering myeloma: An analysis of patients developing overt disease. Blood 58:501, 1982 (suppl 1) (abstr)
23. Durie BGM, Salmon SE: A clinical staging system for multiple myeloma. Correlation of measured myeloma cell mass with presenting clinical features, response to treatment, and survival. Cancer 36:842–854, 1975
24. Nathans D, Fahey JL. Potter M: The formation of myeloma protein by a mouse plasma cell tumor. J Exp Med 108:121–129, 1958
25. Salmon SE, Smith BA: Immunoglobulin synthesis and total body tumor cell number in IgG multiple myeloma. J Clin Invest 49:1114–1121, 1970
26. Sullivan PW, Salmon SE: Kinetics of tumor growth and regression in IgG multiple myeloma. J Clin Invest 51:1697–1708, 1972
27. Bataille R, Morlock G, Rosenberg F, et al: Appreciation de la masse tumorale et de sa regression sous traitment dans le myelome multiple des os. Commentaries critiques a propos de 22 malades. Rev Rhumatol 45:1, 1978
28. Klener P, Donner L, Sak P, et al: Prognosticke factory u plazmocytomu. Shornik Lekasrky 10:331–336, 1980
29. Woodruff RK, Wadsworth J, Malpas JS, et al: Clinical staging in multiple myeloma. Br J Hematol 42:199–205, 1979
30. Salmon SE, Wampler SE: Multiple myeloma: Quantitative staging and assessment of response with a programmable pocket calculator. Blood 49:379–389, 1977
31. Merlini G, Waldenstrom JG, Jayakar SD: A new improved clinical staging system for multiple myeloma based on analysis of 123 treated patients. Blood 55:1011–1019, 1980
32. Alexanian R, Salmon S, Gutterman J, et al: Chemoimmunotherapy for multiple myeloma. Cancer 47:1923–1929, 1981
33. Bergsagel DE, Langley GR, Bailey AJ, et al: The chemotherapy of plasma cell myeloma and the incidence of acute leukemia. N Engl J Med 301:743–748, 1979
34. Cohen HJ, Silberman HR, Larsen WE, et al: Combination chemotherapy with intermittent 1-3-Bis (2-chloroethyl) 1-nitrosourea (BCNU), cyclophosphamide, and prednisone for multiple myeloma. Blood 54:824–836, 1979
35. Cuzick J, Galton DAG, Petro R, et al: Treatment comparisons in the third MRC myelomatosis trial. Br J Cancer 42:831–840, 1980
36. Harley JB, Pajak TF, McIntyre OR, et al: Improved survival of increased-risk myeloma patients on combined triple-alkylating-agent therapy: A study of the CALGB. Blood 54:13–22, 1979
37. Salmon SE, Haut A, Bonnet J, et al: Alternating combination chemotherapy improves survival in multiple myeloma. A Southwest Oncology Group Study. J Clin Oncol 1:453–461, 1983
38. Durie BGM, Dixon DO, Carter S, et al: Improved survival duration with combination chemotherapy induction for multiple myeloma. A Southwest Oncology Group Study. J Clin Oncol 4, 1986 (in press)
39. Durie BGM, Young LA, Salmon SE: Human myeloma in vitro colony growth: Interrelationship between drug sensitivity, cell kinetics, and patient survival duration. Blood 61:929–934, 1983
40. Drewinko B, Alexanian R: Growth kinetics of plasma cell myeloma. JNCI 58:1247–1253, 1977
41. Drewinko B, Alexanian R, Boyer H, et al: The growth fraction of human myeloma cells. Blood 57:333–338, 1981
42. Durie BGM, Russell DH, Salmon SE: Reappraisal of plateau phase in myeloma. Lancet 2:65, 1980
43. Durie BGM: Is myeloma really a monoclonal disease? Br J Haematol 57:357–363, 1984
44. Pileri A, Barnengo MG, Boccadoro M, et al: Early recruitment in the human myeloma cell population after cytostatic treatment. Hematologica 61:184, 1976
45. Salmon SE: Expansion of the growth fraction in multiple myeloma with alkylating agents. Blood 45:119–129, 1975
46. Pileri A, Carmagnola AL, Boccadoro M: Immunobiology and kinetics of human myeloma. Ettore Majorana, Centre for Scientific Culture. International School of Medical Sciences, 15th Course. Adv Lymphoprolif Dis 15:295–301, 1981
47. Bergsagel DE: Plasma cell neoplasms and acute leukaemia, in Salmon SE (ed) Clinics in Haematology. London, Saunders, 1982, pp 221–234
48. Mellstedt H, Holm G, Pettersson D, et al: Idiotype-bearing lymphoid cells in plasma cell neoplasia, in Salmon SE (ed): Clinics in Haematology. London, Saunders, 1982, pp 65–86
49. Mellstadt H, Holm G, Pettersson D, et al: T cells in monoclonal gammopathies. Scand J Hematol 29:57–64, 1982
50. Durie BGM, Grogan TM: CALLA-Positive myeloma: An aggressive subtype with poor survival. Blood 66:229–232, 1985
51. Kronland R, Grogan T, Spier C, et al: Immunotopographic assessment of lymphoid and plasma cell malignancies in the bone marrow. Hum Pathol 16:1247–1254, 1985
52. Rodriguez MA, Durie BGM, Richter L, et al: Immu-

nohistologic studies of bone marrow accessory cell populations in patients with multiple myeloma: Correlations with other prognostic parameters. 1986 (submitted for publication)

53. Pettersson D, Mellstedt H, Holm G: Monoclonal B lymphocytes in multiple myeloma. Scand J Immunol 12:375–382, 1980

54. Boccadoro M, Gavarotti P, Fossati G, et al: Kinetics of circulating B lymphocytes in human myeloma. Blood 61:812–814, 1983

55. Pettersson D, Mellstedt M, Holm G, et al: Monoclonal blood lymphocytes in benign monoclonal gammopathy and multiple myeloma in relation to clinical stage. Scand J Hematol 27:287–293, 1981

56. Ludwig H, Kumpan W, Sinzinger H: Radiography and bone scintigraphy in multiple myeloma: A comparative analysis. Br J Radiol 55:173–181, 1982

57. Wahner HW, Kyle RA, Beabout JW: Scintigraphic evaluation of the skeleton in multiple myeloma. Mayo Clin Proc 55:739–746, 1980

58. Woolfenden JM, Pitt MJ, Durie BGM, et al: Comparison of bone scintigraphy and radiography in multiple myeloma. Radiology 134:723–728, 1980

59. Bataille R, Chevalier J, Rossi M, et al: Bone scintigraphy in plasma-cell myeloma. A prospective study of 70 patients. Radiology 145:801–804, 1982

60. Waxman AD, Siemsen JK, Levine AM, et al: Radiographic and radionuclide imaging in multiple myeloma: The role of gallium scintigraphy: Concise communication. J Nucl Med 22:232–236, 1981

61. Barlogie B, Alexanian R, Gehan EA, et al: Marrow cytometry and prognosis in myeloma. J Clin Invest 72:853, 1983

62. Barlogie B, Latreille J, Alexanian R, et al: Quantitative cytology in myeloma research, in Salmon SE (ed): Clinics in Haematology. London, Saunders, 1982, pp 19–46

63. Bunn PA, Krasnow S, Makuch RW, et al: Flow cytometric analysis of DNA content of bone marrow cells in patients with plasma cell myeloma: Clinical implications. Blood 59:528–535, 1982

64. Latreille J, Barlogie B, Johnston D, et al: Ploidy and proliferative characteristics in monoclonal gammopathies. Blood 59:43–51, 1982

65. Latreille J, Barlogie B, Dosik G, et al: Cellular DNA content as a marker of human multiple myeloma. Blood 55:403–408, 1980

Laboratory Monitoring of Myeloma Proteins

Robert A. Kyle and John P. Garton

ANALYSIS of the serum and urine for monoclonal proteins requires a sensitive, rapid, dependable screening method to detect a monoclonal protein and a specific assay to identify its heavy chain class and light chain type. Electrophoresis on cellulose acetate membrane is satisfactory for screening but may not detect small monoclonal proteins. The high-resolution agarose gel electrophoretic technique is more sensitive than the cellulose acetate electrophoretic technique in detecting small monoclonal proteins.[1] Either immunoelectrophoresis or immunofixation or both should be used to confirm the presence of monoclonal protein and to distinguish the heavy chain class and light chain type.

ANALYSIS OF SERUM FOR MONOCLONAL PROTEINS

Electrophoresis for Detection

Serum protein electrophoresis should be done in all cases in which multiple myeloma, macroglobulinemia, or amyloidosis is suspected. In addition, the test is indicated in any case of unexplained weakness or fatigue, anemia, elevation of the erythrocyte sedimentation rate, back pain, osteoporosis, osteolytic lesions or fracture, immunoglobulin deficiency, hypercalcemia, Bence Jones proteinuria, renal insufficiency, or recurrent infections. Serum protein electrophoresis also should be performed in cases of peripheral neuropathy, carpal tunnel syndrome, refractory congestive heart failure, nephrotic syndrome, orthostatic hypotension, or malabsorption, because a localized band or spike is strongly suggestive of primary amyloidosis. Electrophoresis is an excellent screening test because it can be done easily, rapidly, and cheaply.

The constituents of the major components of the serum electrophoretic pattern are listed in Table 1.

A monoclonal protein (having a single heavy chain class and single light chain type) usually is seen as a narrow peak (like a church spire) on the densitometer tracing or as a dense, discrete band on the cellulose membrane in the γ, β, or α_2-globulin regions (Fig 1 A). In contrast, an excess of polyclonal immunoglobulins (having one or more heavy chain classes and an increase in both κ and λ light chains) makes a broad-based peak or broad band (Fig 1 B) and usually is limited to the γ region. In approximately 2% of sera tested, there is an additional monoclonal protein of different immunoglobulin class, and this situation is designated biclonal gammopathy.[3] Immunoglobulins (IgG, IgA, IgM, IgD, and IgE) make up the γ component, but it must be emphasized that they are also found in the β-γ and β regions and that IgG extends to the α_2-globulin region. Thus, an IgG monoclonal protein may migrate from the slow γ region to the α_2-globulin region. A monoclonal protein is most suggestive of monoclonal gammopathy of undetermined significance (MGUS), multiple myeloma, Waldenström's macroglobulinemia, or other lymphoproliferative disease or of primary systemic amyloidosis (AL).

Hypogammaglobulinemia (γ globulin <0.6 g/dL) is characterized by a definite decrease in the gamma component, and the diagnosis should be confirmed by quantitative determination of the immunoglobulin levels. Hypogammaglobulinemia is seen in about 15% of patients with multiple myeloma and in approximately one third of patients with primary systemic amyloidosis. In this situation, proteinuria of the Bence Jones type is often present, and immunoelectrophoresis or immunofixation of the serum and urine is necessary for identification.

Other shapes may misleadingly suggest a monoclonal protein in the serum. For example, a large, broad peak in the α_2-globulin region may represent hemoglobin-haptoglobin complexes resulting from hemolysis. Fibrinogen may be seen as a band in the β-γ region in a plasma specimen or in a specimen from a patient on anticoagulation therapy. Large amounts of transferrin in

---

From the Division of Hematology and Internal Medicine, Mayo Clinic and Mayo Foundation, Rochester, Minn.

Supported in part by research grant CA-16835 from the National Institutes of Health, Public Health Service, and the Toor Myeloma Research Fund.

Address reprint requests to Robert A. Kyle, MD, Mayo Clinic, 200 First St SW, Rochester, MN 55905.

0093-7754/86/1303-0007$05.00/0

Table 1. Constituents of the Major Components of the Serum Electrophoretic Pattern

+ (anode) Albumin	α_1-Globulin	α_2-Globulin	β-Globulin	− (cathode) γ-Globulin
Albumin	α_1-Antitrypsin	α_2-Macroglobulin	β-Lipoprotein	IgG
	α_1-Lipoprotein	α_2-Lipoprotein	Transferrin	IgA
	α_1-Acid glycoprotein (orosomucoid)	Haptoglobin	Plasminogen	IgM
		Ceruloplasmin	Complement	IgD
		Erythropoietin	Hemopexin	IgE

NOTE. Immunoglobulins may migrate from the slow γ region to the α_2-globulin region.
Reprinted with permission.[2]

patients with iron deficiency anemia may produce a localized band in the β region. Occasionally, the application artifact in the cathodal region actually represents a monoclonal protein.[4] A monoclonal protein may appear as a rather broad band on the cellulose acetate membrane or as a broad peak on the densitometer tracing, and either can be mistaken for a polyclonal increase in immunoglobulins. Presumably, this broad band or peak is due to a complex of monoclonal protein with other plasma components, aggregates of IgG, polymers of IgA, or dimers of IgM. Immunoelectrophoresis or immunofixation is required for identification.

It must be emphasized that a patient can have a monoclonal protein when the total protein concentration, β and γ globulin levels, and quantitative immunoglobulin values are all normal. One must also look at the cellulose acetate strip even when the β or γ globulin values are normal,

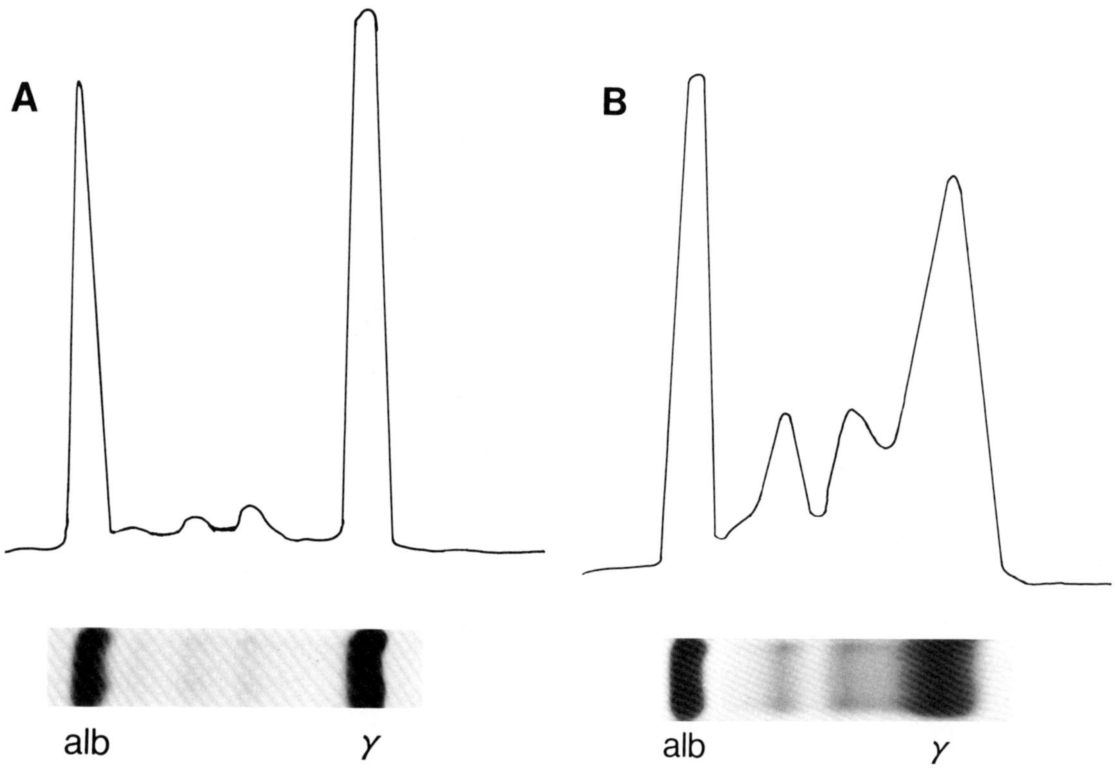

Fig 1 (A) Top, monoclonal pattern of serum protein from densitometer tracing after electrophoresis on cellulose acetate (anode on left): Tall, narrow-based peak of γ mobility; bottom, monoclonal pattern from electrophoresis of serum on cellulose acetate (anode on left): dense, localized band representing monoclonal protein in γ area. (B) Top, polyclonal pattern of serum protein from densitometer tracing after electrophoresis on cellulose acetate (anode on left): Broad-based peak of γ mobility; bottom, polyclonal pattern from electrophoresis of serum on cellulose acetate (anode on left): γ band is broad.

because a small monoclonal protein may be present and not detectable on the densitometer tracing. A small monoclonal peak may be concealed among the β or γ components and be missed. The cellulose acetate pattern and densitometer tracing may seem to be normal even though a monoclonal protein is present. A monoclonal light chain (Bence Jones proteinemia) is rarely seen on the cellulose acetate tracing. In some cases of IgD myeloma, the monoclonal protein has a small peak or is not evident at all. Often the monoclonal protein is not apparent in the heavy chain diseases. Thus, immunoelectrophoresis or immunofixation is necessary for recognition.

For follow-up after the diagnosis of a monoclonal protein in the serum, we recommend using cellulose acetate electrophoresis to detect changes in the amount of the M protein. Repeated immunoelectrophoresis is usually not required unless significant changes in the pattern have occurred.

Immunoelectrophoresis for Identification

Immunoelectrophoresis is a useful technique for the identification of a monoclonal protein. It should be performed in all cases in which a sharp peak or band is found in the cellulose acetate tracing or when myeloma, macroglobulinemia, amyloidosis, or a related disorder is suspected. Immunoelectrophoresis is usually helpful in the differentiation of a monoclonal from a polyclonal increase in immunoglobulins.

Potent antiserum to whole human serum produces more than 30 precipitin arcs and causes difficulty in interpretation. Therefore, one should use monospecific antisera to IgG, IgA, IgM, IgD, and IgE as well as to κ and λ light chains. It is always useful to have antisera from various sources available when typing monoclonal proteins, because the antigenic determinants of some monoclonal proteins are so restricted that they may not be recognized by all antisera.

In multiple myeloma, monospecific antisera to IgG, IgA, IgD, IgE, or κ and λ produce a localized thickening or bowing of a heavy chain arc and a similar thickening or bowing of a light chain arc. The alterations in the heavy chain and light chain arcs should be about the same distance from the well. The presence of an additional light chain arc (double bowing) without a similar bowing of a heavy chain arc indicates a free monoclonal light chain (Bence Jones proteinemia). However, the apparently free light chain may actually represent a component of a biclonal gammopathy in which the heavy chain arc is not detected on immunoelectrophoresis. The immunoelectrophoretic pattern of an IgG κ monoclonal protein is shown in Fig 2. The abnormality in the precipitin arc may occur anywhere from the slow γ region to the α_2-globulin region. A polyclonal increase of a single immunoglobulin often produces a rather localized thickening of the heavy chain arc, but there is no corresponding localized thickness of a single light chain because both κ and λ light chain arcs are increased.

In Waldenström's macroglobulinemia, IgM antiserum and κ or λ produce a dense localized arc (Fig 3). Sometimes the monoclonal IgM protein does not show an accompanying light chain abnormality, and thus misleadingly suggests μ heavy chain disease. Immunofixation is often helpful in this situation. An alternative is to add a reducing agent, such as dithiothreitol (DTT), and this often makes an IgM κ or IgM λ monoclonal protein identifiable.

The monoclonal protein may precipitate near

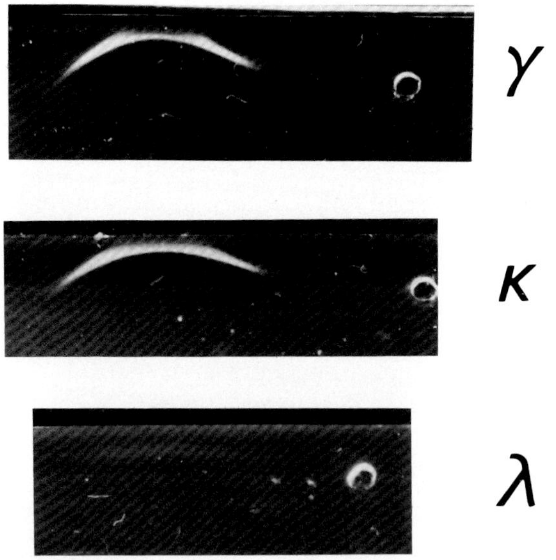

Fig 2. Immunoelectrophoretic pattern of serum. Top, antiserum to IgG (γ) shows a thickened arc; middle, antiserum to κ chains shows a thickened arc similar to the IgG arc; bottom, antiserum to λ chains shows a faint normal arc. The patient's serum contains a monoclonal IgG κ protein.

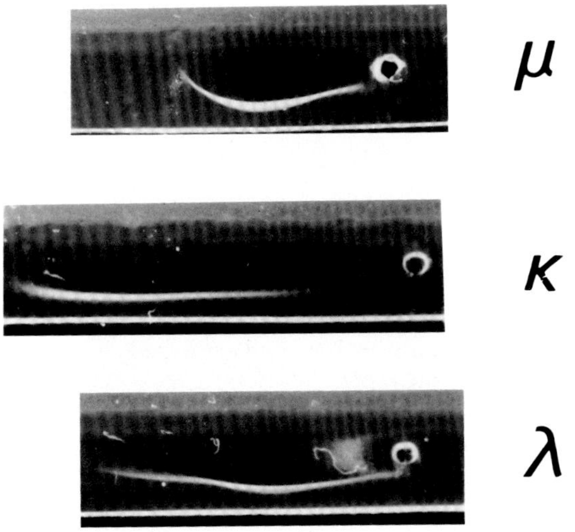

Fig 3. Serum immunoelectrophoretic pattern. Top, antiserum to IgM (μ) shows a thickened arc; middle, antiserum to κ chains shows a normal-appearing arc; bottom, antiserum to λ light chains shows bowing corresponding to the IgM arc. The patient's serum contains an IgM λ protein.

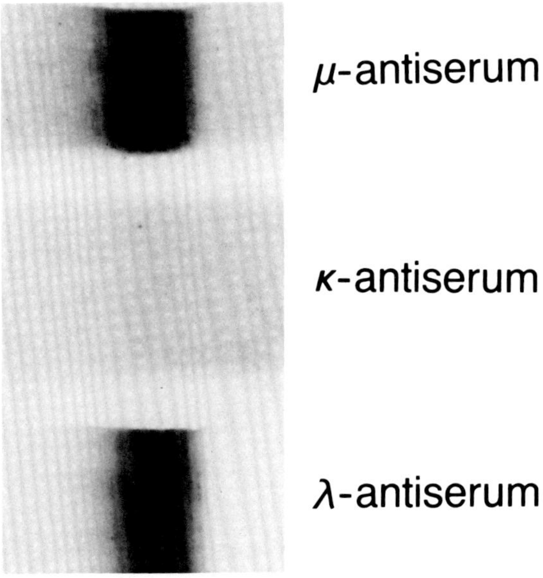

Fig 4. Serum immunofixation. Top, dense localized band with IgM (μ) antiserum; middle, no band with κ antiserum; bottom, dense band with λ antiserum corresponding to the IgM band. This patient has an IgM λ monoclonal protein.

the application well (euglobulin) and produce no diagnostic arcs. Repetition with a lower–ionic-strength buffer or addition of a reducing agent may resolve the problem. Immunofixation may also be useful.

Immunofixation

This technique is useful when results of immunoelectrophoresis are equivocal.[5] The appropriately diluted serum or concentrated urine sample is placed in a small trough in 1% agarose. Electrophoresis is performed, and, immediately afterward, cellulose acetate strips impregnated with monospecific antisera are placed over the electrophoresed protein. The strips are removed after incubation, excess protein is removed by washing in saline, and bands corresponding to an antigen-antibody complex remain. This is stained with Coomassie blue and read (Fig 4). A sharp, well-defined band of a single heavy chain class and light chain type is seen in monoclonal gammopathy, whereas broad, diffuse, heavily stained bands with heavy and light chain antisera are characteristic of a polyclonal gammopathy. Interpretation is sometimes difficult because overdilution of a serum sample will result in loss of the monoclonal band. However, inadequate dilution of a specimen may obscure the recognition of a small monoclonal heavy or light chain in a sample with a normal background of immunoglobulins, and it may produce a dense polyclonal band that may be misinterpreted as a monoclonal protein. Consequently, technical and interpretive expertise is necessary for the proper diagnosis.

Immunofixation is helpful when one suspects a monoclonal protein and finds only bowing of a single heavy chain or a single light chain on immunoelectrophoresis, especially in cases of monoclonal IgM protein in which the bowing of the light chain is often not apparent on immunoelectrophoresis. Immunofixation is also useful in detecting a small monoclonal protein in the presence of normal background immunoglobulins or a polyclonal increase in immunoglobulins. It is particularly advantageous in treated myeloma or macroglobulinemia, when one is looking for a small monoclonal serum protein after the band has disappeared on electrophoresis; in suspected amyloidosis, when one is trying to detect a small monoclonal protein; or in apparently solitary plasmacytoma or extramedullary plasmacytoma after treatment with radiation. It is also helpful in recognition of a biclonal gammopathy (Fig 5).

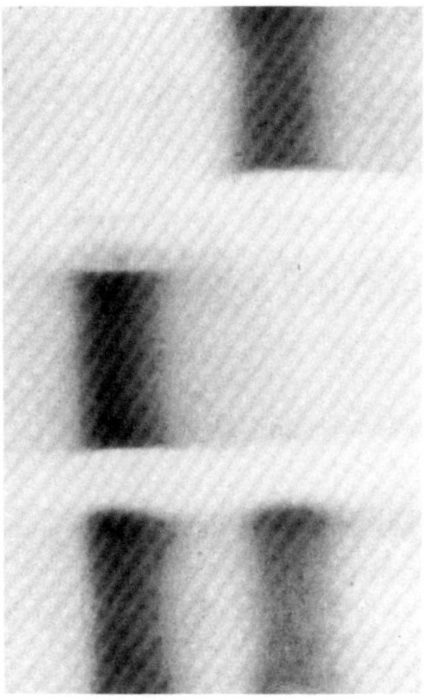

Fig 5. Immunofixation of serum. Top, dense band with IgG (γ) antiserum; middle, dense band with IgA (α) antiserum; bottom, two dense bands with κ antiserum. This patient has biclonal gammopathy (IgG κ and IgA κ).

Despite the advantages of immunofixation, immunoelectrophoresis is recommended as the initial procedure, because it is technically easier and the results generally are satisfactory. In addition, interpretation of immunofixation may be misleading, and one can overdiagnose or underdiagnose monoclonal proteins because the dilution of the serum or urine specimen is crucial.

A rate nephelometer using monospecific anti-κ and anti-λ antisera to identify the light chain component may be used to detect the light chain type of large monoclonal gammopathies. However, small monoclonal proteins will have a normal κ to λ ratio and consequently will not be recognized.[6]

Immunodiffusion (Ouchterlony)

All sera should be screened for the possibility of IgD or IgE monoclonal proteins. This screening is essential when bowing of the κ or the λ arc is seen on immunoelectrophoresis without an accompanying abnormality of the IgG, IgA, or IgM arcs. It is economical to screen the sera of all patients by Ouchterlony immunodiffusion, using antisera to IgD and IgE against each patient's serum. Dense precipitin bands form if the patient has an increased concentration of IgD or IgE. All sera forming a precipitin band are then studied further by immunoelectrophoresis with monospecific antisera to IgD or IgE as well as κ and λ. Because most sera do not produce a reaction on immunodiffusion, immunoelectrophoresis is not necessary.

Quantitation of Immunoglobulins

Quantitation of immunoglobulins is more useful than immunoelectrophoresis or immunofixation in the detection of hypogammaglobulinemia. Usually, quantitation is performed by radial immunodiffusion.[7]

The use of a rate nephelometer is practical for quantitation of immunoglobulins. In this system, the degree of turbidity produced by antigen-antibody interaction is measured by nephelometry in the near ultraviolet region. Because the method is not affected by molecular size of the antigen (as is radial immunodiffusion), the nephelometric technique measures 7S IgM, polymers of IgA, or aggregates of IgG accurately.

Serum Viscometry

Serum viscometry should be done in every case with >3 g/dL of IgM monoclonal protein or >4.0 g/dL of IgA or IgG protein and in any case of oronasal bleeding, blurred vision, or neurologic symptoms suggestive of a hyperviscosity syndrome. The Ostwald-100 viscometer is a satisfactory instrument for this purpose, but a Wells-Brookfield viscometer (Brookfield Engineering Laboratories, Stoughton, Mass) is preferred because it is more accurate, requires less serum (about 1.0 mL), and can perform at different shear rates and at different temperatures. In addition, determinations can be made much more rapidly, especially if the viscosity of the serum sample is high. Symptoms of hyperviscosity are rare unless the value is >4 centipoises. Some patients with a value of 10 centipoises or more do not have symptoms of hyperviscosity.

Cryoglobulins

The serum should be evaluated for the presence of cryoglobulins. Cryoglobulins are proteins that precipitate when cooled and dissolve when heated. Five milliliters of fresh, centrifuged serum kept at 37 °C are placed in a graduated centrifuge tube and incubated at 1 °C (in an ice bath in a refrigerator or cold room) for seven days. If a precipitate or gel is seen, the tube is centrifuged and the cryocrit read. The precipitate is washed in cold saline and then placed in a 37 °C water bath. Immunoelectrophoresis is performed on the resuspended cryoprecipitate with monospecific antisera to IgG, IgA, IgM, κ and λ.

In most cases, monoclonal cryoglobulins (type I) are IgM or IgG, but IgA and Bence Jones cryoglobulins have been reported. Surprisingly, many patients with large amounts of cryoglobulin are completely asymptomatic, whereas others with small monoclonal cryoglobulins in the range of 1 to 2 g/dL have pain, purpura, Raynaud's phenomenon, cyanosis, and even ulceration and sloughing of skin and subcutaneous tissues on exposure to cold. The temperature at which the cryoglobulin precipitates is much more important than the amount of protein.[8]

Cryoglobulinemia may produce a spurious elevation of the leukocyte count on the model S Coulter counter. This elevation is due to particles formed by combination of the cryoglobulin and fibrinogen.[9]

Most commonly, mixed cryoglobulins (type II) consist of IgM-IgG, but IgG-IgG and IgA-IgG combinations have been reported. Usually, the quantity of mixed cryoglobulin is <0.2 g/dL and may not reach maximal amounts for seven days. The serum protein electrophoretic pattern shows normality or diffuse hypergammaglobulinemia. Patients with mixed cryoglobulinemia frequently have vasculitis, glomerulonephritis, lymphoproliferative processes, hepatitis, or other chronic infections.[10]

ANALYSIS OF URINE FOR MONOCLONAL PROTEINS

When patients who have gammopathies are studied, analysis of urine is essential. The use of sulfosalicylic acid, or Exton's test, is best for the detection of protein.

Dipstick tests are used in many laboratories to screen for protein. However, they are often insensitive to Bence Jones protein and should not be used when the possibility of Bence Jones proteinuria exists.

Almost from the time of the discovery of the unique thermal properties of urinary light chains, screening tests for their detection have been in use. All have shortcomings, but the heat test of Putnam et al[11] is the simplest. Most, but not all, monoclonal light chains in the urine precipitate at 40 °C to 60 °C, dissolve at 100 °C, and reprecipitate on cooling to between 40 °C and 60 °C. Occasionally, the result of the heat test is positive even though the patient's urine reveals no sharp peak or localized globulin band on electrophoresis and no evidence of a single monoclonal light chain on immunoelectrophoresis. Such urine usually produces a broad-based γ band and normal-appearing κ and λ arcs. Presumably, the positive result of the test is due to an excess of polyclonal light chains. Such false-positive results occur most often in cases of renal insufficiency, connective tissue disease, or non-plasma-cell neoplastic diseases. However, the results of the Bence Jones heat test have been negative in some cases in which urinary electrophoresis has shown a dense globulin band or spike and immunoelectrophoresis has demonstrated a monoclonal light chain. It is obvious that the heat test for Bence Jones protein has many shortcomings and should not be used except as a rough screening procedure. The recognition of Bence Jones proteinuria depends on the demonstration of a monoclonal light chain by immunoelectrophoresis or immunofixation of an adequately concentrated urine specimen.

Electrophoresis

Electrophoresis, as well as immunoelectrophoresis or immunofixation, should be done in all instances of multiple myeloma, macroglobulinemia of Waldenström, amyloidosis, monoclonal gammopathy of undetermined significance, heavy chain diseases, or suspicion of these entities. Immunoelectrophoresis or immunofixation of urine should also be done in evaluation of older patients with an idiopathic nephrotic syndrome.

First, a 24-hour collection of urine must be made for determination of the total amount of protein excreted each day. This is important when following the course of a patient with a monoclonal light chain in the urine, because the amount of protein correlates directly with the size of the plasma cell burden. Then an aliquot of the 24-hour urine specimen must be concentrated to approximately 3 g/dL (Minicon-B15 concentrator, Amicon Corp, Lexington, Mass). Rarely, one specimen may be contaminated by another because of a leak in the concentrator.

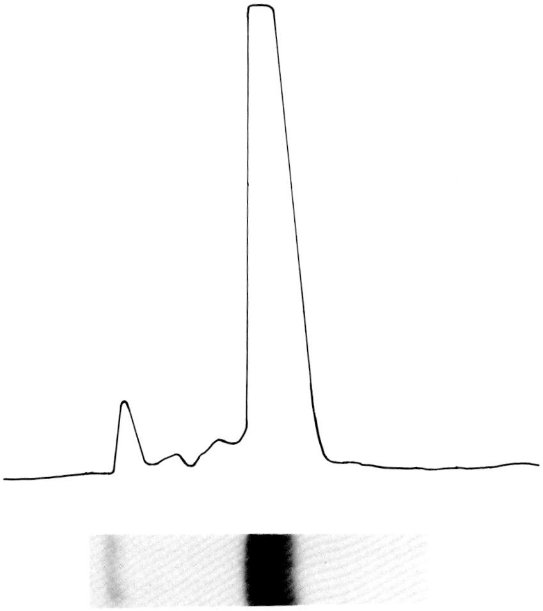

Fig 6. Monoclonal urine protein. Top, densitometer showing a tall, narrow-based peak of β mobility; bottom, cellulose acetate electrophoretic pattern showing a dense band of β mobility. This is consistent with a monoclonal urine protein (Bence Jones protein).

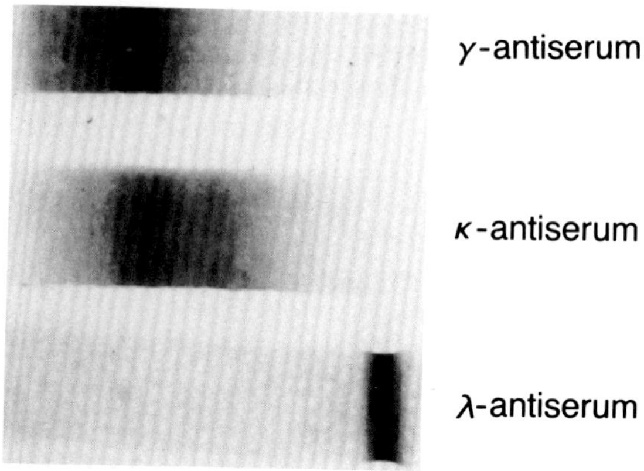

Fig 8. Immunofixation of urine. Top, normal-appearing band with IgG (γ) antiserum; middle, normal-appearing band with κ antiserum; bottom, dense, narrow band with λ antiserum. This patient has a monoclonal λ protein (Bence Jones protein).

A urinary monoclonal protein is seen as a dense, localized band on the cellulose strip or a tall, narrow, homogeneous peak on the densitometer tracing (Fig 6). Occasionally, two discrete globulin bands may be seen in the cellulose acetate tracing of the urine. These bands may be a monoclonal light chain plus a monoclonal immunoglobulin fragment from the serum, or they may be monomers and dimers of the monoclonal light chain. Therefore, immunoelectrophoresis or immunofixation with the appropriate heavy and light chain antisera is necessary. Rarely, two monoclonal light chains (κ and λ) have been noted in the urine.

A polyclonal increase of light chains is seen as a broad band extending through most of the γ region; and it has fuzzy, indistinct cathodal and anodal borders. The densitometer tracing is broad based, and immunoelectrophoresis shows both κ and λ arcs.

Immunoelectrophoresis

Immunoelectrophoresis establishes the presence or absence of light chains and determines whether they are monoclonal or polyclonal. It is not unusual to get a negative reaction for protein,

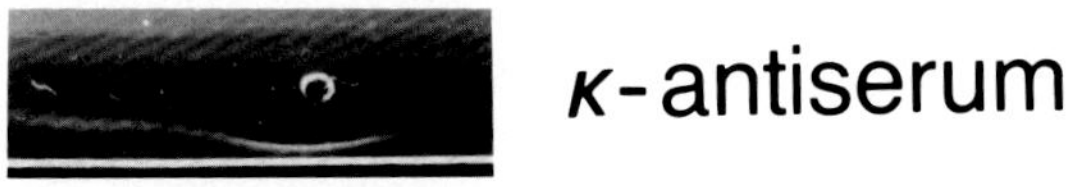

Fig 7. Immunoelectrophoresis of urine. Bowed arc with κ antiserum. This is indicative of a monoclonal κ protein (Bence Jones protein).

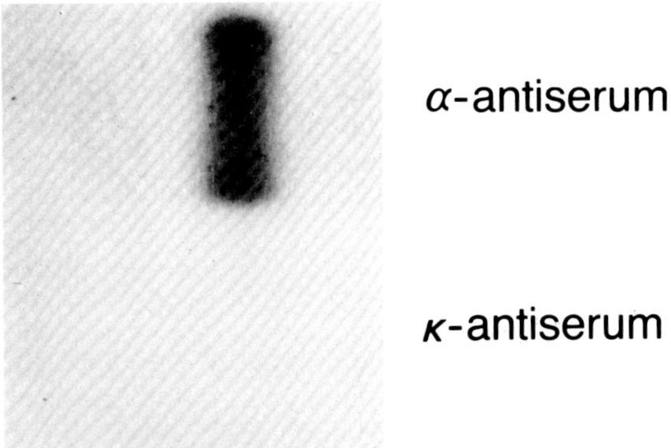

Fig 9. Immunofixation of urine. Top, narrow, localized band with IgA (α) antiserum; middle, no reaction with κ antiserum; bottom, two discrete bands with λ antiserum. This patient has a monoclonal λ protein plus an IgA λ fragment.

and immunoelectrophoresis of concentrated urine reveals a monoclonal light chain. In a number of cases in which electrophoresis of urine shows a large amount of albumin and insignificant amounts of globulin, the urine contains a monoclonal light chain. Most of these patients have primary systemic amyloidosis, although some have multiple myeloma or light chain deposition disease.[12] A monoclonal light chain in the urine is sometimes the first clue that the nephrotic syndrome is due to amyloidosis or related disorders. Immunoelectrophoresis should be done in all cases in which there is a sharp peak or band in the globulin region of the cellulose acetate tracing.

Immunoelectrophoresis of appropriately concentrated urine is performed with antisera to κ and λ and the appropriate heavy chain. If electrophoresis of the urine reveals a localized globulin spike but immunoelectrophoresis with κ and λ antisera does not demonstrate a monoclonal light chain, the presence of γ heavy chain disease should be suspected. Immunoelectrophoresis should then be done with antisera to IgG (γ heavy chains).

A monoclonal protein forms an arc with κ or λ antisera that is bowed locally or restricted (Fig 7), whereas a polyclonal increase of light chains causes elongation and fuzziness of both κ and λ arcs. In cases of renal insufficiency, faint, fuzzy, elongated κ and λ arcs are often seen, but if there is an underlying multiple myeloma or amyloidosis, an additional bowed or restricted arc with either κ or λ antisera may be seen.

Immunofixation

Immunofixation may be helpful in detecting monoclonal Bence Jones proteins and is more sensitive than immunoelectrophoresis (Fig 8).[13] Immunofixation is most helpful when a monoclonal light chain occurs in the presence of a polyclonal increase in light chains. It is also useful in detecting monoclonal heavy chains or fragments in the urine (Fig 9).

The need for collection of a 24-hour urine specimen cannot be overemphasized. Such a collection allows the amount of the monoclonal protein excreted in the urine to be measured, and this value is a reliable indication of the effect of chemotherapy or evidence of progression of the disease and is also very useful in following the course of a patient who has amyloidosis and the nephrotic syndrome.

For demonstrating a monoclonal protein in the urine, electrophoresis and either immunoelectrophoresis or immunofixation of an adequately concentrated aliquot from a 24-hour specimen are the appropriate techniques.

REFERENCES

1. Reichert CM, Everett DF Jr, Nadler PI, et al: High-resolution zone electrophoresis, combined with immunofixation, in the detection of an occult myeloma paraprotein. Clin Chem 28:2312–2313, 1982

2. Kyle RA, Greipp PR: Immunoglobulins and laboratory recognition of monoclonal proteins, in Wiernik PH, Canellos GP, Kyle RA, et al (eds): Neoplastic Diseases of the Blood, vol 1. New York, Churchill Livingstone, 1985, p 431

3. Kyle RA, Robinson RA, Katzmann JA: The clinical aspects of biclonal gammopathies: Review of 57 cases. Am J Med 71:999–1008, 1981

4. Garrison CP, Deegan MJ, Conn RB: Undetected IgM paraproteins on serum protein electrophoresis. Am J Clin Pathol 75:553–557, 1981

5. Ritchie RF, Smith R: Immunofixation. III. Application to the study of monoclonal proteins. Clin Chem 22:1982–1985, 1976

6. Deegan MJ, Perry M, Hayashi H: A rapid method for identifying the light chain component of a monoclonal protein. Blood 66:186a, 1985 (suppl 1) (abstr)

7. Fahey JL, McKelvey EM: Quantitative determination of serum immunoglobulins in antibody-agar plates. J Immunol 94:84–90, 1965

8. Letendre L, Kyle RA: Monoclonal cryoglobulinemia with high thermal insolubility. Mayo Clin Proc 57:629–633, 1982

9. Luzar MJ, Camisa C, Neff JC: Essential mixed cryoglobulinemia (type II) with pseudoleukocytosis. Arthritis Rheum 27:353–355, 1984

10. Gorevic PD, Kassab HJ, Levo Y, et al: Mixed cryoglobulinemia: Clinical aspects and long-term follow-up of 40 patients. Am J Med 69:287–308, 1980

11. Putnam FW, Easley CW, Lynn LT, et al: The heat precipitation of Bence-Jones proteins. I. Optimum conditions. Arch Biochem Biophys 83:115–130, 1959

12. Fang LST: Light-chain nephropathy. Kidney Int 27:582–592, 1985

13. Whicher JT, Hawkins L, Higginson J: Clinical applications of immunofixation: A more sensitive technique for the detection of Bence Jones protein. J Clin Pathol 33:779–780, 1980

Chemotherapy of Previously Untreated Multiple Myeloma Patients: An Analysis of Recent Treatment Results

Jonathan R. Sporn and O. Ross McIntyre

OVER THE LAST few years, several large studies testing various chemotherapeutic regimens in previously untreated patients with multiple myeloma have been reported. A number of these have been discussed in published reviews.[1,2,3] During this same interval there have been advances in our understanding of factors important in determining the prognosis for newly diagnosed patients. Durie's report in this issue of the *Seminars* provides a detailed review of this subject.

This report describes the results of several studies testing various regimens for the initial treatment of myeloma patients. We also offer some observations on the natural history of the disease and attempt to relate these to the decision regarding treatment. Therapy for the advanced or refractory patient with myeloma is discussed in the review by Kyle et al in this issue.

CLINICAL AND BIOLOGIC FACTORS INFLUENCING TREATMENT OUTCOME

The clinical stage of the disease at presentation correlates well with duration of response and survival. It should be noted, however, that other factors may be important in determining treatment outcome and survival. We have pointed out[4] that response to treatment is a more important determinant of survival than initial tumor stage, and that the character and amount of tumor products elaborated may determine disease complications and outcome quite independently of tumor load.

Feinstein pointed out that the duration of the preclinical phase of the tumor predicts the survival subsequent to the clinical recognition and treatment.[5] This characteristic of neoplasia as applied to multiple myeloma explains the different presentations and outcomes of the disease ranging from those presenting with smoldering[6] or indolent disease[7] to those with rapidly progressive disease including the leukemic variants. Joshua et al[8] have suggested that "stable disease" as defined by a low labeling index or by the presence of isotype suppression of surface immunoglobulin on peripheral blood lymphocytes and the presence of increased suppressor T cells in the peripheral blood[9] defines a population of myeloma patients who may not need initial treatment irrespective of stage.

With the increased availability of information on the labeling index or DNA content in myeloma cells provided by cytofluorographic techniques[10] it may soon be possible to characterize this important parameter in most patients at the time of presentation. If such measurements are shown to correlate with disease activity, they may supplant the period of observation that many hematologists use to assess the rate of disease progression in patients who present without hypercalcemia, azotemia, pancytopenia, or threatening pathologic fracture.

Although a number of patients present with indolent disease or are diagnosed incidental to their routine checkups or care of other medical conditions, at least an equal number of myeloma patients present with critical complicatons of advanced disease. These patients do not often appear in reports of clinical trials, which may exclude patients who are not expected to survive the first several weeks of treatment. As one reviews the various reports of treatment it is important to devote some attention to the fraction of patients succumbing to disease during the early weeks of the study. The number of early deaths from disease alone, before any contribution of treatment-related toxicity, is a good measure of the severity of illness of those entered in the study.

In evaluating the efficacy of a given treatment regimen, criteria employed for the assessment of response must be carefully considered. A reduction of serum or urine M protein subsequent to treatment is generally used as objective evidence

From the Dartmouth Hitchcock Medical Center, Hanover, NH.

Supported in part by Grants CA 04326 and CA 23108, from the National Cancer Institute and by Scholar Grant 140 from the American Cancer Society.

Address reprint requests to O. Ross McIntyre, MD, Norris Cotton Cancer Center, Hanover, NH 03756.

0093-7754/86/1303-0008$05.00/0

for a tumor response. One should not dismiss the possibility that therapy, especially with corticosteroids, could change the rate of catabolism of M protein without effecting production. In addition, non-M-protein secreting myeloma clones may emerge during treatment, so that even a marked reduction in M protein does not always correspond to a reduction in tumor load. Many studies report objective responses according to the criteria developed by the Chronic Leukemia-Myeloma Task Force in 1973.[11] In brief, these criteria define an objective response as a 50% or greater reduction in serum M protein concentration; 50% or greater reduction in urinary M protein excretion; more than a 50% decrease in the cross sectional area of a plasmacytoma, or recalcification of bone lesions without the appearance of new lesions. The Southwest Oncology Group (SWOG) has defined an objective response as a 75% reduction in the *production* of myeloma protein.[12] A nomogram relating the serum concentration of IgG M protein to the synthetic index has been prepared that facilitates the calculation of changes in M protein production.[13] This is necessary because the fractional catabolic rate for IgG increases as plasma IgG concentrations increase until the half-life reaches a lower limit of about 11 days as shown in Fig 1.[14] In practice, however, there may be little difference in the percentage of objective responses as defined by the two methods. For instance, Bergsagel has compared the frequency of objective responses as measured for previously untreated patients receiving melphalan and prednisone in eight series, five of which used SWOG criteria and three of which used Myeloma Task Force criteria for response measurement.[2] Responses were observed in 32% to 53% of patients in series using SWOG criteria and in 33% to 56% using Task Force Criteria.

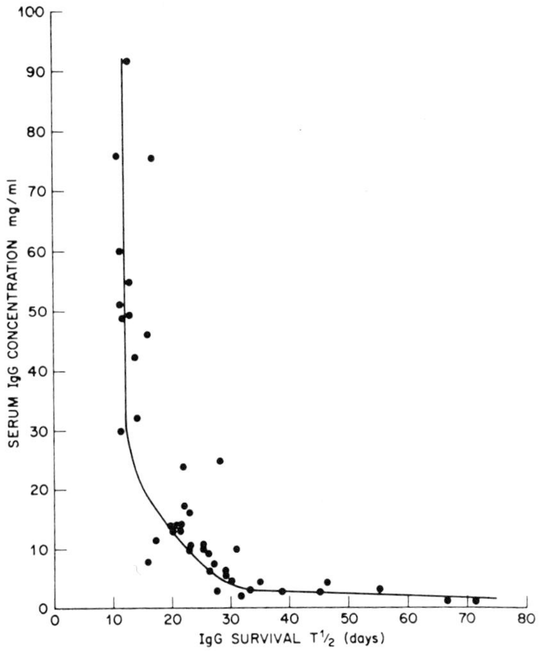

Fig 1. The relationship between the survival half time of IgG and the serum IgG concentration obtained from turnover studies performed in patients with a wide range of IgG concentrations. Reprinted with permission from S. Karger and A.G. Basel.[14]

The quality of supportive care may also influence the outcome of therapy. An analysis of the results of the several melphalan prednisone regimens included as control arms of Cancer and Leukemia Group B (CALGB) protocols from 1972 to 1977 shows progressive improvement in patient survival during this interval.[15] This suggests that supportive therapy, or our ability to apply it to the benefit of the patient, has improved over this period.

ALKYLATING AGENTS AND PREDNISONE

The activity of phenylalanine mustard in myeloma was reported by Blokhin et al in 1958.[16] These results were extended by the report of 165 patients treated with melphalan (L-phenylalanine mustard) by Bergsagel et al in 1962.[17] Shortly thereafter, Korst et al[18] reported the effectiveness of cyclophosphamide in myeloma. When prednisone was added to either melphalan or cyclophosphamide, improved responses were seen as indicated in Table 1. It is important to emphasize that corticosteroids alone produce short-term responses in up to 44% of good risk patients with myeloma.[26]

For the most part, melphalan and prednisone schedules have been of two general types in the various reported series. Intermittent schedules have been most popular but differ in amount and frequency of drug administration as shown in Table 2. Daily treatment after the nadir of cell counts produced by a loading dose of melphalan has been used by the CALGB. As may be seen from Table 1 there is little difference in response or survival on these schedules.

Although the risk of developing acute non-

Table 1. Results of Treatment-Early Series

Author	Treatment	No. of Patients	Percent Responding M Protein*	Median Survival (Months)
Feinleib[19]	None (retrospective)	214	NA	10
Holland et al[20]	Placebo	15	0	12
	Urethane (oral)	15	0	5
Bergsagel et al[17]	Melphalan	165	14	25
Korst et al[18]	Cyclophosphamide	207	—	24
Hoogstraten et al[21]	Melphalan (daily)	64	45b	23
Hoogstraten et al[22]	Melphalan (intermittent)	48	45b	26
Alexanian et al[23]	Melphalan (daily)	31	19c	18
	Melphalan (intermittent)	63	73c	18
Costa et al[24]	Melphalan (daily)			
	good risk	35	20c	30
	poor risk	25	16c	21
	Total	60		26
	Melphalan (daily) plus prednisone			
	good risk	42	43c	53
	poor risk	29	31c	9
	Total	71		35
	Melphalan (daily), prednisone and testosterone			
	good risk	37	46c	36
	poor risk	21	33c	4
	Total	58		24
Medical Research Council[25]	Cyclophosphamide	124	—	20
	Melphalan intermittent	128	—	20
	Melphalan intermittent plus prednisone	120	—	20
McIntyre et al[26]	Prednisone (good risk)	32	44c	21

Abbreviation: NA, not applicable.
*Percent achieving M protein response as defined: b, 2 g/dL decrease; c, Myeloma Task Force Criteria.[11]
Adapted from McIntyre[26a] with permission.

lymphocytic leukemia is probably increased in patients with multiple myeloma as evidenced by the occurrence of patients in whom the two diagnoses are made simultaneously, it is clear that standard alkylating-agent therapy substantially increases that risk.[31,32] The actuarial risk of developing leukemia by 50 months of treatment in one series was 17%.[33] It has been suggested that bolus (intravenous [IV]) administration of melphalan may be associated with a lower risk of leukemia, at least during the early years of treatment, when compared with daily oral or intermittent 4 to 6 day courses of the drug.[34] This observation requires further confirmation.

COMBINATION THERAPY

Table 3 summarizes the results of selected clinical trials, including tests of combination therapy, that have been carried out over the last several years. The rationale for the use of combined therapy is based upon the hypothesis that nonoverlapping drug toxicities and lack of cross resistance to the drugs used in the combination would allow for greater tumor cytoreduction

Table 2. Various MP Schedules Used in Selected Series

Author	Melphalan Dose	Prednisone Dose
Alexanian et al[23]	0.25 mg/kg/d × 4 every 6 wks	1 mg/kg every MWF, 1 mg/kg/d × 4 (+4 d taper)
Harley et al[27]	0.15 mg/kg/d × 7, then 0.05 mg/kg/d when counts rise	1.2 mg/kg/d × 4 (not to exceed 100 mg), 8 d taper
Salmon et al[28]	8 mg/m² orally d 1–4 every 3 wks	60 mg/m² orally d 1–4
Medical Research Council[29]	10 mg/d × 7 orally every 3 wks	40/mg/d × 7
Cornwell et al[30]	0.15 mg/kg/d × 7, then 0.05 mg/kg continuous when counts rise	0.8 mg/kg/d × 14 (not to exceed 100 mg), 6 wk taper

Abbreviation: MWF, Monday, Wednesday, Friday.

Table 3. Selected Results of Treatment—Combination Therapy

Author	Treatment	No. of Patients	Percent Responding	Median Survival (months)
Alexanian et al[35]	melphalan, doxorubicin, prednisone	67	46*	≈24†
	melphalan, cyclophosphamide, prednisone	74	47*	≈24†
	cyclophosphamide, doxorubicin, prednisone	59	39*	≈24†
	melphalan, cyclophosphamide, BCNU, prednisone	70	49*	30^{+}
	vincristine, cyclophosphamide, doxorubicin, prednisone	74	57*	30^{+}
	vincristine, melphalan, cyclophosphamide, prednisone	77	62*	30^{+}
Case et al[36]	melphalan, prednisone, cyclophosphamide, BCNU, vincristine	73	87*	50^{+}
Oken et al[37]	melphalan, prednisone (intermittent)	131	53‡	29.3
	melphalan, prednisone, cyclophosphamide, BCNU, vincristine	134	74‡	33.4
	melphalan (daily) prednisone (tapering)			
Harley et al[27,38]	good risk	62	57‡	38
	poor risk	64	55‡	12
	IV melphalan, cyclophosphamide carmustine, prednisone (tapering)			
	good risk	71	70‡	30
	poor risk	53	64‡	24
Bergsagel et al[33]	melphalan (intermittent), prednisone followed by BCNU, cyclophosphamide on relapse	125	70*	24
	melphalan (oral), cyclophosphamide, BCNU, prednisone (intermittent)	116	72*	
	melphalan (oral), prednisone, cyclophosphamide, BCNU (alternating)	123	68*	30
Abramson et al[39]	melphalan (intermittent), prednisone	72	43‡	24.6
	BCNU, cyclophosphamide, prednisone	70	50‡	18.8
Pavlovsky et al[40]	semustine, cyclophosphamide, melphalan, vincristine, prednisone	105	46‡	41
	melphalan (intermittent), prednisone	129	38‡	39
Medical Research Council[56]	cyclophosphamide IV every 3 wks	71§	—	7
	cyclophosphamide (oral), melphalan (oral), lomustine (oral) and prednisone	61§	—	7
Cornwell et al[30]	melphalan (oral daily or IV), prednisone (tapering)	295		
	vincristine/prednisone every 28 d at wk 22	188	55‡¶	
	BCNU or lomustine, prednisone tapering	262		
	vincristine/prednisone every 28 d at wk 22	110	48‡¶	
Salmon et al[28]	melphalan/prednisone (intermittent)	77	32*	23
	alternating combinations (VMCP + VCAP, VMCP + VBAP) see text for schedule	160	54*	43
Alexanian et al[42]	melphalan/prednisone (intermittent)	30	53*	36
	alternating combinations (VMCP + VCAP, VMCP + VBAP) see text for schedule	76	57*	27
Cooper et al[15]	melphalan IV/prednisone (tapering)	146	47‡	34
	melphalan, BCNU, cyclophosphamide (all IV), prednisone (tapering)	148	56‡	29
	melphalan, carmustine, cyclophosphamide (all IV), doxorubicin 3 wks following, prednisone (tapering)	157	44‡	26
	melphalan, BCNU, cyclophosphamide (all IV, in sequence), prednisone (tapering)	140	47‡	22

*SWOG criteria.[12]

†Mid-range of curve taken.

‡Myeloma Task Force criteria.[11]

§Azotemic patients only.

¶Percent responders after week 22.

than would occur in single agent treatment. This hypothesis is demonstrably correct in experimental mouse myeloma[43] and initial results in humans suggested that a number of myeloma patients did not develop cross resistance to alkylating agents.[44] However, when more stringent definitions of alkylating-agent resistance are used, the fraction of patients demonstrating non-cross-resistance falls.[45] Nevertheless, several of the clinical trials reported in the last few years emphasize comparisons of various combinations of agents.

In CALGB protocol 7261 patients were treated with either oral melphalan/prednisone (MP) or with IV melphalan, carmustine (BCNU), cyclophosphamide, and prednisone.[27,38] This study demonstrated that poor risk or high tumor-cell load patients had improved responses and survival if randomized to receive the combined IV alkylating-agent treatment.

SWOG protocol 7704 randomized patients to MP administered every 3 weeks or a combination consisting of vincristine, melphalan, cyclophosphamide and prednisone (VMCP) alternating with vincristine, cyclophosphamide, doxorubicin and prednisone (VCAP), or to a regimen in which three cycles of VMCP were followed by three cycles of vincristine, carmustine, doxorubicin, and prednisone (VBAP).[28] The overall response rates were 32% for MP and 54% for the alternating combinations. Median survivals were 23 and 43 months, respectively. However, for those achieving a response, the median duration of remission (30 months) was not influenced by the regimen used to produce the response. The beneficial effect of combination therapy appeared to be displayed principally in the 70% of patients with high tumor loads since response rates were similar for patients with stage I and II disease. Bergsagel has commented upon the possibility that the MP dose schedule (every 3 weeks instead of the more usual every 6 weeks) used in this protocol may have adversely influenced the outcome of treatment on this arm of the study.[2]

A similar trial of alternating combination therapy using the same agents used in SWOG 7704 was reported by Alexanian and Dreicer.[42] In contrast to the results cited above, these investigators report a 53% response rate in the 30 patients treated with MP *v* 55% response rate for the 42 patients assigned to alternating VMCP/VCAP, and a 60% response rate for 34 patients receiving alternating VMCP for three doses followed by VBAP for three doses. Median survival for patients administered the alternating combinations were $<$30 months in this study. Despite the findings on these randomized patients, the authors combined their results with the results of other studies carried out over several years and concluded that combination regimens containing combined alkylating agents plus doxorubicin and vincristine produce improved response rates.

Neither high nor intermediate and low tumor-cell load patients randomized to receive combination alkylating-agent therapy in the trial reported by Canadian investigators showed a response or survival advantage.[33] Similar patients treated with combined alkylating agents in the Medical Research Council's trial also failed to show an advantage for combined therapy.[56] A pilot study in which MP, MP plus BCNU, and VCAP were alternated every three cycles yielded a median survival of only 26 months despite the induction of a complete response in 17% of the 35 patients.[46]

The best reported results of combined therapy are those based upon the M-2 protocol developed by investigators at Memorial Sloan Kettering.[36] This regimen contains vincristine in addition to BCNU, melphalan, cyclophosphamide, and prednisone. In this nonrandomized study a response rate of 87% and a median survival of 50 months were reported. Others using similar programs reported comparable response and survival statistics.[47,48,49]

It should be noted that these good results were obtained in nonrandomized studies. When the five-drug combination used in the M-2 protocol was compared with the combination of melphalan and prednisone alone in a randomized study by the Eastern Cooperative Oncology Group, objective responses were seen in 74% of those receiving the M-2 regimen and in 53% of those receiving the two drug program. The median survival, however, did not differ at 33 and 29 months, respectively.[37] In a randomized multicenter study conducted in Denmark, there was no difference in response or survival for patients randomized to MP, MP/vincristine, or to the five-drug M-2 regimen,[55] (differences in the various schedules tested as "M-2" therapy are summarized in Table 4). In another randomized study (in which MeCCNU was substituted for BCNU in the M-2 regimen) patients receiv-

Table 4. Dosages Used in M-2 Protocol—Various Series

Drug	Case et al[36]	Case et al[49]	Oken et al[37]	Tirelli et al[47]	Hansen et al[55]
Melphalan	0.25 mg/kg × d 1-4*	0.25 mg/kg d 1-4	8 mg/m² d 1-4	0.25 mg/kg d 1-4	0.10 mg/kg × d 1-7†
Prednisone	1 mg/kg d 1-7‡	1 mg/kg d 1-7	60 mg/m² d 1-4	1 mg/kg/d × 7§	0.6 mg/kg d 1-14‖
Vincristine	0.03 mg/kg d 1	0.03 mg/kg d 1	1.2 mg/m² d 1	0.03 mg/kg d 21	0.03 mg/kg d 1
BCNU	0.5 mg/kg d 1	1 mg/kg d 1	20 mg/m² d 1	0.5 mg/kg/d 1	0.5 mg/kg d 1
Cyclophosphamide	10 mg/kg d 1	10 mg/kg d 1	400 mg/m² d 1	10 mg/kg d 1	10 mg/kg d 1

*Or 0.1 mg/kg d 1-7.
†Given every 5 wks.
‡0.5 mg/kg d 7-14, continue as necessary.
§Tapered until d 21.
‖Reduced to 0.3 mg/kg in subsequent courses.

ing the five-drug regimen failed to respond significantly better or survive longer than patients treated with MP alone.[40]

The contribution made by vincristine to any of the above combination chemotherapy schedules is unclear because the combined alkylating-agent schedules have never been concurrently tested with and without vincristine. Information on this point is contributed by several studies, however. The Medical Research Council randomized 530 previously untreated patients to receive a standard MP treatment with or without the addition of vincristine as the only variable.[41] In this trial there was no significant difference in the survival of the two groups. In the Danish trial, mentioned previously, a trend toward improved survival in the group randomized to vincristine in addition to MP did not achieve statistical significance.[55] In a sequential study of the SWOG, the addition of vincristine to a MP/procarbazine schedule did not improve response or survival.[50]

In CALGB protocol 7461 a two-step randomization assigned patients to treatment with one of four alkylating agent regimens (IV melphalan, oral melphalan, BCNU, or CCNU, all with a tapering course of prednisone) followed by a randomization at 22 weeks to continued alkylating agent alone or to the alkylating agent plus pulses of vincristine and prednisone every 8 weeks.[30] The initial analysis of this trial showed no response or survival advantage from the addition of vincristine/prednisone at week 22. Recently, an analysis of data, after an additional 3 years of follow-up and with the inclusion of an additional 195 patients assigned to IV melphalan, has been conducted.[51] This shows a significant increase in responses and survival for the group randomized to receive treatment with melphalan plus vincristine/prednisone, but not for those assigned to nitrosourea plus vincristine/prednisone. The contribution of vincristine to the results in this study cannot be determined since a portion, or all, of the effect could have been due to prednisone which was given concomitantly.

CALGB protocol 7761 randomized patients to one of four regimens: IV melphalan; a combination of IV melphalan, cyclophosphamide, and BCNU; a combination of IV melphalan, cyclophosphamide, and BCNU followed by doxorubicin administered 3 weeks after the combination; and IV melphalan, cyclophosphamide, and BCNU administered sequentially. All patients received the same tapering course of prednisone.[15] The response rate (44% to 56%) and toxicity was similar for all regimens, although the nadir of cytopenia was reached sooner in those receiving IV melphalan. The survival was significantly worse for those patients receiving the alkylating agents in sequence (median, 1.8 years for the sequence, 2.2 for the combination plus doxorubicin, 2.4 for the combination, and 2.8 for the IV melphalan). High tumor-cell load patients who were azotemic and received MP or the IV combination of melphalan, cyclophosphamide and BCNU survived better than those assigned to the other regimens.

Although occasional complete responses measured by disappearance of serum and/or urinary M-protein are found in patients treated with any of the above described programs, even these patients would probably demonstrate residual monoclonal protein levels if sophisticated tests with antibodies to M-protein idiotype were used. The calculated cell kill in most patients is <1 log, which is insufficient cell kill in most patients to produce long-term remissions. Newer therapeutic approaches are discussed by Kyle et al in this issue of the *Seminars*.

MAINTENANCE THERAPY

In view of the leukemogenic potential and other undesirable side effects of continued alkylating therapy, some recommend that treatment be discontinued after maximum tumor reduction. Several series have now shown no advantage to continuing treatment beyond this point and have indicated that 40% to 60% of relapsing patients will respond to additional therapy following disease progression.[52,53,42,29] If therapy is stopped, it is important that patients be observed closely for signs of recrudescent disease. Some patients in these series have relapsed and died of their disease without additional treatment. Obviously, careful follow-up of patients in unmaintained remission is imperative.

PERSPECTIVE

Although major strides have been made in the treatment of multiple myeloma, the median survival for patients randomized to current first line treatment protocols is only 30 to 40 months. The discovery of new agents with improved toxic therapeutic ratios will be necessary to produce additional significant advances in the treatment of this disease.

For the present, the introduction of new agents, including interferon (as described in this issue), to conventional treatment programs will be the major direction in which investigation will flow. For previously untreated patients with low or intermediate tumor loads, combination chemotherapy has not been shown to improve response or survival. Even for patients with high tumor loads, who in some series appear to have improved responses to combination therapy, there is no convincing evidence that combination therapy consistently improves responses or extends survival. Therefore, the complexity, cost, and side effects of multiple-agent treatment should be balanced against the results of simpler and less expensive therapy given with full attention to supportive care. The entry of newly diagnosed patients on the various investigations underway in single institutions and cooperative groups is encouraged.

REFERENCES

1. McIntyre OR: Myeloma, in Calabresi P, Schein PS, Rosenberg SA (eds): Medical Oncology. New York, Macmillan, 1985, pp 496–522
2. Bergsagel DE: Controversies in the treatment of plasma cell myeloma. Postgrad Med J 61:109–116, 1985
3. Woodruff R: Treatment of multiple myeloma. Cancer Treat Rev 8:225–270, 1981
4. McIntyre OR: Current concepts in cancer: Multiple myeloma. New Engl J Med 301:193–196, 1979
5. Feinstein AR: A new staging system for cancer and reappraisal of "early" treatment and "cure" by radical surgery. New Engl J Med 279:747–753, 1968
6. Kyle RA, Greipp PR: Smoldering multiple myeloma. New Engl J Med 302:1347–1349, 1980
7. Alexanian R: Localized and indolent myeloma. Blood 56:521–525, 1980
8. Joshua DE, Wearne A, and Kronenberg H: Indication for therapy in multiple myeloma: Should it be stage or stability. Lancet 2: 210, 1985
9. Wearne A, Joshua DE, Kronenberg H: Light chain isotype associated suppression of surface immunoglobulin expression on peripheral blood lymphocytes in myeloma during plateau phase. Br J Haematol 58:483–89, 1984
10. Witzig TE, Greipp PR, Gonchoroff NJ, et al: Peripheral blood B cell labelling indices are a measure of disease activity in plasma cell disorders. Blood 66:193a, 1985 (suppl 1)
11. Chronic Leukemia-Myeloma Task Force: Proposed guidelines for protocol studies. II. Plasma cell myeloma. Cancer Treat Rep 4:145–158, 1973
12. Alexanian R, Gehan E, Bonnet J, et al: Combination chemotherapy for multiple myeloma. Cancer 30:382–389, 1972
13. Salmon SE: Immunoglobulin synthesis and tumor kinetics of multiple myeloma. Semin Hematol 10:135–147, 1973
14. Waldmann TA, Strober W: Metabolism of immunoglobulins. Prog Allergy 13:1–110, 1969
15. Cooper MR, McIntyre OR, Anderson K, et al: Single sequential and multiple alkylating agent therapy for multiple myeloma: A CALGB study: J Clin Oncol, 1986 (in press)
16. Blokhin N, Larionov LF, Perevodchikova NI, et al: Clinical experiences with sarcolysin in neoplastic disease. Ann NY Acad Sci 68:1128–1132, 1958
17. Bergsagel DE, Sprague CC, Austin C, et al: Evaluation of new chemotherapeutic agents in the treatment of multiple myeloma IV: L-phenylalanine mustard. Cancer Chemother Rep 21:87–99, 1962
18. Korst DR, Clifford GO, Fowler WM, et al: Multiple myeloma. II. Analysis of cyclophosphamide therapy in 165 patients. JAMA 189:758–762, 1964
19. Feinleib M, MacMahon B: Duration of survival in multiple myeloma. J Natl Cancer Inst 24:1259–1269, 1960
20. Holland JF, Hosley H, Scharlau C, et al: A controlled trial of urethane treatment in multiple myeloma. Blood 27:328–342, 1966

21. Hoogstraten B, Sheehe PR, Cuttner J, et al: Melphalan in multiple myeloma. Blood 30:74–83, 1967

22. Hoogstraten B, Costa J: Intermittent melphalan therapy in multiple myeloma. JAMA 209:251–253, 1969

23. Alexanian R, Haut A, Khan AU, et al: Treatment for multiple myeloma. JAMA 208:1680–1685, 1969

24. Costa G, Engle RL Jr, Schilling A, et al: Melphalan and prednisone: An effective combination for the treatment of multiple myeloma. Am J Med 54:589–599, 1973

25. Medical Research Council's Working Party on Leukemia in Adults: Report on the second myelomatosis trial after five years of followup. Br J Cancer 42:813–822, 1980

26. McIntyre OR, Pajak TF, Kyle RA, et al: Response rates and survival in myeloma patients receiving prednisone alone. Med Pediatr Oncol 13:239–243, 1985

26a. McIntyre OR: Myeloma, in Calabresi P, Schein PS, Rosenberg SA (eds): Medical Oncology. New York, Macmillan, 1985, pp 496–522

27. Harley JB, McIntyre OR, Pajak TF: Improved survival of poor risk myeloma patients receiving combination alkylating agent therapy. Blood 50:192, 1977 (abstr)

28. Salmon SE, Haut A, Bonnet JD, et al: Alternating combination chemotherapy and levamisole improves survival in multiple myeloma: A SWOG study. J Clin Oncol 1:453–461, 1983

29. Medical Research Council Working Party on Leukemia in Adults: Treatment comparisons in the third MRC myelomatosis trial. Br J Cancer 42:823–830, 1980

30. Cornwell GG III, Pajak TF, Kochwa S, et al: Comparison of oral melphalan, CCNU and BCNU with and without vincristine and prednisone in the treatment of multiple myeloma: Cancer and Leukemia Group experience. Cancer 50:1669–1675, 1982

31. Kyle RA, Pierre RV, and Bayard ED: Multiple myeloma and acute myelomonocytic leukemia. N Engl J Med 283:1121–1125, 1970

32. Rosner F, Grunwald H: Multiple myeloma terminating in acute leukemia. Am J Med 57:927–939, 1974

33. Bergsagel DE, Bailey AJ, Langley GR, et al: The chemotherapy of plasma-cell myeloma and the incidence of acute leukemia. N Engl J Med 301:743–748, 1979

34. McIntyre OR, Pajak TF, Wiernik P, et al: Delayed acute leukemia in myeloma patients receiving pulsed vs. continuous treatment. Blood 58:167, 1981 (suppl)

35. Alexanian R, Salmon S, Bonnet J, et al: Combination therapy for multiple myeloma. Cancer 40:2765–2771, 1977

36. Case DC, Lee BJ III, Clarkson BD: Improved survival times in multiple myeloma treated with melphalan, prednisone, cyclophosphamide, vincristine and BCNU: M2 protocol. Am J Med 63:897–903, 1977

37. Oken MM, Tsiatis A, Abramson N, Glick J: Comparison of standard MP with intensive VBMCP therapy for the treatment of multiple myeloma (MM). Proc Am Soc Clin Oncol 3:270, 1984 (abstr)

38. Harley JB, Pajak TF, McIntyre OR, et al: Improved survival of increased-risk myeloma patients on combined triple alkylating agent therapy: A study of the CALGB. Blood 54:13–22, 1979

39. Abramson N, Lurie P, Mietlowski WL, et al: Phase III study of intermittent carmustine (BCNU) cyclophosphamide and prednisone versus melphalan and prednisone in multiple myeloma. Cancer Treat Rep 66:1273–1277, 1982

40. Pavlovsky S, Saslavsky J, Pinto MT, et al: A randomized trial of melphalan and prednisone versus melphalan, prednisone, cyclophosphamide, MeCCNU and vincristine in untreated multiple myeloma. J Clin Oncol 2:836–840, 1984

41. Medical Research Council's Working Party on Leukemia in Adults: Objective evaluation of the role of vincristine in induction and maintenance therapy for myelomatosis. Br J Cancer 52:153–158, 1985

42. Alexanian R, Dreicer R: Chemotherapy for Multiple Myeloma. Cancer 53:583–588, 1984

43. Ogawa M, Bergsagel D, McCulloch E: Chemotherapy of mouse myeloma: Quantitative cell cultures predictive of response in vivo. Blood 41:7–15, 1973

44. Bergsagel DE, Cowan DH, Hasselback R: Plasma cell myeloma: Response of melphalan-resistant patients to high-dose cyclophosphamide. Can Med Assoc J 107:851–855, 1972

45. Kyle RA, Seligman BR, Wallace HJ Jr, et al: Multiple myeloma resistant to melphalan (NSC-8806) treated with cyclophosphamide (NSC-26271), prednisone (NSC-10023) and chloroquine (NSC-187208). Cancer Chemother Rep 59:557–562, 1975

46. Morstyn G, Schechter GP, Ihde DC, et al: Therapy for multiple myeloma with alternating non-cross-resistant chemotherapy combinations: heterogeneity of tumor responsiveness: Cancer Treat Rep 68:1439–1446, 1984

47. Tirelli U, Crivellari D, Carbone A, et al: Combination chemotherapy for multiple myeloma with melphalan, prednisone, cyclophosphamide, vincristine and carmustine (BCNU) (M2 protocol). Cancer Treat Rep 66:1971–1973, 1982

48. Paccagnella A, Salvagno L, Sileni C, et al: Response and survival in multiple myeloma with CTX, MEL, BCNU, VCR, PRED. (M-2 protocol). Am Soc Clin Oncol 1:185, 1982 (abstr)

49. Case DC, Sonneborn HL, Paul SD, et al: Combination chemotherapy for multiple myeloma with BCNU, cyclophosphamide, vincristine, melphalan, and prednisone (M-2 protocol). Oncology 42:137–140, 1985

50. Alexanian RA, Balcerzak S, Haut A, et al: Remission maintenance therapy for multiple myeloma. Arch Intern Med 135:147–152, 1975

51. Cornwell GG III, Pajak TF, Kochwa S, et al: Vincristine and prednisone prolongs the survival of patients receiving intravenous or oral melphalan with multiple myeloma: Cancer and Leukemia Group B experience. (submitted for publication)

52. Southwest Oncology Group Study: Remission maintenance therapy for multiple myeloma. Arch Int Med 294:17–23, 1976

53. Alexanian R, Gehan E, Haut A, et al: Unmaintained remissions in multiple myeloma. Blood 51:1005–1011, 1978

54. Belch A, White D, Bergsagel DE: The role of maintenance chemotherapy for multiple myeloma. Proc Am Soc Clin Oncol 3:268, 1984 (abstr)

55. Hansen OP, Clausen NT, Drivsholm A, et al: Phase II study of intermittent 5-drug regimen (VBCMP) versus intermittent 3-drug regimen (VMP), versus intermittent melphalan and prednisone (MP) in myelomatosis. Scand J Haematol 35:518–524, 1985

56. Medical Research Council's Working Party on Leukemia in Adults: Treatment comparisons in the third MRC myelomatosis trial. Br J Med 42:823–830, 1980

Treatment of Refractory Multiple Myeloma and Considerations for Future Therapy

Robert A. Kyle, Philip R. Greipp, and Morie A. Gertz

ALL PATIENTS with multiple myeloma who have a response to chemotherapy will eventually relapse if they do not die of another disease. In addition, approximately one third of the patients treated initially with chemotherapy will not obtain an objective response.

In reviewing response data, it is important to consider factors that may alter the likelihood of response in the population of patients selected for study, such as adequacy of dosage and schedule and number of treatment cycles with the initial chemotherapeutic agents, refractoriness to initial chemotherapy, the number of previous chemotherapy agents and regimens given, and whether the patient relapsed while on therapy or after it was discontinued. Survival of a group of patients entering a chemotherapy trial may be prolonged because of the superiority of the new regimen or the selective entry of good-risk patients into the study. Such data are not readily available in most reported chemotherapeutic trials, and they are rarely considered in the study design. These factors limit the conclusions that can be drawn regarding the relative effectiveness of new chemotherapy regimens in patients with refractory myeloma. Finally, it is important to evaluate the effectiveness of therapy in relation to its toxicity before deciding about the applicability of a newly introduced chemotherapy regimen.

COMBINATION REGIMENS

The highest response rates reported for patients with multiple myeloma who are resistant to alkylating agents have been with vincristine, Adriamycin (doxorubicin) (Adria Laboratories, Columbus, Ohio), and dexamethasone (VAD). Vincristine and Adriamycin in a 4-day continuous infusion through an indwelling catheter, using a Travenol pump, along with dexamethasone, 40 mg daily, produced a response in 14 (70%) of 20 patients with resistant multiple myeloma.[1] Patients who responded had a projected survival exceeding 1 year. Infection represented the most frequent complication. Cytopenias were moderate. In a subsequent study, Alexanian et al[2] reported that approximately 25% of previously unresponsive patients treated either with dexamethasone or with VAD responded. In relapsing patients, the response rate was 65% with VAD, in contrast to 22% with dexamethasone alone. The estimated median survival for responders was 22 months.[2]

A combination of doxorubicin and carmustine (BCNU) produced improvement in seven of 13 patients with myeloma who were unresponsive or who had relapsed after chemotherapy.[3] Six of 14 patients with multiple myeloma resistant to melphalan and prednisone obtained objective response when treated with carmustine, cyclophosphamide, doxorubicin, and prednisone.[4] In a series of 35 patients with multiple myeloma resistant to melphalan, treatment with carmustine, doxorubicin, and prednisone produced objective response in 22% and an increase in hemoglobin level, an improvement in performance score, or a decrease of bone marrow plasma cells in 28%.[5] Forty-one percent of the 35 patients receiving these agents obtained some response. Bonnet et al[6] reported that 39 (26%) of 151 patients with relapsing or resistant multiple myeloma had a response to vincristine, carmustine, doxorubicin, and prednisone (VBAP). Of the 123 patients with relapsing myeloma, 37 (30%) responded, while only two (7%) of 28 patients with resistant myeloma responded. Currently, we frequently use a combination of carmustine (30 mg/m^2), doxorubicin (30 mg/m^2), and vincristine (2 mg)—all given intravenously (IV) on day 1—and prednisone (20 mg) three times daily for five days every 3 to 4 weeks to treat relapsing or refractory myeloma. Doses of carmustine and doxorubicin can be increased by 10-mg increments if leukopenia or thrombocytopenia does not develop.

From the Division of Hematology and Internal Medicine, Mayo Clinic and Mayo Foundation, Rochester, Minn.

Supported in part by research grants CA-16835 from the National Institutes of Health, Public Health Service, and the Toor Fund.

Address reprint requests to Robert A. Kyle, MD, Mayo Clinic, 200 First St SW, Rochester, MN 55905.

0093-7754/86/1303-0009$05.00/0

The M-2 protocol[7] produced a response in only five of 46 patients with melphalan-resistant multiple myeloma. However, Paccagnella et al[8] reported that 22 (88%) of 25 patients who responded to the M-2 protocol and then suffered a relapse responded to a modified M-2 protocol. In a later report, they noted that 65% of patients with relapse again responded to the M-2 regimen.[9] Patients who are truly resistant to melphalan seem to respond infrequently to the M-2 regimen, while patients who have responded to the M-2 regimen and who have a relapse during a treatment-free interval will respond. Broun et al[10] reported that nine of 23 patients with refractory myeloma showed some response to a combination of cisplatin, BCNU, cyclophosphamide, and prednisone. Side effects were significant. The addition of cisplatin and bleomycin (Blenoxane, Bristol Laboratories, Syracuse, NY) to VBAP produced response in 33% of patients with myeloma who were resistant to melphalan or cyclophosphamide. The authors concluded that the addition of cisplatin and bleomycin had greater toxicity, expense, and inconvenience and was not superior to VBAP.[11]

SINGLE AGENTS

Generally, patients who are resistant to melphalan are also resistant to standard doses of cyclophosphamide and vice versa. Bladé et al[12] reported that only one of 12 patients resistant to melphalan-prednisone subsequently responded to cyclophosphamide-prednisone. None of the eight patients resistant to cyclophosphamide subsequently responded to melphalan. In a series of 46 patients with refractory myeloma who had measurable disease, cyclophosphamide (600 mg/m^2 IV daily for four days) produced an objective response in 43%.[13] The duration of the objective response was 3 months, and the survival of the responding patients was 9 months. Sixty-three percent of patients had a subjective response characterized by pain relief and improved performance. Treatment-induced leukopenia contributed to fatal infections in 10%. Severe hemorrhage did not occur. The addition of high-dose prednisone to the high-dose cyclophosphamide did not improve the response rate.[14] When compared with the four-day regimen, cyclophosphamide in an IV dose of 2,400 mg/m^2 did not improve the objective response and was associated with greater leukopenia. Vincristine given on day 1 versus day 9 after high-dose cyclophosphamide did not produce a statistically significant difference in response.[15]

Various chemotherapeutic agents have been used with limited success in patients with refractory myeloma. Hexamethylmelamine produced some improvement in only three of 37 patients.[16] Bisantrene caused a decrease of 46% in urinary light chains, a disappearance of bone pain, and an improved performance in one patient with refractory myeloma.[17] Acronine produced an objective response in one of 16 patients, while two other patients had some decrease in M protein level.[18] Aclarubicin, an analogue of doxorubicin, produced a reduction of >50% in M protein level in one patient and a decrease of between 25% and 49% in M protein level in four others in a group of nine patients with previously treated myeloma.[19] High-dose cytosine arabinoside produced a partial remission in only one of 13 patients with advanced refractory multiple myeloma. Myelosuppression caused two treatment-related deaths, one from infection and the other from bleeding.[20] Two of 62 patients with refractory myeloma who received chlorozotocin obtained an objective response, while four others had a decrease of between 25% and 49% in M protein level.[21] In another series of 22 patients with evaluable refractory myeloma, two had a fair response to chlorozotocin and seven showed no progression of disease.[22] Of 35 patients with advanced multiple myeloma given mitoxantrone, only one had a partial response and that persisted for only 2.5 months.[23] Vincristine as a single agent given as a bolus and followed by a five-day continuous infusion produced objective response in only two of 21 patients with refractory multiple myeloma.[24] Pentostatin (2′-deoxycoformycin), an inhibitor of adenosine deaminase, produced objective response in two of seven patients with previously-treated myeloma who had received at least one cycle of the drug.[25] Relapse occurred at 7 months in one patient and 10 months in the other, but neither patient was on continued therapy. Amsacrine (m-AMSA) produced a good response in two (3%) of 70 patients with refractory myeloma, while three others (4%) had some improvement.[26] Toxicity was significant. In another report, none of 34 patients responded to m-AMSA.[27]

Responses have not been noted in patients with refractory multiple myeloma using the following agents: Vindesine,[28,29] spirogermanium,[30] and diaziquone (AZQ).[31]

Corticosteroids used as a single agent produce objective response in patients with refractory multiple myeloma. Salmon et al[32] reported an objective response in eight of ten patients with refractory myeloma given prednisone (200 mg) as a single dose every other morning. Prednisone (60 mg/m^2) for five days every 3 weeks produced some response in 31% of patients with refractory myeloma.[28] The addition of prednisone to apparently inactive agents has been reported to be helpful. The addition of prednisone to hexamethylmelamine,[16,33] or vindesine[28,29] has been reported to produce benefit. Responses have also been noted in patients with advanced multiple myeloma who were given weekly cyclophosphamide and alternate-day prednisone.[34] The use of vincristine (0.25 mg/m^2 IV, days 1 through 4) plus prednisone (1 g/m^2, days 1 and 3, repeated every 2 weeks) produced partial response in five patients and stable disease in four of 16 patients with refractory myeloma. The median survival of all patients was 10.5 months. Serious toxicity was not seen.[35]

The administration of doxorubicin (Adriamycin) weekly rather than every 3 to 4 weeks may be associated with a lesser incidence of cardiomyopathy.[36] Interferon has produced objective response in patients with refractory myeloma and is discussed in Farhangi et al, this issue.

New chemotherapeutic agents with greater specificity for the plasma cell but without increased toxicity must be found before major progress can be made with chemotherapy.

IRRADIATION THERAPY

Hemibody or total-body irradiation has been used in patients with previously treated multiple myeloma. Coleman et al,[37] using a 3 and 2 total nodal radiation technique, reported a reduction in M protein level in four patients and a decrease in pain in five of six patients previously treated with chemotherapy. In seven patients who were resistant to chemotherapy, sequential upper and lower hemibody irradiation produced reductions of 38% to 80% in the total body myeloma cell mass in the five patients who completed treatment.[38] Tobias et al[39] noted that the M protein level decreased in 12 of 22 patients with previously treated myeloma who were given hemibody irradiation. Twelve of 19 patients with relapsed or resistant multiple myeloma were treated with sequential upper and lower halfbody irradiation. Five had an objective response. Six of 13 patients who received upper body irradiation died of apparent pulmonary infection; some might have had radiation pneumonitis.[40]

NEWER THERAPEUTIC APPROACHES

Currently available agents used in different dosages, combinations, schedules, or routes of administration may provide some benefit. McElwain and Powles[41] reported that a single large IV dose of melphalan (100 to 140 mg/m^2) produced a complete remission in three of five patients with multiple myeloma or plasma cell leukemia who were previously untreated. The M protein disappeared from the peripheral blood and urine, whereas the plasma cell level in the bone marrow decreased to 0%. The therapy produced significant hematologic toxicity.[41] They have now given melphalan (140 mg/m^2) to 30 patients less than 60 years of age who had previously untreated multiple myeloma. Seven patients achieved a complete remission, which was characterized by the disappearance of the M protein in serum and urine and the absence of plasma cells in the bone marrow. None of the seven patients have relapsed after follow-up periods ranging from 4 to 42 months. Seventeen patients achieved partial remission and one patient failed to respond.[42] Moderate nausea, vomiting, diarrhea, and alopecia developed in all patients. Five patients died during the first 2 months—mainly from infection. It is encouraging to see that no relapses have occurred in the seven patients who had a complete remission. Further observation is necessary to determine the duration of the complete response. McElwain's group also gave high-dose melphalan (140 mg/m^2) to 15 patients with myeloma who had extensive previous therapy. This regimen produced three complete remissions and seven partial remissions, but the median duration of the remissions was only 6 months.[42] It appears that high-dose melphalan will not be useful for patients with previously treated myeloma.

Very small doses of alkylating agents may be efficacious for the treatment of multiple myeloma. A single small dose of cyclophosphamide (15 mg/kg) eradicated a large (20 mm) subcutaneous (MOPC-315) plasmacytoma in BALB/c mice.[43] On day 11, the administration of a single small dose (0.75 mg/kg) of melphalan to BALB/c mice bearing a 20 mm MOPC-315 tumor cured 90% of them. The alkylating agents did not effect a cure when given at an earlier stage of the tumor (day 4). The authors postulated that antitumor immunity of the host was augmented by elimination of suppressor elements. Bocian et al[44] subsequently showed that melphalan produced strong antitumor immunity in the animals' hitherto immunosuppressed spleen cells.

Potentiation of the effect of melphalan has been reported. Sheldon et al[45] found that the addition of nitroimidazole, a hypoxic cell radiosensitizer, potentiated the cytotoxicity of melphalan. Horsman et al[46] demonstrated the enhancement of melphalan-induced tumor cell killing by 2-nitroimidazole misonidazole. Verapamil enhanced cellular melphalan uptake in mice with fibrosarcoma but not in human bone marrow.[47] The combination of radiosensitizers and chemotherapeutic agents may have a clinical role in the future.

We have recognized a temporary window in which an increase in the plasma cell labeling index occurred after the administration of hydroxyurea. Among eight patients with serum creatinine <1.5 mg/dL, six had a > two-fold or >2% increase in the labeling index at 12 hours. Four patients with serum creatinine levels >1.5 mg/dL had no increase in labeling index at 12 hours, but two of three studied had an increase of two-fold or greater in labeling index at 36 hours. Chemotherapy with VBAP 12 hours after hydroxyurea priming produced an objective response in five of 12 patients. Two responders were previously resistant to VBAP alone. Furthermore, toxicity was minimal and included mild myelosuppression, gastrointestinal symptoms, and neurotoxicity.

The development of a soft-agar colony-forming assay for human myeloma stem cells has presented an opportunity to determine sensitivity to chemotherapeutic drugs in vitro. The number of kinetically active plasma cells is closely related to the number of clonogenic tumor cells that produce colonies in agar.[48] In a series of trials, the human tumor colony assay had a true-positive rate of 71% for predicting drug sensitivity and a true-negative rate of 91% for predicting drug resistance.[49] A major shortcoming is the low cloning efficiency of most tumors; even with depletion of T lymphocytes and the addition of nonproliferating human fetal lung fibroblasts, enough colonies to analyze were produced in only 60% of the cases.[50] Although this technique holds promise, there are many problems and the assay system must be improved before it will be of practical value.[51,52] An assay of the human tumor stem cell may be useful for the screening of drugs that have antitumor activity. The assay has identified several drugs with potential antitumor activity that were not recognized by the prescreen currently used by the National Cancer Institute.[53]

Bone marrow transplantation from an identical twin has produced objective benefit, though myeloma usually progresses later.[54] At the University of Washington, five patients received bone marrow transplants from their identical twin (syngeneic) after a standard regimen of cyclophosphamide and total-body irradiation. One patient died early. Three patients had initial improvement, but their multiple myeloma relapsed—at 6, 17, and 18 months—after transplantation. One patient is doing well 75 months after transplantation but has a small persistent serum M spike.[55] Allogeneic bone marrow transplantation has been performed in several cases, but the results have been equivocal. Furthermore, the age restriction of allogeneic transplants will limit its application in multiple myeloma.

Autologous bone marrow rescue is potentially applicable to treat far more patients than is allogeneic transplantation because the problems of graft-versus-host disease or graft rejection are circumvented. Initially, the patient is treated with conventional chemotherapy to reduce the myeloma tumor burden, and then autologous bone marrow is collected, frozen, and stored. The patient is then treated intensively and rescued by normal stem cells present in the stored marrow. Two major problems exist for patients with myeloma. First, multiple myeloma is difficult to eradicate from the marrow with any form of treatment, even with large doses of chemotherapy and radiation. The second major problem is that of removing myeloma cells and their precursors from the autologous bone marrow before reinfusion. Theoretically, myeloma cells and their precursors can be removed from the bone marrow by using monoclonal antibodies. However, such antibodies are difficult to develop. Anderson et al[56] reported two monoclonal antibodies (PCA-1 and PCA-2) that recognized plasma cell-associated antigens. Unfortunately, these monoclonal antibodies also reacted with granulocytes and monocytes. The same group reported a monoclonal antibody, PC-1, that recognized only plasma cells at the terminal stage of differentiation.[57] Togawa et al[58] described a monoclonal antibody that reacted with immature B cells and plasma cells but not with T lymphocytes, platelets, red blood cells, monocytes, or granulocytes. Another monoclonal antibody, HAN-PC1, reacted only with plasma cells or myeloma cells.[59] The authors stated that this monoclonal antibody had specificity against a maturation antigen present on plasma cells or their malignant counterpart. Our group has developed a mouse monoclonal antibody against a human plasma cell xenograft.[60] This antibody (R1–3) reacts with a more proliferative subset of plasma cells and B lymphocytes but is nonreactive with granulocytes, normoblasts, thymus, spleen, or T cells. Patients with multiple myeloma who expressed R1–3 antigen in their peripheral blood had a large myeloma tumor burden and high bone marrow plasma cell proliferative activity.[61]

Unfortunately, not all of the neoplastic plasma cells in the bone marrow and circulating lymphocyte precursors in the peripheral blood react with the currently available plasma cell monoclonal antibodies. Perhaps a panel of monoclonal plasma cell antibodies of varying specificities will be effective in removing the malignant plasma cells and their precursors. Neoplastic cells may be removed from the bone marrow by the in vitro use of chemotherapeutic agents such as 4-hydroperoxycyclophosphamide, but care must be taken to preserve the hematopoietic stem cells. A combination of 4-hydroperoxycyclophosphamide and monoclonal antibodies was more effective than either one alone in eliminating clonogenic Burkitt's lymphoma cells.[62]

Other techniques for removing neoplastic cells from the bone marrow are being developed. These include immunotoxin-mediated cytotoxicity in which the monoclonal antibody is conjugated to a potent toxin such as ricin, as well as immunophysical techniques in which monoclonal antibodies are labeled with microspheres or metal colloids.[63] Whole-ricin immunoconjugates synthesized with a pan-T-cell antibody T101 were at least ten times more toxic to T lymphocytes than to progenitor cells in the bone marrow and were effective in mixtures of normal and malignant cells.[64] This suggests that appropriate ricin conjugates may remove the target cell without damaging normal progenitor cells.

The therapeutic use of monoclonal antibodies to plasma cell antigens may be possible in the future, but many hurdles must be overcome. A monoclonal antiidiotype antibody has produced an excellent response in a patient with a nodular, well-differentiated lymphocytic lymphoma.[65] Subsequent experience has not been as impressive. The inadequate response may mainly be due to free circulating idiotype protein.[66] The problems are even greater in multiple myeloma because of the large amount of intravascular and extravascular antigenic materials. The possibility of stimulation rather than suppression of antibody production also exists.[67]

A mouse monoclonal antibody to a differentiation antigen expressed by carcinomas was radiolabeled with iodine-131 and injected into the intrapleural, intrapericardial, or intraperitoneal spaces of three patients with metastatic carcinoma. Subsequently, cytologic examination revealed no neoplastic cells in the pleural and peritoneal washings in two patients, while the pericardial tumor was reduced in the third patient.[68] Iodinated (^{131}I) antiferritin antibody produced some response in 40% of 38 patients with advanced progressive Hodgkin's disease. Thrombocytopenia and leukopenia were the most frequent side effects.[69] A group of patients with hepatoma who previously received irradiation and therapy benefited from ^{131}I-antiferritin.[70] These studies should stimulate efforts to develop other radiolabels and antibodies for the treatment of malignant disease.

Although the potential use of monoclonal antibodies is enticing, much work needs to be done before this technique can be effective. Much more needs to be learned about the biologic basis of multiple myeloma before real progress can be made in therapy.

CONCLUSIONS

The treatment of patients with truly refractory multiple myeloma is discouraging. If the patient is asymptomatic and has stable disease, it is advisable to simply observe the patient. Some patients will remain stable for a significant period. If the patient is resistant to melphalan and prednisone or to cyclophosphamide, we prefer to treat the patient with the VBAP regimen. Patients who have had alkylating agents and VBAP or who have severe cytopenias that prevent further chemotherapy may respond to high-dose corticosteroids such as dexamethasone or methylprednisolone.

REFERENCES

1. Barlogie B, Smith L, Alexanian R: Effective treatment of advanced multiple myeloma refractory to alkylating agents. N Engl J Med 310:1353–1356, 1984
2. Alexanian R, Barlogie B, Dixon D: High dose dexamethasone for resistant multiple myeloma. Blood 66:212, 1985 (suppl 1) (abstr)
3. Alberts DS, Durie BGM, Salmon SE: Doxorubicin/B.C.N.U. chemotherapy for multiple myeloma in relapse. Lancet 1:926–928, 1976
4. Presant CA, Klahr C: Adriamycin, 1,3-bis (2-chloroethyl)-1-nitrosourea (BCNU, NSC #409962), cyclophosphamide plus prednisone (ABC-P) in melphalan-resistant multiple myeloma. Cancer 42:1222–1227, 1978
5. Kyle RA, Pajak TF, Henderson ES, et al: Multiple myeloma resistant to melphalan: Treatment with doxorubicin, cyclophosphamide, carmustine (BCNU), and prednisone. Cancer Treat Rep 66:451–456, 1982
6. Bonnet J, Alexanian R, Salmon S, et al: Vincristine, BCNU, doxorubicin, and prednisone (VBAP) combination in the treatment of relapsing or resistant multiple myeloma: A Southwest Oncology Group study. Cancer Treat Rep 66:1267–1271, 1982
7. Lee BJ, Lake-Lewin D, Meyers JE: Intensive treatment of multiple myeloma, in Wiernik PH (ed): Controversies in Oncology. New York, John Wiley & Sons, 1982, pp 61–79
8. Paccagnella A, Cartei G, Fosser V, et al: Treatment of multiple myeloma with M-2 protocol and without maintenance therapy. Eur J Cancer Clin Oncol 19:1345–1351, 1983
9. Paccagnella A, Salvagno L, Bolzonella S, et al: Second and third response to M2 (BCNU, VCR, CTX, PRED) in multiple myeloma. Proc Annu Meet Am Soc Clin Oncol 4:217, 1985 (abstr)
10. Broun GO Jr, Petruska PJ, Hiramoto RN, et al: Cisplatin, BCNU, cyclophosphamide, and prednisone in multiple myeloma. Cancer Treat Rep 66:237–242, 1982
11. Bonnet JD, Alexanian R, Salmon SE, et al: Addition of cisplatin and bleomycin to vincristine-carmustine-doxorubicin-prednisone (VBAP) combination in the treatment of relapsing or resistant multiple myeloma: A Southwest Oncology Group study. Cancer Treat Rep 68:481–485, 1984
12. Bladé J, Feliú E, Rozman C, et al: Cross-resistance to alkylating agents in multiple myeloma. Cancer 52:786–789, 1983
13. Lenhard RE Jr, Oken MM, Barnes JM, et al: High-dose cyclophosphamide: An effective treatment for advanced refractory multiple myeloma. Cancer 53:1456–1460, 1984
14. Lenhard RE Jr: Personal communication, March 1986
15. Lenhard RE, Tsiatis AA, Oken MM, et al: Timed sequential high dose cyclophosphamide (CY) and vincristine (VCR) treatment of multiple myeloma (MM). Proc Annu Meet Am Soc Clin Oncol 4:217, 1985 (abstr)
16. Oken MM, Lenhard RE Jr, Anderson J, et al: The contribution of prednisone to the effectiveness of hexamethylmelamine (HXM) in multiple myeloma (MM). Proc Annu Meet Am Soc Clin Oncol 1:186, 1982 (abstr)
17. Alberts DS, Mackel C, Pocelinko R, et al: Phase I clinical investigation of 9,10-anthracenedicarboxaldehyde bis[(4,5-dihydro-1 *H*-imidazol-2-yl)hydrazone] dihydrochloride with correlative in vitro human tumor clonogenic assay. Cancer Res 42:1170–1175, 1982
18. Scarffe JH, Beaumont AR, Crowther D: Phase I–II evaluation of acronine in patients with multiple myeloma. Cancer Treat Rep 67:93–94, 1983
19. Sezaki T, Adachi T, Ishii H, et al: Aclarubicin in the treatment of multiple myeloma. Jpn J Clin Oncol 14:353–358, 1984
20. Kantarjian H, Dreicer R, Barlogie B, et al: High-dose cytosine arabinoside in multiple myeloma. Eur J Cancer Clin Oncol 20:227–231, 1984
21. Cornell CJ Jr, Pajak TF, McIntyre OR: Chlorozotocin: Phase II evaluation in patients with myeloma. Cancer Treat Rep 68:685–686, 1984
22. Forman WB, Cohen HJ, Bartolucci AA, et al: Phase II evaluation of chlorozotocin in refractory multiple myeloma. Cancer Treat Rep 68:1409–1410, 1984
23. Alberts DS, Balcerzak SP, Bonnet JD, et al: Phase-II trial of mitoxantrone in multiple myeloma: A Southwest Oncology Group study. Cancer Treat Rep 69:1321–1323, 1985
24. Jackson DV, Case LD, Pope EK, et al: Single agent vincristine by infusion in refractory multiple myeloma. J Clin Oncol 3:1508–1512, 1985
25. Belch AR, Henderson JF, Brox LW: Treatment of multiple myeloma with deoxycoformycin. Cancer Chemother Pharmacol 14:49–52, 1985
26. Greipp PR, Rai K, Coleman M, et al: Phase II trial of amsacrine in patients with multiple myeloma. A Cancer and Leukemia Group B study (submitted for publication)
27. Ahmann FR, Meyskens FL Jr, Jones SE, et al: Phase

II evaluation of amsacrine (*m*-AMSA) in solid tumors, myeloma, and lymphoma: A University of Arizona and Southwest Oncology Group study. Cancer Treat Rep 67:697–700, 1983

28. Alexanian R, Yap BS, Bodey GP: Prednisone pulse therapy for refractory myeloma. Blood 62:572–577, 1983

29. Uhm K, Camacho FJ, Bennett JM, et al: Phase II trial of vindesine (VDS) in patients with previously treated multiple myeloma. Proc Annu Meet Am Soc Clin Oncol 3:268, 1984 (abstr)

30. Riggs SA, Cabanillas F, Alexanian R, et al: Phase II study of spirogermanium hydrochloride with or without cytosine arabinoside in the treatment of advanced recurrent lymphoma and multiple myeloma. Proc Annu Meet Am Assoc Cancer Res 26:184, 1985 (abstr)

31. Vinciguerra V, Anderson K, McIntyre OR: Diaziquone for resistant multiple myeloma: Cancer and leukemia group B. Cancer Treat Rep 69:331–332, 1985

32. Salmon SE, Shadduck RK, Schilling A: Intermittent high-dose prednisone (NSC-10023) therapy for multiple myeloma. Cancer Chemother Rep 51:179–187, 1967

33. Cohen HJ, Bartolucci AA: Hexamethylmelamine and prednisone in the treatment of refractory multiple myeloma. Am J Clin Oncol 5:21–27, 1982

34. Brandes LJ, Israels LG: Treatment of advanced plasma cell myeloma with weekly cyclophosphamide and alternate-day prednisone. Cancer Treat Rep 66:1413–1415, 1982

35. Gomez GA, Han T, Ozer H, et al: Salvage treatment for patient with multiple myeloma refractory to alkylating agents. Med Pediatr Oncol 13:325–329, 1985

36. Weiss AJ: Studies on cardiotoxicity and antitumor effect of doxorubicin administered weekly. Cancer Treat Symp 3:91–94, 1984

37. Coleman M, Saletan S, Wolf D, et al: Whole bone marrow irradiation for the treatment of multiple myeloma. Cancer 49:1328–1333, 1982

38. Thomas PJ, Daban A, Bontoux D: Double hemibody irradiation in chemotherapy–resistant multiple myeloma. Cancer Treat Rep 68:1173–1175, 1984

39. Tobias JS, Richards JD, Smith BJ, et al: Hemibody irradiation in multiple myeloma. Presented at the 3rd Annual Meeting of the European Society for Therapeutic Radiology and Oncology, Jerusalem, Israel, September 9–15, 1984 (abstr)

40. Rostom AY, O'Cathail SM, Folkes A: Systemic irradiation in multiple myeloma: A report on nineteen cases. Br J Haematol 58:423–431, 1984

41. McElwain TJ, Powles RL: High-dose intravenous melphalan for plasma-cell leukaemia and myeloma. Lancet 2:822–824, 1983

42. Selby P, Ayliffe M, Behrens J, et al: High dose treatment with melphalan and methyl prednisolone for multiple myeloma. Proceedings of the EURAGE Symposium on Monoclonal Gammapathies, Clinical Significance and Basic Mechanisms. Brussels, Belgium, September 19–20, 1985 (abstr)

43. Ben-Efraim S, Bocian RC, Mokyr MB, et al: Increase in the effectiveness of melphalan therapy with progression of MOPC-315 plasmacytoma tumor growth. Cancer Immunol Immunother 15:101–107, 1983

44. Bocian RC, Ben-Efraim S, Dray S, et al: Melphalan-mediated potentiation of antitumor immune responsiveness of immunosuppressed spleen cells from mice bearing a large MOPC-315 tumor. Cancer Immunol Immunother 18:41–48, 1984

45. Sheldon PW, Batten EL, Adams GE: Potentiation of melphalan activity against a murine tumour by nitroimidazole compounds. Br J Cancer 46:525–531, 1982

46. Horsman MR, Evans JW, Brown JM: Enhancement of melphalan-induced tumour cell killing by misonidazole: An interaction of competing mechanisms. Br J Cancer 50:305–316, 1984

47. Robinson BA, Clutterbuck RD, Millar JL, et al: Verapamil potentiation of melphalan cytotoxicity and cellular uptake in murine fibrosarcoma and bone marrow. Br J Cancer 52:813–822, 1985

48. Karp JE, Burke PJ, Saylor PL, et al: Correlation of proliferative and clonogenic tumor cells in multiple myeloma. Cancer Res 44:4197–4200, 1984

49. Salmon SE: Human tumor colony assay and chemosensitivity testing. Cancer Treat Rep 68:117–125, 1984

50. Durie BGM, Christiansen JA: Improved human myeloma colony growth. Blood 62:189, 1983 (suppl 1) (abstr)

51. Selby P, Buick RN, Tannock I: A critical appraisal of the "human tumor stem-cell assay." N Engl J Med 308:129–134, 1983

52. Twentyman PR: Predictive chemosensitivity testing. Br J Cancer 51:295–299, 1985 (editorial)

53. Shoemaker RH: New approaches to antitumor drug screening: The human tumor colony-forming assay. Cancer Treat Rep 70:9–12, 1986

54. Osserman EF, DiRe LB, DiRe J, et al: Identical twin marrow transplantation in multiple myeloma. Acta Haematol (Basel) 68:215–223, 1982

55. Feffer A: Personal communication, February 1986

56. Anderson KC, Park EK, Bates MP, et al: Antigens on human plasma cells identified by monoclonal antibodies. J Immunol 130:1132–1138, 1983

57. Anderson KC, Bates MP, Slaughenhoupt B, et al: A monoclonal antibody with reactivity restricted to normal and neoplastic plasma cells. J Immunol 132:3172–3179, 1984

58. Togawa A, Inoue N, Mannoji M, et al: B-cell differentiation antigen expressed on a human myeloma cell line (KMM-1). Jpn J Clin Oncol 13:511–515, 1983

59. Mertens N, Van Camp B: A unique monoclonal antibody defining plasma cells. Br J Haematol 60:361, 1985 (abstr)

60. Gonchoroff NJ, Katzmann JA, Garton JP, et al: A monoclonal antibody reactive with a subset of human plasma cells. Br J Haematol 62:619–630, 1986

61. Ruiz-Argüelles GJ, Katzmann JA, Greipp PR, et al: Multiple myeloma: Circulating lymphocytes that express plasma cell antigens. Blood 64:352–356, 1984

62. De Fabritiis P, Bregni M, Lipton J, et al: Elimination of clonogenic Burkitt's lymphoma cells from human bone marrow using 4-hydroperoxycyclophosphamide in combination with monoclonal antibodies and complement. Blood 65:1064–1070, 1985

63. Jansen J, Falkenburg JHF, Stepan DE, et al: Removal

of neoplastic cells from autologous bone marrow grafts with monoclonal antibodies. Semin Hematol 21:164–181, 1984

64. Leonard JE, Taetle R, To D, et al: Preclinical studies on the use of selective antibody-ricin conjugates in autologous bone marrow transplantation. Blood 65:1149–1157, 1985

65. Miller RA, Maloney DG, Warnke R, et al: Treatment of B-cell lymphoma with monoclonal anti-idiotype antibody. N Engl J Med 306:517–522, 1982

66. Meeker TC, Maloney DG, Thielemans K, et al: Anti-idiotype monoclonal antibody therapy of human B lymphocytic malignancy. Blood 62:214, 1983 (suppl 1)(abstr)

67. Teitelbaum D, Rauch J, Stollar BD, et al: In vivo effects of antibodies against a high frequency idiotype of anti-DNA antibodies in MRL mice. J Immunol 132:1282–1285, 1984

68. A Report from the Hammersmith Oncology Group and the Imperial Cancer Research Fund: Antibody-guided irradiation of malignant lesions: Three cases illustrating a new method of treatment. Lancet 1:1441–1443, 1984

69. Lenhard RE Jr, Order SE, Spunberg JJ, et al: Isotopic immunoglobulin: A new systemic therapy for advanced Hodgkin's disease. J Clin Oncol 3:1296–1300, 1985

70. Order SE, Stillwagon GB, Klein JL, et al: Iodine 131 antiferritin, a new treatment modality in hepatoma: A Radiation Therapy Oncology Group study. J Clin Oncol 3:1573–1582, 1985

Interferons in the Treatment of Multiple Myeloma

M. Robert Cooper and Charles E. Welander

IN VIEW of the relative lack of efficacy of chemotherapy for relapsing or refractory patients with multiple myeloma, attempts have been made to investigate the role of biological response modifiers in this disease. Major work has now been performed both in the laboratory and in clinical trials to define the role of interferons in this disease.

Preclinical investigations testing human recombinant interferon alfa(rIFNα_2) with tumor cells has been difficult, due in part to species specificity of the interferons. This species specificity precludes the use of most experimental animal model systems for testing human interferons. Studies using human tumor xenografts implanted into nude mice have been done, but do raise many questions concerning host response and changes in tumor growth related to a species-specific agent such as interferon.[1] Human myeloma cells are technically difficult to culture in vitro, further complicating attempts to perform preclinical studies of interferon effects on human myeloma cells. These problems have been partially remedied by the use of a clonogenic assay to grow human myeloma cell colonies as was first reported in 1977 by Hamburger et al.[2,3] This colony-forming assay could be used to determine sensitivity of myeloma cell colonies to standard chemotherapeutic agents, with retrospective correlations drawn between in vitro sensitivity and patients response to therapy.[4]

Recently, recombinant DNA technology has made adequate quantities of human interferons available for both in vitro and in vivo testing. Although interferons are in the category of biologic response modifiers, they do have some direct cytotoxic effects on human tumor cells that can be quantitated in this colony-forming assay.[5,6] Using concentrations of rIFNα_2 (Intron A, Schering Plough, Kenilworth, NJ) in vitro that are known to be achievable in vivo, reduction in colony formation of human myeloma cells has been observed.[7] Specific mechanisms of action of interferon are unclear, and are probably multifaceted. In addition, there may be indirect effects of rIFNα_2 on tumor cells in vivo, mediated through other host cells. In order to explore this possibility further and to determine whether macrophages and/or lymphocytes alter the growth of tumor cell colonies in vitro, experiments that add additional types of cells to these clonogenic assay cultures have been done.[8]

The following discussion of in vitro studies, using a colony-forming assay to test the effects of anticancer drugs on human tumor cells, is limited to experiments using rIFNα_2, melphalan, cyclophosphamide, and prednisone on an established cell line of human myeloma cells (RPM-8226).[9] Although a variety of cytotoxic agents has been used to treat patients with both newly diagnosed and refractory myelomas, the choice of drugs in these laboratory studies represents a group of commonly used agents in the clinic. The methods used to clone myeloma cell line RPMI-8226 were modified from the original work of Hamburger et al.[10] A required colony stimulating factor was produced by a feeder layer of cells added to the agar culture plates that enhances the colony formation of the myeloma cells. Feeder cells were derived from a human macrophage cell line, U937.[11]

In the clonogenic assay, RPMI-8226, myeloma cells were tested with each of the four drugs noted previously to determine the dose response curves and the dose resulting in a 50% inhibition in colony growth (ID_{50}). Prednisone has the least cytotoxic effect when tested with these myeloma cells as a single agent. Concentrations of Intron A as low as 1 U/mL (international antiviral activity) show a reduction in colony number to <30% of the untreated control cultures. Both melphalan and cyclophosphamide show measurable cytotoxic activity with the ID_{50} of melphalan at 0.15 μg/mL and cyclophosphamide at 0.4 μg/mL.

The following combinations of drugs were tested: (1) Melphalan + Intron A; (2) cyclophos-

---

From the Division of Hematology/Oncology, Bowman Gray School of Medicine, Winston-Salem, NC.

Address reprint requests to M. Robert Cooper, MD, Bowman Gray School of Medicine, Division of Hematology/ Oncology, 300 S. Hawthorne Rd, Winston-Salem, NC 27103.

0093-7754/86/1303-0010$05.00/0

phamide + Intron A; (3) prednisone + Intron A; (4) melphalan + prednisone + Intron A.

The mathematical model that describes how cytotoxicity can be evaluated has been published previously.[12] In summary, using the additivity model, the recorded fractional colony survivals, when each drug is tested singly, are multiplied together. The product of the two fractional survivals becomes the expected colony survival, and is compared with the observed colony survival when the pair of drugs is tested together in vitro. If the observed survival is equal to the expected colony survival, the drug interactions are additive. If the observed is less than the expected, then the interactions are synergistic. Conversely, observed survival greater than the expected survival suggests either subadditive or antagonistic interactions.

In Figs 1, 2, and 3, the paired drug combinations are shown in graphic form. Additive antiproliferative effects were noted with combinations of Intron A-cyclophosphamide (Fig 1) and Intron A-prednisone (Fig 2). However, the Intron A-melphalan combination showed synergistic effects on tumor cell colony reduction (Fig 3). The combination of melphalan and prednisone was also additive in antiproliferative effect on the myeloma cells (data not shown). Even greater cytotoxic activity was seen with the three-drug combination of Intron A-melphalan-prednisone (Fig 4). Very low concentrations of Intron A in combination with melphalan and prednisone resulted in colony reduction to <30% of control values.

It is apparent that a human myeloma clonogenic assay in vitro can measure antiproliferative effects of interferon, prednisone, melphalan, and cyclophosphamide. Combinations of these agents have additive or occasionally synergistic effects on tumor cell colony reduction. The following discussion will describe the clinical trials that have recently been performed or are in progress

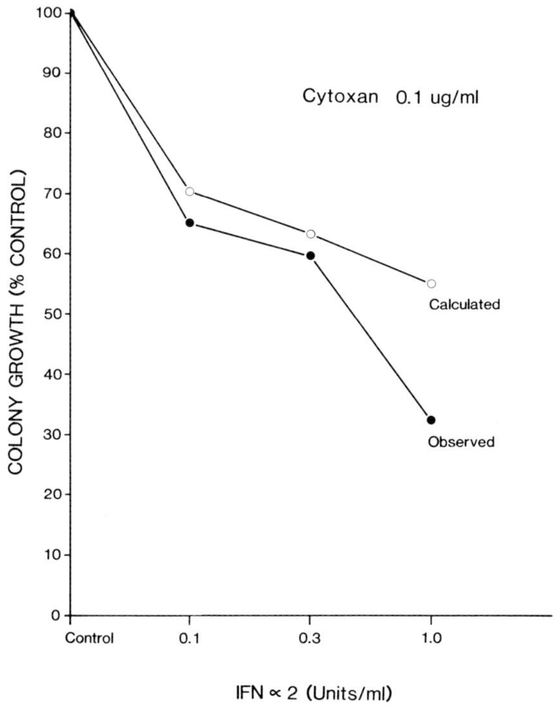

Fig 1. The percent colony reduction of combined cytoxan and interferon is plotted as a function of increasing interferon concentration. Cytoxan concentration is held constant. The observed percent colony survival is compared to the calculated colony survival, using the additivity model. The *P* value for difference between observed and calculated at IFN 1.0 U/mL concentration is not significant.

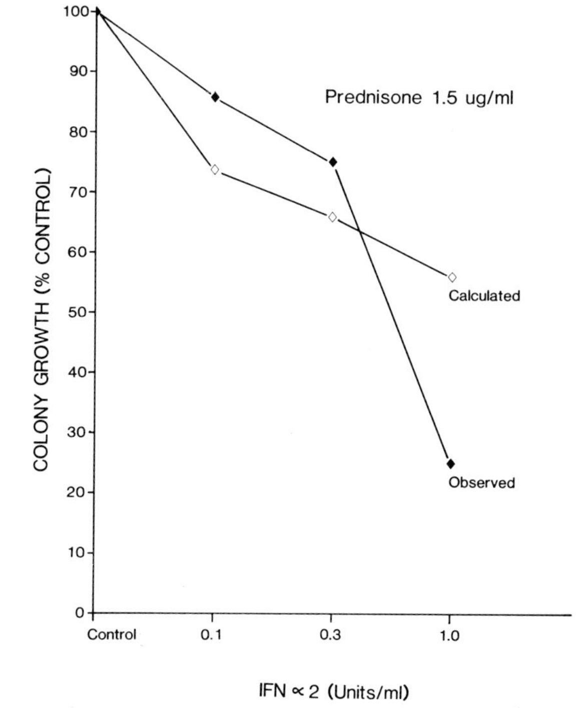

Fig 2. The percent colony reduction of combined prednisone and interferon is plotted as a function of increasing interferon concentration. Prednisone concentration is held constant. The observed percent colony survival is compared to the calculated colony survival, using the additivity model. The *P* value for difference between observed and calculated at IFN 1.0 U/mL concentration is not significant.

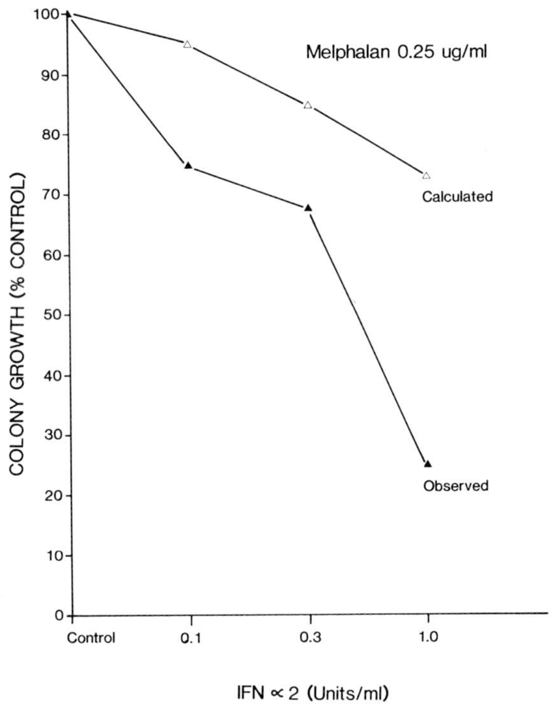

Fig 3. The percent colony reduction melphalan and interferon is plotted as a function of increasing interferon concentration. Melphalan concentration is held constant. The observed percent colony survival is compared to the calculated colony survival, using the additivity model. The *P* value for difference between observed and calculated at IFN 1.0 U/mL is .104.

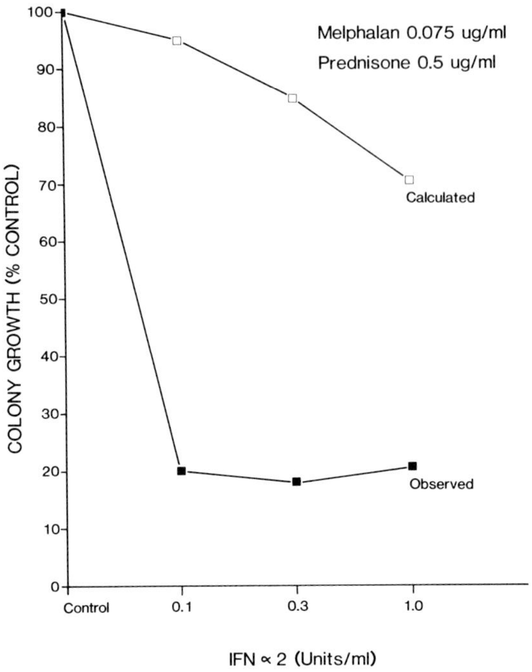

Fig 4. The percent colony reduction of combined melphalan, prednisone, and interferon is plotted as a function of increasing interferon concentration. Melphalan and prednisone concentrations are held constant. The observed percent colony survival is compared to the calculated colony survival, using the additivity model. A *P* value has not been calculated for this three-drug combination.

to determine whether these in vitro effects can be achieved in patients.

Prior results with interferon have been limited but encouraging. Mellstedt administered human leukocyte interferon to four previously untreated patients with multiple myeloma, and all showed a decrease in the percentage of bone marrow plasma cells as well as a decrease in the level of abnormal proteins both in serum and urine.[13] Gutterman et al treated ten myeloma patients with leukocyte interferon; three responded, three improved, and four failed to respond.[14] The responders had decreases in abnormal proteins that lasted up to 63 weeks after therapy was discontinued. Decreases in the percentage of bone marrow plasma cells to 15% or less were also noted. Scandinavian investigators have reported a randomized trial comparing interferon alone with intermittent high dose melphalan and prednisone as first line therapy.[15] Six of 21 evaluable patients in the chemotherapy group and 4 of 22 patients in the interferon group were classified as responders. The acturial survival curves showed no statistically significant difference.

EXPERIENCE IN RELAPSING AND REFRACTORY PATIENTS

A phase II study of Intron A in resistant multiple myeloma recently has been completed and published.[16] Patients entering the study were diagnosed according to the criteria of the myeloma study task force and staged according to the criteria of Durie and Salmon.[17,18] Only patients refractory to prior therapy or relapsing after an initial response to primary treatment were entered. Patients were required to have a life expectancy of at least 4 months and an Eastern Cooperative Oncology Group (ECOG) performance status of 0, 1, 2, or 3. Patients may have received prior radiation therapy but not to a total field encompassing more than 25% of the bone marrow.

Intron A (Schering Sch 30500), the interferon used in this study, is a highly purified human alfa-2b interferon produced by recombinant DNA techniques in *Escherichia coli*.[19] Intron A was administered in three different dose schedules (Table 1). Four centers used a similar schedule of daily intravenous induction followed by subcutaneous 3 times/week maintenance therapy. The fifth center used subcutaneous Intron A from the beginning of therapy. As each schedule had similar toxicity and produced responses at rates not statistically significantly different from each other, results of all studies are combined in this report.

RESULTS

Forty-nine eligible patients were entered into the study of whom 38 were evaluable for efficacy analysis. Patients were considered invalid subjects for response assessment if they had received less than 1 month of treatment. This occurred in 11 patients for the following reasons: One patient was irradiated less than 28 days before Intron A treatment; six patients were removed from study (one refused further treatment, two had intercurrent illnesses not related to Intron A, and three had adverse experiences possibly related to Intron A [severe fatigue, paralytic ileus, and congestive heart failure]); and four patients died (two with disease progression, one with sepsis, and one with pneumonia and respiratory arrest).

Two thirds of the patients entered had been previously treated with multiple drug combinations including agents such as doxorubicin, vincristine, and nitrosoureas in addition to melphalan, cyclophosphamide, and prednisone. At entry, 25 of 49 patients were refractory to all prior chemotherapy, whereas 23 were relapsing after having previously responded to chemotherapy. Of the 38 evaluable patients, there was a total of seven responders (18%). There was one patient with a complete response and six patients who had a partial response (Tables 2 and 3). There were variable response rates among patients with different prognostic subgroups. Among patients who were primary refractory (never responded to prior therapy) there were two of 19 (10.6%) responses, whereas among patients who had previously responded there were five of 19 responses (26%). Three of six patients who had relapsed while off chemotherapy responded to Intron A treatment. The amount of prior treatment also profoundly affected the response rate to Intron A. Two of five patients who received single alkylating agent therapy previously responded to interferon, whereas only three of 25 patients who had failed multiple alkylating agent therapy responded.

Table 1. Intron A—Phase II Myeloma Trials

	Enrolled	Evaluable
3-100 × 10^6 IU/m^2/d IV 3 times/wk × 2 wk then 10 × 10^6 IU/m^2 SC 3 times/wk	23	18
30-50 × 10^6 IU/m^2/d IV, 5 on/9 off × 4 courses then 10 × 10^6 IU/m^2 SC 3 times/wk × 3 mo	12	7
2 × 10^6/m^2/d SC 3 times/wk × 3 mo then 10 × 10^6/m^2/d SC 3 times/wk	14	13
Total	49	38

Abbreviation: SC, subcutaneously.

Table 2. Intron A—Phase II Multiple Myeloma Trials

Results		
Refractory patients	2/19	11%
Relapsing patients (on treatment 2/13, off treatment 3/6)	5/19	26%
Prior treatment: M-P	2/5	40%
M + C + P	2/8	25%
Multiple agents	3/25	12%

NOTE. Strict response criteria, >50% decrease × 4 weeks; follow-up, 3/7 relapses, others remain in remission 52+, 58+, 65+ weeks.

Abbreviations: M, melphalan; C, cytoxan; P, prednisone.

Three of the seven responders continue to respond for >33 months with monoclonal proteins approaching undetectable levels. One patient had a partial response for 40 weeks and then converted to complete response (CR) with disappearance of abnormal M protein and radiographic confirmation of healing lytic bone lesions. This CR now continues at >104+ weeks. Of 29 patients who entered the study with documented bone pain, 18 improved and ten remained unchanged during the course of treatment. Only one patient had worsening of bone pain during Intron A treatment.

Three of the seven responders have had a survival time of >1 year with marked improvement in performance status and one patient has achieved a durable and ongoing complete remission that is rarely seen with either radiation therapy or chemotherapy given for the advanced phase of myeloma.

In a similar study,[20] 23 relapsed or refractory patients were treated with 10 × 10^6 U/m^2 Intron

Table 3. Profile of Responders

Patient No.	Prior Treatment	Stage	Response	Duration of Response (wks)	Best Change in Performance	Best Change in Pain	Paraprotein
1	Melphalan/prednisone	I	PR	62+	No change	No pain*	IgG
2	Multiple drug	III	CR	104+	No change	Improved (mild to none)	IgG
3	Multiple drug	III	PR	21	Improved	Improved (moderate to mild)	IgG
4	Multiple drug	II	PR	56+	No change	Improved (moderate to mild)	IgA
5	Melphalan/prednisone	II	PR	15	Improved	Improved (moderate to mild)	IgA
6	Melphalan/prednisone and cytoxan/prednisone	III	PR	12	No change	No change	LTC(K)
7	Melphalan/prednisone and cytoxan/prednisone	II	PR	16	No change	Improved (moderate to mild)	IgG

Abbreviations: LTC, light chain; PR, partial response; CR, complete response.
*At baseline.

A subcutaneously three times weekly for 12 weeks. Patients with responding or stable disease were continued on treatment until progression. Two of 20 evaluable patients had an objective response to Intron A (50% decrease in plasmacytomas or M protein). Three other patients had objective improvement with 25% to 50% decrease in M protein and a marked decrease in bone pain. Stable disease was observed in two additional patients. Approximately one third of the patients studied appeared to benefit from therapy with alfa-2 interferon.

A more recent study[21] has reported a 20% partial response frequency in previously treated multiple myeloma patients. In this study alfa(r1FNα_2) (Intron A) was given intravenously with escalating dosages during the induction phase to attain a significant degree of myelosuppression. A maintenance schedule of subcutaneous Intron A was then used. Patients not responding after 12 weeks of subcutaneous Intron A then had prednisone added to the treatment. Four of 20 patients achieved a partial remission, three of these occurring before the addition of prednisone. No dose response benefit was noted in this study. Concomitant prednisone reduced the flu-like symptoms of Intron A.

EXPERIENCE IN UNTREATED PATIENTS

In a recent report,[22] recombinant α-interferon clone A (rIFNαA, Roferon, Hoffman LaRoche, Nutley, NJ) 12 $\times$ 10^6U/m^2 was administered daily by intramuscular injection. Seven of 14 previously untreated patients with low to intermediate tumor mass responded to treatment. The response was associated with a rise in polyclonal immunoglobulins. No previously untreated patients with high tumor mass were entered into this study. Among previously treated patients, only two of 15 patients responded.

A pilot study was designed to test the feasibility of combining Intron A with melphalan and prednisone in previously untreated patients with multiple myeloma. The study was designed to determine what dose of interferon could be administered while patients were receiving a standard dose regimen of oral melphalan and prednisone.

Intron A was administered subcutaneously three times/week during week 1 and repeated during week 2. Five dosage levels of alfa-2b interferon were used 0.5, 1.0, 2.0, 5.0, and 10.0 $\times$ 10^6 IU/m^2 administered three times weekly for weeks 1 and 2. Melphalan 9 mg/m^2 orally and prednisone 40 mg/m^2 orally were administered on days 8 through 11 of week 2. The melphalan dose could be escalated until a white blood cell

Table 4. IFN/Melphalan/Prednisone Response by Dose Level

Dose (10^6 IU/m^2)	Entered	Evaluable	PR	NC	PD	%
0.5	6	5	3	0	2	60%
1.0	6	5	3	1	1	60%
2.0	6	5	4	1	0	80%
5.0	5	4	3	1	0	75%
10.0	7	6	4	1	0	67%

Abbreviations: PR, partial response; NC, no change; PD, progressive disease.

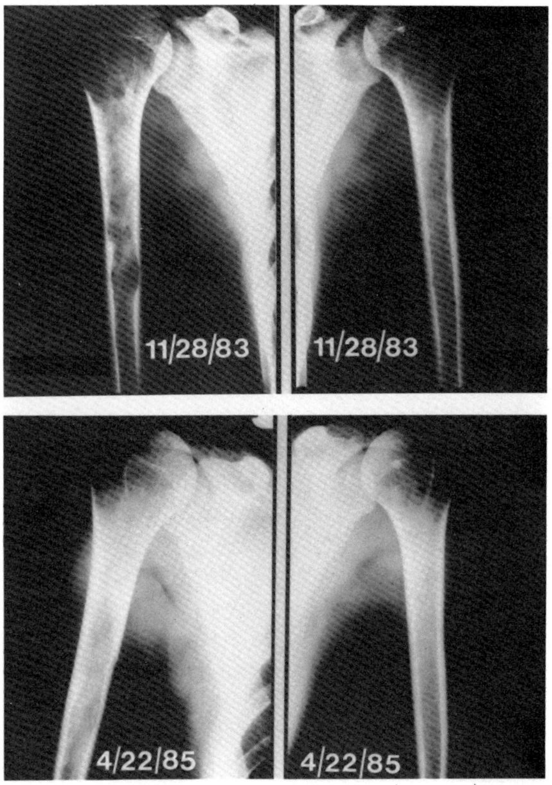

Fig 5. Bone healing in a patient with multiple myeloma treated with melphalan, prednisone, and interferon. Comparison of pretreatment x-rays on 11/28/83 to those of 4/22/85 while on therapy.

count (WBC) of less than 3.000/μL $\times$ $10^6/\mu$L or platelet count of less than 100,000/μL was obtained. No treatment was administered during weeks 3 or 4. A cycle was scheduled to be 28 days and then repeated.

The projected dose of melphalan was analyzed by cycle and dose level of Intron A (Table 4). At low doses of Intron A (0.5 or 1.0 $\times$ $10^6/m^2$) patients received 70% to 105% of the projected dose with the majority of patients receiving 90% or greater. Interferon doses >2.0 $\times$ $10^6/m^2$ led to administration of 37% to 103% of the projected dose of melphalan, with most patients receiving 70% or less of the projected dose.

Although response was not the primary objective of this study, an overall response of 75% was achieved using criteria established by the Chronic Leukemia Task Force.[17] Figure 5 shows bone healing in a patient treated on this pilot study.

Phase II trials conducted thus far have established tumor responsiveness to interferons in human myeloma. It is amply clear that in order to further define the role of these agents in the treatment of myeloma, well planned multicenter studies must be conducted. Cancer and Leukemia Group B, in a randomized trial, is currently testing the effectiveness of melphalan and prednisone compared to melphalan, prednisone and interferon.

REFERENCES

1. Balkwill FR, Moodie EM: Positive interactions between human interferon and cyclophosphamide or Adriamycin in human tumor model system. Cancer Res 44:904–908, 1984

2. Hamburger AW, Kim MB, Salmon SE: The nature of cells generating human myeloma colonies in vitro. J Cell Physiol 98:371–376, 1979

3. Hamburger A, Salmon SE: Primary bioassay of human myeloma stem cells. J Clin Invest 60:846–854, 1977

4. Salmon SE, Hamburger AW, Soehnlen B, et al: Quantitation of differential sensitivity of human tumor stem cells to anticancer drugs. N Engl J Med 298:1321–1327, 1978

5. Salmon SE, Durie BGM, Young L, et al: Effects of cloned human leukocyte interferons in the human tumor stem cell assay. J Clin Oncol 1:217–225, 1983

6. Von Hogg DD, Gutterman J, Protnoy B, et al: Activity of human leukocyte interferon in a human tumor cloning system. Cancer Chemother Pharmacol 8:99–103, 1982

7. Aapro MS, Alberts DS, Salmon SE: Interactions of human leukocyte interferon with vinca alkaloids and other chemotherapeutic agents against human tumors in clonogenic assay. Cancer Chemother Pharmacol 10:161–166, 1983

8. Welander CE, Berens ME, Saito T, et al: In vitro testing of subclones of recombinant interferon alpha using a human tumor clonogenic assay. (submitted for publication)

9. Krueger RG, Staneck LD, Boehlecke JM: Tumor associated antigens in human myeloma. JNCI 56:711–715, 1976

10. Hamburger AW, Salmon SE: Primary bioassay of human tumor stem cells. Science 197:461–463, 1977

11. Sundstrom C, Nilsson K: Establishment and characterization of a human histiocytic lymphoma cell line (U-937). Int J Cancer 17:565–577, 1976

12. Welander CE, Morgan TM, Homesley HD, et al: Combined recombinant human interferon $alpha_2$ and cytotoxic agents studied in the clonogenic assay. Int J Cancer 35:721–729, 1985

13. Mellstedt H, Bjorkholm M, Johansson B: Interferon therapy in myelomatosis. Lancet 1:245–248, 1979

14. Gutterman JU, Blumenschein GR, Alexanian R: Leukocyte interferon-induced tumor regression in human metastatic breast cancer, multiple myeloma, and malignant lymphoma. Ann Intern Med 93:399–406, 1980

15. Mellstedt H, Aahre A, Bjorkholm M: Interferon therapy of patients with myeloma, in Terry WD, Rosenberg SA

(eds): Immunotherapy of Human Cancer. New York, Elsevier, 1982, pp 387–391

16. Costanzi JJ, Cooper MR, Scarffe JH, et al: Phase II study of recombinant alpha-2 interferon in resistant multiple myeloma. J Clin Oncol 3:654–659, 1985

17. Chronic Leukemia-Myeloma Task Force, National Cancer Institute. Proposed guidelines for protocol studies II. Plasma Cell Myeloma. Cancer Chemother Rep 4:145–158, 1973

18. Durie BGM, Salmon SE: A clinical staging system for multiple myeloma. Correlation of measured myeloma cell mass with presenting clinical features, response to treatment, and survival. Cancer 36:842–852, 1975

19. Streuli M, Nagata S, Weissman MC: At least three human type alpha interferons: Structure of $alpha_2$. Science 209:1343, 1980

20. Oken MM, Kyle RA, Kay NE, et al: A phase II trial of interferon $alpha_2$ ($rIFNa_2$) in the treatment of resistant multiple myeloma. Proc Am Soc Clin Oncol 4:215, 1985 (abstract 837)

21. Case DC, Sonneborn HL, Paul SD, et al: Phase II study of rDNA alpha-2 Interferon (INTRON A) in patients with multiple myeloma utilizing an escalating induction phase. Cancer Treat Rep (in press)

22. Quesada JR, Alexanaian R, Hawkins M, et al: Treatment of multiple myeloma with recombinant α-interferon. Blood 67:275–278, 1986

Clinical Implications of Monoclonal Light Chains

Alan Solomon

THE KNOWLEDGE gained over the past two decades of the molecular properties and genetics of immunoglobulin (Ig) light chains has provided the clinician new insights into the pathophysiologic role of the Bence Jones proteins and into the diagnostic, therapeutic, and prognostic importance of these components as biomarkers of cancer. Bence Jones proteins and light chain fragments have long been associated with morphological and functional renal impairment in patients with multiple myeloma. This association is exemplified by tubular cast formation (myeloma kidney), as well as by other types of renal tissue dysfunction related to nodular protein deposits in basement membrane and mesangial tissue (light chain deposition disease) and fibrillar protein deposits in renal and extrarenal sites (primary and myeloma-associated amyloidosis). The salient pathologic and clinical features of these disease entities have been related in detail elsewhere[1–5] and are summarized in Table 1.

LIGHT CHAIN-ASSOCIATED DISEASES

Myeloma Kidney

Although a number of host factors contribute to renal functional impairment associated with Bence Jones proteinuria (eg, dehydration, hypercalcemia, radiographic contrast agents, sepsis, nephrotoxic antibiotics)[6–8] most evidence indicates that the primary culprit is the light chain itself. The pathognomic features of the myeloma kidney are the homogeneous, periodic acid Schiff (PAS)-negative, proteinaceous casts and attendant inflammatory reaction within the renal tubules (Fig 1).[1,3] Such casts are invariably associated with Bence Jones proteinuria, and their presence leads to tubular atrophy with progressive deterioration of renal function. The chief constituent of these casts is the Bence Jones protein as evidenced by immunofluorescent studies. The failure of antilight chain antisera to react with these and other types of light chain-related tissue deposits can be attributed to the specificity of these antisera for κ or λ determinants expressed by the intact light chain—only rarely will such antisera react with light chain fragments.[9]

The fact that tubular cast formation is not an invariable accompaniment of Bence Jones proteinuria or is not necessarily related to the amount of monoclonal light chain synthesized or excreted implies that, in addition to host factors, some, but not necessarily all, Bence Jones proteins are nephrotoxic.[10–13] Bence Jones proteins differ in solubility, isoelectric point, association constant, and their susceptibility to proteolysis.[14–16] These and other unusual structural features may alter light chain renal transport and catabolism. For example, clinical and experimental observations[12,17,18] have related the nephrotoxicity of a Bence Jones protein to its isoelectric point (pI). Based on electrophoretic mobility at pH 8.6, the most electronegative (cationic) proteins have been associated with tubular cast formation and the most electropositive (anionic) proteins with light chain deposition disease and amyloidosis.[12] These findings have been attributed to the enhanced glomerular permeability of light chains with high pIs.[11,12] Because Bence Jones proteins are ampholytic, acidification of the urine can potentiate the insolubility of those proteins having high pI, as shown in an experimental rat model.[17,19] Further, protein-protein complexes may be formed between highly-charged (cationic) Bence Jones proteins and acidic urinary proteins (Tam-Horsfall protein and other urinary glycoproteins)[18,20] or basement membrane constituents as demonstrated for immune complexes.[21] Because the constant (C) region sequence of all κ- (and λ-) type Bence Jones proteins is virtually identical,[22] differences in protein charge must reflect an unusually high variable (V) region content of basic amino acid residues (or a low number of acidic residues).

From the Department of Medicine, University of Tennessee Memorial Research Center and Hospital, Knoxville.

Supported in part by United States Public Health Research grant CA 10056 from the National Cancer Institute and by the Stein Cancer Research Fund.

Address reprint requests to Alan Solomon, MD, University of Tennessee Memorial Research Center and Hospital, 1924 Alcoa Highway, Knoxville, TN 37920.

0093-7754/86/1303-0011$05.00/0

Table 1. Major Forms of Monoclonal Light Chain-Associated Renal Diseases

Entity	Pathognomic Features	Proteinuria: Light Chain	Proteinuria: Albumin	Light Chain Characteristics	Physiological Dysfunction: Glomerular	Physiological Dysfunction: Tubular	Renal Failure: Acute	Renal Failure: Chronic	Supportive	Cytotoxic	Reversibility of Lesions
Meyloma kidney (cast) disease	Tubular casts, inflammatory reaction	++++	++	$\kappa \simeq \lambda$ (insolubility, ↑ pI)	0	++++	+++	++	+++	++	+
Light chain deposition disease	Nodular deposits: basement membrane (glomerular, tubular), mesangium	+	+	$\kappa \gg \lambda$ (abnormal size)	++++	++	++++	+++	+++	+	?
Amyloidosis (AL)	Congo red + (birefringent), fibrillar deposits: glomerular, vascular (mesangium, endothelium)	++	+++	$\lambda > \kappa$ (λVI, light chain fragment)	++++	+	0	++	+	+	?

Further structural characterization of those Bence Jones proteins with exceptionally high pI may provide further insight into their pathophysiologic importance.

Other (as yet unknown) properties of the Bence Jones protein must have pathophysiologic import because tubular cast formation is not invariably correlated with light chain pI.[23] This problem has been addressed experimentally by injecting human Bence Jones proteins into mice[24] or rats[17,19,23] and by in vitro studies.[25–28] Deposits of proteinaceous casts, most prominent in the distal convoluted tubules, were found in the kidneys of mice examined five hours to 14 days after the intraperitoneal injection of a human λ Bence Jones protein.[24] Subsequently, tubular degeneration and atrophy developed, and the extent of pathology was found to be dose-related. Differences in the nephrotoxicity of Bence Jones proteins were evidenced by the fact that only one of three injected λ chains resulted in discernible pathology. Experimental use of the mouse or other types of models[29] may help differentiate which protein and host factors are responsible for the myeloma kidney. Ultimately, this information will provide the clinician new methods for a more effective treatment of this entity.

Bence Jones proteins are associated with other

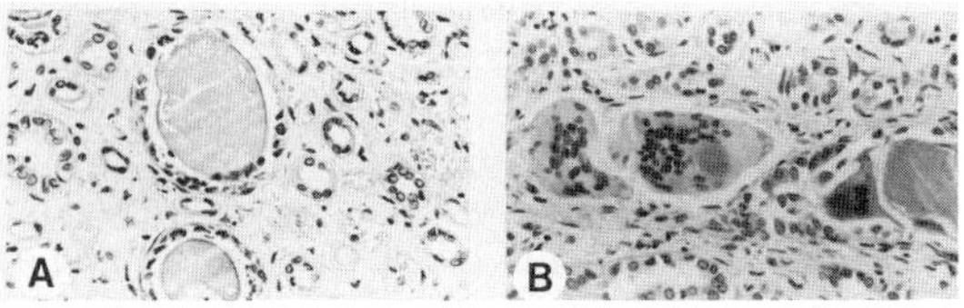

Fig 1. Myeloma (cast) kidney disease. (A) Proteinaceous tubular casts and (B) giant cell reaction (original magnification ×250).

types of renal tubular dysfunction, proximal as well as distal.[5] For example, certain patients with multiple myeloma and Bence Jones proteinuria have an associated adult-type Fanconi syndrome.[30,31] A unique V region sequence has been found for three Fanconi-associated κ Bence Jones proteins.[32] In one case, examination of a renal biopsy specimen by electron microscopy revealed tight junctions between glomerular epithelial cell foot processes.[33] In vitro, the κ Bence Jones protein (one with an unusually high pI) was shown to affect epithelial tight junction structure and permeability. Other defects in proximal and distal tubular function (nephrogenic diabetes insipidus, impairment in urine acidification and concentration, distal renal tubular acidosis) have also been associated with Bence Jones proteinuria.[6,7] Both proximal and distal tubular defects—so-called combined light chain nephropathy—may be manifest.[34] The selective but reversible tubular proteinuria also has been evidenced by excretion of low–molecular-weight urinary proteins (α_1-microglobulin, α_1-acid glycoprotein, β_2-microglobulin) and the renal tubular enzyme β-N-acetyl-D-glucosaminidase.[7,11] The lack of correlation between these physiological aberrations and the amount of Bence Jones proteinuria implicates further the protein itself as responsible for the observed pathology. Since dimeric forms of light chains can serve as antibody,[14,15] similar interactions with specific cellular antigens may be another mechanism for the renal toxicity of Bence Jones protein.

Light Chain Deposition Disease

Another type of renal disease associated with monoclonal light chains is light chain deposition disease. This disorder is distinguished from the more common myeloma kidney by the lack of tubular casts and by the localization as nodular deposits of monoclonal light chains along the basement membrane of renal tubular cells and glomeruli and, additionally, in mesangium (Fig 2).[1-3,5,35-42] Similar types of deposits develop systemically, eg, in lung, liver, and other organs.[35,36,42-45] These deposits often are PAS-positive and are agyrophilic but, in contrast to amyloid, show neither birefringence in polarized light after staining with Congo red nor, when examined by electron microscopy, have a fibrillar structure. The deposits are recognized by immunofluorescence or immunoperoxidase microscopy as containing monoclonal light chains—almost exclusively those of the κ-type.[35,39,42,45] Because patients with this disease often do not have the characteristic findings associated with multiple myeloma (or amyloidosis), light chain deposition disease is rarely recognized clinically. The diagnosis is usually made by immunohistochemical examination of renal biopsy material from patients with unexplained proteinuria or renal failure. Although light chain deposition disease can occur in patients with typical manifestations of multiple myeloma including Bence Jones proteinuria,[42] frequently, there is no evidence of plasma cell malignancy. Thus, the amount of monoclonal light chain in the urine may be miniscule and, therefore, extremely difficult to detect due to the presence of other urinary proteins. Monoclonal serum Igs are rarely present and the concentration of normal serum Igs is not decreased. Only a slight bone marrow plasmacytosis is observed and although atypical cell forms may be noted, sheets of malignant plasma cells are not present, a finding that could possibly account for the small amount of light chain proteinuria. The monoclonal nature of the plasma cells can be demonstrated by immunofluorescence, and there is concordance between the light chain type found in plasma cell cytoplasm and in renal deposits.[35,39,44]

The paucity of monclonal light chains in urine specimens from patients with light chain deposition disease does not reflect the severity of renal failure that most often occurs in such patients. The small amounts of such protein excreted may be attributed either to a low synthetic rate or rapid catabolism, a marked affinity for basement membrane or other tissue components, or an unusual glomerular permeability.[11,42-46] Because of the difficulty in isolating sufficient amounts of monoclonal light chain for detailed chemical and serological analyses, the structural features accounting for their unusual form of tissue deposition are largely unknown. The abnormal nature of these proteins has been evidenced in biosynthetic and other studies that have shown them to be either atypically large or small[35,37,38,42,47]; an ~18,000 dalton κ-chain fragment has also been found in one such patient (Buxbaum JN, Solomon A, unpublished studies). Other types of fibrillary, nonamyloid glomerular disease associated with deposits of polyclonal light chains also have been described.[48,49]

Light Chain-Associated Amyloidosis

The clinical and pathological aspects of amyloidosis—specifically the amyloid disease that occurs in patients with monoclonal B cell proliferative disorders of idiopathic or neoplastic origin, ie, primary or myeloma-associated amyloidosis—are presented in detail elsewhere.[1-4] In such patients, the pathophysiologic manifestations associated with plasma cell or lymphocyte dyscrasias include features that reflect the anatomical site(s) of amyloid deposition and attendant organ dysfunction. The kidneys are commonly involved in the disease process with amyloid deposits found within arterial walls and/or interstitial tissue and in glomeruli. Tubular casts and other hallmarks of the myeloma kidney are less common; the tubular proteinaceous casts rarely have the tinctorial or ultrastructural characteristics of the vascular or mesangial amyloid

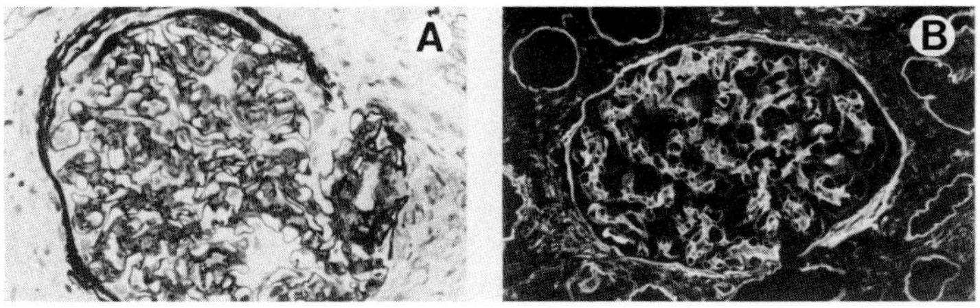

Fig 2. Light chain deposition disease. Periodic acid silver methenamine. (A) Alternations in glomerular mesangium and capillary walls as revealed by PASM-stain. (B) Deposition of κ chains in glomerular capillary walls and capsule and in tubular basement membranes as evidenced by specific immunofluorescence with an anti-κ chain antiserum (original magnification ×250).

deposits. The degree of renal insufficiency is related to the extent of vascular involvement and tubular dysfunction. In contrast, glomerular deposition of amyloid typically results in a nephrotic syndrome. The alteration in glomerular permeability accounts for the presence in urine specimens of serum proteins, which often obscure the detection of Bence Jones protein. The apparent relentless nature of the renal amyloid process, the deposits of amyloid in other organs, and other factors related to malignant B cell disease (when present) results in a relatively poor prognosis.

The pathological diagnosis of amyloidosis requires histochemical and ultrastructural examination of relevant tissue. Although the definitive diagnosis of renal amyloidosis is made by kidney biopsy, its presence can be inferred (especially in adult patients with an idiopathic nephrotic syndrome) by demonstrating vascular amyloid deposits in other readily accessible tissues, eg, rectal valve, gingiva, skin.

Characteristically, the deposits after Congo red staining have an apple green birefringence (Fig 3) when viewed under polarized light microscopy (or fluoresce after thioflavine T staining) and are composed of fine, randomly ordered fibrils when examined by electron microscopy. A major advance in our understanding of the clinical and chemical diversity of amyloidosis came from the ability to extract and analyze the protein constituent of amyloid.[4] The prediction by Isobe and Osserman[50] that monoclonal light chains (Bence Jones proteins and related components) are important in the pathogenesis of certain forms of amyloidosis was borne out through analyses of fibrillar protein isolated from amyloid deposits from patients with primary and myeloma-associated amyloidosis.[4] In such cases, the protein has been found to consist mainly of monoclonal light chains or, more commonly, fragments consisting of the light chain variable domain (V_L), or the V_L and a portion of the constant domain (C_L). Light chain-associated amyloidosis is designated amyloidosis AL.

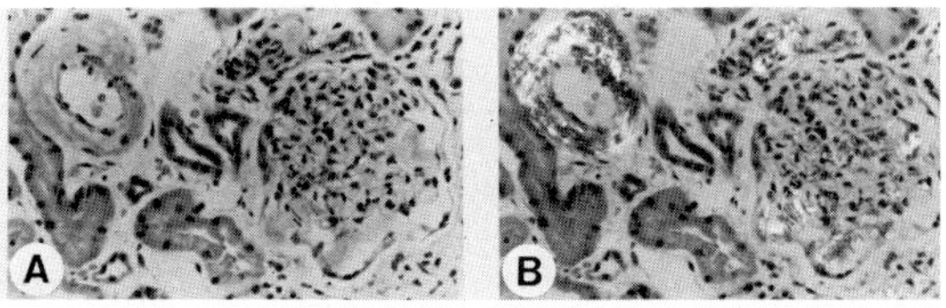

Fig 3. Amyloidosis AL. (A) Congo-red-positive glomerular and vascular deposits showing (B) birefringence under polarized light (original magnification ×250).

A structural basis or predilection for certain types of light chains to be more amyloidogenic than others is implied chemically by the predominance of λ chains over κ chains in amyloidosis AL and by the preferential association of a particular V region subgroup,[22] $V_{\lambda VI}$, with the amyloid process.[49–51] Indeed, λVI-type monoclonal serum and urinary Igs are invariably obtained from patients with amyloidosis AL, and more than 16 such proteins have been identified to date.[51] The frequency of occurrence of λVI light chains in this disease is three- to five-fold higher than expected, based on the ~5% to 11% incidence of λVI light chains among λ-type Igs of normal individuals.[50–52]

Amino acid sequence analyses of the λVI amyloid-associated light chains have shown a two-residue V region insertion between positions 68 and 69—a finding unique to proteins of this subgroup.[51,53–57] The structural implications of the insertion remain unknown but, by comparison with the three-dimensional features of a non-λVI Bence Jones protein,[58] the insertion may cause the V domains of λVI proteins to aggregate in an unusual fashion.[51] Furthermore, λVI light chains are susceptible to a specific site of proteolytic cleavage as evidenced by the molecular weight and the chemical and serological analyses of λVI-related protein extracted from the amyloid fibrils of three patients with amyloidosis AL.[51,53,56,59,60] All three components had a molecular weight of ~18,000 and lacked the ~60 carboxyl-terminal residues of the C region. In one patient, where the intact λVI protein and the λVI amyloid fibril protein fragment were available for comparative analyses, the amino-terminal sequences of both are identical.[51]

Although monoclonal non-λVI proteins occur in patients with amyloidosis AL(λ), the striking association of a particular V region isotype with this process appears limited to λVI proteins; no such association has been evident in patients with amyloidosis AL(κ).[51] Whether amyloid-associated light chains of other V region isotypes possess distinctive structural features[61] that render them amyloidogenic or, alternatively, whether the light chain degradative process is abnormal in patients with amyloidosis AL remains to be established. For example, certain light chains can be readily cleaved by certain types of endopeptidases[62] into Congo red-positive, birefringent, fibrillar V_L-related fragments.[4] Amyloid fibrils have been found extracellularly and within the cytoplasm of bone marrow-derived reticuloendothelial cells from patients with amyloidosis AL.[63,64] An intracellular processing of light chains into amyloid fibrils by lysosomal enzymes was inferred by the presence of both κ chains and fibrils within plasma cells[65] and also by the finding of cytoplasmic amyloid-like material in macrophages cocultured in soft agar with plasma cells from a patient with amyloidosis AL.[66] Despite these observations, whether Bence Jones proteins are actually processed into amyloid intercellularly or extracellularly remains unknown.

Other proteins found in amyloid deposits, chiefly the pentraxin C-reactive protein-related P component,[4] may have etiologic importance. Acquired factor X deficiency has also been noted in association with amyloidosis AL.[60,67–69] Binding of factor X by amyloid fibrils has been demonstrated in one case[70]; however, among 10 amyloid-associated Bence Jones proteins, no evidence of factor X-inhibiting activity was found (Levin J, Solomon A, unpublished studies).

DIAGNOSTIC IMPORTANCE OF BENCE JONES PROTEINS

Bence Jones proteinuria occurs in at least 60% of patients with multiple myeloma. It is also found in association with other B cell-related neoplasms including Waldenström's macroglobulinemia, chronic lymphocytic leukemia, μ heavy chain disease, and other lymphoproliferative neoplasms,[15,71–75] and (as discussed) is an essential constituent of amyloidosis AL.[4] Rarely are Bence Jones proteins found in urine specimens from apparently healthy persons,[76] but when they do occur, the event may be analogous to finding a monoclonal serum Ig in normal individuals, ie, benign monoclonal gammopathy. Such benign Bence Jones proteins may be rendered nonpathogenic by host factors or may lack the structural features of malignant Bence Jones proteins responsible for the light chain-associated renal or systemic diseases.[77] Using the in vivo experimental mouse model,[24] we have obtained correlative evidence for the nephrotoxicity of certain human Bence Jones proteins and for the localization to the V_L of that portion of the light polypeptide chain responsible for the observed renal tubular pathology.[78]

The recognition and classification as κ or λ of Bence Jones proteins in urine or serum specimens are most readily accomplished by immunochemical means—immunoelectrophoresis (Fig 4) or immunofixation as described in detail elsewhere.[52,79,80] These techniques are usually satisfactory for identification of Bence Jones proteins in concentrations >1 mg/mL; the detection of lesser amounts requires appropriate concentration of urine specimens. The failure of certain Bence Jones proteins to give the characteristic heat test—namely, precipitation under specified conditions at 55 to 60 °C, solubilization at 100 °C, and reprecipitation upon cooling—can

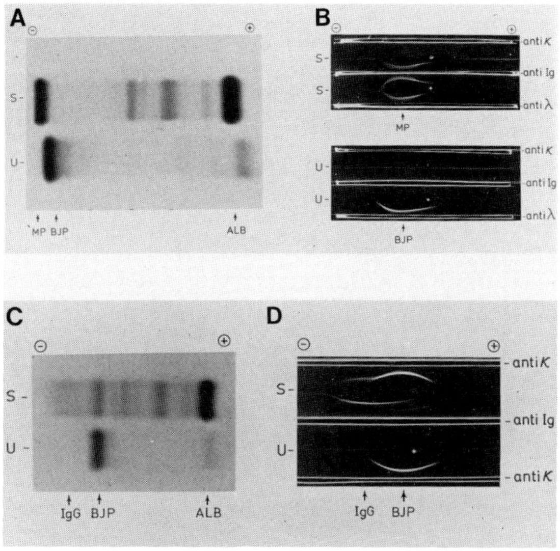

Fig 4. (A and B) Electrophoretic and immunochemical detection of serum myeloma protein and Bence Jones proteinuria. (A) Agarose gel electropherogram of a specimen of serum (*S*) (diluted 1:5) and urine (*U*) (20 mg/mL) from a patient with multiple myeloma. (B). Immunoelectrophoretic analysis. The locations of the IgG myeloma protein (*MP*) in the serum specimen and the λ Bence Jones protein (*BJP*) in the urine specimen are as indicated. (C and D) Bence Jones proteinemia and proteinuria in a patient with multiple myeloma and renal failure. The location of the κ Bence Jones protein (BJP) in the serum and urine specimens is as indicated. Alb: albumin/ anti-κ, anti-Ig, and anti-κ: anti-κ light chain, anti-polyclonal IgG, and anti-λ light chain antisera, respectively.

be attributed to differences in V region structure.[14]

Bence Jones proteins of the λ-type exist primarily as disulfide-linked covalent dimers (molecular weight ~44,000), whereas κ Bence Jones proteins are found more commonly in the form of noncovalent dimers, stable monomers (molecular weight ~22,000), or as mixtures of both.[14] Monoclonal light chains of atypically lower or higher molecular weight (eg, ~88,000 dalton tetramers) or with unusual thermal properties (cryoglobulins) have been described.[14,15,81,82] The clinical importance of such proteins is not known; however, certain forms of nonsecretory myeloma have been attributed to structurally-defective monoclonal light chains.[83,84]

THERAPEUTIC AND PROGNOSTIC IMPORTANCE OF BENCE JONES PROTEIN AS A BIOMARKER OF CANCER

Bence Jones proteins serve as biomarkers for patients with multiple myeloma and related diseases.[85] The importance of detecting these components in urine specimens from patients who apparently have idiopathic renal disease (or where Bence Jones proteins can be obscured by other protein constituents) cannot be overemphasized.[86]

The amount of light chain protein excreted in the urine is dependent on synthetic and catabolic factors[14] but, in general, reflects tumor cell mass. Quantitative measurement of the daily excretion of Bence Jones protein provides an objective index of the response or lack of response to chemotherapy. New methods have been described for protein measurement[87] and for clinical staging of disease.[88] These measurements are of value even for the untreated patient, because an increase in Bence Jones protein excretion may presage tumor growth and lead to eventual clinical relapse. If Bence Jones proteinuria (ie, light chain escape) subsequently develops in patients who initially lacked this constituent, a transition to a more aggressive form of disease usually occurs. Corticosteroid and cytotoxic chemotherapy can have strikingly different effects on Bence Jones protein synthesis.[9] Further, the rate of disappearance of Bence Jones protein posttherapy also has prognostic import.[15] Whether differences in growth rate or sensitivity to chemotherapy of B lymphocytes and plasma cells are related to phenotypic features of the Bence Jones protein products is not known. This relationship, if it does indeed exist, may become evident through a more precise chemical and serological classification of these proteins.

The very presence of Bence Jones proteinuria in patients with multiple myeloma may account for their alleged poorer prognoses, especially those patients with λ- rather than κ-type proteins. However, the ominous significance of λ Bence Jones proteinuria is not always apparent, thus indicating that specific chemical properties of the individual Bence Jones protein may be more important than light chain type.[15,77] Although Bence Jones protein synthesis can be effectively reduced by cytotoxic chemotherapy alternative methods of treatment may be given based on knowledge of why certain Bence Jones proteins are nephrotoxic or amyloidogenic. Plasmapheresis, renal dialysis, and renal transplantation all have alleged benefit in light chain-associated acute and chronic renal failure.[1,5] With appropriate therapeutic measures, the renal failure is often reversible.[8,89–95] Most important are vigorous hydration and treatment of hypercalcemia, anemia, and other factors contributing to renal insufficiency. Alkylinization of the urine, as shown experimentally[17] and clinically,[8] can also be helpful. Therapeutically, cytotoxic regimens used in patients with multiple myeloma have, in some AL-type cases, been associated with clinical improvement and reduction in amyloid deposits.[63,96,97] Such treatment may also benefit patients with light chain deposition disease.[37]

Another important feature of the Bence Jones protein molecule—the idiotypic antigenic determinant formed by a unique V region structure—provides the basis for a new therapeutic strategy for patients with B cell-related neoplasms. In the presence of complement, antiidiotypic monoclonal antisera prepared against human Bence Jones proteins are cytotoxic to target cells.[98] Antiidiotype antisera have been used to induce remission in patients with B cell lymphomas refractory to conventional therapy.[99]

CONCLUSIONS

The continued research by basic scientists and clinical investigators into the chemical and biological properties of Bence Jones proteins and related proteins will furnish new information regarding the pathophysiologic implications of these proteins and their diagnostic, therapeutic, and prognostic importance. This knowledge will provide additional therapeutic approaches essential to reverse or prevent the potentially nephrotoxic or amyloidogenic effect of monoclonal light chains.

ACKNOWLEDGMENT

This article is dedicated to the memory of Henry G. Kunkel, MD. The author thanks Nena Myers and Marty Evers for preparation of the manuscript.

REFERENCES

1. Hill GS: Multiple myeloma, amyloidosis, Waldenström's macroglobulinemia, cryoglobulinemias, and benign monoclonal gammopathies, in Heptinstall RH (ed): Pathology of the Kidney (ed 3). Boston, Little, Brown, 1983, p 993

2. Gallo GR, Feiner HD, Buxbaum JN: The kidney in lymphoplasmacytic disorders. Pathol Annu 17:291–317, 1982

3. Pirani CL, Silva FG, Appel GB: Tubulo-interstitial disease in multiple myeloma and other nonrenal neoplasias, in Cotran RS (ed): Tubulo-Interstitial Nephropathies. Contemporary Issues in Nephrology, vol 10. New York, Churchill-Livingstone, 1982, p 287

4. Glenner GG: Amyloid deposits and amyloidosis: The β-fibrilloses. N Engl J Med 302:1283–1292; 1333–1343, 1982

5. Fang LST: Light-chain nephropathy. Kidney Int 27:582–892, 1985

6. DeFronzo RA, Cooke CR, Wright JR, et al: Renal function in patients with multiple myeloma. Medicine (Baltimore) 57:151–166, 1978

7. Cooper EH, Forbes MA, Crockson RA, et al: Proximal renal tubular function in myelomatosis: Observations in the fourth Medical Research Council trial. J Clin Pathol 37:852–858, 1984

8. MRC Working Party on Leukaemia in Adults. Analysis and management of renal failure in the fourth MRC myelomatosis trial. Br Med J 288:1411–1416, 1984

9. Solomon A: Bence Jones proteins and light chains of immunoglobulins. XV. Effects of corticosteroids on synthesis and excretion of Bence Jones protein. J Clin Invest 61:97–108, 1978

10. Clyne DH, Pollak VE: Renal handling and pathophysiology of Bence Jones proteins. Contrib Nephrol 24:78–87, 1981

11. Scarpioni L, Ballocchi S, Bergonzi G, et al: Glomerular and tubular proteinuria in myeloma. Relationship with Bence Jones proteinuria. Contrib Nephrol 26:89–102, 1981

12. Hill GS, Morel-Maroger L, Méry J-P, et al: Renal lesions in multiple myeloma: Their relationship to associated protein abnormalities. Am J Kidney Dis 2:423–438, 1983

13. Coward RA, Mallick NP, Delamore IW: Tubular function in multiple myeloma. Clin Nephrol 24:180–185, 1983

14. Solomon A: Bence-Jones proteins and light chains of immunoglobulins. N Engl J Med 294:17–23; 91–98, 1976

15. Solomon A: Current developments in immunoglobulins, in Silber T, Gordon AS, Lobue J, et al (eds): Contemporary Hematology/Oncology, vol. 2. New York, Plenum, 1981, p 399

16. Stevens FJ, Westholm FA, Solomon A, et al: Self-association of human immunoglobulin κI light chains: Role of the third hypervariable region. Proc Natl Acad Sci USA 77:1144–1148, 1980

17. Clyne DH, Pesce AJ, Thompson RE: Nephrotoxicity of Bence Jones proteins in the rat: Importance of protein isoelectric point. Kidney Int 16:345–352, 1979

18. Coward RA, Delamore IW, Mallick NP, et al: The importance of urinary immunoglobulin light chain isoelectric point (pI) in nephrotoxicity in multiple myeloma. Clin Sci 66:229-232, 1984

19. Holland MD, Galla JH, Sanders PW, et al: Effect of urinary pH and diatrizoate on Bence Jones protein nephrotoxicity in the rat. Kidney Int 27:46–50, 1985

20. Clyne DH, Kant KS, Pesce AJ, et al: Nephrotoxicity of low molecular weight serum proteins: Physicochemical interactions between myoglobin, hemoglobin, Bence Jones proteins and Tamm-Horsfall mucoprotein. Curr Prob Clin Biochem 9:299–308, 1979

21. Gauthier VJ, Mannik M, Striker GE: Effect of cationized antibodies in preformed immune complexes on deposition and persistence in renal glomeruli. J Exp Med 156:766–777, 1982

22. Kabat EA, Wu TT, Bilofsky H, et al: Sequences of proteins of immunological interest. Bethesda, Md, National Institutes of Health, 1983

23. Smolens P, Venkatachalam M, Stein JH: Myeloma kidney cast nephropathy in a rat model of multiple myeloma. Kidney Int 24:192-204, 1983

24. Koss MN, Pirani CL, Osserman EF: Experimental Bence Jones cast nephropathy. Lab Invest 34:579–591, 1976

25. Fine J, Rees ED: Renal cytotoxic effects of Bence-Jones protein. Lancet 1:150, 1977 (letter)

26. Weiss JH, Williams RH, Galla JH, et al: Pathophysiology of acute Bence-Jones protein nephrotoxicity in the rat. Kidney Int 20:198–210, 1981

27. Baylis C, Falconer-Smith J, Ross BD: The renal handling of human immunoglobulin light chains (IgLC) in the Munich-Wistar rat. Kidney Int 21:242, 1982 (abstr)

28. Batuman V, Batuman O, Sastrasinh M, et al: Bence-Jones protein (BJP) inhibits glucose and alanine uptake in rat renal brush border membrane vesicles (BBMV). Clin Res 32:441A, 1984 (abstr)

29. Bryan CW, McIntire KR: Effect of sustained diuresis on the renal lesions of mice with Bence Jones protein-producing tumors. J Lab Clin Med 83:409–416, 1974

30. Maldonado JE, Velosa JA, Kyle RA, et al: Feanconi syndrome in adults. A manifestation of a latent form of myeloma. Am J Med 58:354–364, 1975

31. Gailani S, Seon B-K, Henderson ES: κ light chain-myeloma associated with adult Fanconi syndrome: Response of the nephropathy to treatment of myeloma. Med Pediatr Oncol 4:141–147, 1978

32. Seon BK: Unique amino acid sequences of Bence Jones proteins in the urine of patients with adult Fanconi syndrome. Mol Immunol 19:83–86, 1982

33. Alavi N, Lianos EA, Palant CE, et al: Induction of epithelial tight junctions by a light chain protein isolated from a patient with Fanconi's syndrome. Nephron 35:130–135, 1983

34. Smithline N, Kassirer JP, Cohen JJ: Light-chain nephropathy. Renal tubular dysfunction associated with light-chain proteinuria. N Engl J Med 294:71-74, 1976

35. Ganeval D, Mignon F, Preud'homme JL, et al: Visceral deposition of monoclonal light chains and immunoglobulins: A study of renal and immunopathologic abnormalities. Adv Nephrol 11:25–63, 1982

36. Randall RE, Williamson WC Jr, Mullinax F, et al: Manifestations of systemic light chain deposition. Am J Med 60:293–299, 1976

37. Preud'homme JL, Morel-Maroger L, Brouet JC, et al: Synthesis of abnormal immunoglobulins in lymphoplasmatcytic disorders with visceral light chain deposition. Am J Med 69:703–710, 1980

38. Preud'homme JL, Morel-Maroger L, Brouet JC, et al: Synthesis of abnormal heavy and light chains in multiple myeloma with visceral deposition of monoclonal immunoglobulin. Clin Exp Immunol 42:545–553, 1980

39. Gallo GR, Feiner HD, Katz LA, et al: Nodular glomerulopathy associated with nonamyloidotic kappa light chain deposits and excess immunoglobulin light chain synthesis. Am J Pathol 99:621–644, 1980

40. Sølling K, Sølling J, Jacobsen NO, et al: Nonsecretory myeloma associated with nodular glomerulosclerosis. Acta Med Scand 207:137–143, 1980

41. Tubbs RR, Gephardt GN, McMahon JT, et al: Light chain nephropathy. Am J Med 71:263–269, 1981

42. Ganeval D, Noël L-H, Preud'homme JL, et al: Light-chain deposition disease: Its relation with AL-type amyloidosis. Kidney Int 26:1–9, 1984

43. Linder J, Vollmer RT, Croker BP, et al: Systemic kappa light-chain deposition. An ultrastructural and immunohistochemical study. Am J Surg Pathol 7:85–93, 1983

44. Droz D, Noel LH, Carnot F, et al: Liver involvement in nonamyloid light chain deposits disease. Lab Invest 50:683–689, 1984

45. Silver MM, Hearn SA, Ritchie S, et al: Renal and systemic kappa light chain deposits and their plasma cell origin identified by immunoelectron microscopy. Am J Pathol 122:17–27, 1986

46. Palant CE, Bonitati J, Bartholomew WR, et al: Nodular glomerulosclerosis associated with multiple myeloma. Role of light chain isoelectric point. Am J Med 80:98–102, 1986

47. Sølling K, Sølling J, Nielsen JL: Polymeric Bence Jones proteins in serum in myeloma patients with renal insufficiency. Acta Med Scand 216:495–502, 1984

48. Duffy JL, Khurana E, Susin M, et al:Fibrillary renal deposits and nephritis. Am J Pathol 113:279–290, 1983

49. Alpers CE, Hopper J Jr, and Biava CG: Light-chain glomerulopathy with amyloid-like deposits. Human Pathol 15:444–448, 1984

50. Isobe T, Osserman EF: Patterns of amyloidosis and their association with plasma-cell dyscrasia, monoclonal immunoglobulins and Bence-Jones proteins. N Engl J Med 290:473–477, 1974

51. Solomon A, Frangione B, Franklin EC: Bence Jones proteins and light chains of immunoglobulins. Preferential association of the $V_{\lambda VI}$ subgroup of human light chains with amyloidosis AL(λ). J Clin Invest 70:453–460, 1982

52. Solomon A, Kyle RA, Frangione B: Light chain subgroups of monoclonal immunoglobulins in amyloidosis AL, in Glenner GG (ed): Proceedings of the IVth International Symposium on Amyloidosis. New York, Plenum, 1986 (in press)

53. Solomon A: Light chains of human immunoglobulins. Methods Enzymol 116:101–121, 1985

54. Sletten K, Natvig JB, Husby G, et al: The complete amino acid sequence of a prototype immunoglobulin-λ light-chain-type amyloid-fibril protein AR. Biochem J 195:561–572, 1981

55. Takahashi N, Takayasu T, Isobe T, et al: Comparative study on the structure of the light chains of human immunoglobulins. Assignment of a new subgroup. J. Biochem 86:1523–1535, 1979.

56. Frangione B, Moloshok T, Solomon A: Primary structure of the variable region of a human λVI light chain: Bence Jones protein SUT. J Immunol 131:2490–2493, 1983

57. Dwelet FE, Strako K, Benson MD: Amino acid sequence of a λVI primary (AL) amyloid protein (WLT). Scand J Immunol 22:653–660, 1985

58. Ghiso J, Solomon A, Frangione B: Association of human λ light chain V/J/C segments: Serologic analysis and primary structure of the λVI Bence Jones protein THO. J Immunol 136:716–719, 1986

59. Schiffer M, Girling RL, Ely KR, et al: Structure of a λ-type Bence Jones protein at 3.5-Å resolution. Biochemistry 12:4620–4631, 1973

60. Skinner M, Benson MD, Cohen AS: Amyloid fibril protein related to immunoglobulin λ-chains. J Immunol 114:1433–1435, 1974

61. Cohen D, Pras M, Franklin EC, et al: Characterization of amyloid deposits and P component from a patient with Factor X deficiency reveals proteins derived from a lambda VI light chain. Am J Med 74:513–518, 1983

62. Sletten K, Westermark P, Pitkänen P, et al: Amino acid sequences in amyloid proteins of κIII immunoglobulin light-chain origin. Scand J Immunol 18:557–560, 1983

63. Solomon A, McLaughlin CL: Bence-Jones proteins and light chains of immunoglobulins. I. Formation and characterization of amino-terminal (variant) and carboxyl-terminal (constant) halves. J Biol Chem 244:3393–3404, 1969

64. Cohen HJ, Lessin LS, Hallal J, et al: Resolution of primary amyloidosis during chemotherapy. Studies in a patient with nephrotic syndrome. Ann Intern Med 82:466–473, 1975

65. Kjeldsberg CR, Eyre HJ, Totzke H: Evidence for intracellular amyloid formation in myeloma. Blood 50:493–504, 1977

66. Nomura S, Kanoh T, Uchino H: Intracellular formation of amyloid fibrils in myeloma: Cytochemical, immunochemical and electron microscopic observations. Cancer 54:303–307, 1984

67. Durie BGM, Persky B, Soehnlen BJ, et al: Amyloid

production in human myeloma stem-cell culture, with morphologic evidence of amyloid secretion by associated macrophages. N Engl J Med 307:1689–1692, 1982
68. Krause JR: Acquired factor X deficiency and amyloidosis. Am J Clin Pathol 67:170–173, 1977
69. Furie B, Greene E, Furie BC: Syndrome of acquired factor X deficiency and systemic amyloidosis. In vivo studies of the metabolic fate of factor X. N Engl J Med 297:81–85, 1977
70. Greipp PR, Kyle RA, Bowie EJW: Factor X deficiency in primary amyloidosis. Resolution after splenectomy. N Engl J Med 301:1050–1051, 1979
71. Triplett DA, Bang NU, Harms CS, et al: Mechanism of acquired factor X deficiency in primary amyloidosis. Blood 50:285, 1977 (suppl) (abstr)
72. Burke JF Jr, Flis R, Lasker N, et al: Malignant lymphoma with "myeloma kidney" acute renal failure. Am J Med 60:1055–1060, 1976
73. Hannam-Harris AC, Gordon J, Smith JL: Immunoglobulin synthesis by neoplastic B lymphocytes: Free light chain synthesis as a marker of B cell differentiation. J Immunol 125:2177–2181, 1980
74. Pierson J, Darley T, Stevenson GT, et al: Monoclonal immunoglobulin light chains in urine of patients with lymphoma. Br J Cancer 41:681–688, 1980
75. Sølling K, Nielsen JL, Sølling J, et al: Free light chains of immmunoglobulins in serum from patients with leukaemias and multiple myeloma. Scand J Haematol 29:309–318, 1982
76. Deegan MJ, Abraham JP, Sawdyk M, et al: High incidence of monoclonal proteins in the serum and urine of chronic lymphocytic leukemia patients. Blood 64:1207–1211, 1983
77. Kyle RA, Greipp PR: "Idiopathic" Bence Jones proteinuria: Long-term follow-up in seven patients. N Engl J Med 306:564–567, 1982
78. Solomon A: Bence Jones proteins: Malignant or benign? N Engl J Med 306:605–607, 1982 (editorial)
79. Solomon A, Machado E: Nephrotoxicity of human Bence Jones proteins. Clin Res 33:354A, 1985 (abstr)
80. Kyle RA: Analyses of immunoglobulins in urine, in Duarte CG (ed): Renal Function Tests. Boston, Little, Brown, 1980, p 291
81. Norden AGW, Fulcher LM, Flynn FV: Detection of Bence-Jones protein by isoelectricfocussing of unconcentrated urine followed by nitrocellulose blotting and immunoperoxidase staining. Clin Chem Acta 153:149–156, 1985
82. Bouvet J-P, Pillot J, Liacopoulos P: Human myeloma light chains with increased molecular weight: High frequency among λ chains. Mol Immunol 20:397–407, 1983
83. Klein M, Kells DIC, Tinker DO, et al: Thermodynamic and conformational studies on an immunoglobulin light chain which reversibly precipitates at low temperatures. Biochemistry 16:552–560, 1977
84. Mosman TR, Williamson AR: Structural mutations in a mouse immunoglobulin light chain resulting in failure to be secreted. Cell 20:283–292, 1980
85. Wu GE, Hozumi N, Murialdo H: Secretion of a λ_2 immunoglobulin chain is prevented by a single amino acid substitution in its variable region. Cell 33:77–83, 1983
86. Solomon A: Monoclonal immunoglobulins as biomarkers of cancer, in Sell S (ed): Cancer Markers: Diagnostic and Developmental Significance. Clifton, NJ, Humana, 1980, p 57
87. Mallick NP, Dosa S, Acheson EJ, et al: Detection, significance and treatment of paraprotein in patients presenting with 'idiopathic' proteinuria without myeloma. Q J Med 47:145–175, 1978
88. McLeod BC, Viernes A, Kyle RA, et al: Analysis of serum free light chains by crossed immunoelectrophoresis: Comparison with urinary light chains in light chain disease. J Clin Oncol 2:1110–1114, 1984
89. Durie BGM, Cole PW, Chen HG, et al: Synthesis and metabolism of Bence Jones protein and calculation of tumour burden in patients with Bence Jones myeloma. Br J Haematol 47:7–19, 1981
90. Brown WW, Hebert LA, Piering WF, et al: Reversal of chronic end-stage renal failure due to myeloma kidney. Ann Intern Med 90:793–794, 1979
91. Misiani R, Remuzzi G, Bertani T, et al: Plasmapheresis in the treatment of acute renal failure in multiple myeloma. Am J Med 66:684–688, 1979
92. Dahlberg PJ, Newcomer KL, Yutuc WR, et al: Myeloma kidney: Improved renal function following long-term chemotherapy and hemodialysis. Am J Nephrol 3:242–243, 1983
93. Bernstein SP, Humes HD: Reversible renal insufficiency in multiple myeloma. Arch Intern Med 142:2083–2086, 1982
94. Pasquali S, Cagnoli C, Rovinetti C, et al: Plasma exchange therapy in rapidly progressive renal failure due to multiple myeloma. Int J Artif Organs 8:S–2, 27–30, 1984
95. Cohen DJ, Sherman WH, Osserman EF, et al: Acute renal failure in patients with multiple myeloma. Am J Med 76:247–256, 1984
96. Buxbaum JN, Hurley ME, Chuba J, et al: Amyloidosis of the AL type: Clinical, morphologic and biochemical aspects of the response to therapy with alkylating agents and prednisone. Am J Med 67:867–878, 1979
97. Wegeluis O: The resolution of amyloid substance. Acta Med Scand 212:273–275, 1982 (editorial)
98. Tutt AL, Stevenson JF, Smith JL, et al: Antibodies against urinary light chain idiotypes as agents for detection and destruction of human neoplastic B lymphocytes. J Immunol 131:3058–3063, 1983
99. Miller RA, Maloney DG, Warnke R, et al: Treatment of B-cell lymphoma with monoclonal anti-idiotype antibody. N Engl J Med 306:517–522, 1982

Monoclonal Immunoglobulins With Antibody Activity in Myeloma, Macroglobulinemia and Related Plasma Cell Dyscrasias

Giampaolo Merlini, Mehdi Farhangi, and Elliott F. Osserman

IN 1964 WALDENSTRÖM et al[1] stated, "Our understanding of the pathology in myeloma and in similar conditions with an increase in so-called M components would be greatly advanced if we could decide whether this increased globulin is chemically abnormal or whether it is one of the normally occurring gamma globulins and is increased only in quantity." He stated further, "We have reason to believe that the hypergammaglobulinemia in these conditions is caused by increased formation of one, or possibly some closely related, individual gamma globulin(s)." On the basis of evidence accumulated over the past two decades, it now appears virtually certain that all monoclonal immunoglobulins (M-Igs) elaborated in multiple myeloma (MM) and related plasma cell dyscrasias (PCD) are functional antibodies for specific antigens. A logical sequitur of this hypothesis is that Bence Jones (BJ) proteins that are L chain polypeptides produced in excess in certain cases of PCD are pieces of functional antibodies and these pieces may also have the capacity to interact with specific ligands, albeit to a lesser extent than intact immunoglobulins. The purpose of this paper is to review some of the evidence supporting these hypotheses and to consider some of the physiologic and pathologic implications of the antibody specificities of M-Igs. Comprehensive reviews of these topics were published by Metzger in 1969,[2] Potter in 1971,[3] and Seligmann and Brouet in 1973.[4] Emphasis will therefore be given to studies published subsequent to these reviews.

Two principal approaches have been used for the detection and delineation of antibody activity of human monoclonal immunoglobulins: (1) Pursuit of clinical leads, ie, recognition and investigation of unusual clinical and/or laboratory features in patients with myeloma and related plasma cell dyscrasias and the demonstration that these manifestations were either directly or indirectly related to the associated monoclonal protein. Examples of this approach are definition of chronic cold agglutinin syndrome due to monoclonal IgM interaction with the polysaccharide antigens of erythrocytes; peripheral neuropathies due to monoclonal IgM binding myelin associated glycoprotein; and xanthomatosis, and hyper- and hypo-lipidemias due to M-Ig interacting with lipids and/or lipoproteins; (2) screening of monoclonal immunoglobulins with a wide spectrum of potential ligands, eg, dinitrophenyl (DNP), nucleic acids, dextrans, phosporylcholine, and/or derivatives or protein conjugates of these haptens.

Our observation of already-bound ligand on a monoclonal IgGλ with antiflavin antibody activity[5] has suggested another possible approach to the detection and elucidation of M-protein antibody activities: (3) Identification of ligands already bound to monoclonal immunoglobulins, ie, analyses of purified M-Igs for any ligands that may be attached to their active sites (Fab fragments).

Each of these three approaches for the identification of antibody activity has its own particular limitations. Among limitations inherent in the detection of antibody activities in monoclonal immunoglobulins via leads provided by specific clinical-pathologic manifestations in individual cases are (1) the relative infrequency of overt abnormalities, eg, cold agglutinin disease, peripheral neuropathies, lipid disturbances, which can be directly related to M protein antibody activity per se, and (2) the difficulty of precisely identifying the antigen or antigenic

---

From the Department of Medicine and Institute of Cancer Research, Cancer Center, College of Physicians and Surgeons, Columbia University, New York; the Institute of Clinical Medicine, II, I.R.C.C.S., Policlinico S. Matteo, Pavia, Italy; and the Department of Medicine, University of Missouri-Columbia.

Supported by grant CA 21112 of National Cancer Institute, the Amy and Saul Z. Cohen Family Foundation.

Address reprint requests to Giampaolo Merlini, MD, Institute of Clinical Medicine, II, I.R.C.C.S. Policlinico S. Matteo, 27100 Pavia, Italy.

0093-7754/86/1303-0012$05.00/0

determinants involved in apparently specific interactions between M proteins and complex macromolecules such as coagulation factors, IgG, and lipoproteins.

Some of the inherent difficulties in the screening approach are (1) the very large number and variety of reactants that must be tested, and (2) the specificity and sensitivity of the techniques for testing, eg, precipitin reactions detect active IgM and probably miss active IgG and IgA. However, the use of more sensitive techniques such as radioimmune assays and enzyme immune assays (ELISA), combined with immunoblotting has proved extremely efficient in detecting and characterizing M-Ig antibody specificities as, for example, in the case of IgM with antimyelin-associated glycoprotein activity.

Finally, with respect to the possibility of already-bound antigens on monoclonal immunoglobulins, certain assumptions must be made including (1) that the putative ligands are attached with sufficiently high affinity not to be dissociated in the course of immunoglobulin purification, and (2) that the ligands are present in sufficiently high concentration to be detectable and identifiable after dissociation from the immunoglobulin. In the case of the flavin-binding IgG,[5] both of these conditions were met.

As will be emphasized below, the great majority of the ligands that have been identified in the human plasma cell dyscrasias are either autologous components such as red blood cell glycoproteins, IgG, neural glycoproteins, or antigens of common bacterial organisms, eg, *Klebsiella*, which are frequently present in normal intestinal bacteria. In both cases, the ligands have the property of persistence, ie, they are not eliminated by the evoked antibody response.

POLYSACCHARIDES

Red Blood Cell Polysaccharide—Related Antigens

Christenson and Dacie[6] first reported antibody activity in M-Ig. They found that nine out of ten sera containing cold agglutinin (CA) at very high titers presented an abnormal peak in the electrophoretic γ_1 region. Comprehensive reviews on CA have been published by Roelcke[7] and by Pruzanski and Katz.[8] As shown in Table 1, most of the CA belong to the IgM class and have κ light chains. However, IgMλ, IgAκ, and IgGκ CA have also been reported. IgMκ CA are usually directed against I antigen; IgMλ CA toward i or non-I/i antigens.

Capra et al[9] studied the N terminal sequence of isolated κ chains of nine IgM CA and found that six were VkIII subgroup, two VkII, and only one VkI subgroup. They postulated that this unusual subgroup distribution was probably related to the specificity of the monoclonal antibody.

CA with related specificities were shown by Williams et al[10] to have unique shared idiotypic determinants. Absorption of antiidiotypic anti-

Table 1. Monoclonal Immunoglobulins (M-Igs) with Antibody Activity Against Red Blood Cell Polysaccharides—Related Antigens

Specificity	M-Igs	Disease	References
I, i, I-i	IgMκ, IgMλ, IgMκ/IgG, IgGκ	CCAD, WM, RS, HL, NHL, CLL, WAHA + CCAD, AIL	9–27
Not I-i	IgMκ, IgMλ	CCAD, WM	15, 29
Pr antigens	IgAκ, IgMλ, IgMκ, IgGκ	CCAD, RS, MM, WM, CLL + CCAD, Lymphoma	14, 20, 28 30–36
Gd	IgMκ, IgMλ	CCAD, WM	37, 38
Sa	IgMκ	CCAD	39
Fl	IgMκ	CCAD + IB	40
Vo	IgMλ	CCAD + CLL	41
P Pp	IgMκ	WM-NHL	42, 43
Forssman	IgMκ	WM	44
Lacto-N-tetraose	IgMλ	Bronchogenic-Ca	45
Lacto-N-neotetraose	IgMκ	WM	46

Abbreviations: CCAD, chronic cold agglutinin disease; WM, Waldenström's macroglobulinemia; RS, reticulosarcoma; HL, Hodgkin's lymphoma; NHL, non-Hodgkin's lymphoma; CLL, chronic lymphocytic leukemia; WAHA, warm autoimmune hemolytic anemia; AIL, angioimmunoblastic lymphadenopathy; MM, multiple myeloma; IB, immunoblastoma; Ca, carcinoma.

sera with other CA did not inhibit precipitation reaction with the immunizing antigen, proving the existence of individual specificities.[11]

The molecular basis of I and i specificities has been elucidated by Feizi et al.[47] The i antigen is a linear and I a branched carbohydrate chain made up of N-acetyllactosamine Galβ(1 $\rightarrow$ 4) GlcNAc units. Both linear and branched structures serve as precursor chains for the blood group A B H antigens. I antigen is present on adult red cells, the i antigen on cord red cells and in infants younger than 18 months. I/i antigens have been shown in a high proportion of B and T cells[48] and expressed in adenocarcinomas of blood group A B H-secreting tissues.[48a] All known IgA and some IgG CA are directed toward Pr antigenic group. Pr antigens are heterogeneous glycoproteins carrying oligosaccharides with terminal immunodominant N-acetylneuraminic acid. Pr antigens are inactivated by proteases and by neuraminidase.[12] The study of anti-Pr cold agglutinins has allowed the detection of the κ chain variable region subgroup VkIV.[49] An M-IgM cryoglobulin with cold agglutinin specificity toward Pr_2 antigen has been reported by Yeni et al.[28] The Pr_2 antigenic determinant, a GM_3-like ganglioside was demonstrated to be tightly bound to purified M-IgM and could only be extracted by denaturing methods. The authors postulated that the already bound ligand could determine the cryoprecipitability of the M-IgM. A similar mechanism might account for the frequent cryoprecipitability of monoclonal CA. Furthermore, the study by Yeni et al[28] shows that part of the circulating M-Ig could have the binding site occupied by a tightly bound ligand. Previously Roelcke et al[50] reported IgMκ CA Ad reacting with the immunodominant neuroaminyl groups on red cell membrane sialoglycoproteins, but with different animal red cell specificity than anti-Pr CA. Two cases of chronic cold agglutinin disease with M-IgMκ in which the agglutinin reactions were inhibited best by the trisaccharide sialyllactose NeuNAcα(2 $\rightarrow$ 3)*D*Galβ (1 $\rightarrow$ 4)*D*Glc have been reported.[51] This specificity has been termed anti-Gd, denoting glycolipid dependence; and it is sensitive to neuraminidase, resistant to proteases, and expressed at birth on red cells. Four other types of neuraminic acid determined antigens have been reported: Sa,[39] Fl,[40] Lud,[52] and Vo.[41] Several other specificities apparently related to blood group glycoproteins have been documented with other M-IgM cold agglutinins as well as IgMs lacking the cold agglutinin property.[13,42,43,45,46]

Acid Polysaccharides

M-Ig's with apparent specificity for acid polysaccharides have been reported by several authors.[53–61] The specificities extend from carrageenean, agar, heparin, dextran, to polysaccharides present on bacterial cell walls and animal tissues. The M-Ig is usually an IgM, but IgG as well as IgA M-Ig have also been reported.

The studies of Burtin and Gendron[54] and of Levy et al[59] strongly suggest that in several instances the M-Ig interactions with sulfated polysaccharides occur as a result of an electrostatic interaction between cationic sites on certain immunoglobulins and anionic sulfate residues of agaropectin[54] and heparin.[59] However, the overall charge of the protein cannot be the sole explanation for this interaction; it may represent only one criterion for binding that requires, in addition, a specific immunoglobulin conformation or charge distribution.

The immunochemical basis of specific reactions to acidic *Klebsiella* polysaccharides has been extensively characterized. Following the studies of Hannestad and Sletten[62] and Harboe et al,[63] on M-IgM that reacted with specific *Klebsiella* polysaccharides, Savage and Dutton, in 1978[64] defined the *Klebsiella* K12 polysaccharide antigenic determinant as 4,6-pyruvylated-*D*-galactose linked β(1 $\rightarrow$ 4) to *D*-glucuronic acid linked β(1 $\rightarrow$ 6) to a main chain. Immunochemical studies, by Kabat et al[65,66] on six human M-IgMκ reacting with *Klebsiella* polysaccharides, found specificity for 3,4-pyruvylated-*D*-galactose in four and for 4,6-pyruvylated-*D*-glucose in one.

Sherman et al[67] and Kabat et al[68] studied two patients with M-IgM, axonal type polyneuropathy, and epidermolysis. Both the IgMs precipitated with chondroitin sulfates, but with different specificities.[68] The authors speculated that the interaction of the IgM with chondroitin sulfates could cause both the axonal polyneuropathy and the epidermolysis.[67]

Emmrich et al[69] reported in 1985 two IgMs out of 550 serum samples from patients with IgM myeloma and macroglobulinemia binding, with relatively high affinity, to the carbohydrate of group A streptococci (A-CHO). It is noteworthy that naturally occurring anti-A-CHO antibodies of low affinity are found in virtually all normal individuals tested.

BACTERIAL EXOENZYMES, EXTRACELLULAR PROTEINS OF MICROORGANISMS

In 1964, Waldenström et al[1] reported several sera with M-Ig and antistreptolysin O (ASLO) and antistaphylolysin activities. In 1968, Zettervall[70] reported that the activities resided in the Fab fragments of some of these purified M-IgG. In the same year, Seligmann et al[71] reported a cryoprecipitable myeloma IgG1κ with ASLO activity localized to the Fab fragment. Several other authors reported monoclonal components with antibody activity against extracellular proteins of microorganisms: Streptolysin 0,[72–81] α-staphylolysin,[70,82] streptococcal hyaluronidase,[83] and streptococcal deoxyribonuclease B.[84] In some cases the patient's history was positive for previous streptococcal infections,[76,78,79] but in most of the patients, the history was negative. However, most human beings have a low level of ASLO antibodies, which probably reflects natural immunization with hemolytic streptococcal strains. There is no striking heavy or light chain restriction, also IgA[74] and IgD[77] monoclonal ASLO antibodies have been described. Attempts to demonstrate shared idiotypy among ASLO M-IgG have been negative so far.[71,80] Mansa and Kjems in 1978[85] published an abstract claiming weak cross-idiotypic reactions between two out of 16 M-Igs with ASLO activity.

RHEUMATOID FACTORS

Rheumatoid factors (RFs) are autoantibodies reacting with the Fc portion of autologous IgG. They have been extensively studied (see reviews by Johnson and Page Faulk,[86] and by Carson).[87] We do not intend to survey this broad field, but to focus on the monoclonal RF (MRF).

Although most MRFs are IgMκ, there are reports of M-IgG (predominantly IgG3)[88] and IgA RF.[89,90] These proteins may require special conditions to demonstrate RF reactivity, such as reaction in the cold or at low pH. In many instances MRF are cryoglobulins. The cryoprecipitate is constituted by M-Ig and polyclonal IgG, ie, the M-Ig circulates with the ligand, IgG, bound to it. MRFs react with a diverse array of antigenic determinants localized in the Fc portion of the IgG molecule, in both the CH_2 and CH_3 domain.[86] IgG subclass restriction (IgG1, IgG2, and IgG4) specificity has been found for IgM RF[91] and IgA RF.[89] This has been attributed to an isotypic IgG autoantigenic determinant shared by the IgG1, IgG2, and IgG4 subclasses, called Ga antigen.[92] The affinity of MRF for IgG has been determined by several authors to be $\sim 6.10^4\ M^{-1}$ for IgM RF,[93] $10^4\ M^{-1}$ for IgG3 RF,[88] and $\sim 10^6\ M^{-1}$ for IgA RF.[89] The values for IgM and IgG RF are from ten- to 100-fold less than the affinities of common heteroantibodies produced after exogenous immunization. A cross-idiotypic specificity for M-IgM anti-γ-globulins has been demonstrated by Kunkel et al[94] who classified these molecules into two idiotypically distinct groups: Wa and Po; a third group, Bla, was subsequently defined by Agnello et al[95] with both anti-IgG and anti-DNA histone activity. Among the Wa-positive IgMκ, a marked restriction of the light chain was noticed[96]: All of them belong to the subgroup VkIIIb[97,98]; indicating a derivation from a family of closely related VkIII germ line genes.

LIPOPROTEINS

In 1960 Heremans[99] delineated a syndrome consisting of xanthomatosis, hyperlipoproteinemia, and plasma cell dyscrasia with IgA M-component. Kayden et al[100] showed in 1962 that the monoclonal immunoglobulin, not characterized, of a patient with MM, planar xanthomatosis, and hyperlipidemia exhibited antibody activity to β-lipoprotein. As outlined in Table 2, biochemical and clinical features of the cases reported subsequently have been highly variable.[57,101–117] The M-Igs are predominantly IgA and IgG (only one IgMκ)[113]; specificities include high density lipoproteins HDL, low density lipoproteins LDL, very low density lipoproteins VLDL, apo-B and apo-E apoproteins. Beaumont and Beaumont[113,117] introduced the concept of autoimmune hyperlipidemia. They showed that the hyperlipidemia is the end result of action of antibodies that inhibit different stages of the complex lipolytic processes and compensatory acceleration of cellular lipoprotein synthesis and secretion.[112,115,117] The lipid profiles in some

Table 2. Monoclonal Immunoglobulins (M-Igs) with Antibody Activity Against Lipoproteins

Specificity	M-Igs	Disease	References
Lipoproteins (LDL)	IgA	MM, plane, tuberous xanthoma	101, 102
	γ-globulin	MM, plane xanthoma	100
	IgA	BMG, plane and/or tuberous xanthoma	99, 103
	IgAλ	BMG, xanthomatosis, hyperlipidemia	104
	IgGκ	BMG, xanthomatosis, hyperlipidemia	105
LDL-VLDL	IgA	MM and hypolipidemia	106
Choline-chloride of α and β lipoproteins	IgAκ	MM, xanthamotosis, hyperlipidemia	107
HDL	IgGλ	MM, xanthomatosis, hyperlipidemia	108
β and pre β lipoproteins, albumin (Nonimmunologic interactions)	IgGκ	MM, plane xanthomatosis, normal lipid	57
VLDL	IgGκ	BMG, plane xanthomatosis, normal lipid	109
P.G. (phospholipid) on α and β lipoproteins	IgAκ	MM, xanthomatosis, hyperlipidemia	110, 111 112
P.G. (phospholipid) on α and β lipoproteins	IgMκ	BMG, xanthomatosis	113
A.S. (lipid) on α and β lipoproteins	IgGκ	MM, xanthomatosis, hyperlipidemia	114
Apo-B (VLDL, IDL, LDL)	IgG, IgAκ, IgGκ	MM, xanthomatosis, hyperlipidemia	106, 115
Apo-B, Apo-E	IgAκ	MM, hyperlipidemia, no xanthomatosis, hyperviscosity syndrome	116

patients have several features in common with familial type III hyperlipoproteinemia (marked elevation of intermediate-density lipoprotein IDL and VLDL) but without the characteristic apo-E abnormality of the inherited disorder.[118] Cortese et al[115] studied two such patients with myeloma, plane xanthoma, and apparent type III hyperlipoproteinemia. Kinetic studies in both patients clearly demonstrated an impairment of lipid catabolism. No degradation of ^{125}I IDL occurred when this lipoprotein was incubated with patient's lymphocytes or lymphocytes from normal subject, albeit, normally functioning receptor for IDL apoprotein was demonstrated on these cells. The M-Ig bound to IDL seemed to interfere with the binding of IDL to its cellular receptor, resulting in a greatly reduced IDL fractional catabolic rate. VLDL, IDL, and LDL all have apo-B in common.[118] Although not studied, a binding of M-Ig to apo-B would readily explain these findings. Kilgore et al[116] studied a myeloma patient with IgAκ M-Ig and hyperlipidemia. The monoclonal protein was also associated with VLDL and LDL, but not HDL and exhibited antibody activity for apo-B and apo-E. Moreover, it showed affinity for apo-B-containing lipoprotein from all vertebrate sera tested.

The pathogenesis of hyperlipidemia in patients with plasma cell dyscrasias is more complex than what has been already uncovered. In most studies, a binding of M-Ig to lipid rather than apoprotein has been shown (Table 2). Moreover, lipid disturbances due to altered activity of the heparin-dependent lipoprotein lipase, brought about by heparin-binding M-Igs have been described.[55,114] Complexes resulting from hydrophobic interactions between M-Ig and lipid present in membranes of B lymphocytes have been reported in patients with monoclonal gammopathy.[119]

PHOSPHOLIPIDS

In 1967, Killander et al[120] reported a patient with highly positive Wasserman, but a negative Kline and *Treponema pallidum* immobilization (TPI) test. The monoclonal component was an IgMκ, which reacted with lecithin but not with cardiolipin or cholesterol. Other M components with antibody-like activity against phospholipids used in the tests for syphilis, lecithin and cardiolipin, were reported later.[60,121–125] In all instances, the M-Ig was an IgM, κ or λ, and the underlying disease was a lymphoma or Waldenström's macroglobulinemia. In one case, the silica gel chromatography of purified IgM revealed the presence of both sphingomyelin and lecithin.[122] The M-Ig was therefore circulating with ligands bound to it. The false positive tests for syphilis observed in these cases are probably due to hydrophobic interactions between the macroglobulins and phospholipids. Cross reactivity of M-IgM with DNA and phospholipids (cardiolipin) has been reported[126]; the common determinant may be phosphate groups in phosphodiester linkage separated by three carbon atoms.

NEURAL ANTIGENS

In 1980, Latov et al[127] showed that in a patient with distal and symmetrical neuropathy and early sensory involvement slowly progressing to motor neuropathy, the M-IgM reacted specifically with a component of human peripheral nerve. In several patients with this type of neuropathy subsequently studied, it was demonstrated that the antibody specificity was for human myelin-associated glycoprotein (MAG).[128] Many patients having similar clinical and serological characteristics have been later reported.[129,130] The IgM (κ or λ) M-Ig were found to bind to the same or closely related carbohydrate determinants present in central and peripheral MAG[131–133] and in several other glycoproteins and glycolipids in peripheral nerve.[134,135] Some human M-IgM anti-MAG and a rabbit anti-human MAG have been shown to react with human natural killer (HNK) cells.[136–138] However, these anti-MAG antibodies differ in their pattern of reactivity with HNK-1 cells from that of a mouse monoclonal antibody (anti-HNK-1).[137] Also, although HNK-1 could block the binding of anti-MAG, the reverse was not true.[138]

Evans et al[139] showed cross idiotype reactivity in three anti-MAG IgM out of 11 tested; while Saito et al[140] did not find any shared idiotype in 13 anti-MAG IgM.

The specificity of M-IgM from patients with polyneuropathy that do not bind to MAG remains unknown in most of the cases. In two patients with axonal type of neuropathy and epidermolysis the M-IgMs bound to chondroitin sulfates.[67,68] An M-IgM that did not react with MAG from a patient with demylinating neuropathy reacted with gangliosides containing disialosyl residues.[141]

Rowland et al[142] described a patient with pure motor neuropathy, or lower motor neuron disease, and M-IgM. Subsequently additional cases with similar neuropathy have been identified. In one patient, the M-IgM bound to the galactosyl β(1,3) N-acetylgalactosaminyl moiety of the gangliosides GM1 and GD1b, and possibly to glycoproteins sharing the same determinant.[143]

The $F(ab')_2$ fragments of an M-IgG from a patient with polyneuropathy was found to bind to nerve tissue, but the antigenic determinant was not defined.[202]

To date there are two reports of the passive transfer of demyelinating neuropathy to experimental animals using the purified M-Ig (one IgG and one IgM) from patients with peripheral neuropathy.[144,145] Besinger et al[144] also demonstrated that the Fab, but not Fc, fragment of the M-IgG caused neuropathy. In experiments conducted by Hays et al,[145] intraneural injection of M-IgM with binding affinity for MAG caused local demyelinating changes. Control serum or M-Ig unassociated with neuropathy did not produce such lesion.

NITROPHENYL LIGANDS

Since the first report by Eisen et al,[146] several human monoclonal immunoglobulins binding mono-, di-, or trinitrophenyl groups, either as free haptens or conjugated to proteins, have been reported.[58,60,147–154] Nitrophenyl haptens have been extensively investigated since the immunoglobulin-nitrophenyl ligand interactions can be quantitatively and qualitatively studied by several sensitive immunochemical techniques. The frequency of DNP-binding activity among human monoclonal immunoglobulins is about 1.5%,[149,152] but the affinity of the anti-DNP M-Ig is usually low (10^3–$10^4 M^{-1}$).[58,147] In several instances, nonspecific hydrophobic interactions were found.[60,149] The crystallographic studies of a DNP binding λ Bence Jones dimer established the primary role of hydrophobic residues (phenylalanine and tyrosine) in this function.[153] Subsequent studies on two DNP-binding-BJ from patients with amyloidosis indicated particular involvement of phenylalanine and tyrosine in the first hypervariable region.[154] These studies and others on murine myeloma proteins raised the question of a nonspecific binding of the hapten to hydrophobic sites of the M-Ig.[146,153,155] Many DNP reactive M-Igs cross-react with apparently structurally unrelated ligands, principally IgG[148,150,151] and nucleic acid derivatives.[58,60,152]

The presently available evidence indicates that a number of M-Igs with various antibody specificities may bind DNP on the basis of similarities in stereochemical configuration, hydrophobicity, and charge of the combining site.

SERUM ALBUMIN

Binding of serum albumin to M-Ig has been reported by several investigators; in some instances, as demonstrated by Mannik,[156] the binding was shown to be covalent via disulfide interchange and therefore not immunologically specific.[157,158] There are a few reports of M-Ig-specific binding to albumin.[159–163] In two cases, the IgGλ reacted with a calcium-dependent antigenic site on human albumin, the resulting immune complexes crystallized in the cold probably causing the purpura and necrotizing vasculitis observed in these patients.[163] This is a further example of M-Ig circulating with an already bound ligand.

ALPHA-2-MACROGLOBULIN

Seligmann et al[164] reported an IgG1k myeloma protein that specifically precipitated with α_2-macroglobulin from horse, rabbit, pig, but not human. The patient had received two injections of horse antitetanus serum about 30 to 40 years before developing MM. Fujita et al[165] also described an M-IgG1k reacting specifically (Fab fragment) with α_2-macroglobulin from horse and rabbit in a patient with BMG who never received injections of horse antitetanus serum.

TRANSFERRIN

Westerhausen et al[166] described a patient with high serum iron level, hemochromatosis, and a monoclonal IgG1k with $F(ab')_2$ fragment reacting with transferrin. More recently, Hilgard et al[167] reported a myeloma patient with widespread thrombosis of the small arteries and veins of the skin and muscles probably caused by the intravascular precipitation of a Fab-related fragment of the M-IgGλ complexed with transferrin. However, it is questionable if the association was due to an antibody activity of the M-Ig fragment because the complete M-Ig did not interact with transferrin.

COAGULATION FACTORS

Upon clotting of plasma from patients with myeloma, not uncommonly, friable bulky, gelatinous fibrin clot is obtained. Some studies have shown that the M proteins, when present in high concentrations, inhibit fibrin polymerization by nonspecific protein—protein interaction and, possibly, by binding of bivalent cations; in some studies, however, such interactions appear to be specific.[168–171] Coleman et al[171] showed that $F(ab')_2$ and Fab fragments of five IgG1λ myeloma proteins of patients showing gelatinous blood clots inhibited fibrin polymerization probably by interacting with hidden determinants of fibrinogen.

M-Ig as factor VIII inhibitor has been reported.[172–174] Zettervall and Nilsson[175] reported a patient with malignant lymphoma and M-IgGk and acquired von Willebrand's disease. The purified IgG complexed with the factor VIII molecule in vitro. These complexes were probably rapidly removed in vivo explaining the rapid turnover of all activities combined with the factor VIII protein complex. This study also confirms the presence of circulating M-Ig complexed with the ligand. A similar condition has been described by Bovill et al[176] in a patient with IgGk myeloma protein directed against von Willebrand factor causing an acquired von Willebrand's disease-like syndrome. Many other cases of acquired von Willebrand factor deficiency associated with monoclonal gammopathy have been reported, but attempts to implicate the M-Ig were unsuccessful. Thiagarajan et al[177] reported a patient with macroglobulinemia and a lupus-type anticoagulant (impaired conversion of prothrombin to thrombin) resulting from the specific reaction of the IgMλ paraprotein with acidic phospholipids. An IgG1k myeloma protein with specificity for platelet glycoprotein IIIa has been found in a patient with fatal massive gastrointestinal bleeding.[178]

THYROGLOBULIN AND THYROID HORMONES

In their survey for antibody activity in M-Ig, Waldenström et al[1] found two sera of patients with PCD (a slowly progressing myeloma and an asymptomatic patient) with high titer (1/2,500 and 1/250,000 respectively) of antithyroglobulin activity. Other investigators have subsequently reported antithyroglobulin activity in an IgGλ myeloma protein,[74] in an IgG1k transient monoclonal component,[179] and in an IgG of a patient with B cell lymphoma.[180] Dighiero et al found four M-Ig (IgMk, IgGk, IgGλ, IgAλ) binding strongly to thyroglobulin and tubulin.[181] It is not known whether thyroglobulin specificity is related to tubulin specificity in all M-Ig binding thyroglobulin. No sign of altered thyroid function was reported in patients with antithyroglobulin M-Ig but hypothyroidism was reported in patients with M-Ig binding to T_3 and T_4 (an M-IgM plus polyclonal IgG[182]; and an IgGλ[183]).

CYTOSKELETON PROTEINS AND CELLS

M-Ig with activity against cytoskeleton proteins actin, tubulin[180,181,184] (including antismooth muscle),[74,185] and intermediate filaments[186] have been reported. Natural human antibodies against tubulin, actin, thyroglobulin, and other proteins have been detected in normal subjects and Dighiero et al[181] emphasize the shared antibody specificities between M-Ig and these so called natural antibodies. Micouin et al[187] reported an IgAk myeloma protein with activity against gastric parietal cells in a patient with past history of peptic ulcer disease and gastrectomy. Kiprov and Miller[188] reported three patients with polymyositis and serum IgGk monoclonal proteins. Muscle biopsy in all three patients revealed, by immunofluorescence, linear deposits of IgGk along the sarcolemmal basement membranes of individual fibers. M-IgM with antibody activity toward kidney glomerular antigens was reported in a patient with nephrotic syndrome.[189] Two macroglobulinemia patients without skin lesions with IgMs that reacted with skin basal cells in vitro have been reported.[190] By contrast Vincendeau et al[191] described a patient with myeloma, bullous dermatosis and IgG3λ that bound exclusively to basal cell layer of epidermis. Undoubtedly there are several factors that determine the pathogenic potential of any specific M-Ig, including the precise specificity, isotype, affinity, and complement activation.

NUCLEAR ANTIGENS

As noted previously, Riesen and Morell[152] reported an IgM myeloma protein cross-reacting with DNP-protein conjugates and single stranded DNA. Several M-Ig cross-reacting with DNP and denatured DNA were found by Freedman et al[60] in their survey, and an IgMk cross-reacting with denatured DNA and several other ligands, DNP, dextran, etc, has also been reported.[58] Dighiero et al[180] and Fermand et al[126] reported a patient with Waldenström's macroglobulinemia, pernicious anemia, and IgMλ with antibody activity for the phosphate-sugar backbone of DNA and phospholipids (mainly cardiolipin).

VIRUSES

Gibaud et al[192] reported an IgGk myeloma protein with antirubeola activity located in the Fab fragment. Seigneurin et al[193] reported a monoclonal IgG3k cryoimmunoglobulin with anticytomegolovirus (CMV) activity in a patient with chronic T cell lymphocytic leukemia and subclinical CMV infection. The authors suggest that the uncontrolled proliferation of IgG3K plasma cell clone may reflect the absence of suppressor mechanisms due to immunosuppressive treatment and the underlying leukemia.

DRUGS AND CONTRAST MEDIA

Several years ago we described[194] an elderly man with IgGk M protein and Bence Jones proteinuria, marrow plasmacytosis, and pancytopenia developed after therapy with a sulfonamide (sulfisoxazole) for urinary tract infection. Discontinuation of the drug resulted in prompt recovery from pancytopenia and disappearance of IgG and Bence Jones proteinuria within six months. Del Carpio et al[195] described two patients who developed M proteins in association with reaction to semisynthetic penicillin and cephalosporin. In these two cases and in our case, attempts to demonstrate binding of drugs by M-Ig were unsuccessful. Although this might indicate that the M gammopathy is unrelated to antigenic stimulus by the sensitizing drug, more sensitive and specific tests for drug:M-Ig interactions are needed. An example of lethal consequences of antibody activity exerted by an M protein was reported by Bauer et al.[196] The monoclonal IgM reacted as a precipitating antibody[197] against meglumineioglycamide, the contrast medium used for cholecystoangiography performed in the patient. The infusion of contrast medium caused massive intravascular precipitation of the antigen-antibody complexes with sudden death of the patient.

RIBOFLAVIN

In 1976 Farhangi and Osserman[5] described a patient with MM and xanthoderma due to a flavin binding monoclonal IgGλ (IgG^{GAR}). Purified IgG^{GAR} was bright yellow, and the acid-dissociated chromophore was identified as riboflavin by chromatography and absorption spectroscopy. Native IgG^{GAR} contained 1.45 mol of flavin per mol of IgG, and increased to 2 mol with addition of riboflavin to saturation. The flavin was localized to the Fab fragment and was bound to IgG^{GAR} with high affinity. IgG^{GAR} showed strongest affinities for riboflavin, flavin mononucleotide, and flavin adenine dinucleotide, and lower affinities for dinitrophenyl derivatives and naphthoquinone. More recently, a similar case (DOT) with clinical and biochemical features like GAR has been found by Dr Robert Kyle at the Mayo Clinic, and studied in our laboratory. The interesting point about these cases is that the color of the hapten bound to monoclonal immunoglobulin advertised its presence; thousands of uncolored substances may be bound to M-Ig and also to normal immunoglobulins without being noticed.

IONS

There have been several isolated reports (reviewed by Merlini et al[198]) of patients with MM and asymptomatic increases in total serum calcium with normal ionized serum calcium values. The elevated total serum calcium level was due to binding of calcium to the patient's myeloma protein, invariably IgG. In all the cases tested, the calcium-binding activity was localized to the Fab region. Probably a specific arrangement of negatively charged amino acid residues on Fab fragment is necessary for calcium-binding activity. Baker and Hultquist[199] described a copper-binding IgG1λ protein from the serum of a hypercupremic myeloma patient.

DISCUSSION

Characteristics of the Ligands

The most striking characteristic of the ligands reacting with M-Igs is that the vast majority of them are autologous components present on cells (red cells, neurons, other tissue cells), cell constituents (cytoskeleton proteins, nuclear components), plasma proteins (IgG, apolipoproteins, coagulation factors), and ubiquitous phospholipids. Activities against synthetic ligands, such as DNP and drugs, may represent cross reactions to some autologous components, IgG or nucleic acids, as shown in several instances.[58,148,151,152]

Some antigens are heterologous, present on bacteria cell wall (*Klebsiella, Pneumococcus*) or bacteria products. In most of the cases, the ligand has the characteristic of persistence, eg, autologous components, antigens from commensal bacteria and essential vitamins.

Considering the chemical composition of ligands, the majority of them are carbohydrates (red cell antigens, acidic polysaccharides, carbohydrate determinant of MAG and possibly, carbohydrate of glycoproteins such as IgGs). Proteins (IgG and few other plasma proteins) and lipids (lipoproteins and phospholipids) are less common. Small ligand-like drugs are rarely reported. However, bias in the detecting system cannot be excluded. For instance, most of the M-Ig against carbohydrates cause clinical symptoms such as hemolytic anemias or polyneuropathies thus facilitating the detection of the M-Ig activity. Furthermore, small ligands, such as flavin[5] or gangliosides[28] can pass unnoticed unless the ligand itself reveals its own presence, like the bright yellow riboflavin.

Characteristics of the M-Igs

In M-Igs with antibody activity against I/i red blood cell antigens, IgG, and MAG, there is a predominance of IgMk. Serologic analysis of M-IgM cold agglutinins and rheumatoid factors showed that there is a correlation between idiotype and specificity.[10,11,94,95] Amino acid sequence studies showed that restricted classes of Ig chains (μ and κIII) were selected for these autoantibodies.[9,96,97,98] In M-IgM anti MAG, cross reactive idiotypes were not found[140] or were found in a low percentage of cases,[139] and, to our knowledge, no amino acid sequence has been performed. These class restricted antibodies have been useful in studying the structure-function relationship: M-Ig with similar amino acid sequences in the complementarity determining regions (hypervariable) share the same idiotype and antibody specificity. However, the autoantigens I/i, IgG, and MAG present several determinants. It is not known why only clones reacting with a specific determinant, as indicated by idiotype and sequence similarities among specific antibodies, expand. Furthermore, natural polyclonal antibodies against I, rarely i, antigens,[8] IgG,[87] myelin basic protein[200] along with many others against tubulin, actin, etc.[181] have been reported. The persistence of the antigen (chronic immunostimulation)[3] is important for the onset of a monoclonal gammopathy: In the cases where the antigen exposure is transient, like for drugs or uncommon infectious agents, the reactive M-Ig is also transient.

Characteristics of Reactions between M-Ig and Ligands

Studies of valency and affinity of M-Ig are rather few.[88,89,93] The data available for monoclonal RF show that IgM and IgG RF have rather low affinity, $\sim 10^4 M^{-1}$,[88,93] while IgA RF have higher affinity, $10^6 M^{-1}$.[89] The binding affinity among the M-Ig with autoantibody activity is comparable to that found in a study on polyclonal or monoclonal autoantibodies: 10^4-$10^5 M^{-1}$,[201] which is consistently lower than the affinities of common heteroantibodies produced after exogenous immunization.

Based on their finding of riboflavin tightly bound to myeloma IgG^{GAR}, Farhangi and Osserman[5] have postulated that this type of association, ie, already bound ligand, may be operative with many other M-Igs. In effect this has been shown by Yeni et al[28] for an IgM cryoglobulin with a cold agglutinin specificity toward Pr_2 antigen. In this case, it was shown that a GM_3-like ganglioside could be extracted from purified M-IgM only by drastic methods, implying very high affinity binding.

It should be recognized that the already bound ligand (ABL) concept, as we are presently implying, does not differ from well-established concept of immune complexes, such as rheumatoid factors and DNA-anti-DNA, except with respect to size and pathophysiologic effects. Thus occupancy of the combining site of IgG^{GAR} by riboflavin apparently produced no change in solubility, or complement binding and therefore should be regarded as a clinically-silent immune complex that would have been certainly overlooked if not for its color. We suggest that a systematic study for comparably small ABL should be made on other M-Ig.

Finally, the role of ABL in the induction and perpetuation of plasma cell dyscrasias requires elucidation: Thus the persistence of a ligand in the antibody combining site as opposed to free antigen may play different roles in B cell regulatory mechanisms.

ACKNOWLEDGMENT

We would like to thank Dr Cesare Bergonzi for advice and cooperation, Betty Moore for bibliographic assistance and Ophelia B. Allison for most valuable secretarial assistance.

REFERENCES

1. Waldenström JG, Winblad S, Hallén J, et al: The occurrence of serological "antibody" reagins or similar γ-globulins in conditions with monoclonal hypergammaglobulinemia, such as myeloma, macroglobulinemia, etc. Acta Med Scand 176:619–631, 1964

2. Metzger H: Myeloma proteins and antibodies. Am J Med 47:837–844, 1969

3. Potter M: Myeloma proteins (M-components) with antibody-like activity. N Engl J Med 284:831–838, 1971

4. Seligmann M, Brouet JC: Antibody activity of human myeloma globulins. Semin Hematol 10:163–177, 1973

5. Farhangi M, Osserman EF: Myeloma with xanthoderma due to an IgGλ monoclonal antiflavin antibody. N Engl J Med 294:177–183, 1976

6. Christenson WN, Dacie JV: Serum proteins in acquired haemolytic anaemia (auto-antibody type). Br J Haematol 3:153–164, 1957

7. Roelcke D: A review. Cold agglutinins. Antibodies and antigens. Clin Immunol Immunopathol 2:266–280, 1974

8. Pruzanski W, Katz A: Cold agglutinins. Antibodies with biological diversity. Clin Immunol Rev 3:131–168, 1984

9. Capra JD, Kehoe JM, Williams RC Jr, et al: Light chain sequences of human IgM cold agglutinins. Proc Natl Acad Sci USA 69:40–43, 1972

10. Williams RC, Kunkel HG, Capra JD: Antigenic specificities related to cold agglutinin activity of gamma M globulins. Science 161:379–381, 1968

11. Lecomte J, Feizi T: A common idiotype on human macroglobulins with anti-I and anti-i specificity. Clin Exp Immunol 20:287–302, 1975

12. Roelcke D, Ebert W, Metz J, et al: I-, MN-, and Pr_1/Pr_2 activity of human erythrocyte glycoprotein fractions obtained by ficin treatment. Vox Sang 21:352–361, 1971

13. Rochant H, Tonthat H, Etievant MF, et al: Lambda cold agglutinin with anti-A_1 specificity in a patient with reticulosarcoma. Vox Sang 22:45–53, 1972

14. Feizi T: Lambda chains in cold agglutinins. Science 156:1111–1112, 1967

15. Cooper AG, Worlledge SM: Light chains in chronic cold haemagglutinin disease. Nature 214:799–800, 1967

16. Baumgarten A, Curtain CC, Golab T, et al: Endemic autoimmunity: Cold auto-agglutinins in melanesia. Br J Haematol 15:567–577, 1968

17. Edman P, Cooper AG: Amino-acid sequence of N-terminal end of a cold agglutinin kappa chain. FEBS Lett 2:33–35, 1968

18. Ambrus M, Bajtai G: A case of an IgG-type cold agglutinin disease. Haematologia 3:225–235, 1969

19. Feizi T, Kabat EA: Immunochemical studies on blood groups. LIV. Classification of anti-I and anti-i sera into groups based on reactivity patterns with various antigens

related to the blood group A, B, H, Le^a, Le^b and precursor substances. J Exp Med 135:1247–1258, 1972

20. Gergely J, Wang AC, Fudenberg HH: Chemical analyses of variable regions of heavy and light chains of cold agglutinins. Vox Sang 24:432–440, 1973

21. Pruzanski W, Cowan DH, Parr DM: Clinical and immunological studies of IgM cold agglutinins with lambda type light chains. Clin Immunol Immunopathol 2:234–245, 1974

22. Pruzanski W, Farid N, Keystone E, et al: The influence of homogeneous cold agglutinins on human B and T lymphocytes. Clin Immunol Immunopathol 4:248–257, 1975

23. Pruzanski W, Sutton DCM, Pantalony D: Angioimmunoblastic lymphadenopathy: An immunochemical study. Clin Immunol Immunopathol 6:62–76, 1976

24. Kay NE, Douglas SD, Mand JJ: Hemolytic anemia with serum and erythrocytic-bound low molecular-weight IgM. Clin Immunol Immunopathol 4:216–220, 1975

25. Kay NE, Gordon LI, Douglas SD: Autoimmune hemolytic anemia in association with monoclonal IgM(k) with anti-i activity. Am J Med 64:845–850, 1978

26. Crookston JH: Hemolytic anemia with IgG and IgM autoantibodies and alloantibodies. Arch Intern Med 135:1314–1318, 1975

27. Fingerle RE, Check IJ: Diclonal gammopathy in chronic cold agglutinin disease. Am J Clin Pathol 78:867–870, 1982

28. Yeni P, Harpin ML, Habibi B, et al: Cryoprecipitation of an anti-Pr_2 monoclonal IgM cold agglutinin in the presence of GM_3 ganglioside. J Clin Invest 74:1165–1172, 1984

29. Kuenn JW, Weber R, Teague PO, et al: Cryopathic gangrene with an IgMλ cryoprecipitating cold agglutinin. Cancer 42:1826–1833, 1978

30. Angevine CD, Andersen BR, Barnett EV: A cold agglutinin of the IgA class. J Immunol 96:578–586, 1966

31. Roelcke D, Ebert W, Geisen HP: Anti-Pr_3: Serological and immunochemical identification of a new anti-Pr subspecificity. Vox Sang 30:122–133, 1976

32. Tonthat H, Rochant H, Henry A, et al: A new case of monoclonal IgAκ cold agglutinin with anti-Pr_1d specificity in a patient with persistent HB antigen cirrhosis. Vox Sang 30:464–468, 1976

33. Tsai CM, Zopf DA, Yu RK, et al: A Waldenström macroglobulin that is both a cold agglutinin and a cryoglobulin because it binds N-acetylneuraminosyl residues. Proc Natl Acad Sci USA 74:4591–4594, 1977

34. Pascali E, Pezzoli A, Melato M, et al: Nodular lymphoma eventuating into lymphoplasmocytic lymphoma with monoclonal IgM/λ cold agglutinin and Bence-Jones proteinuria. Acta Haematol 64:94–102, 1980

35. Dellagi K, Brouet JC, Schenmetzler C, et al: Chronic hemolytic anemia due to a monoclonal IgG cold agglutinin with anti-Pr specificity. Blood 57:189–191, 1981

36. Saurat JH, Chavaz P, Carraux P, et al: A human monoclonal antibody reacting with Merkel cells: Immunofluorescence, immunoperoxidase and immunoelectron microscopy. J Invest Dermatol 81:249–253, 1983

37. Roelcke D, Riesen W, Geisen HP, et al: Serological identification of the new cold agglutinin specificity anti-Gd. Vox Sang 33:304–306, 1977

38. Weber RJ, Clem LW: The molecular mechanism of cryoprecipitation and cold agglutination of an IgMλ Waldenström macroglobulin with anti-Gd specificity: Sedimentation analysis and localization of interacting sites. J Immunol 127:300–305, 1981

39. Roelcke D, Pruzanski W, Ebert W, et al: A new human monoclonal cold agglutinin Sa recognizing terminal N-acetylneuraminyl groups on the cell surface. Blood 55:677–681, 1980

40. Roelcke D: A further cold agglutinin, F1, recognizing an N-acetylneuraminic acid-determined antigen. Vox Sang 41:98–101, 1981

41. Roelcke D, Kreft H, Pfister AM: Cold agglutinin Vo - An IgMλ monoclonal human antibody recognizing a sialic acid determined antigen fully expressed on newborn erythrocytes. Vox Sang 47:236–241, 1984

42. Naiki M, Marcus DM: Binding of N-acetylgalactosamine-containing compounds by a human IgM paraprotein. J Immunol 119:537–539, 1977

43. Von Dem Borne AEG Jr, Mol JJ, Joustra-Maas N, et al: Autoimmune haemolytic anaemia with monoclonal IgM(k) anti-P cold autohaemolysins. Br J Haematol 50:345–350, 1982

44. Alving CR, Joseph KC, Wistar R: Influence of membrane composition on the interaction of a human monoclonal "Anti-Forssman" immunoglobulin with liposomes. Biochem 23:4818–4824, 1974

45. Kabat EA, Liao J, Shyong J, et al: A monoclonal IgMλ macroglobulin with specificity for lacto-N-tetraose in a patient with bronchogenic carcinoma. J Immunol 128:540–544, 1982

46. Tsai CM, Zopf DA, Wistar R Jr, et al: A human cold agglutinin which binds lacto-N-neotetraose. J Immunol 117:717–721, 1976

47. Feizi T, Childs RA, Watanabe K, et al: Three types of blood group I specificity among monoclonal anti-I autoantibodies revealed by analogues of a branched erythrocyte glycolipid. J Exp Med 149:975–980, 1979

48. Feizi T, Kapadia A, Yount WJ: I and i antigens of human blood lymphocytes cocap with receptors for concanavalin A. Proc Natl Acad Sci USA 77:376–380, 1980

48a. Feizi T, Turberville C, Westwood JH: Blood-group precursors and cancer-related antigens. Lancet 2:391–393, 1975

49. Wang AC, Fudenberg HH, Wells JV, et al: A new subgroup of the kappa chain variable region associated with anti-Pr cold agglutinin. Nature New Biol 243:126–127, 1973

50. Roelcke D, Forbes IJ, Zalewski PD, et al: A further subspecificity within human monoclonal anti-Pr cold agglutinins. Blut 45:109–114, 1982

51. Roelcke D, Brossmer R, Riesen W: Inhibition of human anti-Gd cold agglutinins by sialyl-lactose. Scand J Immunol 8:179–185, 1978

52. Roelcke D: The Lud cold agglutinin: A further antibody recognizing N-acetylneuraminic acid-determined antigens not fully expressed at birth. Vox Sang 41:316–318, 1981

53. Miller D: Heparin precipitability of the macroglobulin in a patient with Waldenström macroglobulinemia. Blood 16:1313–1317, 1960

54. Burtin P, Gendron MC: A precipitation reaction

between certain human G immunoglobulins and sulfated galactans. Immunochemistry 8:423–429, 1971

55. Glueck HI, MacKenzie MR, Glueck CJ: Crystalline IgG protein in multiple myeloma: Identification effects on coagulation and on lipoprotein metabolism. J Lab Clin Med 79:731–744, 1972

56. Pogliani E, Cofrancesco E, Praga C: Anti-heparin activity of a macroglobulin from a patient with breast adenocarcinoma. Acta Haematol 53:249–255, 1975

57. Wilson DE, Flowers CM, Hershgold EJ, et al: Multiple myeloma, cryoglobulinemia and xanthomatosis. Distinct clinical and biochemical syndromes in two patients. Am J Med 59:721–729, 1975

58. Tolleshaug H, Hannestad K: Binding of ligands to a monoclonal IgM macroglobulin with multiple specificity. Immunochemistry 12:173–182, 1975

59. Levy DE, Horner AA, Solomon A: Immunoglobulin-sulfated polysaccharide interactions. Binding of agaropectin and heparin by human IgG proteins. J Exp Med 153:883–896, 1981

60. Freedmann M, Merrett R, Pruzanski W: Human monoclonal immunoglobulins with antibody-like activity. Immunochemistry 13:193–202, 1976

61. Riesen W, Noseda G, Rudikoff S, et al: An IgM Waldenström protein with anti-phosphorylcholine specificity, in Peeters H (ed): Protides of the Biological Fluids, XX Colloq. Oxford and New York, Pergamon, 1973, p 201

62. Hannestad K, Sletten K: Multiple M-component in a single individual. III: Heterogeneity of M-components in two macroglobulinemia sera with antipolysaccharide activity. J Biol Chem 246:6982–6990, 1971

63. Harboe M, Deverill J, Eriksen J: Capsular swelling and passive haemagglutination induced by monoclonal IgM reacting with acid polysaccharides of *Klebsiella*. Acta Pathol Microbiol Scand Sect C Immunol 83:97–105, 1975

64. Savage AV, Dutton GGS: Structural investigation of *Klebsiella* serotype K12 polysaccharide. Am Chem Soc Mtgs 1:176, 1978 (abstr)

65. Kabat EA, Liao J, Bretting H, et al: Human monoclonal macroglobulins with specificity for *Klebsiella* K polysaccharides that contain 3,4-pyruvylated-*D*-galactose and 4,6-pyruvylated-*D*-galactose. J Exp Med 152:979–995, 1980

66. Rao AS, Liao J, Kabat EA, et al: Immunochemical studies on human monoclonal macroglobulins with specificities for 3,4-pyruvylated-*D*-galactose and 4,6-pyruvylated-*D*-glucose. J Biol Chem 259:1018–1026, 1984

67. Sherman WH, Latov N, Hays AP, et al: Monoclonal IgMκ antibody precipitating with chondroitin sulfate C from patients with axonal polyneuropathy and epidermolysis. Neurology 33:192–201, 1983

68. Kabat EA, Liao J, Sherman WH, et al: Immunochemical characterization of the specificities of two human monoclonal IgM's reacting with chondroitin sulfates. Carbohydr Res 130:289–297, 1984

69. Emmrich F, Bundle D, van der Zee J, et al: Two human IgM myeloma proteins with unusual specificities for streptococcal carbohydrate-associated epitopes. Scand J Immunol 21:119–126, 1985

70. Zettervall O: Antibody activity in monoclonal immunoglobulin G. Acta Med Scand 492:1–64, 1968 (suppl)

71. Seligmann M, Danon F, Basch A, et al: IgG myeloma cryoglobulin with antistreptolysin activity. Nature 220:711–712, 1968

72. Kronvall G: Ligand-binding sites for streptolysin O and staphylococcal protein A on different parts of the same myeloma globulin. Acta Pathol Microbiol Scand 69:619–621, 1967

73. Raynaud M, Alouf JE, Mihaesco C, et al: Étude quantitative de l'activité anti-streptolysine O d'une protéine myelomateuse IgG humaine. Ann Inst Pasteur 118:448–458, 1970

74. Wager O, Räsänen JA, Haltia K, et al: M components with antibody activity anti-smooth muscle, anti-thyroglobulin and streptolysin-O activity in five M component sera. Ann Clin Res 3:86–97, 1971

75. Holm SE, Kaijser B: Extreme ASO activity in an IgG kappa myeloma protein, in Peeters H (ed): Protides of the Biological Fluids, XX Colloq. Oxford and New York, Pergamon, 1973, p 207

76. Sauvezie B, Missioux D, Leroy V, et al: Une nouvelle observation de myélome dont la paraprotéine possede l'activité anti-streptolysine O. Rev Rhum Mal Osteoartic 41:449–453, 1974

77. Swierczynska Z, Wozniczko-Orlowska G, Maldyk H: An IgD myeloma protein with anti-streptolysin O activity. Immunochemistry 13:379–382, 1976

78. Lusterman FAT, Klein F: Two cases of monoclonal immunoglobulins with antistreptolysin activity: Clinical and laboratory study. J Clin Pathol 30:851–856, 1977

79. Kalliomäki JL, Granfors K, Toivanen A: An immunoglobulin G myeloma with antistreptolysin activity and a lifelong history of cutaneous streptococcal infection. Clin Immunol Immunopathol 9:22–27, 1978

80. Michaelsen TE, Førre Ø, Høyby A, et al: Streptolysin O neutralizing capacity and idiotypic properties of fragments, subunits and reassociated H and L chains from three human IgG monoclonal proteins. Mol Immunol 17:1143–1153, 1980

81. Leroux-Roels GG, Machtelinckx LJ, Van Hove WZ, et al: Monoclonal immunoglobulin G with antistreptolysin-O antibody activity in a patient with multiple myeloma. Acta Clin Belg 37:211–215, 1982

82. Mansa B, Kjems E: Extremely high contents of anti-α-staphylolysin in serum samples from a patient with multiple myeloma. Acta Pathol Microbiol Scand 65:303–310, 1965

83. Videbaek A, Mansa B, Kjems E: A human IgA-myeloma protein with anti-streptococcal hyaluronidase (ASH) activity. Scand J Haematol 10:181–185, 1973

84. Hederstedt B, Holm SE, Norberg R: Extremely high titers of serum antibodies against the streptococcal exoenzyme deoxyribonuclease B. J Clin Microbiol 11:720–723, 1980

85. Mansa B, Kjems E: Investigation on idiotypic determinants of 16 human M-components with anti-streptolysin O (-SLO) activity. Scand J Immunol 8:164, 1978 (abstr)

86. Johnson PM, Page Faulk W: Rheumatoid factor: Its nature, specificity and production in rheumatoid arthritis. Clin Immunol Immunopathol 6:414–430, 1976

87. Carson DA: Rheumatoid factor, in Kelley WN, Harris ED, Ruddy S, et al (eds): Textbook of Rheumatology. Philadelphia, Saunders, 1985, p 664

88. Grey HM, Kohler PF, Terry WD, et al: Human monoclonal γG-cryoglobulins with anti-γ-globulin activity. J Clin Invest 47:1875–1884, 1968

89. Abraham GN, Clark RA, Vaughan JH: Characterization of an IgA rheumatoid factor: Binding properties and reactivity with subclasses of human γG globulin. Immunochemistry 9:301–315, 1972

90. Farhangi M, Luger AM, Morris AD: Pathogenic role of a monoclonal IgA(k) anti-IgG paraprotein associated with hemorrhagic diathesis, rheumatoid arthritis, vascular purpura, and acute membranoproliferative glomerulonephritis. J Clin Immunol 2:75–85, 1982

91. Franklin EC, Frangione B: Common structural and antigenic properties of human γM anti-γ-globulins. J Immunol 107:1527–1534, 1971

92. Allen JC, Kunkel HG: Hidden rheumatoid factors with specificity for native γ globulins. Arthritis Rheum 9:758–768, 1966

93. Stone MJ, Metzger H: Binding properties of a Waldenström macroglobulin antibody. J Biol Chem 243:5977–5984, 1968

94. Kunkel HG, Agnello V, Joslin G, et al: Cross-idiotypic specificity among monoclonal IgM proteins with anti γ globulin activity. J Exp Med 137:331–342, 1973

95. Agnello V, Arbetter A, de Kasep GI, et al: Evidence for a subset of rheumatoid factors that cross-react with DNA-histone and have a distinct cross-idiotype. J Exp Med 151:1514–1527, 1980

96. Kunkel HG, Winchester RJ, Joslin FG, et al: Similarities in the light chains of anti-gamma-globulins showing cross-idiotypic specificities. J Exp Med 139:128–136, 1974

97. Ledford DK, Goñi F, Pizzolato M, et al: Preferential association of KIIIb light chains with monoclonal human IgMκ autoantibodies. J Immunol 131:1322–1325, 1983

98. Goñi F, Chen PP, Pons-Estel B, et al: Sequence similarities and cross-idiotypic specificity of L chains among human monoclonal IgMκ with anti-γ-globulin activity. J Immunol 135:4073–4079, 1985

99. Heremans J: Les Globulines Sériques du Système Gamma: Leur Nature et Leur Pathologie. Paris, Masson et Cie, 1960, p 227

100. Kayden HJ, Franklin EC, Rosenberg B: Interaction of myeloma gamma globulin with human beta lipoprotein. Circulation 20:659, 1962 (abstr)

101. Lennard-Jones JE: Myelomatosis with lipaemia and xanthomata. Br Med J 1:781–783, 1960

102. Aubert L, Arroyo H, Detolle P, et al: Étude clinique et cytologique d'un deuxième cas d'IgA myélome xanthomateux avec auto-anticorps circulant anti-lipoprotéine. Semin Hôp Paris 43:3014–3021, 1967

103. Nir MA, Osserman EF: The cutaneous plasma cell dyscrasias, in Safai B, Good RA (eds): Immunodermatology. New York, Plenum, 1981, p 577

104. Lewis LA, de Wolfe VG, Butkus A, et al: Autoimmune hyperlipidemia in a patient. Atherosclerotic course and changing immunoglobulin pattern during 21 years of study. Am J Med 59:208–218, 1975

105. Kodama H, Nakagawa S, Tanioku K: Plane xanthomatosis and antilipoprotein autoantibody. Arch Dermatol 105:722–727, 1972

106. Riesen W, Noseda G, Bütler R: Anti-β-lipoprotein activity of human monoclonal immunoglobulins. Vox Sang 22:420–431, 1972

107. Mullinax F, Himrod B, Berry EF: Myeloma protein with specific binding of choline. Clin Res 18:83–90, 1970

108. Marien KJC, Smeenk G: Plane xanthomata associated with multiple myeloma and hyperlipoproteinaemia. Br J Dermatol 93:407–415, 1975

109. Groszek E, Abrams JJ, Grundy SM: Normolipidemic planar xanthomatosis associated with benign monoclonal gammopathy. Metabolism 30:927–935, 1981

110. Beaumont JL, Jacotot B, Beaumont V, et al: Myélome, hyperlipidemie et xanthomatose. Nouv Rev Fr Hematol 5:507–517, 1965

111. Beaumont JL: Une spécificité commune aux α et β lipoprotéines du serum révèlée par un auto-anticorps de myélome. C R Acad Sci (Paris) 264:183–186, 1967

112. Baudet MF, Dachet C, Beaumont JL: Interaction between fibroblasts, lipoproteins and three anti-lipoproteins IgA kappa. Clin Exp Immunol 39:455–460, 1980

113. Beaumont JL, Beaumont V: Immunological factors of atherosclerosis, Schettler G, Weizel A (eds): Atherosclerosis III. Berlin, Springer Verlag, 1974, p 579

114. Beaumont JL, Beaumont V, Antonucci M, et al: Les auto-anticorps anti-lipoprotéines de myélome. Etude comparée de deux types: l'IgA anti-Lp P.G. et l'IgG anti-Lp A.S. Ann Biol Clin 28:387–395, 1970

115. Cortese C, Lewis B, Miller NE, et al: Myelomatosis with type III hyperlipoproteinaemia: Clinical and metabolic studies. N Engl J Med 307:79–83, 1982

116. Kilgore LL, Patterson BW, Parenti DM, et al: Immune complex hyperlipidemia induced by an apolipoprotein-reactive immunoglobulin A paraprotein from a patient with multiple myeloma. J Clin Invest 76:225–232, 1985

117. Beaumont JL, Beaumont V: Autoimmune hyperlipidemia. Atherosclerosis 26:405–418, 1977

118. Mahley RW, Angelin B: Type III hyperlipoproteinemia: Recent insights into the genetic defect of familial dysbetalipoproteinemia. Adv Intern Med 29:385–411, 1984

119. Manaster J, Aviram M, Silvian I, et al: Serum immunoglobulin-lipid complexes in plasma cell dyscrasia. Scand J Immunol 22:425–431, 1985

120. Killander A, Killander J, Philipson L, et al: A monoclonal gamma-macroglobulin complexing with lecithin, in Killander J (ed): Nobel Symposium 3. Gamma Globulins. New York, Interscience, 1967, p 359

121. Gisler R, Pillot J: Activité anticardiolipide liée à un complexe macroglobuline de Waldenström-IgG cryoprécipitant. Immunochemistry 5:543–555, 1968

122. Pruzanski W, Warren RE, Goldie JH, et al: Malabsorption syndrome with infiltration of the intestinal wall by extracellular monoclonal macroglobulin. Am J Med 54:811–818, 1973

123. Cooper MR, Cohen HJ, Huntley CC, et al: A monoclonal IgM with antibodylike specificity for phospholipids in a patient with lymphoma. Blood 43:493–504, 1974

124. Drusin LM, Litwin SD, Armstrong D, et al: Waldenström macroglobulinemia in a patient with a chronic biologic false-positive serologic test for syphilis. Am J Med 56:429–432, 1974

125. Merlini G, Forsgren A, Turesson I, et al: An IgM

monoclonal protein with multiple serological specificities. Clin Exp Immunol 37:276–282, 1979

126. Fermand JP, Danon F, Brouet JC: Characterization of a human monoclonal IgM with antibody activity to dsDNA. Clin Exp Immunol 59:467–474, 1985

127. Latov N, Sherman WH, Nemni R, et al: Plasma cell dyscrasia and peripheral neuropathy with a monoclonal antibody to peripheral nerve myelin. N Engl J Med 303:618–621, 1980

128. Braun PE, Frail DE, Latov N: Myelin associated glycoprotein is the antigen for a monoclonal IgM in polyneuropathy. J Neurochem 39:1261–1265, 1982

129. Latov N: Immunological abnormalities associated with chronic peripheral neuropathies: Plasma cell dyscrasia and neuropathy, in Behan P, Spreafico E (eds): Neuroimmunology. New York, Raven, 1984, p 261

130. Gregson NA, Leibowitz S: IgM paraproteinaemia, polyneuropathy and myelin-associated glycoprotein (MAG). Neuropathol Appl Neurobiol 11:329–347, 1985

131. Ilyas AA, Quarles RH, MacIntosh TD, et al: IgM in human neuropathy related to paraproteinemia binds to carbohydrate determinant in the myelin-associated glycoprotein and to a ganglioside. Proc Natl Acad Sci USA 81:1225–1229, 1984

132. Frail DE, Edwards AM, Braun PE: Molecular characteristics of the epitope in myelin-associated glycoprotein that is recognized by a monoclonal IgM in human neuropathy patients. Mol Immunol 21:721–725, 1984

133. Shy ME, Vietorisz T, Nobile-Orazio E, et al: Specificity of human IgM M-proteins that bind myelin-associated glycoprotein: Peptide mapping, deglycosylation, and competitive binding studies. J Immunol 133:2509–2512, 1984

134. Nobile-Orazio E, Hays HP, Latov N, et al: Specificity of mouse and human monoclonal antibodies to myelin-associated glycoprotein. Neurology 34:1336–1342, 1984

135. Freddo L, Ariga T, Saito M, et al: The neuropathy of plasma cell dyscrasia: Binding of IgM M-proteins to peripheral nerve glycolipids. Neurology 35:1420–1424, 1985

136. Murray N, Steck AJ: Indication of a possible role in a demyelinating neuropathy for an antigen shared between myelin and NK cells. Lancet 1:711–713, 1984

137. Dellagi K, Brouet JC: Antigen shared between myelin and NK cells. Lancet 1:1244, 1984

138. Tanaka M, Sato S, Miyatake T: Identification of myelin-associated glycoprotein (MAG) on the cell surface of mononuclear cells in human peripheral blood by a heterologous antiserum. Jpn J Exp Med 54:9–15, 1984

139. Evans SW, Gregson NA, Leibowitz S, et al: Investigation of the idiotypic determinants of IgM monoclonal proteins associated with neuropathy. Clin Exp Immunol 57:621–625, 1984

140. Saito T, Sherman WH, Latov N: Specificity and idiotype of M-proteins that react with MAG in patients with neuropathy. J Immunol 130:2496–2498, 1983

141. Ilyas AA, Quarles RH, Dalakas MC, et al: Monoclonal IgM in a patient with paraproteinemic polyneuropathy binds to gangliosides containing disialosyl groups. Ann Neurol 18:655–659, 1985

142. Rowland LP, Defendini R, Sherman W, et al: Macroglobulinemia with peripheral neuropathy simulating motor neuron disease. Ann Neurol 11:532–536, 1982

143. Donofrio PD, Greenberg HS, Albers JW, et al: IgM monoclonal protein binding to spinal cord and peripheral nerve glycolipids in a patient with motor neuron disease. Ann Neurol 18:161, 1985 (abstr)

144. Besinger UA, Toyka KV, Anzil AP, et al: Myeloma neuropathy: Passive transfer from man to mouse. Science 213:1027–1030, 1981

145. Hays AP, Takatsu M, Latov N, et al: Focal demyelination of cat sciatic nerve induced by intraneural injection of serum from patients with polyneuropathy and monoclonal IgM reactive with MAG. J Neuropathol Exp Neurol 42:349, 1983 (abstr)

146. Eisen HN, Little JR, Osterland CK, et al: A myeloma protein with antibody activity. Cold Spring Harbor Symp Quant Biol 32:75–81, 1967

147. Ashman RF, Metzger H: A Waldenström macroglobulin which binds nitrophenyl ligands. J Biol Chem 244:3405–3414, 1969

148. Hannestad K: Monoclonal and polyclonal γM rheumatoid factors with anti-di and anti-trinitrophenyl activity. Clin Exp Immunol 4:555–578, 1969

149. Terry WD, Boyd MM, Rea JS, et al: Human M-proteins with antibody activity for nitrophenyl ligands. J Immunol 140:256–259, 1970

150. Andersen BR, McAninch JR, Patterson R: The incidence of precipitating activity in monoclonal proteins. Clin Exp Immunol 8:263–269, 1971

151. Warner NL, McKenzie MR, Fudenberg HH: Anti-antibody activity of a monoclonal macroglobulin. Proc Natl Acad Sci USA 68:2846–2851, 1971

152. Riesen W, Morell A: A human myeloma protein with specificity against dinitrophenyl and nucleic acid derivatives. Immunochemistry 9:979–985, 1972

153. Edmundson AB, Ely KR, Girling RL, et al: Binding of 2,4-dinitrophenyl compounds and other small molecules to a crystalline λ-type Bence-Jones dimer. Biochemistry 13:3816–3827, 1974

154. Bertram J, Gualtieri RJ, Osserman EF: Amyloid-related Bence Jones proteins bind dinitrophenyl L-lysine, in Glenner GG, Costa PP, Freitas AF (eds): Amyloid and Amyloidosis. Amsterdam, Excerpta Medica, 1980, p 351

155. Parker CW, Osterland CK: Hydrophobic binding sites on immunoglobulins. Biochemistry 9:1074–1082, 1970

156. Mannik M: Binding of albumin to γA-myeloma proteins and Waldenström macroglobulins by disulfide bonds. J Immunol 99:899–906, 1967

157. Heremans JF, Heremans MT: Immunoelectrophoresis. Acta Med Scand 170:27–59, 1961 (suppl 367)

158. Gallango ML, Caldera LH, Suinaga R, et al: Cooccurrence of albumin complexes with IgE and IgG in the serum of an IgE myeloma patient. Acta Haematol 68:295–299, 1982

159. Harboe M, Følling I: Complex formation between monoclonal IgM and albumin. Scand J Immunol 3:51–60, 1974

160. Hauptman S, Tomasi TB: A monoclonal IgM protein with antibody-like activity for human albumin. J Clin Invest 53:932–940, 1974

161. Bernier GM, Brettman LR: Crystalline complex of monoclonal IgG and albumin. Clin Res 25:614A, 1977 (abstr)

162. Zlotnick A, Mlynek Y: Coexistence of a circulating IgG-albumin complex and a γ heavy chain in the same patient. Isr J Med Sci 16:126–129, 1980

163. Mills LE, Brettman LR, Jentoft JE, et al: Crystallocryoglobulinemia resulting from human monoclonal antibodies to albumin. Ann Intern Med 99:601–604, 1983

164. Seligmann M, Sassy C, Chevalier A: A human IgM myeloma protein with anti-α_2 macroglobulin antibody activity. J Immunol 110:85–90, 1973

165. Fujita K, Sakurabayashi I, Kawai T, et al: A human IgG1κ type M-protein with antibody activity against horse and rabbit $\alpha_2$macroglobulin. Clin Chim Acta 149:205–214, 1985

166. Westerhausen M, Kickhöfen B, Wernet P, et al: Transferrin-Autoimmunsyndrom. Ein neues pathogenetisches Prinzip. Verh Dtsch Ges Inn Med 78:901–904, 1972

167. Hilgard P, Linder KH, Wetter O: Monoclonal cyroglobulin of IgG(λ) type interacting with transferrin. Blut 43:217–225, 1981

168. Sanchez-Avalos J, Soong BCF, Miller SP: Coagulation disorders in cancer. II. Multiple myeloma. Cancer 23:1388–1392, 1969

169. Lackner H, Hunt V, Zucker MB, et al: Abnormal fibrin ultrastructure, polymerization, and clot retraction in multiple myeloma. Br J Haematol 18:625–636, 1970

170. Cohen I, Amir J, Yehuda BS, et al: Plasma cell myeloma associated with an unusual myeloma protein causing impairment of fibrin aggregation and platelet function in a patient with multiple malignancy. Am J Med 48:766–770, 1970

171. Coleman M, Vigliano EM, Weksler ME, et al: Inhibition of fibrin monomer polymerization by lambda myeloma globulins. Blood 39:210–223, 1972

172. Niléhn JE: On symptomatic antihaemophilic globulin (AHF) deficiency: Its modification by penicillin. Acta Med Scand 171:491–505, 1962

173. Castaldi PA, Penny R: A macroglobulin with inhibitory activity against coagulation factor VIII. Blood 35:370–376, 1970

174. Glueck HI, Hong R: A circulating anticoagulant in γ1A-multiple myeloma. J Clin Invest 44:1866–1881, 1965

175. Zettervall O, Nilsson IM: Acquired von Willebrand's disease caused by a monoclonal antibody. Acta Med Scand 204:521–528, 1978

176. Bovill EG, Ershler WB, Golden EA, et al: A human myeloma-produced monoclonal protein directed against the active subpopulation of von Willebrand factor. Am J Clin Pathol 85:115–123, 1986

177. Thiagarajan P, Shapiro SS, DeMarco L: Monoclonal immunoglobulin Mλ coagulation inhibitor with phospholipid specificity. Mechanism of a lupus anticoagulant. J Clin Invest 66:397–405, 1980

178. DiMinno G, Coraggio F, Cerbone AM, et al: A myeloma paraprotein with specificity for platelet glycoprotein IIIa in a patient with a fatal bleeding disorder. J Clin Invest 77:157–164, 1986

179. Michaelsen TE, Gaarder PI, Kornstad L: A transient monoclonal human IgG1κ protein with anti-thyroglobulin activity: Lack of cross-idiotypy with polyclonal anti-thyroglobulin antibodies. Clin Exp Immunol 46:268–276, 1981

180. Dighiero G, Guilbert B, Fermand JP, et al: Thirty-six human monoclonal immunoglobulins with antibody activity against cytoskeleton proteins, thyroglobulin, and native DNA: Immunologic studies and clinical correlations. Blood 62:264–270, 1983

181. Dighiero G, Guilbert B, Avrameas S: Naturally occurring antibodies against nine common antigens in humans sera. II. High incidence of monoclonal Ig exhibiting antibody activity against actin and tubulin and sharing antibody specificities with natural antibodies. J Immunol 128:2788–2792, 1982

182. Trimarchi F, Benvenga S, Fenzi G, et al: Immunoglobulin binding of thyroid hormones in a case of Waldenström's macroglobulinemia. J Clin Endocrinol Metab 54:1045–1050, 1982

183. Moroz LA, Meltzer SJ, Bastomsky CH: Thyroid disease with monoclonal (immunoglobulin G λ) antibody to triiodothyronine and thyroxine. J Clin Endocrinol Metab 56:1009–1015, 1983

184. Toh BN, Ceredig R, Cornell FN, et al: Multiple myeloma and monoclonal IgA with anti-actin reactivity. Clin Exp Immunol 30:379–383, 1977

185. Krulik M, Vittecoq D, Abuaf N, et al: Anti-smooth-muscle activity of the monoclonal IgM in a patient with Waldenström disease. Semin Hopitaux 59:1737–1741, 1983

186. Dellagi K, Brouet JC, Perreau J, et al: Human monoclonal IgM with autoantibody activity against intermediate filaments. Proc Natl Acad Sci USA 79:446–450, 1982

187. Micouin C, Rivat C, Bensa JC, et al: A human immunoglobulin in a myeloma protein with anti-gastric parietal cell autoantigen activity. Clin Exp Immunol 27:78–84, 1977

188. Kiprov DD, Miller RG: Polymyositis associated with monoclonal gammopathy. Lancet 2:1183–1186, 1984

189. Lindström FD, Hed J, Eneström S: Renal pathology of Waldenström's macroglobulinaemia with monoclonal antiglomerular antibodies and nephrotic syndrome. Clin Exp Immunol 41:196–204, 1980

190. Fernandez-Alonso GI, Victorero CO, Meiss RP, et al: Anti-squamous basal cell antibody activity in Waldenström's macroglobulinemia. J Cutan Pathol 11:154–157, 1984

191. Vincendeau P, Claudy A, Thivolet J, et al: Bullous dermatosis and myeloma. Monoclonal anticytoplasmic antibody activity. Arch Dermatol 116:681–682, 1980

192. Gibaud A, Dorche G, Poncet MJ, et al: Une globuline myelomateuse γG à haute activité dans le test d'hémagglutination de la rubéole. Rev Eur Et Clin Biol 12:700, 1972

193. Seigneurin JM, Renversez JC, Baccard M, et al: Monoclonal cryoimmunoglobulin with anti-cytomegalovirus activity associated with T cell chronic lymphocytic leukaemia. Clin Exp Immunol 41:317–325, 1980

194. Osserman EF: Plasma cell dyscrasias. Am J Med 44:256–279, 1968

195. Del Carpio J, Espinoza LR, Lauter S, et al: Transient monoclonal proteins in drug hypersensitivity reactions. Am J Med 66:1051–1056, 1979

196. Bauer K, Tragl KH, Bauer G, et al: Intravasale Denaturierung von Plasmaproteinen bei einer IgM-Paraproteinämie, ausgelöst durch ein intravenös verabreichtes Röntgenkontrastmittel. Wien Klin Wochenschr 86:766–769, 1974

197. Harboe M, Følling I, Haugen OA, et al: Sudden death caused by interaction between a macroglobulin and a divalent drug. Lancet 2:285–288, 1976

198. Merlini G, Fitzpatrick LA, Siris ES, et al: A human myeloma immunoglobulin G binding four moles of calcium associated with asymptomatic hypercalcemia. J Clin Immunol 4:185–196, 1984

199. Baker BL, Ultquist DE: A copper-binding immunoglobulin from a myeloma patient. Purification, identification and physical characterization. J Biol Chem 253:1195–1200, 1978

200. Paterson PY, Day ED, Whitacre CC, et al: Endogenous myelin basic protein-serum factors (MBP-SFs) and anti-MBP antibodies in humans. J Neurol Sci 52:37–51, 1981

201. Wager O, Teppo AM: Binding affinity of human autoantibodies: Studies of cryoglobulin IgM rheumatoid factors and IgG autoantibodies to albumin. Scand J Immunol 7:503–509, 1978

202. Sewell HF, Mattheus JB, Gooch E, et al: Autoantibody to nerve tissue in a patient with a peripheral neuropathy and an IgG paraprotein. J Clin Pathol 34:1163–1166, 1981

The Clinical Implications of Monoclonal Immunoglobulins

Mehdi Farhangi and Giampaolo Merlini

WALDENSTRÖM, in reporting the first three patients with macroglobulinemia, noted a marked elevation of serum viscosity that set his patients apart from usual cases of myelomatosis.[1] Christenson and Dacie found a $\gamma 1$ mobility protein band that was responsible for the high cold agglutinin titers in some patients with acquired hemolytic anemia.[2] Since these early observations, a great deal has been learned regarding the clinical consequences of the monoclonal immunoglobulins (M-Igs).

Based on pathophysiology, M–Ig-associated clinical manifestations can be classified into three groups. (Table 1). In the first group, the clinical disorders are the result of the physicochemical properties of M-Igs, and protein-protein or protein-cell interactions. The hyperviscosity syndrome, cryoglobulinemia, and certain anomalies of coagulation and acid base balance are examples. In the second group, the antibody activity of the M-Igs is the cause of the disorders. For example, the affinity of the M-Igs to red cell antigens produces hemolysis in patients with chronic cold agglutinin disease or M-Igs against lipoproteins[63] can cause hyperlipidemia and xanthomatosis. In the third group, there is an association between M-Ig and the clinical disorders but the pathophysiologic mechanisms are largely unknown. The systemic capillary leak syndrome,[17–22] pyoderma gangrenosum[32–35] and lichen myxedematosus are prototype conditions.[23–31]

In some circumstances, both the antibody activity and the physicochemical properties of the M-Igs appear to participate in the clinical syndrome. For example, the M-Igs with rheumatoid factor activity almost invariably form cryoprecipitate upon complexing with IgG.[63] Thus, immune complex-mediated manifestations (vasculitis, nephritis) and cold sensitivity (Raynaud's phenomenon, vascular occlusion) as well as hyperviscosity may manifest simultaneously or in sequence.

From the Department of Medicine, University of Missouri-Columbia, the Department of Medicine and Institute of Cancer Research-Cancer Center, College of Physicians and Surgeons, Columbia University, New York, and the Institute of Clinical Medicine, II, IRCCS, Policlinico S. Matteo, Pavia, Italy.

Address reprint requests to Mehdi Farhangi, MD, Department of Medicine, University of Missouri at Columbia, Columbia, MO 65201.

0093–7754/86/1303–0013$05.00/0

THE HYPERVISCOSITY SYNDROME

Both plasma proteins and formed elements contribute to the viscosity of blood. A linear relationship between blood viscosity and the hematocrit has been demonstrated.[64] Two other contributing factors are protein-cell interaction and the varying shear rate in the vasculature. The viscosity rises markedly in small vessels with low shear rate[64–66] and most tissue injuries are attributed to defective capillary perfusion.

The viscosity of normal serum or plasma falls within a narrow range (normal viscosity relative to water: 1.4 to 1.8) and may be altered by changes in protein size, molecular asymmetry, and concentration.[67–70] In IgG myeloma patients, the hyperviscosity syndrome only occurs when the serum M-Igs are quite high. Somer reviewed 36 myeloma patients with symptomatic hyperviscosity syndrome and the mean serum monoclonal IgG was 9.2 ± 3.7 g/dL. Only two patients had a monoclonal IgG <5.0 g/dL.[68] The IgG_3 M-components are somewhat an exception, due to their tendency to form large protein-protein complexes[69] and symptoms of hyperviscosity manifest at lower concentrations. The IgA M-Igs, in their polymeric forms, can raise viscosity in a manner disproportionate to their concentration. The hyperviscosity syndrome is most common in macroglobulinemia where it constitutes an important cause of morbidity and mortality. Usually the hyperviscosity syndrome is associated with IgM >5g/dL.[70]

Protein-cell interaction may be important in viscosity elevation. A case in point was a patient with myeloma and sickle cell anemia reported by Anderson et al.[71] At low shear rate, the patient's blood exhibited far greater viscosity than blood from normal subjects or patients with sickle cell anemia without paraprotein. Hyperviscosity due to immune complexes has also been documented.[72,73] Clearly, the clinical expression of

Table 1. Clinical Disorders Associated With Monoclonal Immunoglobulins

Group 1: Clinical disorders primarily due to physicochemical properties and protein-protein or protein-cell interactions
The Hyperviscosity syndrome
Cryoglobulinemia (type I, II Cryo-Ig)
Hemostatic abnormalities
Apparent acid/base perturbances
Group 2: Clinical disorders primarily due to antibody activity of the M-Igs*
Hemolytic anemia with monoclonal cold agglutinins (red cell I, i, Ii, non I-i, and others†)
Bleeding diathesis (Factor VIIIC,[3-5] Factor VIII-R[6-8])
Polyneuropathy (Myelin-associated-glycoprotein,[9] chondroitin sulfate.[10,11])
Cryoglobulinemia (Type II Cryo-Ig) with nephritis, vascular purpura (IgG)
Xanthomatosis (Apo-B, apoE, lipoproteins,† Heparin[12])
Xanthoderma (Riboflavin[13])
Hemochromatosis (Transferrin[14-16])
Group 3: Clinical disorders due to unknown or partially understood pathophysiologic mechanisms
SCLS[17-22]
Lichen myxedematosus[23-31]
Pyoderma gangrenosum[32-35]
Erythema elevatum diutinum[36]
Subcorneal pustular dermatosis[37]
Necrobiotic xanthogranuloma[38]
Xanthomatosis unassociated with lipoprotein or heparin binding M-Ig[39]
Corneal crystalline deposition[40-46]
POEMS syndrome[47-57]
Polyneuropathy with M-Ig nonreactive to nerve constituents
Hypercupremia[58-62]

*The corresponding antigens are shown in parentheses.
†For references, see Tables 1 and 2, respectively, of the preceding chapter.[63]

hyperviscosity is dependent on several variables. Fahey et al[74-76] have emphasized the role of a symptomatic threshold viscosity, different from patient to patient, above which symptoms occur with regularity. Moreover, most patients develop symptoms of hyperviscosity when the relative viscosity reaches 6 or 7.[75]

The clinical manifestations of hyperviscosity are summarized in Table 2. Anemia results from a physiologic adaptation to blood viscosity elevation.[77,78] The measurement of red cell and plasma volumes often discloses apparent rather than real anemia and transfusion in such circumstances may aggravate the hyperviscosity syndrome.[64]

Plasmapheresis is the treatment of choice for the hyperviscosity syndrome. In patients with IgM M-Igs, approximately 80% of paraproteins are in the circulating compartment. Removal of 2 to 4 L of plasma is often sufficient to ameliorate symptoms.[79-81] Further treatment with chemotherapeutic agents usually obviates the need for long-term plasmapheresis except in drug-resistant cases.

Table 2. Signs and Symptoms of the Hyperviscosity Syndrome

Ocular	Distension and tortuosity of retinal veins, string-of-sausage appearance, retinal hemorrhage, papilledema
	Disturbance in vision to complete blindness
Hematologic	Oozing of blood from oral mucous membranes
	Bleeding from nose and urinary and GI tracts
	Prolonged bleeding at sites of minor surgical procedures
	Anemia
Neurologic	Headache, dizziness, vertigo, nystagmus, postural hypotension
	Somnolence, stupor, and coma
	Generalized seizures, EEG changes
Cardiovascular	Congestive heart failure
	Expanded plasma volume
Renal	Glomerular deposits possibly attributable to the hyperviscosity syndrome
	Diminished concentrating and diluting ability, perhaps attributable to the hyperviscosity syndrome
Subjective	Weakness, fatigue, anorexia

CRYOGLOBULINEMIA

Cryoimmunoglobulins (Cryo-Igs) precipitate on cooling and redissolve upon rewarming. Some Cryo-Igs precipitate at above room temperature, thus blood must be drawn using a warmed syringe and tube and clotting allowed at 37° C. One to several days of refrigeration may be necessary for cryoprecipitation to occur at 1 to 4° C. Cryoprecipitate is quantitated by centrifugation and expressed as cryocrit. The normal serum contains less than 0.2% cryoprecipitate.

Comprehensive reviews of Cryo-Igs have been published.[82,83] The classification by Brouet et al based on immunochemical analysis has been generally accepted.[84] The type I Cryo-Igs consist of monoclonal IgM, IgG, IgA, or Bence Jones proteins. This type occurs with Waldenström's macroglobulinemia (WM), multiple myeloma (MM), lymphoproliferative disorders, monoclonal gammopathy of undetermined significance (MGUS), and chronic cold agglutinin disease (CCAD). Type II, mixed Cryo-Igs, are associated with a monoclonal immunoglobulin component with rheumatoid factor activity. Thus, IgM-IgG, IgG-IgG, and IgA-IgG complexes are found in the cryoprecipitate. The associated diseases are similar to type I. In type I and II Cryo-Igs, the levels of cryoprecipitable proteins are usually high (1 to 30 mg/dL) and cryoprecipitation occurs readily. Type III, mixed polyclonal Cryo-Igs, are composed of one or more classes of polyclonal immunoglobulins. Occasionally, other serum proteins such as complement components, nucleic acid, or lipoproteins coprecipitate. The associated diseases are chronic inflammation, infections, autoimmune disease and essential cryoglobulinemia. The concentration of cryoprecipitable fraction is low (0.1 to 1.0 mg/dL) and a prolonged cooling, one to seven days, may be necessary to uncover the presence of Cryo-Ig. Table 3 shows the frequency of clinical manifestations observed in 178 patients with cryoglobulinemia.

BLEEDING DISORDERS

Bleeding diatheses are observed more often in macroglobulinemia (36%) or IgA myeloma (33%) than IgG myeloma (15%).[87] The pathophysiologic mechanisms of coagulation abnormalities are complex and only partially understood. M-Ig interaction with platelets and clotting proteins results in a panorama of abnormal test results but the bleeding appears to correlate best with abnormal platelet function tests such as prolonged bleeding time and abnormal platelet adhesiveness. Prolongation of thrombin time, prothrombin time, and partial thromboplastin time, low fibrinogen and poor clot retraction have less predictive significance.[87] A common observation in myeloma patients is the occurrence of abnormal fibrin clot that is excessively friable, gelatinous, and nonretracting that may be partially corrected by the addition of calcium.[88] A study by Coleman et al[88] of the defective clot showed inhibition of fibrinogen α-chain polymerization by the Fab but not the Fc fragment of five λ-bearing M-Igs. The abnormality of clot retraction is, in part, due to platelet dysfunction. Moreover, in some studies the unavailability of the fibrinogen receptor sites for factor XIII has been implicated.[89,90]

Prolonged bleeding time as a measure of abnormal platelet function has been repeatedly demonstrated.[91] Abnormal platelet adhesiveness to glass beads and the unavailability of platelet factor 3 have also been demonstrated.[91] Although not clearly documented, a protein-protein interaction between M-Ig and various clotting proteins is suspected to be the cause of the reduced clotting factors. Occasionally, monoclonal proteins have specific inhibitory activity; bleeding due to M-Ig with antifactor VIII-C activity[3–5] and acquired von Willebrand's disease due to M-Ig with anti-von Willebrand factor (VIII-R)[6–8] have been reported.

In addition, four distinct bleeding diatheses can occur in patients with plasma cell dyscrasias: The hyperviscosity syndrome, AL-type amyloidosis, factor X deficiency, and cryoglobulinemia. Retinal hemorrhage, epistaxis, and bleeding from other mucosal sites are characteristic of the hyperviscosity syndrome. In patients with amyloidosis, hemorrhage in dependent and traumatized areas of the skin is a frequent finding. Periorbital hemorrhage after proctoscopic examination[92] and the development of ecchymosis after gentle stroking of the skin with a gauze pad are highly suggestive of skin amyloidosis. Occult and overt gastrointestinal bleeding are also common. Capillary fragility due to amyloid deposits in the vessel walls seems to be the main cause of bleeding in amyloidosis. Rarely, patients with amyloidosis may exhibit severe bleeding due to

Table 3. Incidence of Signs and Symptoms in 178 Patients With Cryoglobulinemia

Manifestations	Incidence (%)
Cutaneous	80
Vascular purpura	60
Raynaud's phenomenon	50
Distal necrosis	14
Urticaria	10
Livedo	10
Acrocyanosis	10
Leg ulcers	5
Arthralgia/arthritis	35
Nephritis	20
Neurologic	17
Hemorrhage	7
Abdominal pain	2
Arterial thrombosis	1

Reprinted with permission from W.B. Saunders Co.[85]

factor X or combined factor IX and X deficiency.[93–98] It has been repeatedly shown that the infusion of a large volume of plasma is ineffective because of the rapid clearance of factor X after intravenous infusion due to its adsorption to amyloid deposits.[99,100] Infusion of factor IX concentrate, which contains factor X, may only transiently ameliorate bleeding. In one patient, splenectomy was effective for the control of bleeding,[98] presumably because of the removal of large bulk of amyloid deposits in the spleen. Finally, in patients with cryoglobulinemia, purpuric lesions are common. Immune–complex-mediated vasculitis often accounts for the skin lesions.

SYSTEMIC CAPILLARY LEAK SYNDROME

This rare and usually fatal illness of recurrent shock, generalized angioedema, and hemoconcentration is due to rapid extravasation of plasma fluid, electrolytes, and proteins.[17] Atkinson et al[18] called attention to the occurrence of monoclonal IgG in five previously reported cases and a patient of their own. These investigators found a major shift of water, electrolytes, albumin, and several other plasma proteins from intravascular to extravascular compartment. Moreover, a rise in the concentration of serum IgM and a drop in albumin and IgG during the attack provided an estimate of the size of the capillary defect. Although rare, new cases continue to be reported.[19,20,22]

The pathogenesis of this syndrome and the role of monoclonal IgG have remained enigmatic. The activation of classic and alternate complement pathways was studied by Atkinson et al[18] and George et al[19] and no abnormalities were detected. Lofdahl et al[20] however, found low C4 and disproportionality among C1 subcomponents, suggesting activation of the classic complement pathway. Electron microscopic study of the capillaries obtained by muscle biopsy during and after the attacks, have shown changes attributed to complement activation.[21]

It should be noted that a capillary leak syndrome can occur postpartum and following surgical trauma.[101,102] But it is unlikely that such cases are examples of systemic capillary leak syndrome (SCLS) because two important features of SCLS, the repetitiveness of the attacks and the presence of monoclonal IgG, have not been demonstrated. Treatment of attacks with fluid and volume expanders such as albumin is generally unsuccessful due to rapid transfer of these macromolecules across the capillary walls. The usefulness of vasopressor agents has been questioned.[18] In one patient, treatment with terbutaline and prednisone decreased the number of attacks.[20]

APPARENT ACID/BASE DISTURBANCES

Myeloma proteins at physiologic pH behave as cations. It has been postulated that chloride, bicarbonate, or both are retained, leading to a low anion gap. Murray et al[103] demonstrated that the low anion gap in myeloma patients is related to the cationic property and the concentration of the M-Igs. IgGs are more often associated with this type of apparent acid/base disturbance than IgAs, which are usually less cationic than IgGs.[104] Hypercalcemia and hypoalbuminemia, if present, will further narrow the anion gap. A similar observation has been made in patients with asymptomatic plasma cell dyscrasias[105] and polyclonal hypergammaglobulinemia.[106] Hyperviscosity, for technical reasons, can produce a falsely low anion gap.[107]

HEMOLYTIC ANEMIA ASSOCIATED WITH MONOCLONAL COLD AGGLUTININS

Cold agglutinins (CAs) occurring with infections such as mycoplasma pneumonia and infectious mononucleosis are, with rare exceptions, polyclonal antibodies[108] and, as a rule, transient in nature. In contrast, persistent CAs are almost invariably monoclonal (IgM κ much more than IgM λ, or IgA and IgG M-Igs).[109–111] CAs exhibiting cryoprecipitation are nearly always associated with B cell malignancies.[108] Crisp and Pruzanski reviewed 78 patients with persistent CAs previously reported in literature and from their own institutions: Thirty-one had lymphoma, 13 had WM, six had chronic lymphocytic leukemia and 28 had CCAD.[112] The antibody activity of most CAs in patients with CCAD was directed toward I antigen (70%). In lymphoma/leukemia patients, CA showed affinity for i and non–I-i antigens. The serum levels of M-Ig in patients with CCAD remain stable for a prolonged period of time.[113] Only occasionally will a picture of lymphoma emerge.

The hematologic manifestation associated with CAs has been amply described.[108] The hemolysis appears to occur when the thermal amplitude for red cell agglutination and complement activation (20 to 25 °C) overlap. Consequently, CAs with relatively high thermal amplitudes cause sustained hemolysis and those with low thermal amplitude produce bursts of intravascular hemolysis and hemoglobinuria after exposure to low temperatures. Complement activation also occurs and results in red cell opsonization by C_3b fragments and removal by the reticuloendothelial system.[108]

Treatment is directed toward management of underlying B cell neoplasms. To redue hemolysis, cold exposure should be minimized. Alkylating agents, cytoxan, and leukeran are occasionally effective, while corticosteroids and splenectomy are less effective. Plasmapheresis has been attempted with short-term control of hemolysis.[114] Washed red cells are recommended for transfusion.

PERIPHERAL NEUROPATHY AND THE POEMS SYNDROME

Patients with multiple myeloma and macroglobulinemia occasionally present with polyneuropathy unrelated to amyloidosis. In such patients, the neurologic symptoms are often the earliest clinical manifestations. In patients with MGUS, the incidence of neurologic disease is about 6%.[115,116] Kelly et al[117] found a monoclonal component in 10% of patients with peripheral neuropathy compared with 1% of the age-matched general population.

Nerve biopsy in M-Ig-associated neuropathy, shows demyelinating changes or axonal degeneration. A number of clinical and experimental observation seem to favor the concept that M-Igs are directly involved in the development of the neural lesion. The demonstration of M-Igs with antibody activity for myelin-associated glycoprotein (MAG)[9] in patients with neuropathy and induction of demyelinating lesion by passive transfer of M-Ig into experimental animals[118,119] can be regarded as the strongest evidence. The absorption of serum M-Ig by peripheral nerve or its constituents has also been shown.[10,120] Other lines of support for this concept are derived from clinical observations, notably, the return of some neurologic functions following plasmapheresis and treatment with corticosteroids or cytotoxic agents.[122] The deposition of immunoglobulin in nerve tissue has been noted repeatedly, suggesting an in vivo immunologic interaction. This interpretation, however, has been disputed.[123]

With regard to the clinical presentation of neuropathy, recent data suggest that the antigen-binding specificity of M-Ig is a determinant factor. For example, patients with MAG-binding monoclonal proteins[9,120] are predominantly elderly men with distal symmetrical slowly progressive sensory neuropathy without central nervous system involvement.[121] In two cases with axonal neuropathy and epidermolysis, the M-Igs reacted with chondroitin sulfates[10,11]; and in a case with pure motor neuropathy,[123a] the M-Ig bound to the carbohydrate moiety of some gangliosides[123b]; but in the majority of cases, the antigenic specificity remains undetermined.

Patients with multiple myeloma and peripheral neuropathy exhibit features that set them apart from the usual cases. The frequency of organomegaly was found to be distinctly higher in this group of patients.[124] Other features include a lower incidence of anemia, the absence of hypercalcemia, a strikingly high incidence of osteosclerotic or mixed osteosclerotic-osteolytic bone lesions (61%), and an increased cerebrospinal fluid (CSF) protein (90%) with a low cell count. Although, similar to most patients with myeloma, the IgG M components are twice as common as IgA, the predominance of λ light chain (83%) is quite remarkable.[124]

A rare syndrome of slowly progressive polyneuropathy, endocrinopathy, and skin changes with plasma cell dyscrasia was first described by Crow in 1956[47a] and subsequently Japanese physicians.[47,48] Bardwick et al[55] suggested the acronym POEMS (polyneuropathy, organomegaly, endocrine disorder, M component, skin changes) to describe the most consistent features of this syndrome. This condition appears to occur more frequently in Japan. These patients, generally younger than myeloma subjects, present with symptoms of sensory amd motor peripheral neuropathy that becomes progressively disabling. Leg edema at the early stage, ascites and pleural effusion in the more advanced phase of the disease occur quite frequently. Skin hyperpigmentation, thickening, and hypertrichosis are also prevalent features. Angiomatous verrucae have been observed commonly in the Japanese cases.[49] Endocrinopathy in the form of gynecomastia, hypogonadism, hyperprolactinemia, hyperestrogenemia, and diabetes constitutes another important aspect of this syndrome. An enlarged liver with minimal histologic changes, lymphadenopathy, and splenomegaly occur with high frequency. Lymph node biopsy shows follicular and vascular hyperplasia and monoclonal plasma cell infiltration.[49] A low grade fever, anemia, polycythemia, and thrombocytosis are noted in some patients. Characteristically there is a low percentage of bone marrow plasma cells ($<10\%$) and a low concentration of M-Ig, predominantly IgG or IgA with λ light chain (λ/k ratio of 9 to one). In some typical cases however, no monoclonal protein was identified.[50,51] The skeletal findings are particularly remarkable with a high incidence of osteosclerotic changes and a rarity of pure osteolytic lesions.[52]

The role of M component in the pathogenesis of this syndrome has not been established. Occasionally, a remarkable reversal of neuropathy and endocrinopathy has occurred after treatment with corticosteroids, cytotoxic agents, or irradiation of the involved bone.[53–55] Deposition of paraprotein in neural tissue was observed in one patient.[53] In light of the recent discovery that hybridoma-derived human monoclonal autoantibodies originating from patients with autoimmunity have binding affinity for multiple endocrine organs,[125] it is tempting to speculate that M-Igs in the POEMS syndrome may possess affinity for determinants on neural and endocrine tissues.

Intense plasma exchange is reported to be effective in reversing the motor and, to a lesser extent, the sensory disturbances in patients with polyneuropathy associated with M-Ig. Sherman et al[122] treated ten such patients with plasma exchanges. Overall, six of ten patients responded to treatment. The benefit was more marked in patients with motor disturbances and in patients with IgG M components. The response also correlated with the degree of M-Ig decrease following pheresis. Improvement in electrophysiologic parameters was documented in only one patient. Plasma exchange at present, appears to be a reasonable treatment modality for patients with disabling motor neuropathy. Corticosteroids and cytotoxic chemotherapy, at times, have been rewarding.

NEPHROPATHIES ASSOCIATED WITH M-IGS

The monoclonal light chains account for most acute and chronic renal failure in myeloma patients. Cast nephropathy (myeloma kidney), systemic light chain deposition disease, AL-amyloid nephropathy and tubular dysfunction syndromes (Fanconi and renal diabetes incipidus with metabolic acidosis) have been discussed (see "Clinical Implications of Monoclonal Light Chains" by Alan Solomon, this issue).

Cryo-Igs type I and II are the second most significant monoclonal proteins in regard to renal complications. The actual process of cryoprecipitation probably plays little role in the development of nephritis, although acute oliguric renal failure was reported to occur in a patient with a prolonged exposure to low ambiant temperature in the operating room.[126] Proliferative glomerular lesions including membranoproliferative glomerulonephritis can occur in type I Cryo-Ig.[127]

The type II Cryo-Igs exhibit many features of immune complex-mediated disorders. Acute and chronic vasculitis and hypocomplementemia often accompany the renal glomerular lesions. Moreover, extrarenal manifestations, such as vascular purpura, leg ulcers, Raynaud's phenomenon, arthralgia, arthritis, and peripheral neuropathy may precede or coincide with the kidney disease. In one of our patients with monoclonal IgA, rheumatoid factor, vascular purpura, and arthritis indistinguishable from rheumatoid arthritis occurred several years before the development of an acute membranoproliferative glomerulonephritis.[128] Nephritis in this patient developed when the paraprotein had declined markedly, and free, unbound IgG exceeded the bound fraction. This clinical situation is somewhat comparable to the experimentally-induced nephritis when a diminishing antibody production in the face of excess antigen favors the deposition of immune complexes.[129]

Electron microscopy of the kidney in patients with type II Cryo-Ig may show subendothelial deposits occasionally extending to the mesangium and subepithelium. An inflammatory process, characterized by endocapillary proliferation, with participation by mesangeal and endothelial elements, polymorphonuclear cells, and monocytes follows the immune complex deposition. Kidney biopsies in reported cases have been diagnosed as membranoproliferative glomerulonephritis, mesangeal proliferative glomerulonephritis, focal glomerulitis, and rapidly-progressive glomurulonephritis.[127]

The clinical presentation of renal disease in patients with Cryo-Ig can be limited to an asymptomatic microscopic hematuria or proteinuria. At times however, an acute nephritic syndrome with oliguria and renal failure or nephrotic syndrome with heavy proteinuria is seen with hypertension as a likely associated feature in both. A progression toward an end-stage renal failure is the rule rather than the exception.

Not enough is known about the conditions required for the development of glomerular lesions. The ratio of M-Ig (antibody) to polyclonal IgG (antigen), the size of immune complexes, and the clearance capacity of reticuloendothelial system, as well as the antibody activity of polyclonal IgG,[130] may all be important factors.

Plasmapheresis in conjunction with cytotoxic agents and corticosteroids has been used for treatment, particularly of the acute nephritic syndrome. An increase in creatinine clearance and, occasionally, sustained improvement in renal function have resulted.[131] These clinical observations have been attributed to restoration of the splenic reticuloendothelial cell function resulting in an accelerated rate of immune complex clearance.[132] Attempts have been made to remove only the cryoprecipitable proteins thus avoiding the need for plasma replacement.[133–135] Although no randomized trial of plasmapheresis in this group of patients has ever been conducted, prolonged renal functional improvements and better survival have been reported.[136]

Table 4. Cutaneous Manifestations Associated with M-Igs

Manifestations	Prevalent M components	Biologic Properties and Pathogenic Mechanisms
Cutaneous amyloidosis	Amyloidogenic light chains ($\lambda > \kappa$ λVI subgroup)	AL-amyloid deposits Increased capillary fragility
Purpura Raynaud's phenomenon Urticaria and angioedema Digital infarct, peripheral gangrene, necrosis of the exposed areas Skin ulceration	Types I, and II Cryo-Igs, monoclonal cold agglutinins, IgM > IgG and IgA	Cryoprecipitation and vascular occlusion Rheumatoid factor activity Complement activation Immune-mediated vasculitis Antibody activity for red cell antigen[82–86]
Xanthomatosis	IgA and IgG	Lipoprotein binding affinity[63] Heparin binding affinity[12]
Xanthoderma	IgG_2 λ	Flavin binding affinity[13]
Hemochromatosis	IgG	Transferrin binding affinity[14–16]
Lichen myxedematosus	Extremely catodal IgG	Unknown[23–31]
Pyoderma gangrenosum	IgA $\gg$ IgG, IgM	Unknown (possibly altered granulocyte and monocyte function[32–35])
Erythema elevatum diutinum	IgA	Unknown[36]
Subcorneal pustular dermatosis	IgA	Unknown[37]
Necrobiotic xanthogranuloma	IgG	Unknown[38]
Generalized angioedema of SCLS	IgG	Unknown (possibly complement activation)[17–22]
Hyperpigmentation hypertrichosis of POEMS syndrome	M components with λ-light chain	Unknown[47–57]

CUTANEOUS MANIFESTATIONS

A spectrum of cutaneous manifestations occurs in patients with plasma cell dyscrasias. In Table 4, a list of skin disorders, the prevalent M components, their known biologic properties, and pathogenic mechanisms are tabulated.

Cutaneous Amyloidosis

AL-type amyloid deposits in the skin can be a diffuse infiltration or in the form of papules, plaques, and nodules with a predilection for periorbital, perioral, and perianal regions. Skin lesions are often accompanied by macroglossia, the carpal tunnel syndrome, and symptoms of peripheral neuropathy. In contrast to AL-type amyloid skin disease, the amyloidotic lesions limited to the skin such as the lichen amyloidosis, the macular amyloidosis, and the skin tumor-associated amyloidosis are nonimmunoglobulin in origin.[137] In recent years the diagnosis of amyloidosis has been greatly facilitated by aspiration of abdominal wall fat, which can be readily stained with congo red dye and examined with a polarizing light microscope.[138]

Cryoglobulinemia

Type I and II Cryo-Ig,[84] and occasionally monoclonal cold agglutinins, are responsible for an array of dermal manifestations (Table 3). Purpuric lesions, Raynaud's phenomenon, urticaria/angioedema, skin ulcerations, digital infarction, peripheral gangrene, and necrosis of the exposed areas have all been observed. Among monoclonal Cryo-Igs, type II proteins are most accountable for serious complications. Although cryoprecipitation is intimately associated with most clinical features, at times a non-cryo M component may be present. It is likely that the majority of skin lesions are due to immune-mediated rather than temperature-mediated mechanisms. Activation of the classic complement pathways by IgM and IgG and the alternate pathway by IgA M components, as well as immune complex-mediated vasculitis, are all contributing elements.[139]

Xanthomatosis and Hyperlipidemia

Hypocholesterolemia, rather than hyperlipidemia, is common in untreated patients with myeloma.[140] This has been attributed to an elevated low density lipoprotein receptor activity on the malignant cells.[141] Occasionally, xanthomatosis with or without hyperlipidemia occurs in patients with plasma cell dyscrasias. The majority of reported patients have exhibited overt myeloma but some were classified as MGUS. Commonly, the xanthomatosis is generalized with large flat lesions (plane xanthoma), yellow-golden in color, involving the palm of the hands, eyelids, face, lateral side of the neck, and the upper trunk.[39,142] The eruptive and tuberous forms of xanthoma are seen less frequently. In some patients, symptoms related to hyperviscosity or cryoglobulinemia dominate the clinical presentation. Kilgore et al[143] reported a striking patient with polymeric monoclonal IgA, xanthoma and hyperlipidemia, in whom the ophthalmoscopic examination revealed discrete, white globules flowing through the retinal vessels. The patient, disoriented on arrival, soon lapsed into a coma but regained consciousness after plasmapheresis.

Treatment is directed toward the underlying disease. Dietary measures and clofibrate, which are generally effective in lowering cholesterol in type III familial hyperlipidemia, are ineffective in these patients.[144] Plasmapheresis may be required for the control of hyperviscosity.

Xanthoderma

Intense yellow coloration of the skin without hyperbilirubinemia in a patient with multiple myeloma called our attention to a unique functional property of the M component. The isolated monoclonal $IgG_2\lambda$ exhibited a strong affinity for riboflavin, flavin mononucleotide (FMN), and flavin adenine dinucleotide (FAD).[13] Withdrawal of riboflavin previously prescribed as a vitamin supplement and treatment of myeloma by melphalan resulted in a decrease in paraprotein-bound riboflavin and gradual normalization of the skin and hair color in the ensuing months. No signs of riboflavin deficiency occurred as a result of trapping of this vitamin by the M component.

Hemochromatosis

Westerhausen et al[14] studied a patient with a unique iron overload syndrome. A markedly elevated serum iron, bronzed skin with siderosis, pigmented cirrhosis, and diabetes mellitus were paradoxically associated with absence of marrow iron and a decreased radioiron use by erythroid precursors.[15] An IgG (κ) monoclonal protein with antibody activity for transferrin was subsequently demonstrated.[16]

Lichen Myxedematosus

Lichen myxedematosus (scleromyxedema) is a rare but well-defined dermatologic entity characterized by mucinous infiltrates containing acid mucopolysaccharides (glycosaminoglycans) rich in hyaluronic acid.[145,146] Mucinous infiltrates are not unique to the disease, but occur in several other dermatologic lesions.[146] The absence of thyroid disorders and regular occurrence of an M component, however, distinguish this entity from the skin lesions of hypo- and hyperthyroidism and pretibial myxedema.

Since the initial discovery of the association of an extremely basic monoclonal IgG[23,24] with lichen myxedematosus, a similar M component has been found, with few exceptions, in subsequent observations.[25,26] The plasma cell dyscrasia in these patients remains occult throughout the course of the illness. Occasionally, cases of myeloma or MGUS converting into myeloma have been reported.[26,27] The M component, typically an IgG 1 with a λ light chain[26] is a basic protein due to the high number of lysine residues in the structure of the light chain.[28] No shared idiotype was demonstrated in a study of several such proteins,[29] thus making them unlikely candidates for being antibodies to a single antigenic determinant. Immunoglobulin deposition in the skin lesions has been observed in some cases,[23,25] although, an affinity of the M components for the acid mucopolysaccharide has not been established. A serum factor unrelated to the M component capable of promoting fibroblast proliferation in vitro was demonstrated in patients with scleromyxedema and a less severe form of the disease, papular mucinosis.[30] In a recent report, increased production of hyaluronic acid and prostaglandin E were demonstrated when serum from the affected individual was added to a fibroblast culture.[31] The role of paraprotein in this biologic stimulation remains to be ascertained.

A low-dose melphalan regimen administered continuously was effective in reducing or totally eliminating the skin lesions in six of eight patients treated at the Mayo Clinic.[25] No response was observed when the drug was administered in a cyclic intermittent fashion. In one patient with myeloma and scleromyxedema, a combination of melphalan, cytoxan, prednisone, vincristine, and fluoxymesterone resulted in near complete resolution of the skin lesions.[27]

Pyoderma Gangrenosum

Pyoderma gangrenosum (PG) is a chronic recurring skin ulceration that involves primarily the lower extremities and the trunk, without specific histologic features. Its association with inflammatory bowel disease, arthritis, and a host of other diseases has long been recognized. Monoclonal gammopathy in association with PG has been repeatedly described.[32] Nine of 86 patients with PG seen at the Mayo Clinic had a monoclonal gammopathy and one had myeloma.[33] IgA M components are the most commonly reported M-Igs (>70%) without λ or κ chain predominance.[34] Although the M components are generally recognized after the diagnosis of PG has been made, the priority of events remains uncertain. In cases of myeloma, a rapid healing of PG after an induction of remission has been observed.[35]

The pathogenic events leading to the skin ulceration and the role of the M components have remained obscure. No consistent microorganism has been identified in the ulcerated lesions. In one study,[33] thickening of the vessel walls with a lymphocytic infiltrate and the deposition of immunoglobulins and C3 were demonstrated in biopsies taken from the erythematous marginal zone of the ulcers. Recently, defects have been described of leukocyte motility,[147] phagocytic and chemotactic functions,[35,148] and monocyte phagocytic activity.[35] Thus, it is possible that M components may alter monocyte and granulocyte function and contribute to the development of the skin ulceration.

Erythema Elevatum Diutinum, Subcorneal Pustular Dermatosis, and Necrobiotic Xanthogranuloma

Erythema elevatum diutinum,[36] subcorneal pustular dermatosis,[37] and necrobiotic xanthogranuloma[38] are rare skin disorders in which an association with predominantly IgA or IgG M components has been documented. Hyperpigmentation and hypertrichosis occur frequently with the POEMS syndrome and generalized angioedema occur during the attacks in patients with SCLS.

OCULAR MANIFESTATIONS

Some ocular manifestations in plasma cell dyscrasias are directly related to the neoplastic growth. As an example, proptosis due to orbital plasmacytoma is a well-recognized clinical presentation in myeloma. Paraprotein-related ocular lesions are quite diverse.[149]

Corneal Crystalline Deposition

Crystal-like, electron dense protein deposits in the cornea, conjunctiva, and lens have been observed in patients with prolonged monoclonal gammopathy[40–42] and with rapidly evolving plasma cell neoplasia.[44] The immunoglobulin nature of these deposits has been documented by immunohistochemical methods.[40,41] Electron micrographic studies have shown periodicity of the structure without amyloid fibrils.[40,42,44] Of nine patients in whom the M components were identified by immunoelectrophoresis, seven had an IgG (κ), one IgG (λ), and one IgA (κ).[40–43,45,46] In some patients, crystal-like structures were also seen in the bone marrow plasma cells.[42,44]

Chemotherapy administered for treatment of the underlying myeloma or plasmapheresis[40,43] has been associated with a reduction in corneal deposits and improvement in visual acuity, consistent with the reversible nature of these protein deposits.

Hypercupremia and Ocular Copper Pigment Deposition

The corneal deposition of copper pigment in patients with hepatolenticular degeneration (Kayser-Fleischer ring) is characteristically peripheral in location and starts at the limbus. When similar pigments are distributed throughout the corneal endothelium and Descemet's membrane, another alteration in copper metabolism should be considered. Since the first report by Goodman et al[58] describing golden brown corneal and lenticular pigment deposition in a patient with myeloma associated with a phenomenally high serum copper (3350 ± 235 μg/mL; normal: <30 μg/mL), at least three additional cases have been reported.[59–61] All four had an IgG monoclonal immunoglobulin and two had symptoms of multiple myeloma. A tight binding of copper to the γ globulin fraction of serum proteins was demonstrated.[58,62] Moreover, a marked difference in serum clearance of ^{64}Cu was observed in comparison to a control subject when a tracer amount was administered orally or by intravenous route.[62]

The nature of copper binding affinity (immune binding *v* nonimmune interaction) of these highly unusual monoclonal proteins is still unknown and requires furher investigation.

REFERENCES

1. Waldenström J: Incipient myelomatosis or "essential" hyperglobulinemia with fibrinogenopenia: A new syndrome. Acta Med Scand 117:216–247, 1944
2. Christenson WN, Dacie JV: Serum proteins in acquired haemolytic anaemia (auto-antibody type). Br J Haematol 3:153–164, 1957
3. Niléhn JE: On symptomatic anti-haemophilic globulin (AHF) deficienty. Acta Med Scand 171:491–505, 1962
4. Castaldi PA, Penny R: A macroglobulin with inhibitory activity against coagulation factor VIII. Blood 35:370–376, 1970
5. Glueck HI, Hong R: A circulating anticoagulant in γ1A-multiple myeloma. Its modification by penicillin. J Clin Invest 44:1866–1881, 1965
6. Brody JI, Haider ME, Rossman RE: A hemorrhagic syndrome in Waldenström's macroglobulinemia secondary to immunoadsorption of factor VIII. N Engl J Med 300:408–410, 1979
7. Zettervall O, Nilsson IM: Acquired von Willebrand's disease caused by a monoclonal antibody. Acta Med Scand 204:521–528, 1978
8. Bovill EG, Ershler WB, Golden EA, et al: A human myeloma-produced monoclonal protein directed against the active subpopulation von Willebrand factor. Am J Clin Pathol 85:115–123, 1986
9. Braun PE, Frail DE, Latov N: Myelin associated glycoprotein is the antigen for a monoclonal IgM in polyneuropathy. J Neurochem 39:1261–1265, 1982
10. Sherman WH, Latov N, Hays AP, et al: Monoclonal IgMκ antibody precipitating with chondroitin sulfate C from patients with axonal polyneuropathy and epidermolysis. Neurology 33:192–201, 1983
11. Kabat EA, Liao J, Sherman WH, et al: Immunochemical characterization of the specificities of two human monoclonal IgM's reacting with chondroitin sulfates. Carbohydr Res 130:289–297, 1984

12. Glueck HI, MacKenzie MR, Glueck CJ: Crystalline IgG protein in multiple myeloma: Identification effects on coagulation and on lipoprotein metabolism. J Lab Clin Med 79:731–744, 1972

13. Farhangi M, Ossermann EF: Myeloma with xanthoderma due to an IgG λ monoclonal anti-flavin antibody. N Engl J Med 294:177–183, 1976

14. Westerhausen M, Kickhöfen B, Wernet P, et al: Transferrin-autoimmune syndrom. Ein neues pathogenetisches. Prinzip Verh Dtsch Ges Inn Med 78:901–904, 1972

15. Westerhausen M, Meuret G: Transferrin-immune complex disease. Acta Haematol 57:96–101, 1977

16. Wernet P, Kickhöfen B, Westerhausen M, et al: A monoclonal IgG protein with antibody-like activity for transferrin and with κ chains of an unusual molecular size. Scand J Immunol 3:859–864, 1974

17. Clarkson B, Thompson D, Horwith M, et al: Cyclical edema and shock due to increased capillary permeability. Am J Med 29:193–216, 1960

18. Atkinson JP, Waldmann TA, Stein SF, et al: Systemic capillary leak syndrome and monoclonal IgG gammopathy. Medicine 56:225–239, 1977

19. George C, Regnier B, Le Gall JR, et al: Hypovolemic shock with oedema due to increased capillary permeability. Intens Care Med 4:159–163, 1978

20. Lofdahl CG, Solvell L, Laurell AB, et al: Systemic capillary leak syndrome with monoclonal IgG and complement alterations. Acta Med Scand 206:405–412, 1979

21. Johansson BR, Lofdahl CG: Ultrastructure of microvessels in skeletal muscle in a case of systemic capillary leak syndrome. Acta Med Scand 206:413–416, 1979

22. Maestracci P, Benoit P, Dupeyrat J, et al: Choc hypovolemique par augmentation de la permeabilite capillaire. Nouv Press Med 10:329–330, 1981

23. Osserman EF, Takatsuki K: Role of an abnormal, myeloma-type, serum gamma globin in the pathogenesis of the skin lesions of papular mucinosis (lichen myxedematosus). J Clin Invest 42:962, 1963 (abstr)

24. McCarthy JT, Osserman E, Lombardo PC, et al: An abnormal serum globulin in lichen myxedematosus. Arch Dermatol 89:446–450, 1964

25. Harris RB, Perry HO, Kyle RA, et al: Treatment of scleromyxedema with melphalan. Arch Dermatol 115:295–299, 1979

26. Lang E, Zabel M, Schmidt H: Skleromyxodem Arndt-Gottron und assoziierte phänomene. Dermatologica 169:29–35, 1984

27. Muldrow ML, Bailin PL: Scleromyxedema associated with IgG lambda multiple myeloma. Cleve Clin Q 50:189–195, 1983

28. Lawrence DA, Tye MJ, Liss M: Immunochemical analysis of the basic immunoglobulin in papular mucinosis. Immunochemistry 9:41–49, 1972

29. Wells JV, Fudenberg HH, Epstein WL: Idiotypic determinants on the monoclonal immunoglobulins associated with papular mucinosis. J Immunol 108:977–983, 1972

30. Harper RA, Rispler J: Lichen myxedematosus serum stimulated human skin fibroblast proliferation. Science 199:545–547, 1978

31. Yaron M, Yaron I, Yust I, et al: Lichen myxedematosus (scleromyxedema) serum stimulates hyaluronic acid and prostaglandin E production by human fibroblasts. J Rheumatol 12:171–175, 1985

32. Powell FC, Schroeter AL, Su WPD, et al: Pyoderma gangrenosum and monoclonal gammopathy. Arch Dermatol 119:468–472, 1983

33. Powell FC, Schroeter AC, Su WPD, et al: Pyoderma gangrenosum: A review of 86 patients. Q J Med 55:173–186, 1985

34. Kanoh T, Sakurai M, Ikai K, et al: Studies on the combination of pyoderma gangrenosum and monoclonal gammopathies. Nippon Ketsueki Gakkai Zasshi 43:828–833, 1980

35. Jones RR, Black AK, Donaghy M, et al: Defective monocyte function in pyoderma gangrenosum with IgG kappa paraproteinemia. Clin Exp Immunol 52:685, 1983

36. Kovary PM, Dhonau H, Happle R: Paraproteinemia in erythema elevatum diutinum. Arch Dermatol Res 260:153–158, 1977

37. Sneddon IB, Wilkinson DS: Subcorneal pustular dermatosis. Br J Dermatol 100:61–68, 1979

38. Kossard S, Winkelmann RK: Necrobiotic xanthogranuloma with paraproteinemia. J Am Acad Dermatol 3:257–270, 1980

39. Parker F: Xanthomatosis, in Demis DJ (ed): Clinical Dermatology, ed 12, vol 2. Philadelphia, Harper & Row, Unit 12-1, 1985, pp 1–38

40. Klintworth GK, Bredehoeff SJ, Reed JW: Analysis of corneal crystalline deposits in multiple myeloma. Am J Ophthalmol 86:303–313, 1978

41. Rodrigues MM, Krachmer JH, Miller SD, et al: Posterior corneal crystalline deposits in benign monoclonal gammopathy: A clinicopathologic case report. Arch Ophthalmol 97:124–128, 1979

42. Cherry PMH, Kraft S, McGowan H, et al: Corneal and conjunctival deposits in monoclonal gammopathy. Can J Ophthalmol 18:142–149, 1983

43. Firkin FC, Lee N, Ramsay R, et al: Visual loss caused by corneal crystals in myeloma: Rapid improvement after plasm exchange and chemotherapy. Med J Aust 2:677–678, 1979

44. Pinkerton RMJ, Robertson DM: Corneal and Conjunctival changes in dysproteinemia. Invest Ophthalmol 8:357–364, 1969

45. Barr CC, Gelender H, Font RL: Corneal crystalline deposits associated with dysproteinemia: Report of two cases and review of the literature. Arch Ophthalmol 98:884–889, 1980

46. Nik NA, Martin NF, Berler DK: Corneal crystalline deposits and drusenosis associated with IgA-kappa chain monoclonal gammopathy. Ann Ophthalmol 17:303–307, 1985

47. Shimpo S: Solitary plasmacytoma with polyneuritis and endocrine disturbances. Nippon Rinsho 26:2444, 1968

47a. Crow RS: Peripheral neuritis in myelomatosis. Br Med J 2:802–804, 1956

48. Takatsuki K, Uchiya T, Sagawa K, et al: Plasma cell dyscrasia with polyneuropathy and endocrine disorder: A review of 32 patients, in Seno S, Takaku F, Irino S (eds): Topics in Hematology, Amsterdam, Excerpta Medica, 1970, p 454

49. Takatsuki K, Sanada I: Plasma cell dyscrasia with polyneuropathy and endocrine disorder: Clinical and laboratory features of 109 reported cases. Jpn J Clin Oncol 13:543–556, 1983

50. Meshkinpour H, Myune CG, Kramer LS: A unique multi-systemic syndrome of unknown origin. Arch Intern Med 137:1719–1721, 1977

51. Trentham DE, Masi AT, Marker HW: Polyneuropathy and anasarca. Evidence for a new connective-tissue syndrome and vasculopathic contribution. Ann Intern Med 84:271–274, 1976

52. Resnick D, Greenway GD, Bardwick PA, et al. Plasma cell dyscrasia with polyneuropathy, organomegaly, endocrinopathy, M-protein, and skin changes: The POEMS syndrome. Radiology 140:17–22, 1981

53. Tobin JT, Fitzgerald MX: The Japanese plasma cell dyscrasia syndrome: Case report and theory of pathogenesis. Postgrad Med J 58:786–789, 1982

54. Moya-Mir MS, Barbadillo R, Martin-Jimenez T, et al: Plasma cell dyscrasia with polyneuritis and dermato-endocrine alterations. Review of a new case outside Japan. Postgrad Med J 56:427–430, 1980

55. Bardwick PA, Zvaifler NJ, Gill GN, et al: Plasma cell dyscrasia with polyneuropathy, organomegaly, endocrinopathy, M-protein, and skin changes: The POEMS syndrome. Medicine 59:311–322, 1980

56. Arenson AM, Rubenstein JD, McKee JD: Renal ultrasound in POEMS syndrome. J Clin Ultrasound 13:208–209, 1985

57. Waldenström JG, Adner A, Gydell K, et al: Osteosclerotic 'plasmocytoma' with polyneuropathy, hypertrichosis and diabetes. Acta Med Scand 203:297, 1978

58. Goodman SI, Rodgerson DO, Kauffman J: Hypercupremia in a patient with multiple myeloma. J Lab Clin Med 70:57–62, 1967

59. Ellis PP: Ocular deposition of copper in hypercupremia. Am J Ophthalmol 68:423–427, 1969

60. Lewis RA, Falls HF, Troyer DO: Ocular manifestations of hypercupremia associated with multiple myeloma. Arch Ophthalmol 93:1050–1053, 1975

61. Martin NF, Kincaid MC, Stark WJ, et al: Ocular copper deposition associated with pulmonary carcinoma, IgG monoclonal gammopathy and hypercupremia: A clinicopathologic correlation. Ophthalmol 90:110–116, 1983

62. Lewis RA, Hultquist DE, Baker BL, et al: Hypercupremia associated with a monoclonal immunoglobulin. J Lab Clin Med 88:375–388, 1976

63. Merlini G, Farhangi M, Osserman EF: Monoclonal Immunoglobulins with antibody activity in myeloma, macroglobulinemia and related plasma cell dyscrasias. Semin Oncol (this issue)

64. McGrath MA, Penny R: Paraproteinemia: Blood hyperviscosity and clinical manifestations. J Clin Invest 58:1155–1162, 1976

65. Dintenfass L, Somer T: On the aggregation of red cells in Waldenström's macroglobulinaemia and multiple myeloma. Vasc Res 9:279, 1975

66. Mannik M: Blood viscosity in Waldenström's macroglobulinemia. Blood 44:87–98, 1974

67. Martin NH: Macroglobulinemia. Clin Chim Acta 22:15–25, 1968

68. Somer T: Hyperviscosity syndrome in plasma cell dyscrasias. Adv Microcirc 6:1–55, 1975

69. Capra JD, Kunkel JG: Aggregation of λG3 proteins: Relevance to the hyperviscosity syndrome. J Clin Invest 49:610–621, 1970

70. MacKenzie MR, Babcock J: Studies of the hyperviscosity syndrome. II. Macroglobulinemia. J Lab Clin Med 85:227–234, 1975

71. Anderson S, Yeung K, Hillman D, et al: Multiple myeloma in a patient with sickle cell anemia: Interesting effects on blood viscosity. Am J Med 59:568–574, 1975

72. Jasin JE, LoSpalluto J, Ziff M: Rheumatoid hyperviscosity syndrome. Am J Med 49:484–493, 1970

73. Abbruzzo JL, Heimer R, Guiliano V, et al: The hyperviscosity syndrome, polysynovitis, polymyositis and an unusual 13 S serum IgG component. Am J Med 49:258–264, 1970

74. Fahey JL: Serum protein disorders causing clinical symptoms in malignant neoplastic disease. J Chronic Dis 16:703–712, 1963

75. Fahey, JL, Barth WF, Solomon A: Serum hyperviscosity syndrome. JAMA 192:464–467, 1965

76. Solomon A, Fahey JL: Plasmapheresis therapy in macroglobulinemia. Ann Intern Med 58:789–800, 1963

77. MacKenzie MR, Brown E, Fudenberg HH, et al: Waldenström's macroglobulinemia: Correlation between expanded plasma volume and increased serum viscosity. Blood 35:394–408, 1970

78. Tuddenham EGD, Bradley J: Plasma volume expansion and increased serum viscosity in myeloma and macroglobulinaemia. Clin Exp Immunol 16:169, 1974

79. Lawson NS, Nosanchuk JS, Oberman HA, et al: Therapeutic plasmapheresis in treatment of patients with Waldenström's macroglobulinemia. Transfusion 8:174–183, 1968

80. Schwab PJ, Fahey JL: Treatment of Waldenström's macroglobulinemia by plasmapheresis. N Eng J Med 263:574–579, 1960

81. Godal HC, Borchgrevink CF: The effect of plasmapheresis on the hemostatic function in patients with macroglobulinemia Waldenström and multiple myeloma. Scand J Clin Lab Invest. 17:133, 1965

82. Grey HN, Kohler PF: Cryoimmunoglobulins. Semin Hematol 10:87–111, 1973

83. Malchesky PS, Eng D, Clough JD: Cryoimmunoglobulins. Cleve Clin Q 52:175–192, 1985

84. Brouet JC, Clauvel JP, Danon F, et al: Biologic and clinical significance of cryoglobulins. A report of 86 cases. Am J Med 57:775–788, 1974

85. Winfield JB: Cryoglobulinemia. Human Pathol 14:350–354, 1983

86. Brouet JC, Clauvel J-P, Danon F: Cryoglobulins: Clinicobiological Correlations, In Chenais F (ed): Cryoproteines. LaTronche, France, F. Chenais, 1978, p 159

87. Perkins HA, Mackenzie MR, Fudenberg HH: Hemostatic defect dysproteinemias. Blood 35:695–707, 1970

88. Coleman M, Vigliano EM, Weksler ME, et al: Inhibition of fibrin monomer aggregation by lambda myeloma globulins. Blood 39:210–223, 1972

89. Klingemann HG, Egbring R, Havemann K: Incom-

plete fibrin formation and highly elevated factor XIII activity in multiple myeloma. Scand J Haematol 27:253, 1981

90. Jeannette S, Soria C, Samama M, et al: Analysis of a fibrin formation abnormality in a case of multiple myeloma. Scand J Haematol 15:207–218, 1975

91. Lackner H: Hemostatic asbnormalities associated with dysproteinemias. Semin Hematol 10:125–133, 1973

92. Kyle RA, Bayrd ED: Amyloidosis, in the Monoclonal Gammopathies, Multiple Myeloma and Related Plasma-Cell Disorders. Springfield, Ill, Charles C. Thomas, 1976, p 241

93. Barth WF, Willerson JT, Waldmann TA, et al: Primary amyloidosis. Am J Med 47:259–273, 1969

94. Howell M: Acquired factor X deficiency associated with systematized amyloidosis: A report of a case. Blood 21:739–744, 1963

95. Korsan-Bengtsen K, Kjort PF, Ygge J: Acquired factor X deficiency in a patient with amyloidosis. Thromb Diath Haemorh 7:558–566, 1962

96. Pechet L, Kastrul JJ: Amyloidosis associated with factor X (Stuart) deficiency. Ann Intern Med 61:315–318, 1964

97. McPherson RA, Onstad JW, Ugoretz RF, et al: Coagulopathy in amyloidosis: Combined deficiency of factor IX and X. Am J Hematol 3:225–235, 1977

98. Greipp PR, Kyle RA, Bowie EJW: Factor X deficiency in amyloidosis: Resolution after splenectomy. N Engl J Med 301:1050–1051, 1979

99. Furie B, Greene E, Furie BC: Syndrome of acquired factor X deficiency and systemic amyloidoisis: In vivo studies of the metabolic fate of factor X. N Engl J Med 297:81–85, 1977

100. Furie B, Voo L, McAdam KPWJ, et al: Mechanism of factor X deficiency in systemic amyloidosis. N Engl J Med 304:827–830, 1981

101. Luke IW, Rubinstein E: Fatal postpartum shock due to massive angioneurotic edema. Am J Obstet Gynecol 83:322–327, 1962

102. Smullens SN, Templeton JY: Fatal hypovolemic shock due to massive edema following cardiopulmonary bypass. J Thorac Cardiovasc Surg 61:348–351, 1972

103. Murray T, Long W, Narins RG: Multiple myeloma and the anion gap. N Eng J Med. 292:574–575, 1975

104. Troyer Ad, Stolarczyk A, Zegers De Beyl D, et al: Value of anion-gap determination in multiple myeloma. N Engl J Med 296:858–860, 1977

105. Schnur MJ, Appel GB, Karp G, et al: The anion gap in asymptomatic plasma cell dyscrasias. Ann Intern Med 86:304–305, 1977

106. Keshgegian AA: Decreased anion gap in diffuse polyclonal hypergammaglobulinemia. N Engl J Med 299:99–100, 1978

107. Gabow PA: Disorders associated with an altered anion gap. Kidney Int 27:472–483, 1985

108. Packman CH, Leddy JP: Cryopathic hemolytic anemia, in Williams WJ, Beutler E, Erslev AJ, et al (eds): Hematology, ed 3. New York, McGraw-Hill, 1983

109. Tonthat H, Ronchant A, Henry A, et al: A new case of monoclonal IgA kappa cold agglutinin with anti-Pr_1d specificity in a patient with persistent HB antigen cirrhosis. Vox Sang 30:464–468, 1976

110. Ambrus M, Bajtai G: A case of an IgG-type cold agglutinin disease. Haematologia 3:225–235, 1969

111. Pruzanski W, Katz A: Cold agglutinins. Antibodies with biological diversity. Clin Immunol Rev 3:131–168, 1984

112. Crisp D, Pruzanski W: B cell neoplasms with homogeneous cold-reacting antibodies (cold agglutinins). Am J Med 72:915–922, 1982

113. Harboe M, Torsvik H: Protein abnormalities in the cold hemagglutination syndrome. Scand J Haematol 6:461–462, 1969

114. Taft EG, Propp RP, Sullivan SA: Plasma exchange for cold agglutinin hemolytic anemia. Tranfusions 17:173–176, 1977

115. Isobe T, Osserman EF: Pathologic conditions associated with plasma cell dyscrasias: A study of 806 cases. Ann NY Acad Sci 190:507–517, 1972

116. Kyle RA: Monoclonal gammopathy of undetermined significance (MGUS). A review. Clin Haematol 11:123–150, 1982

117. Kelly JJ, Kyle RA, O'Brien PC, et al: Prevalence of monoclonal protein in peripheral neuropathy. Neurology 31:1480–1483, 1981

118. Besinger UA, Toyka KV, Anzil AP, et al: Myeloma neuropathy: Passive transfer from man to mouse. Science 213:1027, 1981

119. Hays AP, Takatsu M, Latov N, et al: Focal demyelination of cat sciatic nerve induced by intraneural injection of serum from patients with polyneuropathy and monoclonal IgM reactive with MAG. J Neuropathol Exp Neurol 42:349, 1983 (abstr)

120. Latov N, Sherman WH, Nemni R, et al: Plasma-cell dyscrasia and peripheral neuropathy with a monoclonal antibody to peripheral nerve myelin. N Engl J Med 303:618–621, 1980

121. Hafler DA, Johnson D, Kelly JJ, et al: Monoclonal gammopathy and neuropathy: Myelin associated glycoprotein reactivity and clinical characteristics. Neurology 36:75–78, 1986

122. Sherman W, Olarte MR, McKiernan G, et al: Plasma exchange treatment of peripheral neuropathy associated with plasma cell dyscrasia. J Neurol Neurosurg Psychiatry 47:813–819, 1984

123. Swash M, Perrin J, Schwartz MS: Significance of immunoglobulin deposition in peripheral nerve in neuropathies associated with paraproteinaemia. J Neurol Neurosurg Psychiatry 42:179, 1979

123a. Rowland LP, Defendini R, Sherman W, et al: Macroglobulinemia with peripheral neuropathy simulating motor neuron disease. Ann Neurol 11:532–536, 1982

123b. Donofrio PD, Greenberg HS, Albers JW, et al: IgM monoclonal protein binding to spinal cord and peripheral nerve glycolipids in a patient with motor neuron disease. Ann Neurol 18:161, 1985 (abstr)

124. Bergsagel DE, Pruzanski W: Some unusual manifestations of plasma cell neoplasia, in Wiernik PH, Canellos GP, Kyle RA, et al (eds): Neoplastic Disease of the Blood, vol 1. New York, Churchill Livingston, 1985, pp 553–573

125. Satoh J, Probhakar BS, Haspel MV, et al: Human monoclonal autoantibodies that react with multiple endocrine organs. N Eng J Med, 309:217–220, 1983

126. Carloss HW, Tavassoli M: Acute renal failure from precipitation of cryoglobulins in a cool operating room. JAMA 244:1472–1473, 1980

127. Hill GS: Multiple myeloma, amyloidosis, Waldenström's macroglobulinemia, cryoglobulinemia, and benign monoclonal gammopathies, in Heptinstall RH (ed): Pathology of the Kidney, ed 3. Boston, Little, Brown, 1983, pp 993–1067

128. Farhangi M, Lugar AM, Morris AD: Pathogenic role of a monoclonal IgA(κ) anti-IgG paraprotein associated with hemorrhagic diathesis, rheumatoid arthritis, vascular purpura, and acute membranoproliferative glomerulonephritis. J Clin Immunol 2:75–85, 1982

129. Cochrane CG, Hawkins D: Studies on circulating immune complexes. III. Factors governing the ability of circulating complexes to localize in blood vessels. J Exp Med 127:137–154, 1968

130. Gamble CN, Ruggles SW: The immunopathogenesis of glomerulonephritis associated with mixed cryoglobulinemia. N Engl J Med 299:81–84, 1978

131. Geltner D, Kohn RW, Gorevic P, et al: The effect of combination therapy (steroids, immunosuppressives, and plasmapheresis) on 5 mixed cryoglobulinemia patients with renal, neurologic, and vascular involvement. Arthritis Rheum 24:1121–1127, 1981

132. Lockwood CM, Worlledge S, Nicholas A, et al: Reversal of impaired splenic function in patients with nephritis or vasculitis (or both) by plasma exchange. N Engl J Med 300:524–530, 1979

133. L'Abbate A, Paciucci A, Bartolomeo F, et al: Selective removal of plasma cryoglobulins in cryoglobulinaemia. Proc Eur Dial Transplant Assoc 14:486–494, 1977

134. McLeod BC, Sassetti RJ: Plasmapheresis with return of cryoglobulin-depleted autologous plasma (cryoglobulinpheresis) in cryoglobulinemia. Blood 55:866–870, 1980

135. Malchesky PS, Asanuwa Y, Zawicki I, et al: On-line separation of macromolecules by membrane filtration with cryogelatin, in Sieberth HG (ed): Plasma Exchange: International Symposium in Cologne, June 6–7, 1980. Stuttgart, FRG, Schattauer, 1980, pp 133–139

136. Sinico RA, Fornasieri A, Fiorini G, et al: Plasma exchange in the treatment of essential cryoglobulinemia nephropathy. Long-term follow-up. Int J Artificial Org 8:15–18, 1985 (suppl 2)

137. Hashimoto K: Progress in cutaneous amyloidoses. J Invest Dermatol 82:1–3, 1984 (editorial)

138. Libbey JA, Skinner M, Cohen AS: Use of abdominal fat tissue aspirate in the diagnosis of systemic amyloidosis. Arch Intern Med 143:1549–1552, 1983

139. Russell Jones R: The cutaneous manifestations of paraproteinemia. Part I. Br J Dermatol 103:335–344, 1980; Part II. Br J Dermatol 104:209–220, 1981

140. Van Hove W, Rottiers R, Hamers J: Hypercholesterolemia in multiple myeloma before and after treatment. Acta Clin Belg 28:198–205, 1973

141. Vitols S, Bjorkholm M, Gahrton G, et al: Hypocholesterolemia in malignancy due to elevated low-density-lipoprotein-receptor activity in tumor cells: Evidence from studies in patients with leukemia. Lancet 2:1150–1153, 1985

142. Lynch PJ, Winkelmann RK: Generalized plane xanthoma and systemic disease. Arch Dermatol 93:639–646, 1966

143. Kilgore LL, Patterson BW, Parenti DM, et al: Immune complex hyperlipidemia induced by an apolipoprotein-reactive immunoglobuln A paraprotein from a patient with multiple myeloma. J Clin Invest 76:225–232, 1985

144. Cortese C, Lewis B, Miller NE, et al: Myelomatosis with type III hyperlipoproteinemia. Clinical and metabolic studies. N Engl J Med 307:79–83, 1982

145. Steigleder GK, Kuchmeister B: Cutaneous mucinous deposits. J Cutan Pathol 12:334–347, 1985

146. Matsuoka LY, Wortsman J, Carlisle KS, et al: The acquired cutaneous mucinoses. Arch Intern Med 144:1974–1980, 1984

147. Zielinski CC, Dremsek PA, Ahmad R, et al: Recurrent pyoderma in a family with a defect in leucocyte locomotion. Br Med J 289:1561–1563, 1984

148. Petrini N, Acampa D, Modi G, et al: Leukocyte chemotaxis and pyoderma gangrenosum. Int J Dermatol 25:45–47, 1985

149. Orellana J, Friedman AH: Ocular manifestations of multiple myelomas Waldenström's macroglobulinemia and benign monoclonal gammopathy. Surv Ophthalmol 26:157–169, 1981

SUBJECT INDEX

Acid polysaccharides, 352–353
Aclarubicin, 327
Acronine, 327
Adriamycin, 326, 328
AL amyloidosis, 271–272
Alkylating agents and prednisone, 319–320
Allotypes, 263
Alpha-2-macroglobulin, 356
Already bound ligand (ABL) concept, 359
3-Amino-l-hydroxypropane-l (APD), 296
Amsacrine (m-AMSA), 327
Amyloidosis AL, 343–345
Amyloidosis, cutaneous, 373
Antibody activity of monoclonal immunoglobulins, 350–359
Antistreptolysin (ASLO), 353
Apparent acid/base disturbances, 369
Autologous bone marrow rescue, 329–330
Azotemia, 283

Bacillus subtilis, 287
Bacterial exoenzymes, 353
Bacterial infections and multiple myeloma, 282–287
B cells
  immunoglobulins and, 264–265, 266
  multiple myeloma and, 285
BCNU (Carmustine), 322, 323, 326, 327
Bence Jones (BJ) proteins, 341–343, 344, 350
  benign, 345
  diagnostic importance of, 345–346
Biphosphonates, 296
Bisantrene, 327
Bleeding disorders, 368–369
Bleomycin, 327
B-lymphocyte-plasma cell lineage, c-*myc* locus and, 278–279
Bone destruction
  evaluation of in multiple myelona, 305–306
  in plasma cell myeloma, 291–297
Bone marrow precursors and mineral oil, 275–276
Bone marrow transplantation, 329
Bone pain, treatment for, 297
Bone resorbing activity
  hypercalcemia and, 294–295
  in myeloma, 292, 293
Bone scans in myeloma, 291

Calcitonin and corticosteroids, 295–296
Calcium, 358
  and hypercalcemia, 294–295
Carmustine (BCNU), 322, 323, 326, 327
Cephalosporin, 357
Chlorozotocin, 327
Chromosome 15, nonrandom translocations in, 277–278
Cisplatinum, 296, 327
Class switching in immunoglobulin genes, 266
Clinical findings in multiple myeloma, 282–283
Clonogenic assay for human myeloma cell colonies, 334
C-*myc* oncogene in plasmacytoma, 278–279
Coagulation factors, 356
Cold agglutinins (CA), 369–370
Combination therapy, 320–324
  for refractory multiple myeloma, 326–327
Complementarity determining regions (CDR), 260
Corneal crystalline deposition, 375
Corticosteroids, 328
  for bone resorption in myeloma, 295–296
Cryoglobulinemia, 315, 367
  cutaneous manifestations of, 373
Cryoglobulins, 314–315
Cryoimmunoglobulins (Cryo-Igs), 367–368
Cutaneous amyloidosis, 373
Cutaneous manifestations and M-Ig, 372(*t*), 373–375
Cyclophosphamide, 319–324, 327, 329, 334–335
Cytosine arabinoside, 327
Cytoskeleton proteins, 357
Cytotoxic drug therapy for hypercalcemia, 295–297

Dexamethasone, 326
Diaziquone, 328
Diffuse osteopenia, 291
DNA, 263, 268, 306
Doxorubicin, 326, 328

Electrophoresis, 310–312, 315–316
Erythema elevatum diutinum, 375
Escherichia coli, 282, 293
Ethane-l-hydroxy-l, l-diphosphonate (EHDP), 296

Factor X, 345
Flow microfluorometry in multiple myeloma, 306–307
Fluoride, 296
Freund's Adjuvants (FA), 275

Gallium nitrate, 296
Gamma globulin, 287
Gene structure of immunoglobulins, 263–266
Genetic polymorphisms, 263
Germline gene families, 263–264
Glucocorticoids and calcitonin, 296
Granulocyte function in multiple myeloma, 286

Haemophilus influenza, 283
H chain, 263
  genes, 264
  variants, 266–269
Hemochromatosis, 374
Hemolytic anemia and monoclonal cold agglutinins, 369–370
Hexamethylmelamine, 327
Human heavy chain disease (HCD), 266–268
Human leukocyte interferon, 336
Human recombinant interferon alpha, 334
Humoral immune suppression, multiple myeloma and, 283
Hydroxyurea, 329
Hypercalcemia in plasma cell myeloma, 291–297
Hypercupremia, 375
Hyperlipidemia, 373
Hyperviscosity syndrome, 366–367
Hypocholesterolemia, 373
Hypogammaglobulinemia, 310

Seminars in Oncology, Vol 13, No 3 (September), 1986: pp 380–382

Idiotypes, 263
Immunization for multiple myeloma, 286–287
Immunodiffusion, 314, 316–317
Immunoelectrophoresis, 312–313, 316–317
Immunofixation, 313–314, 317
Immunoglobulin A (IgA), 262. *See also* Immunoglobulins
Immunoglobulin D (IgD), 262. *See also* Immunoglobulins
Immunoglobulin E (IgE), 262–263. *See also* Immunoglobulins
Immunoglobulin G (IgG), 261–262. *See also* Immunoglobulins
Immunoglobulin M (IgM), 262. *See also* Immunoglobulins
Immunoglobulins, 283. *See also* Monoclonal immunoglobulins
  gene structure of, 263–266
  structure of, 260–264
Immunosuppression in multiple myeloma, 282–287
Immunotoxin-mediated cytotoxicity, 330
Indomethacin, plasmacytoma and, 277
Infection
  from chemotherapy, 283
  in multiple myeloma, 282–287
Inflammation in plasmacytoma development, 276, 277
Interferons, 334–339
  bone destruction and, 294
Interleukin 1 (Ill), 293–294
Intron A, 334–335
  resistant multiple myeloma and, 336–338
  untreated multiple myeloma and, 338–339
Ions, 358
Irradiation therapy, 328
Isotypes, 260

J chain, 262

Kinetics of multiple myeloma, 300–307
Klebsiella polysaccharides, 352–353

L chain
  genes, 263, 264, 265
  variants, 269–270
Lichen myxedematosis, 374
Ligands reacting with M-Igs, 358, 359
Light chain-associated amyloidosis, 343–345
Light chain deposition disease, 342–343
Lipoproteins, 353–354
Lymphocyte populations in myeloma, 285, 305
Lymphosarcoma cell leukemia, bone resorbing activity in, 292–293
Lymphotoxin, 293
Lysozyme, 287

Macroglobulinemia, 366
Macrophages in plasmacytoma development, 276
Maintenance therapy, 324
Man, plasma cell tumor formation in, 279
Melphalan, 319–324, 328, 329, 334–335, 336, 338–339
Melphalan/prednisone (MP), 322, 323
MGUS. *See* Monoclonal gammopathy of undetermined significance
Mice, plasmacytomas in, 275–280

M-Igs. *See* Monoclonal immunoglobulins
Mineral oil to induce plasmacytomas, 275
Mithramycin, 295
Monoclonal antibodies, 330
Monoclonal gammopathy of undetermined significance (MGUS), 280, 310
  diagnostic features of, 300–301
Monoclonal immunoglobulin deposition disease (MIgDD), 271–272
Monoclonal immunoglobulins (M-Igs). *See also* Immunoglobulins
  antibody activity in, 350–359
  clinical implications of, 366–375
Monoclonal light chains, 341–347
Monoclonal proteins, electrophoresis for, 310–312
Monoclonal rheumatoid factors (MRFs), 353
Myeloma kidney, 341–342
Myeloma proteins, 310–317

Necrobiotic xanthogranuloma, 375
Nephropathies associated with M-Igs, 371–373
Neural antigens, 355
Neutropenia, chemotherapy-induced, 283
Neutrophils in plasmacytoma development, 276–277
New therapeutic approaches, 330–331
Nitrophenyl ligands, 355–356
Nonsecretory myeloma, 270–271
Nonspecific host mechanisms in multiple myeloma, 285–286
Nuclear antigens, 357

Ocular copper pigment deposition, 375
Ocular manifestations, 375
Oil granuloma (OG), 275–280
Osteoclast activating factor (OAF), 292–294
Osteoclast activity in myeloma, 292
Osteosclerosis, 291
Ouchterlony, 314, 316–317

Parasitic infestations, plasmacytoma and, 277
Penicillin, semisynthetic, 357
Pentostatin, 327
Periodic acid Schiff (PAS) reaction, 341, 343
Peripheral neuropathy, 370
Peritoneal plasmacytomas (PCTs), 279–280
Phagocytosis in plasmacytoma development, 276–277
Phenylalanine mustard, 319
Phospholipids, 354–355
Plasma cell myeloma, bone destruction in, 291–297
Plasmacytoma (PC), 275–280, 284
Plicamycin for bone resorption in myeloma, 295
Pneumococcal bacteremia and multiple myeloma, 282
Pneumococcal vaccine for multiple myeloma, 286–287
Pneumonia and multiple myeloma, 282–283
Pneumovax, 287
POEMS syndrome, 370–371
Polysaccharides, 351–353
Prednisone, 319–324, 328, 334–335, 336, 338, 339
Preneoplastic plasma cell lesions in OG, 276
Previously untreated MM, Intron A and, 338–339
Previously untreated myeloma, chemotherapy of, 318–324
Pristane, 275–276

Prognostic factors in multiple myeloma, 301–304
Pyoderma gangrenosum (PG), 374–375

Quantitation of immunoglobulins, 314

Red blood cell polysaccharides-related antigens, 351–352
Refractory multiple myelona, treatment of, 326–331
Regions of Ig chain, 260, 262, 263
Renal calcium excretion in myeloma, 296–297
Renal diseases, monoclonal light chain-associated, 341–345
Renal function, hypercalcemia and, 295
Resistant multiple myeloma and Intron A, 336
Rheumatoid factors (RE), 353
Riboflavin, 357–358, 359
RNA, 306
RNA polymerase, 263

Saline diuresis for myeloma, 296, 297
Scleromyxedema, 374
Secretory IgG (SIgA), 262
Serum albumin, 356
Serum protein electrophoresis, 310–312, 315–316
Serum viscometry, 314
Soft-agar colony-forming assay for human myeloma, 329
Spirogermanium, 328
Spontaneous plasmacytoma and chronic inflammation, 277
Staging of multiple myeloma, 300–307
Streptococcus pneumonia, 282
Subcorneal pustular dermatosis, 375
Sulfonamide, 357
Systemic capillary leak syndrome, 369

T cells
  immunoglobulin genes and, 264
  multiple myeloma and, 284–285
Thyroglobulin, 356–357
Thyroid hormones, 356–357
Transcript processing of immunoglobulin genes, 265–266
Transferrin, 310–311, 356
Tumor necrosis factor, 293
Tumor regression in multiple myeloma with chemotherapy, 304–305

Urine analysis for monoclonal proteins, 315–317

Vaccine for multiple myeloma, 286–287
VAD, 326
Variants, H and L chain, 266–270
VBAP, 326, 327
Vincristine, 326, 327
Vindesine, 328
Viruses, 357

Waldenström's macroglobulinemia, 312–313

Xanthoderma, 373–374
Xanthomatosis, 373

VOL XIII, NO 4 DECEMBER 1986

Seminars in Oncology

Breast Cancer
Part I

Gianni Bonadonna, *Guest Editor*

Contributors

Gianni Bonadonna • G. Saccani Jotti
J.Y. Petit • G. Contesso • Ann Thor • Maureen O. Weeks
Jeffrey Schlom • Stephen A. Feig • Paul P. Carbone
Douglass C. Tormey • Bernard Fisher • Norman Wolmark
Abram Recht • James L. Connolly • Stuart J. Schnitt • Blake Cady
Susan Love • Robert T. Osteen • W. Bradford Patterson • Robert Shirley
William Silen • Steven Come • I. Craig Henderson
Barbara Silver • Jay R. Harris

GRUNE & STRATTON
Harcourt Brace Jovanovich, Inc.

"...cisplatin has become one of the most important agents used in clinical oncology today."[1]

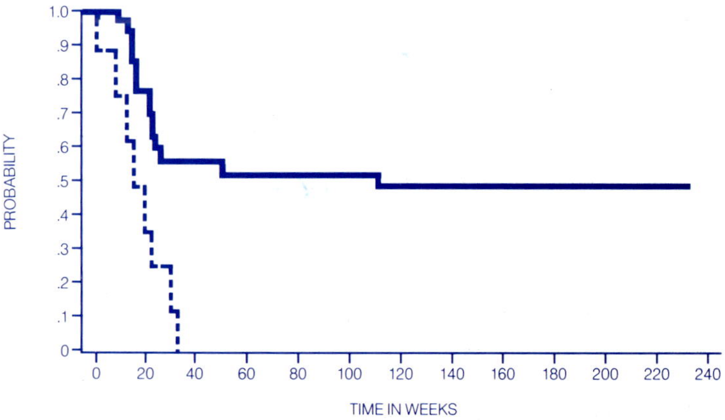

Survival of patients with refractory germinal neoplasms (Indiana-Vanderbilt series): VP-16—containing regimens versus control regimens. ▬▬, VP-16; - - - -, control[2]

- Expanding clinical applications
- Measurable impact on response and survival
- Predictable and manageable toxicities
- Acceptable for outpatient administration

PLATINOL®
Cisplatin for Injection

Please see adjoining page for brief summary of prescribing information.

References:

1. Loehrer PJ, Einhorn LH: Cisplatin. *Ann Intern Med* 100:704-713, 1984.
2. Hainsworth JD, Greco FA, Williams SD, Einhorn LH: VP-16 in the treatment of refractory germinal neoplasms, in Issell BF, Muggia FM, Carter SK (eds): *Etoposide (VP-16): Current Status and New Developments*, pp 243-252. Copyright © 1984 by Academic Press, Inc.

Seminars in Oncology

Vol 13, No 4 **December 1986**

Introduction: Breast Cancer

HUMAN MAMMARY carcinoma is often being used to measure the pace of progress in cancer treatment. Actually, several biological and clinical aspects contribute to the indication of breast cancer as the neoplastic disease par excellence. Its increasing frequency in numerous countries stimulates epidemiologists to further study the importance of exogenous factors such as estrogens, diet, and nutrition; the marked heterogeneity of tumor cell populations puzzles basic scientists and greatly concerns medical oncologists; the frequent systemic nature of what appears to be a localized disease encourages testing of various forms of multidisciplinary approaches; last but not least, an increasing number of surgeons have begun to substitute biological concepts for anatomic principles.

The strong research component in recent treatment efforts is gradually but consistently displacing anecdotal information with results derived from properly conceived trials having biological endpoints. Following a flare of great enthusiasm for the first trials with systemic adjuvant therapy, our demanding audience appears perplexed if not disappointed, by the lack of breakthrough and the consequent prompt reduction in the overall mortality rate. However, physicians, as well as statisticians, should become more aware that several lines of evidence now support that the term "breast cancer" includes many subsets, if not many diseases. Therefore, some subsets benefit more or less than others, and the disparate therapeutic outcome is in keeping with the biological heterogeneity between and within breast cancers. Even more important, the time required from the introduction of a potentially curative treatment to the recognition and confirmation that such treatment has, in fact, yielded positive results is substantial; additional time is then required for the transfer of the new technology to the community to detect a decrease in tumor mortality.

From the strategic point of view, high propensity for early metastatic spread, tumor cell heterogeneity, and primary drug resistance represent the crucial aspects upon which elaborate new working hypotheses rest. The tactic should not neglect that innovative forms of therapy aimed at increasing cure or quality of life, and time for thorough treatment evaluation will remain the essential ingredients of all clinical trials. Thus, the pace of progress will mainly consist in hypotheses modification based on positive and negative research findings. The cycle of testing will continue, and rather than the traditional competing forces, sound research information will influence clinical practice.

Gianni Bonadonna
Istituto Nazionale Tumori
Milan, Italy
Guest Editor

Minimal Breast Cancer: A Clinically Meaningful Term?

G. Saccani Jotti, J.Y. Petit, and G. Contesso

ONE OF THE MAJOR factors that may improve the prognosis of breast cancer could be its earlier detection, ie, before the disease becomes histologically invasive and/or clinically palpable. In recent years, due to the widespread use of mammography and mammographic screening programs, the number of small-size breast carcinomas, including nonpalpable lesions, has increased considerably. High survival rates reflect the importance of detecting breast cancer in early stages of development. The main benefit of identifying small tumors also lies in the resulting possibility of more cosmetic operative intervention. In fact, recent findings have demonstrated convincingly that for tumors of relatively small size, breast-saving procedures can yield relapse-free and total survival rates comparable to those achieved through mutilating surgical procedures.

For many years, pathologists have argued about the definition and the biologic reasons of what is early, minimal, and occult breast cancer. Whether these terms really identify entities that can be meaningful today to clinicians, and whether the prognostic significance of breast cancer measuring 1 cm or less in diameter should have implications in the treatment decision making will be the subject of this review.

DEFINITION

The term "minimal breast cancer" (MBC) was first introduced into the medical literature in 1971 by Gallager and Martin.[1] This term was defined histopathologically as "including noninvasive carcinoma, either ductal or lobular, and invasive carcinoma having a volume no greater than that of a sphere 0.5 cm in diameter" (0.065 cm^3).[2] MBC, as originally conceived on precise mammographic and pathologic studies, is actually (as for cancer of uterine cervix) a stage in progression between atypical hyperplasia and invasive carcinoma and not a special kind of cancer.[3] Later, the same authors clarified the differences among MBC, early, and occult breast cancer.[2] In 1978, McDivitt[4] suggested that the term MBC could be restricted to those infiltrating carcinomas measuring less than 1.0 cm in diameter. In addition, Hutter[5] expanded on MBC by adding certain histologic types of infiltrating carcinoma that could be considered as minimal in relation to their usual excellent prognosis. These histologic types comprise medullary, colloid, and tubular carcinomas of any size as well as other peculiar forms of carcinoma, such as those of the axillary tail, noninfiltrating Paget's disease of the nipple, and carcinoma in fibroadenoma. The lengthening of this list, as well as confusion, reached the apex with the report of Wanebo et al[6] who included within MBC a number of low-grade infiltrating cancers (adenoid cystic, colloid, intracystic papillary, and low-grade tubular carcinomas) as well as several cases with malignant cystosarcoma phyllodes.

In 1981, the American College of Surgeons[7] published a survey of 16,894 pathologically confirmed carcinomas of the female breast, in situ or infiltrative, with negative (N−) or positive (N+) axillary lymph nodes. Of these, 323 cases (1.9%) were in situ carcinomas of any size, and 869 cases (8.4%) were minimal invasive carcinomas 1 cm or less in diameter. The most important conclusions from this study were as follows: (1) There was no significant 5-year survival difference between women with in situ tumors of any size and women with minimal invasive tumors $\leq$1 cm having negative axillary nodes; (2) survival and recurrence rates were significantly superior in N− women with minimal invasive cancer than rates of N− women with invasive tumors $>$1 cm; (3) survival and recurrence rates observed in N+ women with invasive cancers $<$1 cm suggested that nodal status rather

From the Institute of Pathology, University of Parma School of Medicine, Parma, Italy; and the Departments of Surgery and Pathology Institut Gustave Roussy, Villejuif, France.

Supported in part by a grant from the Italian National Research Council, Project "Oncology," Contract No. 85 02351 44 and in part by a grant from the Reggio Emilia section of the Italian League Against Cancer.

Address reprint requests to G. Saccani Jotti, MD, Institute of Pathology, University of Parma School of Medicine, Via Gramsci, 16, Parma 63100, Italy.

0093-7754/86/1304-0002$05.00/0

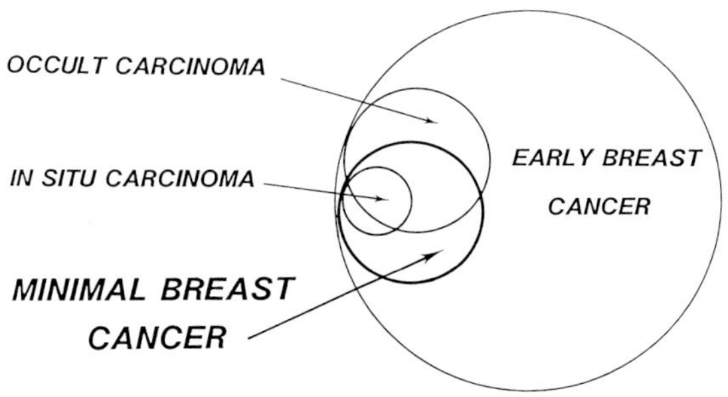

Fig 1. Diagram showing schematically the relation among early breast cancer, occult carcinoma, in situ carcinoma, and minimal breast cancer.

than tumor size alone may determine whether a small invasive tumor below 1 cm should be considered as MBC.

Following the above-mentioned publication all invasive carcinomas ≤1 cm in diameter were included in the definition of MBC[8,9] in addition to lobular carcinoma in situ (LCIS) and intraductal carcinoma (IDC). In terms of postsurgical classification of TNM system (pTNM),[10] MBC would include pTIS (carcinoma in situ), pTi (tumor <0.5 cm), and pTii (tumor >0.5 cm but not >1 cm).

Figure 1 illustrates the relationship between MBC and other similar groups of breast cancer. It is therefore appropriate to state that the term "early breast cancer" indicates a neoplastic lesion detected at an early stage of its development and limited to the breast; this term at times was also applied to carcinomas of any size with no axillary or distant metastases. Whereas most MBC are early, the overwhelming majority of early cancers are not minimal. It is not easy to determine the length of the preclinical phase because cell kinetic studies have demonstrated frequent variations of tumor growth.[11] Furthermore, a limited number of minimal carcinomas can be expected to produce nodal metastases and are not, in that sense, early. The term "occult breast cancer" indicates a nonpalpable cancer,[12] asymptomatic, and for some authors, not even mammographically demonstrable. Most, but not all, minimal cancers are also occult. The term "in situ carcinoma" (or "intraepithelial carcinoma" or "preinvasive carcinoma") can only be used after histopathologic diagnosis. It corresponds to a proliferation of neoplastic elements that remain in the lumen of ducts or lobules. No evidence of tumor development beyond the basement membrane is detectable by light microscopic examination. The borderline difference between in situ and microinvasive carcinomas is often very difficult to distinguish, but it can be shown by electron microscopy.[13]

FREQUENCY AND AGE DISTRIBUTION

According to published data, the frequency of MBC is somewhat variable and ranges from 5% to 10% (Table 1). In the survey of the American College of Surgeons,[7] of 1,489 tumors ≤1 cm, 4.4% were in situ carcinomas, 75.3% were localized N− invasive carcinomas, and 20.3% were N+ invasive carcinomas. In the series of 1,770 cases with breast cancer diagnosed at the Institut Gustave Roussy between 1967 and 1970, 163 (9%) were considered as MBC. Of these, 11 tumors were LCIS, 56 IDC, and 96 infiltrating carcinomas ≤1 cm (minimal invasive cancer [MIC]).

The survey of the American College of Surgeons[7] showed that women with in situ carcinomas were significantly younger than women with infiltrating tumors. At the Institut Gustave Roussy patients with LCIS had a mean age of

Table 1. Frequency of Minimal Breast Cancer in Various Case Series

		LCIS		IDC		MIC		Total With MBC	
First Author or Institution	No. of Patients	No. of Patients	(%)	No. of Patients	(%)	No. of Patients	(%)	No. of Patients	(%)
Peters[14]	2,010	5	(0.2)	71	(4)	20*	(1)	96	(5)
Smart[15]	8,587	127	(2)	268	(3)	326	(4)	721	(9)
Rosen[16]	1,175	59	(5)	60	(5)	nr	(nr)	nr	(nr)
Rosner[17]	10,054	121	(1)	202	(2)	869	(9)	1,192	(12)
Dubin[18]	1,074	19	(2)	35	(3)	59	(5.5)	113	(10.5)
Institut Gustave Roussy	1,770	11	(1)	56	(3)	96	(5)	163	(9)

Abbreviation: nr, not reported.

*Only microinvasive types.

48.5 ± 3 years while the highest mean age (54.6 ± 1 years) was observed in patients with MIC. The mean age of IDC (54.0 ± 2 years) was superimposable on that of patients with infiltrating carcinomas.

DIAGNOSIS

The epidemiologic study of Dubin et al[18] among women screened in New York indicated that several important risk factors may differ between MBC and clinical breast cancer. Women who gave birth at an early age (<20 years), who nursed two or more children, as well as black women, were more likely to be diagnosed with MBC. In addition, unlike clinical breast cancer, MBC failed to exhibit the usual positive relationship with family history of breast cancer or obesity.

The frequency of MBC is directly correlated to the diagnostic procedures used. Mammography is the most consistently accurate means for detecting small-size breast tumors and thus represents the most widely used of the many currently available breast imaging techniques.[19] The equipment and procedures required to produce the images have been considerably refined over the years, and the radiation dose of the examination has been reduced to clinically acceptable safe levels.

The radiographic changes of MBC or noninvasive breast cancer are not specific and include increased vascularity, increased breast density, locally dense stroma, local stroma distortion, enlarged or prominent ducts, and punctate or clustered microcalcifications. The presence of this latter finding is an excellent radiographic marker and should increase the suspicion that a MBC is present and the abnormal area should be removed for histopathologic examination.

The capability of mammography in the detection of breast cancer in early or minimal stages of development was recently shown by the 5-year summary report of the Breast Cancer Detection Demonstration Project.[20] Table 2 summarizes the essential findings on 3,024 cancers under 1 cm in diameter, 68% of which were noninvasive and 32% were in women under the age of 50 years. As one can see, the sensitivity of mammography in the detection of MBC is about 60%.

Table 2. Potential of Mammography in Detection of MBC: Essential Results of Breast Cancer Detection Demonstration Project[20]

	% of All Cancers of Known Size (3,024 Cases)	% of Cancers ≤1 cm (1,149 Cases)	% of Noninfiltrating Cancers (781 Cases)
Mammography alone	43.6	58.4	60.4
Physical examination alone	8.7	6.6	5.6
Positive mammography and physical examination	48.5	35.0*	
True-positive detection rate by mammography	92.0	93.4*	

*Infiltrating and noninfiltrating cancers.

A great diagnostic contribution has also been provided by localization techniques with probes or metal needles[19,21,22] that are increasingly used to help the surgeon in the precise and efficient excision of the suspicious area. Following preoperative needle placement in the breast, confirmatory mammogram images are taken, properly labeled, and immediately sent with the patient to surgery. After surgical excision, specimen radiography confirms that the entire abnormal or suspicious area has indeed been removed. In the experience of the Institut Gustave Roussy, the histologic diagnosis of noninfiltrating carcinoma by frozen section is not reliable because the sensitivity of this histologic examination is about 30% for IDC, 0% for LCIS. The frequency of in situ carcinomas detected histologically depends on the surface and number of specimens actually examined. Depending on the size of the surgically removed fragment, the recommended number of specimens ranges from 6 to 25.[17,23-27] This will often allow detection of minimal changes in the myoepithelial layer with neoplastic cellular interruptions in the surrounding connective tissue, thus enabling the identification of microinvasive carcinomas; microfractures can also be detected for in situ carcinomas by means of electron microscopy.[13]

Multicentricity of noninvasive carcinoma is well known, especially for IDC. At the Institut Gustave Roussy, multicentricity has been observed in most mastectomy specimens removed for IDC (76%).[28] In a previous study, microfoci of IDC distant from the primary tumor (ie, in a different quadrant) were observed in

Table 3. Minimal Breast Cancer: Cumulative Nodal and Bilateral Involvement From Four Case Series[6,14,29,30]

	% of Involved Axillary Nodes	% of Bilaterality (Simultaneous or Subsequent)
Total	5.5*	21.0†
LCIS	2.8	42.4
IDC	1.7	13.4
MIC	13.3	9.9

*On 415 patients who had nodes removed.
†On 429 patients from whom data were available.

69% of cases whereas this finding occurred in only 24% of infiltrating carcinomas ($P = .001$). Such high incidence of multicentricity for noninvasive carcinoma explains the known perplexity of many surgeons to abandon total mastectomy in favor of breast-saving procedures.

NODAL AND BILATERAL INVOLVEMENT

It is well known that among noninvasive carcinomas the incidence of axillary nodal metastasis is low and the rate of bilaterality, especially subsequent bilaterality, is high.

Table 3 shows the histopathologic involvement of axillary lymph nodes in a cumulative series of 415 women with MBC who had nodes removed at the time of primary surgery.[6,14,29,30] The rate of axillary metastases for the entire series was about 5%, and the frequency was higher for microinvasive carcinoma compared to LCIS and IDC. A similar comparative frequency of nodal metastases was observed in the series of 163 women evaluated at the Institut Gustave Roussy (MIC, 37%; IDC, 6%; and LCIS, none). Somewhat intermediate results were reported in the survey of the American College of Surgeons.[7] In fact, axillary node metastases were present in 23% of 157 patients with minimal invasive carcinomas measuring 0.1 to 0.5 cm, and in 20.9% of 964 patients whose tumors measured 0.6 to 1.0 cm.

Bilateral breast carcinoma, either simultaneous or subsequent, occurred in 21% of 429 patients reported in Table 3. The rate was greater among women with LCIS but it was not negligible in women with IDC or MIC. Bilaterality was found most frequently in women in whom multiple contralateral blind biopsies were performed routinely at the time of mastectomy. Among women whose contralateral biopsies were negative, subsequent contralateral carcinomas were extremely rare. In the series of the Institut Gustave Roussy, the frequency of bilateral carcinoma was not significantly different among the three histopathologic types (LCIS, 9%; IDC, 7%; and MIC, 7%).

TREATMENT AND PROGNOSIS

Presently there is insufficient information to indicate what form of treatment can be recommended for MBC. The main reason is the frequent inconsistency of the treatments applied. They have ranged from wedge excision or wide local excision, to simple mastectomy, and to more extensive surgical procedures with axillary node dissection (total mastectomy, modified radical, classical radical mastectomy, or extended radical with internal mammary dissection) with and without postoperative irradiation.

In general, and somewhat regardless of the extent of local-regional therapy, treatment outcome is good.[31] In the cumulative series of 484 women quoted by Gallager,[32] and subjected to a heterogeneous treatment approach, the relapse-free survival for all evaluable patients (average follow-up of 5.3 years) was 96.8%. There was no difference in the survival rate among patients with LCIS, IDC, and microinvasive carcinoma, nor between N− and N+ groups. The actuarial survival curves for the case series of the Institut Gustave Roussy are displayed in Figs 2 and 3. The relapse-free survival rates for patients with LCIS (88%) and IDC (91%) were significantly higher to those of patients with infiltrating carcinoma ≤ 1 cm (75%, $P = .01$). A significantly lower relapse-free survival rate (55%) was found for women with infiltrating cancer >1 cm in diameter ($P = 10^{-4}$). The overall survival curves of the three subgroups with MBC were almost superimposable while the comparative survival of infiltrating carcinomas <1 cm and of in situ carcinoma was not significant ($P = .14$).

The survey of the American College of Surgeons[7] related the treatment outcome to the status of axillary lymph nodes. The 5-year relapse-free survival and recurrence rates in patients with tumors ≤ 1 cm are reproduced in Table 4. The prognostic influence of histologically positive nodes is evident. The total survival of patients with in situ tumors was not significantly different to that of N− patients with minimally invasive tumors <1 cm. Furthermore,

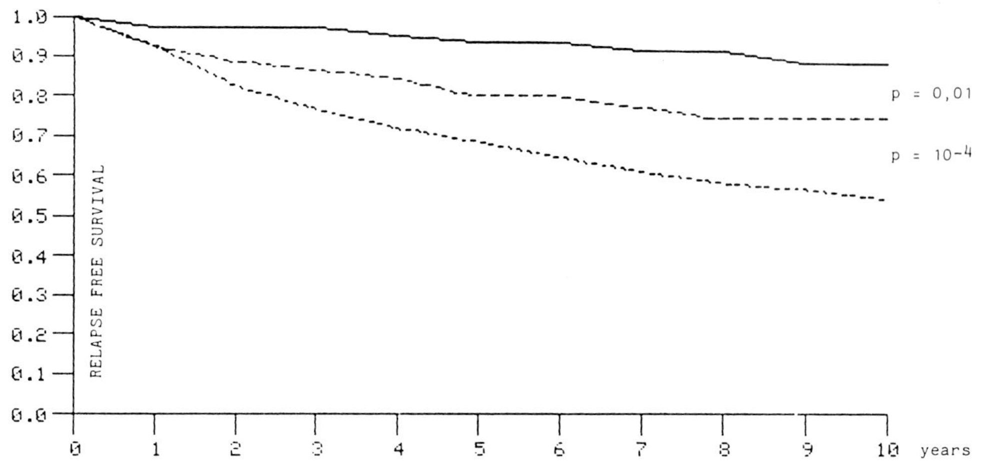

Fig 2. Comparative relapse-free survival among patients with lobular carcinoma in situ and intraductal carcinoma (LCIS + IDC), minimal invasive carcinoma (MIC), and infiltrating cancer (other). Data from the Institut Gustave Roussy.

among N− patients, total survival was not different between women with tumors 0.5 cm or less and those measuring 0.6 to 1.0 cm. In contrast, for N− patients both recurrence and total survival rates were significantly higher in women with minimal invasive cancer compared to invasive tumors >1 cm.

The surgical protocol of the Institut Gustave Roussy makes a clear distinction between treatment for infiltrating minimal and noninvasive breast cancer. Infiltrating carcinomas ≤1 cm are systematically treated by wide tumor resection supplemented by axillary dissection and postoperative radiotherapy to remaining portions of the gland. The radiation dose is 45 Gy plus 15 Gy as a boost dose. Until recently for noninvasive carcinoma, simple mastectomy with or without low axillary dissection has been carried out because of the high multicentricity rate. Immediate breast reconstruction was usually offered to patients to decrease the psychologic distress caused by the mutilating procedure. More recently, total mastectomy with immediate breast reconstruction has remained only for IDC while LCIS are being treated by wide tumor resection alone.

The relative merits of mastectomy (classical radical, modified radical, simple) versus conservative surgical procedures (excision, segmental mastectomy with or without axillary node dissec-

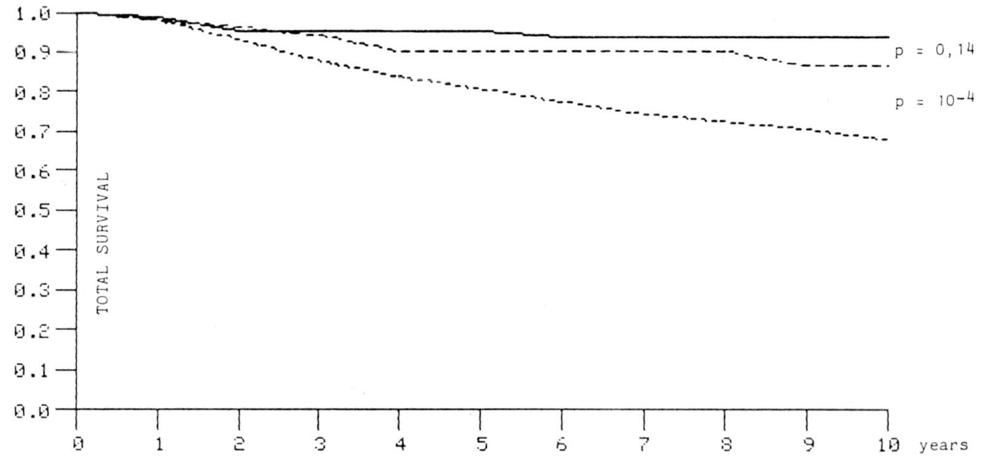

Fig 3. Comparative total survival among patients with lobular carcinoma in situ and intraductal carcinoma (LCIS + IDC), minimal invasive carcinoma (MIC), and infiltrating cancer (other). Data from the Institut Gustave Roussy.

tion) plus irradiation was retrospectively evaluated by Montague at the MD Anderson Hospital.[33] From 1955 through 1979, 121 patients having MBC were treated with mastectomy and all had N− tumors. During the same period of time, 40 other women with MBC were treated with tumor excision followed by radiotherapy. This latter treatment consisted of high-energy irradiation to the breast and adjacent chest wall, axilla (to 36 of 40 patients without axillary dissection), supraclavicular, and internal mammary areas. The 10-year relapse-free survival of the entire series with MBC was about 95% with no difference between patients treated with mastectomy and conservative surgery plus irradiation. The cosmetic results following conservative approach improved as the surgical and radiotherapeutic techniques became more refined and as the irradiated volume was lessened.

Recht et al[34] have recently published the results of excisional biopsy and irradiation in 40 women with IDC treated between 1976 and 1983. The median age was 53 years (range, 28 to 77 years) and the median follow-up time since initiation of irradiation was 44 months (range, 14 to 97 months). Twenty-seven women presented with a palpable mass; in eight cases, the tumor was measuring <1 cm in diameter; and in 13 cases, the tumor was detected only by mammography. A limited axillary dissection was performed in 13 patients, and all lymph nodes were histologically negative. Treatment was administered to the breast and adjacent chest wall to a dose of 4,600 to 5,000 rad. Twenty-six patients also received a boost dose of 1,000 to 2,000 rad to the site of primary tumor. The 5-year actuarial rate of local recurrence was 10%, and no patient developed distant metastases. Cosmetic results are excellent. Little or no fibrosis was noted in the breast following a 5,000-rad tumor dose.

CRITICAL REMARKS

All above described findings, implicating a model of natural history, indicate that there is a stage in the development of breast carcinoma in which invasion is nonexistent or of near microscopic dimension. At this stage, simple methods of treatment might provide long-term control and even cure if regional lymph nodes are not involved. Thus collectively, minimal breast cancer is an expression that connotates curability as

Table 4. Five-Year Relapse-Free Survival and Recurrence Rates in Patients With Breast Cancer ≤ 1 cm

	Patients		5-Year RFS		Recurrence	
Stage	No.	(%)	No.	(%)	No.	(%)
Total	1,489	(100)	1,001	(67.2)	239	(16.0)
In situ	66	(4.4)	53	(80.3)	2	(3.0)
Node negative	1,121	(75.3)	788	(70.3)	143	(12.8)
Node positive	302	(20.3)	160	(50.0)	94	(31.8)

Abbreviation: RFS, relapse-free survival.
Data from the American College of Surgeons.[7]

well as earliness. However, this term may eventually become insidious for clinicians because it groups at least three major entities (lobular carcinoma in situ, noninfiltrating intraductal carcinoma, and minimal infiltrating carcinoma) whose different natural history may require different therapeutic approaches. The following critical remarks will attempt to clarify a few important clinical aspects that may lead to the conclusion that the popular term "minimal breast cancer" lacks specificity and should probably be abandoned.

Is minimal breast cancer an indolent form of carcinoma that never becomes life threatening? Many studies on LCIS and on IDC would confirm that this is not true. For instance in women with LCIS, Rosen et al,[35] in a long-term follow-up study of 99 patients treated only with biopsy, reported that the frequency of subsequent invasive carcinoma was nine times the expected rate, and mortality due to the disease was 11 times greater than expected. The risk of later invasive carcinoma appeared to involve both breasts equally. About 10 years earlier, McDivitt et al[36] had shown that the total risk of developing a homolateral invasive carcinoma was 15% at 10 years and 35% at 20 years. Wheeler et al[37] indicated a comparatively lower risk (9.7%) at 10 years. In two similar studies performed in patients with IDC, Betsill et al[38] and Page et al[26] noticed a 28% frequency of subsequent invasive carcinoma. These data imply that these two forms of minimal breast cancer represent indeed a stage in progression to invasive carcinoma.[32] Thus, detection and treatment are capable of reducing the incidence of more advanced (ie, invasive) disease.

Is minimal breast cancer an early biologic stage of the disease? Considering the natural history of breast cancer through the analysis of tumor doubling times, the answer is no because what is clinically early is actually biologically late. In fact, most breast tumors are detected when their diameter is >1 cm, which is about the limit of palpability. To reach the diameter of 1 cm (equal to one billion cells), it requires 30 population doubles from the initial single cell. Since the doubling time encompasses 30 to 200 or more days, it would take 7 to 9 years to reach this stage, at which many breast cancers have already metastatized. Furthermore, evidence suggests that metastases may occur within the first 10 to 20 doubling times, ie, at a stage in which the tumor is undetectable. Once the early tumor is detected by physical examination, it can cause the death of the host in another 10 to 15 doubles. A small, 0.5 cm breast cancer detected at mammography, although regarded as very early clinically, has already passed through 27 doubles, and is again biologically a late tumor. Thus early detection by mammography does not guarantee cure. The recognized heterogeneity of breast cancer cell populations would in part explain why some tumors may metastasize or exhibit rapid growth characteristics or may be drug sensitive, while other tumors may not. In particular, the long survival of some patients treated only with local-regional modalities would probably reflect slow tumor growth rather than cure.

Which is the optimal treatment strategy for minimal breast cancer? In spite of the inconsistency of treatments applied so far to most published series, it appears advisable to separate minimal invasive cancer from noninvasive cancer (LCIS and IDC). The main reasons are listed below.

In all patients with invasive cancers of small dimensions (≤1 cm) there is now documented evidence from two prospective randomized trials[39,40] that limited surgical procedures to include full axillary dissection and supplemented by local radiotherapy are as effective as Halsted or modified radical mastectomy. In particular, there is no longer a specific reason to keep tumor ≤0.5 cm separate from those of 0.6 to 1.0 cm since prognosis and management will be the same. In all women with histologically involved axillary nodes, systemic drug therapy is now indicated because it has been proven to favorably affect both relapse-free and total survival rates.[41]

Controversy still surrounds the treatment of LCIS, mainly because it appears that the risk of subsequent cancer is equally divided between both breasts. Thus, the treatment choices are among bilateral mastectomy, ipsilateral mastectomy (including low axillary node dissection and controlateral biopsy), subcutaneous mastectomy, or clinical follow-up after limited breast resection. Because indiscriminate bilateral mastectomy is not an attractive alternative and ipsilateral mastectomy does not represent a radical preventive operation, we believe that a sound policy is close clinical follow-up. Of course the patient must be informed about her future risks.[31]

Most surgeons feel that the appropriate treatment for IDC is simple mastectomy supplemented by axillary dissection because of the risk of multicentricity, occult invasion, or metastases. This was also the policy of the Institut Gustave Roussy until recently, leading to the performance of mutilating surgery for noninvasive carcinoma and of a breast-saving procedure for invasive carcinoma. Such a contradictory approach is somewhat difficult to maintain. The question is whether to evaluate the ability of radiotherapy to eradicate the neoplastic microfoci lying within the breast but distant from the primary tumor. Montague,[33] Recht et al[34] and Zafrani et al[42] have already shown that modern radiotherapy can provide acceptable local control and excellent survival after conservative treatment for IDC, when suitable precautions of patient selection and evaluation are taken. However, carefully designed clinical trials are needed to prove whether breast-conservative surgery, with or without postoperative local radiation therapy, or radiotherapy following lumpectomy, is effective in the treatment of IDC as an alternative to mutilating surgery.[43]

In conclusion, the features of what constitutes an early cancer have not been well identified. Breast cancer appears, at least structurally, to evolve from a sequence of changes designated by pathologists as hyperplasia, atypical hyperplasia, carcinoma in situ, and invasive cancer. Such a progression may be nonobligate or discontinuous.[32,44] From the therapeutic point of view, the main benefit of recognition of small tumors, termed minimal breast cancer, will lie in the resulting possibility of more cosmetic operative interventions rather than in biologic reasons. Within this context, the histopathologic entities included in the term "minimal breast cancer" may become academic if clinical experience will confirm that they can be satisfactorily managed by conservative forms of treatment. It is also important to reiterate that in the presence of small size cancer, clinicians should not neglect the concept of multidisciplinary approach.

ACKNOWLEDGMENT

The authors are indebted to H. Mouriesse, PhD, for the statistical evaluation of data from the Institut Gustave Roussy included in this review. The authors are also grateful to E. Ferri for her skillful cooperation in typing the manuscript.

REFERENCES

1. Gallager HS, Martin JE: An orientation to the concept of minimal breast cancer. Cancer 28:1505–1507, 1971

2. Gallager HS: Pathogenesis of early breast cancer, in Zander J, Baltzer J (eds): Early Breast Cancer—Histopathology, Diagnosis and Treatment. Berlin, Springer-Verlag. 1985, pp 14–19

3. Westbrook KC, Gallager HS: Intraductal carcinoma of the breast. A comparative study. Am J Surg 130:667–670, 1975

4. McDivitt RW: Breast carcinoma. Hum Pathol 9:3–21, 1978

5. Hutter RVP: The pathologist's role in minimal breast cancer. Cancer 28:1527–1536, 1971

6. Wanebo HJ, Huvos AG, Urban JA: Treatment of minimal breast cancer. Cancer 33:349–357, 1974

7. Bedwani R, Vana J, Rosner D, et al: Management and survival of female patients with "minimal" breast cancer: as observed in the long-term and short-term surveys of the American College of Surgeons. Cancer 47:2769–2778, 1981

8. Brinton LA, Hoover R, Fraumeni JF: Epidemiology of minimal breast cancer. JAMA 249:483–487, 1983

9. Hartmann WH: Minimal breast cancer. An update. Cancer 53:681–684, 1984

10. TNM Classification of breast cancer. Geneva, UICC, 1982

11. Koscielny S, Tubiana M, Lé MG, et al: Breast cancer: Relationship between the size of primary tumor and the probability of metastatic dissemination. Br J Cancer 49:709–715, 1984

12. Schwartz GF, Patchefsky AS, Feig SA, et al: Clinically occult breast cancer. Multicentricity and implications for treatment. Ann Surg 191:8–12, 1980

13. Ozzello L: Ultrastructure of intra-epithelial carcinomas of the breast. Cancer 28:1508–1515, 1971

14. Peters TG, Donegan WL, Berg EA: Minimal breast cancer: A clinical appraisal. Ann Surg 186:704–710, 1977

15. Smart CR, Myers MH, Gloeckler LA: Implications from SEER data on breast cancer management. Cancer 41:787–790, 1978

16. Rosen PP, Senie R, Schottenfeld D, et al: Noninvasive breast carcinoma. Frequency of unsuspected invasion and implications for treatment. Ann Surg 189:377–382, 1979

17. Rosner D, Bedwani RN, Vana J, et al: Noninvasive breast carcinoma: Results of a national survey by the American College of Surgeons. Ann Surg 189:377–382, 1979

18. Dubin N, Hutter UP, Strax P, et al: Epidemiology of minimal breast cancer among women screened in New York City. JNCI 73:1273–1279, 1984

19. Sickles EA: Breast imaging: A view from the present to the future. Diagn Imag Clin Med 54:118–125, 1985

20. Baker LH: Breast cancer detection demonstration project: Five-year summary report. CA 32:194–225, 1982

21. Le Gal M, Chavanne D, Pellier D: Valeur diagnostique des microcalcifications groupées découvertes par mammographies. A propos de 227 cas avec vérification histologique et sans tumeurs du sein palpable. Bull Cancer (Paris) 71:57–64, 1984

22. Lanyi M: Microcalcifications in the breast—a blessing or a curse? A critical review. Diagn Imag Clin Med 54:126–145, 1985

23. Contesso G, Petit JY: Les adénocarcinomes intracanalaires non infiltrants du sein. Bull Cancer (Paris) 66:1–88, 1979

24. Patchefsky AS, Potok J, Hoch WS, et al: Increased detection of occult breast carcinoma after more thorough histologic examination of breast biopsies. Am J Clin Pathol 60:799–804, 1973

25. Ashikari R, Huros AG, Snyder RE: Prospective study of non-infiltrating carcinoma of the breast. Cancer 39:435–439, 1977

26. Page DL, Dupont WD, Rogers LW, et al: Intraductal carcinoma of the breast: Follow-up after biopsy only. Cancer 49:751–758, 1982

27. Rilke F: Influence of pathologic factors on management, in Bonadonna G (ed): Breast Cancer: Diagnosis and Management. New York, Wiley, 1984, pp 35–62

28. Contesso G, Bertin F, Petit JY, et al: Les carcinomes in situ du sein: Anatomie Pathologique. XXXII Assises Françaises de Gynecologie. Paris, Masson. 1985, pp 159–172

29. Frazier TG, Copeland EM, Gallager HS, et al: Prognosis and treatment in minimal breast cancer. Am J Surg 133:697–701, 1977

30. Nevin JE, Pinzon G, Moran TJ, et al: Minimal breast carcinoma. Am J Surg 139:357–359, 1980

31. Veronesi U: Surgical approach to breast cancer of limited extent, in Hoogstraten B, McDivitt RW (eds): Breast Cancer. Boca Raton, FL, CRC. 1982, pp 172–183

32. Gallager HS: Minimal breast cancer: Definition and prognosis, in Ames FC, Blumenschein GR, Montague ED

(eds): Current Controversies in Breast Cancer. Austin, University of Texas. 1984, pp 79–83

33. Montague ED: Radiation therapy for minimal breast cancer, in Ames FC, Blumenschein GR, Montague ED (eds): Current Controversies in Breast Cancer. Austin, University of Texas Press. 1984, pp 93–100

34. Recht A, Danoff BS, Solin LJ, et al: Intraductal carcinoma of the breast: Results of treatment with excisional biopsy and irradiation. J Clin Oncol 3:1339–1343, 1985

35. Rosen PP, Leiberman PH, Braun DW, et al: Lobular carcinoma in situ of the breast: Detailed analysis of 99 patients with average follow-up of 24 years. Am J Surg Pathol 2:225–251, 1978

36. McDivitt RW, Hutter RVP, Foote FW Jr, et al: In situ lobular carcinoma. A prospective follow-up study indicating cumulative patient risks. JAMA 201:96–100, 1967

37. Wheeler JE, Enterline HT, Roseman JM, et al: Lobular carcinoma in situ of the breast. Long-term follow-up. Cancer 34:554–563, 1974

38. Betsill WL Jr, Rosen PP, Lieberman PH, et al: Intraductal carcinoma. Long-term follow-up after treatment by biopsy alone. JAMA 239:1863–1867, 1978

39. Veronesi U, Saccozzi R, DelVecchio M, et al: Comparing radical mastectomy with quadrantectomy, axillary dissection, and radiotherapy in patients with small cancers of the breast. N Engl J Med 305:6–11, 1981

40. Fisher B, Wallmark N: Conservative surgery: The American experience. Semin Oncol 1986 (this issue)

41. Bonadonna G, Valagussa P: Current status of adjuvant chemotherapy for resectable breast cancer. Semin Oncol 14, 1987 (in press)

42. Zafrani B, Fourquet A, Vilcoq JR, et al: Conservative management of intraductal breast cancer with tumorectomy and radiation therapy. Cancer 57:1299–1301, 1986

43. Fisher ER, Sass R, Fisher B, et al: Pathologic findings from the national surgical adjuvant breast project (protocol 6) 1. Intraductal carcinoma (DCIS). Cancer 57:197–208, 1986

44. Fisher ER: What is early breast cancer? in Zander J, Baltzer J (eds): Early Breast Cancer—Histopathology, Diagnosis and Treatment. Berlin, Springer-Verlag. 1985, pp 1–13

to be unique with respect to percent of reactive mammary tumors, percent of reactive cells within tumors, location of reactive antigen within the tumor cell, degree of reactivity with nonmammary tumors as well as normal tissues, and use in a variety of immunologic methods.

An intensely studied group of MoAbs reactive with human breast carcinoma are those generated using membrane-enriched or crude extracts of metastatic breast tumors as immunogens (Table 1). MoAb B72.3 is reactive with a high molecular weight glycoprotein complex (TAG-72) found in a variety of epithelial derived tumors, particularly adenocarcinomas. It has recently been shown to be reactive with up to 84% of invasive ductal carcinomas, and demonstrates minimal reactivity, if any, with benign breast lesions (one exception being focal reactivity with apocrine metaplasia) and a wide variety of normal tissues.[23,59] This selective reactivity (no reactivity to lymphocytes, myeloid or mesothelial cells has been demonstrated) was recently used to detect and phenotype cell populations from a variety of cytology preparations (discussed below). Fetal gastrointestinal tissues have also been shown to be immunoreactive with MoAb B72.3, indicating that the TAG-72 antigen is oncofetal in nature.[59]

Another common class of MoAbs reactive with breast carcinoma are directed against milk fat globule membrane antigens (derived from the apical epithelial membrane during reverse pinocytosis). Of those listed in Table 1, antiepithelial membrane antigen (anti-EMA) has often been used with immunohistochemical techniques to differentiate epithelial from nonepithelial cell types. However, recent investigations have demonstrated that a variety of nonepithelial-derived neoplasias including mesotheliomas, synovial sarcomas, plasma cell tumors, histiocytic lymphomas, and occasional T cell lymphomas may be immunoreactive with anti-EMA.[32] This lack of specificity is clinically relevant, in that EMA may no longer be safely used to differentiate epithelial from nonepithelial tumors.

MoAbs reactive with breast carcinoma cell lines have demonstrated variable reactivity with resected human tumors. MoAb MBR 1, raised against the MCF-7 human breast cancer cell line, reacts with specific types of nonneoplastic epithelial cells and a number of epithelial tumors including adenocarcinomas and squamous carcinomas from different sites.[39] Human antibreast MoAbs have been developed in our laboratory and in others, however, production and maintenance of secreting human hybridomas has classically been more difficult. The MoAbs developed thus far include MBE6, CLNH5, HM Ab 1 and HM Ab 2.[44–48]

Antibodies reactive with keratins (19 species have been described) can be divided into two types: (1) A broadly reactive group that recognizes many members of the keratin family (not listed in Table 1), and (2) MoAbs with more selective reactivity to individual members of the keratin family. Antikeratin heteroantisera are also widely available. Those antikeratin MoAbs listed in Table 1 are immunoreactive with human mammary carcinoma and have been used by some to confirm the epithelial nature of poorly differentiated tumor masses.

Recent investigations have demonstrated the utility of MoAbs directed against specific receptors. Antiestrogen receptor MoAbs have long been sought in an attempt to simplify estrogen receptor (ER) analysis of individual breast tumors. Those MoAbs produced (D547Spγ, D75P3γ, H222)[53–55] have been used with immunohistochemical techniques to visualize the presence or absence of ER. These assays have the advantage of defining reactivity with specific cell types (ie, the malignant breast epithelial cell) and to overcome the criticism that values obtained from standard assays of tumor extracts may reflect the percent of tumor cells present in the sample rather than an actual amount of ER per tumor cell. Further studies to correlate quantitative ER levels with semiquantitative data obtained with immunohistochemical assays are in progress. In addition, these MoAbs may be adapted to other systems such as radioimmunoassay (RIA) or enzyme linked immunosorbant assay (ELISA). MoAbs directed against the epidermal growth factor receptor and laminin receptor have recently been used to further define biologic features of breast carcinoma cells and cell lines (discussed below).

SERUM ASSAYS

The use of MoAbs to detect tumor-associated antigens in serum may eventually find use in early detection of tumor masses, monitoring for disease recurrence, or therapeutic efficacy. Although no MoAb is currently available to screen mass numbers of asymptomatic individuals as an early diagnostic test, several MoAbs have been reported that recognize circulating breast carcinoma TAAs. For example, MoAb DF3, which reacts with a 300,000 dalton antigen, has been shown in a double determinant enzyme-linked immunoassay to detect ≥30 U/mL DF3 antigen in only six of 111 age-matched normal subjects while 42 of 58 (72%) of breast cancer patients had levels equal to or above this value.[23] Although elevated serum levels of DF3 antigen were also detected in patients with hepatoma and ovarian carcinoma, their results indicate that measurement of DF3 antigen levels may provide a useful marker for following the clinical course of patients with mammary carcinoma. Further studies with this and other MoAbs, either used alone or as part of a MoAb cocktail, are currently being evaluated to monitor serum levels of TAA and concommitant disease progression.

IMMUNOHISTOCHEMICAL APPLICATIONS OF MoAbs

Some of the most immediate applications of MoAbs in the study of breast carcinoma are detection of occult tumor cells (in cytology preparations, bone marrow samples, and lymph nodes) and phenotyping of carcinoma cell populations. Recognition of metastatic breast carcinoma in cytology preparations of serous effusions (from the pleural, pericardial, or peritoneal spaces) is currently based on strict cytomorphologic criteria using routine histochemical stains, and can be difficult, particularly if the tumor cells are rare, single without clusters, or admixed with reactive mesothelial cells. In a recent study at Duke University Medical Center, 5,888 consecutive pleural effusions were evaluated and approximately 10% contained recognizably malignant cells. Of these, 15% contained metastatic breast carcinoma.[60]

MoAb B72.3 (reactive with a high molecular weight mucin-like glycoprotein)[61] has a selective reactivity with carcinoma (particularly adenocarcinoma) versus nonepithelial-derived malignancies and normal cell types including mesothelium. This differential reactivity has been used in two recent studies that demonstrated the usefulness of MoAb B72.3 as an immunohistochemical adjunct for the detection of breast carcinoma cells in various cytology preparations. Johnston et al evaluated formalin-fixed cell block preparations of serous effusions by routine cytologic criteria as well as immunocytochemical staining with MoAb B72.3.[62] The reactive antigen TAG-72 was found on carcinoma cells in 22 of 23 samples from 21 breast cancer patients. Mesothelial, lymphoid, and erythroid cells consistently failed to stain with B72.3, as did 41 benign effusions and nine preparations containing lymphoma or leukemia. In those cases where tumor cells were sparse or difficult to identify by cytologic criteria, MoAb utilization appeared to complement routine cytologic staining. In a study by Martin et al,[63] cytospin preparations of serous effusions were evaluated for B72.3 reactivity. All of 12 metastatic breast carcinoma preparations were immunoreactive, while mesothelial cells, lymphoid elements, and ten of ten benign effusions were negative. Hence, the diagnostic applications of MoAb B72.3, either by itself or in a panel with other MoAbs, as an adjunct for the reliable detection and differentiation of adenocarcinoma from mesothelial or lymphoid elements in cell block or cytospin preparations of human effusions was demonstrated.

Fine needle aspiration biopsies (FNAB) lie somewhere between surgically-obtained tissue specimens and exfoliative cytology preparations; this is because architectural patterns are often poorly preserved and malignant cells may be difficult to identify (particularly in a hypocellular sample) by FNAB. The identification of MoAb probes to aid in the recognition of malignant breast epithelial cells has been difficult, as most MoAbs reactive with breast carcinoma also react with benign breast epithelium. Analyses of FNAB preparations with B72.3 have demonstrated that one of ten benign samples was immunoreactive (although staining was confined to metaplastic apocrine epithelium) while 17 of 21 breast carcinomas stained. In nearly every case, the immunoreactivity obtained by fine needle aspiration biopsy was similar (percent cell reactivity as well as staining pattern) to the reactivity of surgically resected tissues from the same patients.[64] Further studies with a wide variety of histologic breast lesions are now in progress to evaluate the specificity of MoAb B72.3 with

FNAB breast specimens. Eventually, however, a panel of MoAbs may be useful in the detection or phenotyping of breast carcinoma cells in FNAB preparations.

PROGNOSTIC STUDIES

The subclassification of tumors (of a given histologic type) based on MoAb reactivity and antigen expression may eventually provide prognostic information that could be used in patient management. Presently, tumor size, histologic type, histologic and nuclear grade, lymph node metastases, and estrogen receptor status are all used to predict probable patient outcome.[65–70] Nonetheless, 25% to 35% of patients with stage I disease eventually die from metastatic carcinoma,[71–72] and it is impossible at this time to determine which of the stage I patients (particularly those with ER negative tumors) might benefit from more aggressive therapeutic regimens. It would appear that more subtle changes in levels of individual proteins, or the glycoprotein determinants (ie, degree or type of glycosylation of individual proteins), would provide a more accurate assessment as to the degree (or lack thereof) of differentiation or other biologic features of cells within a given tumor mass.

MoAbs that might eventually be useful to predict prognosis may be directed against (1) TAAs, (2) oncogene or protooncogene products, (3) differentiation antigens, (4) proteins associated with the metastatic process, or (5) normal cellular proteins or glycoproteins that are increased or decreased in level during the process of dedifferentiation and cellular transformation. Recent investigations have demonstrated the production of placental and pregnancy-associated glycoproteins by breast carcinoma cells, and several investigators have suggested that the production of these substances may correlate with prognosis.[73–79] Kuhajda et al[79] have demonstrated significant pairwise correlations between recurrence and clinicopathologic features including extensive necrosis, nuclear atypia, mitoses, and tumor marker immunostaining with a polyclonal antibody reactive with pregnancy-associated plasma protein A (PAPP-A) in 40 patients with stage I ER negative breast cancer. Lundy et al[27] have described a MoAb DF3 (reactive with a 300 K glycoprotein molecule) that reacts with breast cancer cells using immunohistochemical techniques. The staining reactivity has been shown to correlate with nuclear grade, histologic grade, and estrogen receptor status, although it is an independent marker of cellular differentiation. MoAbs directed against proteins associated with the metastatic process (attachment) and invasion may also be useful. Various receptors (including the laminin receptor), enzymes (particularly type IV collagenase), oncogene products, and growth factors are being considered for their potential use in predicting the ability of a tumor to metastasize.

IN SITU LOCALIZATION OF TUMOR LESIONS USING RADIONUCLIDE-CONJUGATED MoAbs

A major issue in the management of breast cancer patients is the definition of regional lymph node and distant metastases, both in terms of temporal occurrence and anatomic location. Regardless of the nodal status of a patient at the time of surgery, the patient as well as physician must wait at least ten years before ruling out metastatic spread. The use of a radionuclide-conjugated intact MoAb or labeled fragments reactive with breast tumor associated antigen, administered intravenously (IV) at regular intervals, could prove quite useful in a situation such as this; several MoAbs are being evaluated for this type of use. The choice of radionuclide-conjugated antibody immunoglobulin fragments (for more rapid clearance), and their potential complications, such as the patient developing antiimmunoglobulin antibodies, all are under investigation. Other parameters that will have to be considered individually as well as in combination include the following: (1) Dose and specific activity of radiolabeled MoAb, (2) affinity of the MoAb for a specific antigen, as well as the stability of radionuclide-MoAb complex, (3) route of antibody administration, (4) use of immunoglobulin versus immunoreactive fragments, (5) choice of radionuclide, (6) metabolism and clearance of MoAb-radionuclide complexes, (7) location, vascularization, and viability of each tumor mass, (8) tumor size and degree of antigen expression on the individual cell membranes, (9) the appearance of human antiimmunoglobulin antibodies, and (10) the presence of circulating tumor antigen (Table 2). Every MoAb to be used in vivo must be evaluated in a systematic fashion for optimal results.

Table 2. Factors in MoAb Use for Tumor Localization or Therapy[80]

1.	Tumor size.
2.	Percent of cells expressing reactive antigen in a tumor mass.
3.	Number of cell surface antigen molecules.
4.	Fate of antigen-antibody complex (cell surface stability, internalization, capping, shedding).
5.	Tumor vascularity.
6.	Tumor infiltration or necrosis.
7.	Levels and reactivity of antigen in the circulatory system.
8.	MoAb binding to cell surface (affinity and antigen turnover, see also No. 4).
9.	Immunoglobulin isotype.
10.	Intact immunoglobulin versus reactive fragments.
11.	Blood clearance of MoAb (excretion, reticulo-endothelial system).
12.	MoAb dose.
13.	Route of inoculation of MoAb.
If Radiolabeled MoAb Used	
14.	Isotopes that can be used to label an MoAb.
15.	Specific activity of radiolabeled MoAb.
16.	Changes in affinity of radiolabeled MoAb.
17.	Distance of tumor from body surface (for localization studies).
18.	Scanning time (localization studies).

THERAPY

Tumor therapy may be effected by MoAbs in several ways, including effector cell mechanisms, complement mediated immune response, toxin or drug conjugation, or conjugation with radionuclides. The use of MoAbs for effective tumor killing, however, is clearly a difficult task due to two factors: (1) A very strong degree of selective reactivity of the MoAb for tumor versus normal or benign tissues must be achieved; and (2) all tumor cells of a given tumor mass must express antigen and thus bind to MoAb. The use of MoAb coupled to a killer isotope with the ability to kill five to 50 cell diameters may help circumvent this later situation. Furthermore, multiple factors, as listed in Table 2, No. 2 must also be taken into consideration.

One novel approach to cancer therapy involves the use of antiidiotype MoAbs. Although these reagents are still in the conceptual phase of development for breast cancer, their potential utility and results of preliminary studies using antiviral and antitumor systems are intriguing. This approach involves the use of an experimentally derived antiidiotypic MoAb to stimulate the patient's immune system to produce antibodies directed against endogenous TAA that would not normally be immunogenic.

ONCOGENES AND GROWTH FACTORS

Oncogenes were first identified as potential etiologic factors for neoplasia using viral systems. These oncogenes and protooncogenes (normal cellular homologues) have been defined by their ability to induce cellular transformation via DNA transfection assays in the established 3T3 murine fibroblast system and this has led to the identification of such phenomena as chromosome translocation, gene amplification, or enhanced gene transcription as being characteristic of cellular transformation. The identification of oncogenes or protooncogenes (normal cellular homologues) and structurally or functionally related growth factors has obviously been an exciting area of investigation in the field of cancer research.

Recent studies focusing on the *ras* oncogene family (Harvey-, Kirsten-, and N-*ras*)[81] have demonstrated that a single point mutation at specific sites in the *ras* protooncogene can cause cellular transformation; however, such a mutation does not appear to be involved in mammary carcinogenesis.[82] Enhanced expression of the *ras* gene product, which can occur as a result of gene amplification or enhanced transcriptional activity, can also mediate transformation; the majority of human breast carcinomas have been shown to contain elevated levels of p21 in comparison to normal breast and most benign breast lesions.[82] Other studies have shown a synergism of action between *ras* and a second oncogene *myc* resulting in neoplasia in experimental systems, but the temporal involvement of *ras* in the multistep process of carcinogenesis is still unclear.[83]

Tumor growth factors are substances secreted by transformed cells, and, while growth factors and tumor growth factors are similar in many ways, growth factors are mitogenic and not transforming.[84] Both factors act via a cell surface receptor mechanism, and, in fact, partial homology has been shown between some growth factors or growth factor receptors and oncogene products.[84] The exact roles these genes and gene products play in either mammary differentiation or carcinogenesis is unknown, but it is hoped that exploitation of developing technology such as gene cloning and in situ hybridization will be able to clarify this matter. However, the development and use of MoAbs to various developmental and growth factors, as well as to oncogene and protooncogene products should add to the elucidation of the role these factors play in the etiology of breast cancer by the careful evaluation of translational values via RIA or at the single cell level via immunohistochemical techniques.

CONCLUSION

The MoAbs developed thus far against human breast carcinomas have led to a more systematic study of specific human carcinoma systems. For the first time, one now has tools other than morphology or the presence of hormone receptors to distinguish between two different tumors, or among different cell populations within a given tumor mass. The number of these "fingerprints" for breast cancer is increasing, and further evaluation of their potential uses is in progress. Many new gene products including those of oncogenes have been identified, and remain to be studied with respect to involvement with human mammary carcinoma; new techniques including gene cloning and in situ hybridization may facilitate the examination of breast cancer on a molecular level. Synthetic peptides can now be produced from known DNA sequences, and these have been used to generate MoAbs directed against specific gene products. These techniques will undoubtedly provide insights in the field of tumor biology and immunology, and hopefully, will foster developments in two directions simultaneously—one toward the mechanisms of oncogenesis and its basis in cell biology, and the other toward more immediate clinical applications.

REFERENCES

1. Harris JR, Hellman S, Canellos GP, et al: Cancer of the breast, in DeVita VT, Hellman S, Rosenberg SA (eds): Cancer Principles and Practice. Philadelphia, Lippincott. 1985, pp 1119–1177

2. Kelsey JL: A review of the epidemiology of human breast cancer. Epidemiol Rev 1:74–109, 1979

3. Anderson DE: Some characteristics of familial breast cancer. Cancer 28:1500–1504, 1971

4. Lilienfeld AM: The epidemiology of breast cancer. Cancer Res 23:1503–1513, 1963

5. Li FP, Fraumeni JF: Soft tissue sarcomas, breast cancer, and other neoplasms. A familial syndrome? Ann Intern Med 71:747–752, 1969

6. Patel R, Habal MB, Wilson RE: Histocompatibility (HL-A) antigens and cancer of the breast. Am J Surg 124:31–34, 1972

7. Morosini P, Lee EG, Jones MN: Breast cancer and the S blood group system. Lancet 1:411–412, 1972

8. Armstrong B: Recent trend in breast cancer incidence and mortality in relation to changes in possible risk factors. Int J Cancer 17:204–211, 1976

9. MacMahon B, Cole P, Lin M, et al: Age at first birth and breast cancer risk. Bull WHO 34:209–221, 1970

10. Valaoras VG, MacMahon B, Trichopoulous D, et al: Lactation and reproductive histories of breast cancer patients in greater Athens, 1965–1967. Int J Cancer 4:350–363, 1969

11. Yuasa S, MacMahon B: Lactation and reproductive histories of breast cancer patients in Tokyo, Japan. Bull WHO 42:195–204, 1970

12. Staszewski J: Age at menarche and breast cancer. JNCI 47:935–940, 1971

13. Kiaer W: Relation of Fibroadenomatosis (Chronic mastitis) to Cancer of the Breast. Copenhagen, Munksgaard. 1954

14. Lilienfeld AM: The relationship of cancer of the female breast to artificial menopause and marital status. Cancer 9:927–934, 1956

15. Bulbrook RD, Hayward JL, Spicer CC, et al: Urinary steroid excretion of normal women and women with advanced breast cancer. Lancet 2:1235–1237, 1962

16. Feinleib M: Breast cancer and artificial menopause: A cohort study. JNCI 41:315–329, 1968

17. McGregor DH, Land CE, Choi K, et al: Breast cancer incidence among atomic bomb survivors. Hiroshima and Nagasaki, 1950–69. JNCI 59:799–811, 1977

18. Mackenzie I: Breast cancer following multiple fluoroscopies. Br J Cancer 19:1–8, 1965

19. Myrden JA, Hiltze JE: Breast cancer following multiple fluoroscopies during artificial pneumothorax treatment of pulmonary tuberculosis. Can Med Assoc J 100:1032–1034, 1969

20. Higginson J: The role of geographical pathology in environmental carcinogenesis, in Twenty-fourth Annual Symposium on Fundamental Cancer Research: Environment and Cancer. Baltimore, Williams and Wilkins. 1972, pp 69–71

21. Haenszel W, Kurihara M: Studies of Japanese migrants I. Mortality from cancer and other diseases among Japanese in the United States. JNCI 40:43–68, 1968

22. Colcher D, Horan Hand P, Nuti M, et al: A spectrum of monoclonal antibodies reactive with mammary tumor cells. Proc Natl Acad Sci USA 78:3199–3203, 1981

23. Nuti M, Teramoto YA, Mariani-Costantini R, et al: A monoclonal antibody (B72.3) defines patterns of distribution of a novel tumor-associated antigen in human mammary carcinoma cell populations. Int J Cancer 29:539–545, 1982

24. Colcher D, Hand P, Wunderlich D, et al: Potential diagnosis and prognostic applications of monoclonal antibodies to human mammary cancer, in Wright GL Jr (ed): Monoclonal Antibodies and Cancer. New York, Marcel Dekker. 1983, pp 121–159

25. Colcher D, Horan Hand P, Nuti M, et al: Differential binding to human mammary and nonmammary tumors of monoclonal antibodies reactive with carcinoembryonic antigen. Cancer Invest 1:127–138, 1983

26. Kufe D, Inghirami G, Abe M, et al: Differential reactivity of a novel monoclonal antibody (DF3) with human malignant versus benign breast tumors. Hybridoma 3:223–232, 1984

27. Lundy J, Thor A, Maenza R, et al: Monoclonal antibody DF3 correlates with tumor differentiation and hormone receptor status in breast cancer patients. Breast Cancer Res Treat 5:269–276, 1985

28. Sekine H, Ohno T, Kufe DW: Purification and characterization of high molecular weight glycoprotein detectable in human milk and breast carcinoma. J Immunol 135:3610–3615, 1985

29. Hayes DF, Sekine H, Ohno T, et al: Use of a murine monoclonal antibody for detection of circulating plasma DF3 antigen. J Clin Invest 75:1671–1678, 1985

30. Ellis IO, Robbins RA, Elston CW, et al: A monoclonal antibody, NC RC-11 raised to human breast carcinoma. Histopathology 8:501–516, 1984

31. Taylor-Papadimitriou J, Peterson JA, Arklie J, et al: Monoclonal antibodies to epithelium-specific components of the human milk fat globule membrane: Production and reaction with cells in culture. Int J Cancer 28:17–21, 1981

32. Pinkus GS, Kurtin PJ: Epithelial membrane antigen—A diagnostic discriminant in surgical pathology. Hum Pathol 16:929–940, 1985

33. Sloane JP, Ormerod MG: Distribution of epithelial membrane antigen in normal and neoplastic tissues and its value in diagnostic tumor pathology. Cancer 17:1786–1795, 1981

34. Arklie J, Taylor-Papadimitriou J, Bodmer WF, et al: Differentiation antigens expressed by epithelial cells in the lactating breast are also detectable in breast cancers. Int J Cancer 28:23–29, 1981

35. Foster CS, Dinsdale EA, Edwards PAW, et al: Monoclonal antibodies to the human mammary gland: II. Distribution of determinant in breast carcinomas. Virchows Arch (A) 394:295–305, 1982

36. Rasmussen BB, Hilkens J, Hilgers J, et al: Monoclonal antibodies applied to primary human breast carcinoma: Relationship to menopausal status, lymph node status, and steroid hormone receptor content. Breast Cancer Res Treat 2:401–405, 1982

37. Menard S, Tagliabue E, Canevari S, et al: Generation of monoclonal antibodies reacting with normal and cancer cells of human breast. Cancer Res 43:1295–1300, 1983

38. Canevari S, Fossati G, Balsari A, et al: Immunohistochemical analysis of the determinant recognized by monoclonal antibody MBrl which specifically binds to human mammary epithelial cells. Cancer Res 43:1301–1308, 1983

39. Mariani-Costantini R, Androla S, Rilke F: Tumour-associated antigens in mammary and extramammary Paget's disease. Virchows Arch (A) 405:333–340, 1985

40. Thompson CH, Jones SL, Whitehead RH, et al: A human breast tissue-associated antigen detected by a monoclonal antibody. JNCI 70:409–419, 1983

41. Papsidero LD, Croghan GA, O'Connell MJ, et al: Monoclonal antibodies (F36/22 and M7/105) to human breast carcinoma. Cancer Res 43:1741–1747, 1983

42. Croghan GA, Papsidero LD, Valensuela LA, et al: Tissue distribution of an epithelial and tumor-associated antigen recognized by monoclonal antibody F36/22. Cancer Res 43:4980–4988, 1983

43. Adams DJ, Hajj H, Edwards DP, et al: Detection of a Mr 24,000 estrogen-related protein in human breast cancer by monoclonal antibodies. Cancer Res 43:4297–4301, 1983

44. Schlom J, Wunderlich D, Teramoto YA: Generation of human monoclonal antibodies reactive with human mammary carcinoma cells. Proc Natl Acad Sci USA 77:6841–6845, 1980

45. Wunderlich D, Teramoto YA, Alford C, et al: The use of lymphocytes from axillary lymph nodes of mastectomy patients to generate human monoclonal antibodies. Eur J Cancer Clin Oncol 17:719–730, 1981

46. Teramoto YA, Mariani-Costantini R, Wunderlich D, et al: The immunohistochemical reactivity of a human monoclonal antibody with tissue sections of human mammary tumors. Cancer 50:241–249, 1982

47. Glassy MC, Handley HH, Hagiwara, H, et al: HC 729-6, a human lymphoblastoid B-cell useful for generating antibody-secreting human-human hybridomas. Proc Natl Acad Sci USA 80:6327–6331, 1983

48. Imam A, Taylor CR, Tokes ZA: Hybridizing and selective closing of human lymphocytes which are involved in the hosts immune recognition of tumor cells. Fifteenth International Leucocyte Culture Conference, December 5–10, 1982, Pacific Grove, CA, University of Southern California Cancer Center, 1982 (abstr)

49. Tseng SCG, Jarvinen MJ, Nelson WG: Correlation of specific keratins with different types of epithelial differentiation: Monoclonal antibody studies. Cell 30:361–372, 1982

50. Battifora H: Recent progress in the immunohistochemistry of solid tumors. Semin Diagn Pathol 1:251–269, 1984

51. Cooper D, Schermer A, Pruss R, et al: The use of aIF, AE1 and AE3 monoclonal antibodies for the identification and classification of mammalian epithelial keratins. Differentiation 28:30–35, 1984

52. Makin CA, Bobrow LG, Bodmer WF: Monoclonal antibody to cytokeratin for use in routine histopathology. J Clin Pathol 37:975–983, 1984

53. Poulsen H, Ozzello L, King WJ, et al: The use of monoclonal antibodies to estrogen receptors (ER) for immunoperoxidase detection of ER in paraffin sections of human breast cancer tissue. J Histochem Cytochem 33:87–92, 1985

54. Greene GL, Nolan C, Engler JP, et al: Monoclonal antibodies to human estrogen receptor. Proc Natl Acad Sci USA 77:5115–5119, 1980

55. Shimada A, Kimura S, Abe K, et al: Immunocytochemical staining of estrogen receptor in paraffin sections of human breast cancer by use of monoclonal antibody: Comparison with that in frozen sections. Proc Natl Acad Sci USA 82:4803–4807, 1985

56. Sainsbury JRC, Farndon JR, Sherbet GV, et al: Epidermal-growth factor receptors and oestrogen receptors in human breast cancer. Lancet 1:364–366, 1985

57. Sainsbury JRC, Farndon JR, Harris AL, et al: Epidermal growth factor receptors on human breast cancers. Br J Surg 72:186–188, 1985

58. Horan Hand P, Thor A, Schlom J, et al: Expression of laminin receptor in normal and carcinomatous human tissues

as defined by a monoclonal antibody. Cancer Res 45:2713–2719, 1985

59. Thor A, Ohuchi N, Szpak C: Distribution of oncofetal antigen tumor-associated glycoprotein-72 defined by monoclonal antibody B72.3. Cancer Res 46:3118–3124, 1986

60. Johnston WW: The malignant pleural effusion: A review of cytopathological diagnoses on 584 specimens from 472 consecutive patients. Cancer 56:905–909, 1985

61. Johnson VG, Schlom J, Paterson AJ, et al: Analysis of a human tumor-associated glycoprotein (TAG-72) identified by monoclonal antibody B72.3. Cancer Res 46:850–857, 1986

62. Johnston WW, Szpak CA, Lottich SC, et al: Use of a monoclonal antibody B72.3 as an immunocytochemical adjunct to diagnosis of adenocarcinoma in human effusions. Cancer Res 45:1894–1900, 1985

63. Martin SE, Moshiri S, Thor A: Identification of adenocarcinoma in cytospin preparations of effusions using MAb B72.3. Am J Clin Pathol 86:10–18, 1986

64. Johnston WW, Szpak CA, Thor A: The use of monoclonal antibody (B72.3) as a novel immunohistochemical adjunct for the diagnosis of carcinomas in fine needle aspiration biopsies. Hum Pathol (in press)

65. Antman KH, Blum RH, Greenberger JS, et al: Multimodality therapy for malignant mesothelioma based on a study of natural history. Am J Med 68:356–362, 1980

66. Legha SS, Muggia FM: Pleural mesothelioma: Clinical features and therapeutic implications. Ann Intern Med 87:613–621, 1977

67. Wang N, Huang SN, Gold P: Absence of carcinoembryonic antigen-like material in mesothelioma. An immunohistochemical differentiation from other lung cancer. Cancer 44:937–943, 1979

68. Corson JM, Pinkus GS: Mesothelioma: Profile of keratin proteins and carcinoembryonic antigen. An immunoperoxidase study of 20 cases and comparison with pulmonary adenocarcinomas. Am J Pathol 108:80–87, 1982

69. Said JW, Nash G, Tepper G, et al: Keratin proteins and carcinoembryonic antigen in lung carcinoma: An immunoperoxidase study of 54 cases, with ultrastructural correlations. Hum Pathol 14:70–76, 1983

70. Holden J, Churg A: Immunohistochemical staining for keratin and carcinoembryonic antigen in the diagnosis of malignant mesothelioma. Am J Surg Pathol 8:277–279, 1984

71. American Joint Committee for Cancer: Manual for Staging of Cancer, Chicago, Whiting, 1978

72. Keys HM, Bakemeier RF, Savlov ED: in Rubin P (ed): Clinical Oncology: A Multidisciplinary Approach. Rochester, American Cancer Society, 1983, pp 120–151

73. Horne CHW, Reid N, Milne GD: Prognostic significance of inappropriate production of pregnancy proteins by breast cancers. Lancet 1:279–282, 1976

74. Inaba N, Renk T, Wurster K, et al: Ectopic synthesis of pregnancy specific glycoprotein (SP-1) and placental specific tissue proteins (PP5, PP10, PP11, PP12) in nontrophoblastic malignant tumors: possible markers in oncology. Klin Wochenschr 58:789–791, 1980

75. Kuhajda FP, Abeloff MD, Eggleston JC: Pregnancy associated protein A (PAPP-A): A clinically significant predictor of early recurrence in stage II breast carcinoma. Hum Pathol 16:228–235, 1985

76. Kuhajda FP, Offutt LE, Mendelsohn G: The distribution of carcinoembryonic antigen in breast carcinoma: Diagnostic and prognostic implications. Cancer 52:1257–1264, 1983

77. Sorensen S, Andersen J, Norgaard T: Pregnancy-specific beta-1 glycoprotein (SP-1) in serum and tissue from patients with benign and malignant breast tumours. Br J Cancer 49:663–667, 1984

78. Walker RA: Biological markers in human Breast carcinoma. J Pathol 137:109–117, 1982

79. Kuhajda FP, Eggleston JC: Pregnancy-associated plasma protein A and extensive necrosis. Lab Invest 53:101–107, 1985

80. Schlom J, Weeks M: Potential clinical utility of monoclonal antibodies in the management of human carcinomas, in DeVita V, Hellman S, Rosenberg SA (eds): Important Advances in Oncology 1985. Philadelphia, Lippincott, 1985, pp 170–192

81. Shih TY, Weeks MO: Oncogenes and Cancer: The p21 *ras* genes. Cancer Invest 2:109–123, 1984

82. Horan Hand P, Thor A, Wunderlich D, et al: Monoclonal antibodies of predefined specificity detect activated *ras* gene expression in human mammary and colon carcinoma. Proc Natl Acad Sci USA 81:5227–5231, 1984

83. Marx JD: Cooperation between oncogenes. Science 222:602–604, 1983

84. Weinberg RA: The action of oncogenes in the cytoplasm and nucleus. Science 230:770–776, 1985

The Role of New Imaging Modalities in Staging and Follow-up of Breast Cancer

Stephen A. Feig

IMAGING PROCEDURES have assumed an increasingly important role in the initial evaluation and subsequent follow-up of the breast cancer patient because of advances in imaging methods, the expanded number of treatment options available to many patients, and widespread use of the two-stage surgical procedure in which a biopsy specimen is obtained and permanent histologic sections are evaluated before definitive treatment.

The 20-year survival of breast cancer patients relative to normal life expectancy will depend on the pathologic stage of disease at time of initial diagnosis: Minimal carcinoma (93%), negative axillary nodes (62%), positive axillary nodes (23%), distant metastases (0%).[1,2] Therefore, the frequency of eventual metastases for each respective stage will be somewhat more than 7%, 38%, 77%, and 100%. According to Cutler,[3] the most common sites of distant metastases among 210 patients with only one site of metastatic involvement were bone (58%), lung and pleura (26%), and lymph nodes other than ipsilateral axillary nodes (16%). Initial involvement of the liver and brain are less frequent.[4,5]

SKELETAL SYSTEM

Most radiographically demonstrable skeletal metastases from breast carcinoma are osteolytic. Mixed osteolytic and osteoblastic lesions are less common. Purely osteoblastic metastases are least frequent. Occasionally, small lytic areas do not appear as discrete lesions, but produce patchy areas of decalcification that can be confused with osteoporosis. Another kind of metastasis, the intertrabecular type, may not be radiographically demonstrable because it fills the bone marrow spaces but leaves the trabeculae intact. For a lytic lesion to be visualized on x-ray, it must be greater than 1.5 cm diameter and demineralization of at least 50% must occur.[6–8] Early bone metastases are clinically silent too. Patients remain asymptomatic until the lesions extend to the periosteum causing pain and tenderness from periosteal distension or invasion.

The radionuclide bone scan performed with technetium-99m labeled phosphate compounds is considerably more sensitive than the radiographic skeletal survey in detection of metastases.[9] The bone scan can detect early metastatic disease months or years before it is evident on skeletal x-ray. In patients with advanced disease and multiple lesions, an increased number of lesions may be seen on bone scan compared with skeletal radiographs. The bone scan is, therefore, the procedure of choice for the initial screening for bone metastases.

On the bone scan, metastases are usually seen as areas of increased radioactivity. The mechanism for visualization of these "hot" lesions is new bone formation or increased vascularity.[10]

Because this finding may also result from many other abnormalities including osteomyelitis, Paget's disease, fractures, osteoarthritis, bursitis, and degenerative disc disease, scan abnormalities must be correlated with radiographs to make the examination more specific. In fact, over one third of solitary abnormalities seen on bone scans of patients with primary extraosseous malignancies are the result of benign processes or normal variants.[11] Rarely, breast metastases may present as focal areas of decreased radionuclide activity, "cold" lesions. These are due to focal replacement of bone tumor or obliteration of the local blood supply by tumor.

False-negative bone scans are infrequent but can occur with rapidly growing metastases, slow growing metastases, therapeutically arrested metastases or very small metastatic deposits where there is little bone repair. False-negative scans may also be caused by radionuclide activity in the bladder when it obscures an underlying lesion in the bony pelvis. For this reason, inclusion of an anteroposterior radiograph along with the bone scan has been suggested even though bladder activity can be partially diminished if the

From the Department of Radiology, Jefferson Medical College, Philadelphia.

Address reprint requests to Stephen A. Feig, MD, Department of Radiology, Jefferson University Hospital, 111 S. 11th St, Philadelphia, PA 19107.

0093–7754/86/1304–0004$05.00/0

patient voids immediately before the scan.[12] Another means to eliminate overlying activity such as bladder would be the use of single photon emission computed tomography (SPECT) because it can provide images of radioactive distribution at various levels of the body.[13] Diffuse metastatic disease may also lead to the impression of a negative scan if the radionuclide distribution is nearly uniform. This condition may be suspected if radionuclide activity is diffusely increased in the bones, the so-called "super scan," but absent in the kidneys, bladder, and soft tissues.

Diagnosis

Because it is less expensive, easily performed, and has higher spatial resolution, the skeletal radiograph is the initial procedure of choice for evaluation of a symptomatic site. Once metastases are shown on the skeletal x-ray, these lesions are followed more effectively by this means rather than by bone scan. However, after metastatic disease is demonstrated on the skeletal x-ray, an initial bone scan should also be performed in order to identify other metastatic sites requiring prophylactic treatment, to identify suspicious areas to be followed by x-ray, and to serve as a baseline for subsequent diagnostic radionuclide scans.

If the initial bone x-ray is negative in a symptomatic patient, a bone scan should then be performed since false-negative results frequently occur in conventional skeletal radiography. In fact, the combination of an abnormal bone scan and a normal roentgenogram in a breast cancer patient is highly suggestive of early metastasis.[14] Gold[12] suggests several alternative means of handling the problem of a positive bone scan in combination with a negative skeletal x-ray: (1) Perform a percutaneous needle biopsy; (2) repeat the scan in 4 to 6 weeks to determine if the abnormality was transient and therefore due to trauma or inflammation; (3) repeat the radiograph in 4 to 6 weeks. Some radiographic abnormalities such as stress fracture may not be evident until then. (4) follow the abnormal scan site with radiographs alone. (x-ray evidence of bone metastases may not follow the scan abnormality for up to 18 months).[15]

The following diagnostic indications for radionuclide bone scan have been suggested by Gold[12]: (1) Examination of the patient with clinically suspected bone metastases when radiographs are negative or equivocal. (2) determination of the extent of skeletal metastases when radiographs are abnormal. (3) evaluation of bones that are difficult to study by conventional radiography such as sternum and scapula. (4) differentiation of pathologic from traumatic fractures by disclosing additional sites of involvement not detected by radiographs. (5) planning of radiation treatment portal. (6) monitoring response to chemotherapy or radiation.

Screening

Roentgenographic skeletal surveys are normal in almost all patients with operable breast cancer. In one study of 85 such patients, Gibbons et al[16] could detect no x-ray evidence of skeletal metastases. Similarly, Roberts et al[17] found only two patients with radiographic signs of skeletal metastases among 114 patients with T1 and T2 lesions.

The incidence of true positive bone scans on initial screening is extremely low for stage I and stage II patients, but considerably more for higher stage patients. In published series, positive scans occur in approximately 5% of patients with clinical stage I or stage II[14,18-25] and approximately 35% of stage III patients.[17,18,21,22,25-28]

The frequency of false-positive bone scans will vary according to the radiologist interpreting the exam and the patient population. In one study, 40% of patients with positive bone scans showed no evidence of recurrence on 8-year follow-up.[29] The false-positive rate will be higher for patients with a single lesion than for those with multiple lesions. In one series of patients with proven metastases, only about 15% had a single lesion.[30] Among patients with extraskeletal malignancies, a single focus of increased activity was found to be due to metastatic disease in 64% of patients and secondary to a benign process in 36% of patients.[11] The proportion of positive scans that are due to malignancy will also vary according to the stage of disease. The yield of true-positive scans will be lower for earlier stage disease whereas the percentage of false-positive scans should be unaffected by stage of disease. In two series of stage I and stage II patients, the percentage of true-positive scans and of false-positive scans were both about 2%.[21,24] Because the true-positive and false-positive yields may be approximately equal for stage I or stage II breast cancer, pathologic confirmation of bony metastatic disease is essential in these patients.

Based on such data and the observation that early detection of metastatic disease probably has little effect on survival, it has been suggested that bone scan screening of asymptomatic patients should be reserved only for those with stage III and stage IV disease unless an elevated alkaline phosphatase suggests bone metastasis.[2,29,31]

Other investigators maintain that screening of stage I and stage II patients is also appropriate because many of them will eventually develop bone metastases and because early treatment with radiation therapy or orthopedic surgery may prevent pathologic fractures and their painful disabling sequellae.[32] They also argue that such screening should not be restricted to those with an elevated alkaline phosphatase. Up to 40% of patients with malignant disease and positive bone scans will not have an elevated alkaline phosphatase.[33]

According to McNeil et al, the rate of eventual conversion from negative to positive scans is 7% for stage I, 45% for stage II, and 58% for stage III.[24] When such conversion occurs, it is usually within two years postdiagnosis. Similar data have been reported by other investigators. Among stage I and stage II patients, Lentle et al[23] reported a 19% conversion rate on 12 month follow-up. Citrin et al[34] recorded a 23% conversion rate by 36 months and Gerber et al[21] cited a 26% conversion rate at 24 months.

Because positive bone scans may result from processes other than metastatic disease, an initial baseline scan can be helpful for accurate future interpretation. The subsequent appearance of an abnormal bone scan in a breast cancer patient with a normal baseline study usually indicates metastasis. Based on these factors, McNeil et al[24] recommend that all patients should have bone scans at 6, 12, 18, and 24 months following the baseline study. If the bone scan remains negative after 2 or 3 years, scans are performed only on symptomatic patients. Gerber et al recommend that asymptomatic patients have bone scans for 5 years postdiagnosis.[21] Other physicians maintain that comparison of radionuclide scans with radiographs can sufficiently increase sensitivity and specificity to obviate the need for a baseline study.

Support for screening can be provided by the studies of Hoffman and Marty,[26] Citrin et al,[34] Sklaroff and Sklaroff,[35] Roberts et al,[17] and Campbell et al,[27] who reported an incidence of positive bone scans on initial screening of stage I or stage II patients of 40%, 14%, 14%, 23%, and 36%, respectively. Differences between the results of these studies and those reported by others may result from the diversity of tumor and nodal involvement that may be found in stage I and stage II disease. According to the TNM classification,[36] a 5 cm tumor with nonfixed axillary nodes considered to contain metastases can still be classified as stage II. Thus, it would seem that if only true early cancers are considered, the incidence of positive bone scans on initial study will be very low. For example, axillary node metastases were present in 78% of Hoffman's patients and 100% of those of Sklaroff.

Prognosis

A number of reports have shown that patients with positive bone scans have a poorer prognosis.[26,28,34,37] Interestingly, when metastases were later clinically documented, the bones were frequently not the major site. Accordingly, Galasko maintains that a positive scan should affect decisions regarding primary treatment in these early stage patients.[37] Other investigators believe that these prognostic differences are primarily a reflection of stage of disease.[12] To them, it seems that when scan results are normalized according to lesion size and lymph node status, they become less important predictors. It is their opinion that a positive bone scan should not, in the absence of histologic proof of disseminated disease, preclude an attempt at primary curative treatment. They note that prolonged asymptomatic survival is common among many patients with abnormal preoperative bone scans.[35,38]

Treatment Response

On a skeletal radiograph, healing of a lytic lesion is initially seen as progressive filling in or sclerosis.[9,39] With continued healing, the lesion will gradually fade. Normal or near normal bone density and architecture may eventually be restored. As blastic lesions heal, they remain densely sclerotic or attain the appearance of normal bone.

On bone scan, healing metastases may initially show an increase in isotope activity associated with the increased blood flow. This so-called "flare phenomenon" should not be misconstrued as progressive disease.[40] With complete healing, activity should ultimately return to normal. Other bone metastases will show a prompt reduction in isotope activity from the beginning of treatment.

Diminished focal uptake on sequential scintiscans does not necessarily indicate healing. Reliability is limited by several technical factors. The intensity of a lesion is not only relative to adjacent normal bone, but can vary on a daily basis with the intensity setting selected by the technologist for the gamma camera. Therefore, comparison of how hot a lesion is compared with a previous study is not always a valid indicator of healing or tumor growth. In one study,[41] radiologists were asked to evaluate improvement or deterioration of lesions on serial radionuclide bone scans. Interobserver variation was considerable. Changes of at least 40% in bone scans were necessary before they were recognized with 95% confidence. Quantitating these changes with computer assistance had moderate value. Also, the appearance of new lesions had more significance than changed uptake in older lesions.

Bone scans may have a place in assessment of response to systemic chemotherapy and hormone therapy in patients with disseminated breast cancer, particularly if a return to normal isotope activity can be demonstrated. The value of sequential scans in monitoring the effect of systemic treatment over the short term is not yet clear. Although several series show a general correlation with tumor response,[42,43] the changes are not always sufficiently consistent and reproducible to be a meaningful indicator of tumor response in the individual patient.

Skeletal radiographs are therefore the imaging modality of choice for monitoring treatment response of known lesions. Compared with bone scans, they provide more specific assessment as well as a better detailed image of the metastatic site. Correlaton with sequential bone scan imaging can sometimes be helpful because in some instances, change from a lytic to a blastic appearance can result from either healing or progressive disease. The combination of a dense sclerotic lesion on x-ray and a normal bone scan indicates healed inactive disease. However, for most lesions, the simple clinical observation of relief of bone pain along with appropriate monitoring by skeletal radiography provides the best method of assessing tumor response.

THORAX

Breast metastases may present as pleural effusions, pulmonary nodules, hilar and mediastinal adenopathy, and lymphangitic spread. The chest x-ray is the imaging procedure of choice for initial evaluation of these types of intrathoracic tumor spread. It is reasonably sensitive, relatively inexpensive, universally available, and easily performed.

Pleural effusions are the commonest initial manifestation of intrathoracic metastasis. Approximately 50% of patients with metastatic breast cancer will develop a pleural effusion during the course of their disease.[44] The effusion is ipsilateral in 83% of patients and may represent local chest wall involvement rather than distant metastases.[45,46]

Lymphangitic metastases are most likely the result of hematogenous dissemination.[47,48] They are the most difficult to specifically recognize. Their appearance may be mimicked by other entities such as congestive heart failure and the idiopathic interstitial fibrosis frequently seen among older patients. However, lymphangitic metastases rarely occur in the absence of symptoms such as cough and dyspnea. Change from a previous chest radiographic may be an important observation.

Pulmonary nodules result from blood-borne metastases that penetrate the capillary wall to grow into nodular masses. They usually produce no symptoms until the lung is largely replaced with metastatic tumor. Pulmonary nodules can be demonstrated by chest x-ray, conventional tomography, and computed tomography (CT). On these imaging methods, the chest x-ray is the least sensitive and CT is the most sensitive.[49–53] Chest radiography for detection of metastatic nodules is best performed with high (120 to 150) kilovoltage in order to penetrate the overlying bones, heart, diaphragm, and vasculature and to minimize exposure times. With this technique, almost all lesions larger than 15 mm should be visible. Lesions smaller than 3 mm will not be seen. In the intermediate size range, detection will depend on such factors as presence of overlying structures and lesion location. Visualization of the smaller nodules by conventional tomography and CT is attributable to elimination of overlying obscuring structures and enhancement of soft tissue density differences. In addition, the transverse orientation of CT may help to visualize chest wall lesions and other lesions located near the pulmonary apices, costophrenic angles, retrosternal and retrocardiac regions, and to better indicate their size and extent.

Despite these relative advantages, neither conventional tomography nor CT should be used in place of the chest x-ray for initial screening for chest metastasis. Breast cancer has a relatively low propensity to present with pulmonary nodules as the initial presentation of distant metastases. Therefore, the increased detection yield of pulmonary nodules with conventional tomography or CT will not be sufficient to justify this use.[54,55] In addition, it is unlikely that demonstration of these metastatic nodules will alter the patient's therapeutic regimen. Pulmonary metastases tend to occur late in the disease when distant metastases to other parts of the body are already evident. Moreover, both conventional tomography and CT are more expensive and more time consuming. Accordingly, these procedures are best reserved for confirmation of questionable abnormalities seen on the plain chest film and to define multiple pulmonary nodules in a patient with an apparently solitary nodule on the plain chest film.[56]

A solitary nodule, hilar, or mediastinal node mass alone is rarely observed as a sign of metastatic breast cancer. The breast cancer patient with a single pulmonary lesion is more likely to have a granuloma or neoplasm other than metastatic breast cancer.[57] When such a lesion is found on chest x-ray and was not previously present, CT should be routinely used. The absence of additional nodules on CT raises the possibility of a new primary cancer that should then be investigated and treated aggressively rather than assumed to represent a metastasis.

Not all such nodules demonstrated by CT are necessarily due to metastatic disease. Noncalcified granulomas, which may represent 25% of all occult nodules in endemic areas, may be indistinguishable from pulmonary metastases.[56] However, multiplicity and variation in size favor the diagnosis of metastatic disease. Demonstration of interval growth on a 6 week follow-up CT scan can provide further confirmation. Certain abnormalities such as rib fracture, atelectasis, and pneumonia, which can sometimes superficially resemble pulmonary nodules on chest x-ray, can be better evaluated by conventional tomography than by CT.

Mediastinum

CT has many advantages in the investigation of the mediastinum where conventional tomography is relatively insensitive.[58,59] However, studies to date suggest there is no significant gain when CT is compared to chest radiography and conventional tomography in detection of hilar adenopathy.

CT can increase the accuracy of treatment planning for patients with local recurrence. According to Meyer and Munzenrider,[58] physical examination and chest x-ray underestimated the extent of internal mammary adenopathy in 50% of patients with locally recurrent disease. CT provided better documentation of retrosternal adenopathy and thereby insured more adequate tumor coverage by radiation treatment portals. Although lymphoscintigraphy allows accurate determination of nodal location, Meyer and Munzenrider believe that CT provides more precise definition of subtle enlargement and accurate cross-sectional display.

Because it is concentrated in normally functioning reticuloendothelial cells, subcostal injection of technetium-99m-radiocolloid will be taken up by the internal mammary lymph node chain.[60–62] Internal mammary lymphoscintigraphy can thus provide 3-dimensional localization of the lymph node chain for planning radiation therapy portals by defining nodal depth, distance from the midline, and cross-drainage of parasternal lymphatics.[63,64] As opposed to this technique, the use of an arbitrary reference to estimate nodal depth and location may either not include some nodes or lead to radiation of contiguous normal lung and heart tissue. Two recent studies indicate that in approximately 50% of cases, one or more lymph nodes would have been underdosed if the internal mammary nodes had not been precisely localized by lymphoscintigraphy before treatment.[65,66]

CT appears to be less efficacious in identifying

functionally normal nodes. It found only 29% of those seen on lymphoscintigraphy.[66] Also, CT cannot distinguish nodes from blood vessels. Nevertheless, CT may play a complementary role by identifying enlarged nodes which, because they are totally replaced by tumor, are not seen on lymphoscintigraphy. However, because of shortcomings of each, their role in treatment planning has not been precisely defined.

The role of lymphoscintigraphy including immunoscintigraphy in identifying metastatic disease of both the axillary and internal mammary nodes is currently under investigation.[67] Although certain signs such as decreased uptake, interruption in sequence of lymphatics and alternate pathways suggest tumor involvement, this study cannot reliably rule out the presence of metastatic carcinoma in lymph nodes.[68,69]

Lymphoscintigraphy may represent a prognostic indicator. When normal, there was a 34% incidence of recurrence whereas an abnormal lymphoscintigram was associated with a 67% recurrence.[70] It may also advance our knowledge of the natural history of the disease. Lymphoscintigraphy suggests a similar frequency of involvement of the internal mammary nodes among patients with outer quadrant lesions (57%) as among patients with inner quadrant lesions (48%).[70,71] Internal mammary metastases may be present even if the axillary nodes are negative. Both Dionne et al[71] and Ege[72] found lymphoscintigraphic evidence of internal mammary node involvement in 17% to 18% of breast carcinoma patients who had histologically negative axilla. Ege and Elhakim said that such patients should be considered to have stage II disease and should be offered adjuvant therapy.[73]

Pericardium

Pericardial effusions are not uncommon in patients with widespread intrathoracic metastases. Breast and lung are the most common primary malignancies that metastasize to the pericardium. Ultrasound should be the primary imaging method for pericardial effusion because it is highly sensitive, specific, and cost-effective.[74] Ultrasound can reveal small and medium-sized pericardial effusions that are not apparent on chest x-ray. Effusions as small as 15 mL can be consistently detected by echocardiography.[75] This exam can also provide a rough estimate of the volume of fluid, ie, small (less than 100 mL), moderate (100–500 mL), or large (greater than 500 mL).[74] Misdiagnosis of pericardial effusions by ultrasound can be caused by fat anterior to the heart simulating loculated anterior pericardial effusion.[76]

Enlargement of the cardiac silhouette and a water bottle shaped heart due to effacement of the normal cardiac border on chest x-ray as well as decreased cardiac pulsations on chest fluoroscopy constitute the classical roentgen signs of pericardial effusion. Although these signs are accurate from the descriptive standpoint, their value is limited because they are nonspecific and mainly displayed in moderate or large size effusions. Nevertheless, an abrupt increase in the heart size that cannot be accounted for by intrinsic cardiac disease should suggest the diagnosis of pericardial effusion. The epicardial fat pad sign consists of posterior displacement of the epicardial fat pad line shadow and widening of the pericardial space by increased fluid on the lateral film. This sign is of limited diagnostic value because it requires a rather large amount of fluid and is present in less than 50% of cases of pericardial effusion.[77]

Pericardial effusions as small as 50 mL can be shown by CT.[78,79] CT may also be of help in evaluating the nature of the effusion. Transudates tend to have lower CT attenuation numbers than do bloody or exudative pericardial effusions. Loculated pericardial effusion and pericardial thickening with or without effusion can be detected more successfully with CT than with echocardiography.[80]

Radionuclide angiocardiography following intravenous injection of technetium-99m-labeled albumin is less sensitive than ultrasound or CT. A pericardial effusion of 200 mL or more is necessary for detection.[81]

LIVER

The relative efficacy of CT, ultrasound, and radionuclide scintigraphy in detection of hepatic metastases is difficult to assess. Some studies reveal conflicting results. Most studies involve a single modality rather than several modalities and are hard to compare because of differences in study design, patient population, and rapid changes in technology of any one modality between the time of each study. Two recent studies by Knopf et al[82] and Brendel et al[83] suggest that the detection sensitivity of CT is greater than that of the radionuclide scan (98% *v* 79% and 91% *v* 80%, respectively).

Two other recent studies by Alderson et al and Snow et al that compared all three modalities in a single series of patients with liver metastases found CT to be the most sensitive (93% and 96%), radionuclide scintigraphy to be slightly less sensitive (86% and 94%), and ultrasound to be the least sensitive (82% and 75%) respectively.[84,85] Moreover, many positive interpretations on ultrasound[84] and radionuclide scintigraphy[83] fell into the "possible" (low confidence positive) category. It should also be recognized that the accuracy of ultrasound is highly dependent on operator skills and technical factors such as overlying gas and bony structures.[85–87] The sensitivity of scintigraphy is highly dependent on lesion size. Focal hepatic lesions missed on scintigraphy but detected by CT are frequently those that measure less than 2 cm in size.[82]

One recent innovation in nuclear medicine is a rotating gamma camera system for performing SPECT studies. This process is similar in principle to conventional x-ray transmission CT except that SPECT involves an internal rather than an external source of radiation. Because SPECT is tomographic, it can provide better three-dimensional views of abnormalities than conventional radionuclide imaging. Although one study suggests that the sensitivity of SPECT is similar to that of conventional radionuclide imaging,[88] most studies indicate that the sensitivity of SPECT is better.[83,89,90] However, two of the studies indicate that even with SPECT, radionuclide scintigraphy of the liver is less sensitive than CT.[83,89] In addition, there is as yet no evidence that SPECT will result in increased diagnostic specificity.

The false-positive rates found in the studies of Alderson et al[84] (breast cancer only) and Snow et al[85] (all focal metastases) were lowest for CT (8% and 12%), higher for ultrasound (29% and 17%) and highest for scintigraphy (33% and 26%). The relatively high false-positive rate for scintigraphy has also been noted by others.[91]

A major reason for the relatively low specificity of radionuclide imaging is that focal defects may not only result from metastases but also from pressure defects from the gallbladder, right kidney, and hepatic vein.[92] Diffuse heterogeneous distribution of radionuclide seen in carcinomatosis can also be seen in diffuse parenchymal diseases such as cirrhosis.[93,94] Diffuse defects that cannot be otherwise explained, particularly when unaccompanied by other evidence of disturbed hepatic function, may require histologic confirmation before it can be concluded that they represent metastases. Although the sensitivity of the liver scan in detection of metastatic disease will increase if diffuse abnormalities are included, the number of false-positive studies will also increase. Despite these shortcomings, some physicians prefer radionuclide scintigraphy as the initial screening procedure because of its lower cost and shorter examination time.

Thus, if radionuclide scintigraphy or ultrasound is negative in a patient with clinical or biochemical evidence for liver metastasis, CT may be necessary to detect the lesion. If radionuclide scintigraphy or ultrasound is used as the initial screening procedure, focal defects suspicious for metastasis should be further investigated by CT or biopsy to exclude benign conditions. In most centers, an unenhanced (precontrast) CT is performed followed by a postcontrast CT study. A small percentage of metastases (less than 5%) will only be visible on postcontrast scans and conversely a small number of metastases will become isodense after contrast medium and therefore invisible.[95]

Preliminary studies suggest that magnetic resonance (MR) is currently able to detect hepatic metastasis with a degree of accuracy close to CT.[96–98] Although MR can distinguish vascular from nonvascular hepatic structures without the use of intravenous contrast, CT is still the preferred method of imaging hepatic tumors because of its shorter imaging time (20 *v* 60 minutes), lower cost, and greater spatial resolution.[96]

Screening

An elevated alkaline phosphatase may result from either hepatic or osseous metastases. However, if the heat stable fraction is greater than 35%, liver metastases are probably present. Whereas, if it is less than 35%, bone metastases are more likely. An abnormal alkaline phosphatase value in a breast cancer patient signals hepatic involvement with 85% certainty. False-positive values may be due to laboratory error, hepatitis, cirrhosis, and other liver abnormalities.

Additional serologic tests may result in increased specificity. If the alkaline phosphatase, SGOT, and albumin are all abnormal, hepatic metastases will be present in 92% of cases. If these serologic tests as well as the liver scan are abnormal, hepatic metastases will be present in 99% of cases.[91,99–101]

It has been estimated that up to 10% to 15% of hepatic metastases may not be associated with an abnormal physical examination or abnormal serologic tests.[102] However, because the yield of true-positive pretreatment liver scans is even smaller than that of bone scans, it is generally recommended that they be reserved for patients with appropriate symptoms, abnormal liver chemistry, hepatomegaly or stage III and stage IV disease.[100–104] In one series of 234 breast cancer patients, preoperative liver scans were positive in 11 (5%). However, eight of the 11 represented false-positive diagnoses so that only 1% of the scans yielded correct evidence of metastatic disease.[103] The small increment in detection hardly justifies the false-positive rate of 4%. Similarly, among 100 patients with breast cancer undergoing a liver scan, Sears et al reported that only 1 had metastases documented on the scan.[100]

Treatment Response

Decreased size of a lesion on sequential liver scanning[105] or ultrasound[106] can indicate tumor response. Although carcinoembryonic antigen (CEA) level appears to be a less accurate reflection of such response, both exams have been suggested because absence of change in an intrahepatic focal defect on scan has been noted occasionally in patients who show both clinical response and a decrease in CEA levels.[107] Another misleading finding, an inhomogeneous pattern of isotope distribution resembling that seen in carcinomatosis or cirrhosis has been reported in conjunction with short-term chemotherapy.[108] On the other hand, an increase in size of a lesion on liver scan or the appearance of new focal lesions strongly suggests progressive disease.

BRAIN

Virtually all patients with cerebral metastases will be symptomatic or have abnormalities on routine physical examination. In a study of 116 patients with metastatic breast cancer but no symptoms of intracranial disease, only one abnormal brain scan was found by Muss et al.[109] In addition, the brain is an extremely uncommon site of initial distant recurrence from breast cancer. Among patients with metastatic disease, Winchester et al found brain metastases to be the initial presentation in only 2.4%.[5] Accordingly, asymptomatic breast cancer patients should not be screened for metastatic brain deposits.

The sensitivity of CT is superior to that of radionuclide scanning for detection of brain metastases.[110,111] Administration of intravenous contrast material before CT will result in a slightly increased detection of metastases but a moderate decrease in the number of equivocal scans.[111] A single contrast scan has the same degree of sensitivity as both pre- and postcontrast scans.[111,112] Because the elimination of the preliminary noncontrast enhanced scan will decrease cost and examination time, the current brain imaging procedure of choice is a single contrast-enhanced CT scan.

Preliminary clinical studies with MR imaging clearly indicate that it is the imaging method of choice for evaluation of many types of cerebral disorders such as multiple sclerosis, subcortical arteriosclerotic encephalopathy, posterior fossa infarcts, and tumors.[113] Prospective clinical trials will be necessary to determine the relative efficacy of CT and MR in detection of cerebral metastases. Although the relatively high cost of examination and limited availability of equipment restrict the present use of MR, rapid advances in MR technology and the use of special contrast agents may influence its effectiveness in screening for metastases.

BREAST

Mammographic evaluation before biopsy of a palpable cancer can provide important information regarding the characteristics of the mass and the multiplicity of lesions. These factors can influence the decision between mastectomy and more conservative treatment. Detection of multiple foci of carcinoma is more reliably accomplished at this time rather than following biopsy since edema and hemorrhage may hinder mammographic interpretation. Breast tenderness and fear of partial wound dehisence or bleeding that usually lasts for 3 to 4 weeks postbiopsy will prevent adequate breast compression necessary for a technically satisfactory study. If conservative treatment is planned, mammographic evaluation of the cancerous breast following excisional biopsy may also be useful in demonstrating the presence of residual tumor mass or microcalcifications.[114]

Patients treated by segmental mastectomy and radiation therapy should be evaluated by mammography at 6 months following treatment. At this time, all of the anatomic changes that occur as a result of radiation therapy, except for skin thickening, which may persist for years, have stabilized. Thereafter, annual bilateral mammograms should be obtained. Residual mass or density may represent postbiopsy scarring or sterilized tumor. Tumor calcifications may remain the same, diminish, or disappear. Persistence of density or tumor calcifications following treatment does not necessarily indicate the presence of residual viable tumor.[115] However, an increase in density and/or calcifications in the treated area or development of a new breast mass or tumor calcifications usually indicate recurrent carcinoma.[116]

Mammographic evaluation of the opposite normal breast is also essential. In a study by Kopans et al, mammography was able to detect clinically occult synchronous carcinoma in 3% of patients.[117] Among breast cancer patients treated by mastectomy, there is a 7% cumulative incidence of carcinoma in the remaining opposite breast.[118,119] Mammographic screening of the remaining breast will result in earlier detection and improvement in the stage at the time of detection. Senofsky et al compared two populations of patients with bilateral breast cancer who entered into the system before effective mammographic monitoring (BEM) during the years 1969 to 1975 and after effective mammographic monitoring (AEM) during the years 1977 to 1984.[120] There was a distinctly earlier detection rate of second breast cancers in the AEM group (1.5 years in AEM *v* 4.75 years in BEM). The staging percentage of second breast cancers in both groups is shown in Table 1. The improvement in staging was most noted in the number of in situ lesions: 6.1% of the BEM *v* 50.0% of the AEM group. Because the cumulative incidence of second breast cancers were similar in each group (7.4% of the BEM patients *v* 6.5% of the AEM patients), the authors predict an improved survival rate for the AEM patients.

Table 1. Stage of Second Breast Cancer in Populations Before (BEM) and After (AEM) Mammographic Monitoring

Stage	Percent of 33 (BEM) Patients	Percent of 38 (AEM) Patients
0	6.1	50.0
I	51.5	23.7
II	6.1	15.8
III	21.2	7.9
IV	15.1	2.6

Adapted with permission.[120]

Support for such screening of women with treated and potentially curable breast cancer can also be based on results of studies involving mass population screening. In a randomized trial conducted by the Health Insurance Plan of New York, a 40% mortality reduction was found among women age 50 and over screened by mammography and physical examination.[121] A recent Swedish randomized screening study found a 40% mortality reduction among women screened above age 50 by mammography alone.[122] Results from the Swedish study as well as the American Breast Cancer Detection Demonstration Projects suggest that a similar mortality reduction from screening women below age 50 is a reasonable expectation.[123,124]

CONCLUSION

Recommendations for imaging procedures for breast cancer staging and follow-up should be based on our understanding of the natural history of the disease as well as the accuracy, cost, and

Table 2. Imaging Recommendations

Modality	Staging	Follow-up
Chest x-ray	Yes	Annual
Mammogram	Yes	Annual (plus initial 6 months for 1° rt patients)
Radionuclide bone scan	Only if alkaline phosphatase is elevated, axillary metastases are present, or primary tumor measures more than 2 cm	Every 6 months × 3 years, annually for next 2 years on patients where staging scan was indicated.
Ultrasound or CT (preferably)	Only if liver chemistry values are abnormal	Only if liver chemistry values abnormal
CT brain scan	Only if symptomatic	Only if symptomatic

availability of the studies themselves. While chest roentgenogram and bone scan may uncover metastases in asymptomatic patients, radionuclide scans of the liver and brain have a very low yield in patients clinically free of organ involvement. Although treatment of asymptomatic metastases may possibly result in improved palliation, there is no evidence that such treatment prolongs survival more than does treatment provided when symptoms appear.[2,56]

On the other hand, although the cumulative incidence of carcinoma of the contralateral breast is only 7%, there is strong evidence that early detection of primary breast cancer results in a substantial prolongation of survival. Accordingly, annual screening by mammography and physical examination is advised for patients who have had potentially curable carcinoma of the ipsilateral breast. With these considerations in mind, recommendations for the use of imaging procedures in breast cancer staging and follow-up are provided in Table 2.

REFERENCES

1. US Department of Health and Human Services, Public Health Service, National Institutes of Health, National Cancer Institute: Cancer Patient Survival, A Report from the Cancer Surveillance, Epidemiology and End Results (SEER) Program. Bethesda, MD, NIH Publication No. 77-992, 1976
2. Frazier TG, Copeland EM, Gallager HS, et al: Prognosis and treatment in minimal breast cancer. Am J Surg 133:697–701, 1977
3. Cutler SJ, Asire AJ, Taylor SG: Classification of patients with disseminated cancer of the breast. Cancer 24:861–869, 1969
4. Bruce J, Carter DC, Fraser J: Patterns of recurrent disease in breast cancer. Lancet 1:433–435, 1970
5. Winchester DP, Sener SF, Khandekar JD, et al: Symptomatology as an indicator of recurrent or metastatic breast cancer. Cancer 43:956–960, 1979
6. Shackman R, Harrison CV: Occult bone metastases. Br J Surg 35:385–389, 1948
7. Bachman AL, Sproul EE: Correlation of radiographic and autopsy findings in suspected metastases in spine. NY Acad Med Bull 31:146–148, 1955
8. Edelstyn GA, Gillespie PJ, Grebbell FS: The radiological demonstration of osseous metastases. Experimental observations. Clin Radiol 18:158–162, 1967
9. Citrin DL, Bessent RG, Grieg WR: A comparison of the sensitivity and accuracy of the 99m-Tc-phosphate bone scan and skeletal radiograph in the diagnosis of bone metastases. Clin Radiol 28:107–117, 1977
10. Charkes ND: Mechanisms of skeletal tracer uptake. J Nucl Med 20:794–795, 1979
11. Corcoran RJ, Thrall JM, Kyle RW, et al: Solitary abnormalities in bone scans of patients with extraosseous malignancies. Radiology 121:663–667, 1976
12. Gold RH: Imaging for staging and follow-up of breast cancer, in Ames FC, Blumenschein GR, Montague ED (eds): Current Controversies in Breast Cancer. Austin, TX, University of Texas, 1984, pp 185–195
13. Early PJ, Sodee D: Principles and Practice of Nuclear Medicine. St Louis, Mosby, 1985, pp 241–251
14. Baker RR, Holmes ER, Alderson PO, et al: An evaluation of bone scans as screening procedures for occult metastases in primary breast cancer. Ann Surg 186:363–368, 1977
15. Galasko CSB: The detection of skeletal metastases from mammary carcinoma by gamma camera scintigraphy. Br J Surg 56:757–764, 1969
16. Gibbons J, Holleb A, Farrow JH: An evaluation of routine preoperative skeletal survey for the patient with operable breast cancer. NY J Med 61:4219–4220, 1961
17. Roberts JG, Gravelle IH, Baum M, et al: Evaluation of radiography and isotopic scintigraphy for detecting skeletal metastases in breast cancer. Lancet 1:237–239, 1976
18. Clark DG, Painter RW, Sziklas JJ: Indications for bone scans in preoperative evaluation of breast cancer. Am J Surg 135:667–670, 1978
19. Davies CJ, Griffiths PA, Preston BJ, et al: Staging breast cancer. Role of scanning. Br Med J 2:603–605, 1977
20. Butzelaar RM, Van Dongen JA, Van Der Schoot JB, et al: Evaluation of routine preoperative bone scintigraphy in patients with breast cancer. Eur J Cancer 13:19–21, 1977
21. Gerber FH, Goodreau JJ, Kirchner PT, et al: Efficacy of preoperative and postoperative bone scanning in the management of breast carcinoma. N Engl J Med 29:300–303, 1977
22. El-Domeiri AA, Shroff S: Role of preoperative bone scan in carcinoma of the breast. Surg Gynecol Obstet 142:722–724, 1976
23. Lentle BC, Burns PE, Dierich H, et al: Bone scintiscanning in the initial assessment of carcinoma of the breast. Surg Gynecol Obstet 141:43–47, 1975
24. McNeill BJ, Pace PD, Gray EB, et al: Preoperative and follow-up bone scans in patients with primary carcinoma of the breast. Surg Gynecol Obstet 147:745–748, 1978
25. O'Connell MJ, Wahner HW, Ahmann DL, et al: Value of preoperative radionuclide bone scan is suspected primary breast carcinoma. Mayo Clin Proc 53:221–226, 1978
26. Hoffman HC, Marty R: Bone scanning. Its value in the preoperative evaluation of patients with suspicious breast masses. Am J Surg 124:194–199, 1972
27. Campbell DJ, Banks AJ, Oates GD: The value of preliminary bone scanning in staging and assessing the prognosis of breast cancer. Br J Surg 63:811–816, 1976
28. Hammond N, Jones SE, Salmon SE, et al: Predictive value of bone scans in an adjuvant breast cancer program. Cancer 41:138–142, 1978
29. Lee YT: Bone scanning in patients with early breast carcinoma: Should it be a routine staging procedure? Cancer 47:486–495, 1981

30. Wilson MA, Calhoun FW: The distribution of skeletal metastases in breast and pulmonary cancer: Concise communication. J Nucl Med 22:594–597, 1981

31. Lee Y-T: Bone scans are of sufficient accuracy and sensitivity to be part of the routine work-up prior to definitive surgical treatment of cancer: Opposed, in Van Scoy-Mosher MB (ed): Controversies in Cancer Treatment. Boston, Hall, 1981, pp 53–68

32. Waxman AD: Bone scans are of sufficient accuracy and sensitivity to be part of the routine work-up prior to definitive surgical treatment of cancer: In favor, in Van Scoy-Mosher MB (ed): Controversies in Cancer Treatment. Boston, Hall, 1981, pp 69–76

33. Cowan RJ, Young KA: Evaluation of serum alkaline phosphatase determination in patients with positive bone scans. Cancer 32:887–889, 1973

34. Citrin DC, Furnival CM, Bessent RG, et al: Radioactive technetium phosphate bone scanning in preoperative assessment and follow-up study of patients with primary cancer of the breast. Surg Gynecol Obstet 143:360–364, 1976

35. Sklaroff RB, Sklaroff DM: Bone metastases from breast cancer at the time of radical mastectomy as detected by bone scan. Eight-year follow-up. Cancer 38:107–111, 1976

36. American Joint Committee on Cancer: Manual for Staging of Cancer. Philadelphia, Lippincott, 1983

37. Galasko CSB: The significance of occult skeletal metastases, detected by skeletal scintigraphy in patients with otherwise "early" mammary carcinoma. Br J Surg 62:694–697, 1975

38. Robbins GF, Knapper WH, Barrie J, et al: Metastatic bone disease developing in patients with potentially curable breast cancer. Cancer 29:1702–1704, 1972

39. Libshitz HI, Hortobayg GN: Radiographic evaluation of therapeutic response in bony metastases of breast cancer. Skeletal Radiol 7:159–165, 1981

40. Alexander JL, Gillespie PJ, Edelstyn GA: Serial bone scanning using technetium-99m-diphosphonate in patients undergoing cyclical combination chemotherapy for advanced breast cancer. Clin Nucl Med 1:13–17, 1976

41. Condon BR, Buchanan R, Garvie NW, et al: Assessment of progression of secondary bone lesions following cancer of the breast or prostate using serial radionuclide imaging. Br J Radiol 54:18–23, 1981

42. Galasko CSB, Doyle FH: The response to therapy of skeletal metastases from mammary cancer. Assessment by scintigraphy. Br J Surg 59:85–88, 1972

43. Gillespie PJ, Alexander JL, Edelstyn GA: Changes in 87-Sr concentration in skeletal metastases in patients responding to cyclical combination chemotherapy for advanced breast cancer. J Nucl Med 16:191–193, 1975

44. Fracchia AA, Knapper WH, Carey JT, et al: Intrapleural chemotherapy for effusion from metastatic breast carcinoma. Cancer 26:626–629, 1970

45. Raju RN, Kardinal CG: Pleural effusion in breast carcinoma: Analysis of 122 cases. Cancer 48:2524–2527, 1981

46. Weichselbaum R, Marck A, Hellman S: Pathogenesis of pleural effusion in carcinoma of the breast. Int J Radiat Oncol Biol Phys 2:963–965, 1977

47. Janower ML, Blennerhassett JB: Lymphangitic spread of metastatic cancer to the lung. Radiology 101:267–273, 1971

48. Spencer H: Pathology of the Lung, ed 4. Oxford, Pergamon, 1985, pp 1085–1096

49. Libshitz HI, North LB: Pulmonary metastases. Radiol Clin North Am 20:437–451, 1982

50. Mintzer RA, Malave SR, Neiman HC, et al: Computed vs. conventional tomography in evaluation of primary and secondary pulmonary neoplasms. Radiology 132:653–659, 1979

51. Muhm JR, Brown LR, Crowe JK, et al: Comparison of whole lung tomography and computed tomography for detecting pulmonary nodules. AJR 131:981–984, 1978

52. Schaner EG, Chang AE, Doppman JL, et al: Comparison of computed and conventional whole lung tomography in detecting pulmonary nodules. AJR 131:51–54, 1978

53. Aronberg DJ, Sagel SS: Pulmonary metastases, in Eisenberg RI, Ambert JR (eds): Critical Diagnostic Pathways in Radiology. An Algorithmic Approach. Philadelphia, Lippincott, 1981, pp 359–366

54. Curtis AM, Ravin CE, Collier PE, et al: Detection of metastatic disease from carcinoma of the breast. Limited value of full lung tomography. AJR 134:253–255, 1980

55. Bragg DG: Radiologic detection of breast metastases, in Feig SA, McLelland R (eds): Breast Carcinoma: Current Diagnosis and Treatment. Chicago, Year Book, 1983, pp 495–503

56. Zerhouni EA, Sitik FP: Controversies in computed tomography of the thorax. Radiol Clin North Am 23:407–426, 1985

57. Cahan WG, Castro EB: Significance of a solitary lung shadow in patients with breast cancer. Ann Surg 181:137–143, 1975

58. Meyer JE, Munzenrider JE: Computed tomographic demonstration of internal mammary lymph node metastasis in patients with locally recurrent breast carcinoma. Radiology 139:661–663, 1981

59. Chiles C, Ravin CE: Intrathoracic metastasis from an extrathoracic malignancy: A radiographic approach to patient evaluation. Radiol Clin North Am 23:427–438, 1985

60. McKusick KA: Radionuclide lymphography, in Clous ME, Wallace S (eds): Lymphatic Imaging. Lymphography, Computed Tomography and Scintigraphy. Baltimore, Williams and Wilkins, 1985, pp 95–111

61. Ege GN: Internal mammary lymphoscintigraphy. The rationale, technique, interpretation, and clinical application. A review based on 848 cases. Radiology 118:101–107, 1976

62. Ege GN: Lymphoscintigraphy-techniques and applications in the management of breast carcinoma. Semin Nucl Med 13:26–34, 1983

63. Manji MF: Internal mammary lymphoscintigraphy in breast carcinoma: Possible significance in relation to current treatment. J Can Assoc Radiol 33:10–14, 1982

64. Dufresne EN, Kaplan WD, Zimmerman RE, et al: The application of internal mammary lymphoscintigraphy to radiation therapy planning. J Nucl Med 21:697–699, 1980

65. Rose CM, Kaplan WD, Marck A, et al: Parasternal lymphoscintigraphy: Implications for treatment planning of internal mammary lymph nodes in breast cancer. Int J Radiat Oncol Biol Phys 5:1849–1853, 1979

66. Collier BD, Palmer DW, Wilson JF, et al: Internal mammary lymphoscintigraphy in patients with breast cancer. Radiology 147:845–848, 1983

67. Thompson CH, Lichtenstein M, Stacker SA, et al: Immunoscintigraphy for detection of lymph node metastases from breast cancer. Lancet 2:1245–1247, 1984

68. Peyton JW, Crosbie J, Bell TK, et al: High colloidal uptake in axillary nodes with metastatic disease. Br J Surg 68:507–509, 1981

69. Hill NS, Ege GN, Greyson ND: Predicting nodal metastases in breast cancer by lymphoscintigraphy. Can J Surg 26:507–509, 1983

70. Ege GN, Clark R: IML in conservative management of breast carcinoma. Clin Radiol 31:55–63, 1980

71. Dionne L, Freide J, Blais R: Internal mammary lymphoscintigraphy in breast carcinoma. A surgeon's perspective. Semin Nucl Med 13:35–41, 1983

72. Ege GN, Elhakim T: The relevance of internal mammary lymmphoscintigraphy in the management of breast carcinoma. J Clin Oncol 2:774–781, 1984

73. Ege GN: Internal mammary lymphoscintigraphy in breast carcinoma—A study of 1071 patients. Int J Radiat Oncol Biol Phys 2:755–761, 1977

74. Moncada R, Kotler MN, Steiner RM: Multimodality approach to pericardial imaging. Cardiovasc Clin 17:408–440, 1986

75. Horowitz MS, Schultz CS, Stinson EB, et al: Sensitivity and specificity of echocardiographic diagnosis of pericardial effusion. Circulation 50:239–246, 1974

76. Walinsky P: Pitfalls in the diagnosis of pericardial effusion. Cardiovasc Clin 9:111–122, 1978

77. Carsky EW, Maucer RA, Azimi F: The epicardial fat pat sign. Radiology 137:303–308, 1980

78. Moncada R, Baker M, Salinas M, et al: Diagnostic role of computed tomography in pericardial heart disease: Congenital defects, thickening, neoplasms and effusions. Am Heart J 100:263–282, 1982

79. Wong BYS, Lee KR, MacArthur RI: Diagnosis of pericardial effusion by computed tomography. Chest 81:177–181, 1982

80. Isner JM, Carter BL, Bankoff MS: Computed tomography in the diagnosis of pericardial heart disease. Ann Intern Med 97:473–479, 1982

81. Kriss JP: Diagnosis of pericardial effusion by radioisotopic angiocardiography. J Nucl Med 10:133–241, 1969

82. Knopf DR, Torres WE, Fajman WJ, et al: Liver lesions: Comparative accuracy of scintigraphy and computed tomography. AJR 138:623–627, 1982

83. Brendel AJ, Leccia F, Drouillard J: Single photon emission computed tomography (SPECT), planar scintigraphy, and transmission computed tomography: A comparison of accuracy in diagnosing focal hepatic disease. Radiology 153:527–532

84. Alderson PO, Adams DF, McNeill BJ, et al: Computed tomography, ultrasound, and scintigraphy of the liver in patients with colon or breast carcinoma. A prospective comparison. Radiology 149:225–230, 1983

85. Snow JH, Goldstein HM, Wallace S: Comparison of scintigraphy, sonography and computed tomography in the evaluation of hepatic neoplasms. AJR 132:915–918, 1979

86. Biello DR, Levitt RG, Siegel BA: Computed tomography and radionuclide imaging of the liver. A comparative evaluation. Radiology 127:159–163, 1978

87. Bryan PJ, Dinn WM, Grossman ZD, et al: Correlation of computed tomography, gray scale ultrasonography, and radionuclide imaging of the liver in detecting space-occupying processes. Radiology 124:387–393, 1977

88. Keyes JW, Singer D, Satterlee W, et al: Liver-spleen studies with the rotating gamma camera II: Utility of tomography. Radiology 153:537–541, 1984

89. Yumoto Y, Tokuyama K, Zinno K, et al: Detection of hepatic tumor by means of single photon emission computed tomography, gray scale ultrasonography and computed tomography, in Raynaud C (ed): Nuclear Medicine and Biology. Proceedings of the Third World Congress of Nuclear Medicine and Biology. Paris, Pergamon, 1982, pp 2870–2873

90. Strauss L, Bostel F, Clorius JH, et al: Single-photon emission computed tomography (SPECT) for assessment of hepatic lesions. J Nucl Med 23:1059–1065, 1982

91. Sugarbaker PH, Beard JO, Drum JE: Detection of hepatic metastases from cancer of the breast. Br J Radiol 45:851–854, 1977

92. Chaudhuri TK, Stadalnik RC, Chaudhuri TK: Juxtahepatic structures causing false positive liver scintiscan. Semin Nucl Med 11:61–63, 1981

93. Drum DE, Beard JM: Scintigraphic criteria for hepatic metastases from cancer of the colon and breast. J Nucl Med 17:677–680, 1976

94. Borja ER, Hori JM, Pugh RP: Metastatic carcinomatosis of the liver mimicking cirrhosis: Case report and review of the literature. Cancer 35:445–449, 1975

95. Foley WD, Smith DF, Thorsen MK: Liver, in Greenberg M, Greenberg BM, Greenberg IM (eds): Essentials of Body Computed Tomography. Philadelphia, Saunders, 1983, pp 131–135

96. Heiken JP, Lee JKT, Glazer HS, et al: Hepatic masses studied with MR and CT. Radiology 156:423–427, 1985

97. Moss AA, Goldberg HI, Stark DB, et al: Hepatic tumors: Magnetic resonance and CT appearance. Radiology 150:141–147, 1984

98. Haaga JR: Magnetic resonance imaging of the liver. Radiol Clin North Am 22:879–890, 1984

99. Castagna J, Benfield JR, Yamada H, et al: The reliability of liver scans and function tests in detecting metastases. Surg Gynecol Obstet 134:463–466, 1972

100. Sears HF, Gerber FH, Sturtz DL: Liver scan and carcinoma of the breast. Surg Gynecol Obstet 140:409–411, 1975

101. Liewendahl K, Schauman KO: Statistical evaluation of liver scanning in combination with liver function tests. Acta Med Scand 192:395–400, 1972

102. Felix EL, Bagley DH, Sindelar WF, et al: The value of the liver scan in preoperative screening of patients with malignancies. Cancer 38:1137–1141, 1976

103. Wiener SN, Sachs H: An assessment of routine liver scanning in patients with breast cancer. Arch Surg 113:126–127, 1970

104. Tempero MA, Petersen RJ, Zetterman RK, et al: Detection of metastatic liver disease. JAMA 248:1332–1339, 1982

105. Witik JT, Spencer RP: Scan evidence of decrease in

size of intrahepatic tumors after chemotherapy. Gastroenterology 67:516–518, 1974

106. Bernardino ME, Green B: Ultrasonographic evaluation of chemotherapeutic response in hepatic metastases. Radiology 133:437–441, 1979

107. Bronstein BR, Steele GD, Ensminger W, et al: The use and limitations of serial plasma carcinoembryonic antigen (CEA) levels as a monitor of changing metastatic liver tumor volume in patients receiving chemotherapy. Cancer 46:266–272, 1980

108. Kaplan WD, Drum DE, Lokich JJ: The effect of cancer chemotherapeutic agents on the liver-spleen scan. J Nucl Med 21:84–87, 1980

109. Muss HB, White DR, Cowan RJ: Brain scanning in patients with recurrent breast cancer. Cancer 38:1574–1576, 1976

110. Buell U, Niendorf HP, Kazner E, et al: Computerized transaxial tomography and cerebral serial scintigraphy in intracranial tumors—rates of detection and tumor-type identification: Concise communication. J Nucl Med 19:476–479, 1978

111. Potts DG, Abbott GF, von Sneidern JV: National Cancer Institute study: Evaluation of computed tomography in the diagnosis of intracranial neoplasms. Radiology 136:657–664, 1980

112. Butler AR, Kricheff I: Non-contrast CT scanning: Limited value in suspected brain tumor. Radiology 126:689–693, 1978

113. Bradley WG, Waluch V, Yadley RA: Comparison of CT and MR in 400 patients with suspected disease of the brain and cervical spinal cord. Radiology 152:695–702, 1984

114. Gefter WB, Friedman AK, Goodman RL: The role of mammography in evaluating patients with early carcinoma of the breast for tylectomy and radiation therapy. Radiology 142:77–80, 1982

115. Paulus DD, Libshitz HI: Breast, in Libshitz HI (ed): Diagnostic Roentgenology of Radiotherapy Change. Baltimore, Williams and Wilkins, 1979, pp 55–68

116. Paulus DD: Conservative treatment of breast cancer: mammography in patient selection and follow-up. AJR 143:483–487, 1984

117. Kopans DB, Meyer JE, Cohen AM, et al: Palpable breast masses. The importance of preoperative mammography. JAMA 246:2819–2822, 1981

118. McSweeney MB, Egan RL: Bilateral breast cancer, in Brünner S, Langfeldt B, Andersen PE (eds): Early Detection of Breast Cancer. New York, Springer-Verlag, 1984, pp 41–48

119. Hermann JB: Management of the contralateral breast after mastectomy for unilateral carcinoma. Surg Gynecol Obstet 136:777–779, 1973

120. Senofsky GM, Wanebo HJ, Wilhelm MC, et al: Has monitoring of the contralateral breast improved the prognosis in patients treated for primary breast cancer? Cancer 57:597–602, 1986

121. Shapiro S, Venet W, Strax P, et al: Ten-to-fourteen year effect of screening on breast cancer mortality. JNCI 69:349–355, 1982

122. Tabar LK, Gad A, Fagerberg CJG: Reduction in breast cancer mortality by mass screening with mammography. First results of a randomized trial in two Swedish counties. Lancet 1:829–832, 1985

123. Tabar L, Gad A, Holmberg L, et al: Significant reduction in advanced breast cancer. Results of the first seven years of mammography screening in Kopparberg, Sweden. Diag Imag Clin Med 54:158–164, 1985

124. Feig SA: Low-dose mammography, application to medical practice. JAMA 242:2107–2109, 1979

The Clinical Investigator and the Evolution of the Treatment of Primary Breast Cancer

Paul P. Carbone and Douglass C. Tormey

THE EVOLUTION of the modern treatment of breast cancer can be traced to a rather limited number of incisive clinical observations over the past 100 years. In the 19th century, the major concepts in therapy came from individual clinicians who deduced therapeutic principles from their experiences. The laboratory contributions were late 20th century events and have included methodological assays and other findings that have explained or modified some of the clinical concepts. In the second half of the 20th century, the observational derivation of hypotheses was supplemented and enhanced by the use of clinical trials developed through the early cooperative trial groups. In the last 10 years, the laboratory has begun to make important contributions to therapy by defining concepts such as hormone receptors, and by developing primary human cancer cultures and monoclonal antibodies, as well as uncovering paracrine and autocrine growth factors. Even in the case of hormonal receptors, a recognized major laboratory advance, one of the first demonstrations of the localization of radiolabeled estrogens in human tumors was a clinical experiment, based on histological examination of biopsies of patients infused with tritiated estrogens undergoing adrenelectomies.[1] This report will attempt to define the origins and development of some of the important therapeutic concepts. Many of the more recent developments will also be described in the other reports in this special issue of the *Seminars*.

Before beginning the discussion on the evolution of the modern concepts of breast cancer treatment, we must comment on the idea of trying to attribute advances to specific individuals. Rarely are important advances in therapeutic concepts made by single individuals. They are often the logical conclusion of work performed over a period of time by many, with the false starts being almost as important as correct deductions. The elimination of alternative hypotheses is as important as the derivation of new ones. Also, many initial observations are reported with relatively few patients, often without adequate controls or statistical validity. The confirmation of the results is done by others. The contributions of the confirmatory investigators are often overlooked. In addition, only positive pilot studies are published. We remember the ones that are confirmed, and the many unconfirmed observations are quickly forgotten. The ebb and flow of research advances requires repetitive confirmation or disproof of unique observations. The repeated reporting of impressions and uncontrolled findings that are not confirmed with appropriate clinical trials does not result in a solid foundation for the science of cancer treatment. Instead, these impressions may become ingrained into therapeutic strategies and become difficult to alter. Finally, the authors' perceptions of origins and originators may not be the same as others.

Advances must be confirmed and repeatable by others. Thus, in this report, we have placed major emphasis not necessarily on those studies that were first, but primarily on those studies that were definitive and based on good well-controlled trials. The topics to be covered in this report include the biology of cancer metastasis, the hormonal regulation of breast cancer cells, the treatment of metastases, and the development of potential prevention strategies. Each of these topics will be defined and an historical basis established (Table 1).

THE OUTCOME OF PRIMARY TREATMENT IS NOT RELATED TO THE EXTENT OF SURGERY

Breast cancer has been recognized for centuries. Before the 19th century, therapy included rather crude and rarely effective methods of extirpation of the breast and tumor. Without anesthesia and the understanding of asepsis, advances that occurred in the 19th century, the

From the University of Wisconsin Clinical Cancer Center, Madison.

Supported by Grant Nos. CA14520 and CA21115.

Address reprint requests to Paul P. Carbone, MD, University of Wisconsin Clinical Cancer Center, 600 Highland Ave, Madison, WI 53792.

0093-7754/86/1304-0005$05.00/0

Table 1. Evolution of Therapeutic Concepts in Breast Cancer

Outcome of treatment is not related to the extent of surgery or radiation.
Minimal surgery is equivalent to more radical surgery.
Hormones from the ovaries and adrenals can alter the growth of breast cancer.
Laboratory tests can predict the hormonal sensitivity of cancer cells.
Hormonal action can be affected by chemical antagonism or enzymatic blockade of synthesis.
Micrometastases are eliminated by adjunctive hormones or cytotoxic treatment.
Drug resistance can be overcome by increasing the intensity or dose rate of treatment.

ability of surgery to cure cancer was limited. Though it was well understood that cancer cells could spread by way of the vascular system, emphasis in controlling breast cancer was placed on removing the bulk of the primary and the regional lymph nodes en bloc. Good cancer surgery required a high degree of anatomical understanding of the lymphatics. As late as 1942, in a major textbook of surgery, the following admonition is iterated: "There are occasions when less than a radical operation may be indicated, but they should be rare occasions. . . . It should be borne in mind that it took years of careful observation for the pioneers in surgery to realize the necessity for thorough and radical operation. . . . the optimistic operator . . . who thinks that less than a thorough radical operation is adequate . . . is absolutely wrong and is liable and responsible for the loss of a number of lives before he comes to learn this lesson all over again."[2]

In 1894, Halsted reported 50 cases of carcinoma of the breast treated surgically and commented, "There are undoubtedly many surgeons still in active practice who have not cured a cancer of the breast." Of his 50 patients, only three had local recurrences. About 50% were alive and disease free with a maximum follow-up of approximately 2 years, a remarkable result.[3,4] Over the next 10 years, Halsted devised increasingly more aggressive local operation, with dissection of the neck, and supraclavicular and mediastinal lymph nodes. These operations were repopularized in the 1950s as the super-radical procedures. The main tenet of his operative technique was that cancer spread centrifugally through the lymphatics. Liver, spine, and bone metastases were explained by lymphatic extensions. He categorically denied in his operative strategies that tumor cells could spread through the blood.

Despite a rather more advanced disease state for most of Halsted's patients, the local recurrence rate would be acceptable today, namely 6% to 9%. It was implicit in his argument that the en bloc dissection removed the lymph nodes, which were barriers and channels for tumor dissemination. Except in a few places, these results were not challenged until the middle of the 20th century. Experiments in the laboratory of Fishers clearly demonstrated that tumor cells could easily traverse the lymph nodes and disseminate via the blood vessels.[5] Other investigators also showed the importance of blood-borne metastases. These findings, as well as the clinical impressions from observational studies, began to suggest alternative hypotheses of cancer spread and encourage less radical surgery.

One of the earliest challenges to the Halsted approach to cancer therapy, namely the radical mastectomy, was reported by McWhirter from Scotland in 1948.[6] In a sequential series of patients, he noted that simple mastectomy followed by radiation to the axilla gave comparable results to the more radical procedures. His observational results suggested that the more aggressive approach to breast cancer treatment was not necessarily better. Others, such as Crile[7] and Mustakallio,[8] began to champion the use of even less radical surgery. However, the cries of comparability of the lesser procedures to the more traditional radical mastectomy were not accompanied by good data from randomized trials. Up until the early 1970s there was much discussion, but little hard data to support the lesser surgery approach.

The National Surgical Adjuvant Breast Project (NSABP) over the years has performed several key clinical trials that have not only failed to confirm some of Halsted's concepts of surgery, but also have opened up new conceptual areas of breast cancer biology. In a study of recurrence and survival of over 2,000 patients, the results clearly showed that the parameters of outcome were independent of the number of nodes removed at the time of surgery. Whether the patient had five or 30 nodes removed, the prognosis associated with two positive nodes was the same.[9] In a subsequent study comparing a total mastectomy with and without axillary dissection, the NSABP clearly showed that prognosis was not affected by leaving in or removing the axillary lymph nodes. In 1981, Fisher noted that these results failed to confirm the efficacy of en bloc dissection and supported the hypothesis that while the involvement of the lymph nodes does relate to prognosis, the removal of the lymph nodes did not affect outcome.[10] Furthermore, failure was related to the growth of occult distant micrometastases disseminated through the blood stream.

MINIMAL SURGERY IS EQUIVALENT TO MORE RADICAL SURGERY

While there have been many reports on the apparent value of limited surgery and radiation therapy in the primary treatment of breast cancer, in 1981, Veronesi from the Milan Cancer Institute, reported the first well-performed controlled clinical trial comparing radical surgery to quadrantectomy with radiation to the breast.[11] He summarized the apparent pressures to develop this technique as follows. Firstly, there was a better understanding of the biology of breast cancer and the realization that failure occurs irrespective of the extent of local treatment. Secondly, he attributed the availability of mammograms to detect smaller primary lesions as important. Thirdly, the increasing public desire to be involved in decisions of therapy was translated into pressure for less mutilating procedures. Finally, he stated that the use of minimal surgery would encourage increased emphasis on self screening and earlier diagnosis. The report by Veronesi, showing the equivalence of the quadrantectomy to the more radical surgery, was a hallmark study and convincingly disavowed the Halstedian approach to breast surgery.

A similar trial performed in the United States by the NSABP examined the role of segmental mastectomy alone and with radiation therapy to a total mastectomy.[12] All patients had an axillary dissection. One of the major differences of this study as compared with the Veronesi protocol was the addition of the study arm using segmental mastectomy without radiation. The overall disease-free survival at 5 years were comparable in the three groups. This study clearly showed the value of radiation to the breast in decreasing local recurrences and obviating the subsequent mastectomy. In both of these studies, treatment was performed with discontinous dissection of the primary tumor and the draining axillary lymph nodes, a clear prohibition in the Halsted approach to cancer surgery.

In the field of radiotherapy, Baclesse had shown that patients treated with radiotherapy alone could be salvaged.[13] However, the limitation of the equipment's output of energy and the relative lack of referral of patients prevented the adequate testing of this modality. Despite this, some centers in Europe were able to collect large series of patients and began to note good results. Calle, at the Curie Foundation in Paris, treated 314 patients from 1960 to 1975 by tumorectomy and radiotherapy.[14] The local recurrence rate was 10% and local failure treated with salvage mastectomy was effective in 57% of patients.

Later investigators at the Joint Center for Radiotherapy at Harvard reported 176 consecutive patients who were treated with primary excisional biopsy and breast irradiation.[15] Patients were either stage 1 or 2. Median follow up was 47 months. The overall relapse rate in the breast was 7%. Patients with interstitial radiation had only a 1% relapse rate in the breast. Patients with incisional or needle biopsies had higher local relapse rates.

Clark et al, at the Princess Margaret Hospital in Toronto, reported a 71% 10-year survival for 688 patients treated with conservative surgery and radiation to the breast and axilla in some patients.[16] The study was not controlled for the primary surgery or subsequent radiation. However, they reported that breast radiation did decrease local recurrence, whereas axillary radiation failed to improve the results. In either case, survival was not affected by radiation. The reason for equivalence in survival, the authors report, is that breast recurrence does not adversely impact on survival. Salvage mastectomy in the 20% of breast recurrences is able to favorably influence outcome, unlike local recurrence after mastectomy. These studies added to the depth of data that the radical mastectomy was not the only justified approach to primary therapy, especially for lesions <5 cm in size. It is of note that all these studies were uncontrolled nonrandomized efforts. Credibility was lacking until the studies reported in 1985. It was the

Veronesi and NSABP studies that really provided a high degree of acceptance in the western world for the limited surgeries.

THE HORMONES SECRETED BY THE OVARIES AND ADRENALS CAN ALTER THE GROWTH OF BREAST CANCER

According to Hayward, in 1889 the German physician Albert Schinzinger was the first to suggest that mammary cancer might be ameliorated by oophorectomy.[17] However, Beatson, a Scottish surgeon, performed the first reported therapeutic oophorectomy in 1895 in two premenopausal patients and both responded.[18] Based on his observations that prolonged lactation occurred in cows following a second pregnancy or oophorectomy, Beatson postulated that the induction of differentiation in mammary cancer cells like those of the normal breast in lactation could be induced by removing the ovaries. We now know that this is not the mechanism of regression following ovarian removal. Within 5 years, Boyd postulated a trophic effect of the ovary on maintaining cancer cell growth and he reported the results in 54 patients, with about one third responding to this new treatment.[19] It is noteworthy that Boyd recommended removal of the ovaries even in postmenopausal women, since he postulated that cessation of menses was not necessarily associated with loss of all ovarian function. Although subtotal removal of the adrenals to decrease estrogen production was described in 1947 by Atkins,[20] Huggins and Bergenstal reported the first successful total adrenalectomy in the 1950s,[21] successful primarily because of the use of effective cortisone replacement. These hallmark studies were the basis of the endocrine ablative approach to cancer treatment.

Major milestones in the use of oophorectomy as adjunctive therapy were achieved by the studies of Nissen-Meyer[22] and Cole.[23] In the former study, the results appeared to show a significant delay in recurrence in both pre- and postmenopausal women. Likewise, Cole showed a delay in recurrences. However, both studies failed to confirm a significant increase in survival with the use of prophylactic adjuvant oophorectomy, except possibly in some subsets. Based on the available data, in 1974, Burn stated that there was no basis to use or study further adjuvant oophorectomy.[24]

Definition of the treatment concepts using additive hormone therapy can be traced to the laboratory studies of Haddow and Robinson, who showed that certain polycyclic hydrocarbons with carcinogenic potential could inhibit the growth of mammary cancers.[25] Others reported the estrogenic activity of polycyclic hydrocarbon derivatives of ethylene and their ability to inhibit Walker carcinoma.[26] Diethylstilbesterol was a potent estrogen that belonged to the ethylene family of compounds. This led Haddow in 1944 to initiate a clinical trial in advanced breast cancer with three synthetic ethylenes including diethylstilbesterol.[27] Tumor regressions were seen particularly in the women over 60.

Likewise, the effect of androgens on mammary cancers were first noted in experimental animals. In 1939, it was found that testoterone propionate suppressed the development of spontaneous cancers in female R3 mice by Lacassagne and Raynaud[28] and in C3H mice by Nathanson and Andervont.[29] Within the same year, the activity was confirmed in humans by Loeser.[30] Two large cooperative groups were formed in the United States: American Medical Association Council on Drugs, and the Cooperative Breast Group to study hormonal treatment. Using strict standards, they were able to establish the all important standard of testing and evaluating of hormone compounds. Their studies led to important concepts of tumor flare, sequential use of hormones, and clinical predictive parameters.

LABORATORY TESTS CAN PREDICT THE HORMONAL SENSITIVITY OF CANCER CELLS

Estrogen Receptor

The basic finding that hormones were able to affect the growth of breast cancer in approximately 30% of the patients led to defining several clinical conditions that seemed to predict response. A series of predictive parameters were outlined encompassing the size of the tumor, anatomical distribution, age of the patient, menstrual status, the time from initial therapy, and prior response to hormonal therapy. The development of the laboratory test for estrogen receptor

(ER) was an important advance. In 1961, Folca et al found that the uptake of tritiated estrogens in the tumors were increased as compared with muscle and were the greatest in women who responded to adrenalectomy.[1] This, along with animal studies, led Jensen et al to develop the first human assays of receptors.[31] The basic development of the concepts of hormone receptors were extremely important to the clinical development of the ER test and beyond the scope of this review. However, it was the foresight of Elwood Jensen to work with clinical materials, using a time-consuming and complicated technique to look at the clinical correlations of the test, that makes this effort truly remarkable. The clinical correlative studies done by Jensen and his colleagues firmly established the predictive value of the receptor status of the primary tumor. Early in the clinical experiences with receptors, it became clear that the receptor content of the tumor predicted for response for additive, as well as ablative therapy.[32] Later it was appreciated that prognosis was also related to the ER content. Certainly the ability to defer major ablative surgery in the ER negative patient was important. Likewise, the ability to predict high response rates would be important to the clinician. Curiously, in the mid 1980s while the receptor is still being measured and used to direct therapy, the advent of tamoxifen and aminoglu-thethimide, medical hormone blockers, has become so easy that ablative surgery is not done with any frequency. The result is that hormone therapy has had a resurgence, particularly in the postmenopausal patient. The use of additive hormonal agents is clearly first-line treatment in postmenopausal metastatic disease.

Progesterone Receptors

The interaction of estrogens and progestins on breast cancer cells is complex, but well studied. Progestins not only affect the growth of breast cancer cells directly, but also modify the effects of estrogen and also control the levels of ER. McGuire et al found that progesterone receptor (PR) is under the control of estrogens acting through the receptor.[33] Thus, it is postulated that the presence of PR would imply an intact ER system and, therefore, be more predictive of hormone responsiveness. In another series of studies Clark et al found that the level of PR appears to be more predictive of prognostic variables, such as disease-free survival, than ER.[34] However, there are problems with quality control, and the ultimate utility of measuring both receptors still remains a research question.

HORMONE ACTION CAN BE BLOCKED BY CHEMICAL ANTAGONISM OR ENZYMATIC BLOCKADE OF SYNTHESIS

Antiestrogens

The synthetic triphenylethylene, tamoxifen, was synthesized in the late 1960s by Harper and Walpole as a possible contraceptive.[35] However, this compound was found to induce ovulation in infertile women. Antiestrogens in the clinic were found to cause regressions of human breast cancer at similar rates to other hormone procedures with less toxicity.[36] Undoubtedly, the introduction of the antiestrogen, tamoxifen, has proven to be a major clinical, as well as scientific advance in the biology of breast cancer management. This agent has become first-line therapy in postmenopausal women and is used widely as an adjunctive treatment alone or in combination with other agents. There are still important issues that need to be resolved in the clinic. One of these is the question of duration of tamoxifen treatment. Based on his animal studies, Jordan suggested that long-term duration may be more beneficial.[37] His studies imply that tamoxifen has a primary cytostatic role rather than a cytocidal effect. Tormey and Jordan have published some preliminary clinical results that support this hypothesis,[38] and long-term controlled trials are in progress.

Another potential issue relates to the possible use of tamoxifen in combination with other agents, both hormonal and cytotoxic. Here tamoxifen has been used along with estrogens to synchronize cells for cyotoxic drugs. Likewise, there are many theoretical and clinical reasons why the antiestrogen might be used in combination with other hormonal drugs. However, the clinical proof of this concept still needs evaluation.

A third interesting possibility of the utility of antiestrogens would be to use tamoxifen as a way to prevent breast cancer. Jordan has shown that long-term administration is capable of inhibiting the induction of tumors in rats treated with a carcinogen.[37] This opens up the clinical possibility of suppressing cancer growth by administering the drug in postmenopausal women who have a high risk of developing breast cancer.[39] This approach has been suggested by several investigators and may shortly reach clinical testing. The issues that need to be resolved include the long-term effects on the uterus, bone calcium, and the increased theoretical risk of heart attacks.

Aminoglutethemide

Aminoglutethimide (AG) originally introduced as an anticonvulsant, has become an important addition to the therapeutic options in the treatment of advanced breast cancer.[40] The observation of adrenal insufficiency in the patients receiving this drug led to laboratory studies to define its mechanism of action. AG blocks a series of hydroxylations in the conversion of cholesterol to adrenal steroids. Other studies demonstrated an inhibition of aromatization reactions that cause a change in the A-ring and result in a block of androgen conversion to estrogens. In postmenopausal women this occurs primarily in the extra-adrenal tissues. To prevent the hypoadrenalism, replacement doses of hydrocortisone are administered. Santen showed that about 30% of patients responded to this therapy. They later showed that treatment with AG was equivalent to adrenalectomy. This development opened up a new area of research and greatly reduced the need to do adrenalectomies and hypophysectomies. Another interesting extension of this research is the use of LHRH inhibitors that can suppress FSH and LH pituitary levels.[41] Clinical trials are underway to study the utility of this approach.[42]

TREATMENT OF METASTASIS

Micrometastases Can Be Eliminated in Some Patients by Adjunctive Hormone or Cytotoxic Treatment

Micrometastasis ($<10^6$ cancer cells) are not detectable clinically. Micrometastases are usually more rapidly growing and should be more sensitive to chemotherapy. The biologic principles in attempting to treat these micrometastases include the understanding that chemotherapy drugs kill by first-order kinetics and that treatment should be started as early as possible. Even a few viable cancer cells can develop into lethal tumors, and cure requires the elimination of the last tumor cell. These prinicples were well worked-out in the laboratory experiments of Schabel.[43] Important concepts were also provided by the work of Martin and his colleagues.[44] The data on treatment of experimental mouse mammary tumors have suggested that treatment affected the spontaneous tumor more than the metastatic nodules. This observation suggested the possibility of tumor heterogeneity. These studies supported the idea that treatment should be instituted right after surgery.

Nissen-Meyer et al were the first investigators to explore the role of adjuvant therapy in a randomized clinical trial.[45] Starting in 1964, 1,026 patients treated at a consortium of Scandanavian hospitals, were randomized to receive cylophosphamide or a placebo for a single six-day postoperative course. The data indicated a 10% increase in survival for the chemotherapy treated groups at 10 years.[46] Nissen-Meyer postulated that the differences that occurred at 10 years were highly likely due to cures rather than delays in recurrences.

In the United States, the NSABP was a major clinical trial group that began to explore the use of adjuvant therapy. The NSABP actually began to emply intraoperative drug use.[47] The early trials of adjuvant therapy were studies empirically designed to test available agents against the early residual cells disseminated at the time of primary therapy. The first trials involved the use of thiotepa, and then later fluorouracil. The thiotepa trial, started in 1968, involved a single cycle of chemotherapy administered at the time of surgery and for two days after surgery. The initial 18-month improvement was reviewed after the 10 years of follow-up and found to persist with 21% fewer treatment failures and more survivors. The benefit was in patients under 45 with four or more positive nodes. A follow-up protocol using fluorouracil and thiotepa was not associated with any benefit to fluorouracil and was associated with increased toxicity. Both of these trials showed a benefit for thiotepa. However, the short-term treatment failed to appreciate the concepts of first order kinetics of tumor cell kill. The concept implies that cells are killed in the same proportion and not the same absolute numbers with each dose. Later trials were designed to use longer-term treatment.[48]

The ECOG-NSABP Study

Prolonged adjuvant chemotherapy first was used in a joint NSABP, Eastern Cooperative Oncology Group (ECOG) and Central Oncology Group (COG) study employing 1-PAM, an oral alkylating agent.[49] It was based on the idea that chemotherapy kills by first-order kinetics and, therefore, prolonged adjuvant therapy should be more effective. The study attempted to use melphalan for 18 months. After 2 years of accessions, a significant improvement in disease-free recurrence was seen in the melphalan arm, particularly for premenopausal women. While a trend was similarly seen in the postmenopausal patients, the difference was not significant. This study was subsequently updated and continued to show a relapse-free survival advantage and a slight survival prolongation for patients with one to three nodes positive, even with 10 years of follow-up. A later report showed that the results were still apparent at 5 and 10 years in the subset of premenopausal patients. However, clearly the use of single agents was not associated with a markedly enhanced cure rate.

The use of combination chemotherapy came about along three separate paths. In the United States the NSABP and ECOG groups developed a sequential schema to use two, then three drugs, and later added tamoxifen. In Italy, in several pioneering studies, Bonadonna et al pursued the three-drug combination cyclophosphamide methotrexate 5-fluorouracil (CMF).[50] The results will be described in detail in other chapters. Basically, an improvement was achieved in the relapse-free survival, with total survival benefits demonstrated in some subsets. However, the marked improvement expected in survival based on data from animal studies clearly was not forthcoming. On the other hand, the use of tamoxifen as an adjuvant in other studies indicated a benefit in postmenopausal patients and opened up the whole question of postsurgical endocrine therapy.[51]

In research we must learn from the apparent failures, as well as our successes. The data imply that further achievements are unlikely to come from increasing the number of cytotoxic drugs or duration of treatment. The studies of Bonadonna et al support the value of 6 months of treatment, rather than 12.[50] The current use of multiple drug therapy seems to be concentrating on high intensity or alternating non–cross-resistant combinations. Other tactics include developing strategies to overcome the resistance of the quiescent cells in the tumor. These involve using reinduction attempts or radiation to sites of high recurrences. Another interesting approach is to use the drug tamoxifen for extended periods of time, namely years.

DRUG RESISTANCE CAN BE OVERCOME BY INCREASING THE INTENSITY OR DOSE RATE OF TREATMENT

The development of chemotherapy is beyond the scope of this review. However, there are certain issues that are relevant to breast cancer. Greenspan was among the first to test the idea of combination chemotherapy clinically.[52] Along with Cooper,[53] these two investigators reported observational studies with high response rates. Others, such as the ECOG, showed the value of combinations against advanced-disease patients as contrasted with single agents.[54] A major improvement in treatment occurred with the introduction of Adriamycin (doxorubicin; Adria Laboratories, Columbus, OH) into the clinical armamentarium.[55] It is of note that the survival gains with combination therapy programs has been modest.

The future of chemotherapy attempts will undoubtedly come as we learn more about mechanisms of resistance and how to overcome them. Attempts at trying to increase the cure rate by increasing the intensity of therapy have been evolving at the University of Wisconsin and other centers. Our strategy has been to maximize the use of effective drugs in advanced-disease patients in an intensive high-dose manner to induce remissions and then to consolidate with radiation the major clinical sites of involvement.[56] Others have tried to sequentially administer hormone and chemotherapy agents to increase the sensitivity of the cells to cytotoxic drugs.[57] A third approach has been to administer ultra high-doses of drugs with autologous marrow replacement.[58] All of these attempts are based on the idea that the cells are developing chemoresistance when the drugs are used at conventional doses and the super high-doses will circumvent the resistance. In addition, Tormey and his colleagues are also adding a component of reinduction that is designed to kill cells that might still be sensitive to the drugs, but have been protected during the high-dose treatment and then escape to start growing again. The failures to increase the cure rate with a variety of manipulations of the various drugs at the standard doses have led clinical investigators down these avenues. The initial results of these studies indicate a high response rate with increased percentages of apparent complete clinical remissions. However, the long-term advantages of this high-dose treatment still need to be determined.

FUTURE

The therapy of breast cancer has evolved in a series of steps based on clinical observations, emphasizing extirpation, or hormonal control. The advent of chemotherapy has added significantly to the long-term control of the disease in patients not responding to hormonal therapies. The understanding of the hormone receptors has also added to the ease of disease control. The virtual elimination of ablative measures has occurred with the introduction of tamoxifen, an antiestrogen, and the adrenal-blocking aromatase-inhibitor, aminoglutethimide. However, the long-term cure of breast cancer remains a challenge. The empirical approach of manipulating drugs and duration of treatment seems to have reached a plateau in outcome measured by survival. The new ideas being tested today are relatively few. These are currently related to intensity or duration of therapy. However, there are new possibilities in the area of monoclonal antibodies to identify early metastatic disease and adding specificity to therapy (Table 2). Likewise, we might affect tumor growth by altering the milieu of growth factors or enhancing the differentiation of neoplastic cells.

The laboratory work with autocrine growth factors is exciting, suggesting an important role in cell growth for these agents, particularly in nonhormonally sensitive cells. Both malignant and normal human breast cells are able to be grown in culture. Studies of these cells are going to be important in defining new avenues of approach.

Another approach might be to develop the concepts of prevention, either primary or secondary. The latter implies early diagnosis through cost-effective screening or primary prevention via antiestrogens or other chemoprevention agents. Clinical astuteness and well-designed critical clinical studies tied into good laboratory correlative projects attempting to dissect out the biology of human cancers need to continue. Progress occurs when we examine carefully, not only those things that work clinically, but also determine why treatments are not effective. It is our lack of knowledge of the biology of human breast cancer that is rate-limiting to our successes. The optimal mix of good clinical research and related key biological experiments in the laboratory will undoubtedly win out.

Table 2. Potential New Concepts in Breast Cancer Management

Increasing the specificity of therapy
Monoclonal antibodies
Growth factor antagonism
Induction of differentiation
Preventing breast cancer
Early detection
Antiestrogens
Chemopreventatives
Interfering with progression and metastasis
Dietary manipulations

CONCLUSION

The evolution of the important concepts of breast cancer management have occurred over the past 100 years, primarily through clinical studies. Until the 1950s, most of the concepts were derived from observational studies by individual practitioners. Since 1950, physicians began to talk and write about changes in the approach to breast cancer, then firmly linked to the Halsted radical mastectomies. It was the results of well-designed clinical trials of the 1960s and 1970s that dramatically altered the approach to primary therapy.

The principles of hormone therapy again were derived from observational studies done by surgeons in the late 19th and early 20th centuries. With the identification of hormones in the 1930s, breast cancer management has increasingly become a medical problem. The ablative surgical procedures such as oophorectomy, adrenalectomy, or hypophysectomy have been replaced with antihormones and enzyme inhibitors. The ability to predict hormone action by measuring the estrogen receptor is a real advance based on laboratory, as well as clinical studies. The development of the principles of chemotherapy in leukemias and lymphomas from the early 1960s were applied to breast cancer by individual investigators in the late 1960s. The concepts of adjuvant therapy evolved primarily from clinical trials. However, the expected outcome has not been as dramatic as one might have anticipated based on laboratory studies. Current approaches involve complex regimens and intensive treatment requiring supportive measures, such as autologous marrow transplantation.

The future of breast cancer management undoubtedly lies in increasing the specificity of the therapy through a variety of novel approaches such as monoclonal antibodies and autocrine growth inhibitors. In addition, early detection, through cost-effective screening, has real potential to decrease mortality. Finally, new laboratory studies point to possible ways of preventing the initiation, promotion, or progression of the cancer. These laboratory studies will undoubtedly lead to future clinical trials aimed at having a major impact on breast cancer mortality.

REFERENCES

1. Folca PJ, Glascock RF, Irvine WT: Studies with Tritium-labeled hexoestrol in advanced breast cancer. Lancet 2:796–798, 1961
2. Auchicloss H: Tumors of the breast, in Christopher F (ed): A Textbook of Surgery. Philadelphia, Saunders, 1942, pp 919–920
3. Halsted WS: The results of radical operations for the cure of cancer of the breast performed at The Johns Hopkins Hospital from June 1889 to January 1894. Johns Hopkins Hosp Rep 4:297, 1895
4. Ravitch MM: Carcinoma of the breast. The place of the Halsted radical mastectomy. Johns Hopkins Med 129:202–211, 1971
5. Fisher B: The surgical dilemma in the primary therapy of invasive breast cancer: A critical appraisal, in Ravitch MM, Julian OC, et al (eds): Current Problems in Surgery. Chicago, Yearbook Medical, 1970, pp 1–53
6. McWhirter R: The value of simple mastectomy and radiotherapy in the treatment of cancer of the breast. Br J Radiol 21:599–610, 1948
7. Crile G: Treatment of breast cancer by local excision. Am J Surg 109:400–403, 1965
8. Mustakallio S: Treatment of breast cancer by tumour extirpation and roentgen therapy instead of radical operation. J Fac Radiol 6:23–26, 1964
9. Fisher B, Slack NH: The number of lymph nodes examined and the prognosis of breast cancer. Surg Gynecol Obstet 131:79, 1970
10. Fisher B: A commentary on the role of the surgeon in primary breast cancer. Breast Cancer Res Treat 1:17–26, 1981
11. Veronesi U, Saccozzi R, Del Vecchio M, et al: Comparing radical mastectomy with quadrantectomy, axillary dissection, and radiotherapy in patients with small cancers of the breast. N Engl J Med 305:6–11, 1981
12. Fisher B, Bauer M, Margolese M, et al: Five years of a randomized clinical trial comparing total mastectomy and segmental mastectomy with or without radiation in the treatment of breast cancer. N Engl J Med 312:665–673, 1985
13. Baclesse F: La Roentgentherapie seule dans le traitment des cancers du sein operables et inoperables. Troisieme rapport presente a L'Asso. Franc de Chirurgie 51 eme Congres Francais de Chrurgie, Paris, 1948, pp 125–155, 1948
14. Calle R, Pilleron JP, Schlienger P, et al: Conservative management of operable breast cancer: Ten years experience at the Foundation Curie. Cancer 42:2045–2053, 1978
15. Harris JR, Botnick L, Bloomer WD, et al: Primary radiation therapy for early breast cancer: The experience at the Joint Center for Radiation Therapy. Int J Radiat Oncol Biol Phys 7:1549–1552, 1981
16. Clark RM, Wilkinson RH, Mahoney LJ, et al: Breast cancer: A 21 year experience with conservative surgery and radiation. Int J Radiat Oncol Biol Phys 8:967–975, 1982
17. Hayward J: Hormones and Human Breast Cancer. London, Heineman, 1970
18. Beatson GT: On the treatment of inoperable cases of the mamma. Suggestion for a new method of treatment with illustrative cases. Lancet 2:104–107, 162–167, 1896
19. Boyd S: On oopherectomy in cancer of the breast. Br Med J 2:1161, 1900
20. Atkins H: Carcinoma of the breast. Ann R Coll Surg 38:133, 1966
21. Huggins C, Bergenstal DM: Inhibition of human mammary and prostate cancers by adrenalectomy. Cancer Res 12:134–141, 1952
22. Nissen-Meyer R: Castration as part of the primary treatment for operable female breast cancer: A statistical evaluation of clinical results. Acta Radiol 249:11–12, 1969 (suppl)
23. Cole MP: The place of radiotherapy in the management of early breast cancer. A report of two clinical trials. Br J Surg 51:216–220, 1964
24. Burn I: Endocrine therapy—ablative surgery, in Adtkins A (ed): The Treatment of Breast Cancer. Baltimore, University Park, 1974, pp 87–112
25. Haddow A, Robinson AM: Influence of certain polcyclic hydrocarbons on the growth of rate of transplantable tumours. Proc R Soc Lond. (Biol) 122:442, 1937
26. Badger GM, Elson LA, Haddow A, et al: The inhibition of growth by chemical compounds. Proc R Soc (London) 130:255, 1942
27. Haddow A, Watkinson JM, Paterson E, et al: Influence of synthetic oestrogen upon advanced malignant disease. Br Med J 2:393–398, 1944
28. Lacassagne A, Raynaud A: Sur le mechanisme d'une

action preventive de la testosterone sur le cancer mammaire de la souris. CR Soc Biol (Paris) 131:586–588, 1939

29. Nathanson IT, Andervont HB: Effect of testosterone propionate on development and growth of mammary carcinoma in female mice. Proc Soc Exp Biol Med 40:421–427, 1939

30. Loeser A: Mammary carcinoma: Response to implantation of male hormone and progesterone. Lancet 2:698–700, 1941

31. Jensen EV, Block GE, Smith S, et al: Hormonal dependancy of breast cancer, in, Griem ML, Jensen EV, Wissler RW (eds): Recent Results in Cancer Research: Breast Cancer: A Challenging Problem. New York, Springer-Verlag, 1973, pp 55–62

32. McGuire WL, Carbone PP, Sears ME, et al: Estrogen receptors in human breast cancer: An overview, in Carbone PP, Volmer EP (ed): Estrogen Receptors in Breast Cancer. New York, Raven, 1975, pp 1–8

33. McGuire WL, Horwitz KB, Pearson OH, et al: Current status of estrogen and progesterone receptors in breast cancer. Cancer 39:2934–2947, 1977

34. Clark GM, McGuire WL, Hubay CA, et al: Progesterone receptors as a prognostic factor in stage II breast cancer. N Engl J Med 309:1343–1347, 1983

35. Harper MJK, Walpole AL: Contrasting endocrine activities of cis and trans isomers in a series of substituted triphenyl ethylenes. Nature 212:87, 1966

36. Furr BJA, Jordan VC: The pharmacology and clinical uses of tamoxifen. Pharmacol Ther 25:127–205, 1984

37. Jordan VC: Laboratory studies to develop general principles for the adjuvant treatment of breast cancer with antiestrogens: Problems and potential for future clinical applications. Breast Cancer Res Treat 3:73–86, 1983 (suppl 1)

38. Tormey DC, Jordan VC: Long-term tamoxifen adjuvant therapy in node-positive breast cancer: A metabolic and pilot clinical study. Breast Cancer Res Treat 4:297–302, 1984

39. Carbone PP: Breast cancer 1984: Role of tamoxifen, in Jordan VC (ed): Estrogen/Antiestrogen Action and Breast Cancer Therapy. Madison, University of Wisconsin, 1986 (in press)

40. Santen RJ: Suppression of estrogens with aminoglutethimide and hydrocortisone (medical adrenalectomy) as treatment for advanced breast cancer. Breast Cancer Res Treat 1:183–202, 1981

41. Matnard PV, Nicholson RI: Effects of high doses of a new series of luteinizing hormone-releasing hormone analogues in intact female rats. Br J Cancer 39:274–379, 1979

42. Harvey HA, Lipton A, Max DT, et al: Medical castration produced by the GnRH analogue leuprolide to treat metastatic breast cancer. J Clin Oncol 3:1068–1072, 1985

43. Schabel FM: Concepts for treatment of micrometastases developed in murine systems. Am J Roentgenol Rad Ther Nucl Med 126:500–511, 1976

44. Martin DS: An appraisal of chemotherapy as an adjuvant to surgery for cancer. Am J Surg 97:685, 1959

45. Nissen-Meyer R, Kjellgren K, Malmio K, et al: Surgical adjuvant chemotherapy. Results with one short course with cyclophosphamide after mastectomy for breast cancer. Cancer 41:2088–2098, 1978

46. Nissen-Meyer R: Comparison effects obtained with various types of adjuvant treatments—A commentary. Cancer Treat Rev 6:101–104, 1979 (suppl)

47. Fisher B, Slack N, Katrych D, et al: Ten year follow-up results of patients with carcinoma of the breast in a co-operative clinical trial evaluating surgical adjuvant chemotherapy. Surg Gynecol Obstet 140:528–534, 1975

48. Carbone PP: Adjuvant therapy of breast cancer 1971–1981. Ten years of progress. Breast Cancer Res Treat 2:75–84, 1982

49. Fisher B, Carbone P, Economou SG, et al: L-Phenylalanine mustard (L-PAM) in the management of primary breast cancer. A report of early findings. N Engl J Med 292:117–122, 1975

50. Bonadonna G, Rossi A, Valagussa P: Adjuvant CMF chemotherapy in inoperable breast cancer: Ten years later. World J Surg 9:707–713, 1985

51. Rose C, Thorpe SM, Anderson KW, et al: Beneficial effect of adjuvant tamoxifen therapy in primary breast cancer patients with high oestrogen receptor values. Lancet 1:16–19, 1985

52. Greenspan EM: Regression of metastatic hepatomegaly from mammary carcinoma. Cytotoxic combination chemotherapy with 5-FU. NY State J Med 64:2442–2449, 1964

53. Cooper RG: Combination chemotherapy in hormone resistant breast cancer. Proc Am Assoc Cancer Res 10:15, 1969 (abstr)

54. Canellos GP, Pocock SJ, Taylor SG III, et al: Combination chemotherapy for metastatic breast carcinoma. Prospective comparison of multiple drug therapy with L-phenylalanine mustard. Cancer 38:1882–1886, 1976

55. Tormey DC: Adriamycin (NSC-123127) in breast cancer: An overview of studies. Cancer Chemother Rep 6:319–327, 1975

56. Tormey DC, Kline JC, Palta M, et al: Short term high density systemic therapy for metastatic breast cancer. Breast Cancer Treat 5:177–188, 1985

57. Allegra JC, Woodcock TM, Richman Sp, et al: A phase II trial of tamoxifen, premarin, methotrexate and 5-fluorouracil in metastatic breast cancer. Breast Cancer Res Treat 2:93–99, 1982

58. Eder JP, Antman KH, Elias A, et al: High dose combined alkylating agents (HDCA) with autologous bone marrow transplantation (ABMT) in metastatic breast cancer. Breast Cancer Treat 6:286, 1985 (abstr)

Conservative Surgery: The American Experience

Bernard Fisher and Norman Wolmark

SEVERAL DECADES AGO, as a result of the efforts of a few individuals who deviated from the use of the Halsted radical mastectomy, conservative breast cancer treatment began to be infrequently used in the United States and Canada. Surgeons can take little credit for the departure from tradition. But for several exceptions, radiation therapists were responsible. Anecdotal descriptions of personal experiences with breast conservation in America began to be published in the mid-1960s and have continued to the present time. The few surgeons who attracted attention by their writings were Crile et al,[1-4] Cope et al,[5] and Adair.[6] Reports by Peters,[7-9] Prosnitz et al,[10] Montague et al,[11] and Hellman et al[12-16] are representative of the activities of American radiation therapists who were early advocates of breast preservation. They promulgated the thesis of "primary treatment of breast cancer by radiation"—a misleading description of therapy because the radiation was administered following tumor excision. The rationale used by those surgeons and radiation therapists to justify use of the conservative approach is not clear from their reports. What is most certain is that no clear biological principle prompted their efforts. Breast preservation was used either because patients refused to have a recommended radical mastectomy, were elderly and infirm, had medical contraindications to more extensive surgery, or had locally advanced disease unsuitable for mastectomy. Those publications of retrospectively collected information from small heterogenous patient populations are by today's standards inadequate to permit appropriate evaluation. Consequently, as a result of those experiential reports, important questions regarding the efficacy of breast conserving procedures were unanswered. The reports did, however, demonstrate that survival free of disease for many years was possible in at least some patients after limited surgery and radiation therapy; whether to the same extent as following more radical therapy continued to remain uncertain.

The introduction of prospective randomized controlled clinical trials represents a major medical advance of the last 50 years. Such trials supply more definitive data regarding the efficacy of treatments than do past anecdotal reports. The only randomized trials in America from which data have been provided to determine the efficacy of alternative local and regional treatments of primary breast cancer are the two studies carried out by the National Surgical Adjuvant Breast and Bowel Project (NSABP). Those investigations have attempted to resolve existing controversies relative to the local/regional management of primary breast cancer and simultaneoulsy to redefine the biological basis for cancer surgery.

The first study (protocol B-04) was begun in 1971 to determine whether the outcome of patients with clinically negative axillary nodes treated by either total mastectomy followed by delayed axillary dissection in those who subsequently had positive axillary nodes, total mastectomy followed by postoperative regional irradiation, or total mastectomy was equivalent. For patients with clinically positive nodes, the objective was to ascertain whether radical mastectomy and total mastectomy followed by radiation produced an equivalent outcome.

When early findings from that trial[3,4] failed to indicate that patients treated by total mastectomy without axillary node dissection were at higher risk of distant disease or death than were those undergoing a Halsted radical mastectomy, it was considered justifiable to begin a new study (protocol B-06) to evaluate the worth of breast conservation by local tumor excision with or without breast radiation. Beginning in 1976, patients were randomly assigned to total mastectomy, segmental mastectomy, or segmental mastectomy followed by breast irradiation. Women in all treatment groups had an axillary dissection, and those with positive nodes received

From the National Surgical Adjuvant Breast and Bowel Project (NSABP).

Supported by Public Health Service Grants from the National Cancer Institute (NCI-U10-CA-12017 and NCI-U10-CA-34211) and by a grant from the American Cancer Society (ACS-RC-13).

Address reprint requests to NSABP Headquarters, Room 914 Scaife Hall, 3550 Terrace St, Pittsburgh, PA 15261.

0093-7754/86/1304-0006$05.00/0

chemotherapy. The operation used lumpectomy — abandoned conventional concepts of cancer surgery by removing only enough breast tissue to ensure that margins of the resected surgical specimens were free of tumor. The study was designed to determine the effectiveness of segmental mastectomy for breast preservation, whether radiation therapy reduced the incidence of tumor in the ipsilateral breast after segmental mastectomy, whether breast conservation resulted in a higher risk of distant disease and death than does mastectomy, and the clinical significance of multicentricity.

The terms "segmental mastectomy" and "lumpectomy" are used interchangeably in this presentation to describe the operation used. Neither appellation is entirely satisfactory. The former (segmental mastectomy) is misleading because there are no true segments of breast such as in other anatomic structures, eg, the lung, while the latter (lumpectomy) is inelegant and imprecise. The term "tylectomy," also used, is likewise uninformative. The same may be said for "local excision" or "tumorectomy." Those terms fail to indicate whether the primary tumor has been completely or partially removed and whether an attempt was made to remove the tumor so that the specimen margins were tumor free. In no circumstance was a "quadrantectomy" used.

We have recently published findings from the two NSABP randomized trials, ie, the 10 year results of that (B-04) which compared radical mastectomy with lesser breast removing procedures[17] and the 5 year results from the B-06 trials that compared the lumpectomy and axillary dissection with and without breast radiation to total mastectomy and axillary dissection.[18]

This presentation is limited to a brief overview of the American experience with breast conservation derived from prospective randomized clinical trials. In the United States and Canada that experience entirely relates to the NSABP B-06 study. Attention will therefore be given to the 5 year results from that segmental mastectomy trial derived from a recent update (November 30, 1985) that provides a follow-up time that is 17 months longer than that used in the original publication.[18] The data are derived from patients having a mean follow-up time of 56 months. For information regarding selection of patients, study design, statistical analyses, and evidence of the comparability of patients among treatment groups within each study, the reader is referred to the original publication.

CONCERNING THE NSABP TRIAL

Protocol Design

To ensure credibility of the findings from this trial, a sophisticated experimental design was necessary (Fig 1). The protocol required that, if the margins of specimens removed by segmental mastectomy were not tumor free, a subsequent mastectomy be performed. It also mandated that should tumor occur in the operated breast subsequent to segmental mastectomy, a total mastectomy be carried out. Such a breast tumor occurrence (reoccurrence) was not considered to be a "treatment failure," but because the breast was removed, the patient was regarded as having a "cosmetic failure". It also must be emphasized that when determining event-free survival (EFS), distant disease-free survival (DDFS) and survival (S) in the three treatment groups, it was necessary that all patients in each group be included—even those in the two segmental mastectomy groups who had margins involved and

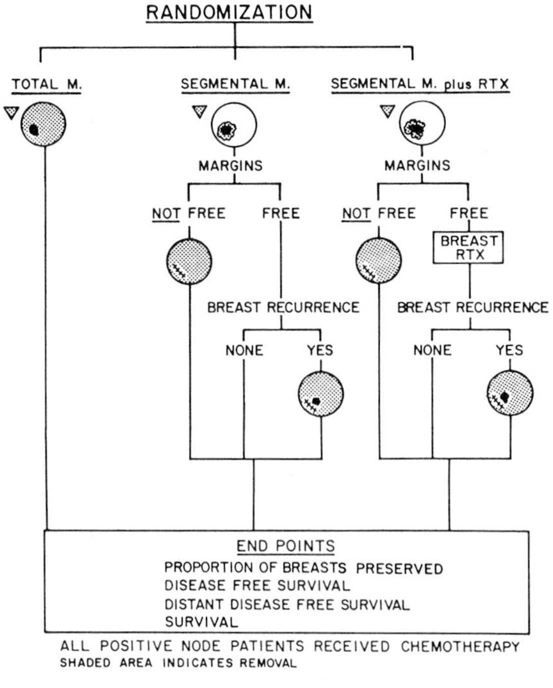

Fig 1. Treatment strategy NSABP B-06.

consequently had a mastectomy. Margin involvement was found to be associated with tumors having a poorer prognosis than tumors associated with free margins. Consequently, to have eliminated those patients from the segmental mastectomy groups would have created a bias because patients with a similarly poor prognosis existed in the total mastectomy group. Their elimination would have resulted in segmental mastectomy patients appearing to have a much more favorable outcome than those who had total mastectomy.

Tumor Specimen Margins

Positive margins were reported in 10% of all patients after lumpectomy, approximately the same incidence of each of the two groups (10% in the lumpectomy alone group and 9.5% in the group that received radiation). Those with larger tumors, positive nodes, and centrally located tumors were more apt to have margin involvement.

The original protocol design required that it be demonstrated pathologically that specimen margins were free of tumor, ie, that tumor was not transected so that a portion remained in the patient. When a previous biopsy was carried out and no attention was paid to specimen margins by the initial surgeon, it was obligatory that at the time of axillary node dissection a reresection be performed to ensure free margins. Thus, it is to be emphasized that the results obtained in the NSABP lumpectomy study relate to patients who, as far as could be reasonably determined, had free specimen margins. Since publication of our findings, it is frequently asked whether a mastectomy really needs to be done if margins are involved with tumor. There are currently no data to resolve that question. Because of the infrequency of margin involvement in a properly carried out lumpectomy in which attention is paid to the obtaining of free margins, it may be difficult to obtain an answer resulting from quantitative information. While in our publication (based on findings by institutional pathologists) we reported 10% margin involvement, another review of all pathologic specimens by the NSABP headquarters pathologist indicates that tumor was present at the time of resection in only about 7% of cases. Some institutional pathologists were reluctant to call margins free if a tumor was only several millimeters or even a greater distance from the specimen edge.

Perhaps radiation therapy will be adequate to eliminate microscopic residual tumor, obviating the need for mastectomy, and perhaps as noted for some head and neck cancers[19] and as has long been appreciated with basal cell carcinoma of the skin, involvement of specimen margins may not universally signify that reoccurrence will occur. It continues to remain NSABP policy, however, that all patients treated by lumpectomy have tumor-free specimen margins. It is also our opinion that in no circumstance is there justification for surgeons to not make every effort to obtain tumor-free margins. Nor, is it justifiable for a radiation oncologist to dismiss the importance of free margins because "radiation therapy will take care of it." It is to be emphasized that abandonment of Halstedian principles of cancer surgery does not imply that sloppy surgery can be condoned. We have also advocated that every breast biopsy be carried out as if a lumpectomy were being done, ie, that specimen margins be clear of tumor.[20] The NSABP is collecting information from patients who, despite appropriate lumpectomy by surgeons who make every effort to obtain tumor-free margins, have margin involvement and are treated by breast radiation instead of mastectomy. That effort should provide information regarding the effectiveness of such an approach for local/regional tumor control when margins are involved.

Tumor Reoccurrence in the Operated Breast

Findings demonstrating the probability of patients remaining free of tumor in the ipsilateral breast after 5 years support the worth of radiation (Fig 2). Whereas 93% of those treated by segmental mastectomy and radiation were free of tumor, only 68% of those having a lumpectomy and no radiation were tumor free. That a higher percentage of positive-node patients treated by segmental mastectomy and radiation (96%) remained free of tumor than did similarly treated negative-node patients (91%) is of special interest because the former (those with positive nodes) received adjuvant chemotherapy in addition to radiation therapy.

The question is often asked whether mastectomy is necessary for breast tumor reoccurrence or whether "relumpectomy" could be used. Just

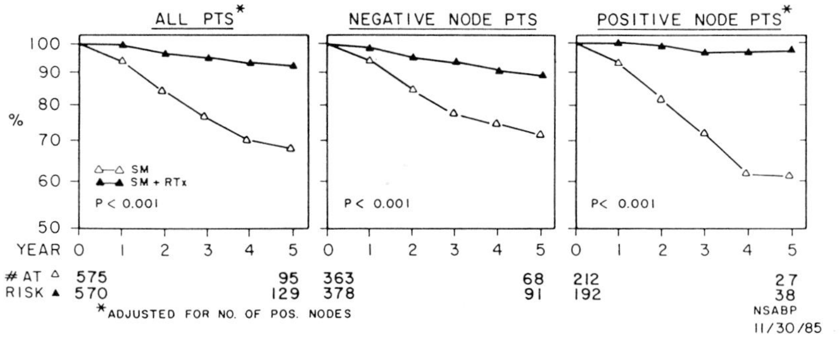

Fig 2. Breast recurrence following segmental mastectomy (lumpectomy) with and without breast radiation.

as with margin involvement, no data exist to answer the question. Because the reoccurrence rate at 5 years was only 7% overall following segmental mastectomy plus radiation (4% in those with positive nodes), the number of patients and follow-up time necessary to obtain such information makes such a study impossible using such patients. The high incidence of reoccurrence in the lumpectomy group without radiation precludes using that group of patients to study the issue.

A recent pathologic review of breast tumor reoccurrences revealed that 95% involved the mammary parenchyma and the remaining 5% were in the skin and/or nipple of the breast.[21] All but one of the latter appeared within the scar of the prior lumpectomy. All reoccurrences were in or close to the quadrant of the removed tumor. In 14% it not only involved the same quadrant but was more diffuse within the breast extending to remote areas. This type was characterized pathologically by marked intralymphatic extension as well as involvement of the overlying skin and/or nipple after the fashion of so-called "inflammatory" or "occult inflammatory" breast cancer. The reoccurrences noted in the skin and/or nipple only were also pathologically characterized by intralymphatic involvement in the majority of instances. These two forms appear to reflect the localized growth of highly aggressive invasive breast cancers.

Of interest was the observation that 10% of the breast reoccurrences were noninvasive intraductal (DCIS). In 86% of the reoccurrences demonstrating tumor invasion, the histologic types and grades of the reoccurrences were identical to those in the initial lesion. In 14% the histologic type was dissimilar. In 9% of the latter, the recurrent cancer could have represented one portion of a combination tumor type. Contingency table analyses disclosed that reoccurrences in the lumpectomy group that received breast radiation were related only to intralymphatic extension in the primary tumor ($P = .07$). In the group treated by lumpectomy alone (no radiation), those having tumors ≥2.0 cm ($P = .02$), poor histologic grade ($P = .01$), poor nuclear grade ($P = .002$) and/or intralymphatic extension ($P = .004$) were associated with breast reoccurrence. Disappointing in view of the meticulous follow-up program used was the observation that the mean largest diameters of the initial and recurrent cancers were 2.5 ± 1.3 cm and 2.4 ± 1.4 cm, respectively. Our experience differs from that of Schnitt et al[22–24] who related reoccurrence following biopsy and irradiation of breast cancer to anaplasia and a marked or moderate intraductal component of the initial

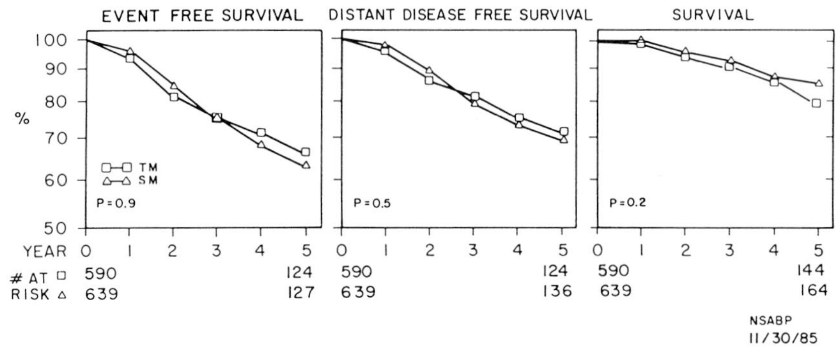

Fig 3. Total mastectomy *v* segmental mastectomy (lumpectomy)—all patients (adjusted for number of positive nodes).

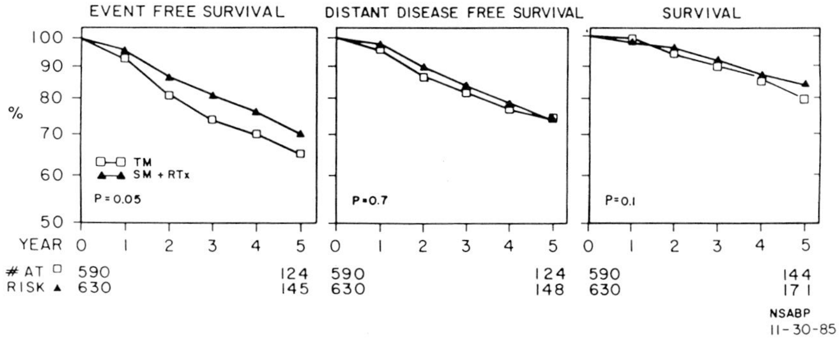

Fig 4. Total mastectomy *v* segmental mastectomy (lumpectomy) plus breast radiation—all patients (adjusted for number of positive nodes).

cancer. Our failure to recognize this association may be due to our frequent (44%) observation of an intraductal component at the periphery of all invasive breast cancers. It is our conclusion that there are no pathologic discriminants that contraindicate lumpectomy and radiation. The failure to as yet discern any adverse effect of local reoccurrence on survival indicates to us that some of these events, particularly those mimicking occult inflammatory cancer represent local manifestations of highly aggressive cancers whose prognosis would not be influenced by any form of local control.

Event-Free Survival, Distant Disease-Free Survival and Survival

Life table analyses revealed that at the end of 5 years of follow-up there was no significant difference in EFS, DDFS, or S (Fig 3) between patients treated by total mastectomy and axillary dissection and those subjected to segmental mastectomy and axillary dissection without breast radiation. When breast conservation followed by breast radiation and axillary dissection was compared with the total mastectomy group, there was a better EFS ($P = .05$) in the lumpectomy radiation group (Fig 4). There was no significant difference between the two groups, however, in DDFS or S. When a comparison was made between the two segmental mastectomy groups, ie, those with and without breast radiation, the EFS was significantly better ($P = .02$) in the group receiving radiation (Fig 5). DDFS and S were not significantly different.

Operative Considerations

The following describes the surgical technique used by NSABP investigators. It is the procedure that we recommend as the result of our experience with the 1,269 patients having segmental mastectomy.

Incisions and Skin Removal

We use curvilinear incisions no matter where in the breast a lesion occurs (Fig 6). Such incisions should be used even when tumors are in the upper-outer quadrant of the breast near the axilla. A separate incision for the axillary dissection is almost always made even when a tumor is in that portion of the breast. To achieve the best cosmetic results, radial incisions are *not* recommended. Some NSABP surgeons prefer radial incisions for lesions at the 6 o'clock position in the breast. Our own preference is for curvilinear

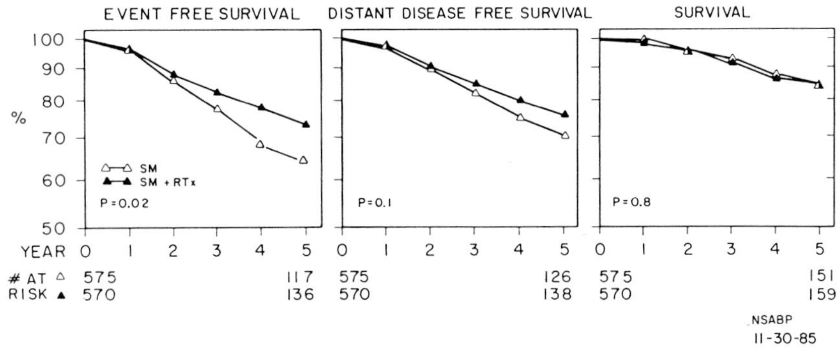

Fig 5. Segmental mastectomy (lumpectomy) *v* segmental mastectomy (lumpectomy) plus breast radiation—all patients (adjusted for number of positive nodes).

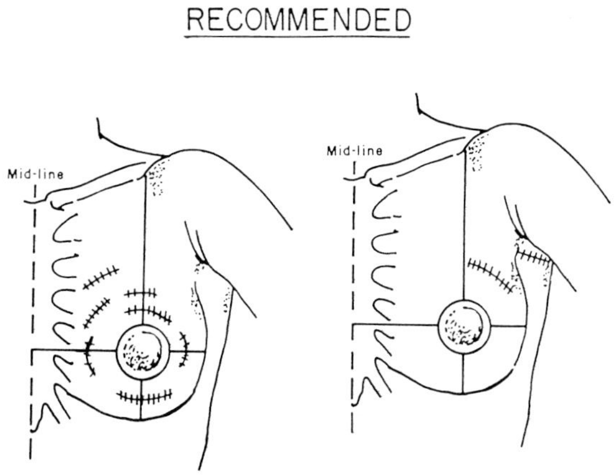

Fig 6. Recommended incisions.

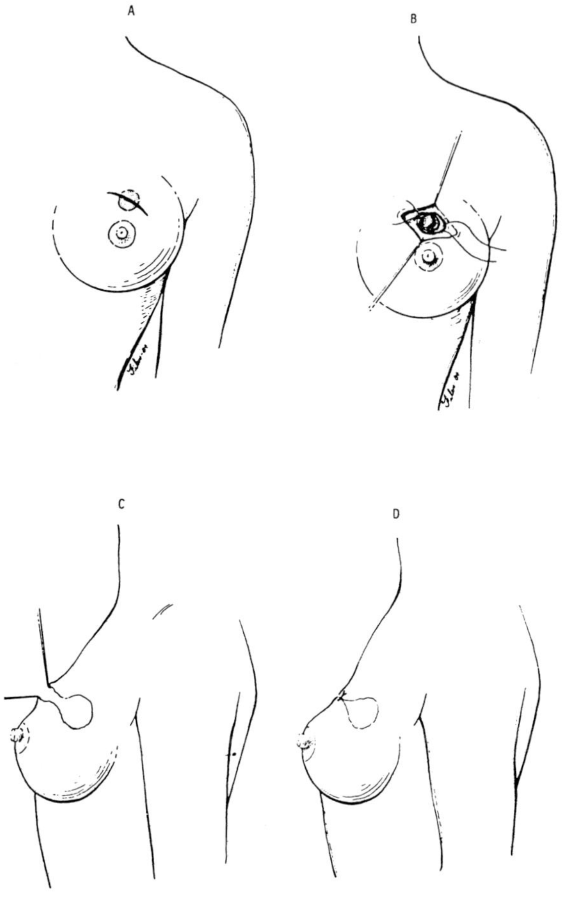

Fig 7. Technique of lumpectomy.

incisions even when tumors are in that location. To perform a satisfactory lumpectomy, it is essential that the incision be placed directly over the tumor (Fig 7A). The use of a circumareolar incision for removal of a lesion that is not in proximity to the areola is inappropriate. Reexcision of the tumor site to obtain tumor-free specimen margins is difficult and often impossible when such an incision is made.

Because lumpectomy is not a Halstedian operation and patients with tumor involving the overlying skin are apt not to be candidates for the operation, skin removal is not a requisite of the operation. We do not ordinarily remove skin because the quality of cosmesis is inversely related to the amount of skin removed. If a prior biopsy is performed, skin encompassing the biopsy is removed when doing the lumpectomy.

Tumor Removal

The tumor is removed so that it is completely enveloped in normal fat and/or breast tissue. This does not necessitate removal of a predefined amount of normal tissue around the lesion. The aim is to remove just the amount that is adequate to achieve specimen margins grossly free of tumor (Fig 7B). A special point to be emphasized is that when the excision is being carried out, skin edges are not undermined, ie, thin skin flaps are not desirable. Undermining of skin, just as with skin removal, results in an unfavorable cosmetic result. No special effort is made to include pectoral fascia in the specimen unless the lesion lies in close proximity to it. Our practice is to tag the specimen before it leaves the operating field (Fig 7B). Any system for doing this may be used. A long silk suture is use by us to mark the lateral surface, a short suture to identify the medial aspect of the specimen and two short tags close together to identify the top of the specimen, ie, the anterior or superficial margin. Additional tags may be placed to designate the superior or cephalad margin and the inferior or caudal border. The pathologist's role is to confirm or establish the diagnosis of cancer, aid the surgeon in deciding intraoperatively whether the specimen margins are *grossly* free of tumor, and take an aliquot of tumor for estrogen and progesterone receptor analyses. Rarely will there be a subsequent report of microscopic tumor at margins that have been reported to be grossly free. Almost never do we carry out frozen sections to determine if the margins are free of tumor. If on gross examination, tumor is found to be close to a portion of the resected tissue margin, the resection in that area is extended by removal of an additional rim of breast tissue and fat. The new true margin of the area that was considered to be close is identified for the pathologist by placing methylene blue on the surface of the reresected portion of tissue that is farthest from the initial resection site.

To achieve optimal cosmesis, after meticulous hemostasis of the biopsy site, no attempt is made to obliterate the dead space in the breast by approximating breast tissue or fat, nor is a drain of any type placed in the wound (Fig 7C). Within the past year we have routinely approximated the subcuticular fat (not the deep fat) by the use of interrupted fine stitches. This has resulted in an improvement in cosmesis. The skin is then carefully approximated by the use of a fine continuous subcuticular suture (Fig 7D).

Lumpectomy for Subareolar Tumors or for Tumors >4 cm

The aim of the NSABP lumpectomy protocol was to carry out the operation so that a normal-appearing breast resulted in all patients. Since subareolar tumors or those close to that position might require removal of the nipple and areola to ensure tumor-free specimen margins with a resultant cosmetic defect, lesions in such a location were considered not to be amenable to lumpectomy. When tumor-free margins could be obtained without removal of the nipple and areola and a satisfactory cosmetic result obtained, patients with subareolar or periareolar lesions were considered candidates for the operation. Particularly was this the case in women with large breasts and posteriorly located tumors. Recent experience has indicated that the removal of subareolar lesions with the nipple and areola can be carried out with a satisfactory cosmetic result. The breast mound resulting is more normal than that achieved by breast reconstruction following total mastectomy.

Following publication of the results of our trial, the impression was erroneously created that lumpectomy was only appropriate for patients with very small tumors. This occurred despite the fact it was clearly stated that women with tumors ≤4 cm were eligible. That tumor size was originally selected because it had been demonstrated by us that the incidence of multicentricity was apt to be greater in tumors >4 cm. We have recently liberalized the tumor size requirement so as to make patients with tumors ≤5 cm eligible for our present protocols, providing they have an ample-sized breast so that a favorable cosmetic result can be obtained. Thus, patients with clinical stage I and II tumors are eligible for lumpectomy regardless of their location. It has long been our opinion that, when technically feasible, women with larger tumors and/or clinically positive nodes are better served by lumpectomy because they are at such great risk for the development of distant metastases and death regardless of what operation is performed.

Axillary Dissection

Axillary "sampling" as a substitute for axillary dissection is not recommended. The purpose of an axillary dissection is to achieve local/regional disease control and to use the information relative to nodal involvement for determining prognosis and for staging relative to the use of adjuvant chemotherapy. We have demonstrated that the qualitative status of axillary lymph node involvement, ie, either positive or negative, may be accurately determined by examining relatively few nodes. For accurately determining the number of nodes involved, a more complete dissection is required.[25] Since patient outcome is significantly related to the number of positive nodes present, ie, one to three, four to nine, ≥10, a sufficient number must be obtained to quantitate patient prognosis more accurately.[26] In all NSABP breast protocols, an axillary dissection includes nodes from at least axillary levels I and II. While the surgical site in the breast is not drained, a drain in the axilla is present for several postoperative days.

Comments Regarding Radiation Therapy

Radiation used by the NSABP in protocol B-06 was aimed at eliminating occult tumor foci remaining in the ipsilateral breast. The dose level used in the NSABP trial was that which was considered to be cancericidal and not likely to produce distortion and fibrosis of the breast or other undesirable sequelae. The efficacy of the dose used relative to those requirements has been met as is indicated by the findings from the study.[18] The marked reduction in breast occurrence following radiation, the failure to observe undesirable cosmetic sequelae, and the absence of complications such as fractures of ribs and pneumonitis that have been reported by others attests to the propriety of the techniques of radiation administered.

The intent of the radiation therapy was to treat the skin, breast tissue, muscle, lymphatics, and entire scar of the breast. No attempt was made to include axillary, supraclavicular, interpectoral, and internal mammary lymph nodes. Since the latter lie at the medial edge of the treatment field, they were sometimes either partially or wholly included. No special attempt was made to exclude them because that would interfere with irradiation of the entirety of the breast. Our findings over the years indicate no advantage for axillary radiation when an axillary dissection has been carried out and radiation of the internal mammary nodes has resulted in no survival benefit in any of the NSABP trials.

When segmental mastectomy and axillary dissection were performed through separate incisions, if the scar of the axillary dissection was extrinsic to the breast, no irradiation was directed to that scar. If the axillary dissection scar was in continuity with that of the segmental mastectomy, no special attempt was made to irradiate that portion of the scar that was beyond the breast tissue.

Radiation therapy was initiated during the time in which healing of the surgical incision was taking place, ie, about ten to 14 days following surgery. However, when certain adjuvant chemotherapy regimens are used, radiation therapy may be postponed until one or more courses of chemotherapy have been administered. A minimum dose of 5,000 rad was administered. The dose was given at a rate of 1,000 rad per week (daily increments of 200 rad per day, 5 days per week). Dry desquamation with pigmentation and/or erythema at the end of treatment were considered desirable; limited patches of moist desquamation were acceptable. Extensive areas of moist desquamation were avoided.

The worth of radiation therapy following lumpectomy has been demonstrated by our findings. Of greatest importance is the fact that those results were achieved using radiation therapy that did not include the use of radiation boosts, either external beam or interstitial implants. Since our incidence of breast reoccurrence approximated that observed by proponents of such additive therapy, it would seem that the need for a radiation boost to the excision site is not necessary when attention is paid to specimen margins. The size of the patient population that would be required to conduct a clinical trial for the evaluation of boost versus no boost or between external beam boost and boost by interstitial implant makes such an undertaking almost impossible. Moreover, considering such a trial a high priority might be questioned. We are currently evaluating our data with respect to patient and tumor characteristics associated with tumor reoccurrence following radiation in an attempt to indicate which patients might benefit from a boost. If despite our findings indicating the lack of need for a boost there are circumstances in which the radiation therapist would feel more comfortable using one, in view of the need for additional hospitalization, morbidity, imprecision of the radiation dose delivered, and lack of data demonstrating its superiority, an external beam boost would seem appropriate.

CONCLUSION

Findings from the American randomized clinical trial—NSABP Protocol B-06—continue to indicate, as previously reported, that segmental mastectomy (lumpectomy) followed by breast irradiation in all patients and adjuvant chemotherapy in women with positive nodes is appropriate therapy for stage I and II breast tumors. Despite continued effort, it has as yet not been possible to define a subset of lumpectomy patients who would not need to receive breast radiation. Similarly, it has not been possible to determine subsets of stage I and II patients who are *not* candidates for breast conservation. We continue to emphasize that surgeons make every effort to ensure that resected specimen margins are not involved with tumor. When margins are free the overall reoccurrence of tumor following lumpectomy and breast radiation without the use of any boost, external beam or interstitial, is only 7% through 5 years. Moreover, there continues to be no significant difference in DDFS or S between patients subjected to lumpectomy with or without breast radiation and axillary dissection and total mastectomy with axillary dissection. To the present time, there is no evidence that multicentricity is a clinical problem following lumpectomy because no breast reoccurrence in either of the lumpectomy groups has as yet appeared in a breast quadrant other than that which contained the primary tumor.

REFERENCES

1. Crile G Jr: Treatment of breast cancer by local excision. Am J Surg 109:400–403, 1965
2. Crile G Jr, Hoerr SO: Results of treatment of carcinoma of the breast by local excision. Surg Gynecol Obstet 132:780–782, 1971
3. Crile G Jr, Esselstyn CB Jr, Hermann RE, et al: Partial mastectomy for carcinoma of the breast. Surg Gynecol Obstet 136:929–933, 1973
4. Crile G Jr, Cooperman A, Esselstyn CB Jr, et al: Results of partial mastectomy in 173 patients followed for from five to ten years. Surg Gynecol Obstet 150:563–566, 1980
5. Cope O, Wang CA, Chu A, et al: Limited surgical excision as the basis of a comprehensive therapy for cancer of the breast. Am J Surg 132:400–406, 1976
6. Adair FE: The role of surgery and irradiation in cancer of the breast. N Engl J Med 121:553–560, 1943
7. Peters MV: Wedge resection and irradiation, an effective treatment in early breast cancer. JAMA 200:134–135, 1967
8. Peters MV: Cutting the "Gordian Knot" in early breast cancer. Ann R Coll Phys Surg Can 8:186–192, 1975
9. Peters MV: Wedge resection with or without radiation in early breast cancer. Int J Radiat Oncol 2:1151–1156, 1977
10. Prosnitz LR, Goldenberg IS, Packard RA, et al: Radiation therapy as initial treatment for early stage cancer of the breast without mastectomy. Cancer 39:917–923, 1977
11. Montague ED, Guiterrez AE, Barker JL, et al: Conservative surgery and irradiation for the treatment of favorable breast cancer. Cancer 43:1058–1061, 1979
12. Weber E, Hellman S: Radiation as primary treatment for local control of breast carcinoma. A progress report. JAMA 234:608–611, 1975
13. Levene MBF, Harris JR, Hellman S: Treatment of carcinoma of the breast by radiation therapy. Cancer 39:2840–2845, 1977
14. Harris JR, Levene MR, Hellman S: Results of treating stage I and II carcinoma of the breast with primary radiation therapy. Cancer Treat Rep 62:985–991, 1978
15. Harris JR, Botnick L, Bloomer WD, et al: Primary radiation therapy for early breast cancer: The experience at the joint center for radiation therapy. Int J Radiat Oncol Biol Phys 7:1549–1552, 1981
16. Harris JR, Hellman S: Primary radiation therapy for early breast cancer. Cancer 52:2547–2552, 1983
17. Fisher B, Redmond C, Fisher ER, et al: Ten year results of a randomized clinical trial comparing radical mastectomy and total mastectomy with or without radiation N Engl J Med 312:674–681, 1985
18. Fisher B, Bauer M, Margolese R, et al: Five year results of a randomized clinical trial comparing total mastectomy and segmental mastectomy with or without radiation in the treatment of breast cancer. N Engl J Med 312:665–673, 1985
19. Bauer WC, Lesinski SG, Ogura JH: The significance of positive margins in hemilaryngectomy specimens. Laryngoscope 85:1–13, 1985
20. Fisher B: Reappraisal of breast biopsy prompted by the use of lumpectomy: A position paper on surgical strategy. JAMA 253:3585–3588, 1985
21. Fisher ER, Sass R, Fisher B, et al: Pathologic findings from the national surgical adjuvant breast project (protocol 6). II. Relation of local breast recurrence to multicentricity. Cancer 57:1717–1724, 1986
22. Schnitt SJ, Connolly JL, Harris JR, et al: Pathologic predictors of early local recurrence in stage I and II breast cancer treated by primary radiation therapy. Cancer 53:1049–1057, 1984
23. Harris JR, Connolly JL, Schnitt SJ, et al: Clinical pathologic study of early breast cancer treated by primary radiation therapy. J Clin Oncol 1:184–189, 1983
24. Connolly JL, Schnitt SJ, Harris J, et al: Pathologic correlates of local tumor control following primary radiation therapy in patients with early breast cancer, in Harris J, Hellman S, Silen W, (eds): Conservative Management of Breast Cancer. Philadelphia, Lippincott, pp 123–136, 1983
25. Fisher B, Wolmark N, Bauer M, et al: The accuracy of clinical nodal staging and of limited axillary dissection as a determinant of histologic nodal status in carcinoma of the breast. Surg Gynecol Obstet 152:765, 1981
26. Fisher B, Bauer M, Wickerham L, et al: Relation of number of positive axillary nodes to the prognosis of patients with primary breast cancer—an NSABP update. Cancer 52:1551, 1983.

Conservative Surgery and Radiation Therapy for Early Breast Cancer: Results, Controversies, and Unsolved Problems

Abram Recht, James L. Connolly, Stuart J. Schnitt, Blake Cady, Susan Love, Robert T. Osteen, W. Bradford Patterson, Robert Shirley, William Silen, Steven Come, I. Craig Henderson, Barbara Silver, and Jay R. Harris

THE COMBINATION of conservative surgery and radiation therapy (sometimes called "primary radiation therapy") has become an increasingly accepted alternative to mastectomy for the treatment of clinical stages I and II breast cancer. This mode of therapy may be defined as a combination of conservative surgery for resection of the primary tumor ("lumpectomy," "partial mastectomy," "segmental mastectomy," or "quadrantectomy"), with or without surgical staging of the axilla, followed by radiation therapy for the eradication of residual microscopic disease in the breast and, in some cases, draining nodal tissues. Patients treated with breast-conserving therapy have a more positive body image[1,2] and less fear of recurrence of cancer[1] than do patients treated with radical mastectomy (RM). The goal of this treatment is to provide highly satisfactory cosmetic results, without compromising local tumor control or survival compared with radical surgical procedures.

The rationale for and results of conservative surgery plus radiation therapy were discussed in this journal in 1978.[3] There has been increasing support for the use of this approach in the years since then. In this report, we will review both retrospective and prospective studies of primary radiation therapy for early breast cancer, including the cosmetic results and complications of such treatment. We will then examine some current controversies and unresolved questions concerning patient selection, surgical and radiotherapeutic techniques, management of the regional lymph nodes, integration with adjuvant systemic therapy, and the management of recurrences after primary radiation therapy. We will be concerned primarily with those series that have used excision of the primary tumor, rather than radiotherapy alone. We will not examine the treatment of patients with noninvasive ductal or lobular carcinomas or with locally advanced breast cancers who are not candidates for radical surgery, which has been discussed elsewhere.[4,5]

From the Joint Center for Radiation Therapy, Department of Radiation Therapy, the Departments of Pathology, Surgery, and Medicine, Beth Israel Hospital, the Department of Surgery, New England Deaconess Hospital, the Departments of Surgery and Obstetrics and Gynecology, Brigham and Women's Hospital, and the Department of Medicine, Dana-Farber Cancer Institute, Harvard Medical School, Boston.

Address reprint requests to Abram Recht, MD, Joint Center for Radiation Therapy, 50 Binney St, Boston, MA 02115.

0093-7754/86/1304-0007$05.00/0

LOCAL-REGIONAL RECURRENCE IN PATIENTS TREATED WITH MASTECTOMY OR CONSERVATIVE SURGERY ALONE

Before reviewing the results of conservative surgery and radiation therapy, it is important (as a base for comparison) to examine the local-regional recurrence rates in patients with operable breast cancers treated with either radical surgery or with conservative surgery without radiation therapy.

The incidence of recurrence in the chest wall, axillary nodes, supraclavicular or infraclavicular nodes, and/or internal mammary nodes after mastectomy depends on many factors. The most important of these appears to be whether or not the axillary lymph nodes are pathologically involved. The chance of a local-regional recurrence following RM for a patient with pathologically uninvolved ("negative") lymph nodes is from 3% to 8%. However, when the axillary lymph nodes are involved by tumor ("positive"), the incidence of local-regional recurrence increases to 19% to 27%.[6-8] Approximately two thirds of these are isolated recurrences, and the remainder are simultaneous with or following the appearance of distant metastases. Such local-regional recurrences can produce significant morbidity, despite aggressive treatment. The initial complete response rate to aggressive radiotherapy in these patients is 63% to 97%. However, one third to one half of such responders will suffer further local-regional recurrences, of which 66% to 75% are within the radiation fields.[6,9-16] Even when local-regional disease is eradicated, almost all of these patients will eventually develop distant metastases. The 5-year survival rate in patients with isolated local-regional recurrence in recent series ranges from 35% to 50%, with only 20% to 30% disease-free survival.[12-15] The 10-year survival is 23% to 30%, but disease-free survival is only 7% to 15%. Thus, local-regional recurrence after radical surgery is both difficult to control in the area of recurrence and is associated with a poor prognosis.

Several groups have also treated patients who have early breast cancer with conservative surgery alone. Selection of patients and length of follow-up varies substantially between these series. Such treatment has been associated with a recurrence rate in the breast of 15% to 37%.[17-21] As yet, it is unclear whether these patients have a lower survival rate than those treated initially with mastectomy or primary radiation therapy. There is only one published randomized study comparing conservative surgery alone with either conservative surgery with radiation or with mastectomy—the National Surgical Adjuvant Breast Project (NSABP) B-06 trial.[21] In this study, all patients underwent axillary dissection, and patients with involved lymph nodes received chemotherapy. Ten percent of patients who originally were randomized to undergo segmental mastectomy, but in whom the margins of the excision specimen were involved, were excluded from conservative treatment and underwent mastectomy. Excluding these latter patients, the incidence of distant metastases in patients with pathologically uninvolved axillary nodes who were treated with segmental mastectomy alone was significantly greater than in patients who received irradiation or total mastectomy (27% *v* 18%, $P < .05$). However, there was no statistical difference between treatment arms in the incidence of distant metastases at 5 years in those patients who had pathologically involved lymph nodes (Table 1). While some of the patients excluded from conservative management in this study may have had more aggressive tumors with a higher incidence of distant metastases, the distribution of such tumors should have been equal between the different arms allocated to segmental mastectomy with or without radiation therapy. As yet, there are no differences in overall survival between these patients, but the mean follow-up of this series is only 39 months. This trend suggests that the effectiveness of local control techniques may in fact have an impact on patient survival, particularly for patients whose cancer is of an early stage. Patients with uninvolved nodes likely have the greatest potential for cure by effective local-regional treatment alone. Patients with involved nodes appear much more likely to have systemic subclinical disease at initial presentation, and the effectiveness of local treatment may have less of an impact on their survival. These data provide support for a position midway between the classical Halstedian view of breast carcinoma as a predominantly local-regional disease, and the idea that breast cancer is almost inevitably a systemic disease.

Table 1. Actuarial 5-Year Incidence of Distant Metastases, NSABP B-06

	TM	*SM*	*SM + XRT*
Negative Nodes	19%	27%	18%
Positive Nodes	41%	34%	35%

TM: patients assigned to total mastectomy arm (negative nodes, 362; positive nodes, 224)

SM: patients assigned to and actually receiving segmental mastectomy alone (assigned, but excluded because of margins: negative nodes, 32 of 390 [8%]; positive nodes, 35 of 242 [14%])

SM + XRT: patients assigned to and actually receiving segmental mastectomy and radiotherapy (assigned, but excluded because of margins: negative nodes, 23 of 396 [6%]; positive nodes 36 of 229 [16%])

Abbreviations: TM, total mastectomy; SM, segmental mastectomy; XRT, radiation therapy.

Data from Fisher et al.[21]

RETROSPECTIVE STUDIES OF PRIMARY RADIATION THERAPY

Since the mid-1950s, there have been numerous reports from centers in Europe and North America on the use of primary radiation therapy to treat patients with clinical stage I and II breast carcinomas. Table 2 summarizes the results of series in which treatment was administered with (predominantly or exclusively) supervoltage equipment, and in which at least 100 patients were explicitly listed as available for assessment of breast recurrence at 5 or more years after treatment. Many other series with fewer patients or shorter follow-up have also been reported.[23-33]

Table 2. Modern Large Retrospective Studies of Primary Radiotherapy (Less-than-Excisional Biopsy Excluded)

Institution	Dates	No. of Breasts	Evaluable at 5 (10) Yrs	Crude/5(10)-Yr Actuarial Breast Recurrence	Crude/5(10)-Yr Actuarial Total LR Recurrence
Institut Curie[66]	1960–1976	268	240 (143)	6%/—	7.5%/—
Marseilles[77]	1960–1971	276	Minimum 10-yr follow-up	16%/—	17%/—
Princess Margaret[89]	1958–1980	605	351 (106)	—*/ 9% (13%) —†/13% (21%)	—*/21% (25%)
MD Anderson[22]	1955–1980	345	118 (25)	5%/—	6%/—
Gustave-Roussy[69]	1970–1981	436	171 (22)	3%/ 5% (7%)	5.5%/ 7% (10%)
JCRT[34,35]	1968–1980	510	148 (10)	6%/ 7% (18%)	7%/—

*Radiation given to breast alone (252).

†Radiation given to breast and some or all regional nodes (353); total local-regional recurrence not calculated for this grouping.

Comparison of these series to one another is difficult for many reasons, including differences in patient selection, treatment machines, delivered dose and dose distributions, and surgical and clinical staging of patients, as well as differing methods of data presentation and analysis, and changes in treatment policies and techniques with time. For example, in the series of patients treated at the Joint Center for Radiation Therapy (JCRT) from 1968 to 1980, the actuarial 5-year breast recurrence rate for 411 patients treated with excisional biopsy and supplementary irradiation ("boost") to bring the dose to the primary site to over 6,000 cGy (1 cGy = 1 rad) was 6% for clinical stage I and 8% for clinical stage II patients (23 breast recurrences) (Fig 1).[34,35] There were only three patients with isolated nodal failures. In contrast, 211 patients with clinically uninvolved axillary lymph nodes treated in the Royal Marsden Hospital series were found to have a (crude) local-regional recurrence rate of 14.5% at 5 years, and 21.5% at 10 years.[36] The breast recurrence rate at 10 years was 18%, the remainder being isolated regional nodal failures. There were several differences in technique between these series, which could account for these differing results. Patients in the JCRT series were treated with supervoltage linear accelerators to a dose of 4,500 to 5,000 cGy delivered over 4½ to 5 weeks, with five fractions per week to the entire breast and often to lymph nodes. This was followed by a boost with external photons or electrons or an interstitial iridium implant. Most patients also underwent axillary dissection. Patients in the Royal Marsden series were treated with orthovoltage or cesium 137 (a relatively low-energy isotope), receiving on average a dose to the breast and draining lymph nodes of 4,500 cGy in 20 fractions over 8 weeks, followed by a boost of 1,000 cGy in five fractions over 2 weeks. No axillary dissections were performed. The differences in the total dose and fractionation between these institutions most likely account for the differences in results.

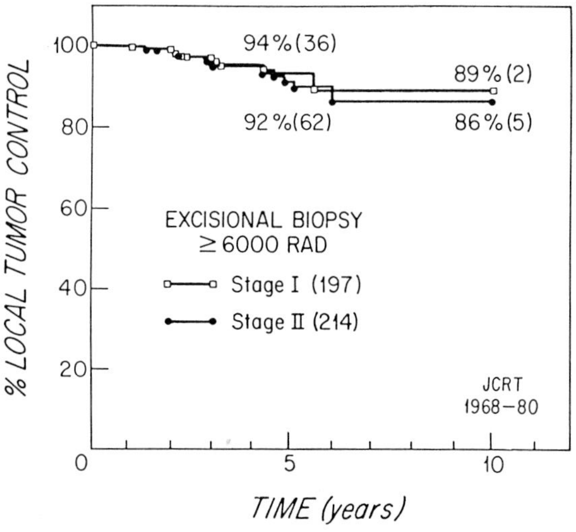

Fig 1. Local control, JCRT: excisional biopsy and dose to primary site ≥ 6,000 cGy, 1968 to 1980.

One important conclusion to be drawn from these retrospective analyses concerns the time course to local recurrence. Whereas most local-regional recurrences after mastectomy will be present within the first several years, patients treated with primary radiation therapy must be observed for local recurrence for a much longer period of time. A collaborative retrospective review was recently done of the results of treatment of 152 patients irradiated before 1967 at the Institut Curie, the Marseilles Cancer Institute, or the Princess Margaret Hospital.[37] Minimum follow-up time was 15 years. The techniques and doses used during this period were less satisfactory than current ones. Although most breast recurrences occurred during the first 5 years after treatment, the actuarial risk of local recurrence was nearly constant for 14 years after treatment. No local recurrences were seen between 15 to 20 years. The 15-year actuarial risk of developing a breast recurrence was 29%. However, this incidence was different for each of the three institutions, and was lowest for the center that gave the highest average doses of radiation. The actuarial 15-year freedom from distant metastases and overall survival rates were 71% and 52%, respectively. The salvage of patients who developed a local-regional recurrence with subsequent surgery (usually mastectomy) yielded 58% freedom from distant metastases at 5 years, and 50% at 10 years. Salvage rates did not vary significantly as a function of the time to recurrence after initial therapy. These data suggest both the likelihood of higher local control with higher dose of radiation therapy and the high rate of long-term salvage of these patients who develop local failure after primary radiation therapy as compared with those who fail in local-regional areas following mastectomy. Similar long-term data have recently been reported by others.[38]

RANDOMIZED PROSPECTIVE STUDIES OF PRIMARY RADIATION THERAPY *v* MASTECTOMY

The critical issue regarding primary radiation therapy is whether it yields survival equal to mastectomy. This issue can only be answered by randomized prospective trials in which the treatment arms are well balanced in terms of prognostic features. There have now been several such studies.

The earliest such trial was that of Guy's Hospital, London, beginning in 1961.[39–41] Patients with T1-2, N0-1 breast cancer were allocated randomly to receive either RM or wide excision (WE), with both groups receiving postoperative radiation. Premenopausal patients were excluded from the study. All patients treated before 1968 also received adjuvant thiotepa. Patients in the WE group were treated on a 6-meV machine, receiving 3,500 to 3,800 cGy in 3 weeks to the breast and internal mammary nodes, and 2,500 to 2,700 cGy in 12 days to the axilla and supraclavicular nodes. None of the WE patients had an axillary dissection. As a result, an excess of axillary recurrences was noted in the group treated with WE. In the WE group, the actuarial incidence of local-regional recurrence at 10 years was 33% in the patients without initially palpable axillary nodes, as compared with 63% in those with clinically enlarged axillary lymph nodes. By comparison, 15% and 24% of the patients with, respectively, clinically uninvolved and involved axillary nodes treated with RM and post operative radiation developed a local-regional recurrence. The incidence of freedom from distant metastases and the likelihood of survival were the same in both arms for the N0 patients. There was a survival advantage at 10 years for the N1 patients treated with radical mastectomy, but with further follow-up at 15 years, freedom from distant relapse was similar in these groups (26% in the WE group *v* 22% in the RM group). A second trial with the same randomization and similar inadequate radiotherapy doses was later performed, but was restricted to patients with clinically uninvolved nodes. This second series of patients showed an advantage in local-regional control, freedom from distant relapse, and survival for the RM group. However, the median follow-up in this series is 8 years, and it was only on longer follow-up of the first series of patients that the treatment results converged.

Since 1970, there have been four prospective randomized trials using better radiation therapy techniques. One such trial (abbreviated "QUART") was performed at the National Cancer Institute of Milan, Italy.[42,43] From 1973 to 1980, 701 evaluable patients with primary tumors ≤ 2 cm in size and clinically uninvolved axillary nodes (T1N0) were entered. Patients were randomized to receive RM or conservative surgery and radiotherapy. Conservative surgery consisted of a resection of the entire involved quadrant of the breast (quadrantectomy) and a full axillary dissection. Radiotherapy was then administered to the breast alone through two opposing tangential fields, giving a dose of 5,000 cGy in 5 weeks. Another 1,000 cGy was then administered to the tumor site using orthovoltage radiation. From 1973 to 1975, patients with involved lymph nodes were further randomized to receive radiotherapy either to the breast alone or to the breast and to the draining lymph node areas as well. After 1975, all patients with involved lymph nodes were treated with 12 cycles of chemotherapy. The two arms were well balanced with regard to age, tumor size, and axillary nodal status. Microscopically involved axillary nodes were found in 25% of the radical mastectomy group compared with 27% of the conservatively treated group. Five patients from the mastectomy group and five in the quadrantectomy group had developed a local recurrence at last report.[43] Seven additional cases of a second primary cancer in the remnant ipsilateral breast were found in the group that was treated conservatively. The number of deaths in each treatment group since the start of treatment was the same, and relapse-free and overall survival rates were similar between the two groups. Patients with involved axillary nodes had better relapse-free survival if treated with quadrantectomy and radiotherapy than mastectomy (87% *v* 72% at 5 years, $P = .02$). Adjuvant chemotherapy was administered simultaneously with radiotherapy without major problems or the need for significant dose reductions.[44]

The NSABP began a three-arm trial (Protocol B-06) in 1976 comparing mastectomy with segmental mastectomy, with or without radiotherapy.[21] A total of 1,843 evaluable patients with clinical stage I or II carcinoma, with the primary clinically measuring up to 4 cm in size, were entered. One hundred seventy-four patients (8%) refused their assigned treatment and were excluded from analysis. All patients underwent axillary dissection. Those with involved lymph nodes underwent adjuvant chemotherapy with melphalan and 5-fluorouracil (L-PAM/5-FU), with one cycle administered before radiotherapy began. Whereas in the Milan trial an entire quadrant of the breast was removed, segmental mastectomy as performed in the NSABP trial included a resection of the tumor with only enough normal tissue removed around it to attempt to insure that the specimen margins were tumor-free. It was considered impossible to obtain tumor-free margins in 10% of the patients randomly assigned to segmental mastectomy, and total mastectomy was carried out in these patients. Radiotherapy was delivered to the breast alone with supervoltage equipment, using opposed tangential fields (often without wedge filters to compensate for the slope of the breast), to a dose of 5,000 to 5,300 cGy in 5 to 6 weeks. The regional lymph nodes were not treated, and no boost was given to the tumor site. Of the patients who received radiotherapy, the 5-year actuarial incidence of recurrence in the breast was 8%, compared with 28% of patients who did not have radiotherapy ($P < .001$). This marked difference was seen both in patients with histologically involved and uninvolved lymph nodes. Of note, patients with involved lymph nodes treated with segmental mastectomy and adjuvant chemotherapy (but without radiotherapy) had a greater risk of breast recurrence (36%) than did patients with uninvolved nodes treated only with segmental mastectomy (24%). However, patients with involved nodes who received radiotherapy, as well as chemotherapy, had a smaller risk of breast recurrence (2%) than did patients with uninvolved nodes treated with segmental mastectomy and radiotherapy (10%). This suggests that chemotherapy by itself does little to prevent breast recurrence, but that radiotherapy and chemotherapy may be additive or synergistic in reducing tumor recurrence in the breast.

Another trial was conducted from 1972 to 1979 at the Institut Gustave Roussy in Villejuif, France, under the sponsorship of the World Health Organization (WHO).[45] This included 179 patients with tumors pathologically 2 cm or smaller, with either clinically involved or uninvolved lymph nodes. Patients were randomized to receive either modified RM or conservative surgery. This consisted of removal of the tumor with a surrounding margin of 2 cm of grossly normal breast tissue ("tumorectomy"). All patients underwent low axillary dissection; if involved lymph nodes were detected, this was extended to a complete axillary dissection. Patients randomized to either mastectomy or tumorectomy who had involved lymph nodes were further randomized to receive postoperative axillary, supraclavicular, and internal-mammary nodal irradiation or no further treatment. Adjuvant chemotherapy was not used. Radiotherapy was given with cobalt 60 to a dose of 4,500 cGy in 18 fractions over 1 month, treating the breast four times weekly. A boost of 1,500 cGy was given to the tumor bed in six fractions. The total length of irradiation was 6 weeks. With a median follow-up of 4.5 years, there was no statistically significant difference in freedom from distant metastases or overall survival between the two treatment groups; however, there was a trend in favor of the tumorectomy group. The local recurrence rates were 5% and 12% in the tumorectomy and mastectomy groups, respectively, at 5 years.

The fourth and most recent prospective randomized trial was begun by the US National Cancer Institute in 1979. By September 1984, 165 patients with clinical stage I or II breast cancers had been entered and randomized to receive either modified RM or conservative excision, full axillary dissection, and radiotherapy to the breast. Patients with histologically involved nodes also receive doxorubicin plus cyclophosphamide chemotherapy. With a median follow-up of 27 months, there was no significant difference in outcome between these two groups.[46]

These randomized prospective trials demonstrate two important points. First, the techniques of radiation therapy have an important bearing on the likelihood of local recurrence, and this in turn appears likely ultimately to have an impact on survival, at least in some patient groups. Second, when adequate treatment techniques are used, there is no significant difference in survival between patients treated with radical surgery and those treated with primary radiation therapy. Although longer follow-up will be necessary to verify these results, at present they confirm the evidence of the retrospective trials as to the value of using primary radiation therapy for patients with early breast cancer.

COSMETIC RESULTS OF RADIOTHERAPY

The cosmetic results after treatment with conservative surgery and radiotherapy have generally been good to excellent, with nearly all patients being satisfied with their results. The results of the JCRT are typical of other series using modern equipment and currently accepted doses.[47,48] Measured parameters included breast edema, retraction, telangiectasias, arm edema, and overall cosmetic appearance as judged by the physician. In a series of 239 patients treated from 1976 to 1980 (four with bilateral tumors treated), none of whom received chemotherapy adjuvantly, the overall cosmetic results declined during the first 3 years after treatment, but then stabilized (Fig 2). At 5 years, the overall cosmetic results were judged as excellent (little or no observable change) in 77% of patients, good (minimal, but identifiable changes) in 9%, fair (significant results of radiation therapy noted) in 9%, and poor (severe normal tissue sequelae) in 5%. The results were found to depend on the dose and technique of radiotherapy, with increasing doses of external beam radiation to the entire breast (>5,000 cGy) being associated with greater degrees of retraction and fibrosis. Poorer cosmetic results were also associated with very large implants (>100 seeds) and implant doses over 1,800 cGy, and with higher overall doses to the primary volume. Breast and arm edema were rarely cosmetically significant, but were more common in patients who underwent axillary dissection than among those who did not. Factors that did not influence cosmetic outcome in our series were the age of the patient, the site of the primary tumor, the size of the primary, and the use of axillary dissection.[47] The use of chemotherapy (especially when given concurrently with irradiation) appears to cause a decrease in the overall cosmetic results, but further follow-up of these patients will be needed to be certain of this effect.[48] Greater breast size has been associated with increased retraction after primary radio-

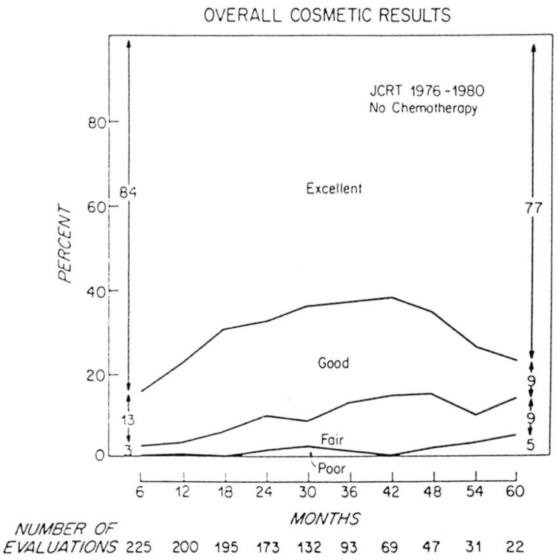

Fig 2. Overall cosmetic results, JCRT: no chemotherapy, 1968 to 1980. Reprinted with permission.[47]

therapy in other series in which this has been measured.[49]

COMPLICATIONS OF PRIMARY RADIATION THERAPY

The acute complications of radiotherapy for early breast cancer include fatigue, irritation and erythema of the skin, and occasionally moist desquamation. However, these are self-limited and resolve within 1 to several weeks after treatment.

The development of significant long-term complications is highly unusual. At the JCRT, transient or mild complications occur in a small number of patients. The most common are rib fractures (5%), cosmetically (though rarely functionally) significant arm edema (4%), radiation pneumonitis (2%), and rarely paresthesias or brachial plexus disorders. Other rare complications in our experience have been radiation pericarditis (one patient), soft tissue necrosis (one patient), and occasionally fibrosis of the pectoral muscles. Similar results have been reported by others.[25]

The risk of arm edema in our population appears most strongly related to the extent of axillary surgery and axillary irradiation.[50] The actuarial risk of arm edema at 6 years was 4% for patients who did not undergo axillary surgery, and 13% for patients who did have axillary dissection ($P = .006$). Nearly all patients had irradiation of the full axilla. Patients who underwent an axillary dissection that included stripping of the axillary vein had a 37% risk of arm edema at 6 years, as compared with only 7% in patients who had a lesser axillary procedure ($P < .001$). Arm edema in our series has been either mild or moderate, with no patients having severe edema.

A potential complication of treatment of the axillary and supraclavicular regions is injury to the brachial plexus. The classic chronic radiation-induced injury rarely occurs with doses <5,000 cGy.[51,52] This syndrome is stable or progressive, and is characterized by mild discomfort in the shoulder and by paresthesias and weakness of the upper arm and hand. A reversible brachial plexopathy can sometimes be seen even at doses <4,500 cGy.[53] This was observed in eight patients treated between 1975 and 1978 (approximately 3% of the total) and was more common when patients received adjuvant chemotherapy. Instances of this syndrome have been rare since 1978, and the relation to the use of adjuvant chemotherapy suggests a potential infectious etiology during this period.

A detailed study was recently undertaken at the JCRT of the effects of primary radiotherapy on the heart and pericardium for 20 patients with left-sided breast cancer.[54] Electrocardiogram (EKG) changes included rightward shift of the frontal plane QRS and T axes and T-wave inversion of one or more of leads V2-V6. However, these changes resolved within a 2-year period. Four of 20 patients were found to have asymptomatic pericardial effusions, only one of which was persistent. At 5 years, none of the evaluable patients had any decrease in ventricular function on noninvasive cardiac evaluation. The reason for this low rate of cardiac complication in our patients may be due to treatment technique, as we do not use the so-called hockey-stick field, which results in greater irradiation of the heart.[55]

Another potential long-term complication of primary radiotherapy is carcinogenesis. In the JCRT series of 525 patients treated between 1968 and 1980, there has been only one case of acute nonlymphocytic leukemia. This occurred in a patient who received 2 years of adjuvant chemotherapy that included an alkylating agent. No patient treated with radiation alone has developed leukemia. Also of some concern is whether the scattered radiation to the contralateral breast from primary radiotherapy will cause an increase in contralateral breast cancer. No significant increase has been seen to date, and we feel this is unlikely to occur. The actuarial incidence of contralateral metachronous breast cancers in the JCRT patients is 5% at 5 years, increasing to 9% at 10 years (with a small number of patients at risk).[56] This is similar to patients treated with radical surgery alone.[8,17,57–58] Further, in two series with long follow-up, there is no detectable increase in the number of contralateral primaries in patients who received postoperative chest-wall irradiation after mastectomy.[59,60] However, it is possible that we would be unable to detect any increase at present, for two reasons. First, the latency period between radiation and the development of clinically detectable carcinoma is at least 5 years and probably closer to 10 years.[61] Second, the magnitude of the added risk in patients receiving therapeutic irradiation is likely to be quite small. If the estimate of six cancers per million person-cGy-years is used,[61] and the dose to the opposite breast is 3% to 8% of the prescribed dose,[62] then the added risk of contralateral breast carcinoma would be *at most* 1% at 5 years. Further, the likelihood of inducing a breast cancer is strongly influenced by the age of the individual at the time of exposure, and appears extremely unlikely in individuals over age 35,[61] so even this estimate is likely to be much too large.

Another form of carcinogenesis is the induction of sarcomas of the bones or soft tissues in the treatment fields. These are well recognized following radiation given after mastectomy and have now been reported following primary radiotherapy as well.[38,62] However, these are likely to be rare. In one series, only one such case was reported in 289 patients surviving at least 10 years after radiation.[38]

CONTROVERSIES AND UNSOLVED PROBLEMS IN THE USE OF PRIMARY RADIATION THERAPY FOR EARLY BREAST CANCER

Patient Selection and Surgery for the Primary

The major criteria for patient selection for primary radiation therapy are the ability to resect the primary without causing major cosmetic deformities and the likelihood of breast recurrence. Whether the former is possible is determined by several factors, such as the size of the primary tumor, the size of the breast, the location of the tumor, and the extent of the surgical margin felt to be necessary. These factors and others, such as the histology of the tumor, may also be related to the risk of breast recurrence. However, there is disagreement over the relative importance of some of these.

Patients with two nonadjacent primaries in the same breast (demonstrated either by palpation or mammographically) are poor candidates for breast-conserving treatment for two reasons. First, the cosmetic results of multiple wide local excisions and radiation boosts are likely to be undesirable. Second, these patients may well have other relatively large concentrations of tumor cells within the breast. Another group of patients in whom similar concerns obtain is that in which mammograms reveal extensive microcalcifications. Just over half of the patients in each of these groups will have more than one quadrant of the breast involved pathologically when mastectomy is performed.[64] We would expect the rate of breast recurrence in these patients to be substantially higher than usual because the radiation dose tolerated by the entire breast is less likely to control the greater numbers of residual tumor cells probably present in these patients (after excisional biopsy) than in patients with a single gross lesion.

There is general agreement about the importance of mammography in selecting patients for primary radiation therapy. Modern film-screen mammography often provides critical information in the initial evaluation of these patients and should be done routinely before accepting patients for this treatment. Mammography should be performed before biopsy if possible, in order to avoid obscuring potentially important details by postoperative scarring or hematoma.

The location of the tumor is a consideration of treatment selection for patients with subareolar primaries. Patients with noninvasive ductal carcinomas who present with nipple discharges and subareolar lesions have been found to have a high breast failure rate.[4] Whether this is also true of invasive cancers is unclear. However, in one series, many of these patients were found to have extensive spread of disease along the ducts that might not have been excised had conservative resection been done.[64] We feel that for such patients to be treated successfully with primary radiation therapy resection of the nipple-areola complex may be necessary. Whether the individual patient would be willing to consider this relatively deforming surgery as acceptable is an equally important question.

Breast recurrence is clearly more frequent among patients who do not have a complete gross excision of the primary. At the JCRT, the 5-year actuarial incidence of recurrence in the breast in 26 breasts having incisional biopsy was 31% compared with 7% in a group of 510 breasts treated with excision of the tumor from 1968 to 1980.[34,35] Similar (and even higher) local failure rates have been seen in other series of patients treated with radiotherapy alone without an excision of the primary.[65–67] It is possible that increasing the dose of radiation could improve this to the level of patients treated with excision. For example, Pierquin found that patients with T2 tumors treated to 8,300 cGy (including an iridium implant) to the primary site had a 7% local failure rate at 10 years.[68] Others have found a similar phenomenon.[67] However, the cosmetic results of such treatment are likely to be substantially poorer than those that combine more modest doses of radiotherapy with surgical excision. Hence, complete gross excision of the primary appears mandatory. However, that being the case, controversy then arises concerning the maximum size of the primary acceptable for treatment. Tumor size itself has not been shown to be a significant risk factor for local recurrence after excisional biopsy and radiotherapy. In the JCRT series, local recurrence rates were similar for all sizes up to 5 cm.[56] In the NSABP B-06 trial, local recurrence was 6.5% for T1 patients and 9.6% for T2 tumors.[21]

The extent of surgical resection required before radiotherapy has been controversial. Some centers have advocated a wide resection, removing up to 2 cm of unaffected breast tissue around the primary mass (eg, the Institut Curie[65]) or even removal of the entire affected quadrant. Such wide margins do not appear necessary to achieve excellent local rates provided an adequate dose of radiation is given. The high level of local tumor control in the JCRT series was obtained following the removal of only a small rim of normal tissue around the primary. At the Institut Gustave Roussy, where a boost dose was also typically used, local-regional recurrence was seen in 4 of 47 or 9% of patients treated with quadrantectomy, compared with 20 of 389 or 5% of patients treated with excisional biopsy.[69] Similarly Chu et al[24] did not find an advantage to quadrantectomy over excisional biopsy for patients treated with radiotherapy, including a boost to the primary site. It appears likely that an inverse relationship of sorts links these two aspects of therapy—that is, equal results can be achieved with wider excisions and lower doses of radiation, or with smaller gross total excisions and higher doses.

A related controversy exists as to whether patients who have microscopically involved (or "positive") margins can be treated as successfully as can patients with microscopically uninvolved margins. The experience at the JCRT and the Institut Gustave Roussy suggests that by the use of a boost to the primary site to doses of at least 6,000 cGy local tumor control can be achieved in patients with close or involved margins (with the possible exception of patients in certain pathologic subgroups, discussed below). Whether a boost is always needed in patients with uninvolved margins remains unclear and will be dealt with in more detail. In addition, there are technical problems in assessing the margins. It is essential that the pathologist inks the margins of resection before cutting the specimen, so that they can be clearly identified on microscopic examination. However, there is no clear definition of what constitute "involved margins." This can imply that cancer is seen either directly at an inked surface or within some arbitrary distance from an inked margin. Such a definition is obviously influenced by the number of sections assessed for involvement.

Investigators at the JCRT have studied the influence of other pathologic features in the excision specimen on the subsequent risk of local recurrences.[70–74] The most recent report examined the risk of local recurrence in 356 patients with infiltrating ductal histology treated from 1968 to 1980 in whom there was sufficient adjacent breast tissue for pathologic review.[74] The median follow-up in this group is 63 months (range, 29 to 167 months). In the large majority of patients, the tumor was excised grossly, with a small rim of adjacent breast tissue without regard to the microscopic margins of resection. The margins of resection were not routinely inked or labeled during this period and, therefore, were not evaluable in most cases on review. Many factors, such as dose to the primary site, nuclear grade, the size of the primary, clinical axillary status, lymphatic vessel invasion, and blood vessel invasion were examined. However, the only feature shown to have a statistically significant impact on the local recurrence rate was the presence of what we have called an "extensive intraductal component" (EIC). Tumors were described as being in this category when two features were simultaneously present: intraductal carcinoma comprising 25% or more of the area of the primary mass; and intraductal carcinoma clearly extending beyond the infiltrating margin of the tumor or present in sections of grossly normal adjacent breast tissue. Such extensive intraductal carcinoma was found in 38% of patients. This group with extensive intraductal involvement had a 23% actuarial risk of breast recurrence at 5 years, compared with only 2% for other patients ($P < .0001$). The presence of both substantial intraductal carcinoma "within" the primary and "adjacent" to it were necessary to cause this increased risk of local recurrence (Fig 3). Of importance, the 5-year risk of distant failure was similar for patients either with or without EIC (20% *v* 21%). Tumors with high nuclear grade and extensive intraductal involvement tended to recur sooner than those with low nuclear grade and EIC, but with longer follow-up failure rates were similar. Of the 24 local recurrences in patients with extensive intraductal involvement, 22 were either within or at the edge of the boost field, and, therefore, we feel likely to represent a recurrence of the original primary tumor. Only two patients in this group developed a recurrence elsewhere in the breast (ie, probably due to a preexisting subclinical second primary tumor present during the initial treatment, or a new primary that originated after radiotherapy). Of the three breast recurrences in patients without EIC, two were within the boost field, and one was elsewhere in the breast. Patients with extensive intraductal involvement who received <6,000

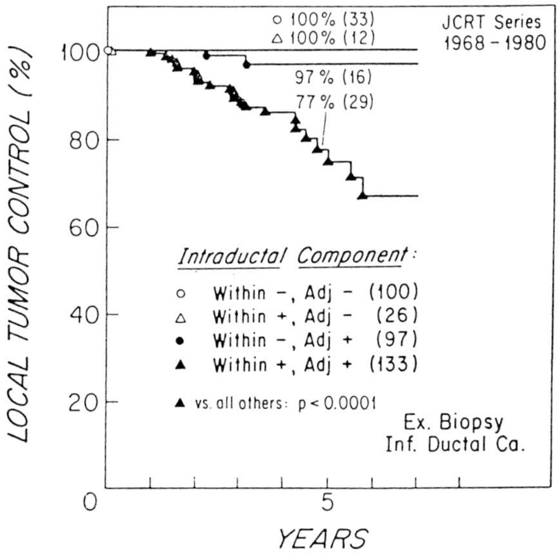

Fig 3. Effect of the intraductal component on local tumor control, JCRT: excisional biopsy, infiltrating ductal histology only, 1968 to 1980.

cGy to the primary site tended to fail directly at the site of the primary (ie, true recurrence), and patients who received a boost of radiation to the primary site to >6,000 cGy tended to fail at the edge of the boost (ie, marginal miss).

The reason for the association of EIC with a high risk of local recurrence is not entirely clear. It seems likely that these patients have a greater residual tumor burden following gross excision than do other patients. We have found that in a group of patients who underwent re-excision of the primary site, patients with extensive intraductal carcinoma in the initial specimen were more likely to have residual cancer or re-excision than other patients.[75] The likelihood of finding substantial intraductal cancer in the re-excision specimen was 37% for patients with EIC in the initial excision, compared with only 7% for other patients. The presence of extensive intraductal carcinoma has not predicted for local recurrence in the Milan series (Veronesi, personal communication, 1984) or the Villejuif series,[69] in which quadrantectomy or very wide excision were used. At present, our policy in patients with EIC is to carefully review the specimen and mammograms to be certain that the areas of intraductal spread have been adequately excised. The specimen should be closely examined to see if any microcalcifications present were associated with benign or malignant processes. If EIC is present and the margins are microscopically involved or equivocal, then a re-excision of the biopsy site should be performed if primary radiotherapy is to be considered further. If the margins of the re-excision specimen are also involved, then the patient should understand that she may still be at greater risk of local recurrence if treated by radiotherapy than if treated by mastectomy, despite the re-excision. While the rates of distant metastases and survival to date have been the same in both the groups at low and high risk of recurrence in the breast, this may change with further follow-up, and hence mastectomy may be preferable. In a situation where re-excision is not technically possible or cannot be done without severe deformity of the breast, then mastectomy may also be more desirable.

The results at the JCRT suggest that the optimal extent of resection may depend on the extent of associated intraductal carcinoma. Patients without extensive intraductal involvement are well treated with excisional biopsy, while patients with extensive intraductal involvement probably require a wide resection in order to achieve an equal rate of local control.

In practice, we are also influenced strongly by the status of the axillary nodes. When axillary nodes are pathologically involved, the potential long-term risks of breast recurrence may be of relatively less importance to the overall outcome of therapy, as shown by the NSABP B-06 study. Further, the rate of local-regional recurrence after mastectomy in these patients is substantial, making mastectomy a less effective option than in patients with uninvolved nodes.

Radiotherapy Techniques and Doses

The importance of the time-dose factors of the radiotherapy as a risk factor for local recurrence has been suggested in a number of studies. Kurtz et al[77] found that local recurrence was greater when 800 cGy or less was administered per week (a crude incidence of 28%) than when more than 800 cGy was given (13%). At the Royal Marsden Hospital, a high rate of local recurrence was also noted with a weekly dose of 800 cGy or less.[36] At the Institut Gustave Roussy, the local-regional recurrence rate was 14 of 153 or 8% when treatment was protracted compared with ten of 269 or 4% when it was not ($P < .05$).[69]

There is not universal agreement as to the need for a radiation boost dose to the primary site. As noted above, the utility of a boost must be considered in relation to the extent of surgical resection. It is likely that a boost is more important after routine excisional biopsy than after very wide excision or quadrantectomy. The major evidence against the use of a boost as a standard part of treatment is the results of the NSABP B-06 trial, in which no boost was used. This study resulted in a 5-year risk of a breast relapse after excision and radiotherapy of 8%, which is comparable to that found at other institutions when a boost was used.[21] However, the approximately 3-year median follw-up time in the NSABP trial may not be adequate to assess fully the risk of local recurrence. Further, the absence of the routine and uniform use of tissue compensators as part of the radiotherapy technique of the NSABP trial may have resulted in an increased inhomogeneity of the dosage of radiation and a greater effective dose to the tumor site than the nominal dose of 5,000 to 5,300 cGy. At the JCRT patients have received a boost to the primary site. Since the morbidity of a boost of moderate size and dose is small,[47] we believe that the combination of local excision (for primaries without EIC) and radiotherapy, including a boost, provides both an excellent level of local tumor control and highly satisfactory cosmetic results.

The Role and Extent of Axillary Surgery

Another area of controversy in the management of patients with primary radiation therapy concerns the extent of axillary dissection. Axillary dissection serves several functions. Since patients with involved axillary nodes are at greater risk for distant relapse, they are currently considered for adjuvant systemic therapy (either chemotherapy or hormonal therapy). Axillary dissection is also indicated in all patients with clinically suspicious axillary nodes as part of the overall treatment of their local-regional disease. The dose of radiation required to control such grossly involved nodes is considerably greater than that required to control subclinical involvement and is associated with a much greater risk of complications. The information obtained from axillary dissection also yields information concerning the risk of involvement in the internal mammary and supraclavicular regions. Further, axillary dissection itself is an effective means of preventing tumor recurrence in the axilla. Therefore, an axillary dissection should be extensive enough to detect axillary metastases reliably when present and to provide a high level of local tumor control. The dissection itself should also be easily integrated with subsequent radiotherapy and should not result in a significant risk of complications or cosmetic deformities.

The surgical technique which best meets these requirements is described as a "level I/II dissection."[78] The boundaries of this dissection are the latissimus dorsi laterally, the pectoralis minor muscle medially, the axillary vein superiorly, and the tail of the breast inferiorly. This provides as high a detection rate of lymph nodes involvement as does a full dissection (which includes removal of the apical nodes and skeletonization of the axillary vein), without the morbidity of a full dissection. In a group of 541 patients from the JCRT and the University of Pennsylvania who underwent such limited axillary surgery, the incidence of histologically involved nodes was 36% when more than five nodes were obtained, similar to the incidence seen following complete dissection.[79] Similar results have been reported by the NSABP.[80] To many, but not all surgeons, the level I/II dissection includes stripping of the adventitial tissue from the vein as well. In our experience, removal of the level III nodes and/or stripping of the axillary vein has increased the actuarial likelihood of arm edema from 6% to 36% at 6 years when full axillary irradiation is also given.[50] This compares with a 4% risk of arm edema for patients who did not have axillary surgery, but did receive full axillary irradiation. Thus, the combination of axillary dissection and full axillary irradiation results in a significant risk of arm edema. Since reports of axillary recurrence after adequate level I/II dissection are uncommon, we feel that routine irradiation of the full axilla after adequate dissection is unnecessary and likely to increase morbidity. However, such a risk may be worthwhile in order to assure local tumor control in patients who have more than 50% of nodes involved and/or substantial extracapsular extension of disease, or in patients who have gross residual disease after axillary dissection.

Treatment of Other Regional Lymph Nodes

Patients who have involved axillary nodes or medial lesions are known to be at significant risk for subclinical involvement of the internal mammary and supraclavicular nodal areas, and some radiotherapists favor treatment of these in order to prevent tumor recurrence. At present, there are no data indicating that such treatment improves overall survival rates. The results in the randomized trials of Milan and of the NSABP comparing mastectomy with conservative surgery and radiation therapy were achieved with irradiation of the breast alone. Further, significant technical requirements must be met in order to avoid overlapping of fields and to minimize irradiation of the underlying lung.[81–83] For patients with left-sided lesions, substantial doses to the heart may accompany irradiation of the internal mammary nodes with certain radiotherapy techniques.[55] At present, we feel that treatment to the breast alone is acceptable in all situations, but that it is reasonable to treat the internal mammary and supraclavicular areas in patients who have involved axillary nodes or in whom the primary tumor is located medially, provided that the treatment techniques available to the radiotherapist allow this to be done with only limited potential morbidity.

Integration with Adjuvant Systemic Therapy

The optimal sequencing and timing of radiation and chemotherapy is unknown. Possibilities include giving the entire course of chemotherapy before radiation, the entire course of chemotherapy after radiation, giving both concurrently, or giving a portion of the chemotherapy before irradiation and then completing chemotherapy afterward ("sandwich technique"). Several studies have assessed the results of giving chemotherapy after radiation.[44,46,84–87] With the exception of one retrospective study,[85] these groups have shown that patients receiving primary radiation can receive adequate (≥85%) doses of chemotherapy. However, an increased incidence of lymphocytopenia has been generally seen in patients treated after radiotherapy.[44,86] As a result, dose modifications in patients who receive chemotherapy after irradiation should be based on the granulocyte count, rather than on the total WBC count.

At present there is no consensus as to the optimal timing of chemotherapy and radiation. In order to resolve this controversy, we have begun a prospective randomized trial at our member institutions for patients who will receive primary radiotherapy. Patients with involved axillary nodes are randomized to receive four cycles, each lasting 3 weeks, consisting of cyclophosphamide, Adriamycin (Adria Laboratories, Columbus, Ohio), methotrexate, 5-FU, and prednisone (CAMFP) either before or following completion of radiotherapy. So far this regimen has been well tolerated both symptomatically and hematologically, but as yet there are insufficient numbers of patients and follow-up to draw significant conclusions. When patients do receive chemotherapy first, we prefer not to give more than 3 months of chemotherapy before beginning irradiation, in order to minimize the likelihood of tumor growth within the breast should chemotherapy prove ineffective. We also prefer to avoid concurrent administration of chemotherapy and irradiation because of the higher incidence of acute (but reversible) skin and hematological toxicities than when these modalities are used sequentially.

Salvage of Breast Failure. Is Mastectomy Always Necessary?

Recurrence in the breast following primary radiation therapy has a much better prognosis than a chest-wall recurrence after mastectomy, with approximately 50% of such patients being alive and free of distant metastases at 5 years.[22,25,34,35,37,56,66,77] Salvage may be as high as 75% of those patients who can undergo potentially curative mastectomy (ie, who do not have simultaneous distant metastases or inoperable breast recurrence).[34,35]

Whether a mastectomy is superior to lesser procedures in the setting of an isolated breast recurrence is unclear. Patients in this situation have occasionally refused mastectomy or have been medically inoperable. At least some of these patients appear to be cured by conservative excision alone. Four of eight patients treated only with excisional biopsy after failing primary radiation therapy at the JCRT are alive without disease, as is one patient treated only with an iridium implant. However, follow-up on these patients is only 0 to 69 months among the survivors.[35] Fifty-five patients have been treated with WEs for a breast recurrence at the Marseilles Cancer Institute. These patients had mobile lesions smaller than 3 cm and no skin involvement (this group constituted only 35% of all patients undergoing salvage procedures between 1961 and 1979). With a median follow-up time of 4 years (range 1 to 13), the actuarial 5-year survival rate was 82%. The actuarial disease-free survival rates were 79% at 5 years and 66% at 8 years. Eight patients (14.5%) had further breast or regional recurrences 9 to 50 months following the first recurrence. Further surgery was able to control disease locally in five of eight patients, but two patients were inoperable at that time.[88] Therefore, it is possible that after careful clinical and radiological evaluation to rule out multifocal disease, selected patients might be treated equally well with wide local excision as with mastectomy. However, at present, we feel that mastectomy is the treatment of choice for all operable patients with breast recurrence following primary radiation therapy.

CONCLUSION

The results at 5 and 10 years from prospective randomized trials indicate that survival following primary radiation therapy for early breast cancer is equivalent to that following mastectomy. Because breast cancer has a long natural history, further follow-up of these patients will be required for ultimate proof of the relative merits of these treatments. However, long-term results of retrospective studies suggest that, for the great majority of individuals, mastectomy or conservative surgery plus radiation therapy will be equally effective. When competently performed, primary radiation therapy gives highly satisfactory cosmetic results and acceptably low rates of local tumor recurrence. A number of controversial issues remain concerning patient evaluation and selection and the optimal techniques of treatment, both surgical and radiotherapeutic. In addition, further work is needed to clarify the best way to integrate primary radiotherapy with adjuvant systemic treatment. Further experience is also necessary to determine whether the small number of patients with breast recurrences can be managed with an operation less than mastectomy. With the increasing numbers of patients being treated with primary radiation therapy, it appears likely that many of these questions will be answered in time for the centennial of Roentgen's discovery of x-rays in 1895.

REFERENCES

1. Bartelink H, Van Dam F, Van Dongen J: Psychological effects of breast conserving therapy in comparison with radical mastectomy. Int J Radiat Oncol Biol Phys 11:381–385, 1985

2. Schain E, Edwards B, Gorrell CR, et al: Psychosocial and physical outcomes of primary breast cancer therapy: Mastectomy vs. excisional biopsy and irradiation. Breast Cancer Res Treat 3:377–382, 1983

3. Harris JR, Levene MB, Hellman S: The role of radiation therapy in the primary treatment of carcinoma of the breast. Semin Oncol 5:403–416, 1978

4. Recht A, Danoff BS, Solin LJ, et al: Intraductal carcinoma of the breast: Results of treatment with excisional biopsy and irradiation. J Clin Oncol 3:1339–1343, 1985

5. Harris JR, Hellman S: The role of radiation therapy in the management of locally advanced carcinoma of the breast. Cancer 53:758–761, 1984

6. Donegan WL, Perez-Mesa CM, Watson FR: A biosta-

tistical study of locally recurrent breast carcinoma. Surg Gynecol Obstet 122:529–540, 1966

7. Haagensen CD: Diseases of the Breast, (ed 2 revised). Philadelphia, Saunders, 1971

8. Valagussa P, Bonadonna G, Veronesi U: Patterns of relapse and survival following radical mastectomy: Analysis of 716 consecutive patients. Cancer 41:1170–1178, 1978

9. Chen KKY, Montague ED, Oswald MJ: Results of irradiation in the treatment of loco-regional breast cancer recurrence. Cancer 56:1269–1273, 1985

10. Chu FCH, Lin FJ, Kim JH, et al: Locally recurrent carcinoma of the breast: Results of radiation therapy. Cancer 37:2677–2681, 1976

11. Patanaphan V, Salazar OM, Poussin-Rosillo H: Prognosticators in recurrent breast cancer: A 15-year experience with irradiation. Cancer 54:228–234, 1984

12. Bedwinek JM, Fineberg B, Lee J, et al: Analysis of failures following local treatment of isolated local-regional recurrence of breast cancer. Int J Radiat Oncol Biol Phys 7:581–585, 1981

13. Toonkel LM, Fix I, Jacobson LH, et al: The significance of local recurrence of carcinoma of the breast. Int J Radiat Oncol Biol Phys 9:33–39, 1983

14. Aberizk WJ, Silver B, Hellman S, et al: The results of radiation therapy for locally recurrent breast carcinoma after mastectomy. Cancer, 1986 (in press)

15. Beck TM, Hart NE, Woodard DA, et al: Local or regionally recurrent carcinoma of the breast: Results of therapy in 121 patients. J Clin Oncol 1:400–405, 1983

16. Danoff BF, Coia LR, Cantor RI, et al: Locally recurrent breast carcinoma: The effect of adjuvant chemotherapy on prognosis. Radiology 147:849–852, 1983

17. Crile G: Multicentric breast cancer: The incidence of new cancers in the homolateral breast after partial mastectomy. Cancer 35:475–477, 1975

18. Peters MV: Wedge resection with or without radiation in early breast cancer. Int J Radiat Oncol Biol Phys 2:1151–1156, 1977

19. Lagios MD, Richards VE, Rose ME, et al: Segmental mastectomy without radiotherapy: Short-term follow-up. Cancer 52:2173–2179, 1983

20. Montgomery AC, Greening WP, Levene AL: Clinical study of recurrence rate and survival time of patients with carcinoma of the breast treated by biopsy excision without any other therapy. J R Soc Med 71:339–342, 1978

21. Fisher B, Bauer M, Margolese R, et al: Five-year results of a randomized clinical trial comparing total mastectomy and segmental mastectomy with or without radiation in the treatment of breast cancer. N Engl J Med 312:665–673, 1985

22. Montague ED: Conservation surgery and radiation therapy in the treatment of operable breast cancer. Cancer 53:700–704, 1984

23. Cedermark B, Askergren J, Alveryd A, et al: Breast-conserving treatment for breast cancer in Stockholm, Sweden, 1977 to 1981. Cancer 53:1253–1255, 1984.

24. Chu AM, Cope O, Russo R, Lew R: Patterns of local-regional recurrence and results in stages I and II breast cancer treated by irradiation following limited surgery. Am J Clin Oncol (CCT) 7:221–229, 1984

25. Danoff BF, Pajak TF, Solin LJ, et al: Excisional biopsy, axillary node dissection and definitive radiotherapy for stages I and II breast cancer. Int J Radiat Oncol Biol Phys 11:479–483, 1985

26. Hery M, Namer M, Verschoore J, et al: Conservative treatment of breast cancer: A report on 108 patients. Int J Radiat Oncol Biol Phys 10:2185–2190, 1984

27. Hunig R, Walther E, Harder FH, et al: The Basel lumpectomy protocol—five-year experience with a prospective study for conservative treatment of breast cancer, in Harris JR, Hellman S, Silen W (eds): Conservative Management of Breast Cancer. Philadelphia, Lippincott, 1983, pp 23–33

28. Kuske RR, Compaan PJ, Aron BS, et al: Breast conservation therapy for breast cancer: A report on 215 patients. Int J Radiat Oncol Biol Phys 11:184, 1985 (suppl 1) (abstr)

29. Gerard JP, Montbarbon JF, Chassard JL, et al: Conservative treatment of early carcinoma of the breast: Significance of axillary dissection and iridium implant. Radiother Oncol 3:17–22, 1985

30. Weissberg JB, Hartman PV, Mate TP, et al: Primary radiation therapy in operable breast cancer. Int J Radiat Oncol Biol Phys 10:140, 1984 (suppl 2) (abstr)

31. Nobler MP, Venet L: Prognostic factors in patients undergoing curative irradiation for breast cancer. Int J Radiat Oncol Biol Phys 11:1323–1331, 1985

32. Pierquin B, Otmezguine Y, Lobo PA: Conservative management of breast carcinoma. The Creteil experience. Acta Radiol Oncol 22:101–107, 1983

33. Pierquin B: Conservative treatment for carcinoma of the breast: Experience of Creteil—ten-year results, in Harris JR, Hellman S, Silen W (eds): Conservative Management of Breast Cancer. Philadelphia, Lippincott, 1983, pp 11–14

34. Harris JR, Recht A, Schnitt S, et al: Current status of conservative surgery and radiotherapy as primary local treatment for early carcinoma of the breast. Breast Cancer Res Treat 5:245–255, 1985

35. Recht A, Silver B, Harris JR: The patterns of failure within the treated breast following primary radiation therapy. Int J Radiat Oncol Biol Phys 10:79, 1984 (suppl 2) (abstr)

36. Osborne MP, Ormiston N, Harmer CL, et al: Breast conservation in the treatment of early breast cancer. Cancer 53:349–355, 1984

37. Harris JR, Recht A, Amalric R, et al: Time course and prognosis of local recurrence following primary radiation therapy for early breast cancer. J Clin Oncol 2:37–41, 1984

38. Kurtz JM, Amalric R, Delouche G, et al: The second ten years: Long-term risks of breast conservation. Int J Radiat Oncol Biol Phys 11:184–185, 1985 (suppl 1) (abstr)

39. Atkins H, Hayward JL, Klugman DJ, et al: Treatment of early breast cancer: A report after ten years of a clinical trial. Br Med J 2:423–429, 1972

40. Hayward JL: The Guy's trial of treatments of "early" breast cancer. World Surg 1:314–316, 1977

41. Hayward JL: The Guy's hospital trials on breast conservation, in Harris JR, Hellman S, Silen W (eds): Conservative Management of Breast Cancer. Philadelphia, Lippincott, 1983, pp 77–90

42. Veronesi U, Saccozzi R, Del Vecchio M, et al: Comparing radical mastectomy with quadrantectomy, axillary

dissection, and radiotherapy in patients with small cancers of the breast. N Engl J Med 305:6–11, 1981

43. Veronesi U: Randomized trials comparing conservation techniques with conventional surgery: An overview, in Tobias JS, Peckham MJ (eds): Primary Management of Breast Cancer: Alternatives to mastectomy. London, Edward Arnold, 1985, pp 131–152

44. Bonadonna G, Valagussa P, Zucali R, et al: Feasibility of adjuvant chemotherapy plus radiotherapy in operable breast cancer, in Harris JR, Hellman S, Silen W, (eds): Conservative Management of Breast Cancer. Philadelphia, Lippincott, 1983, pp 321–328

45. Sarrazin D, Le M, Rouessé J, et al: Conservative treatment *versus* mastectomy in breast cancer tumors with macroscopic diameter of 20 millimeters or less: The experience of the Institut Gustave Roussy. Cancer 53:1209–1213, 1984

46. Findlay P, Lippman M, Danforth D, et al: A randomized trial comparing mastectomy to radiotherapy in the treatment of stage I-II breast cancer: A preliminary report. Proc Am Soc Clin Oncol 4:C–230, 1985

47. Beadle GF, Harris JR, Silver B, et al: Cosmetic results following primary radiation therapy for early breast cancer. Cancer 54:2911–2918, 1984

48. Beadle GF, Come S, Henderson IC, et al: The effect of adjuvant chemotherapy on the cosmetic results after primary radiation treatment for early stage breast cancer. Int J Radiat Oncol Biol Phys 10:2131–2137, 1984

49. Pezner RD, Patterson MP, Hill LR, et al: Breast retraction assessment: An objective evaluation of cosmetic results of patients treated conservatively for breast cancer. Int J Radiat Oncol Biol Phys 11:575–578, 1985

50. Larson D, Weinstein M, Goldberg I, et al: Arm edema is influenced by the extent of axillary surgery in patients treated with primary radiation therapy. Int J Radiat Oncol Biol Phys 10:78, 1984 (suppl 2) (abstr)

51. Bagley FH, Walsh JW, Cady B, et al: Carcinomatous versus radiation-induced brachial plexus neuropathy in breast cancer. Cancer 41:2154–2157, 1978

52. Match RM: Radiation-induced brachial plexus paralysis. Arch Surg 110:384–386, 1975

53. Salner AL, Botnick LE, Herzog AG, et al: Reversible brachial plexopathy following primary radiation therapy for breast cancer. Cancer Treat Rep 65:797–802, 1981

54. Loeffler JS, Goldberg ID, Risser TA, et al: Noninvasive cardiac evaluation after definitive radiation therapy for carcinoma of the breast. Int J Radiat Oncol Biol Phys 11:103, 1985 (abstr) (suppl 1)

55. Danoff BF, Galvin JM, Cheng E, et al: The clinical application of CT scanning in the treatment of primry breast cancer, in Ames FC, Blumenschein GR, Montague ED (eds): Current Controversies in Breast Cancer. Austin, University of Texas, 1984, pp 391–397

56. Recht A, Silver B, Schnitt S, et al: Breast relapse following primary radiation therapy for early breast cancer. I. Classification, frequency, and salvage. Int J Radiat Oncol Biol Phys 11:1271–1276, 1985

57. Slack NH, Bross ID, Nemoto T, et al: Experiences with bilateral primary carcinoma of the breast. Surg Gynecol Obstet 136:433–440, 1973

58. Robbins GF, Berg SW: Bilateral primary breast cancers—a prospective clinicopathological study. Cancer 17:1501–1527, 1967

59. Schell SR, Montague ED: Bilateral breast cancer in patients with initial stage I and II disease. Cancer 50:1191–1194, 1982

60. McCredie JA, Inch WR, Alderson M: Consecutive primary carcinomas of the breast. Cancer 35:1472–1477, 1975

61. Committee on the Biological Effects of Ionizing Radiations: The effects on populations of exposure to low levels of ionizing radiation. Washington, DC, National Academy, 1980, pp 269–284

62. Svensson GK, Kase KR, Chin LM, et al: Dose to the opposite breast as a result of primary radiation therapy for carcinoma of the breast. Int J Radiat Oncol Biol Phys 7:1209, 1981 (abstr)

63. Kuten A, Sapir D, Cohen Y, et al: Postirradiation soft tissue sarcoma occurring in breast cancer patients: Report of seven cases and results of combination chemotherapy. J Surg Oncol 28:168–171, 1985

64. Danoff B, Goodman RL: Identification of a subgroup of patients with breast cancer in whom conservative surgery and radiation is contraindicated. Int J Radiat Oncol Biol Phys 11:104, 1985 (suppl 1) (abstr)

65. Calle R, Pilleron JP, Schlienger P, et al: Conservative management of operable breast cancer: Ten years experience at the Foundation Curie. Cancer 42:2045–2053, 1978

66. Calle R, Vilcoq JR, Pilleron P, et al: Conservative treatment of operable breast carcinoma by irradiation with or without limited surgery—ten-year results, in Harris JR, Hellman S, Silen W (eds): Conservative Management of Breast Cancer. Philadelphia, Lippincott, 1983, pp 3–10

67. Amalric R, Santamaria F, Robert F, et al: Radiation therapy with or without primary limited surgery for operable breast cancer: a 20-year experience at the Marseilles Cancer Institute. Cancer 49:30–34, 1982

68. Pierquin B, Owen R, Maylin C, et al: Radical radiation therapy of breast cancer. Int J Radiat Oncol Phys 6:17–24, 1980

69. Clarke DH, Le MG, Sarrazin D, et al: Analysis of local-regional relapses in patients with early breast cancers treated by excision and radiotherapy: Experience of the Institut Gustave Roussy. Int J Radiat Oncol Biol Phys 11:137–145, 1985

70. Schnitt S, Connolly J, Recht A, et al: Breast relapse following primary radiation therapy for early breast cancer. II. Detection, pathologic features, and prognostic significance. Int J Radiat Oncol Biol Phys 11:1277–1284, 1985

71. Schnitt SJ, Connolly JL, Harris JR, et al: Pathologic predictors of early local recurrence in stage I and II breast cancer treated by primary radiation therapy. Cancer 53:1049–1057, 1984

72. Harris JR, Connolly JL, Schnitt SJ, et al: The use of pathologic features in selecting the extent of surgical resection necessary for breast cancer patients treated with primary radiation therapy. Ann Surg 201:164–169, 1985

73. Recht A, Schnitt S, Connolly J, et al: The use of pathologic features in selecting the extent of surgery for early breast cancers treated by primary radiation therapy. Proc Am Soc Clin Oncol 4:60, 1985 (abstr)

74. Schnitt SJ, Connolly JL, Silver B, et al: Updated

results on the influence of pathologic features on treatment outcome in stage I and II breast cancer patients treated by primary radiation therapy. Int J Radiat Oncol Biol Phys 11:104–105, 1985 (suppl 1) (abstr)

75. Brenner MJ, Schnitt SJ, Connolly JL, et al: The use of reexcision in primary radiation therapy for stage I and II breast carcinoma. Int J Radiat Oncol Biol Phys 11:151, 1985 (abstr) (suppl 1)

76. Durand JC, Poljicak M, Lefranc JP, et al: Wide excision of the tumor, axillary dissection, and postoperative radiotherapy as treatment of small breast cancers. Cancer 53:2439–2443, 1984

77. Kurtz JM, Spitalier JM, Amalric R: Late breast recurrence after lumpectomy and irradiation. Int J Radiat Oncol Biol Phys 9:1191–1194, 1983

78. Harris JR, Hellman S, Kinne DW: Limited surgery and radiotherapy for early breast cancer. N Engl J Med 313:1365–1368, 1985

79. Rose CM, Botnick LE, Goodman RL, et al: The role of limited axillary dissection in the treatment of breast cancer by primary irradiation, in Harris JR, Hellman S, Silen W (eds): Conservative Management of Breast Cancer. Philadelphia, Lippincott, 1983, pp 155–162

80. Fisher B, Wolmark N, Bauer M, et al: The accuracy of clinical nodal staging and of limited axillary dissection as a determinant of histologic nodal status in carcinoma of the breast. Surg Gynecol Obstet 152:765–772, 1981

81. Svensson GK, Bjarngard BE, Larson RD, et al: A modified three-field technique for breast treatment. Int J Radiat Oncol Biol Phys 6:689–694, 1980

82. Siddon RL, Buck BA, Harris JR, et al: Three-field technique for breast irradiation using tangential field corner blocks. Int J Radiat Oncol Biol Phys 9:583–588, 1983

83. Siddon RL, Chin LM, Zimmerman RE, et al: Utilization of parasternal lymphoscintigraphy in radiation therapy of breast carcinoma. Int J Radiat Oncol Biol Phys 8:1059–1063, 1982

84. Botnick LE, Come S, Rose CM, et al: Primary breast irradiation and concomitant adjuvant chemotherapy, in Harris JR, Hellman S, Silen W (eds): Conservative Management of Breast Cancer. Philadelphia, Lippincott, 1983, pp 321–328

85. Levine JF, Coleman CN, Cox RS, et al: The effect of postoperative and primary radiation therapy on delivered dose of adjuvant cyclophosphamide, methotrexate, and 5-fluorouracil (CMF) chemotherapy in breast cancer. Cancer 53:237–241, 1984

86. Lippman ME, Lichter AS, Edwards BK, et al: The impact of primary irradiation treatment of localized breast cancer on the ability to administer systemic adjuvant chemotherapy. J Clin Oncol 2:21–27, 1984

87. Danoff BF, Goodman RL, Glick JH, et al: The effect of adjuvant chemotherapy on cosmesis and complications in patients with breast cancer treated by definitive irradiation. Int J Radiat Oncol Biol Phys 9:1625–1630, 1983

88. Kurtz JM, Amalric R, Brandone H, et al: A second chance to preserve the breast: Results of wide excision for breast recurrence after lumpectomy and irradiation. Int J Radiat Oncol Biol Phys 11:103, 1985 (suppl 1) (abstr)

89. Clark RM: Alternatives to mastectomy—the Princess Margaret Hospital experience, in Harris JR, Hellman S, Silen W (eds): Conservative Management of Breast Cancer. Philadelphia, Lippincott, 1983, pp 35–46

AUTHOR INDEX

Allen, J.C., 110

Beaney, R.P., 83
Berd, D., 186
Bertolini, D.R., 291
Bigner, D.D., 94
Blasberg, R.G., 70
Bloom, J., 110
Bonadonna, G., 383
Borden, E.C., 144
Brooks, D.J., 83
Bullard, D.E., 94
Burger, P.C., 16
Buxbaum, J.N., 260

Cady, B., 434
Carbone, P.P., 415
Come, S., 434
Conlon, P.J., 218
Connolly, J.L., 434
Contesso, G., 384
Cooper, M.R., 334
Cosman, D., 218

Dower, S.K., 218
Durie, B.G.M., 300

Enck, R.E., 128
Ertel, I., 110
Evans, A., 110

Farhangi, M., 259, 350, 366
Feig, S.A., 402
Fisher, B., 425
Frangione, B., 260

Gabrilove, J.L., 228
Garton, J.P., 310
Gertz, M.A., 326
Gillespie, G.Y., 94
Gillis, S., 218
Greipp, P.R., 326
Groothuis, D.R., 70
Gutin, P.H., 46

Hammond, D., 110
Harris, J.R., 434
Hawkins, M.J., 132, 144
Henderson, I.C., 434
Herberman, R.B., 195
Hopp, T.P., 218
Hoth, D.F., 132
Houghton, A.N., 165

Jacobson, D.R., 282
Jenkin, D., 110
Jones, H., 110

Kelly, P., 27
Krown, S.E., 207
Kyle, R.A., 310, 326

Laws, E., 27
Levin, V., 110
Love, S., 434

Maguire, H., Jr, 186
Mahaley, M.S., 94
Mastrangelo, M.J., 186
McIntyre, O.R., 318
Merlini, G., 350, 366
Mihich, E., 234
Mochizuki, D.Y., 218
Morton, D.L., 180
Mundy, G.R., 291

Nelson, D.F., 46

Osserman, E.F., 350
Osteen, R.T., 434

Patterson, W.B., 434
Petit, J.Y., 384
Pinsky, C.M., 131, 141
Potter, M., 275
Price, V., 218

Ransohoff, J., 27
Recht, A., 434
Reisfeld, R.A., 153
Rosen, S.M., 260
Rosenberg, S.A., 200

Saccani Jotti, G., 384
Saunders, W.M., 46
Scheinberg, D.A., 165
Schlom, J., 393
Schnitt, S.J., 434
Shapiro, J.R., 4, 56
Shapiro, W.R., 1, 38, 56
Sheline, G.E., 46
Shirley, R., 434
Silen, W., 434
Silver, B., 434
Solomon, A., 341
Sporn, J.R., 318
Sposto, R., 110

Thomas, D.G.T., 83
Thor, A., 393
Tormey, D.C., 415

Urdal, D.L., 218
Urtasun, R.C., 46

Wara, W., 110
Weeks, M.O., 393
Welander, C.E., 334
Wittes, R.E., 132
Wolmark, N., 425

Zolla-Pazner, S., 282

SUBJECT INDEX

Adrenals, 418
Adriamycin, 445
AG, 420
Age distribution in MBC, 385–386
American College of Surgeons, 384, 385
Aminoglutethimide (AG), 420
Anti-EMA, 394–395
Antiepithelial membrane antigen (anti-EMA), 394–395
Antiestrogens, 419–420
Antiidiotype MoAbs, 398. *See also* Monoclonal antibodies
Arm edema, 439, 440
Autocrine growth factors, 422
Axillary dissection, 431
  radiation therapy and, 444–445
Axillary lymph nodes. *See* Axillary dissection; Nodal involvement

Basement membrane, 385
Bilateral involvement in MBC, 387
Bilateral mastectomy, 390
B lymphocytes, 393
Body image, 434. *See also* Cosmetic results of radiation therapy
Brachial plexus, 440
Brain, 409

CAMFP, 445
Carcinogenesis from radiation therapy, 440–441
Cardiac complication from radiation therapy, 440
CMF, 421
Combination chemotherapy, 421
Conservative *v* radical surgery, 417–418, 425–432
Cosmetic results of radiation therapy, 439–440. *See also* Body image
Cyclophosphamide, 420
  radiation and, 439, 445

Diagnosis of MBC, 386–387
Doubling times of tumor, 390
Doxorubicin, 439
Drug resistance, 421

Early breast cancer
  definition of, 385
  radiation therapy and, 434–446
Early detection, 384
Edema, 439, 440
Estrogen, 418–419
Estrogen receptor test, 418–419

Family history of breast cancer, 386
Fine needle aspiration biopsy (FNAB), 396–397
5-Fluorouracil, 420
  radiation and, 438, 445
FNAB, 396–397
Frequency of MBC, 385–386
5-FU. *See* 5-Fluorouracil
Future trends in therapy, 422

Growth factors, 398–399

Halsted radical mastectomy, 425, 430
High-dose treatment, 421–422
Hormones, 418–419

IDC, 390
Imaging procedures, 402-411
Immunohistochemical applications of MoAbs, 396-397
Injury, radiation-induced, 440
In situ carcinoma, 385
Institut Gustave Roussy, 388
Intermediate filaments and MoAbs, 394–395
Intraductal carcinoma (IDC), 385, 386–387
Intraepithelial carcinoma, 385

JCRT, 436
Joint Center for Radiation Therapy (JCRT), 436

LCIS, 385, 386, 387, 389, 390
Left-sided breast cancer and radiation therapy, 440
Liver, 407–409
Lobular carcinoma in situ (LCIS), 385, 386, 387, 389, 390
Local-regional recurrence, 434–435
Lumpectomy, 426. *See also* Surgery
Lymph nodes. *See also* Nodular involvement
  MoAbs and, 394–395

Mammary carcinoma metastasis and MoAbs, 394–395
Mammography
  MBC and, 386
  occult breast cancer and, 385
MBC. See Minimal breast cancer
Mediastinum, 406–407
Melphalan, 421
  radiation and, 438
Methotrexate, 445
Micrometastasis, treatment for, 420
Milk fat globule membranes and MoAbs, 394–395
Minimal breast cancer (MBC), 384–391
  definition of, 384
MoAbs, 393–399
Monoclonal antibodies (MoAbs), 393–399

National Surgical Adjuvant Breast and Bowel Project (NSABP), 425–432
Nodal involvement, 384–385, 387. *See also* Axillary dissection
NSABP, 425–432

Obesity, 386
Occult tumor
  definition of, 385
  MoAbs and, 396
Oncogenes, 398–399
Oophorectomy, 418

PAPP-A, 397
Pericardium, 407
Pleural effusion, 396
Postsurgical classification of TNM system (pTNM), 385
Prednisone, 445

Pregnancy-associated plasma protein A (PAPP-A), 397
Preinvasive carcinoma, 385
Progesterone receptors, 419
Prognosis for MBC, 387–389
Prognostic studies with MoAbs, 397

Radiation therapy, 431–432
  chemotherapy and, 445–446
  early breast cancer and, 434–446
Radical *v* conservative surgery, 417–418, 425–432
Radionuclide-conjugated MoAbs, 397–398

Segmental mastectomy, 426. *See also* Surgery
Serum assays and MoAbs, 395–396
Skeletal system, imaging procedures for, 402–405
Subareolar tumor, 431
Subsets, 383
Surface receptors and MoAbs, 394–395
Surgery
  history of, 415–417
  radical *v* minimal, 417–418, 425–432

TAAs, 393, 396, 397
Tamoxifen, 419–420, 421
Testosterone propionate, 418
Thiotepa, 420
Thorax, imaging procedures for, 405–407
Treatment. *See also* specific treatment
  evolution of, 415–423
  for MBC, 387–389
Tumor-associated antigens, 393, 396, 397

MUTAMYCIN®
Mitomycin For Injection

This is the full text of the latest Official Package Circular dated December 1985 [3001DIM-21].

WARNING

Mutamycin should be administered under the supervision of a qualified physician experienced in the use of cancer chemotherapeutic agents. Appropriate management of therapy and complications is possible only when adequate diagnostic and treatment facilities are readily available.

Bone marrow suppression, notably thrombocytopenia and leukopenia, which may contribute to overwhelming infections in an already compromised patient, is the most common and severe of the toxic effects of Mutamycin (see "WARNINGS" and "ADVERSE REACTIONS" sections).

Hemolytic Uremic Syndrome (HUS)–A serious, and often fatal, syndrome consisting of microangiopathic hemolytic anemia, thrombocytopenia, renal failure and hypertension has been reported in patients receiving Mutamycin. Most of these patients received long-term therapy (6 to 12 months) with Mutamycin in combination with fluorouracil; however, some patients received Mutamycin in combination with other drugs or were treated for less than 6 months.

DESCRIPTION

Mutamycin (also known as mitomycin and/or mitomycin-C) is an antibiotic isolated from the broth of *Streptomyces caespitosus* which has been shown to have antitumor activity. The compound is heat stable, has a high melting point, and is freely soluble in organic solvents.

ACTION

Mutamycin selectively inhibits the synthesis of deoxyribonucleic acid (DNA). The guanine and cytosine content correlates with the degree of Mutamycin-induced cross-linking. At high concentrations of the drug, cellular RNA and protein synthesis are also suppressed. In humans, Mutamycin is rapidly cleared from the serum after intravenous administration. Time required to reduce the serum concentration by 50% after a 30 mg bolus injection is 17 minutes. After injection of 30 mg, 20 mg, or 10 mg I.V., the maximal serum concentrations were 2.4 mcg/ml, 1.7 mcg/ml, and 0.52 mcg/ml, respectively. Clearance is effected primarily by metabolism in the liver, but metabolism occurs in other tissues as well. The rate of clearance is inversely proportional to the maximal serum concentration because, it is thought, of saturation of the degradative pathways.

Approximately 10% of a dose of Mutamycin is excreted unchanged in the urine. Since metabolic pathways are saturated at relatively low doses, the percent of a dose excreted in urine increases with increasing dose. In children, excretion of intravenously administered Mutamycin is similar.

Animal Toxicology–Mutamycin has been found to be carcinogenic in rats and mice. At doses approximating the recommended clinical dose in man, it produces a greater than 100 percent increase in tumor incidence in male Sprague-Dawley rats, and a greater than 50 percent increase in tumor incidence in female Swiss mice.

INDICATIONS

Mutamycin is not recommended as single-agent, primary therapy. It has been shown to be useful in the therapy of disseminated adenocarcinoma of the stomach or pancreas in proven combinations with other approved chemotherapeutic agents and as palliative treatment when other modalities have failed. Mutamycin is not recommended to replace appropriate surgery and/or radiotherapy.

CONTRAINDICATIONS

Mutamycin is contraindicated in patients who have demonstrated a hypersensitive or idiosyncratic reaction to it in the past.

Mutamycin is contraindicated in patients with thrombocytopenia, coagulation disorder, or an increase in bleeding tendency due to other causes.

WARNINGS

Patients being treated with Mutamycin must be observed carefully and frequently during and after therapy.

The use of Mutamycin results in a high incidence of bone marrow suppression, particularly thrombocytopenia and leukopenia. Therefore, the following studies should be obtained repeatedly during therapy and for at least eight weeks following therapy: platelet count, white blood cell count, differential, and hemoglobin. The occurrence of a platelet count below 150,000/mm^3 or a WBC below 4,000/mm^3, or a progressive decline in either is an indication for interruption of therapy.

Patients should be advised of the potential toxicity of this drug, particularly bone marrow suppression. Deaths have been reported due to septicemia as a result of leukopenia due to the drug.

Patients receiving Mutamycin should be observed for evidence of renal toxicity. Mutamycin should not be given to patients with a serum creatinine greater than 1.7 mg percent.

Usage in Pregnancy–Safe use of Mutamycin in pregnant women has not been established. Teratological changes have been noted in animal studies. The effect of Mutamycin on fertility is unknown.

ADVERSE REACTIONS

Bone Marrow Toxicity–This was the most common and most serious toxicity, occurring in 605 of 937 patients (64.4%). Thrombocytopenia and/or leukopenia may occur anytime within 8 weeks after onset of therapy with an average time of 4 weeks. Recovery after cessation of therapy was within 10 weeks. About 25% of the leukopenic or thrombocytopenic episodes did not recover. Mutamycin produces cumulative myelosuppression.

Integument and Mucus Membrane Toxicity–This has occurred in approximately 4% of patients treated with Mutamycin. Cellulitis at the injection site has been reported and is occasionally severe. Stomatitis and alopecia also occur frequently. Rashes are rarely reported. The most important dermatological problem with this drug, however, is the necrosis and consequent sloughing of tissue which results if the drug is extravasated during injection. Extravasation may occur with or without an accompanying stinging or burning sensation and even if there is adequate blood return when the injection needle is aspirated. There have been reports of delayed erythema and/or ulceration occurring either at or distant from the injection site, weeks to months after Mutamycin, even when no obvious evidence of extravasation was observed during administration. Skin grafting has been required in some of the cases.

Renal Toxicity–2% of 1,281 patients demonstrated a statistically significant rise in creatinine. There appeared to be no correlation between total dose administered or duration of therapy and the degree of renal impairment.

Pulmonary Toxicity–This has occurred infrequently but can be severe. Dyspnea with a non-productive cough and radiographic evidence of pulmonary infiltrates may be indicative of Mutamycin-induced pulmonary toxicity. If other etiologies are eliminated, Mutamycin therapy should be discontinued. Steroids have been employed as treatment of this toxicity, but the therapeutic value has not been determined.

Hemolytic Uremic Syndrome (HUS)–A serious, and often fatal, syndrome consisting of microangiopathic hemolytic anemia, thrombocytopenia, renal failure and hypertension has been reported in patients receiving Mutamycin. Most of these patients received long-term therapy (6 to 12 months) with Mutamycin in combination with fluorouracil; however, some patients received Mutamycin in combination with other drugs or were treated for less than 6 months.

Acute Side Effects Due to Mutamycin were fever, anorexia, nausea and vomiting. They occurred in about 14% of 1,281 patients.

Other Undesirable Side Effects that have been reported during Mutamycin therapy have been headache, blurring of vision, confusion, drowsiness, syncope, fatigue, edema, thrombophlebitis, hematemesis, diarrhea, and pain. These did not appear to be dose related and were not unequivocally drug related. They may have been due to the primary or metastatic disease processes.

DOSAGE AND ADMINISTRATION

Mutamycin should be given intravenously only, using care to avoid extravasation of the compound. If extravasation occurs, cellulitis, ulceration, and slough may result.

Each vial contains either mitomycin 5 mg and mannitol 10 mg or mitomycin 20 mg and mannitol 40 mg. To administer, add Sterile Water for Injection, 10 ml or 40 ml respectively. Shake to dissolve. If product does not dissolve immediately, allow to stand at room temperature until solution is obtained.

After full hematological recovery (see guide to dosage adjustment) from any previous chemotherapy, the following dosage schedule may be used at 6 to 8 week intervals:

20 mg/M^2 intravenously as a single dose via a functioning intravenous catheter.

Because of cumulative myelosuppression, patients should be fully reevaluated after each course of Mutamycin, and the dose reduced if the patient has experienced any toxicities. Doses greater than 20 mg/M^2 have not been shown to be more effective, and are more toxic than lower doses.

The following schedule is suggested as a guide to dosage adjustment:

Nadir After Prior Dose		
Leukocytes	**Platelets**	**Percentage of Prior Dose to be Given**
> 4000	> 100,000	100%
3000-3999	75,000-99,999	100%
2000-2999	25,000-74,999	70%
< 2000	< 25,000	50%

No repeat dosage should be given until leukocyte count has returned to 3,000 and platelet count to 75,000.

When Mutamycin is used in combination with other myelosuppressive agents, the doses should be adjusted accordingly. If the disease continues to progress after two courses of Mutamycin, the drug should be stopped since chances of response are minimal.

STABILITY

1. **Unreconstituted** Mutamycin is stable for at least 4 years at room temperature. Avoid excessive heat (over 40°C).
2. **Reconstituted** with Sterile Water for Injection to a concentration of 0.5 mg per ml, Mutamycin is stable for 14 days refrigerated or 7 days at room temperature.
3. **Diluted** in various I.V. fluids at room temperature, to a concentration of 20 to 40 micrograms per ml:

I.V. Fluid	Stability
5% Dextrose Injection	3 hours
0.9% Sodium Chloride injection	12 hours
Sodium Lactate Injection	24 hours

4. The combination of Mutamycin (5 mg to 15 mg) and heparin (1,000 units to 10,000 units) in 30 ml of 0.9% Sodium Chloride Injection is stable for 48 hours at room temperature.

Procedures for proper handling and disposal of anti-cancer drugs should be considered. Several guidelines on this subject had been published.[1-6] There is no general agreement that all of the procedures recommended in the guidelines are necessary or appropriate.

References:

1. Recommendations for the Safe Handling of Parenteral Antineoplastic Drugs. NIH Publication No. 83-2621. For sale by the Superintendent of Documents, U.S. Government Printing Office, Washington, D.C. 20402.
2. AMA Council Report. Guidelines for Handling Parenteral Antineoplastics. JAMA, March 15, 1985.
3. National Study Commission on Cytotoxic Exposure–Recommendations for Handling Cytotoxic Agents. Available from Louis P. Jeffrey, Sc.D., Director of Pharmacy Services, Rhode Island Hospital, 593 Eddy Street, Providence, Rhode Island 02902.
4. Clinical Oncological Society of Australia: Guidelines and Recommendations for Safe Handling of Antineoplastic Agents. Med. J. Australia 1:426-428, 1983.
5. Jones, R.B., et. al. Safe Handling of Chemotherapeutic Agents: A Report from the Mount Sinai Medical Center. Ca–A Cancer Journal for Clinicians Sept./Oct., 258-263, 1983.
6. American Society of Hospital Pharmacists Technical Assistance Bulletin on Handling Cytotoxic Drugs in Hospitals. Am. J. Hosp. Pharm. 42:131-137, 1985.

SUPPLY

Mutamycin (mitomycin) for Injection

NDC 0015-3001-20–Each vial contains 5 mg mitomycin.

NDC 0015-3002-20–Each vial contains 20 mg mitomycin.

Proven effective in a number of tumor types

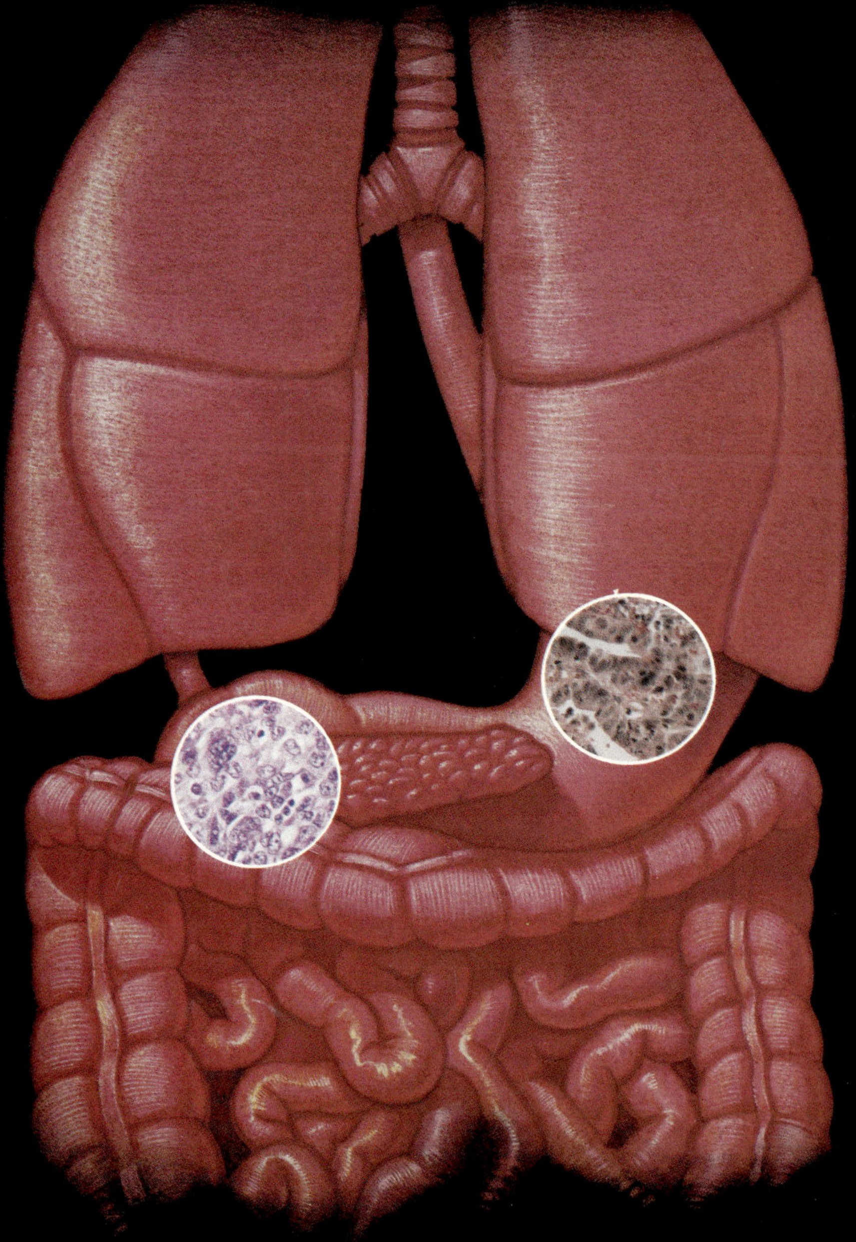

BRISTOL LABORATORIES™

ONCOLOGY PRODUCTS
Bristol-Myers Oncology Division
Evansville, Indiana 47721-0001

MUTAMYCIN®
(mitomycin for injection)

UA-383-1

7/86

VOL XIII, NO 1, SUPPL 1 MARCH 1986

Seminars in Oncology

Prednimustine

Contributors

Philip S. Schein
Franco Cavalli • Beryl Hartley-Asp
Martin R. Berger • Michael Habs • Dietrich Schmähl
David R. Gandara • Howard G. Wold • John Redmond • Marsha Kohler
Ralph Reynolds • Peter Wong • James Forsythe • Karen Fisher
Brian Lewis • Eva Cavallin-Ståhl • Torgil R. Möller • A. Santoro
S. Viviani • P. Valagussa • V. Bonfante • G. Bonadonna
H.T. Mouridsen • Manfred Lehnert • Georg Biffl • Harald Wascher
Konstantin Jordis-Lohausen • Svante Wåhlby • Matti S. Aapro
Michel Forni • Felix Krauer • Pierre Alberto
M. Andersson • L. Pederson
Joseph Allegra

Grune & Stratton, Inc.

Harcourt Brace Jovanovich, Publishers

Seminars in
Oncology

Prednimustine

VOL XIII, NO 1, SUPPL 1 **MARCH 1986**

Table of Contents

Prednimustine: The Rationale for Clinical Development ...... *Philip S. Schein and Franco Cavalli* 1

The Antitumor Effect of Prednimustine in Vitro and in Vivo .... *Beryl Hartley-Asp* 3

Long-Term Toxicology Effects of Prednimustine in Comparison With Chlorambucil, Prednisolone, and Chlorambucil Plus Prednisolone in Sprague-Dawley Rats
Martin R. Berger, Michael Habs, and Dietrich Schmähl 8

Prednimustine in Refractory Non-Hodgkin's Lymphoma: A Phase II Study of the Northern California Oncology Group
David R. Gandara, Howard G. Wold, John Redmond, Marsha Kohler, Ralph Reynolds, Peter Wong, James Forsythe, Karen Fisher, and Brian Lewis 14

Prednimustine *v* Cyclophosphamide-Vincristine-Prednisolone in the Treatment of Non-Hodgkin's Lymphoma With Favorable Histopathology: Results of a National Cancer Care Program in Sweden
Eva Cavallin-Ståhl and Torgil R. Möller, With the Swedish Lymphoma Study Group 19

CCNU, Etoposide, and Prednimustine (CEP) in Refractory Hodgkin's Disease
A. Santoro, S. Viviani, P. Valagussa, V. Bonfante, and G. Bonadonna 23

Prednimustine in Advanced Breast Cancer: A Review .... *H.T. Mouridsen* 27

A Preliminary Analysis of Combination Therapy With Vincristine, Adriamycin, and Prednimustine (VAP) in Advanced Breast Cancer: A Phase II Study
Manfred Lehnert, Georg Biffl, Harald Wascher, Konstantin Jordis-Lohausen, and Svante Wählby 32

Preliminary Analysis of Combined Treatment With Prednimustine and 4′Epidoxorubicin in Advanced Breast Cancer
Matti S. Aapro, Michel Forni, Felix Krauer, Pierre Alberto, and Svante Wählby 35

Combined Cytotoxic and Endocrine Treatment of Postmenopausal Patients With Advanced Breast Cancer: Preliminary Results of a Phase II Study of the Combination of Prednimustine, Novantrone, Methotrexate, 5-Fluorouracil, and Tamoxifen
H.T. Mouridsen, M. Andersson, and L. Pederson 39

A Randomized Comparative Study of Prednimustine and Doxorubicin in Patients With Metastatic Breast Cancer
Joseph Allegra for the Prednimustine Collaborative Study Group 42

Seminars in Oncology

Seminars in Oncology (ISSN 0093–7754) is published quarterly at 6277 Sea Harbor Drive in Orlando, FL 32821. Months of issue are March, June, September, and December. Second class postage paid at Orlando, FL, and at additional mailing offices.

Editorial correspondence should be addressed to Dr John W. Yarbro, MD, PhD, School of Medicine, University of Missouri at Columbia, Columbia, MO 65201.

Business correspondence (subscriptions, change of address) should be addressed to the Publisher, Grune & Stratton, Inc., Journal Subscription Fulfillment Department, 6277 Sea Harbor Drive, Orlando, FL 32821.

Customer Service: (305) 345-2777.

Subscription rates: one volume of four issues, $58.00 within the United States and Canada; elsewhere, $83.00. Libraries and institutions: $75.00 within the United States and Canada; elsewhere, $83.00. Single Copies, $19.50 within the United States and Canada; elsewhere, $22.50. Students, Fellows, Interns, and Residents in the United States, Canada, and Australia may subscribe at a discount rate of $34.00 per year. A letter giving qualifying data must accompany such orders. Subscriptions are accepted on a calendar-year basis. Prices are subject to change. Current prices are in effect for back volumes and back issues. Single issues, both current and back, exist in limited quantities and are offered for sale subject to availability. Journal orders are payable in advance.

Advertising representative: Cunningham Associates, PO Box 308, Park Ridge, NJ 07656, telephone (201) 767-4170.

Agents for Great Britain: Grune & Stratton, Ltd., 24–28 Oval Rd, London NW1 7DX, England. Agents for Australia and New Zealand: Grune & Stratton Australia, PO Box 300, North Ryde, NSW 2113, Australia. Publication of an advertisement in *Seminars in Oncology* does not imply endorsement of its claims by the Editor(s) or Publisher of the journal.

Postmaster: Send change of address to *Seminars in Oncology,* c/o Grune & Stratton, Inc., Journal Subscription Fulfillment Department, 6277 Sea Harbor Drive, Orlando, FL 32821. Return postage guaranteed.

G&S

Orlando, FL 32887

HARCOURT BRACE JOVANOVICH, Publishers

Seminars in Oncology

Prednimustine

Seminars in Oncology

Seminars in Oncology

VOL XIII, NO 1, SUPPL 1 MARCH 1986

Prednimustine: The Rationale for Clinical Development

Philip S. Schein and Franco Cavalli

PREDNIMUSTINE was synthesized in 1969 at A.B. Leo Research Laboratories as part of an investigative program in hormone-cytotoxic agent conjugates. Preclinical studies in a variety of animal systems indicated both high antitumor activity and a favorable therapeutic/toxic ratio, which led to the initiation of clinical trials. As an ester of chlorambucil and prednisolone, agents that are active in lymphoproliferative disease, prednimustine was first evaluated in patients with non-Hodgkin's lymphoma (NHL) and chronic lymphocytic leukemia. It was found to be highly efficacious when administered orally, and well-tolerated in phase II studies conducted in Europe and the United States. More recently, prednimustine has shown promising results as part of a combination salvage regimen in Hodgkin's disease.

The Swedish Lymphoma Group has conducted a comparison of prednimustine with COP (cyclophosphamide, vincristine, and prednisolone) in 206 evaluable patients. When patients with low-grade or favorable histology non-Hodgkin's lymphoma (according to the Kiel classification) were analyzed, prednimustine achieved a response rate equivalent to that observed with COP. In addition, oral administration and the avoidance of vincristine-induced neuropathy and potential extravasation were considered to be important features favoring prednimustine with regard to quality of life and convenience of care.

Prednimustine has also been studied extensively in patients with breast cancer. The drug showed significant single-agent activity in an initial phase II study. Subsequently, a comparative trial was carried out with the objective of determining whether the efficacy of prednimustine could be attributed to the combined molecule or rather to the two single components of the drug. More than 180 patients were randomized to two different regimens of prednimustine and to doses of chlorambucil and prednisolone selected to produce equivalent toxicity based on pharmacologic considerations. The majority of these patients had previously shown progressive disease while under treatment with alkylating agents containing chemotherapy regimens. This trial showed a doubling in response rate for prednimustine as compared with the two components of the molecule and a lesser degree of toxicity. The continuous administration of prednimustine produced a statistically significant advantage as regards time to progression when compared with chlorambucil and prednisolone. Responses were observed in patients previously treated with alkylating agents, suggesting, at a minimum, incomplete cross-resistance, a theme that is reinforced in many clinical trials of prednimustine. Encouraged by the results with prednimustine as single-agent therapy, further single-agent trials and studies of prednimustine-based regimens of combination chemotherapy have been initiated.

Prednimustine's favorable therapeutic index was originally attributed to a tumor-specific distribution of this drug in relationship to chlorambucil. Recent pharmacokinetic studies in animals and humans, however, have shown that prednimustine is rapidly hydrolyzed in vivo to its two constituents. The plasma concentration *v* time course of chlorambucil released from prednimus-

From Clinical Research and Development, Smith Kline & French Laboratories, and the Department of Medicine and Pharmacology, University of Pennsylvania, School of Medicine, Philadelphia; and the Oncology Service, Ospedale San Giovanni, Bellinzona, Switzerland.

Address reprint requests to Philip S. Schein, MD, Clinical Research and Development, Smith Kline & French Laboratories, PO Box 7929, Philadelphia, PA 19101.

0093–7754/86/1301–1001$05.00/0

tine differs from that observed after direct administration of chlorambucil. Prednimustine produces a lower peak level and a longer elimination phase. The sustained plasma concentrations of drug could allow for a greater proportion of neoplastic cells to enter sensitive phases of the cell cycle and be destroyed. Attentuation of peak plasma chlorambucil levels could also account for the reduction of clinical toxicity observed at therapeutic doses.

The demonstration of prednimustine's improved therapeutic action relative to its constituents and its pharmacokinetic profile provides convincing evidence that prednimustine has unique pharmacologic properties that separate it from chlorambucil. This statement is supported by the repeated demonstration of activity in tumors refractory to alkylating agents and by additional information derived from preclinical and clinical studies. As an example, one of us (Schein) has recently compared the therapeutic activity of prednimustine and chlorambucil in a Walker 256 carcinosarcoma cell line made resistant to chlorambucil. Both drugs required an exposure time of 22 hours for maximum cytotoxicity; with prednimustine, 95% of cells were killed at a concentration of 5 μM, whereas the threshold for cell death with chlorambucil was 75 μM. As a second example, data are presented in this supplement that show that prednimustine is less carcinogenic in rodent systems when compared with chlorambucil, once again suggesting a distinct and improved toxicity profile vis-a-vis chlorambucil.

During the past 5 years, our assessment of the clinical results with new anticancer drugs has become more critical. The severe toxicities associated with many therapeutic agents are no longer acceptable to either patients or their physicians. This is particularly the case where there is no convincing evidence that such toxic treatment results in improved survival relative to what is expected with better-tolerated treatment that preserves quality of life.

In this regard, the emerging pharmacologic profile of prednimustine is more than relevant. Predimustine has therapeutic activity at least equivalent to existing treatment for favorable histology non-Hodgkin's lymphoma and breast cancer. This has been achieved, however, with both a qualitative and quantitative reduction in serious adverse reactions. As an orally active agent, it is both convenient and inexpensive to administer, which makes it a logical choice for the outpatient management. In essence, prednimustine serves as a model drug for the next decade of clinical oncology.

This supplement presents a comprehensive review of the preclinical pharmacology and clinical results of prednimustine in lymphoma and breast cancer. It is hoped that this presentation will increase the awareness of the medical profession about this important drug and its potential for application in clinical practice.

The Antitumor Effect of Prednimustine in Vitro and in Vivo

By Beryl Hartley-Asp

Prednimustine is active against a wide variety of experimental tumors both in vivo and in vitro. In many of these tumor systems, prednimustine exhibits distinct advantages over a mixture of its constituents, chlorambucil and prednisolone. In vitro, a higher cell kill is obtained, and in vivo, at doses that are equally effective, prednimustine is less toxic. These differences could be connected with the different pharmacokinetic profiles found between prednimustine and chlorambucil plus prednisolone.

PREDNIMUSTINE is an orally active 21-prednisolone ester of chlorambucil (Fig 1). The underlying rationale for design of the drug was that the prednisolone moiety of prednimustine would preferentially bind to glucocorticoid receptors and facilitate the intracellular uptake of the alkylating moiety. Subsequent analysis of plasma samples obtained following oral administration of prednimustine in experimental animals and humans demonstrated rapid hydrolysis of the drug to its constituents chlorambucil and prednisolone.[1-3]

However, experimental antitumor data in vitro and in vivo have established that prednimustine differs with regard to both activity and toxicity in comparison with its components.

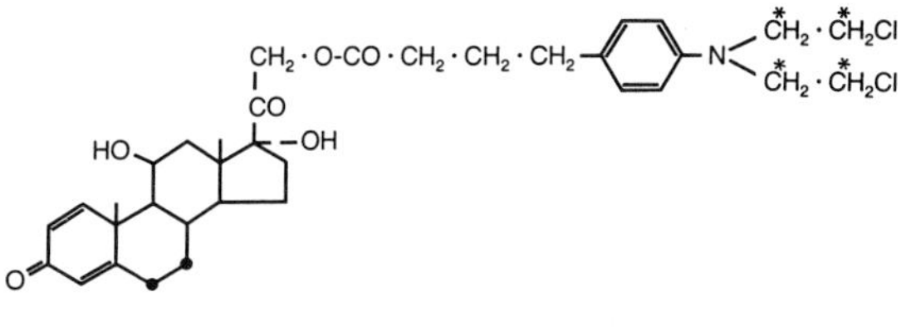

Fig 1. Structural formula and position of radiolabel for prednimustine. Key:*, ^{14}C; ●, ^{3}H.

IN VIVO ANTITUMOR DATA

Prednimustine has demonstrated antineoplastic activity in many transplantable tumor systems in rats and mice, as well as in 7-12 dimethyl benz(a)anthracene (DMBA)–induced rat mammary tumors[4,5] (Table 1). Prednimustine has also shown activity against the 13762 mammary adenocarcinoma and the Mario Negri Institute spontaneous mammary tumor (Garattini S, personal communication, 1973). An interesting observation was that not only was prednimustine highly effective against the normal sensitive Yoshida ascites sarcoma tumor, but it was also effective against a line with a 50-fold acquired resistance to chlorambucil (Table 1). Comcomitant administration of chlorambucil and prednisolone failed to overcome this resistant; however, by delaying the administration of prednisolone for exactly four hours after chlorambucil, a similar cell kill to that of prednimustine was achieved. This potentiation by prednisolone was also found when given four hours after prednimustine, producing an even higher cell kill than for prednimustine alone.[4] This increased activity is borne out in several of the other tumor systems, in which prednimustine was found to be more effective than chlorambucil (Table 2).

One of the major findings in the experimental tumor studies was that prednimustine was less toxic than chlorambucil to the animals.[4,5] This is reflected by the high therapeutic index (TI) found for many of the experimental tumor models (Table 1) and is further exemplified in Figure 2 from the DMBA-induced mammary carcinoma studies.[5] This shows that at equipotent doses, prednimustine caused less mortality than the combination of chlorambucil and prednisolone. The lower toxicity has been examined in detail by Evenaar et al,[6] who tested the effectiveness of subcutaneous (SC) administration of prednimustine on the survival of resting and rapidly proliferating hemopoetic stem cells and L1210 leukemia cells in mice. They found that the relative killing effectiveness of prednimustine for L1210 compared with normal stem cells was higher than for any other alkylating agents (Table 3). This, however, was a consequence of its low bone marrow toxicity and not of an increase in tumor efficacy.

From the Pharmacology Department, Aktiebolaget Leo, Helsingborg, Sweden.

Address reprint requests to Beryl Hartley-Asp, PhD, Pharmacology Department, Aktiebolaget Leo, Box 941, S-251 09 Helsingborg, Sweden.

0093–7754/86/1301–1002$05.00/0

Table 1. The Effect of Prednimustine on Murine Experimental Tumors

Tumor	Mode of Administration	LD50 mg/kg	ED50 mg/kg	TI (LD50/ED50)
Ehrlich ascites	Orally	1 × 470	1 × 265	1.8
Hepatoma AH 130	Orally	1 × 380	1 × 155	2.5
Crocker sarcoma 180	Orally	7 × 159	7 × 10	16
HP melanoma	Orally	11 × 40	11 × 6	6.7
Walker 256 solid	Orally	5 × 64	5 × 1	64
DMBA-induced mammary carcinoma	Orally	20 × 64	20 × 64	2.7
Yoshida sensitive	Subcutaneously	>128	1	>128
Yoshida chlorambucil resistant	Subcutaneously	>128	28	>4.6

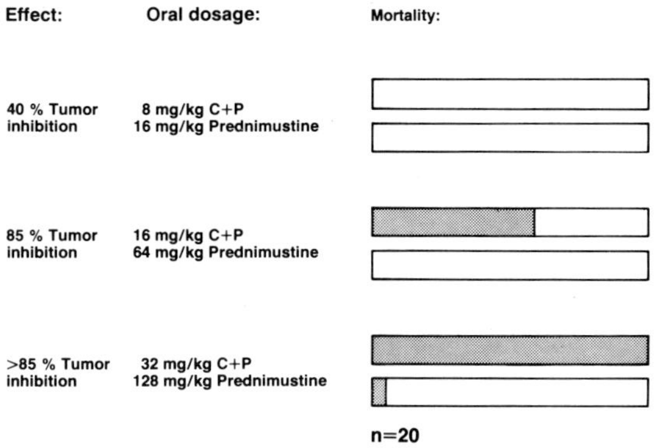

Fig 2. The effect of prednimustine against DMBA-induced mammary tumors. Prednimustine and the mixture chlorambucil (C) and prednisolone (P) were given orally by gavage once daily, five days a week for 4 weeks, to animals bearing tumors of at least 1 cm in diameter. Tumor inhibition is given as a percentage of the control at the end of treatment.

Table 2. The Effect of Prednimustine (S) in Comparison with Chlorambucil (C) in Several Murine Tumors

DMBA	S > C
Yoshida sensitive	S > C
Yoshida resistant	S > C
Ehrlich	S = C
Hepatoma	S > C
Crocker sarcoma	S = C
HP melanoma	S > C

Table 3. Relative Cell Killing Effectiveness of Different Alkylating Agents for L1210 in Comparison with Normal Stem Cell

Drug	Ratio of Slopes of Survival Curves
BCNU	8.0
CCNU	9.2
MeCCNU	18.8
Cyclophosphamide	5.8
DTIC	3.4
TEM	1.5
Prednimustine	23.3

Table 4. The Effect of Prednimustine (S) and Chlorambucil (C) and Prednisolone (P) in Several Tumor Cell Lines

L1210 mouse leukemia	S = C + P
Walker 256 rat mammary carcinoma	S < C + P
S49 mouse lymphoma	S > C
	S = P
V79 Chinese hamster cells	S > C + P
MCF7 human mammary carcinoma	S > C + P

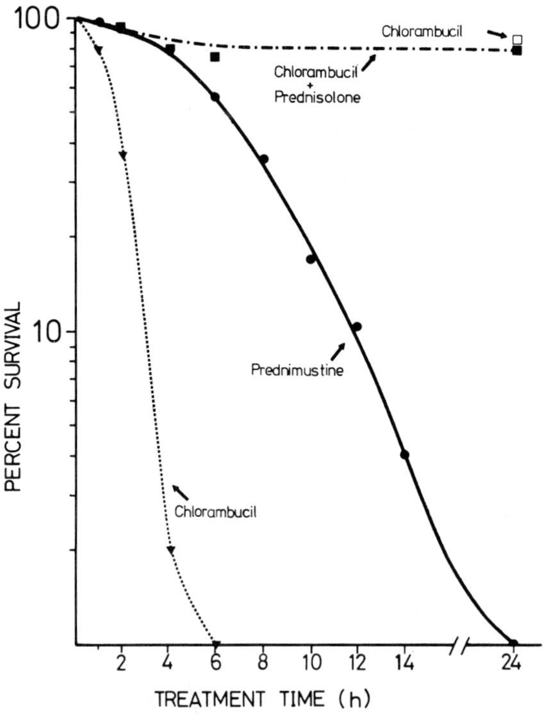

Fig 3. The effect of different lengths of treatment with prednimustine, 30 μg/mL (—●—), chlorambucil, 15 μg/mL (□) and 30 μg/mL (····▼····) and a combination of chlorambucil and prednisolone, 15 + 15 μg/mL (-··■··-) on Chinese hamster V79 cells. The cells were treated in petri dishes 24 hours after subculture. The compounds were washed and the cells allowed to grow for six days. Colonies were stained with methylene blue and then counted. Survival was calculated in respect to the control. Data are the means of two separate experiments.

IN VITRO ANTITUMOR DATA

Prednimustine has been studied in several tumor cell lines in vitro. As can be seen in Table 4, these results were not always in agreement with the data in vivo. However, in both V79 Chinese hamster cells and MCF-7 human mammary carcinoma cells, prednimustine was found to induce more cell death than the combination of chlorambucil and prednisolone. Thus, these two cell lines have been used to examine the mode of action of prednimustine in detail.

Using the clonogenic assay in V79 cells, it was found that prednimustine caused more cell death than chlorambucil with or without prednisolone throughout the whole dose range, as shown in Figure 3 (15 μg/mL chlorambucil *v* 30 μg/mL prednimustine). The effect of prednimustine was found to be very dependent upon the length of treatment time, 24 hours being necessary to obtain full cell kill, whereas chlorambucil reached its maximum cell kill after six hours (Fig 3).

Using radiolabeled compounds, metabolism experiments showed that the release of chlorambucil from prednimustine was very slow, resulting in a higher concentration of chlorambucil during the last 12 hours of treatment than after chlorambucil treatment itself (Fig 4). It was determined that the esterases present in the 10% fetal calf serum addition were responsible for this hydrolysis.[7] The data in Figure 4 suggest that it is the constant presence of chlorambucil, even if only at a low concentration, that is responsible for the increase in cell kill. Experiments in which the rate of hydrolysis was slowed down by substitution of the fetal calf serum supported this hypothesis as no cell kill was found while the prednimustine remained intact.[7]

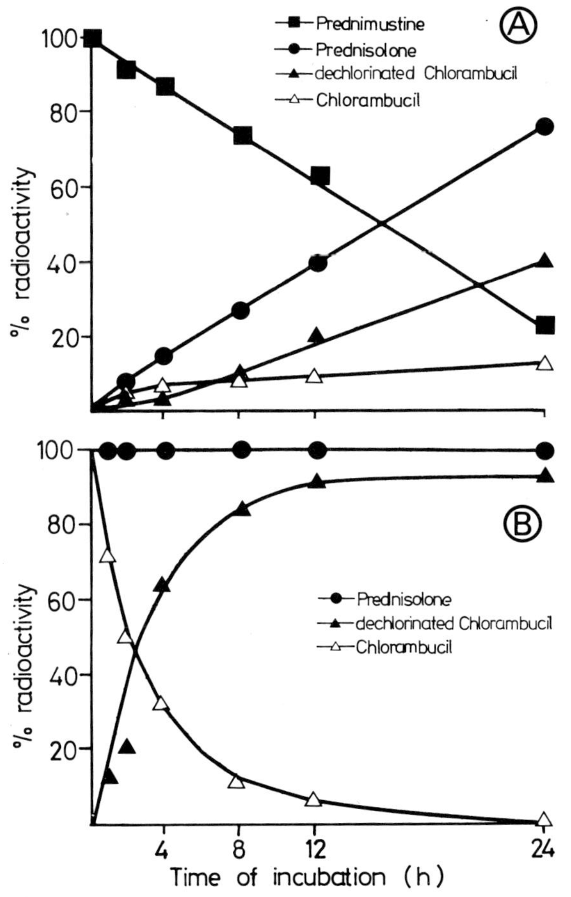

Fig 4. (A) Metabolism of ^{3}H, ^{14}C-prednimustine, 30 μg/mL, in the V79 cell medium system. (B) Metabolism of chlorambucil and prednisolone, 15 + 15 μg/mL, in the V79 cell medium system. Media samples were diluted and injected directly into the high-performance liquid chromatography (HPLC). Authentic compounds were used as standards. Radioactivity was measured in the HPLC fractions, and the percentage of radioactivity in the medium is presented. Data are the means of two independent experiments.

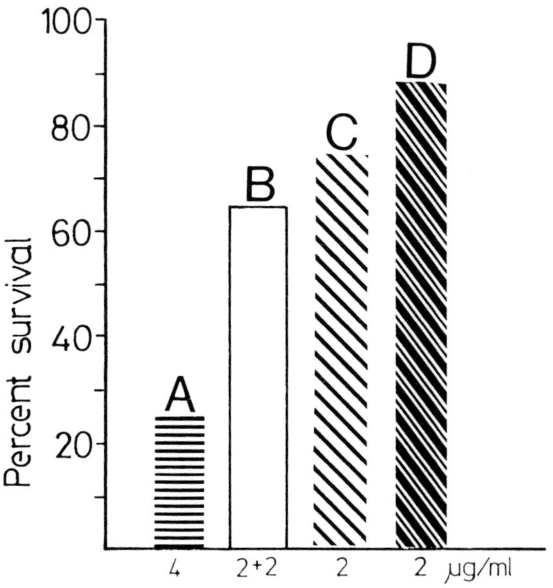

Fig 5. The effect of (A) prednimustine, (B) chlorambucil plus prednisolone, (C) chlorambucil alone, and (D) prednisolone alone on MCF-7 human mammary carcinoma cells. The cells were grown in microwells and treated for 24 hours with the drugs the day after subculture. Viable cells were counted on day 6. Survival is given as a percentage of the control. The results are the means of two independent experiments.

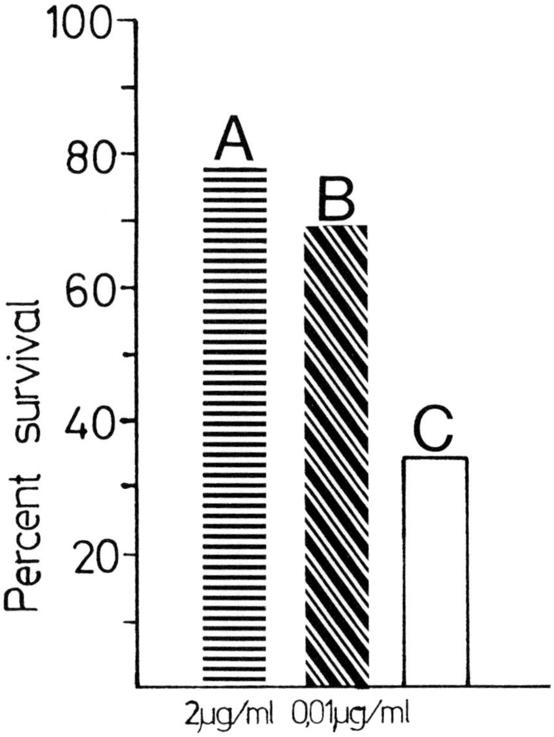

Fig 6. The effect of (A) prednimustine, (B) adriamycin, and (C) prednimustine plus adricamycin on MCF-7 cells in culture. See Figure 5 for experimental details.

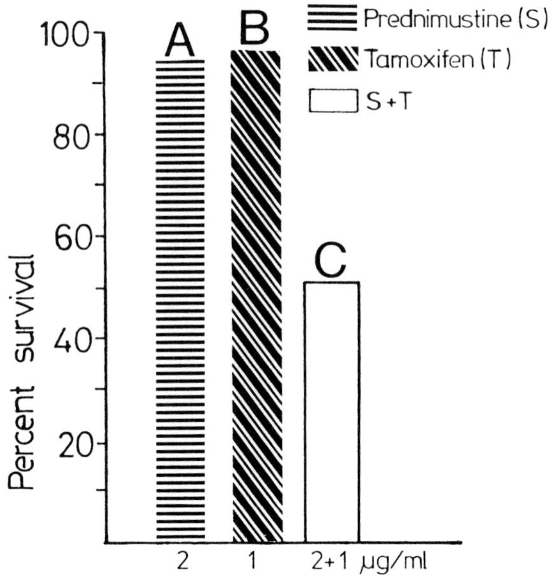

Fig 7. The effect of (A) prednimustine, (B) tamoxifen, and (C) prednimustine plus tamoxifen on MCF-7 cells in culture. See Figure 5 for experimental details.

In human breast cancer trials, prednimustine produced a superior response rate and less toxicity than the combination of chlorambucil and prednisolone.[8] This indicated that prednimustine could be an ideal candidate for inclusion in the combination chemotherapy of breast cancer; therefore, experiments with the human breast carcinoma cell line MCF-7 were carried out. The cell line was adapted for growth in microwells, and the change in the number of cells per well was used as the parameter to measure the inhibition of cell growth.

Dose response data have been obtained for prednimustine, chlorambucil, prednisolone, adriamycin, and tamoxifen. In accordance with the data for V79 Chinese hamster cells, prednimustine was more effective than the mixture of chlorambucil and prednisolone throughout the concentration range. This is demonstrated in Figure 5. As metabolism experiments showed the same profile of hydrolysis as for V79 cells, this was not unexpected. Combined treatments with concentrations of prednimustine and adriamycin that individually produced 20% to 30% cell kill resulted in 65% cell death, indicating an additive reaction (Fig 6). This additive effect was also found at higher concentrations.

Tamoxifen and prednimustine could be a very interesting clinical combination as both of these drugs have a low toxicity profile. As seen in Figure 7, the combination treatment with these two drugs resulted in synergistic cell kill. Preliminary evidence indicates that this is not even the optimum schedule for this combination and demonstrates that this could be a feasible choice for further clinical trials.

In conclusion, prednimustine is an effective antitumor agent in a wide variety of tumor models in vitro and in vivo. In many of these tumor systems, prednimustine demonstrates a distinct advantage over that of its constituents, chlorambucil and prednisolone, especially with respect to its lower toxicity. A lower peak level of chlorambucil and a longer availability after treatment with prednimustine *v* chlorambucil per se has been found in preliminary pharmacokinetic investigations in humans.[9] Therefore, the hypothesis derived from the cell culture work that the longer availability of chlorambucil could be responsible for the increase in cell death may be valid even for the clinic.

REFERENCES

1. Newell DR, Shepherd CR, Harrap KR: The pharmacokinetics of prednimustine and chlorambucil in the rat. Cancer Chemother Pharmacol 6:85–91, 1981

2. Newell DR, Calvert AH, Harrap KR, et al: Studies on the pharmacokinetics of chlorambucil and prednimustine in man. Br J Clin Pharmacol 15:253–258, 1983

3. Plym Forshell G, Gunnarsson PO, Liljekvist J: On the clinical pharmacology of prednimustine. Br J Pharmacol 16:760–761, 1983

4. Harrap KR, Riches PG, Gilby ED, et al: Studies on the toxicity and antitumor activity of prednimustine, a prednisolone ester of chlorambucil. Eur J Cancer 13:873–881, 1977

5. Fredholm B, Gunnarson K, Jensen G, et al: Mammary tumor inhibition and subacute toxicity in rats of prednimustine and its molecular components chlorambucil and prednisolone. Acta Pharmacol Toxicol 42:159–163, 1978

6. Evenaar AH, Wins EHR, van Putten LM: Cell killing effectiveness of an alkylating steroid (Leo 1031). Eur J Cancer 9:773–774, 1973

7. Hartley-Asp B, Gunnarsson PO, Liljekvist J: Cytotoxicity and metabolism of prednimustine, chlorambucil and prednisolone in a Chinese hamster cell line. Cancer Chemother Pharmacol (in press)

8. Lober J, Mouridsen HT, Christiansen IE, et al: A phase III trial comparing prednimustine (Leo 1031) and chlorambucil plus prednisolone in advanced breast cancer. Cancer 52:1570–1576, 1983

9. Ehrsson H, Wallin I, Nilsson SO, et al: Pharmacokinetics of chlorambucil in man after administration of the free drug and its prednisolone ester (prednimustine, Leo 1031). Eur J Clin Pharmacol 24:251–253, 1983

Long-Term Toxicology Effects of Prednimustine in Comparison With Chlorambucil, Prednisolone, and Chlorambucil Plus Prednisolone in Sprague-Dawley Rats

By Martin R. Berger, Michael Habs, and Dietrich Schmähl

Chlorambucil was linked to prednisolone to improve the therapeutic and toxic properties of this potent alkylating agent, which is known to induce second tumors in humans. To compare the carcinogenic potency of the linked compound with that of the respective individual agents and of their unlinked mixture, prednimustine (I), chlorambucil (II), prednisolone (III), chlorambucil plus prednisolone (IV), or vehicle were administered to groups of 120 female Sprague-Dawley rats for 18 months. The following doses were administered nine, four, five, two times, or once a month per subgroup of 30 rats: I, 12 mg/kg; II, 3 mg/kg; III, 3 mg/kg; IV, 3 mg/kg. After natural death of animals, median survival times were analyzed, and percentages of malignant tumors were recorded. An increased tumor risk was found in the following organs compared with those of vehicle-treated controls: I, external auditory canal (EAC); II, mammary gland (MG), central and peripheral nervous tissue (CPNT), hematopoietic and lymphatic tissue (HLT), and EAC; III, none; and IV, MG, CPNT, and EAC. There is evidence of carcinogenic activity of prednimustine compared with untreated controls, but the cancer-inducing potential of the linked compound is distinctly lower than that of the unlinked mixture of chlorambucil plus prednisolone or that of chlorambucil.

THE RESULTS of experimental and clinical studies suggest that little improvement in therapeutic ratios can be expected from currently available cytostatic drugs unless pharmacokinetics and tissue specificity are modified. It is hoped that this will be accomplished by linking compounds with known anticancer efficacy to appropriate carrier molecules. The aim of such an approach is target-oriented drug therapy and concomitant reduction of systemic toxicity. This strategy was first realized successfully by Druckrey and Raabe, who synthesized diethylstilbestrol diphosphate (Honvan®).[1] Many other hormone-linked cytostatics have been developed since then; few, however, have achieved any clinical significance so far.

Recently, a prednisolone ester of chlorambucil [pregna-1,4-diene3,20-dione, 11, 17-dihydroxy, 21-4-p-(bis-(2-chloroethyl)-amino)phenyl-butyrate)], prednimustine, was synthesized to improve the antitumor selectivity of chlorambucil by facilitating uptake into tumors that contain high concentrations of glucocorticoid receptors.[2] Subsequently, the compound was tested successfully in a variety of experimental[3–5] and human tumors.[6–19] Its anticancer activity was different from chlorambucil and the unlinked mixture of chlorambucil plus prednisolone.

After oral administration (the main application route in humans), however, pharmacologic studies revealed distinctly reduced gastrointestinal (GI) absorption rates of prednimustine compared with the individual components chlorambucil and prednisolone.[20–23] Moreover, no intact prednimustine could be detected in serum of animals or patients,[21,22,24–26] thus indicating rapid metabolic decomposition during absorption. These findings thwarted the original concept of this prednisolone ester as a suitable carrier molecule.[27] Surprisingly different ratios of released chlorambucil and prednisolone were detected in blood samples of treated patients.[24,26] These results were confirmed by findings that the chlorambucil moiety of prednimustine was excreted more slowly and less quantitatively than the respective prednisolone moiety.[21,22]

Gunnarsson et al,[28] recently detected a cholesterol ester of chlorambucil originating from acyltransferase-catalyzed transesterification of prednimustine. Such a reaction could explain the different half lives of prednimustine-derived chlorambucil and chlorambucil alone and might be responsible for the qualities of prednimustine that are different from those of chlorambucil or chlorambucil plus prednisolone.

This experiment was guided by the intention to discover possible differences in long-term toxico-

From the Institute of Toxicology and Chemotherapy, the German Cancer Research Center, Heidelberg, Germany.

Address reprint requests to Martin R. Berger, MD, Institute of Toxicology and Chemotherapy, German Research Center, Im Neuenheimer Feld 280, D-6900 Heidelberg, Germany.

0093–7754/86/1301–1003$05.00/0

Table 1. Rationale for Dosing Prednimustine, Chlorambucil, and Prednisolone (Effecting About Equivalent Bioavailability)

Compound	Structure	Molecular Weight	Gastrointestinal Absorption (%)	Individual Dose (mg/kg)
Prednimustine	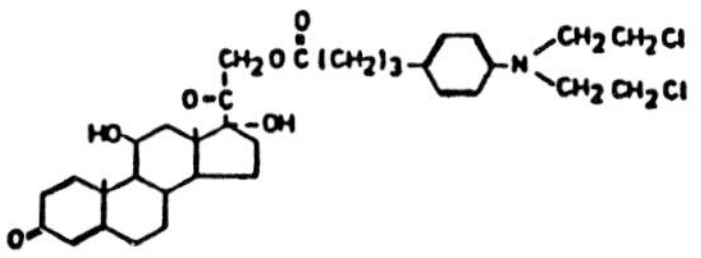	647	40–60	12
Chlorambucil	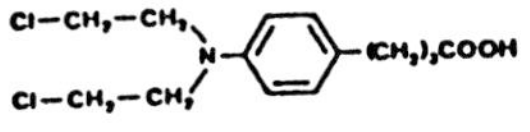	304	70	3
Prednisolone	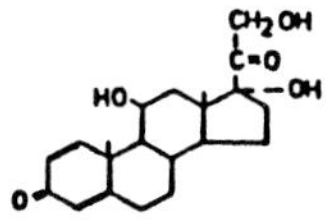	361	80	3

logic qualities among prednimustine and its unlinked individual components. Such differences could be expected to manifest themselves in increased or decreased carcinogenic potency of the linked compound in comparison with chlorambucil or chlorambucil plus prednisolone. Furthermore, new target organs were to be detected.

LONG-TERM TOXICOLOGIC EFFECTS

The rationale for dosing prednimustine and its unlinked moieties either alone or in combination is given in Table 1. The experimental design aimed at a dose-response study and was based on equivalent bioavailability (Table 2).

RESULTS

Median survival time and mean body weight development in each group, as well as overall neoplastic changes after long-term application of prednimustine, chlorambucil, prednisolone, and chlorambucil plus prednisolone in comparison with vehicle-treated controls, are given in Table 3. No symptoms of apparent toxicity could be observed during the experimental period. Regular administration of compounds led to similar weight development in treated and control groups; slightly diminished body weight gain was found only in animals that received prednimustine or the unlinked mixture of chlorambucil plus prednisolone at the highest dose levels (groups 2a and 5a, respectively).

The life expectancy of rats in the highest treatment groups corresponded to that of vehicle-treated controls with the exception of groups 3a and 5a, in which it was significantly lower (alpha < 0.01).[29] Apart from the highest dose level, life expectancy was long enough in all treatment groups to allow sufficient time even for late tumors to develop. Relatively short median survival times (groups 3a and 5a) were correlated with high overall incidences of malignant neo-

Table 2. Experimental Design of a Carcinogenicity Study on Prednimustine, Chlorambucil, Prednisolone, and Chlorambucil Plus Prednisolone Comprising 600 Female Sprague-Dawley Rats

Compound	Group Number*	Scheme of Treatment†
Vehicle	1	9 × 0.3 mL/rat/mo × 18
Prednimustine	2a	9 × 12 mg/kg/mo × 18
	2b	4.5 × 12 mg/kg/mo × 18
	2c	2 × 12 mg/kg/mo × 18
	2d	1 × 12 mg/kg/mo × 18
Chlorambucil	3a	9 × 3 mg/kg/mo × 18
	3b	4.5 × 3 mg/kg/mo × 18
	3c	2 × 3 mg/kg/mo × 18
	3d	1 × 3 mg/kg/mo × 18
Prednisolone	4a	9 × 3 mg/kg/mo × 18
	4b	4.5 × 3 mg/kg/mo × 18
	4c	2 × 3 mg/kg/mo × 18
	4d	1 × 3 mg/kg/mo × 18
Chlorambucil plus prednisolone	5a	9 × 3 mg/kg/mo × 18 each
	5b	4.5 × 3 mg/kg/mo × 18 each
	5c	2 × 3 mg/kg/mo × 18 each
	5d	1 × 3 mg/kg/mo × 18 each

*Each group consisted of 120 rats; each subgroup consisted of 30 rats.

†All treatment was administered orally by gavage.

Table 3. Median Survival Time, Weight Development, and Overall Neoplastic Changes After Long-Term Application of Prednimustine, Chlorambucil, Prednisolone, and Chlorambucil Plus Prednisolone

Group Number	Median Survival Time (Days)*	Percentage of Increase in Animal Weight†	Overall Neoplastic Changes: Malignant Number	Malignant Percentage	Benign Number	Benign Percentage
1	705 (641–761)	+121	13	11	43	36
2a	683 (649–840)	+103	6	20	13	43
2b	755 (704–779)	+118	3	10	12	40
2c	843 (772–905)	+115	9	30	15	50
2d	823 (713–884)	+111	6	20	17	57
3a	593 (545–662)	+113	15	50	15	50
3b	690 (632–768)	+111	15	50	15	50
3c	703 (664–823)	+109	11	33	18	60
3d	831 (705–898)	+115	8	27	18	60
4a	778 (669–826)	+116	2	7	15	50
4b	826 (701–892)	+119	4	13	12	40
4c	820 (683–905)	+118	4	13	12	40
4d	822 (767–892)	+128	5	17	21	70
5a	604 (552–645)	+97	15	50	9	30
5b	650 (506–704)	+107	12	40	13	43
5c	709 (596–772)	+101	15	50	17	57
5d	824 (726–848)	+109	8	27	20	67

*Confidence limits equal 95%.
†Calculated for the whole administration period.

plastic changes and vice versa, whereas overall incidences of benign tumors showed no such correlation; this is in agreement with the relative inferior influence of benign tumors on survival times.

Table 4 summarizes organ-specific incidences of malignant and benign neoplasias of all experimental groups. Benign tumors were recorded in 36% to 70% of the rats. Mostly adenomas or adenofibromas of the mammary glands were diagnosed, followed by leiomyomas of the uterus, adenomas of the adrenal gland, hemangiomas, lipomas, and one incidence each of islet cell tumor of the pancreas, papilloma of the forestomach, meningioma, thymoma, cholangioma, adenoma of the pituitary gland, and adenoma of the external auditory canal. No evidence of any treatment-related influence on tumor development was established by analysis of tumor rates and organ distribution.[30] Higher incidences of benign tumors were found in treatment groups that received less frequent administration of compounds.

Malignant tumors occurred in 11% to 50% of experimental animals. The main histologic types were adenocarcinomas or fibrosarcomas of the mammary gland, neurogenic sarcomas or astrocytomas, myelogenic and mixed-cell leukemias, and squamous-cell carcinomas of the external auditory canal. Less frequently found were fibrosarcomas of the liver, granulosa-cell tumors of the ovary, squamous-cell carcinomas or fibrosarcomas of the uterus, fibrosarcomas or squamous-cell carcinomas of the vagina, squamous-cell carcinomas or histiocytomas of the head and neck region, fibrosarcomas of the lower jaw bone, adenocarcinomas of the adrenal gland, fibrosarcomas of the colon, and local subcutaneous fibrosarcomas. There was one incidence each of mesenchymal tumor of the kidney, adenocarcinoma of the pancreas, and fibrosarcoma of the lung.

The significance of these findings is depicted in Table 5. Tumors found five times or less among all 600 animals (less than 1%) were discarded from analysis. These tumors are known to occur occasionally in Sprague-Dawley rats (the "historical" control in our laboratory), and there was no evidence of any treatment-related influence on their development. Thus, these tumors should be regarded as of spontaneous origin.

Of the four main malignant tumor types observed under the present experimental conditions, administration of prednimustine was related only to an increased incidence of squa-

Table 4. Long-Term Toxicologic Effects of Prednimustine, Chlorambucil, Prednisolone, and Chlorambucil Plus Prednisolone in Comparison With Vehicle-Treated Controls With Respect to Organ Specificity

	Malignant Tumors*					*Benign Tumors			
Group Number	Mammary Gland	Nervous Tissue	Hematopoietic and Lymphatic Tissue	External Auditory Canal	Others†	Mammary Gland	Uterus	Adrenal Gland	Others‡
1	8 (7)	2 (2)	1 (1)	0 (0)	2 (2)	39 (33)	0 (0)	2 (2)	2 (2)
2a	2 (7)	0 (0)	1 (3)	2 (7)	1 (3)	12 (40)	0 (0)	0 (0)	1 (3)
2b	0 (0)	1 (3)	0 (0)	2 (7)	0 (0)	10 (33)	1 (3)	1 (3)	0 (0)
2c	7 (23)	0 (0)	0 (0)	1 (3)	1 (3)	13 (43)	0 (0)	0 (0)	2 (7)
2d	5 (17)	1 (3)	0 (0)	0 (0)	0 (0)	14 (47)	2 (7)	0 (0)	1 (3)
3a	5 (17)	3 (10)	0 (0)	3 (10)	4 (13)	12 (40)	2 (7)	1 (3)	0 (0)
3b	10 (33)	3 (10)	0 (0)	0 (0)	2 (7)	14 (47)	0 (0)	0 (0)	1 (3)
3c	4 (13)	1 (3)	4 (13)	0 (0)	2 (7)	17 (57)	1 (3)	0 (0)	0 (0)
3d	2 (7)	2 (7)	0 (0)	2 (7)	2 (7)	15 (50)	3 (10)	0 (0)	0 (0)
4a	1 (3)	0 (0)	1 (3)	0 (0)	0 (0)	15 (50)	0 (0)	0 (0)	0 (0)
4b	1 (3)	2 (7)	0 (0)	0 (0)	1 (3)	10 (33)	2 (7)	0 (0)	0 (0)
4c	0 (0)	2 (7)	0 (0)	0 (0)	2 (7)	11 (37)	0 (0)	1 (3)	0 (0)
4d	0 (0)	0 (0)	2 (7)	1 (3)	2 (7)	19 (63)	1 (3)	0 (0)	1 (3)
5a	12 (40)	0 (0)	0 (0)	1 (3)	2 (7)	6 (20)	1 (3)	0 (0)	2 (7)
5b	5 (17)	4 (13)	0 (0)	0 (0)	3 (10)	10 (33)	0 (0)	1 (3)	2 (7)
5c	6 (20)	4 (13)	0 (0)	2 (7)	3 (10)	13 (43)	2 (7)	0 (0)	2 (7)
5d	3 (10)	2 (7)	0 (0)	0 (0)	3 (10)	17 (57)	2 (7)	0 (0)	1 (3)

*The first number denotes number of animals; the number in parentheses denotes percentage.

†Malignant tumors of different origin include neoplasias found in the liver (five), ovaries (four), uterus (three), vagina (two), head and neck region (four), adrenal glands (two), gut (two), lungs (one), pancreas (one), kidneys (mesenchymal origin) (one) and local subcutaneous fibrosarcomas (three).

‡Benign tumors of different origin include hemangioma (six), lipoma (two), islet-cell tumor of the pancreas (one), papilloma (one), meningioma (one), thymoma (one), cholangioma (one), and adenomas of the pituitary gland (one) and the external auditory canal (one).

mous-cell carcinomas of the external auditory canal. In contrast to this finding, administration of chlorambucil was found to induce significantly raised incidences of malignant tumors in tissues of the mammary gland, the central and peripheral nervous system, the hematopoietic and lymphatic system, and the external auditory canal. Regular administration of prednisolone effected no increase in manifestation of malignant tumors, whereas administration of the unlinked mixture of chlorambucil and prednisolone was found to cause increased malignancy incidences in tissues of the mammary gland, the central and peripheral nervous system, and the external auditory canal.

When comparing observed *v* expected tumor incidences between prednimustine and chlorambucil plus prednisolone on the one hand and between chlorambucil and chlorambucil plus prednisolone on the other hand, it is interesting to note that the unlinked mixture induced significantly higher tumor incidences in the mammary gland (at nine and four and a half administrations each month) and in the central and peripheral nervous tissue (at two administrations each month). Administering this mixture or chloram-

Table 5. Organs in Which an Increased Tumor Risk was Diagnosed After Long-Term Application of Prednimustine, Chlorambucil, Prednisolon, and Chlorambucil Plus Prednisolone in Sprague-Dawley Rats*

Organ	Prednimustine	Chlorambucil	Prednisolone	Chlorambucil Plus Prednisolone
Mammary gland	−	++	−	++
Nervous tissue	−	+	−	+
Hematopoitic and lymphatic tissue	−	++	−	−
External auditory canal	(+)	++	−	+

Key: −, $P > 0.05$; (+), $P < 0.05$; +, $P < 0.01$; ++, $P < 0.001$.

*Established according to Peto et al.[30]

bucil alone, however, showed no significant difference between the treatment modalities with the exception of a higher malignancy rate in the central and peripheral nervous system at the highest dose level of chlorambucil alone.

CONCLUSIONS

Using doses with bioavailability equivalent to chlorambucil, prednisolone, or the unlinked mixture of the two, long-term administration of prednimustine revealed an elevated risk of developing squamous-cell carcinomas of the external auditory canal only. Simultaneous application of chlorambucil plus prednisolone, however, induced significantly increased rates of adenocarcinomas of the mammary gland, of malignant tumors of the central and peripheral nervous tissues, and of squamous-cell carcinomas of the external auditory canal. Chlorambucil alone caused significantly increased malignancies of the hematopoietic and lymphatic tissue,[31,32] in addition to effects observed after administration of the unlinked mixture of chlorambucil plus prednisolone. In accordance with results reported previously,[32,33] administration of prednisolone was not related to any increased rate of malignancies. These differences in neoplastic effects between the linked agent and the unlinked compounds might well be related to different metabolic pathways and excretion rates after GI absorption. It is concluded that the carcinogenic potential of prednimustine is significantly lower than that of its unlinked individual agents in a rat bioassay. Extrapolating these results to the human situation, therapy with prednimustine should be safer than therapy with chlorambucil or chlorambucil plus prednisolone with regard to the induction of secondary tumors.

REFERENCES

1. Druckrey H, Raabe S: Organspezifische Chemotherapie des Krebs (Prostata-Karzinom). Klin Wochenschr 30:882–884, 1952
2. Könyves I, Liljèkvist J: The steroid molecule as a carrier of cytotoxic groups, in Davis W, Maltoni C (eds): Biological Characterisation of Human Tumours: Advances in tumour prevention, Detection and Characterisation, vol 3. Amsterdam-Oxford, Excerpta Media, 1976, pp 98–105
3. Evenaar AH, Wins EHR, van Putten LM: Cell killing effectiveness of an alkylating steroid (LEO1031). Eur J Cancer 9:773–774, 1973
4. Harrap KR, Riches PG, Gilby ED, et al: Studies on the toxicity and antitumour activity of prednimustine, a prednisolone ester of chlorambucil. Eur J Cancer 13:873–881, 1977
5. Fredholm B, Gunnarson K, Jensen G, et al: Mammary tumour inhibition and subacute toxicity in rats of prednimustine and of its molecular components chlorambucil and prednisolone. Acta Pharmacol Toxicol 42:159–163, 1978
6. Brandt L, Könyves I, Möller TR: Therapeutic effect of LEO1031, an alkylating corticosteroid ester in lymphoproliferative disorders. I. Chronic lymphocytic leukemia. Acta Med Scand 197:317–322, 1975
7. Clinical Screening Cooperative Group of EORTC: A phase II clinical trial of prednimustine. Biomed 27:158–161, 1977
8. Kaufmann JH, Hanjura GL, Mittelman A, et al: Study of LEO1031 (NSC-134087) in lymphocytic lymphoma and chronic lymphocytic leukemia. Cancer Treat Rep 60:277–279, 1976
9. Pedersen-Bjergaard J, Mørk-Hansen M, Geisler CH, et al: Clinical trial of prednimustine, LEO1031 (NSC-134087), in patients with non-Hodgkin lymphomata and chronic lymphocytic leukemia previously treated with steroids and alkylating agents. Acta Med Scand 207:215–220, 1980
10. Håkansson L, Könyves I, Lindberg LG, et al: Continuous treatment of non-Hodgkin's malignant lymphoma with prednimustine (LEO1031). Oncology 35:103–106, 1978
11. Mattsson W, von Eyben F, Turesson I, et al: Prednimustine (NSC-134087, LEO1031) treatment of lymphocytic and lymphocytic-histiocytic lymphomas. Cancer 41:112–116, 1978
12. Möller TR, Brandt L, Könyves I, et al: Therapeutic effect of LEO1031, an alkylating corticosteroid ester, in lymphoproliferative disorders. II. Lymphocytic lymphoma. Acta Med Scand 197:323–327, 1975
13. Brandt L, Könyves I: Therapeutic effect of prednimustine (LEO1031) in various types of leukaemia. Eur J Cancer 13:393–398, 1977
14. Brandt L, Könyves I: Use of prednimustine for remission induction without drug-induced bone marrow aplasia in adult acute non-lymphocytic leukaemia (ANLL). Med Oncol 3:521, 1978
15. Johansson JE, Tropé C, Mattsson W, et al: Phase II study LEO1031 (prednimustine) in advanced ovarian carcinoma. Cancer Treat Rep 63:421–424, 1979
16. Lele SB, Piver MS, Barlow JJ, et al: LEO1031 (NSC-134087) in gynecological malignancies. Oncology 35:101–102, 1978
17. Catane R, Kaufmann JH, Madajewicz S, et al: Prednimustine therapy of advanced prostatic cancer. Br J Urol 50:29–32, 1978
18. Mouridsen HT, Kristensen D, Halskov-Nielsen J, et al: Phase II trial of prednimustine, LEO1031 (NSC-134087), in advanced breast cancer. Cancer 46:253–255, 1980
19. Løber J, Mouridsen HT, Christiansen JE, et al: A phase III trial comparing prednimustine (LEO1031) to chlorambucil plus prednisolone in advanced breast cancer. Cancer 52:1570–1576, 1983
20. Könyves I, Nordenskjöld B, Plym-Forshell G, et al: Preliminary clinical and absorption studies with prednimus-

tine in patients with mammary carcinomas. Eur J Cancer 11:841–844, 1975

21. Kirdani RY, Murphy GP, Sandberg AA: Some metabolic aspects of a nitrogen mustard of prednisolone. Oncology 35:47–53, 1978

22. Gaver RC, Deeb G, Pittman KA, et al: Disposition of orally administered ^{14}C-prednimustine in cancer patients. Cancer Chemother Pharmacol 11:139–143, 1983

23. Plym-Forshell G, Wennberg B: The absorption and excretion of orally administered ^{3}H-prednimustine by rats—A comparison of different dosage forms. Int Res Rep 981, 1976

24. Sayed A, Van Hove W, Vermeulen A: Prednisolone plasma levels after oral administration of prednimustine. Oncology 38:351–355, 1981

25. Newell DR, Calvert AH, Harrap KR, et al: The clinical pharmacology of chlorambucil and prednimustine. Br J Clin Pharmacol 16:762–763, 1983

26. Ehrsson H, Wallin I, Nilsson SO, et al: Pharmacokinetics of chlorambucil in man after administration of the free drug and its prednisolone ester (prednimustine, LEO1031). Eur J Clin Pharmacol 24:251–253, 1983

27. Newell DR, Calvert AH, Harrap KR, et al: Studies on the pharmacokinetics of chlorambucil and prednimustine in man. Br J Clin Pharmacol 15:253–258, 1983

28. Gunnarsson PO, Johansson SA, Svensson L: Cholesterol ester formation by transesterification of chlorambucil: A novel pathway in drug metabolism. Xenobiotica 14:569–574, 1984

29. Dunn OJ: Multiple comparison using rank sums. Technometrics 6:241–252, 1964

30. Peto R, Pike MC, Day NE, et al: Guidelines for simple, sensitive significance tests for carcinogenic effects in long-term animal experiments, in IARC (ed): Monographs on the Evaluation of the Carcinogenic Risk of Chemicals to Humans. Suppl 2: Long-Term and Short-Term Screening Assays for Carcinogens, A Critical Appraisal. Lyon, IARC, 1980, pp 311–426

31. IARC: Monographs on the Evaluation of the Carcinogenic Risk of Chemicals to Humans, Some Antineoplastic and Immunosuppressive Agents, vol 26. Lyon, IARC, 1981

32. Palmer RG, Denman AM: Malignancies induced by chlorambucil. Cancer Treat Rev 11:121–129, 1984

33. Schmähl D: Investigations on the influence of immunodepressive means on the chemical carcinogenesis in rats. Z Krebsforsch 81:211–215, 1974

Prednimustine in Refractory Non-Hodgkin's Lymphoma: A Phase II Study of the Northern California Oncology Group

By David R. Gandara, Howard G. Wold, John Redmond, Marsha Kohler, Ralph Reynolds, Peter Wong, James Forsythe, Karen Fisher, and Brian Lewis

Fifty-six patients with advanced non-Hodgkin's lymphoma (NHL) were entered into a phase II study of prednimustine, an ester of chlorambucil and prednisolone. All patients were refractory to extensive prior combination chemotherapy. Therapy with prednimustine, 100 mg/m^2/day orally, was given for three consecutive days every 2 weeks. The overall response rate in 43 evaluable patients was 30% (13/43), with 9% (4/43) achieving complete response (CR) and 21% (9/43) achieving partial response (PR). In the favorable histology subgroup (23 patients), the response rate was 39% (9/23), with 4% (1/23) achieving CR and 35% (8/23) achieving PR. In the unfavorable histology subgroup (20 patients), responses were seen in 20% (4/20) with 15% (3/20) achieving CR, all in heavily pretreated diffuse histiocytic lymphoma. Toxicity of this regimen was mild, with leukopenia below 3,000/mm^3 in 22% and thrombocytopenia below 90,000/mm^3 in 16% of patients. A positive correlation was observed between response and hematologic toxicity, indicating the potential for a dose-escalation schedule in future trials. These data confirm activity of prednimustine in NHL refractory to standard treatment. In view of its relatively mild toxicity, we conclude that prednimustine is an appropriate agent to test in combination chemotherapy regimens in this group of lymphomas.

THE NON-HODGKIN'S LYMPHOMAS (NHL) are a complex and heterogeneous group of disorders. Appropriate treatment is generally based on extent of disease and histologic subtype, broadly divided into *favorable* and *unfavorable* histologies.[1] Since the majority of patients present with advanced disease, treatment usually consists of chemotherapy, ranging from single-agent alkylator therapy for favorable histology patients to aggressive combination regimens for patients with unfavorable histologies. For those patients developing resistance to standard treatment, attempts at secondary therapy are often compromised because of disease-related or treatment-related cytopenias. New therapeutic agents that are relatively nonmyelosuppressive might benefit this group of patients with refractory disease.

Prednimustine, a prednisolone ester of chlorambucil, is active in several animal tumor systems, including a cell line resistant to standard alkylating agents alone.[2] Early clinical trials have reported responses in a variety of solid tumors and hematologic malignancies, especially chronic lymphocytic leukemia and NHL, and have demonstrated mild toxicity.[3–5] In addition to high response rates for prednimustine used as primary therapy in NHL, several reports have demonstrated activity in patients failing regimens containing alkylating agents and corticosteroids, suggesting a possible lack of cross-resistance.[6,7]

This report describes the results of a Northern California Oncology Group (NCOG) study of prednimustine in patients with refractory NHL, divided into favorable and unfavorable histology subsets. To better define the independent activity of this agent, all patients were refractory to conventional chemotherapy, including standard alkylating agents and corticosteroids.

MATERIALS AND METHODS

Patient selection. Criteria for study entry for NCOG 13-L-80-2 consisted of biopsy-documented advanced NHL (stages III and IV); measurable disease refractory to conventional chemotherapy, including standard alkylating agents and corticosteroids; a Karnofsky performance status of 50% or greater; a granulocyte count more than 1,000/mm^3; a platelet count more than 50,000/mm^3; adequate renal function; and written informed consent.

From the Northern California Oncology Group, Palo Alto, Calif; the Division of Hematology-Oncology, University of California, Davis, and Veterans Administration Medical Center, Martinez, Calif; the Hematology-Oncology Service, Letterman Army Medical Center, San Francisco; the Department of Medicine, Madigan Army Medical Center, Tacoma, Wash; and the Division of Hematology-Oncology, University of California, San Francisco.

The opinions or assertions contained herein are the private views of the authors and are not to be construed as official or as reflecting the view of the Department of the Army or the Department of Defense.

This paper was supported in part by Grants CA35041, CA21744, and NO1-CN-35037 from the National Cancer Institute.

Address reprint requests to David R. Gandara, MD, University of California Service, VA Medical Center 612/111 H, 150 Muir Road, Martinez, CA 94553.

0093-7754/86/1301-1004$05.00/0

Definition of response and toxicity criteria. Standard cooperative group criteria of the NCOG were used for assessment of response and toxicity.

Treatment schedule. Prednimustine, 100 $mg/m^2/day$ orally, was administered in a pulse regimen for three consecutive days every 2 weeks. Therapy was repeated in 2-week cycles until complete response was obtained or progression of disease was observed. Patients with stable disease following six cycles (12 weeks) of therapy were considered treatment failures and were removed from study. A graded dose-reduction schedule was used, based on absolute granulocyte and platelet count and whether initial cytopenia was present due to bone marrow lymphoma or bone marrow hypoplasia from prior therapy.

RESULTS

Patient Characteristics

From September 23, 1981, to March 5, 1985, 56 patients from member institutions of NCOG were entered into this study. Patient characteristics at time of study entry are summarized in Table 1. Of 56 patients entered on study, 26 are registered as favorable histology and 30 as unfavorable histology NHL. The mean age for all patients is 62.2 years, with a range of 22 to 84 years. Karnofsky performance status (KPS) at study entry varied considerably dependent on favorable *v* unfavorable histologic subtype. While only 4% (1/26) of favorable histology patients had a low KPS of 50% to 60%, 33% of patients with unfavorable histology had KPS scores in this range. The great majority of patients (45/56) had stage IV disease including 22 of 26 patients in the favorable category and 23 of 30 in the unfavorable category. In this study, all patients, including all patients in the favorable histology subgroup, were refractory to extensive prior combination chemotherapy.

Using a modified Rappaport classification system, patients were divided into two histologic subgroups: favorable histology (26 patients) and unfavorable histology (30 patients). Characteristics of the two groups are shown in Table 2. The most common histologic subtypes in this study are lymphocytic, well-differentiated (12 patients) and nodular lymphocytic, poorly differentiated (10 patients) in the favorable histology subgroup, and diffuse lymphocytic, poorly differentiated (13 patients) and diffuse histiocytic (12 patients) in the unfavorable histology subgroup.

Response Data

Of 56 patients entered on study, 43 were fully evaluable and form the basis of this report. Following central NCOG pathology review, three patients were deemed ineligible because of histologic misclassification. Four patients in the unfavorable category were inevaluable due to early, non–treatment-related death. One patient was inevaluable because of inadequate data, and one patient never received therapy. At the present time, four additional patients are too early to evaluate. Response data for favorable and unfavorable histologic subtypes are shown in Table 3. The overall response rate is 30% (13/43), with complete response (CR) in 4 out of 43 (9%) and partial response (PR) in 9 out of 43 (21%). In favorable histology patients, there were one CR (4%) and eight PRs (35%) in 23 evaluable patients for an overall objective response (CR and PR) of 9 of 23 (39%). In the unfavorable

Table 1. Patient Characteristics at Study Entry

Patient Characteristic	Patient Category: Favorable	Unfavorable	Total
Number of patients	26	30	56
Age in years			
Mean	60.4	63.7	62.2
Range	(41-84)	(22-80)	(22-84)
Karnofsky performance status at entry			
90%-100%	20	11	31
70%-80%	5	9	14
50%-60%	1	10	11
Stage			
III	4	7	11
IV	22	23	45
Prior therapy			
Extensive	26	30	56
Nonextensive	0	0	0

Table 2. Patient Categories and Histologic Subtypes

Categories and Subtypes	Number of Patients
Favorable histology	
Lymphocytic, well-differentiated	12
Nodular lymphocytic, poorly differentiated	10
Nodular mixed cell	3
Cutaneous T cell	1
Total	26
Unfavorable histology:	
Nodular histiocytic	1
Diffuse lymphocytic, poorly differentiated	13
Diffuse mixed cell	3
Diffuse histiocytic	12
Diffuse undifferentiated	1
Total	30

Table 3. Overall Response Status for Evaluable Patients

Response Categories	Response Rate*		
	Favorable	Unfavorable	Total
Complete Response	1/23	3/20	4/43
	(4)	(15)	(9)
Partial Response	8/23	1/20	9/43
	(35)	(5)	(21)
Overall objective response†	9/23	4/20	13/43
	(39)	(20)	(30)

*Numbers with slashes represent responses out of the total; numbers in parentheses show percentages.

†CR and PR.

Table 4. Hematologic Toxicity

Severity of Toxicity (Grade)	Patients Evaluable for Toxicity*		
	Favorable	Unfavorable	Total
WBC (thousand/mm^3)			
Grade 2 (2.9–2.0)	4	3	7
Grade 3 (1.9–1.0)	2	2	4
Grade 4 (<1.0)	0	0	0
Total (<3.0)	6	5	11†
Platelets (thousand/mm^3)			
Grade 2 (89–50)	2	4	6
Grade 3 (49–25)	2	0	2
Grade 4 (<25)	0	0	0
Total (<90)	4	4	8‡

*N = 49.

†22%.

‡16%.

histology subgroup, there were three CRs (15%) and one PR (5%) for an overall objective response of 4 of 20 (20%).

In favorable histologic subtypes, responses in evaluable patients were as follows: two responses out of nine patients with lymphocytic, well-differentiated NHL; three out of ten with nodular lymphocytic, poorly differentiated; three out of three with nodular mixed cell; and one out of one with cutaneous T cell lymphoma. In the unfavorable histologic subtypes, the following responses were observed: no response in the one case of nodular histiocytic NHL; no response in the six with diffuse lymphocytic, poorly differentiated; one out of two with diffuse mixed cell; and three out of 11 with diffuse histiocytic lymphoma. The median survival time (mst) for all evaluable patients is 5.3 months, with an mst of 3.6 months for nonresponders. For responding patients, the mst is 11.3 months, with a median duration of response of 3.8 months. In two of three patients with diffuse histiocytic lymphoma achieving CR, a long duration of response (9 and 24 months) was observed.

Toxicity

Forty-nine of the 53 eligible patients were evaluable for toxicity analysis: the remaining four patients are too early to evaluate at this point. Hematologic toxicity graded by NCOG criteria is shown in Table 4. No grade 4 hematologic toxicity was observed. Grade 2–3 leukopenia or thrombocytopenia occurred in 22% (11/49) and 16% (8/49) of patients, respectively, and was seen in all histologic subgroups. There were no episodes of treatment-related infection or hemorrhage. Nonhematologic toxicity was mild, with the exception of severe mucositis in one patient.

Correlation of response to hematologic toxicity (grade 2–4) in patients evaluable for response shows that 9 of 15 patients (60%) experiencing either leukopenia or thrombocytopenia, or both, responded to prednimustine. Specifically, response occurred in six of 11 patients with leukopenia and six of eight patients with thrombocytopenia. By contrast, of 28 patients evaluable for response having no significant hematologic toxicity (none or grade 1), responses occurred in only four patients (14%). Response and hematologic toxicity were highly correlated (chi square, P = .0019).

DISCUSSION

Early clinical trials of prednimustine in NHL have reported overall response rates of 50% to 86%, with complete responses comprising over one-half of this total in many series. A review of prior studies using prednimustine as a single agent in NHL is shown in Table 5.[5–9] Most studies contain a variable mixture of different histologic subtypes of NHL. Exceptions are the study of Kaufman et al,[6] which consists of lymphocytic lymphoma only, and the recent study of the Swedish Lymphoma Group reported by Cavallin-Stahl et al,[9] which includes only favorable histology patients.

Most previous trials include patients receiving prednimustine as both primary and secondary therapy. In some cases, a clear distinction has not been made between patients merely relapsing after prior therapy *v* those actually refractory to

Table 5. Prednimustine in NHL: Comparability of Studies

Study	Number of Evaluable Patients	Therapy Type	Drug Schedule	Response Rate (%) CR	PR	CR and PR
Kaufman et al[6]	12	P and S	C, 24 mg/d	25	58	83
Hakansson et al[5]	37	P and S	C, 8–60 mg/d	59	27	86
Pedersen-Bjergaard et al[7]	16	S	C, 80 mg/d, or I, 200 mg/d × 5	13	37	50
Moller et al[9]	43	P and S	C, 40–60 mg/d,	60	15	75
			v I, 150–200 mg/d × 5	57	26	83
Cavallin-Stahl et al[9]	103	P and S	I, 150–200 mg/d × 5	40	23	63

Abbreviations: P, primary; S, secondary; C, continuous; I, intermittent.

therapy. The studies of Kaufman et al and Pederson-Bjergaard et al are of particular interest in regard to the use of prednimustine as secondary therapy. Kaufman and co-workers' series[6] was the first to demonstrate activity of prednimustine in patients actually refractory to alkylating agent and corticosteroid therapy. In the study of Pedersen-Bjergaard et al,[7] responses occurred in the seven of 14 patients with disease progressing during prior therapy.

The most common dose schedules have been a continuous daily regimen and a higher dose intermittent schedule. Favorable response rates have been reported for all doses and schedules. Moller et al,[8] who randomized patients to either continuous or intermittent therapy, found no significant differences in prednimustine's efficacy or toxicity. The diversity of histologic subtypes treated, the mixture of patients receiving prednimustine as primary or secondary therapy, and the different dose schedules used make comparison of previous trials difficult. Thus, despite clear activity demonstrated in NHL, the exact role of prednimustine has remained unclear.

Our objective was to better define the degree of independent activity of prednimustine by limiting eligibility to patients with advanced NHL clearly refractory to conventional chemotherapy, in all cases including standard alkylating agents and corticosteroids. Since NHL is a heterogeneous group of disorders, patients were categorized into favorable and unfavorable subgroups in order to determine differences in response rates. All patients, regardless of subgroup, were treated with an identical pulse regimen of prednimustine. The dose schedule used was selected as an intermediate dose range because of expected poor tolerance in this heavily pretreated population, many with cytopenias present at study entry. Dose escalation was not a feature of our study, since a dose-response relationship has not previously been shown with this agent and because of initial concern regarding myelosuppression in this refractory group of patients.

The response rates in this study (30% overall, 39% in favorable histology, and 20% in unfavorable histology subgroups) confirm previous reports of prednimustine activity in NHL refractory to primary therapy. Responses occurred in several different favorable histology subtypes, including three of three nodular mixed cell lymphomas. In the unfavorable histology subgroup, the three complete remissions seen in diffuse histiocytic lymphoma suggest a greater degree of activity in this subtype than previously reported. While responses were generally of short duration, complete remissions of 9 and 24 months' duration in refractory diffuse histiocytic lymphoma are encouraging. The correlation of response to hematologic toxicity observed in this study is noteworthy. While response occurred in nine of 15 (60%) patients who experienced at least grade 2 toxicity, responses occurred in only four of 28 (14%) patients without hematologic toxicity. Thus, a dose escalation schedule may be important in the design of future trials using prednimustine.

In summary, this study confirms activity of prednimustine in refractory non-Hodgkin's lymphoma, both in favorable and unfavorable histologic subtypes. In an intermittent schedule, prednimustine is well-tolerated, even in pretreated patients. The correlation of response to hematologic toxicity observed in this study suggests the potential for dose escalation. Lastly, prednimustine is an appropriate agent to test in combination chemotherapy regimens in non-Hodgkin's lymphoma.

ACKNOWLEDGMENT

We wish to thank Karen Fisher and Linda Gourley for assistance in data collection, Dee Villaflor for manuscript preparation, and Nina Sanders for manuscript editing.

REFERENCES

1. Rosenberg SA: Non-Hodgkins lymphoma—Selection of treatment on the basis of histologic type. N Engl J Med 301:924–928, 1979

2. Harrap KR, Riches PG, Gilby ED, et al: Studies on toxicity and antitumor activity of prednimustine, a prednisolone ester of chlorambucil. Eur J Cancer 13:873–881, 1977

3. Lober J, Mouridsen HT, Christiansen IE, et al: A phase II trial comparing prednimustine (Leo 1031) to chlorambucil plus prednisolone in advanced breast cancer. Cancer 52:1570–1576, 1983

4. Idestrom K, Kimby E, Bjorkholm M, et al: Treatment of chronic lymphocytic leukemia and well-differentiated lymphocytic lymphoma with continuous low or intermittent high-dose prednimustine versus chlorambucil/prednisolone. Eur J Cancer 18:1117–1123, 1982

5. Hakansson L, Konyves I, Lindberg LG, et al: Continuous treatment of non-Hodgkin's lymphoma with prednimustine (Leo 1031). Oncology 35:103–106, 1978

6. Kaufman JH, Hanjura GL, Mittleman A, et al: Study of Leo-1031 (NSC-134087) in lymphocytic lymphoma and chronic lymphocytic leukemia. Cancer Treat Rep 60:277–279, 1977

7. Pedersen-Bjergaard J, Hansen MM, Geisler CH, et al: Clinical trial of prednimustine, Leo-1031 (NSC-134087), in patients with non-Hodgkin lymphomata and chronic lymphocytic leukemia previously treated with steroids and alkylating agents. Acta Med Scand 207:215–220, 1980

8. Moller T, Hakansson L, Konyves I, et al: Prednimustine in the treatment of non-Hodgkin's lymphomas. Presented at the International Conference on Malignant Lymphomas, Lugano, Switzerland, September 1981

9. Cavallin-Stahl E, Möller TR, et al: Prednimustine *v* cyclophosphamide-vincristine-prednisolone in the treatment of non-Hodgkin's lymphoma with favorable histology: Results of a national cancer care program in Sweden. Semin Oncol 13:19–22, 1986 (suppl 1)

Prednimustine *v* Cyclophosphamide-Vincristine-Prednisolone in the Treatment of Non-Hodgkin's Lymphoma With Favorable Histopathology: Results of a National Cancer Care Program in Sweden

By Eva Cavallin-Ståhl and Torgil R. Möller, With the Swedish Lymphoma Study Group*

In a nationwide multicenter study, single-agent treatment with prednimustine (PM) was compared with combination chemotherapy with CVP (cyclophosphamide, vincristine, and prednisolone) in patients with stage III–IV non–Hodgkin's lymphoma (NHL) with favorable histology (Rappaport groups nodular lymphocytic poorly differentiated, nodular mixed, and diffuse lymphocytic poorly and well-differentiated). From January 1979 to May 1982, 217 evaluable patients were randomized, and at present analysis, the median follow-up time is 42 months. Overall response rate in the PM group was 63% (complete, 40%; partial, 23%) compared with 66% in the CVP group (complete, 32%; partial, 34%). There was no significant difference in relapse-free survival (RFS) or survival between the two groups, median RFS being 30 months and median survival being 42 months, respectively. Reclassification of the lymphomas according to the Kiel system (possible in 80%) revealed high-grade malignant NHL in 22 patients (12 in PM group, 10 in CVP group). Within this small group, there was a marked difference in survival in favor of CVP-treated patients. However, treatment with PM was less toxic and better tolerated than the CVP regimen. It was concluded that for patients with low-grade malignant NHL treatment with PM is equally effective and less toxic than the CVP regimen.

PREDNIMUSTINE (PM) has been used for the treatment of non-Hodgkin's lymphoma (NHL) for more than 10 years. In several small series of patients, PM as single agent has been shown to give an objective (complete or partial) remission in about 75% of previously untreated patients (Table 1).[1–4] In patients with low-grade malignant lymphomas, PM appeared to be equally effective as many combination regimens, and less toxic.

Based on these data, it was decided by the Swedish Lymphoma Study Group to perform a nationwide prospective randomized study in which patients with stage III–IV malignant lymphoma, favorable histology according to Rappaport, were randomized to treatment with either PM or combination chemotherapy with cyclophosphamide, vincristine, and prednisolone (CVP).

This study is a part of a total cancer care program for NHL in Sweden, also including randomized studies in stage I and II disease and stage III–IV high-grade malignant lymphomas (Fig 1).

MATERIAL AND METHODS

Patient Material

According to the care program, all patients with NHL were subject to a standardized work-up comprising hereditary, occupational, and medical histories, physical examination, chest x-ray, liver and spleen scan, bone marrow biopsy, fine needle biopsies of enlarged lymph nodes and of liver and spleen, and surgical excision of lymph nodes. During anesthesia, Waldeyer's ring was inspected and multiple blind biopsies were taken.

Lymphangiography and/or computerized tomography scan and/or ultrasound scanning of the abdomen and pelvis were also performed. Staging was based on the Ann Arbor classification but did not include laparotomy. The histopathological typing was done according to the Rappaport classification.

It was estimated that for four out of the seven health care regions in Sweden, patient accrual to the cancer care program comprised 40% to 50% of all available patients. Patients fulfilling the following criteria were eligible to the trial of PM *v* CVP: age, 15 to 79 years; stage III–IV disease, and favorable histopathology according to Rappaport, viz. nodular lymphocytic well-differentiated (NLWD), diffuse lymphocytic well-differentiated (DLWD), nodular lymphocytic poorly differentiated (NLPD), diffuse lymphocytic poorly differentiated (DLPD), and nodular mixed (NM) types.

From the Department of Oncology, University Hospital, Lund, Sweden.

**Other members of the Swedish Lymphoma Study Group participating in this study included Magnus Björkholm, Danderyd; Karol Landys, Göteborg; Olof Dahl, Karlstad; Leif Håkansson and Hans Zachrisson, Linköping; Anna Johnson and Dick Killander, Lund; Torsten Landberg, Malmö; Bo Johansson and Christina Lindemalm, Stockholm; Per Lenner and Per Westling, Umeå; and Hans Hagberg and Andreas Killander, Uppsala.*

This work was supported by the Swedish Cancer Society, Grants No. 84:211 and 85:84.

Address reprint requests to Torgil R. Möller, Department of Oncology, University Hospital, S-221 85 Lund, Sweden.

0093–7754/86/1301–1005$05.00/0

Table 1. Summary of Reports on Prednimustine as a Single-Agent Treatment in non-Hodgkin's Lymphoma

Study	Number of Evaluable Patients	Number of Responses CR	PR	NR	Total Percentage of CR and PR
Kaufman et al[1]	12	3	7	2	83
Håkansson et al[2]	37	22	10	5	86
Pedersen-Bjergaard et al[3]	16	2	6	8	50
Möller et al[4]	43	25	9	9	79
Total	108	52	32	24	78

From January 1, 1979, to April 30, 1982, a total of 226 patients entered the study of which 217 were evaluable at the time of this analysis. The distribution of number of patients, age, sex ratio, nodality, previous treatment and histopathological types between the two treatment arms is given in Tables 2 and 3.

Treatment Schedules

PM was given orally in a dose of 150 mg (body surface < 1.8 m²) and 200 mg (body surface ≥ 1.8 m²) daily for five consecutive days every 2 weeks for 12 cycles or for as long as progressive disease could not be assessed. When a complete remission was documented, the length of the cycle was prolonged by 2 weeks every third cycle. The total time of therapy was 2 years after achievement of complete remission. In partial remission, the next cycle was always started on day 15.

The CVP regimen consisted of cyclophosphamide, 800 mg/m² intravenously (IV), and vincristine, 1.4 mg/m² (maximum, 2 mg) IV, on day 1 and prednisolone, 25 mg orally three times a day, for five days. The length of the cycle was 3 weeks. The CVP regimen was administered for at least 12 cycles. When a complete remission was assessed, the length of the cycle was successively prolonged by 2 weeks every third cycle. The total time of treatment was 2 years after a complete remission was documented. In partial remission, the next cycle was always started on day 22.

When a relapse or progressive disease occurred, a crossover between CVP and PM was advocated.

Table 2. Clinical Data on 217 Evaluable Patients With Favorable NHL Entering Present Study

	Total Number of Patients	Sex Ratio (M/F)	Age Median	Age Range	Nodal/ Extranodal	Previously Treated
CVP	111	62/49	62.7	17–79	43/68	11
PM	106	66/40	61.7	30–79	51/55	13

Follow-Up

During treatment, patients on the PM regimen were usually seen at start of every second or third cycle, when blood counts were also examined. For CVP patients, blood counts were controlled before the start of each cycle.

Physical examination of involved sites was performed at each follow-up visit; chest x-ray and investigation of any other involved site, such as bone marrow, were performed 4 months after start of treatment and then regularly at 4-month intervals.

Complete remissions were documented by radiography and histopathology, whenever applicable. At the conclusion of therapy, 2 years after a complete remission was achieved, a full work-up identical to the one performed before the start of treatment was carried out.

At the time of the present analysis, the patients have a median follow-up time of 42 months with a minimum follow-up time of 24 months.

RESULTS

In the group of patients treated with PM, the overall response rate was 63% (67/106) with 40% of the patients (42/106) obtaining a com-

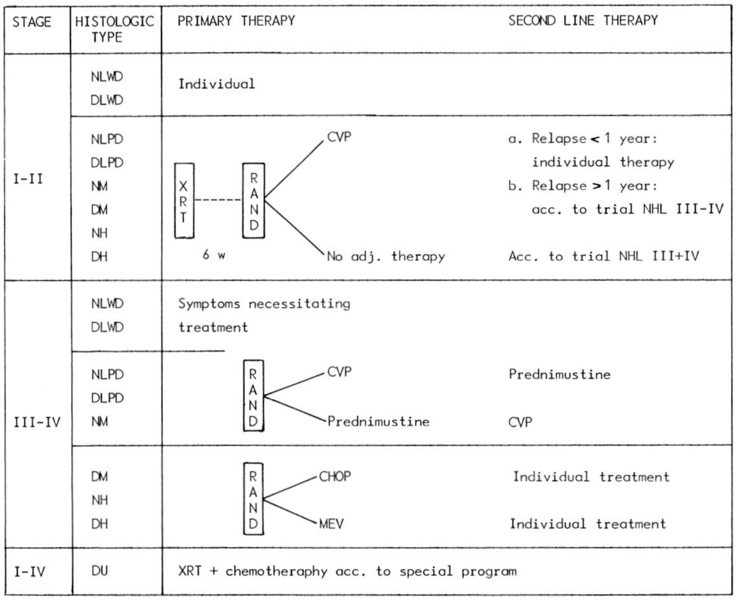

Fig 1. Design of the national cancer care program, effective 1979 through 1983. The program includes three randomized trials.

Table 3. Distribution of Histopathologic Type According to the Rappaport and Kiel Classifications

	Rappaport Classification (N = 217)					Kiel Classification (N = 171)	
	DLPD	DLWD	NLPD	NLWD	NM	Low-Grade	High-Grade
CVP	51	19	25	5	11	77	10
PM	51	14	28	—	13	72	12
Total	102	33	53	5	24	149	22

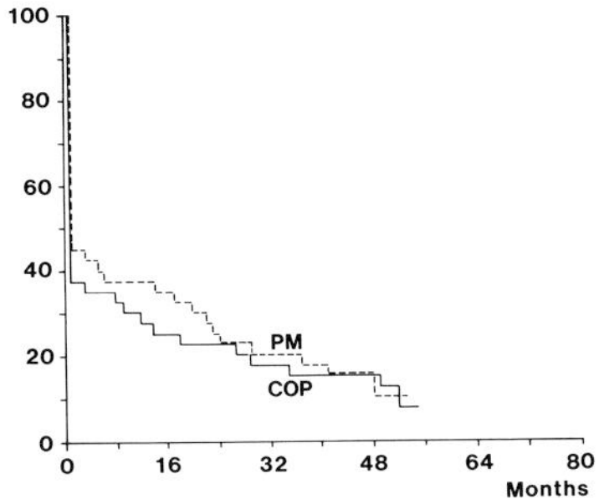

Fig 2. Relapse-free survival of patients with favorable NHL treated with PM and CVP. Median duration of complete remission is approximately 30 months in both groups.

plete remission. The corresponding figures for the CVP-treated group were 66% (73/111) overall response and 32% (36/111) complete remissions. The relapse-free survival (RSF) did not differ significantly between the two treatment groups, the median RFS time being about 30 months (Fig 2). Less than 20% of the total number of patients have a lasting complete remission. Overall survival was also identical, with a median survival of 42 months in each group (Fig 3).

A retrospective reclassification of 171 patients according to the Kiel classification was performed (Table 4). Twelve of the lymphomas in

Table 4. Reclassification of 171 Patients According to Kiel

	Kiel, Low-Grade				Kiel, High-Grade			
Rappaport	CB-CC*	CC	IC	LC	CB	CB-CC-D	IB	LB
DLPD	19	17	19	4	6	6	4	5
DLWD	1	5	8	7	—	—	—	—
NLPD	42	2	—	—	1	—	—	—
NLWD	5	—	—	—	—	—	—	—
NM	20	—	—	—	—	—	—	—
Total	87	24	27	11	7	6	4	5

Abbreviations: CB, centroblastic; CB-CC-D, centroblastic-centrocytic diffuse; CB-CC-F, centroblastic-centrocytic follicular; CB-CC-F + D, centroblastic-centrocytic follicular and diffuse; CC, centrocytic; IB, immunoblastic; IC, immunocytic; LB, lymphoblastic.

*Comprises CB-CC-F and CB-CC-F + D.

the PM group and 10 in the CVP group were considered to be high grade.

Survival analysis showed a marked (but not significant) difference in survival in favor of the CVP regimen for patients with high-grade lymphomas, whereas for the low-grade lymphomas no significant difference in survival was observed (Fig 4).

Toxicity

Treatment with PM was less toxic and better tolerated than the CVP regimen. Dose reduction due to toxicity had to be performed in 28% of the PM patients and 62% of the CVP patients. The reason for dose reduction was bone marrow depression in the PM group while neurotoxicity was a significant problem in the CVP group.

CONCLUSIONS

Treatment with PM is equally effective and less toxic than the CVP regimen for low-grade malignant lymphomas. It is also more feasible

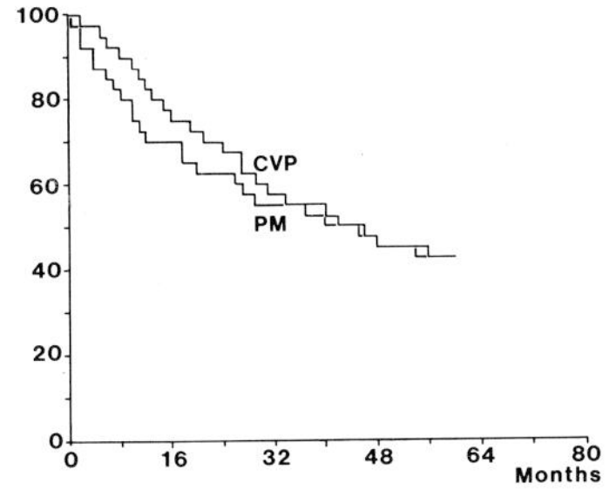

Fig 3. Overall survival of patients with favorable NHL treated with PM (N = 106) and CVP (N = 111). Median survival is 42 months.

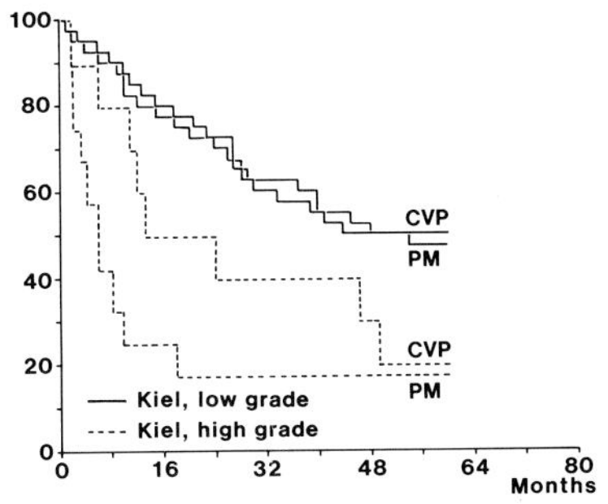

Fig 4. Survival of 171 patients, as reclassified according to Kiel.

for the patients and consumes less hospital care resources. In a new trial, included in the revised version of the national cancer care program for NHL, activated in March 1983, patients with low-grade malignant lymphomas according to the Kiel classification, stage II–IV, are randomized to receive PM either at diagnosis or when general symptoms appear.

REFERENCES

1. Kaufman JH, Hanjura GL, Mittelman A, et al: Study of Leo-1031 (NSC-134087) in lymphocytic lymphoma and chronic lymphocytic leukemia. Cancer Treat Rep 60:277, 1976

2. Håkansson L, Könyves I, Lindberg LG, et al: Continuous treatment of non-Hodgkin's malignant lymphoma with prednimustine (Leo 1031). Oncology 35:103, 1978

3. Pedersen-Bjergaard J, Mørk Hansen M, Geisler CH, et al: Clinical trial of prednimustine, Leo-1031 (NSC-134087), in patients with non-Hodgkin's lymphomata and chronic lymphocytic leukemia previously treated with steroids and alkylating agents. Acta Med Scand 207:215, 1980

4. Möller T, Håkansson L, Könyves I, et al: Prednimustine in the treatment of non-Hodgkin's lymphomas. Presented at the International Conference on Malignant Lymphomas, Lugano, Switzerland, September 1981

CCNU, Etoposide, and Prednimustine (CEP) in Refractory Hodgkin's Disease

By A. Santoro, S. Viviani, P. Valagussa, V. Bonfante, and G. Bonadonna

Starting in February 1980, 58 patients with Hodgkin's disease refractory to both MOPP and ABVD received as third-line chemotherapy a combination of CCNU or lomustine, etoposide, and prednimustine (CEP). Complete response (CR) was achieved in 40% of cases and partial response (PR) in 14%. The median duration of CR was greater than 15 months, and the median survival of complete responders was longer than 24 months. In addition, CEP alternating with ABVD was given to 21 patients refractory to MOPP chemotherapy. In this series, CR was documented in 67% of patients with a median duration of 24+ months and a median survival of 36+ months. Treatment was generally well tolerated, and all acute side effects were reversible. Present findings indicate that CEP is an effective regimen in patients refractory to MOPP and ABVD.

IN RECENT YEARS, attempts have been made to develop new drug combinations to be tested in Hodgkin's disease refractory to primary chemotherapy.[1,2] An additional impetus to this search for new salvage chemotherapy regimens has been the use of potentially non–cross-resistant drug regimens at the outset for newly diagnosed patients.[3–5]

In 1973, the Milan Cancer Institute developed the ABVD (Adriamycin, bleomycin, vinblastine, and dacarbazine) combination[6] to treat MOPP-resistant patients. The updated 7-year results have confirmed the efficacy of ABVD as second-line chemotherapy[1,7] as well its superiority to MOPP (mechlorethamine, vincristine, procarbazine, and prednisone) chemotherapy when ABVD was alternated monthly with MOPP in stage-IV Hodgkin's disease.[1,3]

In 1980, our research group empirically developed a new drug combination utilizing CCNU or lomustine, etoposide, and prednimustine (CEP) to treat refractory Hodgkin's disease.[8] The preliminary results with this third-line chemotherapy in patients failing after MOPP and ABVD administered either in sequential or alternating fashion were recently published.[9] The aim of present report is to update previous results in a larger series of patients and with a longer follow-up. In addition, detailed results of a series of patients refractory to MOPP and treated with alternating ABVD-CEP regimen will also be presented.

MATERIALS AND METHODS

From February 1980 to June 1984, a total of 79 patients with Hodgkin's disease failing after MOPP and/or ABVD chemotherapy were treated with CEP alone (58 cases) or alternating with ABVD (21 cases). Patient characteristics are shown in Table 1. For both regimens, slightly more than half of the patients presented with extranodal disease prior to beginning of salvage treatment. Systemic symptoms were present in only one third of patients treated with ABVD-CEP and in 45% of patients given CEP. In this latter series, 28 patients (48%) were initially treated with alternating MOPP-ABVD, and 30 patients (52%) were treated first with one combination, the other being utilized as first salvage treatment (MOPP ⇌ ABVD). Response to prior chemotherapy was defined as complete remission (CR) lasting longer than 12 months for patients treated with either MOPP alone (12 patients) or MOPP-ABVD (four patients). In addition, seven patients who obtained CR after MOPP and ABVD given sequentially were also categorized as responsive patients. Resistance to prior chemotherapy was defined as induction failure during treatment or as a CR lasting less than 12 months from drug discontinuation. In addition, 15 patients given sequential MOPP ⇌ ABVD and resistant to one of the two regimens were considered as resistant to prior chemotherapy. Median age was 31 years for both CEP (range, 17 to 65) and ABVD-CEP (range, 16 to 54). Nodular sclerosis histology was the single most frequent histopathologic subgroup (CEP, 69%; ABVD-CEP, 62%).

Before CEP chemotherapy was started, the disease extent was accurately reassessed and pathologic restaging was performed in patients initially presenting with involvement of bone marrow and/or liver. The CEP regimen consisted of CCNU, 80 mg/m^2 orally on day 1, etoposide (VP-16), 100 mg/m^2 orally each day from day 1 to 5, and prednimustine, 60 mg/m^2 orally each day from day 1 to 5. Treatment was recycled on day 29. CEP was administered to CR plus two additional consolidation cycles (minimum, six cycles). In individual clinical situations, involved field radiotherapy was delivered either immediately prior to or during chemotherapy in six patients (CEP, four; ABVD-CEP, two). Radiotherapy was also delivered to three patients who achieved maximal tumor shrinkage after CEP and to eight complete responders (CEP, six; ABVD-CEP, two) as consolidation therapy. No other maintenance treatment was given to complete responders (CR$_s$). The median follow-up was 33 months

From the Istituto Nazionale Tumori, Milan, Italy.

Address reprint requests to Dr Armando Santoro, Istituto Nazionale Tumori, Milan, Italy.

0093–7754/86/1301–1006$05.00/0

Table 1. Patient Characteristics

	CEP*		ABVD-CEP†	
	Number	Percentage	Number	Percentage
Disease extent				
Nodal	27	47	9	43
Extranodal ± nodal	31	53	12	57
Systemic symptoms				
Absent	32	55	14	77
Present	26	45	7	33
Prior chemotherapy				
MOPP ⇌ ABVD	30	52	—	
MOPP-ABVD	28	48	—	
MOPP	—		21	100
Response to prior chemotherapy				
Responsive	11	19	12	57
Resistant	47	81	9	43
Median follow-up	33 mo (11–63)		41 mo (11–51)	

*Fifty-eight patients.
†Twenty-one patients.

(range, 11 to 63) in the CEP group and 41 months (range, 11 to 51) in the ABVD-CEP series.

RESULTS

The essential therapeutic results are summarized in Table 2. CEP resulted in CR in 23 patients (40%) previously given both MOPP and ABVD. In addition, partial remission (PR) was documented in eight patients (14%), for an overall response rate of 54%. It is worth noting that of the remaining 27 patients categorized as induction failures, five showed progressive disease after the first treatment cycle. The response rate after ABVD-CEP in patients failing after MOPP was 67%; no PRs were documented, but all 14 patients achieved CR. The achievement of CR was negatively correlated with extranodal disease presentation (CEP, 32%; ABVD-CEP, 50%), presence of systemic symptoms (CEP, 35%; ABVD-CEP, 43%), and resistance to prior chemotherapy (CEP, 30%; ABVD-CEP, 44%). In patients given CEP alone, there was no difference in the CR rate whether prior MOPP and ABVD were given sequentially (40%) or in an alternating fashion (39%).

Median duration of CR has not yet been achieved, and it is estimated to be 15+ months after CEP and 24+ months after ABVD-CEP. Similarly, median survival of CR_s is in excess of 24 and 36 months, respectively. Median overall survival was 17 months after CEP and 34 months after ABVD-CEP. These latter findings largely reflect the different pretreatment characteristics of the two series in terms of resistance to previous regimens (CEP, 81%; ABVD-CEP 43%). It is worth noting, in fact, that in the nine patients resistant to MOPP, the median overall survival after ABVD-CEP was 12 months.

Treatment with either CEP or ABVD-CEP was well-tolerated in general, and only three patients refused to complete the drug therapy. Table 3 lists the percentages of the major toxic manifestations. All toxic signs were reversible, but two patients who received extensive prior irradiation required hospital admission because of severe and prolonged thrombocytopenia after CEP. Slightly more than one tenth of the cycles had to be delayed because of marrow suppression persisting on day 29. Nausea and vomiting were more frequently observed after ABVD-CEP on the day of Adriamycin and dacarbazine administration. Similarly, incidence of hair loss was higher in the Adriamycin-containing regimen. The percentage of optimal dose administered was as follows: CCNU and etoposide, 88%; predni-

Table 2. Response to Salvage Chemotherapy

	CEP		ABVD-CEP
	CR (%)	PR (%)	CR (%)
Total	40	14	67
Disease extent			
Nodal	48	19	89
Extranodal ± nodal	32	10	50
Systemic symptoms			
Absent	44	22	79
Present	35	4	43
Response to prior chemotherapy			
Responsive	82	9	83
Resistant	30	15	44
Median duration of CR	15 + mo		24 + mo
Median survival of CR_s	24 + mo		36 + mo
Median overall survival	17 mo		34 mo

Table 3. Percentages of Major Toxic Manifestations

	CEP (%)	ABVD-CEP (%)
WBC < 1,500/mm^3	10	9.5
Platelets < 50,000/mm^3	16	14
Nausea	84	95
Vomiting	69	95
Hair loss	43	62
Alopecia	29	29
Treatment refusal	4	5
Cycles postponed beyond day 29	12	12
(Postponements/total cycles)	(40/327)	(15/128)

mustine, 87% after CEP alone; CCNU and etoposide, 82%; prednimustine, 81%; Adriamycin and vinblastine, 84%; bleomycin, 97%; and dacarbazine, 88% after ABVD-CEP.

DISCUSSION

The updated results with CEP either alone or alternated with ABVD appear encouraging. After CEP, CR was documented in 40% of patients refractory to both MOPP and ABVD; 56% of CR_s are alive after a median follow-up of 33 months. Present data also showed that, in contrast to preliminary results,[9] CEP therapy was equally effective whether patients were previously treated with MOPP and ABVD sequentially or in an alternating fashion. In patients refractory to MOPP alone, alternating ABVD-CEP yielded CR in 67%, with a median duration in excess of 24 months. A larger series of patients and a longer follow-up are mandatory in this latter subgroup to clearly establish whether the present alternating regimen is superior to ABVD alone in MOPP-resistant Hodgkin's disease.[1,7] In addition, it is worth noting that alternating MOPP-CEP was thus far administered in five patients resistant to ABVD. CR was documented in three patients (60%), and the median survival of CR_s is in excess of 36 months. Toxicity was moderate and reversible, thus allowing treatment administration in the outpatient clinic. The new oral regimen was well-tolerated as also exemplified by the fact that only three of 84 patients refused to complete the treatment program.

In our opinion, the present updated results on the therapeutic index of the CEP combination would suggest that it is beneficial to utilize this combination in clinical practice for Hodgkin's disease patients refractory to two of the most widely utilized drug combinations.

Table 4. Results of Third-Line Salvage Regimens

Institution	Acronym	Number of Cases	Response Rate (%) CR	Response Rate (%) Overall
Milan	CEP	58	40	54
M. D. Anderson[10]	MIME	43	23	60
Stanford[11]	CEM	21	14	43
MSKCC[12]*	CAD	15†	13	46

*Memorial Sloan Kettering Cancer Center.
†Only nine patients were pretreated with MOPP and ABV(D).

As reported in Table 4, our findings with CEP are in line with recently reported third-line salvage regimens, namely methyl-Gag, ifosfamide, methotrexate, and etoposide (MIME)[10]; CCNU, etoposide, and methotrexate (CEM)[11]; and CCNU, Alkeran, and vindesine (CAD).[12] The overall response rate in four series varied from 43% to 60%; beside prior drug therapy, results were affected by disease extent, systemic symptoms, and patient performance status. The relative incidence of unfavorable prognostic factors is probably responsible for the apparent fluctuation in reported findings, especially in terms of CR.

A possible alternative to conventional third-line salvage regimens could be represented by the use of very high-dose chemotherapy with autologous bone marrow transplantation.[13,14] Although preliminary results seem to confirm the efficacy of such programs in heavily pretreated patients, larger series with longer follow-up are required to determine the exact role of autologous bone marrow transplantation in the management of patients with refractory Hodgkin's disease.

REFERENCES

1. Santoro A, Bonfante V, Bonadonna G: Salvage chemotherapy with ABVD in MOPP-resistant Hodgkin's disease. Ann Intern Med 96:139–144, 1982

2. Bonadonna G, Santoro A: ABVD chemotherapy in the treatment of Hodgkin's disease. Cancer Treat Rev 9:21–31, 1982

3. Bonadonna G: Chemotherapy strategies to improve the control of Hodgkin's disease: The Richard and Hinda Rosenthal Foundation Award Lecture. Cancer Res 42:4309–4320, 1982

4. Santoro A, Bonadonna G, Bonfante V, et al: Alternating drug combinations in the treatment of advanced Hodgkin's disease. N Engl J Med 306:770–775, 1982

5. Straus DJ, Myers J, Lee BJ, et al: Treatment of advanced Hodgkin's disease with chemotherapy and irradiation. Controlled trial of two versus three alternating potentially non-cross-resistant drug combinations. Am J Med 76:270–278, 1984

6. Bonadonna G, Zucali R, Monfardini S, et al: Combination chemotherapy of Hodgkin's disease with Adriamycin, bleomycin, vinblastine and imidazole-carboxamide. Cancer 36:252–259, 1975

7. Santoro A, Bonfante V, Viviani S, et al: Salvage chemotherapy in relapsing Hodgkin's disease. Proc Am Soc Clin Oncol 3:254, 1984

8. Santoro A, Bonfante V, Bonadonna G: Third-line chemotherapy with CCNU, etoposide, and prednimustine

(CEP) in Hodgkin's disease resistant to MOPP and ABVD. Proc Am Soc Clin Oncol 1:165, 1982

9. Bonadonna G, Viviani S, Valagussa P, et al: Third-line salvage chemotherapy in Hodgkin's disease. Sem Oncol 12:23–25, 1985 (suppl 2)

10. Tannir N, Hagemeister F, Vellekoop L, et al: MIME: A new effective third-line combination chemotherapy for patients with recurrent Hodgkin's disease. Proc Am Soc Clin Oncol 3:245, 1984

11. Tseng C Jr, Jacobs C, Coleman S, et al: A pilot study utilizing CCNU, VP-16, and methotrexate as third-line chemotherapy for recurrent Hodgkin's disease. Proc Am Soc Clin Oncol 4:204, 1985

12. Straus DJ, Myers J, Koziner B, et al: Combination chemotherapy for the treatment of Hodgkin's disease in relapse. Results with lomustine (CCNU), melphalan (Alkeran), and vindesine (DVA) alone (CAD) and in alternation with MOPP and doxorubicin (Adriamycin), bleomycin and vinblastine. Cancer Chemother Pharmacol 11:80–85, 1983

13. Carella AM, Santini G, Santoro A, et al: Massive chemotherapy with non-frozen autologous bone marrow transplantation in 13 cases of refractory Hodgkin's disease. Eur J Cancer Clin Oncol 21:607–613, 1985

14. Jagannath S, Spitzer G, Dicke KA, et al: High dose chemotherapy and autologous bone marrow transplant in relapsed Hodgkin's disease. Proc Am Soc Clin Oncol 3:252, 1984

Prednimustine in Advanced Breast Cancer: A Review

H.T. Mouridsen

This review summarizes the available data of phase II and phase III single-agent trials with predminustine and one phase II trial of prednimustine in combination with methotrexate, 5-fluorouracil, and tamoxifen in the treatment of advanced breast cancer. The data available so far indicate that the drug is more active than in combined treatment with the two components, chlorambucil and prednisolone. Future trials should be designed to analyze whether this could be ascribed to a sustained release of the components from the parent drug. The data also indicate that prednimustine is as active but less toxic than cyclophosphamide, but this needs to be confirmed in ongoing randomized comparisons. A number of phase II and phase III trials with prednimustine as a part of combinations are in progress. Mature results from these studies are needed to define the future role of prednimustine in the systemic therapy of breast cancer.

PREDNIMUSTINE is an ester of chlorambucil and prednisolone that was initially synthesized with the aim of using the steroid molecule as a carrier for chlorambucil across the tumor cell membrane to achieve a locally higher concentration of the alkylating agent with less systemic toxicity.[1] However, more recent pharmacokinetic studies in humans have failed to demonstrate the presence of the parent drug in blood, whereas prednisolone and chlorambucil and a metabolite from chlorambucil, phenylacetic mustard, are easily detected.[2,3] This indicates that the drug is split into the two components during its passage from the gastrointestinal (GI) tract into the blood or is split immediately after entering the intravascular space.

Antineoplastic activity of prednimustine has been demonstrated in experimental tumors of rats and mice.[1,4] Furthermore, comparing equimolar amounts of prednimustine with chlorambucil plus prednisolone in DMBA rat mammary tumors has shown a higher antitumor activity and a lower hematologic toxicity of the former drug.[5]

In humans, an antineoplastic effect of prednimustine has been observed in non-Hodgkin lymphomas[6–11] and in chronic lymphatic leukemia.[6,8,11–13] In solid tumors, some activity has been observed in cancer of the ovary,[14,15] cancer of the prostate,[16] cancer of the lung, and malignant melanoma.[6]

SINGLE-AGENT, PHASE II TRIALS

Three phase II trials have been published.[17–19] The treatment results of these studies are presented in Table 1. Fifteen patients entered the first study.[17] Patients were all postmenopausal, 14 with locally advanced disease and one with lung metastases. The daily dose of prednimustine was 20–100 mg. Five patients had received prior endocrine and three patients prior endocrine plus cytotoxic therapy. Among the eight patients with prior systemic therapy, two responses were observed compared with five responses among seven patients with no prior therapy. It appeared that the side effects were time dependent; most frequently they were moderate leucopenia and thrombocytopenia.

The subsequent study[18] included 33 patients with advanced breast cancer. Criteria of eligibility were poorly defined. It was indicated in the paper that all the patients were severely ill and that there was nothing to lose and something to gain. The dosage of prednimustine was 20–40 mg daily or 300 mg/day for five days, repeated after an interval of 10 days. No responses were observed among 24 evaluable patients.

The last trial[19] used a schedule of prednimustine, 40 mg/m^2/day given continuously. Fourteen of 35 patients responded with a median duration of response of 5 months. When analyzing the response in relation to prior therapy, it appeared that among six patients with prior endocrine therapy only, four responded compared with 10 responders among 28 patients with prior endocrine therapy and cytotoxic therapy as well. It was remarkable that among the 14 responding patients, 10 were resistant to prior

---

From the Department of Oncology I, Finsen Institute, Copenhagen.

Address reprint requests to H. T. Mouridsen, MD, Department of Oncology I, Finsen Institute, 49 Strandboulevarden, DK-2100 Copenhagen 0, Denmark.

0093–7754/86/1301–1007$05.00/0

Table 1. Treatment Results in Phase II Studies of Prednimustine in Advanced Breast Cancer

Study	Number of Patients	NE	PD	NC	Partial Remission	Complete Remission	Total Remissions
Könyves et al[17]	15	—	3	5	5	2	7
EORTC[18]	33	9	12	12	0	0	0
Mouridsen et al[19]	35	—	6	15	12	2	14

Abbreviations: NE, nonevaluable; PD, progressive disease; NC, no change.

cytotoxic therapy including alkylating agents, which, in eight cases, was cyclophosphamide. Side effects were moderate. Only three of the patients experienced nausea and vomiting, and one patient had hair loss requiring a wig.

The discrepancies among these three phase II studies could probably be ascribed to the different doses, schedules, and criteria of eligibility. However, it could be concluded from these phase II trials that the drug is active in advanced breast cancer and that toxicities are only modest.

SINGLE-AGENT, PHASE III TRIALS

Only one phase III trial has been published.[20] This trial was designed to analyze whether the described efficacy of prednimustine should be attributed to prednimustine itself or to the two single components of the molecule and to compare two different schedules of prednimustine, continuous and intermittent administration.

Initially, data of 195 evaluable patients were published.[20] However, following a later reevaluation of the material, it appeared that the data of some of the patients entered from one of the participating institutions (Malmoe) were unreliable. For this review, therefore, the 15 patients from that institution have been excluded. It should be emphasized that the exclusion of these patients does not change the overall conclusion of the study.

The treatment results are presented in Table 2. Group I received prednimustine continuously, 40 mg/m^2/day; group II, intermittent prednimustine, 160 mg/m^2, days 1 to 5 repeated every 3 weeks; and group III received the two components of prednimustine, chlorambucil, 8 mg/m^2/day, and prednisolone, 8 mg/m^2/day, both administered continuously.

The response rates of the two regimens of

Table 2. Response to Treatment in 180 Evaluable Patients

Treatment Groups	Number of Patients	PD	NC	Partial Remission	Complete Remission	Total Remissions
I	59	28	19	9	3	12 (20%)
II	62	26	22	13	1	14 (23%)
III	59	35	17	7	0	7 (12%)

Abbreviations: PD, progressive disease; NC, no change.

prednimustine are identical ($P > 0.20$) and superior to treatment with the two components (II *v* III, $P = 0.045$; I *v* III, $P = 0.09$).

Median durations of response with the three regimens were 9.4, 5.9, and 5 months, respectively; none of these differences reach the 5% level of significance (I *v* II, $P = 0.12$; I *v* III, $P = 0.11$; II *v* III, $P > 0.2$). As far as time to progression is concerned, there is no difference between the two groups treated with prednimustine ($P > 0.2$) nor between intermittent prednimustine and chlorambucil plus prednisolone ($P > 0.2$). However, the continuous prednimustine was significantly superior to treatment with the two components ($P = 0.041$).

According to the criteria of eligibility, all the patients had received prior systemic therapy for advanced disease. It appears from the data in Table 3 that the rate of respose was higher in patients with prior endocrine therapy only compared with patients who had received prior chemotherapy and endocrine therapy as well. When analyzing response in relation to dominant site, it is also apparent (Table 4) that the highest response rates were observed in patients with soft tissue as the dominant site of disease compared with bone and viscera. In these subgroup analyses, higher response rates are consistently observed in patients treated with prednimustine compared with those treated with the two components.

Table 5 shows toxicity data; 123 patients experienced hematologic toxicity grade II or higher, requiring dose reduction. Treatment with

Table 3. Response (Complete and Partial) in Relation to Prior Therapy

Treatment Groups	Prior Endocrine Therapy Only		Prior Endocrine and/or Cytotoxic Therapy	
	Number	Percentage	Number	Percentage
I	6/15	40	6/44	14
II	4/9	44	10/53	19
III	4/11	36	3/48	6

Table 4. Response Rate (Complete and Partial) in Relation to Dominant Site of Disease

Treatment Groups	Soft-Tissue Number	Soft-Tissue Percentage	Bone Number	Bone Percentage	Viscera Number	Viscera Percentage
I	4/11	36	4/17	24	4/31	13
II	5/14	36	6/19	32	3/29	10
III	3/12	25	0/15	0	4/32	13

Table 6. Average Relative Drug Doses of Prednimustine

Series	Percentage of Dose					
	Cycle 1		Cycle 2		Cycle 3	
	Day 1	Day 8	Day 1	Day 8	Day 1	Day 8
1	98	74	83	75	84	79
2	94	83	84	69	76	69

chlorambucil and prednisolone was significantly more toxic than that with the two prednimustine regimens (I *v* III, $P = 0.05$; II *v* III, $P = 0.006$), whereas there was no difference between the two prednimustine regimens ($P > 0.20$). The most frequent nonhematologic side effects were nausea and vomiting, occurring in 42% of patients with intermittent prednimustine and in 22% in the other two treatment groups. However, in the vast majority of patients this side effect was moderate (grade I–II). Alopecia was observed in only two cases, and a wig was not required.

In conclusion, in addition to the lower hematologic toxicity of prednimustine, the drug was significantly superior to its two components with regard to response rate. Time to progression was also significantly superior with the continuous prednimustine. It should also be emphazised that the drug is well-tolerated and that alopecia requiring a wig was observed in none of the patients.

COMBINATION-THERAPY, PHASE III TRIAL

The obvious objective of studies in advanced breast cancer is to develop regimens with higher efficacy or with less toxicity and at least equal efficacy. Based upon the available data, it seems that prednimustine may be at least as effective as cyclophosphamide and that it probably causes less subjective toxicity and a lower grade of alopecia.

CMF (cyclophosphamide, methotrexate, and 5-fluorouracil) has been one of the most widely used combination therapies in advanced breast cancer, with a response rate of about 50%. Therefore, it would seem reasonable in a randomized trial to compare CMF with a combination of prednimustine, methotrexate, and 5-fluorouracil (PMF). This would require preliminary experience with the PMF combination.

Table 5. Hematologic Toxicity

Toxicity Grade	Leukocytes ($\times 10^9$/L)	Platelets ($\times 10^9$/L)	No. of Patients in Treatment Groups I	II	III
0	≥ 4.0	≥ 150	9	10	4
I	3.0–3.9	100–149	12	13	9
II	2.0–2.9	75–99	12	19	14
III	1.0–1.9	50–74	14	10	13
IV	< 1.0	< 50	11	9	21
Total			58	61	61

For that reason we conducted a study of PMF in patients with advanced breast cancer.[21] Prednimustine was administered at two dose levels, 80 mg/m^2, days 1 to 5 (series I), and 100 mg/m^2, days 1 to 5 (series II). Both groups received methotrexate, 40 mg/m^2 IV, days 1 and 8 and 5-fluorouracil, 600 mg/m^2 IV, days 1 and 8. These cycles were repeated every 4 weeks. In addition, the patients received continuous tamoxifen based upon our recent experience of the superiority of CMF plus tamoxifen to tamoxifen alone in younger postmenopausal women.[22]

It appeared that the WBC counts were depressed significantly more often than the platelet counts, and it further appeared that during the first three cycles 70% of the patients had a WBC count nadir corresponding to toxicity grade II or more. In both series, the doses of prednimustine, methotrexate, and 5-fluorouracil had to be reduced because of toxic effects, more so in series II (Table 6). A total of 38 patients were treated for an additional 1 to 19 months (median, 10.5). No signs of cumulative hematologic toxicity were observed in these patients, and median drug doses in cycles 5, 10, and 15 were 74%, 77%, and 72%, respectively. Three patients developed severe leukopenia and sepsis requiring hospital admission and treatment with antibiotics.

Nausea and vomiting occurred in 40 of the 47 patients; five patients had grade III–IV and 35 had grade I–II. Only one of the patients developed alopecia requiring a wig.

Twenty-eight of the treated patients had evaluable disease (16 in series I and 12 in series II).

Among these, complete remission was observed in 12 cases and partial remission in 9 cases, with a total remission rate of 75% with a median duration of response of 13 months.

In conclusion, it seems that prednimustine can be safely used in combination with methotrexate and 5-fluorouracil.

CONCLUSION

Prednimustine is an alkylating agent of considerable interest in the treatment of advanced breast cancer. The data available so far indicate that the drug is more active than a combined treatment with its two components, chlorambucil and prednisolone. The data also indicate that prednimustine probably is as active but less toxic than cyclophosphamide. This needs, however, to be confirmed in a randomized comparison, and one such study is being conducted in Sweden.

Due to the modest toxicity and the rate of occurrence of alopecia, it would be of interest to include the drug in combinations designed with the aim to achieve less toxic regimes without losing activity. Preliminarily, it seems that prednimustine can be safely combined with methotrexate and 5-fluorouracil; a randomized trial comparing CMF with PMF is being done in the UK.

A number of other phase II and phase III trials with prednimustine in combination with other drugs are in progress. Mature results from these studies are needed to define the future role of prednimustine in the systemic therapy of breast cancer. Future trials should also be designed to analyze whether the superiority of prednimustine to its two components is simply due to a sustained release of the components from the parent drug.

REFERENCES

1. Harrap KR, Riches PG, Gilby ED, et al: Studies on the toxicity and antitumor activity of prednimustine: A prednisolone ester of chlorambucil. Eur J Cancer 13:873–881, 1977

2. Newell DR, Hart LI, Harrap KR: The estimation of chlorambucil, phenyl acetic mustard and prednimustine in human plasma by high performance liquid chromatography. J Chromatogr Biomed Appl 164:114–119, 1979

3. Plym Forshell G, Gunnarsson PO: Plasma concentrations of prednimustine, chlorambucil and phenulacetic mustard in patients treated with prednimustine. Internal report. UPJ Leo 1031, No. 1903, 1978

4. Evenaar AH, Wins EHR, van Putten LM: Cell killing effectiveness of an alkylating steroid (Leo 1031). Eur J Cancer 9:773–774, 1973

5. Fredholm B, Gunnarson K, Jensen G, et al: Mammary tumor inhibition and subacute toxicity in rats of prednimustine and its molecular components chlorambucil and prednisolone. Acta Pharmacol Toxicol 42:159–163, 1978

6. Clinical Screening Cooperative Group of EORTC: A phase II clinical trial of prednimustine. Biomedica 27:158–161, 1977

7. Hôkansson L, Könyves I, Lindberg L-G, et al: Continuous treatment of non-Hodgkin's malignant lymphoma with prednimustine (L-1031). Oncology 35:103–106, 1978

8. Kaufman JH, Hanjura GL, Mittelman A, et al: Study of Leo 1031 in lymphocytic lymphoma and chronic lymphocytic leukemia. Cancer Treat Rep 60:277–279, 1976

9. Mattsson W, von Eyben F, Turesson I, et al: Prednimustine treatment of lymphocytic and lymphocytic-histiocytic lymphoma. Cancer 41:112–116, 1978

10. Moller TR, Brandt L, Könyves I, et al: Therapeutic effect of Leo 1031, an alkylating corticosteroid ester in lymphoproliferative disorders. II: Lymphocytic lymphoma. Acta Med Scand 197:323–327, 1975

11. Pedersen-Bjergaard J, Mørk-Hansen M, Geisler CH, et al: Clinical trial of prednimustine Leo 1031 (NSC-134087) in patients with non-Hodgkin lymphomata and chronic lymphocytic leukaemia previously treated with steroids and alkylating agents. Acta Med Scand 207:215–220, 1980

12. Brandy L, Könyves I, Møller TR: Therapeutic effect of Leo 1031, an alkylating corticosteroid ester, in lymphoproliferative disorders. I: Chronic lymphocytic leukemia. Acta Med Scand 197:317–322, 1975

13. Lutz D, Böhnel J: Die Wirkung von Prednimustine bei chronischen lymphatischen Leukämien. Oestr Zschr Onkol 3:154–159, 1976

14. Johansson J-E, Tropé C, Mattsson W et al: Phase II study Leo 1031 (prednimustine) in advanced ovarian carcinoma. Cancer Treat Rep 63:421, 1979

15. Lele SB, Piver MS, Barlow J, et al: Leo 1031 (NSC-134087) in gynecologic malignancies. Oncology 35:101, 1978

16. Catane R, Kaufman JH, Madajewicz S, et al: Prednimustine therapy for advanced prostatic cancer. Br J Urol 50:29, 1978

17. Könyves I, Nordenskjöld B, Plym Forshell G, et al: Preliminary clinical and absorption studies with prednimustine in patients with mammary carcinoma. Eur J Cancer 11:841–844, 1975

18. Clinical Screening Cooperative Group of EORTC: A phase II clinical trial of prednimustine. Biomedica 27:158–161, 1977

19. Mouridsen HT, Kristensen D, Halskov Nielsen J, et al: Phase II trial of prednimustine, L-1031 (NSC-134087) in advanced breast cancer. Cancer 46:253–255, 1980

20. Løber J, Mouridsen HT, Christiansen IE, et al: A phase III trial comparing prednimustine (Leo 1031) to

chlorambucil plus prednisolone in advanced breast cancer. Cancer 52:1570–1576, 1983

21. Boesen E, Mouridsen HT: Prednimustine in combination with methotrexate and 5-FU (PMF): A pilot study. Cancer Treat Rep 66:2081–2083, 1982

22. Mouridsen HT, Rose C, Engelsman E, et al: Combined cytotoxic and endocrine therapy in postmenopausal patients with advanced breast cancer. A randomized study of CMF vs. CMF plus tamoxifen. Eur J Cancer Clin Oncol 21:291–299, 1985

A Preliminary Analysis of Combination Therapy With Vincristine, Adriamycin, and Prednimustine (VAP) in Advanced Breast Cancer: A Phase II Study

By Manfred Lehnert, Georg Biffl, Harald Wascher, Konstantin Jordis-Lohausen, and Svante Wählby

Between March 1984 and May 1985, 29 patients with metastatic breast cancer and high-risk prognostic factors were treated with vincristine, 1.4 mg/m² IV on day 1, Adriamycin, 40 mg/m² IV on day 1, and prednimustine, 100 mg/m² PO on days 3 to 7. Courses were repeated every 3 weeks. At the present time, 26 patients are evaluable for tumor response; 29 are evaluable for toxicity. Fourteen of 26 patients (53.8%) achieved a partial response lasting 2 to 9 months (median 5.5+). A complete response was not recorded. Ten of 26 patients (38.5%) had stable disease; two patients (7.7%) showed a primary tumor progression. Most common side effects were nausea, vomiting, and alopecia, all generally mild to moderate. Fourteen of 29 patients developed leukocytopenia, mainly of WHO grade 1; thrombocytopenia was registered in one patient only and a fall of hemoglobin in three patients only. In 15 patients, no hematologic toxicity occurred. These preliminary data suggest good antitumor activity and acceptable toxicity for vincristine-Adriamycin-prednimustine in patients with metastatic breast cancer.

FOR SEVERAL YEARS, the results with chemotherapy in metastatic breast cancer could not be improved. Response rates ranged between 40% and 70%; about 20% of patients achieved a complete remission. The median remission duration was 8 to 10 months.[1] Since any treatment in recurrent breast cancer has palliative intent, it appears reasonable to increase the therapeutic index of treatment by decreasing toxicity. Prednimustine (Sterecyt*) was reported to achieve a response rate up to 40% in metastatic breast cancer, objective and subjective side effects being minimal.[2,3] Some of the most common toxic effects, eg, nausea, vomiting, and myelotoxicity, caused by the original vincristine-Adriamycin-cyclophosphamide (VAC) regimen for breast cancer, were due to cyclophosphamide, which in this protocol was administered at rather high oral doses.[4] Thus, we substituted cyclophosphamide with prednimustine in this regimen with the hope of minimizing toxicity while achieving comparable therapeutic results. Some preliminary data are presented in this paper.

MATERIALS AND METHODS

Between March 1984 and May 1985, 29 patients with metastatic breast cancer were entered into the study. Patient and tumor characteristics are listed in Table 1 and 2.

Entry criteria included histologically proven metastatic or recurrent breast cancer; measurable or at least evaluable disease; normal function values of bone marrow, liver, and kidneys; tumor progression under cyclophosphamide-methotrexate-5-fluorouracil; or presence of one of the following indications for first-line systemic therapy with an Adriamycin regimen: liver metastases; extensive lung metastases, each lung metastasis with a short recurrence-free interval; extensive bone metastases with a short recurrence-free interval; metastases in more than two organs; and rapid tumor growth. Essential exclusion criteria were other concurrent malignancy excluding skin cancer and cervical cancer stage 0, brain metastases, severe diabetes, severe cardiac disease, and gastric or duodenal ulcers.

Patients with a WBC of more than $4 \times 10^9/L$ and platelet count of more than $120 \times 10^9/L$ received vincristine, 1.4 mg/m² (maximum, 2 mg) intravenously (IV) on day 1, Adriamycin, 40 mg/m² IV on day 1, and prednimustine, 100 mg/m² orally (PO) on days 3 to 7. Courses were repeated at 3-week intervals. A WBC of 2.5 to $3.9 \times 10^9/L$ and/or a platelet count of 75 to $119 \times 10^9/L$ led to a 50% dosage reduction of all three drugs; lower values for leukocytes, and/or platelets led to a withdrawal of treatment until bone marrow recovery. Tumor responses were assessed according to UICC (International Union Against Cancer) criteria,[5] adverse reactions being classified as recommended by WHO.[6]

RESULTS

At the present time, 26 of the 29 patients are evaluable for tumor response, and all are evaluable for toxicity. One patient had no evaluable disease after surgical removal of a soft-tissue recurrence; one patient developed a long-lasting grade 2 granulocytopenia after the first VAP course leading to withdrawal of treatment; and one is too early to evaluate. Overall results are listed in Table 3. A complete response was not

---

**Trademark AB LEO, Sweden.*

From the Third Medical Department, LKH Graz, Austria.

Address reprint requests to Dr Manfred Lehnert, 3. Medizinische Abteilung, LKH Graz, Auenbruggerplatz 15, A-8036 Graz, Austria.

0093-7754/86/1301-1008$05.00/0

Table 1. Characteristics of 29 Patients Treated With VAP

	Age (Years)	Number of Patients
Median	57	
Range	38–75	
Performance status (ECOG)		
0		10
1		11
2		6
3		1
4		1
Menopausal age		
Premenopausal		5
Perimenopausal		9
Postmenopausal		15
Prior systematic therapy		
Endocrine		5
Cytotoxic		3
Endocrine and cytotoxic		7

registered; 14 of 26 patients (53.8%) achieved a partial remission with a median duration of 5+ months (range, 2 to 9). Twenty-five of 26 patients are alive; one patient died due to malignant disease 8 months after the first VAP course. In Tables 4 and 5, tumor responses are related to dominant site of disease and systemic pretreatment, respectively. Nine of 12 patients (75%) with prior endocrine plus/minus cytotoxic treatment achieved partial responses in contrast to only 5 of 14 patients (36%) without prior endocrine therapy ($P = 0.045$). This marked difference in tumor response was not significantly influenced by other prognostic variables such as type of metastasis, hormonal receptor status, efficacy of prior endocrine therapy, menopausal age, or performance status. Thirty of the total 163 VAP courses (18.4%) were followed by generally moderate and short-lasting leukocytopenia. After the first VAP course, one patient developed a grade 2 granulocytopenia lasting 3 months, without full recovery of the WBC. Bone marrow examination in this patient transiently revealed marked reduction of the granulopoietic system. This patient had not received any previous cytotoxic treatment. Leukocytopenia occurred in 15 of the 29 patients (51.7%), whereas red cells and platelets were rarely influenced.

The most common side effects were alopecia and nausea and vomiting, both usually mild to moderate. Three patients experienced mild and fully reversible peripheral neurotoxicity; one patient developed skin necrosis obviously caused by paravenous injection of adriamycin or vincristine. Hematologic toxicity is listed in Table 6; other side effects are summarized in Table 7.

Table 2. Tumor Characteristics in 29 Patients Treated With VAP

	Number of Patients
Hormonal receptor	
Positive	9
Negative	8
Unknown	12
Sites of recurrence*	
Lymph nodes	6
Skin	9
Bone	9
Lung	7
Liver	6
Malignant effusion	7
Others	3
Mixed	12
Dominant site	
Soft tissue	3
Bone	5
Visceral	21
Recurrence-free interval (years)	
0–1	14
1–5	8
>5	7

*Patients can be listed in more than one category.

Table 3. Overall Results in 26 Evaluable Patients

	Number of Patients	Percentage
Complete response (CR)	0/26	—
Partial responses (PR)	14/26	53.8
No change (NC)	10/26	38.5
Progressive disease (PD)	2/26	7.7
Response rate (RR)	14/26	53.8

DISCUSSION

This preliminary analysis of our VAP data in metastatic breast cancer demonstrated good antitumor activity in this population with high-risk prognostic factors. The response rate of 53.8% is comparable with the experience with other Adriamycin regimens.[7–9] At our institution, the original VAC protocol of the Tucson group

Table 4. Results Related to Dominant Sites of Recurrence

	Soft Tissue	Bone	Visceral
Total Number	2/26	4/26	20/26
PR	1	2	11
NC	1	2	7
PD	—	—	2
RR	1/2 (50%)	2/4 (50%)	11/20 (55%)

Table 5. Results Related to Prior Systemic Therapy

	Endocrine (E)	Cytotoxic (C)	E and C	Number
Total Number	5/26	3/26	7/26	11/26
PR	3	1	6	4
NC	2	2	1	5
PD	—	—	—	2
RR	3/5 (60%)	1/3 (33%)	6/7 (86%)	4/11 (36%)

was used in metastatic breast cancer during the last years.[4] The criteria for treatment with VAC were very similar to the entry criteria for the current study, so patient and tumor characteristics for both series are comparable. In 36 evaluable patients, VAC achieved an overall response rate of 50% (18/36). Five of 36 patients (13.9%) showed a complete response, while 13 of 36 patients (36.1%) showed a partial remission (previously unpublished data). Only three of 13 patients (23%) with endocrine plus/minus cytotoxic pretreatment experienced an objective tumor response to VAC compared with nine of 12 patients (75%) treated with VAP. In contrast, only four of 11 patients (36%) responded to first-line systemic therapy with VAP, while 10 of the 14 patients (71%) of this subgroup did so to VAC. Whether patient selection or distinct clinical efficacy are responsible for this considerable difference in tumor response to VAP and VAC could only be clarified by a randomized and stratified comparison of VAC *v* VAP. As reported for other Adriamycin-containing protocols,[10] visceral metastases responded to VAP, as did other locations.

Table 6. Hematologic Toxicity in 29 Patients Treated With VAP

	Grade*				
	0	1	2	3	4
Leukocytes	14	12	3	—	—
Platelets	28	1	—	—	—
Hemoglobin	26	1	2	—	—

*Grading according to WHO recommendations.[6]

Table 7. Nonhematologic Toxicity in 29 Patients Treated With VAP

	Grade*				
	0	1	2	3	4
Nausea and vomiting	6	12	7	3	1
Hair	5	8	12	4	—
Peripheral neurotoxicity	26	2	1	—	—
Cutaneous	28	—	—	—	1

*Grading according to WHO recommendations.[6]

The overall toxicity of the protocol was moderate. In two patients therapy had to be stopped due to side effects. One patient refused further therapy after the sixth course because of severe gastrointestinal intolerance. One patient developed a long-lasting leukocytopenia grade 2. No life-threatening complications occurred. Both VAC and VAP caused similar myelotoxicity; the subjective tolerance to VAP, however, was markedly improved, especially regarding the severity of nausea and vomiting.

In conclusion, the antitumor activity of VAP was comparable with reported results with other Adriamycin regimens and our own experience with VAC. As the overall toxicity was slightly reduced, the VAP protocol was able to increase the therapeutic index. If this experience is confirmed in a larger series, a randomized comparison of this regimen *v* vincristine-Adriamycin-cyclophosphamide could be of great interest.

ACKNOWLEDGMENT

We gratefully acknowledge the assistance of AB LEO, Sweden, in supplying the prednimustine used in this study.

REFERENCES

1. Henderson IC, Canellos GP: Cancer of the breast: The past decade. N Engl J Med 302:78–90, 1980

2. Mouridsen HT, Kristensen D, Halskov Nielsen J, et al: Phase II trial of prednimustine, L-1031 (NSC-134087), in advanced breast cancer. Cancer 46:253–255, 1980

3. Løber J, Mouridsen HT, Christiansen IE, et al: A phase III trial comparing prednimustine (LEO 1031) to chlorambucil plus prednisolone in advanced breast cancer. Cancer 52:1570–1576, 1983

4. Rainey JM, Jones SE, Salmon SE: Combination chemotherapy for advanced breast cancer utilizing vincristine, adriamycin, and cyclophosphamide (VAC). Cancer 43:66–71, 1979

5. Hayward JL, Carbone PP, Heuson JC, et al: Assessment of response to therapy in advanced breast cancer. Eur J Cancer 13:89–94, 1977

6. Miller AB, Hoogstraten B, Staquet M, et al: Reporting results of cancer treatment. Cancer 47:207–214, 1981

7. Muss HB, Richards F, Jackson DV, et al: Vincristine, doxorubicin, and cyclophosphamide versus low-dose intravenous methotrexate and 5-fluorouracil in advanced breast cancer. Cancer 50:2269–2274, 1982

8. Jones SE, Durie BGM, Salmon SE: Combination chemotherapy with Adriamycin and cyclophosphamide for advanced breast cancer. Cancer 36:90–97, 1975

9. Tranum BL, McDonald B, Thigpen T, et al: Adriamycin combinations in advanced breast cancer. Cancer 49:835–839, 1982

10. Nash CH, Jones SE, Moon TE, et al: Prediction of outcome in metastatic breast cancer treated with Adriamycin combination chemotherapy. Cancer 46:2380–2388, 1980

Preliminary Analysis of Combined Treatment With Prednimustine and 4′Epidoxorubicin in Advanced Breast Cancer

By Matti S. Aapro, Michel Forni, Felix Krauer, Pierre Alberto, and Svante Wählby

In an effort to define a well-tolerated therapeutic regimen for advanced breast cancer, we have studied a combination of 4′epidoxorubicin, 50 mg/m² IV on day 1, and prednimustine, 100 mg/m² PO on days 3 to 7 given every 3 weeks. Twenty-nine patients have been entered, and 22 are presently evaluable for response. Median age of the evaluable patients is 62 (range, 36 to 77), and median performance status (SAKK) is 2. Five patients had received chemotherapy, 16 hormonal therapy, five radiation therapy, and five no prior therapy for advanced disease. Most patients were in a high-risk group, with dominant visceral metastatic sites in 19 out of 22 cases. We have observed eight partial responses, nine no changes, and five progressions. Median response duration is 6 months. It is too early to discuss median overall survival. Toxicity is evaluable in 27 patients who received at least one course with a full dose of chemotherapy. Hematologic toxicity has been low, with only four patients having leukocyte nadirs below 2000/mm³ and three patients with thrombocyte nadirs below 100,000/mm³. Major alopecia (requiring a wig) was observed in eight patients. Emesis (controlled by minor antiemetics) was reported in six cases. This well-tolerated regimen is active in advanced high-risk elderly breast cancer patients, but dosage might be too low for younger patients and nonpretreated patients.

COMBINATION CHEMOTHERAPY is an effective palliative treatment for patients with advanced breast cancer.[1] There is no clear evidence of a superiority of any particular regimen, at least in terms of overall survival. 4′Epidoxorubicin is an anthracycline derivative with activity in breast cancer comparable with doxorubicin. It may have less acute and cumulative anthracycline-related toxicities (alopecia, cardiac toxicity).[2] Prednimustine is an ester of chlorambucil and prednisolone with activity in breast cancer when used as a single agent.[3] As part of our efforts to define a well-tolerated therapeutic regimen for advanced metastatic breast cancer, we have studied a combination of these agents.

MATERIALS AND METHODS

Selection of Patients

Oral informed consent was obtained from patients entering this study, which was approved by the Institutional Review Board. Patients of any age were eligible, provided that they had progressive, objectively evaluable, metastatic disease.[4] Prior chemotherapy without doxorubicin, or with combinations including very low-dose doxorubicin (10 mg/m² every 3 to 4 weeks) was acceptable. Prior or concomitant radiotherapy was acceptable if it did not include marker lesions. Initial leukocyte counts of 4.0×10^9/L and platelet counts of 150×10^9/L were required. Exclusion criteria included active cardiovascular history, another malignant tumor, and/or uncontrolled brain metastases.

Treatment

Chemotherapy consisted of 4′epidoxorubicin, 50 mg/m² intravenously (IV) on day 1, and prednimustine, 100 mg/m² orally (po) in divided doses on days 3 to 7. The first three courses were administered at 21-day intervals and subsequently every 3 to 4 weeks. There was no initial dosage reduction for elderly patients. Dosage increase by 20% was proposed in case of nonresponse after two courses, provided no toxicity had been observed.

Work-up and Follow-up

Initial work-up included history, complete physical examination with documentation of measurable lesions (fine-needle biopsy for soft-tissue masses), complete blood counts, routine chemistry profile, electrocardiogram, chest roentgenogram, and skeletal survey. At follow-up, weekly blood counts were required during the first two courses, and liver function tests were to be checked at each course. Index lesions were followed at every alternate course, at least. Response and toxicity criteria are those adopted by the Swiss Group for Clinical Cancer Research (SAKK), according to WHO guidelines.[5] Patients had to have at least two courses of chemotherapy (6 weeks of treatment) to be evaluable. A no-change situation lasting only 8 weeks or less, ie, progression before the fourth treatment course, was termed a failure.

RESULTS

Twenty-nine patients were registered between May 1984 and April 1985. Twenty-six were eligible for this study. The three noneligible patients were one who had had a mastectomy in

From the Division of Oncology and Clinic of Gynecology, University Hospital, Geneva, and the Division of Cancer Research, Leo Sweden, Helsingborg, Sweden.

Address reprint requests to Matti S. Aapro, MD, Division of Oncology, University Hospital, 1211 Geneva 4, Switzerland.

0093–7754/86/1301–1009$05.00/0

1964, had Waldenström's macroglobulinemia, and presented with a gluteal and iliac mass with a diagnosis of undifferentiated carcinoma; one who was progressing after 2 months of weekly 4'epidoxorubicin, 20 mg/m^2; and one who had active brain metastases at entry. Four patients

Table 1. Patient Characteristics

Number of treated patients	29
Number of eligible patients	26
Noneligibility reasons	
Not breast cancer	1
Brain metastases	1
Prior doxorubicin	1
Number of evaluable patients	22
Nonevaluability reasons	1
Early death	1
Radiotherapy to evaluable lesion	1
Too early	2
Median age	62
Range	36–77
Number of patients younger than 50 years	2
Number of patients 50 or older	20
Performance status	
0	5
1	6
2	9
3–4	2
Disease-free interval (years)	
< 2	10
> 2	12
Hormone receptors status	
ER+/PR+	6
ER+/PR−	3
ER+/PR unknown	1
ER−/PR+	1
ER−/PR−	4
Unknown	7
Prior nonadjuvant treatment	
Radiotherapy	5
Endocrine	16
Chemotherapy	5
Site of relapse	
Skin	6
Lymph nodes	7
Bone	17
Lung	14
Pleural effusion	8
Liver	7
Sites per patient	
1	3
2	4
≥ 3	15
Dominant site	
Soft tissue	0
Bone	3
Viscera	19

Abbreviations: ER+, estrogen receptors above 10 fmol/mg; PR+, progesteron receptors above 10 fmol/mg.

Table 2. Characteristics of Response

	Number of Patients	Number of Patients Progressing After Response	Number of Deaths
Partial response	8	6	3
No change	9	3	2
Progressive disease	5	5	3

are not evaluable for response: two are too early, one died 6 weeks after entry (early death), and one received radiation therapy to the measurable soft-tissue masses (she was treated for 6 months, until pulmonary progression).

Twenty-two patients are evaluable for response. Table 1 gives details of the pretreatment characteristics. Median age was 62 years, with 20 of 22 patients older than 50 years. Performance status was 0 or 1 in 11 patients, 2 in nine, and 3 and 4 in one patient each. Rapidly progressive disease was observed in 10 cases (less than 2 years disease-free interval from primary treatment). Prior therapy included chemotherapy for advanced disease in only five cases and hormonal treatment in 16 instances. The majority of the patients had visceral-dominant disease, with 14 lung, eight pleural, and seven liver sites. Fifteen patients had three or more metastatic sites.

Objective partial responses have been observed in eight patients, all with measurable or evaluable visceral sites. These patients also had other sites of disease that responded. No patient qualifies for a complete response, as there was always at least one site in which all manifestations of disease did not disappear. Similarly, nine patients who are considered to have a no-change situation had a response in one site but stable disease in another (frequently bone). These patients do not qualify for a partial response but might still enter a partial response with longer follow-up. Median duration of response is 24 weeks at the time of this analysis, with six out of

Table 3. Response Duration and Patient Survival

	Time to Progression (Weeks)		Time to Death (Weeks)		Follow-up (Weeks)	
	Median	Range	Median	Range	Median	Range
Partial response	24	14–35	44	33–44	31	8–47
No change	13	12–16	18	16–20	16	7–33
Progressive disease	9	4–11	11	10–26	11	10–26

Table 4. Response by Site

	Responders	Evaluable Cases
Soft tissue	3	8
Bone	3	11
Viscera	8	17
One site	0	3
Two sites	2	4
Three or more sites	6	15

eight patients having relapsed. Six of nine stable disease patients show no signs of progression after a median follow-up time of 16 weeks for this group. Median overall survival is 33 weeks, but only eight out of 22 patients died after a median follow-up time of 18 (range 7 to 47) weeks (Tables 2, 3, and 4; Fig 1).

Treatment was well tolerated. Table 5 gives the details of what we have observed in all patients who received at least one full course of chemotherapy. Two patients, one early death and one evaluable for response (progressed), received 50% and 80% of the doses and are not considered for toxicity. Special mention is needed of the single case of diabetic decompensation. The patient, a diabetic, needed transitory management with insulin for symptomatic hyperglycemia. The anxiety observed in one patient was prednimustine related. Chills and fever were 4'epidoxorubicin related in a patient who received two courses with the agent without side effects, and, during the next two courses, had severe chills and moderate fever (up to 38 °C) starting after injection of the IV drug and lasting a few hours. No other drug or solvent was injected at the same time. Urticaria or pruritus were not observed.[6]

Table 5. Toxic Effects

Number of evaluable patients	27
Leukocyte nadir	
3000–2000	13
2000–1000	2
< 1000	2
Thrombocyte nadir	
50,000–100,000	2
< 50,000	1
Alopecia	
None	9
Minimal	10
Major (wig required)	8
Nausea	
None	8
Nausea only	13
With vomiting	6
Other	
Skin toxicity (injection site)	2
Diarrhea	1
Anxiety	1
Chills and fever	1
Diabetic decompensation	1

DISCUSSION

This is a preliminary evaluation of a simple combination of 4'epidoxorubicin and prednimustine administered every 3 weeks for treatment of advanced metastatic breast cancer. Follow-up is too short to draw any conclusions on patient survival.

We have observed eight partial responses, and

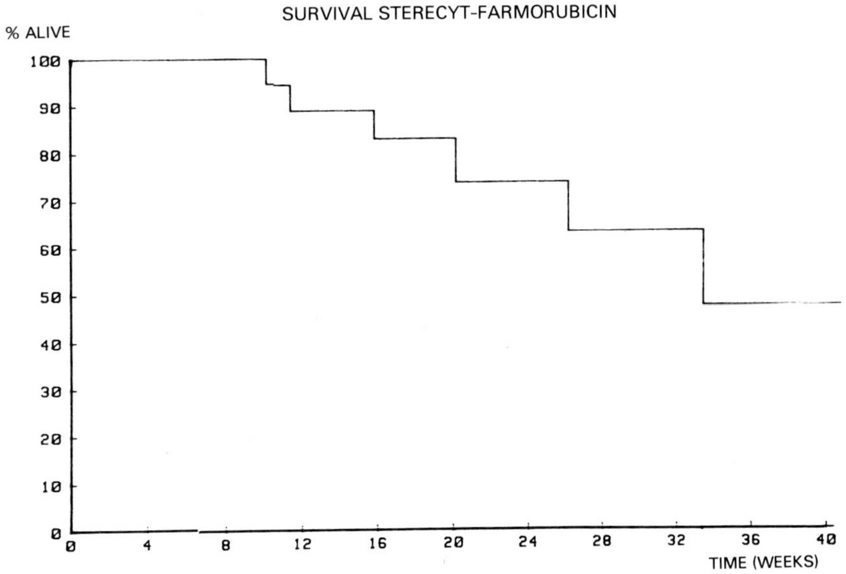

Fig 1. Survival curve, according to the Kaplan-Meier method, of all evaluable patients entered in the study.

nine further patients were stabilized. The poor performance status of the 22 evaluable patients, with 19 having visceral involvement and 15 having three or more sites of disease, does not seem to have adversely affected the response rate. However, only five patients had received prior chemotherapy and most (16) had failed hormonal therapy. These results are comparable with those achieved with many other regimens.[1] The advantage of this regimen, compared with others aimed at reduced toxicity,[7] is its every-3-week schedule, which reduces unnecessary outpatient visits.

Twenty-seven patients were treated at least once according to protocol and can be evaluated for toxicity. Hematotoxicity has been minor, with two cases of leukocyte nadirs below 1000 and one case of thrombopenia below 50,000. The latter occurred in combination with leukopenia in a patient with progressive liver metastases, and the other major leukopenia occurred in a heavily pretreated patient. Six patients experienced vomiting, which was controlled with minor antiemetics. Alopecia requiring a wig was observed in only eight cases. We are presently analyzing the influence of scalp hypothermia on the incidence of this side effect.[8] Diabetic decompensation was actually observed in a patient who was treated with 50% of the recommended dosage and who had an early death; the decompensation, therefore, could be related to the terminal status of the patient rather than to prednimustine.

This regimen has shown activity in an unfavorable-prognosis group of elderly patients. The very moderate hematotoxicity indicates that younger or nonpretreated patients could receive higher doses. Only longer follow-up will allow a better understanding of the impact of this treatment in advanced breast cancer.

ACKNOWLEDGMENT

We wish to thank our colleagues whose patients have been entered into this study. Accurate data management has been possible with the help of Ms F. Misset and Mr P.A. Iten. The outstanding secretarial skills of C. Amez-Droz have been essential to our work.

REFERENCES

1. Bonadonna G, Valagussa P: Chemotherapy of breast cancer: Current views and results. Int J Radiat Oncol Biol Phys 9:279–297, 1982

2. Bonadonna G, Brambilla C, Rossi A, et al: Epirubicin in advanced breast cancer, in Bonadonna G (ed): Advances in Anthracycline Chemotherapy: Epirubicin. Milano, Italy, Masson, 1984, pp 63–70

3. Løber J, Mouridsen HT, Christiansen IE, et al: A phase II trial comparing prednimustine (LEO 1031) to chlorambucil plus prednisolone in advanced breast cancer. Cancer 52:1570–1576, 1983

4. Hayward JL, Carbone PP, Heuson JC, et al: Assessment of response to therapy in advanced breast cancer. Eur J Cancer 13:89–94, 1977

5. WHO: WHO Handbook for Reporting Results of Cancer Treatment. Geneva, WHO, WHO Offset Publication No. 48, 1979, pp 22–24

6. Souhami L, Feld R: Urticaria following intravenous doxorubicin administration. JAMA 240:1624–1625, 1978

7. Jones WG, Mattsson W: Phase II study of weekly low-dose 4′epidoxorubicin in advanced postmenopausal breast cancer. Cancer Treat Rep 68:675–677, 1984

8. Dean JC, Salmon SE, Griffith KS: Prevention of doxorubicin-induced hair loss with scalp hypothermia. N Engl J Med 301:1427–1430, 1979

Combined Cytotoxic and Endocrine Treatment of Postmenopausal Patients With Advanced Breast Cancer: Preliminary Results of a Phase II Study of the Combination of Prednimustine, Novantrone, Methotrexate, 5-Fluorouracil, and Tamoxifen

By H.T. Mouridsen, M. Andersson, and L. Pedersen

Postmenopausal patients with advanced measurable and/or evaluable breast cancer entered a phase II trial of multiple agent cytotoxic therapy combined with endocrine therapy. Cycles of PNMF (prednimustine, novantrone, methotrexate, and 5-fluorouracil) were repeated every 4 weeks as follows: P, 100 mg/m² PO on days 1 to 5; M, 40 mg/m² IV on day 1; F, 600 mg/m² IV on day 1, and N, 14 mg/m² IV on day 8. The endocrine therapy was tamoxifen given continuously, 10 mg three times daily. As of May 1985, 32 eligible patients had entered the study, 20 of whom had been treated for a sufficient time to enable evaluation of response. Ten patients responded (one complete, nine partial), five experienced no change, and five patients experienced progressive disease. The treatment regimen was fairly well tolerated, the dose-limiting factor being the hematologic toxicity. Conclusions from the trial must await the inclusion of more patients and longer time of follow-up.

SEVERAL RANDOMIZED STUDIES have demonstrated cytotoxic multiple-agent therapy to be superior to single-agent therapy in advanced breast cancer in postmenopausal patients.[1,2] The two most frequently used combinations are CMF (cyclophosphamide, methotrexate, and 5-fluorouracil) and CAF (cyclophosphamide, Adriamycin, and 5-fluorouracil), which induce remission in about 50% of patients.[3,4]

As of today, systemic treatment of advanced breast cancer remains palliative, and further progress should include the introduction of more effective drugs as well as the development of regimens with at least similar activity as now but with less toxicity.

Prednimustine is an ester of chlorambucil and prednisolone. In a phase II study including 35 patients, of whom 29 had received prior cytotoxic therapy, a 40% response rate was observed,[5] and in a subsequent large randomized study, prednimustine was demonstrated to be significantly superior (response rate, 21%) to combined treatment with the components of prednimustine, prednisolone and chlorambucil (response rate, 11%).[6] These results indicate that prednimustine is as effective as cyclophosphamide. The studies also demonstrated that prednimustine is probably less toxic in terms of subjective symptoms and alopecia. These were the reasons for a subsequent study in which cyclophosphamide in the CMF plus tamoxifen combination was replaced by prednimustine.[7] Among 28 patients treated with this combination, response was observed in 21. Side effects, including alopecia, were significantly less frequent and less pronounced than reported for CMF plus tamoxifen.[8]

Novantrone is an anthracenedione derivative and thus an agent within the group of antibiotics.[9] In two phase II studies in patients without prior cytotoxic therapy, response rates of 31%[10] and 44%[11] have been reported, ie, response rates comparable with those achieved with Adriamycin. In a randomized study,[12] no significant difference was observed between Adriamycin and Novantrone as far as response rate and response duration is concerned, and preliminary results indicate that a combination of cyclophosphamide, 5-fluorouracil, and Novantrone has efficacy comparable with that of the CAF regimen.[13] Characteristics of these studies of Novantrone has been the general impression of less occurrence of the serious toxicities often associated with treatment with Adriamycin.

The objective of the present study is to evaluate the efficacy and toxicity of a combination of the presently most active drugs in breast cancer, cyclophosphamide, methotrexate, 5-fluorouracil, and Adriamycin, but with the replacement of the

---

From the Department of Oncology I, Finsen Institute, Copenhagen.

Address reprint requests to H.T. Mouridsen, MD, Department of Oncology I, Finsen Institute, 49 Strandboulevarden DK-2100 Copenhagen Ø, Denmark.

0093-7754/86/1301-1010$05.00/0

more toxic agents, cyclophosphamide and Adriamycin, with prednimustine and Novantrone, respectively. Tamoxifen is added to the combination based upon our experience of the superiority of CMF plus tamoxifen to CMF alone in younger postmenopausal patients.[8]

MATERIAL AND METHODS

Criteria of eligibility. Postmenopausal patients less than 65 years of age with advanced measurable breast cancer were eligible for the study, provided that the performance status was 3 or less and that the hematologic values were normal (platelets $\geq$ 100 $\times$ $10^3/\mu L$ and WBC $\geq$ 3 $\times$ $10^3/\mu L$). Patients who had received adjuvant endocrine or cytotoxic therapy within the previous 12 months or who had received prior therapy for advanced disease with any of the study drugs were ineligible. Also, the presence of CNS metastases, other prior or concomitant malignant disease, congestive heart failure, insulin-treated diabetes mellitus, active gastric or duodenal ulcer, or serum-bilirubin $\geq$30 μmol/L not considered to be due to liver metastases was reason not to be included in the study. The patients verbal informed consent had to be obtained prior to entry to the study.

Pretreatment and follow-up investigations. Pretreatment examinations included physical examination, chest x-ray, bone x-ray or bone scintigraphy, clinical chemical tests (serum-creatinine, serum-calcium, serum alkaline phosphatase, serum-transaminase, and serum-bilirubin), ultrasound scanning of the liver, and isotopic cardiography (MUGA). The physical examination, including evaluation of side effects, was repeated every 4 weeks. The other examinations were repeated every 3 months—MUGA only from cycle 9, however.

Therapeutic regimen. Cycles of PNMF (prednimustine, Novantrone, methotrexate, and 5-fluorouracil) were repeated every 4 weeks as follows: P, 100 mg/m^2 orally on days 1 to 5; M, 40 mg/m^2 IV bolus on day 1; F, 600 mg/m^2 IV bolus on day 1; and N, 14 mg/m^2 IV bolus on day 8. Tamoxifen was given continuously, 10 mg three times daily.

Dose modification. The relative dose of PNMF was adjusted according to platelets and WBC counts on the scheduled day of the cycle as follows: platelets $\geq$100 $\times$ $10^3/\mu L$ and WBC $\geq$3 $\times$ $10^3/\mu L$, 100%; platelets 75 to 99 and/or WBC 2.0 to 2.9, 50%; platelets 50 to 74 and/or WBC 1.0 to 1.9, 25%; platelets less than 50 and/or WBC less than 1, 0%.

If the platelet counts were less than 75 and/or WBC less than 2 at the beginning of the 28-day cycle, the cycle was delayed 2 weeks. If on day 8 of the cycle of platelet count was less than 50 and/or the WBC was less than 1, no drug was given on day 8, and in the subsequent cycle the dose was reduced to 50%, even if hematologic values were normal.

Treatment duration. Our aim was to give a minimum of 12 weeks of treatment. If, at that time, disease progression was observed, the patient went off the study. Otherwise, treatment continued until progression.

Definitions of response. Patients were assessed 12 weeks after initiation of therapy and at 1- to 3-month intervals thereafter. Assessment of response, duration of response, time to treatment failure, and duration of survival were done according to the UICC criteria.[15]

Definition of toxicity. Toxicities were graded according to the WHO criteria.[15]

RESULTS

From September 1984 to May 1985, a total number of 37 patients were registered, and among these 32 patients were eligible. Reasons for noneligibility were adjuvant tamoxifen therapy within the last year (two patients), a performance status of 4 (one patient), age more than 65 years (one patient), and premenopausal status (one patient). Twelve patients are not yet evaluable due to treatment and follow-up time of less than 3 months. This leaves 20 patients for evaluation, the characteristics of whom are shown in Table 1.

Among the 20 evaluable patients, 10 responded (one complete, nine partial), five experienced no change, and five had progressive disease. It must be emphasized that the data are very preliminary, as the median time of treatment and follow-up is only 4.5 months. Among the five patients with progressive disease, three died of the malignant disease within 3 months of initiation of treatment, while two patients had relapse after two and three months of treatment, respectively. Among the five patients with no change, one experienced progression after 6 months. The other 14 patients are still in treatment.

The treatment regimen has generally been well tolerated. No patient had to have the treatment discontinued due to side effects, but four patients have been treated for sepsis with no fatal outcome.

Table 1. Characteristics of Evaluable Patients

Characteristics	Median	Range	Number of Patients
Age (years)	61	29–65	
Menopausal age (years)	9	1–25	
Disease-free interval (months)	24	0–108	
Observation time (months)	4.5	1–8	
Dominant site of disease			
Viscera			11
Bones			6
Soft tissue			3
Performance status			
Grade 0			15
Grade 1			1
Grade 2			4
Total			20

Table 2. Number of Patients With Toxicities and Side Effects

	Toxicity Grade				
	0	1	2	3	4
WBC	8	3	9	3	5
Platelets	18	4	4	2	0
Alopecia	12	9	7	0	0
Nausea and vomiting	9	10	7	2	0
Diarrhea	26	2	0	0	0
Stomatitis	22	2	2	2	0
Infection	20	1	2	5	0

*Number of patients is 28; this includes all eligible patients except four who have been in treatment for only 1 month.

In Table 2, the observed maximum toxicities and side effects are listed and graded according to the WHO criteria.[15] The myelosuppression was modest and predominantly affected the WBC. Only two patients experienced severe vomiting, while nine patients suffered no gastrointestinal discomfort at all. Moderate, patchy alopecia developed in seven patients treated for a median of 6 months (range, 1 to 8 months). No patients had total alopecia, and 12 patients treated for 1 to 4 months (median 2 months) had no hair loss at all.

DISCUSSION

The preliminary results from this study of combined treatment with prednimustine, Novantrone, methotrexate, 5-fluorouracil, and tamoxifen show that the regimen is effective in the treatment of advanced breast cancer in postmenopausal patients. It is still too early to calculate response rate, but the results obtained seem promising so far. With regard to the toxic side effects of the treatment, it appears that it is fairly well tolerated and that the dose-limiting factor is the hematologic toxicity, particularly WBC counts.

Conclusions from the trial must await the inclusion of more patient and longer follow-up.

REFERENCES

1. Mouridsen, HT, Palshof T, Brahm M, et al: Evaluation of single-drug versus multiple-drug chemotherapy in the treatment of advanced breast cancer. Cancer Treat Rep 61:47–50, 1977
2. Rozencweig M, Heuson J-C, von Hoff DD: Breast cancer, in Staquet M (ed): Randomized Trials in Cancer. A Critical Review by Sites. New York, Raven Press, 1978, p 31
3. Carter SK: Integration of chemotherapy into combined modality treatment of solid tumors. VII. Adenocarcinoma of the breast. Cancer Treat Rev 3:141–175, 1976
4. Henderson C, Canellos GP: Cancer of the breast. The past decade. N Engl J Med 302:78–90, 1980
5. Mouridsen HT, Kristensen D, Halskov Nielsen J, et al: Phase II trial of prednimustine L-1031 (NSC-134087) in advanced breast cancer. Cancer 46:253–255, 1980
6. Løber J, Mouridsen HT, Christiansen IE, et al: A phase III trial comparing prednimustine (LEO 1031) to chlorambucil plus prednisolone in advanced breast cancer. Cancer 52:1570–1576, 1983
7. Mouridsen HT, Boesen E: Prednimustine in combination with methotrexate and 5-fluorouracil in advanced breast cancer. A phase I–II study. Breast Cancer Res Treat 3:85–89, 1983
8. Mouridsen HT, Rose C, Engelsman E, et al: Combined cytotoxic and endocrine therapy in postmenopausal patients with advanced breast cancer. A randomized study of CMF vs. CMF plus tamoxifen. Eur J Cancer Clin Oncol 21:291–299, 1985
9. Smith IE: Mitoxantrone (Novantrone): A review of experimental and early clinical studies. Cancer Treat Rev 10:103–117, 1983
10. Smith JE, Stuart-Harris R, Pavlidis N, et al: Mitoxantrone (Novantrone) as single agent and in combination therapy in treatment of advanced breast cancer. Cancer Treat Rev 10:37–41, 1983
11. Mouridsen HT, Rose C, Nooy MA, et al: Mitoxantrone as first line cytotoxic therapy in advanced breast cancer. Preliminary results of a phase II study. Cancer Treat Rev. 10:47–52, 1983
12. Neidhart JA, Gochnour D, Roach RW, et al: Mitoxantrone versus doxorubicin in advanced breast cancer. A randomized cross-over trial. Cancer Treat Rev 10:41–47, 1983
13. Yap HY, Esparza L, Blumenschein GR, et al: Combination chemotherapy with cyclophosphamide, mitoxantrone and 5-fluorouracil in patients with metastatic breast cancer. Cancer Treat. Rev 10:53–57, 1983
14. Hayward JL, Carbone PP, Heuson JC, et al: Assessment of response to therapy in advanced breast cancer. Cancer 39:1289–1294, 1977
15. WHO Handbook for Reporting Results of Cancer Treatment. Geneva, WHO Offset Publication No. 48, 1979

A Randomized Comparative Study of Prednimustine and Doxorubicin in Patients With Metastatic Breast Cancer

By Joseph C. Allegra for the Prednimustine Collaborative Study Group

A clinical protocol outline of a study randomizing prednimustine *v* doxorubicin in patients with metastatic breast cancer is presented. The study has just been initiated, and no results are available at the present time. Unique features of this clinical trial are discussed, including the correlation of objective parameters of tumor response with symptomatic improvement as measured by quality of life, performance status, and pain indices as well as alterations in body weight.

SURGERY is the mainstay of breast cancer therapy, but recurrent or metastatic disease after surgical therapy remains a major medical problem. It is fortunate that, in the United States, the majority of women now present with stage I cancer of the breast and are cured by their primary operation; however, 30% to 35% of women still present with stage II operable breast cancer, and only a minority of these women are cured by surgery alone. The remaining 15% to 20% of women present with either stage III or stage IV breast carcinoma.

The medical management of metastatic breast cancer has involved either hormonal manipulation if the patient has a hormone-dependent tumor or combination chemotherapy in hormone-independent disease. The combination of cyclophosphamide, methotrexate, and 5-fluorouracil (CMF), with or without prednisone, is the most widely used first-line chemotherapy for metastatic adenocarcinoma of the breast, with clinical trials yielding response rates of 46% to 65%. However, duration of response is limited to a median of approximately 10 to 12 months, and gains in median survival are small.[1,2]

Usual therapy after failure of CMF chemotherapy consists of doxorubicin as a single agent or in combination with other cytotoxic agents. As first-line cytotoxic therapy, standard regimens of doxorubicin have shown response rates of 40% to 50%, with a median duration of response ranging from 4 to 8 months.[3] When utilized as secondary chemotherapy, response rates have ranged from 20% to 38%, and median survival has been unaffected.[4-8]

The clinical usefulness of doxorubicin is further limited by its toxicity. Myelosuppression is a dose-limiting side effect of particular importance in patients whose bone marrow reserve is impaired by previous chemotherapy, and the possibility of irreversible cardiotoxicity requires monitoring and may be dose limiting. Doxorubicin must be administered intravenously (IV), and care must be taken to avoid extravasation, since local vesicant action and tissue necrosis may result. At recommended doses of 60 to 75 mg/m^2 of doxorubicin administered every 3 weeks, alopecia and severe nausea and vomiting are also common.[9]

As treatment of patients with metastatic breast cancer is pallative rather than curative, a comparably active agent that is orally administered and less toxic than those currently available would be of great benefit to the practicing oncologist.

Prednimustine is a C21-prednisolone ester of chlorambucil and has been studied extensively in Europe. It has been shown to be efficacious in both non-Hodgkin's lymphoma and metastatic breast cancer. Most important, prednimustine is not only therapeutically active in these diseases but presents a relatively limited subjective and objective toxicity profile in comparison with other available therapy.

In breast cancer, pioneering studies in Europe were performed by Konyves et al,[10] who reported seven responses in 15 evaluable patients, with prednimustine-utilizing doses between 20 and 100 mg daily and by Mouridsen et al,[11] who reported a 39% response rate in 35 evaluable patients, all of whom had received either endocrine or chemotherapy prior to treatment with prednimustine. Dosage in the Mouridsen et al

From the University of Louisville School of Medicine, Department of Medicine, Louisville, Ky.

Address reprint requests to Joseph C. Allegra, MD, Professor and Chairman, Department of Medicine, Ambulatory Care Building, University of Louisville, Louisville, KY 40292.

0093-7754/86/1301-1011$05.00/0

study was 40 mg/m^2 daily. In these two clinical trials, toxicity related to prednimustine was acceptable.

These pioneering studies stimulated the prednimustine collaborative study group to embark on the present clinical trial. The goal of our clinical trial, which will compare prednimustine and doxorubicin in patients with metastatic breast cancer, is to compare the effects on tumor response, duration of tumor response, and symptomatic improvement as determined by measurements of pain, weight loss, and performance status. We will also compare the toxicity profiles of prednimustine and doxorubicin as well as the effects of the two cytotoxic agents on overall survival. This clinical trial is also unique in that it admits that objective tumor responses are frequently observed with secondary chemotherapy for advanced breast cancer, but also acknowledges that significant improvement in median survival for treated patients has not generally been demonstrated. Nevertheless, our study group felt that such therapy is generally considered to be providing important palliative benefit to patients responding to therapy. Traditionally, cancer clinical trials have utilized end points related to objective tumor response and/or survival, and palliative benefit has not been addressed as a therapeutic end point nor has a convincing relationship between tumor response and palliative benefit been demonstrated in clinical trials. We felt that in instances in which gains in median survival are not anticipated, such a demonstration of palliative benefit and its relationship to tumor response would be necessary to confirm the clinical usefulness of a study treatment. Hence, this study's secondary objectives are to compare descriptively the general toxicity profiles and quality of life indices associated with each treatment and to correlate objective parameters of tumor response with symptomatic improvement. Specifically, in this clinical trial we will be comparing the quality of life, performance status, and pain indices, as well as body weight, in patients assigned to each treatment group.

Finally, this study is designed to test two major hypotheses: first, that prednimustine and doxorubicin are similar in terms of both objective response and palliative benefit, and second, that prednimustine's toxicity profile is more favorable than that observed with doxorubicin.

MATERIALS AND METHODS

Table 1 lists the membership in the prednimustine collaborative study group. There are currently ten institutions that will be participating in this randomized clinical trial.

The treatment schema is illustrated in Figure 1. After stratification for extent of disease and performance status, patients will be randomized between doxorubicin, 60 mg/m^2, IV every 3 weeks, and prednimustine 20 mg/m^2, orally twice each day. A total of 270 patients evaluable for response is required for this clinical trial. These patients will be studied by the ten centers, each of which will provide at least 16 evaluable patients for analysis. Each center must provide eight evaluable subjects per treatment group to be included in any statistical analysis of efficacy. Each center will keep a log of all subjects for screening, and that log will include the reason for any patient exclusions. Informed consent must be obtained at screening prior to carrying out any of the procedures in this protocol.

Eligibility criteria include female sex with no age restrictions. The patients must have bidimensional measurable histologically documented metastatic or locally recurrent adenocarcinoma of the breast, and an estrogen receptor status of the primary tumor or metastases must be documented. The patients must have exhibited progressive disease during the course of first-line, advanced disease chemotherapy or within 6 months of cessation of adjuvant chemotherapy. The presence of at least one of the following findings is required: (1) combined pain and analgesic use score of greater than 4; (2) documented body weight loss of at least 5% within the past 6 months; or (3) performance status (Eastern Cooperative Oncology Group) of 0, 1, or 2.

These parameters are crucial to this study design since the

Table 1. Prednisone Collaborative Study Group

University of Louisville
University of Kentucky
Medical-Dental University of New Jersey
Georgetown University
University of Pennsylvania
University of Colorado
Duke University
University of Montreal
Vanderbilt University
Dalhousie University

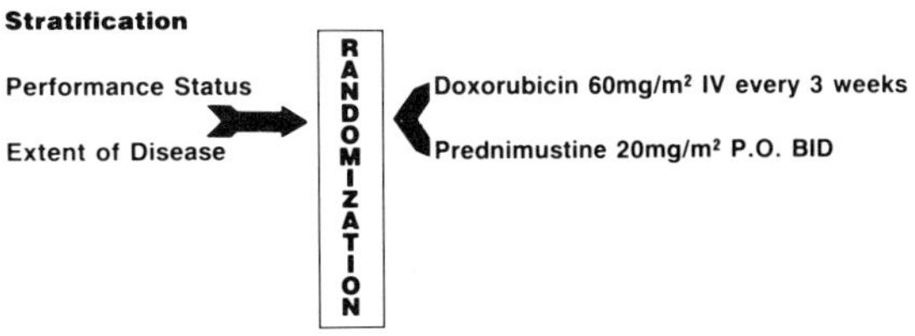

Fig 1. Treatment schema. A third party not involved in the care of the patient, and who is blinded to the medication assignment and disease status, will perform the pain, performance status, and quality of life index assessments.

study will correlate alteration in these parameters with response to therapy. No previous treatment with anthracycline-containing chemotherapy regimen or with an advanced regimen containing corticosteroids is allowed. The patients must have normal bone marrow function and liver function, and total bilirubin must be less than 2 mg/100 mL at the beginning of the study. The patients can have no medical contradictions to corticosteroid administration such as insulin-dependent diabetes mellitus, past history of steroid-induced psychosis, or active peptide ulcer disease. Patients with overt congestive heart failure will not be randomized in this clinical trial, and all patients must have an expected survival of greater than 3 months.

RESULTS AND DISCUSSION

No results are available at the present time.

This manuscript describes in brief outline form a new randomized clinical trial comparing prednimustine and doxorubicin to be performed by ten institutions in North America. A unique feature of this clinical trial involves an attempt to correlate objective parameters of tumor response with symptomatic improvement in the patients receiving therapy. A quality of life evaluation has been developed and will be used, along with a pain and analgesic index and evaluation of alterations in performance status and body weight. It is hoped that data will be available in the near future.

REFERENCES

1. Hellman S, Harris JR, Canellos GP, et al: Cancer of the breast, in DeVita VT, Jr, Hellman S, Rosenberg SA (eds): Cancer Principles and Practice of Oncology. J.B. Lippincott, Philadelphia-Toronto), 1982, pp 914–963

2. Carmo-Periera J, Costa FO, Henriques E: Chemotherapy of advanced breast cancer: A randomized trial of vincristine, Adriamycin and cyclosphosphamide (VAC) versus cyclophosphamide, methotrexate, 5-fluorouracil and prednisone. Cancer 48:1517–21, 1981

3. Creech RH, Catalano RB, Shah MK: An effective low-dose Adriamycin regimen as secondary chemotherapy for metastatic breast cancer patients *Cancer* 46:4433–4437, 1980

4. Brambilla C, DeLena M, Rossi A, et al: Response and survival in advanced breast cancer after two non-cross-resistant combinations. 3:801–807, 1976

5. Gottlieb J, Rivkin S, Spigel S, et al: Superiority of Adriamycin over oral nitrosoureas in patients with advanced breast carcinoma. Cancer 33:519–526, 1974

6. Hoogstraten B, George S, Samal B, et al: Combination chemotherapy and Adriamycin in patients with advanced breast cancer—A Southwest Oncology Group Study. Cancer 38:13–20, 1976

7. O'Bryan R, Baker L, Gottlieb J, et al: Dose response evaluation of Adriamycin in human neoplasia. Cancer 39:1940–1948, 1977

8. Tormey DC: Adriamycin (NSC-123127) in breast cancer: An overview of studies. Cancer Chemother Res 6:319–327, 1975

9. Calabresi P, Parks RE Jr: Antiproliferative agents and drugs used for immunosuppression, in Gilman AG, Goodman LS, Gilman A (eds.): The Pharmacological Basis of Therapeutics (ed 6). New York, MacMillan, 1980, p 1293

10. Konyves I, Nordenskjold B, Plym Forshell G, et al: Preliminary clinical and absorption studies with prednimustine in patients with mammary carcinoma. Eur J Cancer 11:844, 1975

11. Mourisden HT, Kristensen D, Halskov J, et al: Phase II trial of prednimustine, L-1031, (NSC-134087) in advanced breast cancer. Cancer 46:253–255, 1980

Seminars in Oncology
will publish in future issues

Biological Response Modifiers

Myeloma

Breast Cancer

Head and Neck Cancer

Tumor Markers

Endocrine Malignancies

VOL XIII, NO 3, SUPPL 2 SEPTEMBER 1986

Seminars in Oncology

Alpha Interferon Therapy in Oncology: Clinical Update

Contributors

Sydney E. Salmon
Howard Ozer • Paul P. Trotta
M. Robert Cooper • Marc J. Ratain
James W. Vardiman • Harvey M. Golomb • Daniel E. Bergsagel
Rainer H. Haas • Hans A. Messner • Kenneth A. Foon
Mark S. Roth • Paul A. Bunn, Jr • Donald I. Abrams • Paul A. Volberding
John M. Kirkwood • Marc Ernstoff • Frank M. Torti • Bert L. Lum
Jonathan S. Berek • Neville F. Hacker • Alan Lichtenstein • Tyler Jung
Celsa Spina • Reba M. Knox • Jeanine Brady • Teri Greene
Lupe M. Ettinger • Leo D. Lagasse • Eric M. Bonnem • Robert J. Spiegel
Jacob Zighelboim • Daniel D. Von Hoff • Giselle Sarosy • Thomas D. Brown
John G. Kuhn • Daniel L. Kisner • John Torrisi
Christine Berg • Anatoly Dritschilo • Brian G.M. Durie
Lawrence Clouse • Theodore Braich
Meredith Grimm • Aurelia B. Robertone

GRUNE & STRATTON
Harcourt Brace Jovanovich, Inc.

Seminars in Oncology

Alpha Interferon Therapy in Oncology: Clinical Update
Proceedings of a Symposium held April 11–12, 1986, at Johns Island, South Carolina.

Sponsored by Lineberger Cancer Center of the University of North Carolina at Chapel Hill and Schering Corporation

VOL XIII, NO 3, SUPPL 2 **September 1986**

Table of Contents

Introduction .... *Sydney E. Salmon and Howard Ozer* 1

Preclinical Biology of Alpha Interferons .... *Paul P. Trotta* 3

Interferons in the Treatment of Multiple Myeloma .... *M. Robert Cooper* 13

The Role of Interferon in the Treatment of Hairy Cell Leukemia .... *Marc J. Ratain, James W. Vardiman, and Harvey M. Golomb* 21

Interferon Alfa-2b in the Treatment of Chronic Granulocytic Leukemia .... *Daniel E. Bergsagel, Rainer H. Haas, and Hans A. Messner* 29

Alpha Interferon Treatment of Low-Grade B-Cell Non-Hodgkin's Lymphomas, Cutaneous T-Cell Lymphomas, and Chronic Lymphocytic Leukemia .... *Kenneth A. Foon, Mark S. Roth, and Paul A. Bunn, Jr* 35

Alpha Interferon Therapy of AIDS-Associated Kaposi's Sarcoma .... *Donald I. Abrams and Paul A. Volberding* 43

Potential Applications of the Interferons in Oncology: Lessons Drawn from Studies of Human Melanoma .... *John M. Kirkwood and Marc Ernstoff* 48

Superficial Carcinoma of the Bladder: Natural History and the Role of Interferons .... *Frank M. Torti and Bert L. Lum* 57

Intraperitoneal Recombinant α-Interferon for "Salvage" Immunotherapy in Stage III Epithelial Ovarian Cancer: A Gynecologic Oncology Group Study .... *Jonathan S. Berek, Neville F. Hacker, Alan Lichtenstein, et al* 61

Rationale for and Conduct of a Phase I Clinical Trial With Interferon Alfa-2b Plus Doxorubicin .... *Daniel D. Von Hoff, Giselle Sarosy, Thomas D. Brown, John G. Kuhn, and Daniel L. Kisner* 72

The Combined Use of Interferon and Radiotherapy in Cancer Management .... *John Torrisi, Christine Berg, Eric Bonnem, and Anatoly Dritschilo* 78

Interferon Alfa-2b—Cyclophosphamide Combination Studies: In Vitro and Phase I–II Clinical Results .... *Brian G.M. Durie, Lawrence Clouse, Theodore Braich, Meredith Grimm, and Aurelia B. Robertone* 84

Intron® A (Interferon Alfa-2b): Clinical Overview and Future Directions ...... *Robert J. Spiegel* 89

Seminars in Oncology

Alpha Interferon Therapy in Oncology: Clinical Update Proceedings of a Symposium held April 11–12, 1986, at Johns Island, South Carolina

Sponsored by Lineberger Cancer Center of the University of North Carolina at Chapel Hill and Schering Corporation

Seminars in Oncology

VOL XIII, NO 3, SUPPL 2 **SEPTEMBER 1986**

Introduction

SINCE the cloning and expression of the interferon alfa-2b gene in 1980, clinical research with recombinant alpha interferons has proceeded at a rapid pace. In this supplement, investigators who have made important contributions to clinical research utilizing alpha interferons, particularly interferon alfa-2b, present their current studies and describe potential future directions for the use of interferons and related compounds in the treatment of cancer. Basic research is presented regarding the pleiotropic effects of interferon on in vitro tumor cell proliferation and immunomodulation. Evidence is provided from both athymic nude mouse models and human tumor clonogenic assays suggesting the possibility of direct antiproliferative activity of alpha interferon. Such activity would be in addition to interferon's known antiviral and immunologic effects that include modulating cellular functions such as natural killer cell activity.

CLINICAL APPLICATIONS

The marked therapeutic activity of alpha interferon as a single agent for patients with hairy cell leukemia, originally identified by Quesada and his colleagues, is underscored in data presented from a large multicenter trial of interferon alfa-2b (Intron®A) for patients with this disorder. Trials of alpha interferon as therapy for multiple myeloma demonstrate antitumor activity in previously treated patients; they also suggest a potential role for alpha interferon in combination with melphalan and prednisone in previously untreated myeloma patients.

Clinical studies in lymphomatous disorders are presented by investigators describing interferon's antitumor activity in nodular and T-cell–derived lymphomas and in AIDS-associated Kaposi's sarcoma. Additionally, the usefulness of interferon therapy in chronic myeloid leukemia is suggested by the finding that interferon can markedly reduce the self-renewal capacity of myeloid leukemic blasts in vitro, as well as delay the rise in the leukocyte counts after cytoreduction with in vivo administration.

Results of clinical trials for other selected solid tumors are also reviewed. Approximately 20% of patients with malignant melanoma have shown responses to interferon treatment, according to one of the presentations; perhaps one third of these responders achieved durable remissions. Another report reveals that interferon alfa-2b appears to have significant antitumor activity against in situ bladder carcinoma when given by the intravesical route. The potential role of alpha interferon for regional high-dose therapy was further underscored by the demonstration of clinical response in patients with epithelial ovarian carcinoma receiving repeated cycles of interferon administered intraperitoneally. Finally, the potential uses and pitfalls in developing combination therapy with alpha interferon and conventional treatment modalities are suggested by preliminary phase I clinical trials combining interferon and doxorubicin; interferon and radiation therapy; and interferon plus cyclophosphamide.

Throughout this symposium summary, issues of short- and long-term toxicities, dose route and schedule, and potential mechanisms of action of recombinant alpha interferon in malignant disease are emphasized. Importantly, it is noted, antibody formation to interferon alfa-2b appears to be a relatively infrequent event. Finally, the symposium addresses some promising future directions in clinical research as well as problems that may arise in the broad clinical application of the interferons. It is clear from the available data that recombinant alpha interferons will assume a significant role in the treatment of cancer.

Sydney E. Salmon, MD
Department of Internal Medicine,
The Arizona Cancer Center
and
University of Arizona College of Medicine
Tucson, Ariz

Howard Ozer, MD, PhD
Department of Medicine,
Lineberger Cancer Research Center
and
The University of North Carolina
at Chapel Hill
Chapel Hill, NC

Preclinical Biology of Alpha Interferons

Paul P. Trotta

The availability of large quantities of purified recombinant human alpha interferons has permitted an expansion of studies on the preclinical biology of interferon. These purified preparations have definitively established that interferon exhibits pleiotypic effects on cellular function, including antiviral, antiproliferative, and immunomodulatory activities. Thus, interferon can exert therapeutic activity by both direct effects on the growth of the tumor and by modulation of the biologic response of the host. The exact mechanism of action will most probably vary from patient to patient. The variety of biologic activities that interferon displays, as well as the fact that it is highly species-specific, makes it difficult to design preclinical studies that can provide guidance for the clinical application of interferon as an antineoplastic agent. Two models that have provided useful preclinical data on human cell lines or fresh biopsies are reviewed: the human tumor clonogenic assay and human tumor xenografts in immunodeficient mice. These models indicate that interferon is likely to be an effective treatment for a broad range of malignancies, and that the response will be highly dependent on the type of interferon as well as its dose, schedule, and route of administration. Both models have provided evidence that alpha interferon may demonstrate a synergistic or additive interaction with standard chemotherapeutic agents like cyclophosphamide or doxorubicin. The utility of any preclinical model for predicting an individual patient's response to interferon is yet to be established.

ISAACS and Lindenmann[1] demonstrated in 1957 that when chicken egg chorioallantoic membranes were exposed to a heat-inactivated influenza virus, a factor was released that could protect fresh tissues from virus infection with live influenza. They termed this substance "interferon," based upon its ability to interfere with viral infectivity. Viruses from every major category, as well as a variety of nonviral inducers (eg, double-stranded RNA, bacteria, or mitogens) are now known to induce interferon production. Interferon was subsequently demonstrated to consist of a family of related proteins that could inhibit the replication of a broad spectrum of RNA- and DNA-containing viruses, including both oncogenic and nononcogenic strains. Interferon is distinct from other antiviral agents in that it acts directly on the host cell, not on the virus, to induce a state that is resistant to viral replication. Binding to the cell surface has been established as a prerequisite for the establishment of the antiviral state.[2] Binding studies with radiolabeled ligands have definitively established that interferon binds to specific, saturable, high-affinity receptors on the plasma membrane as the first step in the expression of its biologic activity.[3,4]

Three major categories of interferon have been described: alpha (leukocyte), beta (fibroblast), and gamma (immune). These can be distinguished by antigenic and physicochemical properties, as well as by the nature of the interferon inducer and the cell source from which they are derived. Interferon alphas are a family of at least 14 highly homologous species (ie, approximately 75% homology in their amino acid sequences) that are produced by a variety of cell types, including macrophages, null cells (non-B, non-T lymphocytes), and B-cell lines upon exposure to live or inactivated virions, double-stranded RNA, or bacterial products.

Interferon beta, which is produced mainly from fibroblasts and epithelial cells in response to the same inducers that produce interferon alpha, consists predominantly of a single species (interferon beta-1) that shares approximately 30% amino acid sequence homology with interferon alpha.[5] Other human interferon beta genes have also been described.[6] Most data support the observation that interferon alpha and interferon beta (also referred to as type I interferons) compete for the same cell surface receptor.[4,7]

Interferon gamma (type II interferon), the product of a single gene, is derived from T cells that have been stimulated by specific antigens and nonspecific mitogens as well as from natural killer cells. Interferon gamma has a cell surface receptor distinct from that for type I interferons and appears to have unique biochemical effects.[8,9] Interferon gamma has only minor amino acid sequence homology with type I interferons.[10]

From Schering-Plough Corp., Bloomfield, New Jersey.

Address reprint requests to Paul P. Trotta, PhD, Schering-Plough Corp., 60 Orange Street, Bloomfield, NJ 07003.

BIOLOGIC ACTIVITY

Soon after the identification of interferon as an antiviral agent, it was recognized that interferon preparations could exhibit other biologic effects. Thus, Paucker et al[11] first demonstrated that relatively impure preparations of murine interferon exerted an antiproliferative effect on mouse fibroblasts. It was consistent with this observation that murine interferon preparations could display antitumor activity in mice implanted with a variety of tumor cell lines[12] or in which tumors were chemically induced,[13] in addition to an expected prophylactic activity on tumors of viral origin.[14] Early studies by Gresser and colleagues[15] indicated that a leukemic cell line that was not sensitive to the antiproliferative activity of interferon in vitro did respond in vivo when it was grown as a leukemia. These data suggested that interferon is also capable of stimulating the host immune system and that antitumor activity might result from a combination of host-mediated effects and direct anticellular activity. To date, multiple so-called nonantiviral effects have been reported in a variety of histologic cell types (reviewed by Stewart[16] and Taylor-Papadimitriou[17]), as summarized in Table 1.

Most of the diverse biologic effects described in Table 1 were originally described with relatively impure murine or human interferon preparations. It was a serious concern whether other components in the preparations were the true mediators of the response, especially in light of the fact that some of the results were apparently contradictory—eg, both inhibition[18] and activation[19] of suppressor T-lymphocyte generation were observed. The cloning of a single gene for human interferon alpha[20] followed by the purification of large quantities of the expressed protein[21] permitted an unequivocal demonstration that these biologic properties are an inherent property of interferon. The purified recombinant DNA–derived interferon subtypes generally provide a more powerful means of understanding the biology and mechanism of action of interferon than does natural leukocyte interferon, which represents a heterogeneous mixture of interferon alpha subtypes. In addition, the application of recombinant DNA technology has permitted the construction of novel variants and hybrid interferons[22] that have resulted in important insights into the structural basis of interferon's biologic effects.

Table 1. Biologic Activities of Interferon*

Antiviral activity
Inhibition of the replication of a broad spectrum of RNA- and DNA-containing viruses
Anticellular activity
Inhibition of cellular growth
Alterations in the state of cellular differentiation
Effects on the cell cycle
Reversion of the malignant phenotype
Interference with oncogene expression
Immunomodulatory activity
Regulation of cytotoxic effector cells
Alterations in cell surface antigen expression
Effects on antibody production

*References are cited by Taylor-Papadimitriou.[17]

A number of volumes have adequately reviewed the in vitro and in vivo biologic activity of interferon.[23-28] Of special importance are the preclinical models that might provide guidance with respect to the clinical application of interferon as an antineoplastic agent. Ideally, such models would be expected to: identify individual patients most likely to respond to interferon treatment; indicate for each patient which interferon subtype would be the most effective antitumor agent; provide guidance with respect to clinical dosing and scheduling regimens; and establish conditions for combining interferon with standard chemotherapeutic agents for producing synergistic or additive interactions. Reviewed herein are selected studies that relate to recent developments in two preclinical models that have potential for achieving at least some of these goals. These laboratory models for the in vitro and in vivo evaluation are the human tumor clonogenic assay and human tumor xenografts, respectively. Emphasis is given to studies employing highly purified preparations of human interferon alpha.

HUMAN TUMOR CLONOGENIC ASSAY

Hamburger and Salmon[29] and Smith and associates[30] have developed culture conditions for assessing colony formation from tumor cells. This clonogenic assay employs a semisolid agar medium that supports colony growth from fresh human tumor biopsies as well as malignant cell lines but suppresses normal cell proliferation. The use of the clonogenic assay for evaluating the antitumor potential of a drug is based on the so-called stem cell model for cancer, in which both primary tumor growth and metastatic potential are attributed to the rapidly proliferating stem cell populations. This assay has been previously demonstrated to be useful in identifying new antitumor agents as well as in predicting individual patient response.[31,32] The rationale behind its application in evaluating potential antitumor activity is that chemotherapy should be directed to the proliferating stem cell population and that the relatively differentiated cells do not affect long-term tumor development of metastasis.

It has been reported that partially purified natural leukocyte interferon demonstrates antitumor activity in the clonogenic assay.[33-38] Responses were noted in a variety of malignancies, including leukemia and cancers of the ovary, breast, prostate, and lung. Salmon and co-workers[39] have tested 273 fresh human tumor biopsies for sensitivity to purified recombinant interferon alfa-2a. Continuous exposure of the cells to interferon alpha caused a reduction in colony formation to 50% or less of control values for 104 (38.1%) tumor specimens, of which 51 tumors (18.7%) demonstrated reduction in colony number to 30% or less of control values. Responses were observed in a wide variety of solid and hemopoietic tumors; the percentage response for any particular histologic type was 20% to 55%. Melanoma, ovarian cancers, and sarcomas showed the greatest percentage of high responders (ie, 30% or less colony survival) compared with a less marked sensitivity in tumors of breast, lung, and kidney, and acute leukemias.

Another purified recombinant interferon alpha subtype (interferon alpha-D) was tested in the same study against 71 tumors and appeared to be less active than interferon alfa-2a. At the same concentration as that employed for interferon alfa-2a—ie, 4 ng/mL—tumor colony formation was reduced by interferon alpha-D to 50% or less of control values in 12 tumor specimens (16%) and to 30% or less of control values in six tumor specimens (8%). A number of tumors from individual patients were also reported to appear to be more sensitive to one or the other of the subtypes—usually, interferon alfa-2a. These data suggested that: clinical responses might be expected for a broad range of neoplasms; and differences in the number or degree of responses might be expected among different interferon subtypes or combinations of subtypes.

Two general mechanisms can account for the responses observed in the clonogenic assay of fresh tumor biopsies: a direct anticellular effect on the tumor and an indirect effect mediated by stimulation of host cytotoxic effector cells (eg, natural killer cells or cytotoxic T lymphocytes) present in the fresh tumor biopsies. The exact mechanism is likely to be highly variable even among malignancies of the same histologic type. The use of established cell lines has allowed a study of the direct effect on cellular growth. Two independent studies[40,41] have identified cell lines whose growth is inhibited by purified recombinant interferon alpha. As shown in Table 2, this effect is schedule- and concentration-dependent. Although a brief (1 hour) exposure of cells to interferon was not sufficient to demonstrate sensitivity, even at a concentration of 10,000 IU/mL, continuous exposure during the length of the assay (7 to 21 days) revealed a significant anticellular effect (colony reduction $\leq$50%) in four out of six cell lines tested. The demonstration of an anticellular effect by continuous exposure is generally considered to reflect a cytostatic rather than a cytotoxic effect, whereas antiproliferative effects observed after short-term exposure suggest a cytotoxic mechanism.

An ovarian cell line, BG-1, was chosen for studying the potential interaction of recombinant interferon alfa-2b (Intron® A) with eight standard cytotoxic drugs (doxorubicin, cisplatin, vinblastine, 5-fluorouracil, methotrexate, bleomycin, triethylene-thiophosphoramide, and mitoxantrone). Both short-term (1 hour) sequential exposure to interferon alfa-2b followed by doxorubicin and long-term continuous exposure to both agents during the assay were employed. Contrary to the report cited above, synergistic interactions were demonstrated for

Table 2. In Vitro Sensitivity of Cell Lines to Recombinant Human Interferon Alfa-2b*

Cell Lines	Number of Separate Experiments	Concentration of Interferon Alfa-2b: Continuous Exposure 100 IU/mL	Continuous Exposure 10,000 IU/mL	1-Hour Exposure 100 IU/mL	1-Hour Exposure 10,000 IU/mL
BG-1	22	R	S	R	R
SKMEL-28	6	R	S	R	R
ME-180	3	R	S	R	R
CASKI	3	R	S	R	R
CAKI-2	5	R	R	R	R
MCF-7	2	NT	NT	R	R

Abbreviations: R, resistant (>50% colony survival); S, sensitive (≤50% colony survival); NT, not tested.
*Data were obtained from Welander et al.[41]

combinations of interferon alfa-2b and doxorubicin utilizing both methods of exposure at both high and low interferon concentrations, as shown in Table 3. The short-term sequential exposure treatment was also synergistic for two other cell lines and a primary tumor explant. It is interesting that the synergy observed was found to be schedule-dependent in this study, since a 1-hour interferon alfa-2b treatment followed by long-term doxorubicin exposure (or vice versa) produced additive or antagonistic effects. In addition, apparent synergy was observed for combinations of interferon alfa-2b and both cisplatin and vinblastine only under conditions of continuous exposure. The relationship between interferon alfa-2b and the other drugs cited above was generally additive.

Earlier studies of Aapro and co-workers[40] also tested the combination of purified recombinant interferon alfa-2a and various cytotoxic drugs (ie, vinblastine, vincristine, vindesine, vinzolidine, cisplatin, doxorubicin, etoposide, and melphalan) against three human tumor cell lines. The most significant result was the synergy observed when vinblastine and interferon alfa-2a were combined continuously during the assay period. These results appeared to be schedule-dependent, since 1-hour treatment with vinblastine followed by continuous exposure to interferon alfa-2a demonstrated a lower frequency of synergy. Synergy was also observed for continuous simultaneous exposure to interferon alfa-2a and cisplatin; however, 1-hour exposure to cisplatin followed by continuous exposure to interferon alfa-2a did not show synergistic action. The other agents tested generally showed additive or subadditive effects. These data are in general agreement with those of Welander et al,[41] except for the failure of Aapro and co-workers[40] to observe synergy in combinations of interferon alpha and doxorubicin. This discrepancy may be related to the different cell lines employed or differences in the preparations of the purified interferon alpha subtypes.

HUMAN TUMOR XENOGRAFT MODELS

As previously noted, animal interferons have demonstrated potent antitumor activity in a variety of animal tumor models (reviewed by Gresser and Tovey[12] and Balkwill[42]). In general, it is difficult to test human interferons in such models, due to the fact that—with the exception of an artificial hybrid interferon produced by recombinant DNA technology—human interferon generally displays its highest levels of activity on human cells.[22] This phenomenon is referred to as "species specificity." Human tumor xenografts implanted in immunocompromised mice represent an animal model for evaluating that aspect of the antitumor action of interferon that is mediated by direct inhibition of tumor cell proliferation, since modulation of the host immune system is, in general, expected to be low or nonexistent. In support of this conclusion, studies in athymic nude mice have indicated that purified recombinant interferon alfa-2b does not result in significant changes in host

Table 3. Interactions of Recombinant Human Interferon Alfa-2b and Cytotoxic Drugs Employing 1-Hour Sequential Exposure or Continuous Exposure With Ovarian Cell Line BG-1*

Drug (Concentration)	Interferon Concentration (IU/mL)	Exposure Method†	Expected Colony Survival (Standard Error)	Observed Colony Survival (Standard Error)	Combined Effect	*p* Value‡
Doxorubicin	100	1-hour	0.83 (0.194)	0.52 (0.49)	Synergistic	<0.05
(0.006 μg/mL)	10,000	1-hour	0.85 (0.182)	0.38 (0.062)	Synergistic	<0.01
	100	Continuous	0.51 (0.118)	0.11 (0.019)	Synergistic	<0.01
	10,000	Continuous	0.37 (0.073)	0.03 (0.016)	Synergistic	<0.01
Cisplatin	100	1-hour	0.68 (0.154)	0.44 (0.071)	Additive	NS
(0.25 μg/mL)	10,000	1-hour	0.69 (0.144)	0.47 (0.093)	Additive	NS
	100	Continuous	0.43 (0.101)	0.012 (0.004)	Synergistic	<0.01
	10,000	Continuous	0.32 (0.063)	0.02 (0.008)	Synergistic	<0.01
Vinblastine	100	1-hour	0.44 (0.119)	0.33 (0.037)	Additive	NS
(0.0783 μg/mL)	10,000	1-hour	0.45 (0.115)	0.44 (0.056)	Additive	NS
	100	Continuous	0.04 (0.012)	0.01 (0.006)	Additive	NS
	10,000	Continuous	0.03 (0.008)	0.002 (0.002)	Synergistic	<0.05

Abbreviations: NS, not significant.

*Data were adapted from Welander et al.[41]

†Sequential exposure involved 1-hour exposure to interferon alpha-2b followed by 1-hour exposure to the cytotoxic drug prior to culturing of the cells in a soft agar medium. For the continuous exposure methodology, both agents were present simultaneously in the soft agar medium.

‡*p* values are reported only for differences between "expected" and "observed" colony survival that indicate statistically significant drug synergy or antagonism.

natural killer cell activity[43] in this model, and that purified human lymphoblastoid interferon alpha had no apparent effect on the levels of either cytochrome P-450 or glutathione S-transferases.[44] Thus, this model may be useful in comparing the direct antitumor effects of different interferon preparations, alone and in combination, as well as in evaluating potential synergistic interactions with standard chemotherapeutic agents or other cytokines that are mediated through direct effects on the tumor. In addition, information obtained from treatment of xenografts may provide insight into the relative importance of host-mediated *v* direct tumor effects.

A number of reports have indicated that highly purified human interferon alpha displays antitumor activity against human tumor xenografts. For example, intralesional treatment of a human osteosarcoma implanted in athymic mice with recombinant interferon alfa-2b resulted in a significant effect on the rate of tumor growth (Table 4). The number of animals developing tumors within the first 2 weeks following tumor implantation also appeared to be reduced by administration of interferon alpha. An apparent dose response was observed in this study by comparing interferon alfa-2b doses of 2×10^5 IU with those of 8×10^5 IU, each administered for 7 days. In general, reported experiments with human tumor xenografts have employed a variety of tumor types, sites of tumor inoculation, and routes of administration.[45] It is notable that in a number of these studies, the dose of interferon (measured in antiviral units) required to achieve an effect was severalfold greater than the maximally tolerated clinical dose. These results imply that host-mediated effects may play an additional important role in the observed clinical responses. However, other explanations for larger doses apparently being required in the animal models may be invoked—eg, a population of cells that was inherently less sensitive to interferon's antiproliferative action was selected during the growth of the tumor.

The responses to treatment of human tumor xenografts with human interferon alpha have been highly variable. Thus, purified recombinant interferon alfa-2b has been reported to inhibit the growth of renal[43] and osteosarcoma cell lines (Table 4) implanted in athymic nude mice, but failed to affect three other xenografts implanted in immunodeprived mice.[46] Differences in dosing, routes of administration, scheduling, and the characteristics of the host animal might account for the different results. However, in experiments conducted on the same host strain, utilizing identical treatment protocols and dosing, Balkwill et al[47] have reported that daily treatment of six primary human explants with purified lymphoblastoid interferon alpha resulted in responses ranging from no effect to complete tumor eradication. Biochemical characteristics of these cells would have to be known in order to establish a mechanism for these observations (eg, differences in the affinity of interferon for the cell surface receptor or in the total number of receptors per cell). In addition, these authors demonstrated that the model was able to distinguish differences in response among interferon alpha subtypes. Thus, utilizing a primary breast carcinoma xenograft, interferon alpha-D was considerably less effective than interferon alfa-2a. It is notable that neither beta nor gamma interferon inhibited growth of this xenograft.

Human tumor xenografts recently have been shown to have potential for evaluating the interactions between interferon and cytotoxic drugs. As shown in Figure 1, simultaneous administration of cyclophosphamide and varying doses of purified lymphoblastoid interferon alpha resulted in a tumor stasis at relatively low doses and a complete regression at the highest doses.[48] This result was clearly superior to therapy with each agent alone, which resulted only in tumor growth inhibition at the highest dose employed. No apparent bone marrow toxicity was observed in the same study for the combination. Comparable synergistic effects demonstrating tumor stasis and regression were also observed for simultaneous combinations of interferon and doxorubicin.

A number of in vivo studies[49-53] with murine interferon alpha/beta and various cytotoxic drugs have also found a synergistic interaction against murine tumors; however, other data indicate the absence of interaction[54] as well as antagonism.[55] The use of xenografts permits at least a partial elucidation of the mechanisms potentially involved in these interactions. Although it has been reported that interferon depresses the activity of the cytochrome P-450 system,[56] it is unlikely that this effect is relevant to the antitumor effects obtained in the nude mouse model in response to treatment with human interferon alpha, due to the fact that interferon displays a high degree of species specificity. This conclusion is supported by the failure of simultaneous administration of murine interferon to modify the apparent synergy between

Table 4. Treatment of Human Osteosarcoma Tumors Implanted in Nude Balb/c Mice With Two Doses of Recombinant Human Interferon Alfa-2b*

	Mean Tumor Volume (mm^3) at Number of Weeks Following Human Osteosarcoma Tumor Incubation					
	1	2	3	4	5	6
Saline treated	12 (15/15)†	34 (15/15)	101 (15/15)	214 (15/15)	529 (15/15)	1,026 (15/15)
Interferon treated						
Low dose‡	14 (9/15)	24 (14/15)	125 (14/15)	242 (15/15)	364 (15/15)	547 (15/15)
High dose§	8 (10/15)	18 (9/15)	65 (12/15)	131 (13/15)	229 (14/15)	382 (14/15)

*Interferon alfa-2b was injected intralesionally 24 hours after subcutaneous tumor transplantation and continued daily for 7 days. Data were obtained from Douglas K. Kelsey (unpublished observations).

†Numbers in parentheses represent the number of mice with tumors divided by the total number of mice.

‡The dose was 200,000 IU per mouse.

§The dose was 800,000 IU per mouse.

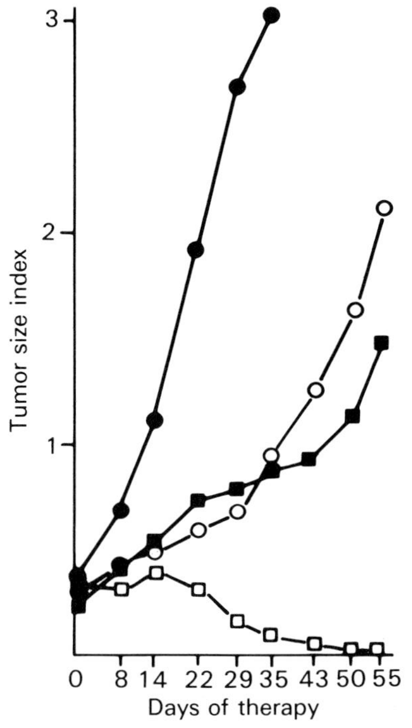

Figure 1. Human lymphoblastoid interferon gamma plus cyclophosphamide therapy of a human breast cancer xenograft. Interferon was administered subcutaneously on a daily basis and cyclophosphamide was given intraperitoneally during 3 of every 4 weeks. The tumor was derived from a mucoid carcinoma of the breast in an untreated postmenopausal woman. It was established and passed solely in nude mice and had a human karyotype. Each experimental group contained four mice. ●, control; ■, cyclophosphamide, 0.25 mg; ○, human lymphoblastoid interferon alpha (2 × 10^5 units); □, human lymphoblastoid interferon alpha (2 × 10^5 units) plus cyclophosphamide (0.25 mg). Reprinted with permission from Balkwill and Moodie.[48]

human interferon alpha and cytotoxic drugs in the nude mouse model or to affect the levels of drug-metabolizing enzyme activities.[44] However, the same study found that the combination of human interferon alpha and either doxorubicin or cyclophosphamide exhibited direct effects on the tumor, as demonstrated by effects on the cell cycle—ie, a delay in G_2 accumulation and an increased number of S-phase cells. In distinction, human interferon alpha alone had only minor effects on the distribution of cells in the cycle, consistent with in vitro data supporting that its principal effect is to increase the length of all phases, not to cause a selective accumulation.[57] Since both doxorubicin and cyclophosphamide exert toxic effects in S phase, the accumulation of malignant cells in this phase may be responsible for the synergistic interaction with interferon. However, other biochemical mechanisms may also be operative—eg, membrane-associated effects of interferon on the flux of the drug into or out of the cell.

SUMMARY AND CONCLUSIONS

The biologic profile of interferon indicates that it has the properties of a classical biologic response modifier—ie, it exerts therapeutic activity by modifying the host's biologic response to malignant cells. Interferon has the capacity to alter the relationship between host and tumor by augmentation of host effector mechanisms or by direct effects on the tumor involving changes in the state of differentiation or in the expression of tumor-associated antigens. However, the mechanism of interferon's antitumor activity is further complicated by the fact that it has direct effects on the proliferation of tumor cells. The relative importance of direct *v* host-mediated effects in the expression of the antitumor activity of interferon in the clinic remains unknown. It is likely that the exact mechanism will vary from patient to patient, depending principally on the immune status of the host and the biochemical characteristics of the tumor (eg, the presence or absence of interferon receptors or the ability of the tumor to inactivate the interferon by release of proteases). It is also apparent from the preclinical studies cited above that the type of the interferon as well as its dose, scheduling, and route of administration will be important factors in determining the nature of the clinical response.

A principal goal of preclinical studies on purified human interferon alpha is to determine which patients would be most likely to respond to interferon alone as well as in combination with other biologic response modifiers or cytotoxic agents. It is hoped that preclinical models will also provide guidance for dosing and scheduling regimens, as well as define broad classes of malignancies responsive to interferon. A former obstacle to accomplishing these goals has been the availability of purified interferon. As previously noted, the application of recombinant DNA technology has solved this problem.

However, the question remains as to which preclinical model is most likely to provide useful information relevant to clinical trials. The species specificity of human interferons implies that the classical animal tumor models for evaluating the activity of chemotherapeutic agents cannot be employed. Human tumor xenografts derived from fresh tumor biopsies may be employed for evaluating direct inhibition of tumor cell growth. The response of human melanoma cells implanted in nude mice to chemotherapeutic agents has been shown to correlate with clinical results.[58] When fresh tumor biopsies are studied in this model, indirect effects may have a role in the response, since infiltrating effector cells (lymphocytes and macrophages) from the patient could also be present in the xenograft. In addition, the question arises whether effects on a biopsy will be representative of the response of the entire tumor. The same concern is applicable to responses observed in the human tumor clonogenic assay. It is notable that results from the latter assay have correctly predicted that interferon alpha would show clinical efficacy against a broad range of tumors with a response rate generally under 50%.[59]

An alternative approach for preclinical models of interferon therapy is to employ purified murine interferon in appropriate murine animal tumor models. Although such experiments may contribute to our understanding of the biology of interferon and its mechanism of action, it is not yet established that such models can provide guidance for the clinical application of human interferon. Similarly, the utility of any of the preclinical models described here in evaluating the antitumor activity of human interferon alpha must still be determined by a direct comparison on an individual basis of the sensitivity of malignant cells in preclinical tests with the observed clinical response.

REFERENCES

1. Isaacs A, Lindenmann J: Virus interference. The interferon. Proc R Soc B 147:258–267, 1957

2. Friedman RM: Interferon binding: The first step in establishment of antiviral activity. Science 156:1760–1761, 1967

3. Zoon KC, Zur Nedden D, Arnheiter H: Specific binding of human alpha interferon to a high affinity cell surface binding site on bovine kidney cells. J Biol Chem 257:4695–4697, 1982

4. Joshi AR, Sarkar FH, Gupta SL: Interferon receptors. Cross-linking of human leukocyte interferon alpha-2 to its receptor on human cells. J Biol Chem 257:13774–13887, 1982

5. Ohno S, Taniguchi T: Structure of a chromosomal gene for human interferon beta. Proc Natl Acad Sci USA 78:5305–5309, 1981

6. Sehgal PB, May LT, Sagar AD: Multiple human B interferon genes, in DeMaeyer E, Schellekens H (eds): The Biology of the Interferon System 1983. New York, Elsevier, 1983, pp 15–20

7. Branca AA, Baglioni C: Binding to human cells of [^{125}I] labelled alpha interferon produced in *E. coli.* Evidence for distinct receptors for type I and II interferons. Nature 294:768–770, 1981

8. Littman SJ, Faltynek CR, Baglioni C: Binding of human recombinant ^{125}I-interferon gamma to receptors on human cells. J Biol Chem 260:1191–1195, 1985

9. Weil J, Epstein CJ, Epstein LB, et al: A unique set of polypeptides is induced by gamma-interferon, in addition to those induced in common with IFN-alpha and IFN-beta. Nature 301:437–439, 1983

10. Gray PW, Leung DW, Pennica D, et al: Expression of human immune interferon cDNA in *E. coli* and monkey cells. Nature 295:503–508, 1982

11. Paucker K, Cantell K, Henle W: Quantitative studies on viral interference in suspended L cells. III. Effect of interfering viruses and interferon on the growth rate of cells. Virology 17:324–334, 1962

12. Gresser I, Tovey MG: Antitumor effects of interferon. Biochim Biophys Acta 516:231–247, 1978

13. Salerno RA, Whitmore CA, Garcia IM, et al: Chemical carcinogenesis in mice inhibited by interferon. Nature New Biol 239:31–32, 1972

14. Atanasiu P, Chany C: Action d'un interferon provenant de cellules malignes sur l'infection experimentale du hamster nouveau-ne par le virus de polyome. Cr Acad Sci (D) Paris 251:1687–1689, 1960

15. Gresser I, Maury C, Brouty-Boye D: Mechanism of the antitumor effect of interferon in mice. Nature 239:167–168, 1972

16. Stewart WE II: Varied biologic effects of interferon, in Gresser I (ed): Interferon 1979. New York, Academic Press, 1979, pp 29–51

17. Taylor-Papadimitriou J: Effects of interferons on cell growth and function, in Billiau A (ed): Interferon 1. General and Applied Aspects. Amsterdam, Elsevier, 1984, pp 139–166

18. Fradelizi D, Gresser I: Interferon inhibits the generation of allospecific suppressor T lymphocytes. J Exp Med 155:610–622, 1982

19. Onsrud M: Enhancement of suppressor cell generation in human mixed lymphocyte cultures by interferon. Int Arch Allergy Appl Immunol 67:315–321, 1982

20. Streuli M, Nagata S, Weissmann C: At least three human type alpha interferons: Structure of alpha$_2$. Science 209:1343–1347, 1980
21. Nagabhushan TL, Surprenant HV, Le HV, et al: Characterization of genetically engineered alpha-2 interferon, in Zoon KC, Noguchi PD, Liu T-Y (eds): Interferon: Research, Clinical Application and Regulatory Consideration. New York, Elsevier, 1984, pp 79–88
22. Streuli M, Hall A, Ball W, et al: Target cell specificity of two species of human interferon-alpha produced in *Escherichia coli* and of hybrid molecules derived from them. Proc Natl Acad Sci USA 78:2848–2852, 1981
23. Stewart WE II: The Interferon System (2nd ed.) New York, Springer-Verlag, 1981
24. Baron S, Dianzani F, Stanton GJ (eds): The Interferon System: A Review to 1982—Part I. Galveston, University of Texas Medical Branch, 1982
25. Baron S, Dianzani F, Stanton GJ (eds): The Interferon System: A Review to 1982—Part II. Galveston, University of Texas Medical Branch, 1982
26. Kirchner H, Schellekens H (eds): The Biology of the Interferon System 1984. New York, Elsevier, 1985
27. Vilcek J, DeMaeyer E (eds): Interferon 2. Interferons and the Immune System, vol 2. New York, Elsevier, 1984
28. Finter NB, Oldham RK (eds): Interferon 4. In Vivo and Clinical Studies, vol 4. New York, Elsevier, 1985
29. Hamburger AW, Salmon SE: Primary bioassay of human tumor stem cells. Science 197:461–463, 1977
30. Smith IE, Courtenay VD, Selby PJ, et al: Growth of human tumor cell colonies from biopsies using two soft-agar techniques. Br J Cancer 38:77–81, 1978
31. Von Hoff DD, Clark GM, Stogdill BJ, et al: Prospective clinical trial of a human tumor cloning system. Cancer Res 43:1926–1931, 1983
32. Shoemaker RH, Wokpert-DeFilippes MK, Makuch RW, et al: Use of the human tumor clonogenic assay for new drug screening. Proc Amer Assoc Cancer Res 24:311, 1983
33. Alberts DS, Chen HSB, Soehnlen B, et al: In vitro clonogenic assay for predicting response of ovarian cancer to chemotherapy. Lancet 2:340–342, 1980
34. Bradley EC, Ruscetti FW: Effect of fibroblast, lymphoid and myeloid interferons on human tumor colony formation in vitro. Cancer Res 41:244–249, 1982
35. Epstein LB, Shen JS, Abele JS, et al: Sensitivity of human ovarian carcinoma cells to interferon and other antitumor agents as assessed by an in vitro semisolid agar technique. Ann NY Acad Sci 350:228–244, 1980
36. Ludwig H, Swetley P: In vitro inhibitory effects of interferon on colony formation of myeloma stem cells. Cancer Immunol Immunother 9:139–143, 1980
37. Salmon SE: Applications of the human tumor stem cell assay to new drug evaluation and screening, in Salmon SE (ed): Cloning on Human Tumor Stem Cells. New York, Alan R Liss, 1980, pp 291–312
38. Von Hoff DD, Gutterman J, Portnoy B, et al: Activity of a human leukocyte interferon in a human tumor cloning system. Cancer Chemother Pharmacol 8:99–103, 1982
39. Salmon SE, Durie BGM, Young Y, et al: Effect of cloned leukocyte interferons in the human tumor stem cell assay. J Clin Oncol 1:217–225, 1983
40. Aapro MS, Alberts DS, Salmon SE: Interactions of human leukocyte interferon with vinca alkaloids and other chemotherapeutic agents against human tumors in clonogenic assay. Cancer Chemother Pharmacol 10:161–166, 1983
41. Welander CE, Morgan TM, Homesley HD, et al: Combined recombinant human interferon alpha$_2$ and cytotoxic agents studied in a clonogenic assay. Int J Cancer 35:721–729, 1985
42. Balkwill FR: Antitumor effects of interferons in animals, in Finter NB, Oldham RK (eds): Interferon 4: In Vivo and Clinical Studies, vol 4. New York, Elsevier, 1985, pp 23–45
43. Heston WDW, Fleischmann J, Tackett RE, et al: Effects of alpha-difluoromethylornithine and recombinant interferon-alpha$_2$ on the growth of a human renal cell adenocarcinoma xenograft in nude mice. Cancer Res 44:3220–3225, 1984
44. Balkwill FR, Mowshowitz Z, Seilman SS, et al: Positive interactions between interferon and chemotherapy due to direct tumor action rather than effects on host drug-metabolizing enzymes. Cancer Res 44:5249–5255, 1984
45. Trotta PP: Summary of preclinical data, in Kisner DL, Smyth JF (eds): Interferon Alpha-2: Preclinical and Clinical Evaluation. Boston, Martinus Nijhoff Medical Division, 1985, pp 13–27
46. Clutterbuck RD, Millar JL, Alexander P: Failure of high doses of alpha interferon to affect the growth of human carcinoma, melanoma and myeloid leukaemia xenografts. Br J Cancer 48:445–447, 1983
47. Balkwill FR, Aldam G, Lee A: The action of interferons on human tumor xenografts growing in nude mice, in Dianzani F, Rossi GB (eds): The Interferon System. New York, Raven, 1985, pp 327–331
48. Balkwill FR, Moodie EM: Positive interactions between human interferon and cyclophosphamide or Adriamycin in a human tumor model system. Cancer Res 44:904–908, 1984
49. Gresser I, Maury C, Tovey M: Efficacy of combined interferon-cyclophosphamide therapy after diagnosis of lymphoma in AKR mice. Eur J Cancer 14:97–99, 1978
50. Tozawa M, Kidowaki T, Tanaka R, et al: Effects of interferon on C1300 mouse neuroblastoma. Cancer Treat Rep 66:1575–1577, 1982
51. Heremans H, Billiau A, DeSomer P: Effect of interferon on the growth of tumors in experimental murine models, in DeMaeyer E, Schellekens H (eds): The Biology of the Interferon System. Amsterdam, Elsevier, 1983, pp 425–430
52. Chirigos MA, Pearson JW: Cure of murine leukemia with drug and interferon treatment. J Natl Cancer Inst 541:1367–1368, 1973
53. Mowshowitz SL, Chin-Bow ST, Smith GD: Interferon and cis-DDP combination chemotherapy for P388 leukemia in CDF 1 mice. J Interferon Res 2:587–591, 1982
54. Slater LM, Setzel MW, Cesario T: Combined interferon antimetabolite therapy of murine L1210 leukemia. Cancer 48:5–9, 1981

55. Marquet RL, Schellekens H, Westbroek DL, et al: Effect of treatment with interferon and cyclophosphamide on the growth of a spontaneous liposarcoma in rats. Int J Cancer 31:223–226, 1983

56. Renton KW, Mannering GJ: Depression of hepatic cytochrome-P-450-dependent mono-oxygenase systems with administered interferon inducing agents. Biochem Biophys Res Commun 73:343–348, 1976

57. Balkwill FR, Watling D, Taylor-Papadimitriou J: Inhibition by lymphoblastoid interferon on growth of cells derived from the human breast. Int J Cancer 22:258–265, 1978

58. Povlsen CO, Jacobsen GK: Chemotherapy of a human malignant melanoma transplanted in the nude mouse. Cancer 35:2790–2796, 1975

59. Kisner DL, Smyth JF (eds): Interferon Alpha-2: Preclinical and Clinical Evaluation. Boston, Martinus Nijhoff Medical Division, 1985

Interferons in the Treatment of Multiple Myeloma

M. Robert Cooper

Recombinant DNA technology has made adequate quantities of human interferons available for both in vitro and in vivo testing. In the clonogenic assay, RPMI-8226 myeloma cells were tested with recombinant interferon alfa-2b (Intron® A), melphalan, cyclophosphamide, and prednisone. Prednisone used as a single agent had the least cytotoxic effect. Concentrations of alfa-2b as low as 1 unit/mL (international antiviral activity) showed a reduction in colony number of <30% of the untreated controlled cultures. Melphalan and cyclophosphamide showed measurable cytotoxic activity, expressed in terms of 50% inhibition of colony growth, at doses of 0.15 μg/mL and 0.4 μg/mL, respectively. Additive antiproliferative effects were noted with combinations of alfa-2b plus cyclophosphamide and alfa-2b plus prednisone. However, the alfa-2b–melphalan combination had a synergistic effect on tumor-cell colony reduction. Even greater cytotoxic activity was seen with the three-drug combination of alfa-2b, melphalan, and prednisone. Clinical trials have shown that alfa-2b may be effective in patients with relapsing and refractory multiple myeloma. Of 38 patients evaluated, seven responded to treatment. Three of the seven responders have continued to respond for over 33 months, with monoclonal proteins approaching undetectable levels. A pilot study of the feasibility of combining alfa-2b with melphalan and prednisone in previously untreated patients with multiple myeloma has been completed. Although response was not the primary objective of this study, an overall response rate of 78% was achieved using criteria established by the Chronic Leukemia Task Force. Phase II trials conducted thus far have established tumor responsiveness to interferons in human myeloma. To clearly define the role of these agents in the treatment of myeloma, well-planned multicenter studies are needed.

IN VIEW of the relative inefficacy of chemotherapy in patients with relapsing or refractory multiple myeloma, attempts have been made to investigate the role of biologic response modifiers in this disease. In particular, both laboratory studies and clinical trials have been conducted to define the role of interferons in multiple myeloma.

SUMMARY OF IN VITRO STUDIES

Testing the effects of human recombinant alpha interferon on tumor cells in preclinical investigations has been difficult, partly because of the species specificity of the interferons, which precludes the use of most experimental animal model systems. Studies using human tumor xenografts implanted into nude mice have been conducted, but they raise many questions concerning host response and changes in tumor growth related to a species-specific agent such as interferon.[1] The technical difficulty of culturing human myeloma cells in vitro further complicates attempts to perform preclinical studies of the effect of interferon on human myeloma cells. These problems have been partially remedied by the use of a clonogenic assay for growing human myeloma-cell colonies first reported by Hamburger, Salmon, and Kim in 1977 and 1979.[2,3] This colony-forming assay could be used to determine the sensitivity of myeloma-cell colonies to standard chemotherapeutic agents, with retrospective correlations drawn between in vitro sensitivity and patient response to therapy.[4]

Recently, recombinant DNA technology has made adequate quantities of human interferons available for both in vitro and in vivo testing. Although interferons are in the category of biologic response modifiers, they have some direct effects on human tumor cells that can be quantitated in the colony-forming assay.[5,6] Using concentrations of recombinant interferon alfa-2b (Intron® A) in vitro known to be achievable in vivo, a reduction in colony formation of human myeloma cells has been observed.[7] The specific mechanisms of action of interferon are unclear and are probably multifaceted. In addition, there may be indirect effects of recombinant alpha interferon on tumor cells in vivo mediated through other host cells. In order to explore this possibility further and to determine whether macrophages and/or lymphocytes alter

From the Division of Hematology/Oncology, Bowman Gray School of Medicine, Winston-Salem, North Carolina.

Address reprint requests to M. Robert Cooper, MD, Bowman Gray School of Medicine, Division of Hematology/Oncology, 300 S Hawthorne Road, Winston-Salem, NC 27103.

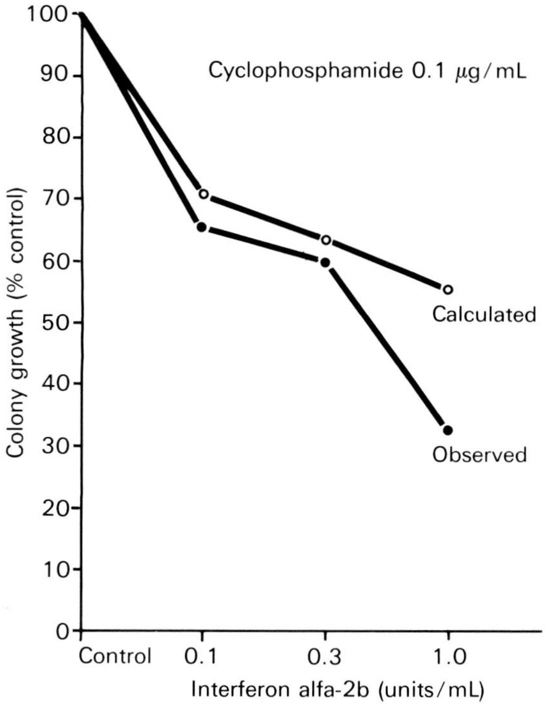

Figure 1. The percent colony reduction achieved with combined cyclophosphamide and interferon plotted as a function of increasing interferon concentration. Cyclophosphamide concentration is held constant. The observed percent colony survival is compared to the colony survival calculated using the additivity model. The *p* value for the difference between observed and calculated survival at an interferon concentration of 1 unit/mL is not significant.

the growth of tumor-cell colonies in vitro, experiments that add additional types of cells to these clonogenic assay cultures have been conducted (Welander CE, Berens ME, Saito T, et al, unpublished data).

The following discussion is limited to in vitro studies using a colony-forming assay to test the effects of recombinant interferon alfa-2b, melphalan, cyclophosphamide, and prednisone on an established cell line of human myeloma cells (RPMI-8226).[8] Although a variety of cytotoxic agents have been used to treat patients with both newly diagnosed and refractory myelomas, these drugs are commonly used in the clinic. The methods used to clone myeloma-cell line RPMI-8226 were modified from the original work of Hamburger and Salmon.[9] A required "colony-stimulating factor" was produced by adding a feeder layer of cells to the agar culture plates, thus enhancing the colony formation of the myeloma cells. Feeder cells were derived from a human macrophage cell line, U937.[10]

In the clonogenic assay, RPMI-8226 myeloma cells were tested with each of the four drugs to determine the dose-response curves and the dose resulting in a 50% inhibition of colony growth (ID_{50}). Prednisone alone had the least cytotoxic effect on these myeloma cells. With concentrations of interferon alfa-2b as low as 1 unit/mL (international antiviral activity), colony number was reduced to <30% of that of the untreated control cultures. Both melphalan and cyclophosphamide showed measurable cytotoxic activity, with ID_{50} values of 0.15 μg/mL and 0.4 μg/mL, respectively. The following combinations of drugs were also tested: melphalan plus interferon alfa-2b; cyclophosphamide plus interferon alfa-2b; prednisone plus

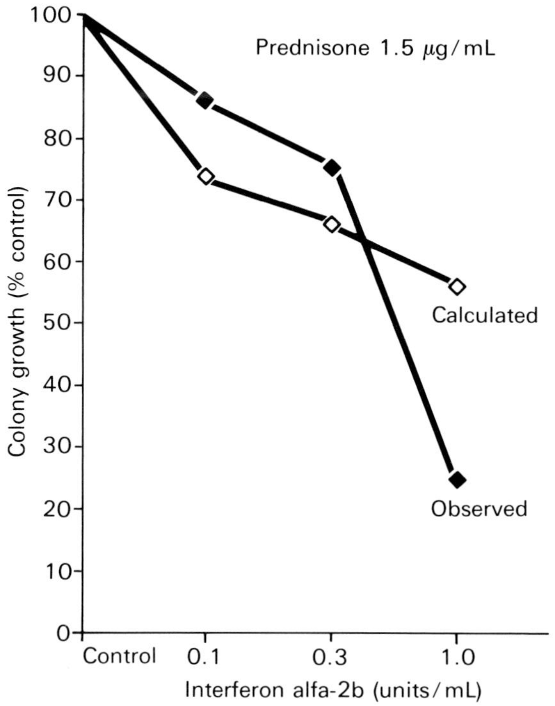

Figure 2. The percent colony reduction achieved with combined prednisone and interferon plotted as a function of increasing interferon concentration. Prednisone concentration is held constant. The observed percent colony survival is compared with the colony survival calculated using the additivity model. The *p* value for the difference between observed and calculated survival at an interferon concentration of 1 unit/mL is not significant.

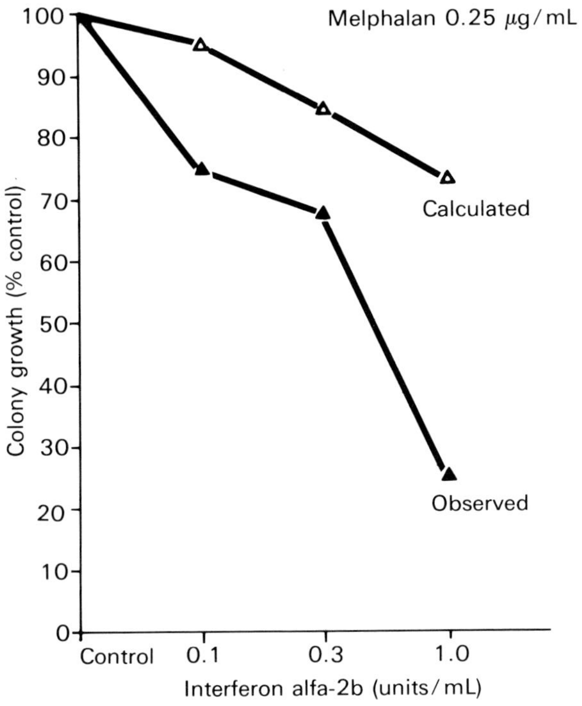

Figure 3. The percent colony reduction of combined melphalan and interferon plotted as a function of increasing interferon concentration. Melphalan concentration is held constant. The observed percent colony survival is compared with the colony survival calculated using the additivity model. The *p* value for the difference between observed and calculated survival at an interferon concentration of 1 unit/mL is 0.104.

interferon alfa-2b; and melphalan plus prednisone plus interferon alfa-2b.

The mathematical model used to evaluate cytotoxicity has been published elsewhere.[11] In summary, using the additivity model, the fractional colony survivals obtained when each drug to be used in a combination is tested singly are multiplied. The product of the two fractional survivals is the expected colony survival. This value is compared with that obtained when the combination of drugs is tested in vitro. If the observed survival is equal to the expected colony survival, the drug interactions are additive. If the observed survival is less than expected, the interactions are synergistic. Conversely, an observed survival greater than the expected survival suggests either subadditive or antagonistic interactions.

Figures 1 to 3 illustrate the effect of various drug combinations on colony survival. Additive antiproliferative effects were noted with interferon alfa-2b plus cyclophosphamide (Figure 1) and interferon alfa-2b plus prednisone (Figure 2). The interferon alfa-2b plus melphalan combination, however, showed synergistic effects on tumor-cell colony reduction (Figure 3). The combination of melphalan and prednisone also had an additive antiproliferative effect on the myeloma cells. Even greater cytotoxic activity was seen with the three-drug combination of interferon alfa-2b, melphalan, and prednisone (Figure 4). The use of very low concentrations of interferon alfa-2b combined with melphalan and prednisone resulted in the reduction of colony size to <30% of control values.

CLINICAL INVESTIGATIONS

It is apparent that an in vitro human myeloma clonogenic assay can measure antiproliferative effects of interferon, prednisone, mel-

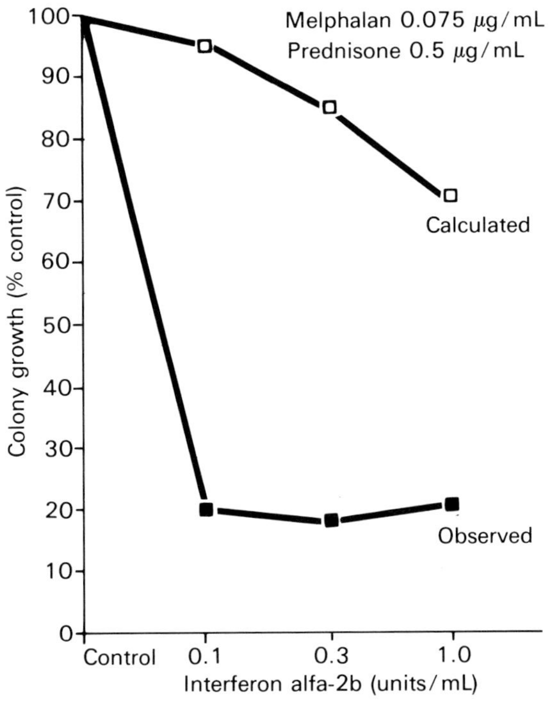

Figure 4. The percent colony reduction of combined melphalan, prednisone, and interferon is plotted as a function of increasing interferon concentration. Melphalan and prednisone concentrations are held constant. The observed percent colony survival is compared with the colony survival calculated using the additivity model. A *p* value has not been calculated for this three-drug combination.

phalan, and cyclophosphamide. Combinations of these agents have additive and, occasionally, synergistic effects on tumor-cell colony reduction. The following discussion describes recently completed or ongoing clinical trials undertaken to determine if these in vitro effects can be achieved clinically.

Prior results with interferon have been limited but encouraging. Mellstedt et al[12] administered human leukocyte interferon to four previously untreated patients with multiple myeloma. All four showed a decrease in the percentage of bone marrow plasma cells as well as a decrease in the level of abnormal proteins both in serum and in urine. Of ten myeloma patients treated with interferon alfa-2a by Gutterman et al,[13] three responded, three improved, and four failed to respond. The responders showed decreases in abnormal proteins that persisted for up to 63 weeks after therapy was discontinued. Decreases in the percentage of bone marrow plasma cells to 15% or less were also noted. A randomized trial conducted in Scandinavia compared interferon alone with intermittent high-dose melphalan and prednisone as first-line therapy.[14] Six of 21 evaluable patients in the chemotherapy group and four of 22 patients in the interferon group were classified as responders. The actuarial survival curves showed no statistically significant difference.

Experience in Relapsing and Refractory Patients

A phase II study of interferon alfa-2b in resistant multiple myeloma recently has been completed and published.[15] Patients entering the study were diagnosed according to the criteria of the Chronic Leukemia-Myeloma Task Force[16] and staged according to the criteria of Durie and Salmon.[17] Only patients who were refractory to prior therapy or who relapsed after an initial response to primary treatment were admitted. Patients were required to have a life expectancy of at least 4 months and an ECOG (Eastern Cooperative Oncology Group) performance status of 0, 1, 2, or 3. Patients who had received prior radiation treatment of a field encompassing more than 25% of the bone marrow were excluded from the study.

Intron® A (Schering Sch 30500), the interferon used in this study, is a highly purified human alfa-2b interferon produced by recombinant DNA techniques in *Escherichia coli.*[18] This agent was administered according to three different dose schedules (Table 1). Four centers used a similar schedule of daily intravenous induction followed by subcutaneous (SC) maintenance therapy three times weekly. The fifth center used SC interferon alfa-2b from the beginning of therapy. Because each regimen had similar toxicity and produced responses at rates not statistically significantly different from the others, results of all studies are combined in this report.

Of the 49 eligible patients who entered the study, 38 were evaluable for efficacy. Eleven patients were considered invalid for response assessment because they had received less than 1 month of treatment: one was irradiated less than 28 days before interferon alfa-2b treat-

Table 1. Treatment Regimens Used in Phase II Myeloma Trials With Interferon Alfa-2b

	Number of Patients	
	Enrolled	Evaluable
3-100 $\times$ 10^6 IU/m^2/day IV TIW for 2 weeks; then, 10 $\times$ 10^6 IU/m^2 SC TIW at least one year or to relapse	23	18
30-50 $\times$ 10^6 IU/m^2/day IV for 5 days at 14-day intervals—4 courses; then, 10 $\times$ 10^6 IU/m^2 SC TIW for 3 months	12	7
2 $\times$ 10^6 IU/m^2/day SC TIW for 3 months; then, 10 $\times$ 10^6 IU/m^2/day SC TIW at least one year or to relapse	14	13
Total	49	38

Abbreviation: TIW, three times weekly.

ment; six were removed from the study (one refused further treatment, two had intercurrent illnesses not related to interferon alfa-2b administration, and three had adverse experiences possibly related to interferon alfa-2b, including severe fatigue, paralytic ileus, and congestive heart failure); and four died (two from disease progression, one from sepsis, and one from pneumonia and respiratory arrest).

Two thirds of the patients who entered the study previously had been treated with multiple drug combinations, including agents such as doxorubicin, vincristine, and nitrosoureas in addition to melphalan, cyclophosphamide, and prednisone. At entry 25 of the 49 patients were refractory to all prior chemotherapy, whereas 24 were relapsing after having previously responded to chemotherapy. Of the 38 evaluable patients, seven (18%) were classified as responders. One of these patients achieved a complete response and six had a partial response (Tables 2 and 3).

Response rates were variable among patients in different prognostic subgroups. A response occurred in two (10.6%) of 19 patients who had never responded to prior therapy and in five (26%) of 19 who had previously responded to treatment. Three of six patients who had relapsed while off chemotherapy responded to interferon alfa-2b treatment. The amount of prior treatment also profoundly affected the response rate to interferon alfa-2b. Two of five patients who previously had been treated with a single alkylating agent responded to interferon, whereas only three of 25 patients who had failed to respond to multiple alkylating agent therapy responded to interferon.

Three of the seven responders continued to respond for more than 33 months, with monoclonal proteins approaching undetectable levels. One of these patients exhibited a complete re-

Table 2. Patient Response* to Interferon Alfa-2b in Phase II Multiple Myeloma Trials

	Responders	
	Number	%
Refractory patients	2/19	11
Relapsing patients	5/19	26
During treatment	2/13	15
Off treatment	3/6	50
Patients receiving prior therapy		
Melphalan + prednisone	2/5	40
Melphalan + cyclophosphamide + prednisone	2/8	25
Multiple agents	3/25	12

*Response = >50% reduction in colony size for at least 4 weeks.

Table 3. Profile of Patients Responding to Interferon Alfa-2b

Patient No.	Prior Treatment	Stage	Response	Duration of Response (weeks)	Change in Performance	Change in Pain	Para protein
1	Melphalan/prednisone	I	Partial	62+	No change	No pain*	IgG
2	Multiple drugs	III	Complete	104+	No change	Improved (mild to none)	IgG
3	Multiple drugs	III	Partial	21	Improved	Improved (2 to 1)	IgG
4	Multiple drugs	II	Partial	56+	No change	Improved (moderate to mild)	IgA
5	Melphalan/prednisone	II	Partial	15	Improved (3 to 1)	Improved (moderate to mild)	IgA
6	Melphalan/prednisone & cytoxan/prednisone	III	Partial	12	No change	No change	Light chain K
7	Melphalan/prednisone & cytoxan/prednisone	II	Partial	16	No change	Improved (moderate to mild)	IgG

*At baseline.

sponse, with disappearance of abnormal M-protein and radiographic evidence of healing lytic bone lesions, after having had a partial response for 40 weeks. Complete remission in this patient has now been maintained for more than 104 weeks. Of 29 patients who entered the study with documented bone pain, 18 improved and ten remained unchanged during the course of treatment. Bone pain worsened in only one patient during interferon alfa-2b treatment. Survival time is greater than 1 year in three of the seven responders who also show marked improvement in performance status; one patient has achieved a durable and ongoing complete remission rarely seen with either radiation therapy or chemotherapy in the advanced phase of myeloma.

In a similar study[19] 23 patients with relapsed or refractory multiple myeloma were treated with 10×10^6 units/m² of interferon alfa-2b administered SC three times weekly for 12 weeks. Patients with responding or stable disease were continued on treatment until disease progression was noted. Two of 20 evaluable patients had an objective response to interferon alfa-2b, as indicated by a 50% decrease in plasmacytomas or M-protein. Three other patients had objective improvement, with a 25% to 50% decrease in M-protein and a marked reduction in bone pain. Disease stabilized in two additional patients. Approximately one third of the patients studied appeared to benefit from therapy with interferon alfa-2b.

In a more recent study (Case DC, Sonneborn HL, Paul SD, et al, unpublished data), a 20% partial response rate was achieved in previously treated multiple myeloma patients. In this study, interferon alfa-2b was given intravenously; dosages were increased during the induction phase to attain a significant degree of myelosuppression. A maintenance schedule of SC interferon alfa-2b was then used. Prednisone was added to the treatment regimen of patients who did not respond after 12 weeks of SC interferon alfa-2b therapy. Four of 20 patients achieved a partial remission. Three of these remissions occurred prior to the addition of prednisone. No dose-response benefit was noted in this study. Concomitant prednisone administration reduced the flu-like symptoms associated with interferon alfa-2b.

Experience in Untreated Patients

A pilot study was designed to determine the dose of interferon alfa-2b that could be administered to previously untreated patients with multiple myeloma who received a standard regimen of oral melphalan and prednisone.

Interferon alfa-2b was administered SC three times weekly during the first and second weeks of treatment. Five dosage levels of interferon alfa-2b were used—0.5, 1, 2, 5, and 10×10^6 IU/m². Interferon alfa-2b was administered three times weekly during the first and second weeks. Oral doses of 9 mg/m² of melphalan and 40 mg/m² of prednisone were administered on days 8 to 11 of the second week. The melphalan dose could be increased until the white blood cell count fell to less than 3×10^6/mm³ or the platelet count fell to less than 100,000/mm³. No treatment was administered during the third and fourth weeks. Each treatment cycle was 28 days in duration.

The projected dose of melphalan was analyzed by cycle and dose level of interferon alfa-2b (Table 3). At low doses of interferon alfa-2b (0.5 or 1×10^6 IU/m²), patients received 70% to 105% of the projected dose of melphalan, with the majority of patients receiving 90% or greater. Interferon doses greater than 2×10^6 IU/m² resulted in administration of 37% to 103% of the projected dose of melphalan, with most patients receiving 70% or less of the projected dose.

Although response was not the primary objective of this study, an overall response rate of 75% was achieved using criteria established by the Chronic Leukemia-Myeloma Task Force.[16] Figure 5 shows bone healing in one patient treated in this pilot study.

Phase II trials conducted thus far have established tumor responsiveness to interferons in human myeloma. In order to clearly define the role of these agents in the treatment of myeloma, well-planned multicenter studies must be conducted. A randomized trial being conducted by the Cancer and Leukemia Group B is comparing the effectiveness of melphalan plus prednisone to that of the combination of melphalan, prednisone, and interferon.

Figure 5. Radiographs from a patient with multiple myeloma obtained prior to (11/28/83) and during (4/22/85) treatment with melphalan, prednisone, and interferon. Bone healing is apparent in the later radiograph.

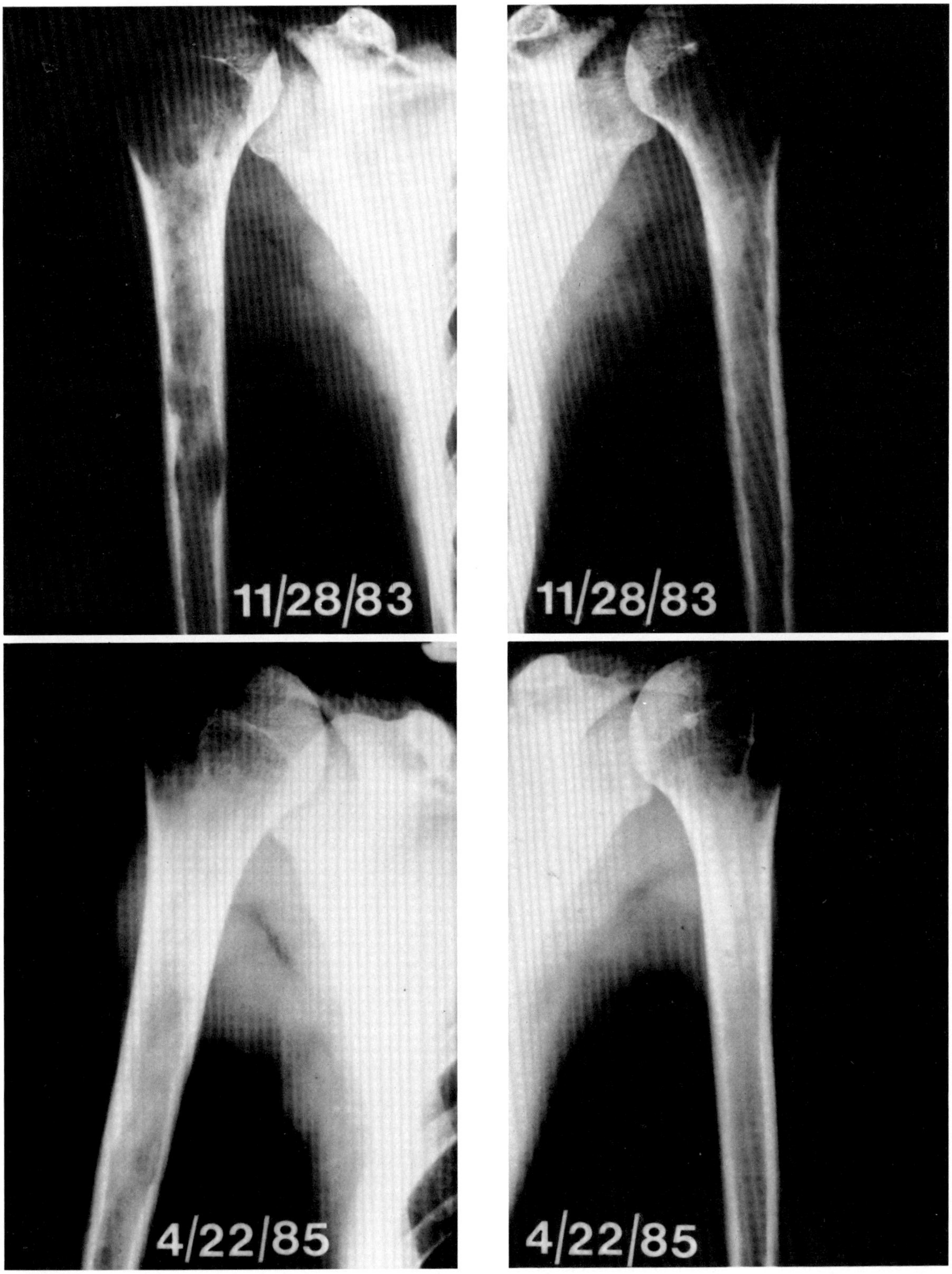

REFERENCES

1. Balkwill FR, Moodie EM: Positive interactions between human interferon and cyclophosphamide or Adriamycin in a human tumor model system. Cancer Res 44:904–908, 1984

2. Hamburger AW, Kim MB, Salmon SE: The nature of cells generating human myeloma colonies in vitro. J Cell Physiol 98:371–376, 1979

3. Hamburger A, Salmon SE: Primary bioassay of human myeloma stem cells. J Clin Invest 60:846–854, 1977

4. Salmon SE, Hamburger AW, Soehnlen B, et al: Quantitation of differential sensitivity of human tumor stem cells to anticancer drugs. N Engl J Med 298:1321–1327, 1978

5. Salmon SE, Durie BGM, Young L, et al: Effects of cloned human leukocyte interferons in the human tumor stem cell assay. J Clin Oncol 1:217–225, 1983

6. Von Hoff DD, Gutterman J, Portnoy B, et al: Activity of a human leukocyte interferon in a human tumor cloning system. Cancer Chemother Pharmacol 8:99–103, 1982

7. Aapro MS, Alberts DS, Salmon SE: Interactions of human leukocyte interferon with vinca alkaloids and other chemotherapeutic agents against human tumors in clonogenic assay. Cancer Chemother Pharmacol 10:161–166, 1983

8. Krueger RG, Staneck LD, Boehlecke JM: Tumor associated antigens in human myeloma. J Natl Cancer Inst 56:711–715, 1976

9. Hamburger AW, Salmon SE: Primary bioassay of human tumor stem cells. Science 197:461–463, 1977

10. Sundstrom C, Nilsson K: Establishment and characterization of a human histiocytic lymphoma cell line (U-937). Int J Cancer 17:565–577, 1976

11. Welander CE, Morgan TM, Homesley HD, et al: Combined recombinant human interferon $alpha_2$ and cytotoxic agents studied in a clonogenic assay. Int J Cancer 35:721–729, 1985

12. Mellstedt H, Bjorkholm M, Johansson B: Interferon therapy in myelomatosis. Lancet 1:245–248, 1979

13. Gutterman JU, Blumenschein GR, Alexanian R: Leukocyte interferon-induced tumor regression in human metastatic breast cancer, multiple myeloma, and malignant lymphoma. Ann Intern Med 93:399–406, 1980

14. Mellstedt H, Aahre A, Bjorkholm M: Interferon therapy of patients with multiple myeloma, in Terry WD, Rosenberg SA (eds): Immunotherapy of Human Cancer, New York, Elsevier-North Holland, Inc., 1982, pp 387–391

15. Costanzi JJ, Cooper MR, Scarffe JH, et al: Phase II study of recombinant alpha-2 interferon in resistant multiple myeloma. J Clin Oncol 3:654–659, 1985

16. Chronic Leukemia-Myeloma Task Force, National Cancer Institute. Proposed guidelines for protocol studies. II. Plasma cell myeloma. Cancer Chemother Reports 4:145–158, 1973

17. Durie BGM, Salmon SE: A clinical staging system for multiple myeloma. Correlation of measured myeloma cell mass with presenting clinical features, response to treatment, and survival. Cancer 36:842–852, 1975

18. Streuli M, Nagata S, Weissman C: At least three human type alpha interferons: Structure of $alpha_2$. Science 209:1343–1347, 1980

19. Oken MM, Kyle RA, Kay NE, et al: A phase II trial of interferon $alpha_2$ ($rIFN_2$) in the treatment of resistant multiple myeloma. Proc Am Soc Clin Oncol 4:215, 1985 (abstr 837)

The Role of Interferon in the Treatment of Hairy Cell Leukemia

Mark J. Ratain, James W. Vardiman, and Harvey M. Golomb

Hairy cell leukemia (HCL) is a rare chronic lymphoproliferative disorder usually manifested by pancytopenia. Prior to the use of interferon in the treatment of this disease, initial therapy most often consisted of splenectomy. Patients with progressive disease after splenectomy often benefited from low-dose chlorambucil, although many other treatment modalities had been tested. Interferon (partially purified) was first reported to be effective in HCL by Quesada et al in 1984, with responses in seven of seven patients. Subsequent studies demonstrated that recombinant interferon was also effective. Major responses (normalization of peripheral blood counts) have been obtained in 50% to 80% of patients treated to date, and virtually all patients show some improvement. There is rapid improvement in the platelet count (1 to 2 months), followed by improvement in absolute neutrophil count (2 to 3 months) and hemoglobin (3 to 6 months). In addition, leukemic patients have a rapid reduction in circulating hairy cells. Interferon alpha also has been demonstrated to reduce the incidence of serious infections and the need for transfusions, as compared to the 6-month period prior to therapy. Bone marrow shows improvement as well, with a reduction in hairy cells and an increase in normal precursors. However, bone marrow remains abnormal, with increased reticulin, decreased myeloid precursors, and, usually, discernible hairy cells. Following discontinuation of therapy, a slow increase in hairy cells may occur. The mechanism of interferon's action is unknown. Interferon induces the synthesis of new proteins and the formation of new organelles. Although natural killer cell activity increases with the introduction of interferon, these changes probably do not mediate the response to the agent. Interferon has been demonstrated in vivo to have a direct antiproliferative effect on hairy cells. We conclude that interferon is highly effective in progressive disease following splenectomy. Its exact role in nonsplenectomized patients remains to be determined, as does its optimal use in the long-term management of HCL.

HAIRY cell leukemia (HCL) is a chronic lymphoproliferative disorder. Described as "leukemic reticuloendotheliosis" by Bouroncle et al[1] in 1958, it was renamed by Schreck and Donnelly eight years later.[2] Few institutions have had large clinical experience with this rare disease.[3-6] However, the initial success of Quesada et al[7] in treating HCL with partially purified interferon has sparked a growing interest in HCL therapy. The purpose of this article is to review the experience to date with interferon in HCL and to clarify the role of interferon in the management of this disorder in relation to both older and newer treatment modalities.

CLINICAL FEATURES OF HCL

There have been several recent reports of large single-institution experiences with HCL.[3-6] The clinical features of this disease at diagnosis are summarized in Table 1. Most patients exhibit pancytopenia or a decrease in two blood counts.[3] However, 10% to 17% of patients present with an elevated white count (Table 1). Approximately one third of patients have more than 50% hairy cells in the peripheral blood at diagnosis.[6]

Diagnosis of HCL sometimes is difficult because bone marrow aspirates frequently are dry. The initial bone marrow biopsy is hypercellular in about half the patients, but approximately 10% of patients present with hypocellular marrows.[3-8] There usually is diffuse infiltration of the bone marrow by mononuclear cells, the nuclei of which are widely separated by abundant cytoplasm; up to 80% replacement occurs in about 50% of the patients studied. Even in advanced cases, there usually are islands of residual erythropoiesis and megakaryocytopoiesis, but granulopoiesis is severely reduced in amount. Bone marrow plasma cells may be numerous in patients with this illness. An increase in stromal reticulin is present in virtually all cases.

From the Joint Section of Hematology/Oncology, Department of Medicine, and the Department of Pathology, University of Chicago Pritzker School of Medicine, and Michael Reese Medical Center, Chicago, Illinois.

Supported in part by grants from the Schering Corporation, the Harry Greenburg Foundation, the Diane Hirsch Greenspan Memorial Fund, and the Iona Moore Memorial Fund.

Address reprint requests to Mark J. Ratain, MD, Division of Hematology/Oncology, Michael Reese Hospital and Medical Center, Lake Shore Drive at 31st Street, Chicago, IL 60616.

Table 1. Summary of Clinical Features of HCL at Presentation

	Series			
	Golomb et al[3]	Flandrin et al[4]	Jansen et al[5]	Bouroncle[6]
Total patients	199	211	74	100
Mean age (range)	52(23–82)	52(23–89)	53*(29–88)	55(NS)
Male:female	4.7:1	3.7:1	5.7:1	4.9:1
Splenomegaly by physical examination (%)				
None	28	28	20	NS
Mild	24	14	18	NS
Moderate	28	40	NS	NS
Marked	21	18	22	NS
Hepatomegaly (%)	10	20	NS	NS
Lymphadenopathy (%)	30†	5	NS	19
Leukemic phase (%)	17	11	10	NS

Abbreviation: NS, not stated.
* Median.
† ≤2 cm.

The presence of tartrate-resistant acid phosphatase (TRAP)-staining lymphocytes in peripheral blood or bone marrow is characteristic of HCL.[9] However, hairy cells usually have diffuse staining, whereas focal cytoplasmic staining may be seen in activated lymphocytes or in other well-differentiated lymphoproliferative disorders, such as macroglobulinemia.[10] In addition, nonhematopoietic cells may stain positive for TRAP. Therefore, careful review of the histologic and cytochemical preparations by an experienced pathologist is essential for diagnosis.

PRE-INTERFERON TREATMENT MODALITIES

Splenectomy

Splenectomy has been considered the initial treatment of choice in HCL for many years.[11] Its purpose is to eliminate the effects of the hypersplenism on pancytopenia.[12] Virtually all patients have an improvement in at least one blood count, with normalization of blood counts occurring in 40% to 60% of patients following surgery.[4,13,14] Prognostic variables for patients with HCL undergoing splenectomy are not well established, but they include the hairy cell index (percent cellularity × percent bone marrow hairy cells/10,000),[13] initial blood counts,[4,15] and spleen size.[6]

Chemotherapy

Because of the successful palliation of cytopenias achieved with splenectomy, chemotherapy traditionally has been reserved for patients with progressive disease following splenectomy or those with the leukemic phase of the disease. Combination chemotherapy has been employed by multiple investigators, but has a high incidence of treatment-related morbidity and mortality.[4,5]

Daily low-dose alkylating agent therapy with chlorambucil has also been demonstrated to be effective palliation, showing significant effects in up to 60% of patients treated with a 6-month trial at 2 to 4 mg/d.[16] However, neutropenia rarely resolved with chlorambucil, and the median actuarial survival was only 48 months. Death was usually due to infection. In addition, one patient developed a myelodysplastic syndrome presumed to be secondary to prolonged alkylating agent therapy.[17]

Other Treatment Modalities

Prior to the introduction of interferon, there was no reliable therapy for advanced HCL other than low-dose chlorambucil administered for a minimum of 6 months. Other treatment modalities have been employed, each in small numbers of patients. Yam et al[18] recently re-

Table 2. Response Rates to Recombinant Alpha Interferon in Advanced HCL

	Series			
	Golomb et al[23]	Quesada et al[24]	Flandrin et al[25]	Foon et al[26]
IFN type	Alfa-2b	Alfa-2a	Alfa-2a* Alfa-2b	Alfa-2a
Evaluable patients (≥ 4 months of IFN)	64	28	17	12
CR (%)†	5	18	6	8
PR (%)	70	61	‡	83
MR (%)	14	21	82	8
Dose schedule	2 MU/m² TIW	3-12 MU QD	3 MU QD or 2 MU/m² TIW	3 MU QD

Abbreviations: IFN, interferon; CR, complete response; PR, partial response; MR, minor response; MU, million units; QD, daily; TIW, thrice weekly.

* Nine patients, alfa-2a; eight patients, alfa-2b (nonrandomized).

†Response criteria defined in Table 3.

‡No distinction made between partial and minor response.

viewed a multicenter experience with leukapheresis involving a total of ten patients. Leukapheresis was carried out two to three times a week for 20 to 120 days. Seven of eight patients treated exclusively with leukapheresis responded. Patients with hyperleukocytosis experienced the greatest benefit, but those with cytopenias often showed improvement as well.

Magee et al[19] recently reported their experience in six patients treated with androgens for progressive HCL after splenectomy. Using oxymetholone, 50 mg three times a day, three of six patients showed improvement in at least one cytopenia.

Although lithium carbonate[20] and syngeneic bone marrow transplantation[21] have also been used in advanced HCL, the experience with these measures is anecdotal. Most of the clinical research in HCL in the last 3 years has focused on the role of interferon.

INTERFERON

The approach to patients with advanced HCL has changed dramatically since 1984, when Quesada et al[7] reported a 100% response rate in the first seven patients they treated with partially purified interferon. Ratain et al[22] demonstrated that synthetic recombinant interferon alfa-2b (Intron® A) was also effective in advanced HCL, enabling this treatment modality to be administered to larger groups of patients.

There are two recombinant interferons currently employed in phase II trials for HCL in the United States: interferon alfa-2a (Hoffman-LaRoche) and interferon alfa-2b (Schering). The two drugs are identical with the exception of amino acid 23: alfa-2a contains a lysine residue, and alfa-2b contains an arginine residue.

Both interferons have been demonstrated to be effective in virtually all patients with advanced HCL (Table 2). Although criteria for response have not been standardized, we use the definitions detailed in Table 3. Because it is difficult to definitely *exclude* the presence of small numbers of hairy cells in the bone marrow, we use the criterion that a complete response is defined by the presence of <5% hairy cells without focal clumping.

Improvement occurs in all three hematologic parameters, usually beginning with the platelet count, as early as 2 weeks after starting interferon therapy.[22] Neutropenia resolves in 2 to 3 months,[7,22] but the hemoglobin may continue to increase for as long as 9 months after starting therapy.[23] Peripheral hairy cells also rapidly decrease, with changes seen within the first week of therapy.[3,25,26] In addition, interferon alfa-2b has been demonstrated to significantly decrease

Table 3. Criteria for Response to Interferon in HCL

Response*	Peripheral Blood Counts	Bone Marrow
Complete	Hb $\geq$ 12 g/dL, ANC $\geq$ 1,500/μL, Plts $\geq$ 100,000/μL No hairy cells	$<$5% hairy cells without focal clumping
Partial	Hb $\geq$ 12 g/dL, ANC $\geq$ 1,500/μL, Plts $\geq$ 100,000/μL	
Minor	Hb $\geq$ 12 g/dL* or ANC $\geq$ 1,500/μL or Plts $\geq$ 100,000/μL or reduction in WBC to $<$10,000/μL†	

Abbreviations: Hb, hemoglobin; ANC, absolute neutrophil count; Plts, platelet count; WBC, white blood count.

* To be evaluable for response, parameter must have been initially abnormal: Hb $<$10 g/dL, ANC $<$1,000/μL, Plts $<$100,000/μL, WBC $>$10,000/μL ($>$50% hairy cells).

†Leukemic patients only.

the incidence of serious infections and the need for red blood cell and platelet transfusions.[23]

The toxicity of interferon has been extensively described elsewhere.[27] The most frequent interferon-related toxicities in 64 patients treated with thrice-weekly injections of interferon alfa-2b are shown in Table 4. Other, less common, toxicities reported in HCL patients treated to date include alopecia,[22,25] gynecomastia,[28] and gonadal failure.[28,29] In addition, most patients with HCL develop transient myelosuppression during the first month of interferon therapy.[22,25] The nadir neutrophil and platelet counts occur at a median of 1 week after starting interferon, usually recovering by the end of the first month.

Although interferon is highly effective in palliating the cytopenias and infectious complications of HCL, it is probably not curative. Complete responses ($<$5% hairy cells in bone marrow) are uncommon (Table 2), even with prolonged therapy.[23] Myeloid hypoplasia (with reduced or inverted myeloid:erythroid ratios) and increased reticulin fibers also persist.[25,30,31]

It is not clear why HCL is so exquisitely sensitive to interferon therapy. Interferon has only marginal activity in chronic lymphocytic leukemia, a related B-cell lymphoproliferative disorder.[32] Because patients with HCL have decreased natural killer cells,[33] and interferon is known to stimulate natural killer cell activity,[34] it was originally speculated that interferon might act indirectly in HCL via natural killer cell stimulation.[22] More recent work has established that natural killer cells are increased in HCL as a consequence of interferon; this finding was based on functional natural killer cell activity,[26,35] morphologic assessment of large granular lymphocytes,[31] and flow cytometric assessment of Leu 11a$^+$ cells.[36] Although the increase in natural killer cells is associated with response to interferon, there is no evidence suggesting that the response is mediated by these cells. In fact, there is evidence against the mediation of the response to interferon by natural killer cells. The increase in these cells is inconsistent,[26,31] and often does not occur until after significant improvement in the platelet count has already taken place.[26,35]

Other investigators have focused their work on structural changes that interferon induces in hairy cells. Recombinant interferon alpha has been demonstrated to induce an 80kDa protein, p80, at concentrations as low as 0.1 IU/mL.[37] A number of other proteins are induced as well; current studies are comparing interferon's effect on hairy cells with its effect on other lymphocytes. It is possible that these induced proteins

Table 4. Most Frequent Interferon-Related Toxicities in 64 Patients Treated With Interferon Alfa–2b*

Toxicity	Percentage of Patients	Percentage With WHO Grade III Toxicity†
Flu-like symptoms (fevers, malaise, fatigue, myalgias, anorexia, dry mouth)	95	19
Skin disorders (dry skin, seborrheic dermatitis)	48	2
Application site disorder (local inflammation)	27	3
Gastrointestinal disorder (diarrhea, constipation)	41	0
Nausea/vomiting	30	0
Central or peripheral nervous system disorder (paresthesias, depression)	20	2

* Adapted from Golomb et al.[23]
†No patient exhibited grade IV toxicity.

are involved in the expression of class II HLA antigens[38] or the formation of tubuloreticular structures or annulate lamellae[39] that recently have been reported to be a consequence of interferon exposure in hairy cells.

Experimental studies of HCL have been hampered by the difficulty of culturing hairy cells in vitro. Paganelli et al[40] recently reported their experience with recombinant interferons in vitro using hairy cells stimulated by B-cell growth factor. In their system, interferon alfa-2b inhibited growth, although it was used at a relatively high concentration (1,000 IU/mL). Interferon gamma had no inhibitory effect. In addition, these investigators demonstrated a high-affinity binding site (Kd of 7.1×10^{-10} M) for interferon alfa-2b on hairy cells, using iodinated interferon alfa-2b. Interferon beta competed for the same binding site, but interferon gamma showed no competition, indicating that it has a separate binding site. These results suggest that type I interferons act directly as antiproliferative agents in HCL, although further studies need to be conducted both using lower interferon concentrations (0.1 to 100 IU/mL) and comparing the effects of interferons on hairy cells with their effects on other malignant lymphocytes.

FUTURE STUDIES

Although interferon is highly effective in inducing responses in HCL, it is not known whether any patients will be cured with interferon alone. The evidence to date is strongly against this possibility. First of all, complete responses to interferon are rare and almost never include complete normalization of the bone marrow. In addition, alpha interferon is primarily a cytostatic agent. Thus, if interferon acts by a direct antiproliferative effect on hairy cells, complete elimination of all hairy cells would not be expected. Instead, interferon may block hairy cells in G_0-G_1,[41] an effect that would be expected to be reversed upon removal of the drug.

Currently there are only limited clinical data regarding the course of responding patients with HCL following interferon therapy. The University of Chicago group[42] has carefully evaluated the peripheral blood counts and bone marrow biopsies of 15 patients who had completed a 12-month course of interferon alfa-2b therapy. There was no deterioration of peripheral blood counts over the first 9 months after the cessation of therapy. However, over the first 3 months off interferon, there was a significant decrease in bone marrow cellularity and an increase in the percentage of bone marrow hairy cells. There was no absolute increase in bone marrow hairy cells, after correction for changes in cellularity; there was no change over the subsequent 3 to 6 months. Only one patient had been restarted on interferon therapy. Based on these results, it was concluded that responses to interferon in HCL are durable for at least 6 to 9 months, although there is a relative increase in bone marrow hairy cells over the first 3 months. This was attributed to a rapid exit from the bone marrow of normal elements after the discontinuation of interferon.

Since interferon is highly effective in patients with progressive disease after splenectomy, should it be used as initial therapy instead of splenectomy? This question currently is being addressed in ongoing cooperative trials. Analysis of prognostic features of patients initially treated with splenectomy may also be helpful. Based on our current knowledge, patients with packed marrows (high hairy cell index) and small (nonpalpable) spleens and those in the leukemic phase of the disease should be considered for initial interferon therapy. Other patients requiring therapy should continue to have splenectomy or should be entered in clinical trials. It must be considered that approximately 50% of patients treated with splenectomy have a prolonged treatment-free survival.[3]

Further trials are also necessary to define the optimal dosing and schedule of this agent. Most trials with interferon alfa-2a have utilized daily doses of 3 MU/m^2, whereas the interferon alfa-2b studies have utilized thrice weekly doses of 2 MU/m^2. Since interferon therapy of HCL is probably not curative, it remains to be determined whether certain patients should receive some form of maintenance therapy to suppress regrowth of the malignant cells.

Interest in the therapy of HCL has also been prompted by the adenosine deaminase inhibitor pentostatin.[43-45] Early results suggested that complete responses, including resolution of bone marrow fibrosis, can be obtained rapidly in up to 50% of patients. Because this agent exhibits significant toxicity, it is too soon to comment regarding its ultimate role in therapy. Its clinical effect on HCL is probably due to the decreased levels of adenosine deaminase activity in hairy cells as compared to other lymphocytes.[46]

CONCLUSION

Alpha interferon is effective palliation for advanced HCL after splenectomy, but it probably does not eradicate the disease. Responses occur in 1 to 4 months; there is little additional improvement after 9 months. An increase in peripheral blood counts is accompanied by a decrease in infectious complications and transfusion requirements. Other parameters of immune function, such as natural killer cell activity, also improve. Following discontinuance of interferon, there is a rapid relative increase in bone marrow hairy cells. However, there is usually no need for further therapy in the first 6 months after stopping interferon. Additional clinical trials need to be conducted in order to define the optimal dose and schedule of interferon and determine the exact role of interferon in relation to splenectomy and pentostatin.

ACKNOWLEDGMENT

We thank Dora Currin for assistance in preparation of this manuscript.

REFERENCES

1. Bouroncle BA, Wiseman BK, Doak CA: Leukemic reticuloendotheliosis. Blood 13:609–629, 1958

2. Schreck R, Donnelly WJ: "Hairy" cells in blood lymphoreticular neoplastic disease and "flagellated" cells of normal lymph nodes. Blood 27:199–211, 1966

3. Golomb HM, Ratain MJ, Vardiman JW: Sequential treatment of hairy cell leukemia: A new role for interferon, in DeVita VT Jr, Hellman S, Rosenberg SA (eds): Important Advances in Oncology 1986. Philadelphia, JB Lippincott Company, 1985, pp 311–321

4. Flandrin G, Signaux F, Sebahoun G, et al: Hairy cell leukemia: Clinical presentation and follow-up of 211 patients. Semin Oncol 11 (suppl 2):458–471, 1984

5. Jansen J, den Ottolander GJ, Holdrinet RSG, et al: Prognosis and therapy in hairy cell leukemia. Semin Oncol 11 (suppl 2):472–478, 1984

6. Bouroncle BA: The history of hairy cell leukemia: Characteristics of long-term survivors. Semin Oncol 11 (suppl 2):479–485, 1984

7. Quesada JR, Reuben JR, Manning JT, et al: Alpha

interferon for the induction of remission in hairy cell leukemia. N Engl J Med 310:15–18, 1984

8. Burke JS, Rappaport H: The diagnosis and differential diagnosis of hairy cell leukemia in bone marrow and spleen. Semin Oncol 11:334–346, 1984

9. Yam LT, Li CY, Lam KW: Tartrate-resistant acid phosphatase isoenzyme in the reticulum cells of leukemic reticuloendotheliosis. N Engl J Med 284:357–360, 1971

10. Yam LT, Phyliky RL, Li CY: Benign and neoplastic disorders simulating hairy cell leukemia. Semin Oncol 11:353–361, 1984

11. Mintz U, Golomb HM: Splenectomy as initial therapy in twenty-six patients with leukemic reticuloendotheliosis (hairy cell leukemia). Cancer Res 39:2366–2370, 1979

12. Lewis SM, Catovsky D, Howes JM, et al: Splenic red cell pooling in hairy cell leukemia. Br J Haematol 35:351–357, 1977

13. Golomb HM, Vardiman JW: Response to splenectomy in 65 patients with hairy cell leukemia. An evaluation of spleen weight and bone marrow involvement. Blood 61:349–352, 1983

14. Jansen J, Hermans J: Splenectomy in hairy cell leukemia: A retrospective multicenter analysis. Cancer 47:2066–2076, 1981

15. Jansen J, Hermans J: Clinical staging system for hairy-cell leukemia. Blood 60:571–577, 1982

16. Golomb HM, Schmidt K, Vardiman JW: Chlorambucil therapy of twenty-four postsplenectomy patients with progressive hairy cell leukemia. Semin Oncol 11 (suppl 2):502–506, 1984

17. Albain K, Le Beau MM, Vardiman JW, et al: Development of dysmelopoietic syndrome in a hairy cell leukemia patient treated with chlorambucil: Cytogenetic and morphologic evaluation. Cancer Genet Cytogenet 8:107–115, 1983

18. Yam LT, Klock JC, Mielke CH: Therapeutic leukapheresis in hairy cell leukemia—Review of literature and personal experience. Semin Oncol 11 (suppl 2):493–501, 1984

19. Magee MJ, McKenzie S, Filippa DA, et al: Hairy cell leukemia: Durability of response to splenectomy in 26 patients and treatment of relapse with androgens in six patients. Cancer 56:2557–2562, 1985

20. Blum SF: Lithium in hairy cell leukemia. N Engl J Med 303:464–465, 1980 (letter)

21. Cheever M, Fefer A, Greenberg PD, et al: Identical twin bone marrow transplantation for hairy cell leukemia. Semin Oncol 11 (suppl 2):511–513, 1984

22. Ratain MJ, Golomb HM, Vardiman JW, et al: Treatment of hairy cell leukemia with recombinant alpha-2-interferon. Blood 65:644–648, 1985

23. Golomb HM, Jacobs A, Fefer A et al: Alpha-2-interferon therapy of hairy cell leukemia; A multi-center study of 64 patients. J Clin Oncol 12:900–905, 1986

24. Quesada JR, Hersh EM, Reuben J, et al: Treatment of hairy cell leukemia with recombinant-DNA derived interferon alpha. Proc Am Soc Clin Oncol 4:222, 1985 (abstr)

25. Flandrin G, Sigaux F, Castaigne S, et al: Treatment of hairy cell leukemia with recombinant interferon alpha. I. Quantitative study of bone marrow changes during the first months of treatment. Blood 67:817–820, 1986

26. Foon KA, Maluish AE, Abrams PG, et al: Recombinant leukocyte A interferon therapy for advanced hairy cell leukemia: Therapeutic and immunologic results. Am J Med 80:351–356, 1986

27. Quesada JR, Talpax M, Rios A, et al: Clinical toxicity of interferon in cancer patients—A review. J Clin Oncol 4:234–243, 1986

28. Thompson JA, Brady J, Kidd P, et al: Recombinant alpha-2-interferon in the treatment of hairy cell leukemia. Cancer Treat Rep 69:791–793, 1985

29. Davidson HS, Schilsky RL, Golomb HM: Gonadal and sexual function following treatment of hairy cell leukemia with recombinant alpha-2-interferon. Proc Am Soc Clin Oncol 4:232, 1985 (abstr)

30. Naeim F, Jacobs AD: Bone marrow changes in patients with hairy cell leukemia treated by recombinant alpha$_2$-interferon. Hum Pathol 16:1200–1205, 1985

31. Bardawil RG, Groves C, Ratain MJ, et al: Changes in peripheral blood and bone marrow specimens following therapy with recombinant alpha$_2$ interferon for hairy cell leukemia. Am J Clin Pathol 85:194–201, 1986

32. Foon KA, Bottino GC, Abrams PG, et al: A phase II trial of recombinant leukocyte A interferon for patients with advanced chronic lymphocytic leukemia. Am J Med 78:216–220, 1985

33. Ruco LP, Procopio A, Maccallini V, et al: Severe deficiency of natural killer activity in the peripheral blood of patients with hairy cell leukemia. Blood 61:1132–1137, 1983

34. Lee SH, Kelly S, Chin H, et al: Stimulation of natural killer cell activity and inhibition of proliferation of various leukemic cells by purified human leukocyte interferon subtypes. Cancer Res 42:1312–1316, 1982

35. Ozer H, Dadey B, Gavigan M, et al: Normalization of defective natural killer activity in hairy cell leukemia correlates with rDNA α-2 interferon therapy in contrast to splenectomy. Blood 64 (suppl 1):171a, 1984 (abstr)

36. Vokes EE, Bitter MA, Ratain MJ, et al: Flow cytometric evidence for increasing natural killer cell activity in patients with hairy cell leukemia treated with α-2 interferon. Proc Am Assoc Canc Res 27:153, 1986 (abstr)

37. Samuels BS, Giometti CS, Brownstein BH, et al: Alpha-interferon induced proteins in hairy cell leukemia. Blood 66 (suppl 1):208a, 1985 (abstr)

38. Baldini L, Cortelezzi A, Polli N, et al: Human recombinant interferon α-2c enhances the expression of class II HLA antigens on hairy cells. Blood 67:458–464, 1986

39. Hiraoka A, Rosner MC, Golomb HM: In vitro response of cells from three patients with hairy cell leukemia to a recombinant leukocyte interferon. Virchows Archiv [Cell Pathol] 49:73–82, 1985

40. Paganelli KA, Evans SS, Han T, et al: B cell growth factor-induced proliferation of hairy cell lymphocytes and inhibition by type I interferon *in vitro.* Blood (in press)

41. Roos G, Leanderson T, Lundgren E: Interferon-induced cell cycle changes in human hematopoietic cell lines and fresh leukemic cells. Cancer Res 44:2358–2362, 1984

42. Ratain M, Golomb H, Vardiman J, et al: Durability of responses to α-2-interferon in advanced hairy cell leukemia. Proc Am Soc Clin Oncol 5:163, 1986 (abstr)

43. Spiers ASD, Parekh SJ, Bishop MB: Hairy-cell leukemia: Induction of complete remission with pentostatin (2′ deoxycoformycin). J Clin Oncol 2:1336–1342, 1984

44. Spiers ASD, Parekh SJ, Ramnes CR, et al: Hairy cell leukemia: Pentostatin is effective both as initial treatment and after failure of splenectomy and alpha interferon. Blood 66 (suppl 1):208a, 1985 (abstr)

45. Kraut EH, Bouroncle BA, Grever MR: Treatment of hairy cell leukemia with low dose 2′ deoxycoformycin. Blood 66 (suppl 1):203a, 1985 (abstr)

46. Ho AD, Dietz G, Hunstein W, et al: Enzymes of purine metabolism in hairy cell leukemia. Blood 66 (suppl 1):223a, 1985 (abstr)

Interferon Alfa-2b in the Treatment of Chronic Granulocytic Leukemia

Daniel E. Bergsagel, Rainer H. Haas, and Hans A. Messner

Studies of the effect of interferon on the growth of colonies of myeloid leukemic blast cells, myeloma colony-forming cells, and normal hemopoietic precursor cells have demonstrated that interferon shows no specificity in inhibiting the growth of these cells in culture (ie, growth of the malignant and normal precursor cells is equally inhibited). However, interferon markedly reduces the self-renewal capacity of acute myeloid leukemic blast cells and myeloma cells. This observation suggested that interferon's ability to prolong rather than induce remissions should be tested. We have studied the ability of interferon alfa-2b (Intron® A) to prolong remissions induced by busulfan (Myleran) in patients with chronic granulocytic leukemia (CGL). The leukocyte doubling time and remission duration among patients receiving no therapy was compared with the values observed during interferon alfa-2b maintenance therapy. Nine patients have begun the study; five have completed 3 months of interferon alfa-2b therapy. In four (80%) of the five patients, there has been a significant slowing of the leukocyte doubling time and prolongation of the remission duration. A larger study, with longer follow-up, will be required to determine whether interferon alfa-2b therapy will slow progression of CGL to the blast phase and prolong survival.

INTERFERONS are known to have both antiviral and antiproliferative biologic activity. Alpha interferon recently has been evaluated in the treatment of chronic granulocytic leukemia (CGL). Satisfactory cytoreduction was achieved in five of the seven initial CGL patients in the chronic phase who were treated with this agent.[1] In addition, alpha interferon has been reported to have temporarily controlled the blast phase in three patients[2,3] and suppressed a secondary Ph′ clone in another.[2] The work of the M. D. Anderson Hospital investigators has been recently updated.[4]

Studies of the effect of interferons on the growth of normal and CGL granulocyte-macrophage precursor cells (CFU-C) in cell culture revealed that neither leukocyte nor fibroblast beta interferon showed any specificity in inhibiting the growth of leukemic cells.[5] Taetle et al[6] found that interferon beta was equally toxic for normal CFU-C and acute myeloid blasts and contributed the important finding that interferon beta reduced the self-renewal capacity of the leukemic blast cells. In unpublished studies, we have also found that interferon alpha and interferon beta inhibit equally the growth of early hemopoietic precursor cells capable of forming mixed colonies of granulocytes, erythroblasts, macrophages, and megakaryocytes (CFU-GEMM) and myeloma colony-forming cells. Additionally, both types of interferon reduced the self-renewal capacity of the myeloma colony-forming cells.

The observation that interferon does not show any specificity in inhibiting the growth of malignant cells in culture but does reduce the self-renewal capacity of at least myeloid blast cells and myeloma cells, suggested to us that interferon should be tested for its capacity to prolong remissions, rather than as a remission-inducing agent. We chose to test the effect of interferon alfa-2b (Intron® A) on busulfan (Myleran)-induced remissions in CGL patients.

CGL is a clonal hemopathy in which malignant transformation probably occurs in an early hemopoietic precursor cell, since most progeny of the hemopoietic stem cell appear to be derived from the leukemic clone in patients with this disease.[7] The course of CGL is marked by a progressive increase in the growth rate of the leukemic population and loss of the leukemic cells' ability to differentiate into functional cells. There is a good correlation of the leukocyte doubling time during relapse from busulfan- or irradiation-induced remission and survival.[8]

In our investigation, we studied the effect of interferon alfa-2b therapy on the leukocyte doubling time and remission duration of busulfan-induced CGL remissions. We found that inter-

---

From the University of Toronto and the Princess Margaret Hospital, Toronto, Canada

Address reprint requests to Daniel E. Bergsagel, MD, DPhil, Princess Margaret Hospital, 500 Sherbourne Street, Toronto M4X 1K9, Canada.

feron alfa-2b prolonged the leukocyte doubling time and the remission duration in four of the five CGL patients who have completed 3 months of interferon alfa-2b therapy.

STUDY DESIGN AND METHODS

The study design is illustrated in Figure 1. Each patient was to be treated with busulfan, 4 to 6 mg/day, until the leukocyte count fell to $<10 \times 10^9$ cells/L. Busulfan would then be stopped, and the leukocyte doubling time during relapse and remission duration (the interval between stopping and restarting busulfan) would be determined. When the leukocyte count rose to $>30 \times 10^9$/L, busulfan would be reinstated and continued until the leukocyte count fell to $<10 \times 10^9$/L.

The effect of interferon alfa-2b on the remission was tested by administering 2 million units (MU)/m² subcutaneously (SC) three times per week until the leukocyte count again rose above 30×10^9/L. During interferon alfa-2b therapy the leukocyte doubling time and the remission duration were compared with the values obtained when no interferon alfa-2b was used. Thus, patients served as their own control.

A second remission was induced in one patient (Figures 4 and 5), and the value of a double dose of interferon alfa-2b (4 MU/m² SC, three times per week) was tested. If interferon alfa-2b were to have no effect on the course of CGL, we would expect an increase in the growth rate of the relapsing leukemic cells and a shortening of the leukocyte doubling time, as illustrated by the dotted line labeled 1 in Figure 1. If interferon alfa-2b slowed relapse, we would

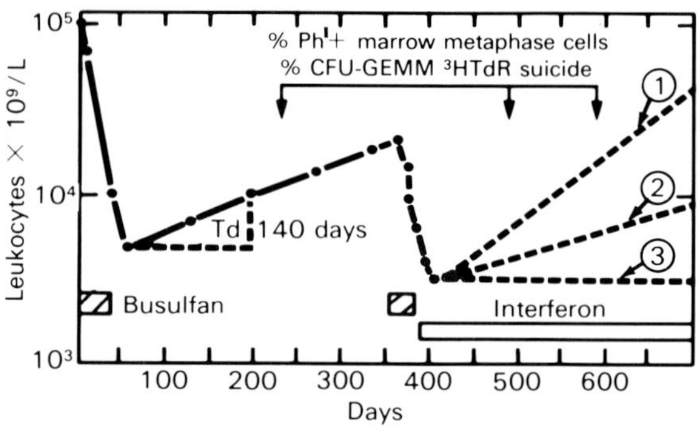

Figure 1. Study design. The leukocyte doubling times (Td) and durations of busulfan-induced remissions are determined first on no therapy, and then during interferon alfa-2b maintenance therapy. If the leukocyte Td shortens (as illustrated by the dotted line labeled 1), interferon alfa-2b will have had no effect. If the leukocyte Td is slowed moderately (line 2) or markedly (line 3), interferon alfa-2b will have interfered with the relapse process.

expect a moderate prolongation of the leukocyte doubling time (dotted line 2) or a flattening of the leukocyte count if interferon alfa-2b were to completely block the relapse (dotted line 3).

In addition, the proportion of marrow metaphase cells containing the Philadelphia chromosome and early hemopoietic progenitor cells (CFU-GEMM) in the DNA synthesis phase of the cell cycle were determined by methods that have been described previously.[9,10] These studies were done prior to initiation of interferon alfa-2b and at various intervals after therapy began.

Nine patients with CGL have been started on study but only five have received interferon alfa-2b for more than 3 months. The clinical features of these patients appear in Table 1.

Table 1. Clinical Features of Five CGL Patients Treated With Interferon Alfa-2b

Case	Age/Sex	Karyotype	Prior Treatment	Phase of CGL	Time from Diagnosis to Interferon (Months)
169799	50/M	46,XY,t(9:22)	Busulfan	Chronic	24
172703	34/F	46,XX,t(9:22)	Busulfan	Chronic	25
174833	67/M	46,XY	None	Chronic	5
174978	54/M	47,XY,+21	None	Chronic	9
180203	42/M	46,XY,t(9:22)	Hydroxyurea	Accelerated	17

Abbreviations: CGL, chronic granulocytic leukemia; M, male; F, female.

RESULTS

The course of a 34-year-old woman with Ph′-positive CGL (patient 172703) is illustrated in Figures 2 and 3. The diagnosis was made in December 1982. She was relatively asymptomatic; the leukocyte count increased slowly. Busulfan was administered February to April 1983. Bone marrow transplantation was considered initially, but the patient did not have an HLA-compatible sibling donor.

Treatment with busulfan 6 mg/day was restarted in March 1984. The leukocyte count promptly fell to $<10 \times 10^9/L$ and then increased slowly. The changes in the leukocyte count during relapse were so erratic that the doubling time could not be estimated.

The leukocyte count reached $34.1 \times 10^9/L$ by October 1984, and busulfan was restarted after a 182-day remission. This patient has now received 3.1 MU interferon alfa-2b SC three times per week for over 1 year, but the leukocyte count has not exceeded $10 \times 10^9/L$. Since June 1985, the count has been rising slowly. If the present trend continues, the leukocyte doubling time will be about 250 days. The interval between stopping and restarting busulfan (when the leukocyte count is estimated to reach $30 \times 10^9/L$) will be about 911 days.

Interferon alfa-2b appears to have greatly slowed the rate of relapse and prolonged the duration of remission for this patient in the early, slowly progressive, chronic phase of CGL.

The course of a patient with Ph′-negative CGL is shown in Figures 4 and 5. The leukocyte doubling time was 32 days; remission duration was 63 days during relapse on no maintenance therapy. With interferon alfa-2b maintenance therapy, the leukocyte doubling time was prolonged to 45 days and the remission duration increased to 141 days. A third remission was induced with busulfan, and the effect of doubling the dose of interferon alfa-2b (to 9.2 MU SC, three times per week) was tested.

The increased dose of interferon did not slow the leukocyte doubling time further, and the remission duration was increased only to 189 days. We concluded that increasing the interferon alfa-2b dose from 2 to 4 MU/m^2 SC three times per week did not increase the effectiveness

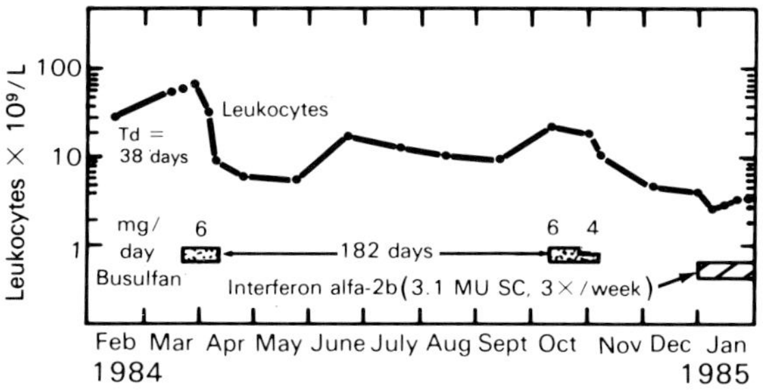

Figure 2. Response of patient 172703, with a slowly progressive CGL, to busulfan therapy.

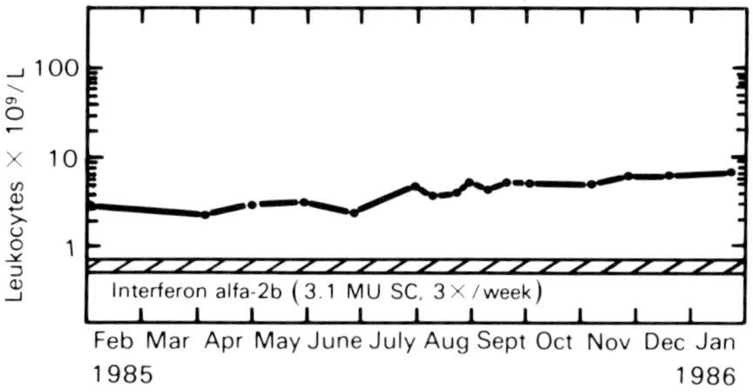

Figure 3. Effect of interferon alfa-2b on the busulfan-induced remission in patient 172703.

of this agent in slowing the rate of relapse or prolonging the duration of remission in this patient.

The course of a third patient—with Ph′-positive CGL in an accelerated phase—is shown in Figure 6. The leukocyte doubling time was very rapid (4 days), and the remission lasted only 41 days when no interferon alfa-2b was given following busulfan treatment. A second busulfan-induced remission was incomplete because splenomegaly continued. A strange cycling of the leukocyte count became evident during the relapse that occurred during interferon alfa-2b maintenance therapy. It is clear that interferon alfa-2b slowed the relapse rate in this patient, but it is difficult to measure a doubling time because of the cycling. The doubling time, estimated by connecting the troughs of the cycles, was 42 days; the remission duration, 255 days.

The effect of interferon alfa-2b on busulfan-induced remissions in patients with CGL is summarized in Table 2. The leukocyte doubling

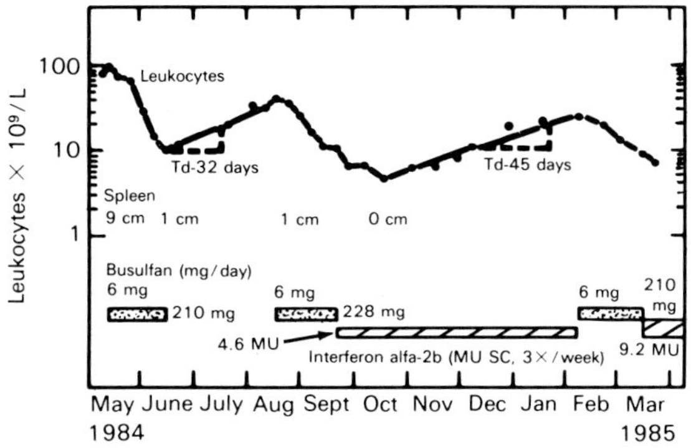

Figure 4. Effect of interferon alfa-2b (2 MU/m² SC, three times per week) on the leukocyte doubling time (Td) and remission duration in patient 174833. After relapse another remission was induced by busulfan and the effect of doubling the dose of interferon to 4.0 MU/m² SC three times per week was tested.

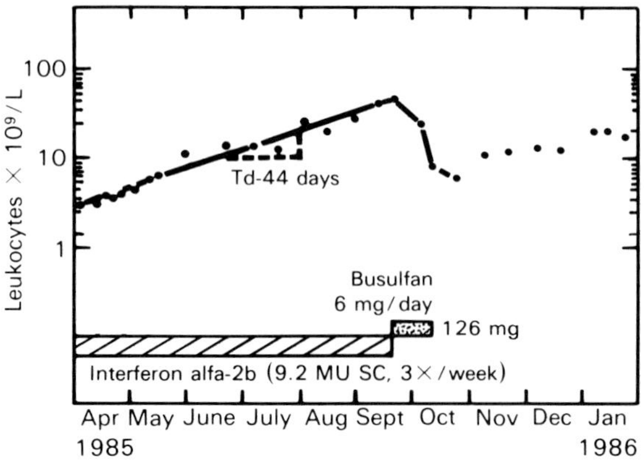

Figure 5. Effect of doubling the interferon alfa-2b dose on the leukocyte doubling time (Td) and remission duration in patient 174833.

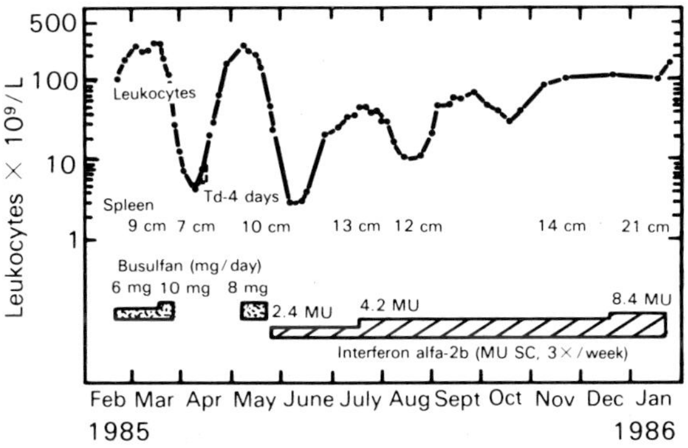

Figure 6. Effect of increasing doses of interferon alfa-2b on the busulfan-induced remission of patient 180203 in the accelerated phase of CGL.

time usually shortens with each relapse following busulfan treatment. However, this did not occur when interferon alfa-2b was administered during remissions. Instead, the leukocyte doubling time was prolonged in four of the five patients, and the remission duration was at least doubled.

We have been able to compare the proportion of early hemopoietic progenitor cells (CFU-GEMM) in the S-phase of the cell cycle before and after interferon alfa-2b therapy in only one patient, who showed a reduction from 100% to 63% after 8 months of treatment.

Karyotypic studies have been repeated on two patients after 7 and 10 months of treatment with interferon alfa-2b. In both cases, all of the metaphase cells continued to carry the Ph′ chromosome.

All patients developed a fever after the first injection of interferon alfa-2b. This reaction to

Table 2. Effect of Interferon Alfa-2b on Busulfan-Induced Remissions in CGL Patients

	Leukocyte Doubling Time (Days)		Remission Duration (Days)
Case	Before Interferon Alfa-2b	On Interferon Alfa-2b	On Interferon Alfa-2b/No Therapy
169799	4	?42	255/41 = 6.2
172703	?	~250	~911/182 = ~5.0
174833	32	45 (4.6 MU)	141/63 = 2.2
		44 (9.2 MU)	189/63 = 3.0
174978	92	92	239/141 = 1.7
180203	19	112	214/109 = 2.0

Table 3. Chronic Toxicity of Interferon Alfa-2b

Case	Muscle Ache	Headache	Weight Change (kg)
169797	Yes	No	−4.7
172703	Yes	No	0
174833	Yes	No	−17.8
174978	Yes	Yes	−7.0
180203	No	No	+2.0

therapy became less marked as treatment progressed and was not detected after 2 to 3 weeks. The chronic toxicity associated with interferon alfa-2b is detailed in Table 3. Toxicity was mild in three patients but required discontinuation of interferon alfa-2b in one (case 174978) because of headache and muscle ache, and another (case 174833) because of severe weight loss.

DISCUSSION

CGL is marked by a progressive increase in the growth rate of the leukemic population, with remissions that become shorter and shorter as the disease progresses from the chronic through the accelerated to the acute blast phase. Marrow failure, marked by severe anemia, thrombocytopenia, and an increasing number of blast cells, develops as the disease enters the blast phase, during which at least 85% of CGL patients die. An agent that slows the rate of progression of CGL to the blast phase would be expected to prolong the survival of patients with this disease. If the action of the agent were strong enough to maintain the disease in the chronic phase and prevent progression, survival to a normal life expectancy would be expected.

Interferon alfa-2b clearly slowed the leukocyte doubling time, and at least doubled the remission duration, in four of the five patients included in this study. These effects are encouraging, but they do not mean that interferon alfa-2b will alter the course of CGL or prolong survival. Our results may be due to a cytotoxic or cytostatic effect of interferon alfa-2b on the leukemic cell population, without altering the progression of the disease.

A larger study, with previously untreated patients and longer follow-up, will be required to show that interferon alfa-2b therapy slows or prevents progression to the blast phase and prolongs survival. The report that interferon therapy temporarily controlled the blast phase in three patients[2,3] and suppressed a secondary Ph′ clone in another[2] lends support to the view that this agent may be capable of regulating the growth of CGL cells. We are encouraged by these preliminary results and will continue this study.

ACKNOWLEDGMENTS

Dr R.H. Haas was supported by Deutsche Krebshilfe e V, Mildred Scheel Stiftung.

We are grateful to Schering for supplying us with the recombinant interferon alfa-2b and for a grant to support the clinical and laboratory investigations.

REFERENCES

1. Talpaz M, McCredie KB, Mavlight GM, et al: Leukocyte interferon-induced myeloid cytoreduction in chronic myelogenous leukemia. Blood 62:689–692, 1983

2. Talpaz M, Trujillo JM, Hittelman WN, et al: Suppression of clonal evolution in two chronic myelogenous leukaemia patients treated with leukocyte interferon. Br J Haematol 60:619–624, 1985

3. Hill NO, Kahn A, Pardue A, et al: Response of a blast crisis of CGL to leukocyte-alpha. Proc Am Soc Clin Oncol 1:C–499, 1982

4. Talpaz M, Kantarjian, HM, McCredie K, et al: Hematologic remission and cytogenetic improvement induced by recombinant human interferon alpha A in chronic myelogenous leukemia. N Engl J Med 314:1065–1069, 1986

5. Oladipupo Williams CK, Svet-Moldavskaya I, Vicek J, et al: Inhibitory effects of human leukocyte and fibroblast interferons on normal and chronic myelogenous leukemic granulocytic progenitor cells. Oncology 38:356–360, 1981

6. Taetle R, Buick RN, McCulloch EA: Effect of interferon on colony-formation in culture by blast cell progeni-

tors in acute myeloblastic leukemia. Blood 56:549–552, 1980

7. Bergsagel DE: Chronic granulocytic leukemia. Curr Hematol 2:1–26, 1983

8. Bergsagel DE: The chronic leukemias: A review of disease manifestations and the aims of therapy. Can Med Assoc J 96:1616–1620, 1967

9. Rowley JD: A new consistent chromosomal abnormality in chronic myelogenous leukemia identified by Quinacrine fluorescence and Giemsa staining. Nature 243:290–293, 1973

10. Lepine J, Messner HA: Pluripotent hemopoietic progenitors (CFU-GEMM) in chronic myelogenous leukemia. International Journal of Cell Cloning 1:230–239, 1983

Alpha Interferon Treatment of Low-Grade B-Cell Non-Hodgkin's Lymphomas, Cutaneous T-Cell Lymphomas, and Chronic Lymphocytic Leukemia

Kenneth A. Foon, Mark S. Roth, and Paul A. Bunn, Jr

The interferons represent an important first member of a family of biologic response modifiers used in treating human malignancies. Activities associated with the interferons include inhibition of viral replication, influence on cellular protein production, direct antiproliferative effects, and a variety of modulatory effects on the immune response. These regulatory functions of interferon underlie the interest in its use as an anticancer agent. Interferon alpha is the most extensively studied interferon species. Although antitumor activity has been seen both in vivo and in vitro in some solid malignancies, the most impressive responses have occurred in the hematologic malignancies. For the low-grade non-Hodgkin's lymphomas, response rates of 50%, with 10% to 15% complete responses, have been reported. A response rate of 15% has been reported for chronic lymphocytic leukemia in studies outside of the National Cancer Institute (NCI); in our phase II trials at the NCI, only two (11%) of 18 patients had brief partial responses to recombinant interferon alpha. For patients with cutaneous T-cell lymphomas (mycosis fungoides and the Sézary syndrome), a response rate of 45%, with 10% complete responses, was seen in patients treated with recombinant interferon alpha. Based on such findings, interferon appears to be one of the most effective single agents for cutaneous T-cell lymphomas. Further phase II trials are being conducted to determine whether lower doses of interferon alpha are as effective as the high doses used in the previously reported studies. Phase III trials will involve the use of interferons in combination with chemotherapeutic agents as well as in the adjuvant setting.

"INTERFERON" was the term originally applied to a soluble factor recognized by its ability to induce interference against viral infection of chick chorioallantoic membrane by influenza A virus.[1] This factor subsequently has been shown to be a family of closely related proteins and glycoproteins that, in addition to exhibiting antiviral activity, are potent regulators of cellular function and structure, and possess direct antiproliferative activities. These latter properties underlie the current interest in interferon as an anticancer agent.

Three major species of human interferon are recognized: interferon alpha, interferon beta, and interferon gamma.[2] Interferon alpha is produced by leukocytes (B cells, T cells, and macrophages) upon exposure to B-cell mitogens, viruses, foreign cells, or tumor cells. Interferon beta is produced by fibroblasts upon exposure to viruses or foreign nucleic acids. Interferon gamma is produced by T lymphocytes upon stimulation with T-cell mitogens, specific antigens, or interleukin-2.[3] By use of recombinant DNA techniques, complete nucleotide and amino acid sequences for alpha, beta, and gamma interferons have been defined.

The genes recognized to code for interferon alpha have been assigned to chromosome 9.[4] Sixteen distinct sequences for interferon alpha have been described. Each is approximately 166 amino acids in length, with an additional 20 amino acid secretory peptides present on the amino-terminal end. The human genes differ by approximately 10% in nucleotide sequences and by 15% to 20% in amino acid sequences.[5] Two recombinant human interferons, alfa-2a and alpha-D, comprise over 60% of interferons present after buffy coat stimulation; these have been extensively studied.[6] Although they possess different antiviral and antiproliferative activity in vitro, similar in vivo effects on immune effector cells have been observed.[6] The interferon alpha used in the first human clinical trials was obtained from Sendai virus-stimulated buffy coat leukocytes, and represented 1% purity (10^6 units/mg protein).[7] Refinement in purification methods by use of high-perform-

From the Department of Medicine, Division of Hematology and Oncology University of Michigan, Ann Arbor, Michigan, and the Department of Medicine, Division of Medical Oncology, University of Colorado Health Sciences Center, Denver, Colorado.

Address reprint requests to Kenneth A. Foon, MD, A. Alfred Taubman Health Care Center, 3119, University of Michigan Medical Center, Ann Arbor, MI 48109.

ance liquid chromatography, two-dimensional polyacrylamide gel electrophoresis, and immunoaffinity chromatography has allowed purification to homogeneity (10^8 units/mg protein).[8-10] The use of recombinant DNA techniques in splicing the interferon alpha gene into *Escherichia coli* has further allowed for pure single-species interferon alpha in larger quantities.

Industrial-scale production of beta and gamma interferons only recently has been accomplished; clinical trials with these are limited in number. In contrast, interferon alpha has been extensively studied for the past decade in both basic science and clinical research; it is among the most potent biologic agents ever administered to man. Although antitumor activity has been seen both in vitro and in vivo and in some solid malignancies (renal-cell cancer, Kaposi's sarcoma, bladder cancer, ovarian cancer, and melanoma),[11,12] the most impressive responses have occurred in the hematologic malignancies.[13] A summary of the results for patients with non-Hodgkin's lymphomas, including cutaneous T-cell lymphoma and chronic lymphocytic leukemia, is presented.

NON-HODGKIN'S LYMPHOMAS

A histologic classification of non-Hodgkin's lymphomas that does not conform with the commonly used Rappaport system[14] has recently been proposed. Based on prognosis and morphology, the histologic types of malignant lymphoma have been grouped into low-, intermediate-, and high-grade malignancy.[15] Although many chemotherapeutic agents produce responses, patients with low-grade non-Hodgkin's lymphomas cannot be cured with currently available treatment. This fact, in combination with the indolent nature of the disease, leads to multiple episodes of treatment and relapse, with the patient eventually dying of unrelated causes, toxicity of therapy, progressive disease, or emergence of a more aggressive histology.

The low-grade non-Hodgkin's lymphomas have shown responsiveness to interferon alpha. Trials with crude interferon alpha preparations have resulted in responses in 11 of 32 patients[16-19]; similar results have been reported with recombinant interferon alpha.[20-23]

In our trial at the NCI (see Table 1), patients were treated with interferon alfa-2a (Hoffmann-La Roche, Nutley, NJ) at a dose of 50×10^6 units/m^2 three times a week.[20] Doses were adjusted downward for toxicity. Thirteen responses were obtained (four complete, nine partial) among 24 evaluable patients with low-grade malignancy. Six of the nine patients with partial responses had nearly complete resolution of "bulky" disease in lymph nodes, liver, and spleen (Figure 1). Most of the responding patients received interferon alfa-2a for 4 to more than 36 months; the median duration of response was 8 months. Of the four patients with complete responses, one had a malignant lymphoma of the follicular mixed small cleaved cell and large cell type, and three had malignant lymphomas that were follicular and predominantly of the small cleaved cell type. One of these patients has maintained a complete remission on interferon therapy for more than 36 months. Before interferon therapy, three of the four patients with complete responses had bone marrow involvement; all patients had extensive lymphadenopathy (one had resolution of disease in lymph nodes as large as 12×12 cm). Responses were documented in all patients by appropriate noninvasive tests and, when indicated, biopsies at sites of previous disease.

Seven of the partially responding patients with low-grade disease had follicular, predominantly small cleaved cell malignant lymphomas; one had a follicular, mixed small cleaved cell and large cell lymphoma, and another had a diffuse small cleaved cell lymphoma. Four of the partial responders had disease progression while receiving a 10% maintenance dose of interferon, and two had progression 3 and 5 months, respectively, after cessation of therapy. One of the patients who had a partial response after the first course of interferon went on to have a partial response with resolution of extensive pulmonary involvement after a second course.[24]

Interferon alpha has shown less effectiveness in patients with the intermediate- and high-grade lymphomas. The treatment of 36 such patients with both crude and recombinant interferon alpha has resulted in only five responses.[16-20,25] In our study at the NCI, one partial response and one complete response

Table 1. Results of Interferon Alpha Trials in Patients With Low-Grade Non-Hodgkin's B-Cell Lymphomas, Cutaneous T-Cell Lymphomas, and Chronic Lymphocytic Leukemia

	Number of Patients	Response		Total Percentage of Patients Responding	References
		Complete	Partial		
Low-Grade Non-Hodgkin's B-Cell Lymphoma					
NCI study	24	4	9	54	20
Published literature	81	7	25	40	16–19,21–23
Cutaneous T-Cell Lymphoma					
NCI study	20	2	7	45	41
Chronic Lymphocytic Leukemia					
NCI study	18	0	2	11	30
Published literature	39	0	6	15	18,19,22,28,29

were noted among six evaluable patients with intermediate-grade non-Hodgkin's lymphomas.[20] Both responders had diffuse small cleaved cell malignant lymphomas. In that same study, only one of seven evaluable patients with high-grade disease responded to interferon therapy. This patient, who had a lymphoblastic malignant lymphoma, had a response lasting 10 weeks; an atypical tumor lysis syndrome developed after the interferon therapy.[26] All the other patients with high-grade disease had large cell immunoblastic malignant lymphomas. In one patient, the disease was stable; in five, it progressed.

CHRONIC LYMPHOCYTIC LEUKEMIA

Chronic lymphocytic leukemia is a hematologic malignancy characterized by proliferation and accumulation of lymphocytes with a relatively mature appearance.[27] Most cases involve a clonal proliferation of B lymphocytes. Chronic lymphocytic leukemia typically occurs in persons over 50 years of age (median age, 60 years) and affects more males than females (by a ratio of 2:1).[27] The disease is usually stable for months or years, but transformation to a more aggressive disease state does occur. Alkylating agents, radiation therapy, and corticosteroids are commonly used to treat patients, although few data show that survival is substantially improved by these measures. Crude and purified interferon alpha preparations were reported to be moderately active in patients with advanced chronic lymphocytic leukemia,[18,22,28] but this is a controversial finding.[19,29,30]

In our phase II trial at the NCI, 19 patients were administered recombinant interferon alpha three times a week at both high and low doses—50×10^6 and 5×10^6 units/m^2 intramuscularly (IM), respectively.[30] Of 18 evaluable patients, only two exhibited responses, which

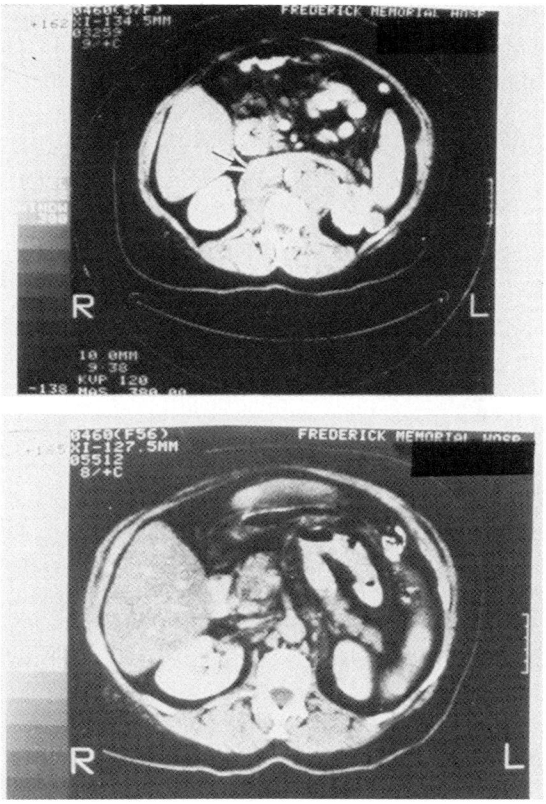

Figure 1. Computerized axial tomography showing enlarged retroperitoneal lymph nodes (arrow) prior to interferon therapy in a patient with non-Hodgkin's lymphoma (upper panel). During therapy with interferon there was complete resolution of the retroperitoneal lymph nodes (lower panel).

were brief and partial. Five patients appeared to have an acceleration of disease while receiving treatment. This finding is in marked contrast to results obtained in patients with chemotherapy-refractory low-grade non-Hodgkin's lymphomas and hairy cell leukemia.[31]

CUTANEOUS T-CELL LYMPHOMAS

The cutaneous T-cell lymphomas (CTCL)—comprising primarily mycosis fungoides and the Sézary syndrome—are indolent T-cell non-Hodgkin's lymphomas.[32] Phenotypic and functional studies have shown that the malignant cells in these disorders are the helper T cells.[33,34] These lymphomas are characterized by initial symptoms in the skin and subsequent spread to peripheral blood, lymph nodes, and other organs. The prognosis for patients with these disorders is highly dependent on the stage, as determined by the type of skin lesions and the presence or absence of peripheral blood, lymph node, and visceral involvement. Overall, the cutaneous T-cell lymphomas are indolent in nature, being associated with a median survival rate of approximately 8 to 10 years (as generally is the case with the B-cell indolent non-Hodgkin's lymphomas). Systemic spread, nearly universal, can be documented by light microscopic examination in up to one half of the patients at the time of diagnosis.[35]

Initial therapies developed for these disorders focused on treatment of the skin. These therapies included the use of topical nitrogen mustard applied daily to the skin,[36] administration of psoralen plus ultraviolet A light irradiation (PUVA) three times a week,[37] and application of electron beam irradiation to the entire body.[38] Such treatment approaches effectively alleviate skin lesions and produce skin clearing in the majority of patients. For all three treatments, the complete response rate is directly related to the disease stage; complete response occurs in the majority of patients with plaque lesions but in a minority of those with tumors or erythroderma. The median duration of response for these therapies is 1 to 2 years; 10% to 20% of patients are disease-free at 3 years. This long disease-free interval occurs exclusively in patients with early plaque lesions. Relapses after 3 years were reported with the use of topical nitrogen mustard, but were not observed with total skin electron irradiation. This observation suggests that some of these patients may in fact be cured of this malignant neoplasm. Long-term data on PUVA therapy are not available, but late relapses appear to be common with this treatment.

Patients with more advanced disease have been treated with chemotherapy, either in single-drug or multiagent form.[39,40] These treatments produced objective remissions in the majority of cases; however, complete remissions occurred in only 20% to 25% of the patients. Furthermore, relapse is universal; there have been no suggestions of cures reported to date.

Because of the propensity for early systemic spread and the lack of cure with known treatments, new systemic approaches to the cutaneous T-cell lymphomas are clearly needed. In response to this need, we studied the maximally tolerated doses of interferon alfa-2a in these neoplasms in our NCI trial. All patients entered in this trial had been treated unsuccessfully with multiple therapies.

Objective antitumor responses were noted in nine of the 20 patients in this study, representing a response rate of 45%, with a 95% confidence interval of 25% to 69%.[41] All objective responses were noted within 1 month and lasted from 3 months to more than 36 months. At 3 months, none of the remissions were complete; however, two patients subsequently developed normal skin biopsy results and were scored as complete responders. Thus, the complete response rate was 10% and the partial response rate was 35%. Responses were seen in extracutaneous and cutaneous sites and did not correlate with prior therapy (Figure 2). Eight of nine responders had received prior systemic chemotherapy. Extracutaneous responses were documented by a decrease in the size of palpable lymph nodes in eight of 16 patients with adenopathy, and by a greater than 50% decrease in the number of circulating malignant cells in two patients as shown by cytologic study and DNA content analysis. The median duration of response was 5.5 months. It is notable that three patients—representing one third of the responders and 15% of all patients—have continued to respond for over 2 years.

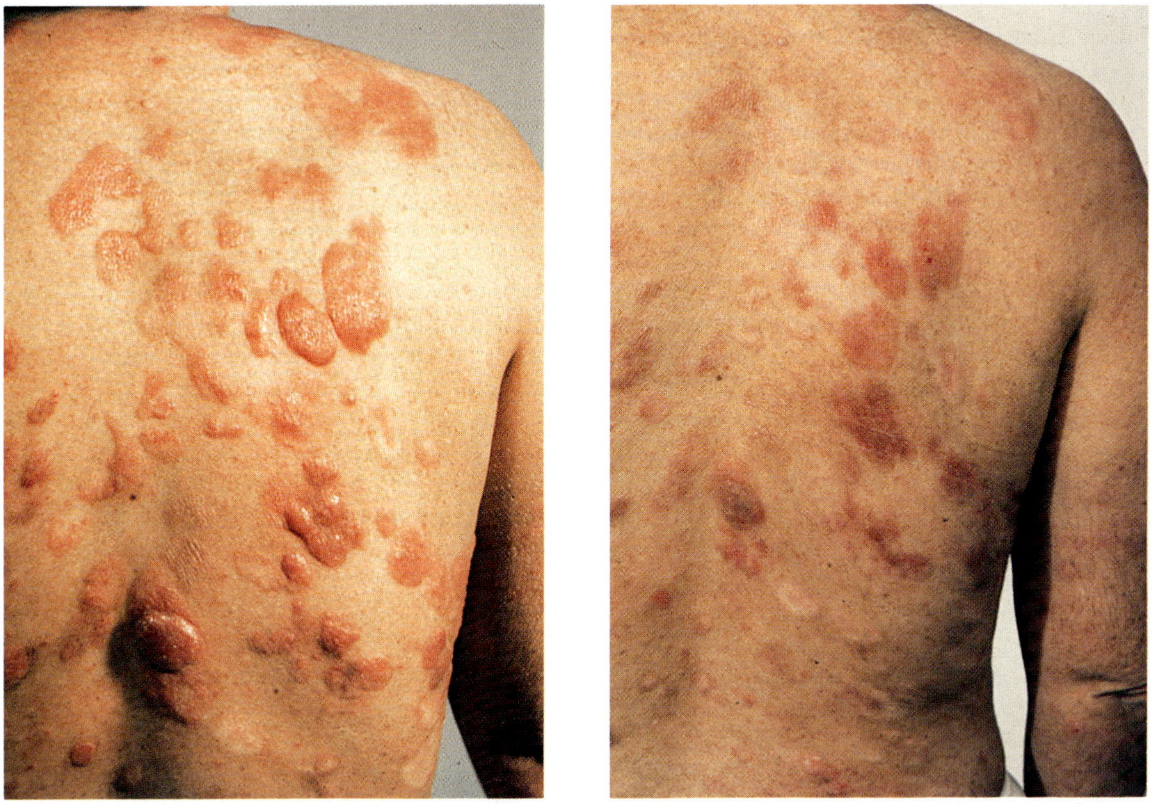

Figure 2. Multiple plaques and tumors on a patient with cutaneous T-cell lymphoma prior to interferon therapy (left panel). During therapy with interferon, there was complete resolution of cutaneous lesions (right panel). Biopsies of the lesions following response to interferon demonstrated no mycosis fungoides tumor cells.

Mixed or minor responses were noted in five patients, and three others remained stable for 3 months; therapy was discontinued in these eight patients at 3 months. Another three patients progressed during the initial 3 months of therapy; one patient received only the initial dose of therapy, and two others progressed after 1 and 2 months, respectively.

TOXICITY OF INTERFERON

The major dose-limiting toxicity of interferon in these trials was a flu-like syndrome consisting of malaise, fatigue, anorexia, and, in rare cases, mental confusion. These were clearly dose-dependent toxic effects, since they were relieved by a dose reduction. In our NCI studies, the average duration of therapy was 4 weeks at the 100% dose of 50×10^6 units/m^2 and 9 weeks at the 50% dose. Fatigue was the most common reason for dose reduction; all but one of the patients required at least a 50% reduction. Febrile responses were noted in all patients, but these were almost always most severe after the first dose and were rarely a problem after the first week of therapy. The peak temperatures ranged from 38 to 42°C. Hematologic toxicity was not dose-limiting. One patient with extensive pulmonary involvement exhibited adult respiratory distress syndrome after receiving 50×10^6 units/m^2 of interferon alfa-2a; he responded rapidly to corticosteroids. Because the patient had previously responded to interferon and had not responded to a number of chemotherapeutic regimens, interferon was carefully reinstituted; he had an excellent partial response.[24] One patient with underlying coronary artery disease had a massive myocardial infarction and died after the first dose of interferon. Reversible elevations in hepatic enzyme levels occurred in a minority of patients. The dose was reduced in all of these patients, and the hepatic enzyme levels returned to normal. One patient developed a reversible nephrotic syndrome and renal failure with minimal-change glomerulonephritis.[42] This syndrome disappeared after discontinuation of the interferon. One patient with the Sézary syndrome developed acute monocytic leukemia after 11 months on interferon therapy; therapy was discontinued at that time. The patient had been heavily pretreated with alkylating agents and electron beam irradiation. He subsequently was treated with high-dose cytosine arabinoside, which produced a complete remission of his leukemia; he has been in remission from the leukemia and the Sézary syndrome since the completion of therapy, more than 16 months ago.

An unexpected toxicity, the reactivation of perioral herpes simplex lesions, occurred in seven of 19 patients with chronic lymphocytic leukemia. In two instances, the severity of this condition was sufficient to require discontinuation of interferon therapy and institution of treatment with acyclovir.[27] One other interesting and unusual side effect was uncontrolled growth of eyelashes and axillary and pubic hair in two of the patients with low-grade B-cell non-Hodgkin's lymphomas.[43] This hair growth ceased when the interferon was discontinued.

DISCUSSION

Much of the initial enthusiasm for interferon as an anticancer agent has been dampened by disappointing clinical results. Recent clinical studies have shown, however, that interferons do have considerable activity in a limited spectrum of diseases. The studies reported here establish the activity of interferon against low-grade non-Hodgkin's lymphomas and cutaneous T-cell lymphomas. All patients involved in these trials had advanced disease refractory to one or more standard treatments, including systemic chemotherapy; interferon was found to be more active in such patients than any other recently evaluated experimental therapy. The high response rate and long duration of response observed in our study suggest that the effect of interferon in earlier disease stages should be evaluated, and that the efficacy of interferon in combination with standard treatment should be investigated and compared with that of standard agents used alone.

The issue whether interferon has any role at all in the treatment of chronic lymphocytic leukemia remains unresolved. Our studies at NCI found only a minimal response and perhaps even a progression of disease in a number of patients treated with either 50×10^6 or 5×10^6 units/m^2 of interferon alfa-2a. Should future studies include patients in earlier stages of disease and employ doses of interferon that have been proven to modify biologic responses, the findings might be more favorable.

The toxicity associated with interferon at high doses has been troublesome. The flu-like syndrome and high fever can be alleviated by initiating therapy at low doses, with subsequent escalation. This "tachyphylaxis" appears to be a consistent finding in most patients. However, the severe fatigue following high doses of interferon is not alleviated by these methods. It seems clear from these studies that acetaminophen should be given to all patients at the initiation of interferon therapy to alleviate fever. Patients with severe cardiac disease and those in whom high temperature is life-threatening should not be placed on interferon at high doses. Renal and hepatic functions should be monitored routinely to detect dose-limiting toxicity, which has been observed in some patients. Lowering of blood counts did not appear to be caused by direct bone marrow suppression. However, this effect should not be ignored when considering combined chemotherapy and interferon trials, because the chemotherapy doses are modified according to the peripheral blood counts. It has been suggested that because chemotherapy is immunosuppressive and interferons may be immunostimulatory, chemotherapy should be given intermittently and interferon given continuously.

In our studies, there was no correlation between the development of antibodies to interferon and response rate or response duration. There was no obvious correlation between in vitro laboratory tests, including phytohemagglutinin stimulation and T-cell subsets, and clinical responses. It appears unlikely that the response to treatment was due to the fever, since there was no correlation with the degree of the febrile response; also, the responses continued long after the patients ceased to have fevers. Direct cytotoxic effects have been proposed as a likely mechanism of interferon activity, particularly in light of the demonstrated effect of interferon on cutaneous T-cell lymphomas: in a number of patients, the disease progressed when the dose was lowered and remitted when the dose was increased.[41] Interferons also increase the expression of tumor-associated and histocompatibility antigens on malignant cells, suggesting that they may be combined with monoclonal antibodies or other biologic response modifers. Future phase II trials will address these issues.

The optimal dose of interferon for any particular malignancy is unknown. The responses observed in our studies were to a high dose of interferon, which was associated with considerable toxicity; dose reduction was necessary in nearly all patients. Lower doses of interferon, such as 3×10^6 units/day, have elicited consistent responses in patients with hairy cell leukemia.[31] Whether lower doses of interferon will be effective in patients with low-grade non-Hodgkin's lymphomas and cutaneous T-cell lymphomas is currently unknown. However, randomized trials of low-dose interferon in such patients have recently begun. Important information regarding efficacy and toxicity should be forthcoming.

REFERENCES

1. Isaacs A, Lindenman J: Virus interference I. The interferon. Proc R Soc Lond [Biol] 147:258–267, 1957

2. Stewart WE II, Blalock JE, Burke DC, et al: Interferon nomenclature. J Immunol 125:2353, 1980 (letter)

3. Fleischmann WR, Klimpel GR, Tyring SK, et al: Interferon and cancer: Current use and novel approaches, in Sunkara PS (ed): Novel Approaches to Cancer Chemotherapy. Orlando Fla, Academic Press, 1984, pp 1–22

4. Sehgal PB: The interferon gene. Biochim Biophys Acta 695:17–33, 1982

5. Borden EC: Progress toward therapeutic application of interferons, 1979–1983. Cancer 54:2770–2776, 1984

6. Hawkins MJ, Borden EC, Merritt JA, et al: Comparison of the biologic effects of two recombinant human interferons alpha (rA and rD) in humans. J Clin Oncol 2:221–226, 1984

7. Cantell K, Hirvonen S: Preparation of human leukocyte interferon for clinical use. Tex Rep Biol Med 35:138–144, 1977

8. Pestka S: The purification and manufacture of human interferons. Sci Am 249:37–43, 1983

9. Lin LS, Stewart WE II: Purification of human leukocyte interferon by two-dimensional polyacrylamide gel electrophoresis. Methods Enzymol 78:481, 1981

10. Berg K, Heron I: Antibody affinity chromatography of human leukocyte interferon. Methods Enzymol 78:487, 1981

11. Kirkwood JM, Ernstoff MS: Interferons in the treatment of human cancer. J Clin Oncol 2:336–352, 1984

12. Bonnem EM, Spiegel RJ: Interferon-α: Current status and future promise. J Biol Response Mod 3:580–598, 1984

13. Roth MS, Foon KA: Alpha interferon in the treatment of hematologic malignancies. Am J Med (in press).

14. Rappaport H, Winter WJ, Hicks EB: Follicular lymphoma: A reevaluation of its position in the scheme of malignant lymphoma, based on a survey of 253 cases. Cancer 9:792–821, 1956

15. The Non-Hodgkin's Lymphoma Pathologic Classification Project, National Cancer Institute sponsored study of classification of non-Hodgkin's lymphomas: Summary and description of a working formulation for clinical usage. Cancer 49:2112–2135, 1982

16. Merigan TC, Sikora K, Bredden JH, et al: Preliminary observations on the effect of human leukocyte interferon in non-Hodgkin's lymphoma. N Engl J Med 299:1449–1453, 1978

17. Louie AC, Gallagher JG, Sikora K, et al: Follow-up observations on the effect of human leukocyte interferon in non-Hodgkin's lymphoma. Blood 58:712–718, 1981

18. Gutterman JU, Blumenschein GR, Alexanian R: Leukocyte interferon-induced tumor regression in human metastatic breast cancer, multiple myeloma, and malignant lymphoma. Ann Intern Med 93:399–406, 1980

19. Horning SJ, Merigan TC, Korwn SE, et al: Human interferon alpha in malignant lymphoma and Hodgkin's disease. Result of the American Cancer Society Trial. Cancer 56:1305–1310, 1985

20. Foon KA, Sherwin SA, Abrams PG: Treatment of advanced non-Hodgkin's lymphoma with recombinant leukocyte A interferon. N Engl J Med 311:1148–1152, 1984

21. Leavitt RD, Kaplan R, Ozer H, et al: Low dose alpha-2 interferon (IFN) treatment for low grade non-Hodgkin's lymphoma (NHL). Blood 64 (suppl 1):182a, 1984 (abstr)

22. O'Connell MJ, Colgan JP, Oken MM, et al: Clinical trials of recombinant leukocyte A interferon in initial therapy for favorable histology non-Hodgkin's lymphoma and chronic lymphocytic leukemia. An Eastern Cooperative Oncology Group pilot study. J Clin Oncol 4:128–136, 1986

23. Quesada JR, Hawkins M, Horning S, et al: Collaborative phase I–II study of recombinant DNA-produced leukocyte interferon (clone A) in metastatic breast cancer, malignant lymphoma, and multiple myeloma. Am J Med 77:427–432, 1984

24. Stevenson HC, Ochs JJ, Halverson L, et al: Recombi-

nant alpha interferon in retreatment of two patients with pulmonary lymphoma: Dramatic responses with resolution of pulmonary complications. Am J Med 77:355–358, 1984

25. Leavitt RD, Ratanatharathorn V, Ozer H, et al: A phase II study of recombinant alpha 2 interferon in patients with malignant lymphoma with unfavorable histology. Proc Am Soc Clin Oncol 2:54, 1983 (abstr)

26. Fer MF, Bottino GC, Sherwin SA, et al: Atypical tumor lysis syndrome in a patient with T-cell lymphoma following recombinant leukocyte interferon therapy. Am J Med 77:953–956, 1984

27. Gale RP, Foon KA: Chronic lymphocytic leukemia: Recent advances in biology and treatment. Ann Intern Med 103:101–120, 1985

28. Misset JL, Mathé G, Gastiabury J, et al: Traitement des leucémies et des lymphomes par les interférons. II Essai phase II de traitement de la leucémie lymphoide chronique par l'interferon α humain. Biomedicine 36:112–116, 1982

29. Schuloff RS, Lloyd MJ, Stallings JJ, et al: Recombinant leukocyte A interferon in B-cell chronic lymphocytic leukemia: In vivo effects on autologous antitumor immunity. J Biol Response Mod 4:310–323, 1985

30. Foon KA, Bottino G, Abrams PG, et al: Phase II trial of recombinant leukocyte A interferon in patients with advanced chronic lymphocytic leukemia. Am J Med 78:216–220, 1985

31. Foon KA, Maluish AE, Abrams PG, et al: Recombinant leukocyte A interferon therapy for advanced hairy cell leukemia: Therapeutic and immunologic results. Am J Med 80:351–356, 1986

32. Lutzner M, Edelson R, Schein P, et al: Cutaneous T-cell lymphomas: The Sézary syndrome, mycosis fungoides, and related disorders. Ann Intern Med 83:534–552, 1975

33. Broder S, Edelson RL, Lutzner MA et al: The Sézary syndrome: A malignant proliferation of helper T cells. J Clin Invest 58:1297–1306, 1976

34. Haynes BF, Metzgar RS, Minna JD, et al: Phenotypic characterization of cutaneous T-cell lymphoma: Use of monoclonal antibodies to compare with other malignant T cells. N Engl J Med 304:1319–1323, 1981

35. Bunn PA, Huberman MS, Whang-Peng J, et al: Prospective staging evaluation of patients with cutaneous T-cell lymphomas: Demonstration of a high frequency of extracutaneous dissemination. Ann Intern Med 93:223–230, 1980

36. Vonderheid EC, Van Scott EJ, Wallner PE, et al: A 10-year experience with topical mechlorethamine for mycosis fungoides: Comparison with patients treated by total-skin electron beam radiation therapy. Cancer Treat Rep 63:681–689, 1979

37. Roenigk HH Jr: Photochemotherapy for mycosis fungoides: Long-term followup study. Cancer Treat Rep 63:669–673, 1979

38. Hoppe RT, Cox RS, Fuks Z, et al: Electron-beam therapy for mycosis fungoides: The Stanford University experience. Cancer Treat Rep 63:691–700, 1979

39. Winkler CF, Bunn PA Jr: Treatment of T-cell lymphomas: Mycosis fungoides and the Sézary syndrome, in Conn HF (ed), Current Therapy 1985. Philadelphia, WB Saunders, p 317, 1985

40. Bunn PA Jr, Carney DN: Treatment of cutaneous T-cell lymphomas. J Dermatol Surg Oncol 6:383–388, 1980

41. Bunn PA, Foon KA, Ihde DC, et al: Recombinant leukocyte A interferon: An active agent in advanced cutaneous T-cell lymphomas. Ann Intern Med 101:484–487, 1984

42. Averbuch SD, Austin HA III, Sherwin SA, et al: Acute interstitial nephritis with nephrotic syndrome following recombinant leukocyte A interferon therapy for mycosis fungoides. N Engl J Med 310:32–35, 1984

43. Foon KA, Dougher G: Increased growth of eyelashes in a patient given leukocyte A interferon. N Engl J Med 311:1259, 1984 (letter)

Alpha Interferon Therapy of AIDS-Associated Kaposi's Sarcoma

Donald I. Abrams and Paul A. Volberding

Alpha interferon has been the most widely studied biologic response modifier for the treatment of Kaposi's sarcoma (KS) associated with acquired immune deficiency syndrome (AIDS). At San Francisco General Hospital's AIDS Clinic, three sequential trials of recombinant interferon alfa-2b (Intron® A) were conducted between August 1982 and April 1984. In the first study, ten patients with early KS were randomized to receive either low-dose (1 MU/m²) subcutaneous (SC) or high-dose (50 MU/m²) intravenous (IV) treatment 5 days per week, every other week, for eight weeks. A perceived advantage of the latter regimen led to a subsequent trial in which 20 subjects received high-dose IV therapy. A 32% objective response rate was achieved, despite the fact that these patients had less favorable disease status and more constitutional symptoms than those in the first trial and had also experienced previous opportunistic infections (OIs). A final 8-week investigation evaluated the use of 30 MU/m² three times per week in 30 subjects. Drug-related toxicity seemed more pronounced with this regimen, but overall objective responses were identical to those seen in the high-dose IV study. None of the trials produced evidence of immune reconstitution on laboratory evaluation. The patients were not protected from developing AIDS-related OI either during or following interferon therapy, although OI was diagnosed less frequently in responders, who also displayed a distinct survival advantage over those with progressive disease. These trends remained evident when the data from the three studies were pooled with those from three parallel trials conducted at the University of California, Los Angeles (UCLA). Studies evaluating the combined use of alpha interferon and chemotherapeutic agents known to be active against AIDS-related KS (such as VP-16 and vinblastine) have thus far failed to demonstrate a synergistic antitumor effect, while toxicity has increased. In light of in vitro evidence that alpha interferon suppresses the AIDS retrovirus and has clinical efficacy in KS comparable to that of cytotoxic agents, additional investigations, focusing on maximizing therapeutic potential, are warranted.

IN THE SAN FRANCISCO area, up to one third of all males diagnosed as having acquired immune deficiency syndrome (AIDS) initially present with Kaposi's sarcoma (KS), a malignant disease characterized by cutaneous and visceral lesions.[1,2] Although some cytotoxic agents are effective against KS, they may further compromise immune responses in patients with AIDS.[3-12] For this reason, alpha interferon, a biologic response modifier, has been widely studied in the treatment of these individuals.[13-20]

INTERFERON ALFA-2b TRIALS

From August 1982 to April 1984, three trials undertaken at the AIDS Clinic of San Francisco General Hospital (SFGH) evaluated the effects of recombinant interferon alfa-2b (Intron® A) in a total of 60 patients with KS.[15,16,21,22] A similar number of patients were enrolled in concurrent trials at the University of California, Los Angeles (UCLA).[15,23] These studies were aimed at determining the agent's ability to control the progression of disease, reconstitute the immune system, and prevent the development of subsequent opportunistic infections (OIs). The study protocols and laboratory tests followed are summarized in Table 1.

The response criteria were defined as follows:

1. Complete response—eradication of all previously detectable disease
2. Partial response—a 50% decrease in the biperpendicular size or number of lesions or nodes
3. Minor response/stable disease—less than a partial response, with no new evidence of disease
4. Progressive disease—an increase in the size or number of lesions or nodes

The second and third definitions allowed for some subjective interpretation regarding the nodularity and pigmentation of lesions.

In the first trial, ten patients with early KS were randomized to receive either low-dose

From the AIDS Clinic, San Francisco General Hospital, San Francisco, and the University of California, San Francisco.

Address reprint requests to Donald I. Abrams, MD, Ward 84, 995 Potrero Avenue, San Francisco, CA 94110.

This work was supported in part by NIH grant U01 CA34980.

D.I.A. is a recipient of an American Cancer Society Career Development Award.

Table 1. Study Designs and Laboratory Tests Used in Interferon Alfa-2b Trials in Patients with AIDS-Related Kaposi's Sarcoma at San Francisco General Hospital (SFGH) and the University of California at Los Angeles (UCLA)

Study designs	Three sequential trials of interferon alfa-2b conducted in parallel at SFGH and UCLA
	1. Randomized: • Low dose SC (1 MU/m², 5 days QD x 8 weeks)
	• High dose IV (50 MU/m², 5 days QD x 8 weeks)
	2. High dose IV (50 MU/m², 5 days QD x 8 weeks)
	3. High dose SC (30 MU x m², SC TIW x 8 weeks)
Laboratory tests	*Candida*-induced mitogenesis
	Endoscopy in earlier patients
	Interferon and interferon neutralizing
	T-lymphocyte subsets

Abbreviations: MU, million units; QD, daily; TIW, three times weekly.

(1 MU/m²) subcutaneous (SC) or high-dose (50 MU/m²) intravenous (IV) alpha interferon 5 days per week, every other week, for 8 weeks.[15,21,22]

The subjects who received the high-dose IV therapy had a 40% overall response rate (combining complete and partial responses), compared to 20% in the low-dose SC group. Furthermore, of four subjects who failed or progressed on the low-dose SC regimen, two achieved objective responses when switched to high-dose IV therapy.

The more favorable outcomes on high-dose treatment prompted a second 8-week study designed to assess the effects of this regimen in another group of 20 patients. A 32% objective response rate was achieved, even though these subjects had less favorable disease status than those in the first study, as evidenced by more lymphatic and visceral involvement, a greater number of constitutional symptoms, and histories of previous OIs.[16,22]

Subsequently, a third trial was undertaken using 30 MU/m² of interferon alfa-2b via the SC, rather than IV, route, to provide ease of administration and allow patients to treat themselves at home. The overall objective response rate in these 30 subjects, who received the agent three times per week for 8 weeks, was identical to that seen in high-dose IV study, but drug-related toxicity appeared more pronounced.[22]

Pooling the results of the three protocols, alpha interferon therapy produced a 35% response rate in the 60 KS patients. When the results of these trials were combined with those of three parallel studies conducted at UCLA, which enrolled the same number of subjects, a 30% to 40% overall response rate was seen.[24] In analyzing the combined SFGH and UCLA results, several trends became evident (Table 2).

In the initial randomized trials at both institutions, higher doses of alpha interferon were found more effective than lower doses. In all the studies, responders tended to have a survival

Table 2. Results of Interferon Alfa-2b Trials in Patients with AIDS-Related Kaposi's Sarcoma at San Francisco General Hospital (SFGH) and the University of California at Los Angeles (UCLA)

Patients	• 20 in randomized trial (high IV v low SC dose)
	• 40 in high-dose IV trial
	• 60 in high-dose SC trial
Results	• 30% to 40% complete plus partial response in Kaposi's lesions
	• Response rate greater with high than with low doses
	• Opportunistic infections occurred, especially in nonresponders
	• No evidence of immune augmentation
Toxicity	• Fever, malaise, and myalgias in all patients
	• Transient paresthesia, mild confusion, insomnia, leukopenia, thrombocytopenia
	• Mild hepatotoxicity; severe hepatotoxicity rare

advantage over nonresponders, even though no evidence of immune-system restoration was observed when laboratory parameters were evaluated. The subjects were not protected from the development of AIDS-related OI either during or following interferon therapy, but the frequency of OI was lower in responders. Whether the interferon itself contributed to the lower incidence of OIs and, consequently, prolonged survival remains unclear. This effect may simply have resulted from the fact that responders were more likely to have more favorable courses from the outset.

In general, the treatment was well tolerated, except for subjective toxicity at higher doses. All the subjects suffered toxicity in the form of fever, malaise, and myalgias. Other side effects included transient paresthesias, mild confusion, insomnia, leukopenia, thrombocytopenia, and mild hepatotoxicity; severe hepatotoxicity was rare. Some toxic effects, such as confusion and insomnia, were slow to resolve, however, and therapy had to be discontinued due to intolerable flu-like symptoms in a small number of patients.

RESULTS OF OTHER STUDIES

The trends noted in the SFGH/UCLA investigations have been reflected in the findings of other studies on the use of alpha interferon in the treatment of AIDS-associated KS.

The advantage of using high doses, for instance, can be confirmed by a review of the literature. Designating 20 MU/m^2 as the dividing line between low and high doses, the results of three low-dose and six high-dose trials performed in the United States have shown that the latter approach is clearly more effective (Table 3).[13-24]

Table 3. Efficacy of Low- *v* High-Dose Therapy with Alpha Interferon in AIDS-Related Kaposi's Sarcoma*

Response	Low Dose ($<$20 MU/m^2) (n = 65)	High Dose ($>$20 MU/m^2) (n = 105)
Complete	1 (2%)	18 (17%)
Partial	3 (5%)	27 (26%)
Minor or stable	13 (20%)	17 (16%)
Progression	48 (74%)	43 (41%)

Abbreviations: MU, million units, n, number of evaluable patients.

* Data compiled from results of three low- and six high-dose studies conducted at San Francisco General Hospital, the University of California at Los Angeles, M.D. Anderson Hospital and Tumor Institute, Memorial Sloan-Kettering Cancer Center, and the National Cancer Institute.

Most investigators have attempted to determine what factors in patients with AIDS-related KS are predictive of response to alpha interferon.[13,14,17,18,20,22,23] The factors that have been suggested include an absence of constitutional symptoms, an absence of a history of previous OI, and a more intact immune system (as demonstrated by a higher number of total T-helper lymphocytes as well as the absence of anergy). In addition, the presence of detectable circulating interferon prior to therapy has been associated with a poorer prognosis and diminished response to the agent.[17,25]

OTHER THERAPEUTIC APPROACHES

Other therapeutic approaches evaluated in patients with AIDS-related KS have included cytotoxic drugs, either alone or in combination with alpha interferon, as well as a host of noncytotoxic agents.

In our experience, the overall objective response rate to alpha interferon has equaled or surpassed that of conventional cytotoxic chemotherapy. At SFGH, the use of weekly IV vinblastine has produced 25% to 28% overall response rates.[8] A regimen consisting of doxorubicin, bleomycin, and vinblastine was abandoned soon after we began treating patients with this disease, because it seemed to cause more rapid deterioration and development of OI.[26]

To date, only two studies have reported on the combined use of alpha interferon and cytotoxic agents. In an investigation at New York University, VP-16 was combined with alpha interferon in two protocols.[27] In the first protocol, interferon was given initially as induction therapy for 8 weeks, followed by VP-16 for 4 months. Of 12 patients treated, only two were able to complete the study, and only one attained a partial response. The therapy did not prevent the development of OIs. In the second protocol, alpha interferon and VP-16 were given

Table 4. Results of Investigational Drug Trials in Patients with AIDS-Related Kaposi's Sarcoma at San Francisco General Hospital

Agent	N	Response		Immune Benefit	Anti-retrovirus	Toxicity
		KS	OI			
Alpha interferon	60	35%	?	No	NT	+ − ++
Gamma interferon	15	No	No	No	NT	++ − +++
Interleukin-2	87	No	No	No	NT	High dose
Suramin	23	No	No	No	22%	+++
HPA-23	16	No	No	NA	NA	+

Abbreviations: OI, opportunistic infection; N, number of evaluable patients; NT, not tested; NA, not available.

concurrently in escalating doses. This regimen was associated with low response rates, and OIs again developed. The investigators noted that the combination regimen produced lower response rates and a higher incidence of OI than has been reported with either agent alone.

Another study, conducted at M.D. Anderson Hospital and Tumor Institute, examined the use of alpha interferon (20 MU/m^2/day intramuscularly) plus vinblastine (5 mg/m^2 every other week) over a period of 60 days in 15 patients with advanced KS.[28] Although two complete and seven partial responses were achieved, these investigators noted marked suppression of host defense mechanisms and, therefore, recommended against the use of this combined regimen.

At our own center, we have studied the use of gamma interferon, interleukin 2 (IL-2), suramin, and HPA-23 in AIDS-related KS (Table 4). Of 15 subjects treated with gamma interferon, none responded and no benefits were noted with regard to immunologic status or development of OI (unpublished). Likewise, no responders were found among 87 patients treated with IL-2.[22,29] When suramin was given to 23 subjects, five cleared their retrovirus, but KS progressed in all patients and OIs developed.[30] Preliminary evaluations of our recent investigation of the use of HPA-23 in 16 KS patients demonstrated neither retardation of the disease process nor decreased incidence of OI (unpublished). Of all the alternatives to cytotoxic therapy that we have evaluated to date in AIDS-associated KS, therefore, only interferon alfa-2b has produced responses.

CONCLUSION

In patients with AIDS-associated KS, overall objective response rates with alpha interferon have equaled or surpassed those seen with conventional cytotoxic chemotherapy. The treatment is well tolerated, except for subjective toxicity at higher doses. Higher doses have produced more favorable response rates than have lower doses, although no reproducible positive effects on immune status have been noted. In light of the fact that other non-cytotoxic agents have not yielded comparable results, and that cytotoxic therapy may further compromise immune status, alpha interferon may be considered a viable front-line treatment for these patients. Further studies are warranted to maximize the agent's therapeutic potential and evaluate its in vivo efficacy against the causative retrovirus.

REFERENCES

1. Hymes KB, Cheung TL, Greene JB, et al: Kaposi's sarcoma in homosexual men: A report of 8 cases. Lancet 2:598, 1981

2. Friedman-Kien AE, Lauberstein LJ, Rubenstein P, et al: Disseminated Kaposi's sarcoma in homosexual men. Ann Intern Med 96 (Part 1):693–700, 1983

3. Volberding P, Conant MA, Stricker RB, et al: Chemotherapy in advanced Kaposi's sarcoma. Am J Med 74:652–656, 1983

4. Krigel RL: The natural history and treatment of epidemic Kaposi's sarcoma, in Selikoff IJ, Teirstein AS, Hirschman SZ (eds): Acquired Immune Deficiency Syndrome, vol 437. New York, The New York Academy of Sciences, 1984

5. Laubenstein LJ, Kreigel RL, Odajnyk CM, et al: Treatment of epidemic Kaposi's sarcoma with etoposide or a combination of doxorubicin, bleomycin, and vinblastine. J Clin Oncol 2:1115–1120, 1984

6. Volberding P: Therapy of Kaposi's sarcoma in AIDS. Semin Oncol 11:60–67, 1984

7. Volberding P, Abrams D, Kaplan L, et al: Therapy of AIDS-related Kaposi's sarcoma with ICRF-159. Proc Am Soc Clin Oncol 4:4, 1985

8. Volberding PA, Abrams DI, Conant MA, et al: Vinblastine therapy of Kaposi's sarcoma in AIDS. Ann Intern Med 103:335–338, 1985

9. Mintzer DM, Real FX, Jovino L, et al: Treatment of Kaposi's sarcoma and thrombocytopenia with vinblastine in patients with the acquired immunodeficiency syndrome. Ann Intern Med 102:200–202, 1985

10. Volberding P: Kaposi's sarcoma and the acquired immunodeficiency syndrome, in Cooney TG, Ward TT (eds): The Medical Clinics of North America, vol 70. Philadelphia, W. B. Saunders Company, 1986, pp 665–675

11. Armentrout SA: Cytotoxic chemotherapy in Kaposi's sarcoma, in Gupta S (ed): AIDS-Associated Syndromes, vol 187. New York, Plenum Press, 1985

12. Volberding PA: The problem of Kaposi's sarcoma in AIDS, in Vaeth JM (ed): Frontiers of Radiation Therapy and Oncology: Cancer and AIDS, vol 19. New York, Karger, 1985, pp 91–98

13. Krown SE, Real FX, Cunningham-Rundles S, et al: Preliminary observations on the effects of recombinant leukocyte a interferon in homosexual men with Kaposi's sarcoma. N Engl J Med 308:1071–1076, 1983

14. Krown SE, Real FX, Krim M, et al: Recombinant leukocyte A interferon in Kaposi's sarcoma. Proceedings of The New York Academy of Sciences, 437:431–438, 1984

15. Groopman JE, Gottlieb MS, Goodman J, et al: Recombinant alpha-2 interferon therapy for Kaposi's sarcoma associated with acquired immune deficiency syndrome. Ann Intern Med 100:671–676, 1984

16. Volberding P, Valero R, Rothman J, et al: Alpha interferon therapy of Kaposi's sarcoma in AIDS, in Selikoff IJ, Teirstein AS, Hirschman SZ (eds): Acquired Immune Deficiency Syndrome, vol 437. New York, The New York Academy of Sciences, 1984

17. Gelmann EP, Preble OT, Steis R, et al: Human lymphoblastoid interferon treatment of Kaposi's sarcoma in the acquired immune deficiency syndrome: Clinical response and prognostic parameters. Am J Med 78:737–741, 1985

18. Krown SE, Real FX, Krim M, et al: Interferons and other biological response modifiers in the treatment of Kaposi's sarcoma, in Vaeth JM (ed): Frontiers of Radiation Therapy and Oncology: Cancer and AIDS, vol 19. New York, Karger, 1985, pp 138–149

19. Rios A, Mansell PWA, Newell GR, et al: Treatment of acquired immunodeficiency syndrome-related Kaposi's sarcoma with lymphoblastoid interferon. J Clin Oncol 3:506–512, 1985

20. Krown SE, Real FX, Vadhan-Raj S, et al: Kaposi's sarcoma and the acquired immune deficiency syndrome. Cancer 57:1662–1665, 1986

21. Volberding PA: Therapy of Kaposi's sarcoma with interferon, in Friedman-Kien AE, Laubenstein LJ (eds): AIDS: The Epidemic of Kaposi's Sarcoma and Opportunistic Infections, New York, Masson Publishing USA, Inc, 1984, pp 63–67

22. Volberding PA, Wofsy CB, Abrams DI: Interferon and interleukin-2 therapy of Kaposi's sarcoma, in Gupta S (ed): AIDS-Associated Syndromes, vol 187. New York, Plenum Press, 1985

23. Mitsuyasu RT, Taylor JMG, Glaspy J, et al: Heterogeneity of epidemic Kaposi's sarcoma: Implications for therapy. Cancer 57:1657–1661, 1986

24. Volberding PA, Mitsuyasu RT, Golando JP, et al: Treatment of Kaposi's sarcoma with alfa-2b interferon (INTRON A). Cancer (in press)

25. Preble OT, Rook AH, Steis R, et al: Interferon-induced 2′–5′ oligoadenylate synthetase during interferon-alpha therapy in homosexual men with Kaposi's sarcoma: Marked deficiency in biochemical response to interferon in patients with acquired immunodeficiency syndrome. J Infect Dis 152:457–465, 1985

26. Lewis BJ, Abrams DI, Ziegler J, et al: Single agent or combination chemotherapy of Kaposi's sarcoma in AIDS. Proc Am Soc Clin Oncol 2:59, 1983

27. Lonberg M, Odajnyk C, Krigel R, et al: Sequential and simultaneous alpha 2 interferon (IFN) and VP-16 in epidemic Kaposi's sarcoma (EKS). Proc Am Soc Clin Oncol 4:2, 1985

28. Rios A, Mansell P, Newel G, et al: The use of lymphoblastoid interferon Hu IFN alpha (LY) and vinblastine in the treatment of acquired immunodeficiency syndrome (AIDS) related Kaposi's sarcoma (KS). Proc Am Soc Clin Oncol 4:6, 1985

29. Volberding P, Abrams D, Beardslee D, et al: Recombinant interleukin-2 (rIL-2) therapy of AIDS. Second International Conference on AIDS, Paris, 1986

30. Kaplan LD, Abrams DI, Wong R, et al: Failure of suramin as treatment for AIDS. Second International Conference on AIDS, Paris, 1986

Potential Applications of the Interferons in Oncology: Lessons Drawn From Studies of Human Melanoma

John M. Kirkwood and Marc Ernstoff

The rationale for application of interferons in the treatment of melanoma is based on evidence suggesting that this tumor exhibits antigens capable of eliciting a host immune response. Agents that act as immunomodulators or that enhance the expression of tumor antigens may have greater therapeutic potential than agents that act solely as direct cytotoxic or antiproliferative agents. Data suggest that interferons may manifest all three categories of antineoplastic function. Early empirical trials with naturally derived leukocyte-lymphoblastoid interferons yielded poor therapeutic results. In contrast, in four subsequent trials conducted using recombinant DNA–synthesized interferon alfa 2's at three independent institutions, an objective response rate of 19% was achieved. Of the 20 responses obtained in the 102 evaluable patients, eight were complete. Three further preliminary reports enlarged the data base to 215 patients, 35 of whom showed an objective response. The response to systemic interferon alfa-2's appears to be associated with several factors including (1) continuous treatment for periods of up to several months at dosages greater than 10 MU/day intravenously (IV) or intramuscularly (IM) or 12.5 MU/m²/day IM on alternate days, and (2) metastatic tumor involving nonvisceral sites and the lung. The analysis of immunologic and other factors that may be related to or predictive of response has been hampered by the low overall frequency of response. New trials currently in progress to determine the efficacy of interferon alfa-2's as an adjuvant to surgery in candidates at high risk of recurrence and the efficacy of interferon alfa-2's when used in combination with gamma interferon, other biological agents, and chemotherapy may allow these questions to be resolved.

THE CLINICAL application of interferons in cancer has followed a more rigorous path than that of most other immunologic approaches to cancer therapy. Yet the empirical study designs used have generally focused *first* on toxicity or clinical response and second on the analysis and optimization of immunologic parameters that distinguish the interferons and other biological response modifiers from conventional chemotherapy. The multiplicity of direct and indirect activities of interferon when administered in vivo has complicated the development of definitive clinical trials of interferon for cancer therapy, and no in vitro parameter has yet been shown to reflect or predict response. Only a few trials have systematically analyzed immune function in patients treated with interferon, and even fewer trials have focused on homogeneous populations of cancer patients with a single malignancy such as melanoma.[1]

Because of its cutaneous origin and pattern of metastasis to the skin and soft tissues, melanoma is particularly well suited to immunologic study and intervention. Histopathology, in vitro laboratory findings, and much circumstantial and direct clinical evidence suggest that this tumor is immunogenic.[2-5] Unfortunately, a further impetus to the evaluation of new immunologic modalities lies in the well-recognized failure of all conventional chemotherapy to alter the survival of patients with metastatic melanoma. No acceptable standard chemotherapy regimen exists either for patients with advanced disease with surgically incurable metastasis or for those at a high risk of postoperative relapse as indicated by deep primary lesions >3 to 4 mm or regional lymph node metastasis.

Although we lack treatments for melanoma, in the last decade prognostic factors have been identified that improve the precision with which we may predict relapse and death from primary melanoma in stage I and regionally (lymph node) metastatic melanoma in stage II.[6,7] More recently, epidemiologic studies of the exponentially rising incidence of melanoma have pointed to a potentially treatable syndrome of dysplastic nevi, which have been identified as

From the Division of Medical Oncology, Department of Medicine, Pittsburgh Cancer Institute and University Health Center of Pittsburgh, Pittsburgh, Pennsylvania.

Supported by Grant IM-433 from the American Cancer Society and Clinical Study Awards from Schering-Plough Corporation, Hoffman-LaRoche Corporation, and Biogen Corporation.

Address reprint requests to John M. Kirkwood, MD, Division of Medical Oncology, Department of Medicine, Pittsburgh Cancer Institute and University Health Center of Pittsburgh, 230 Lothrop Street, Pittsburgh, PA 15213-2592.

direct precursors in familial melanoma.[8,9] While the role of the dysplastic nevus in sporadic melanoma is yet to be established, it appears that the presence of the dysplastic nevus is, at the least, a marker for melanoma susceptibility in this situation. Our options for melanoma prophylaxis in patients with sporadic dysplastic nevi will depend upon the demonstration of their role in non-familial melanoma (direct, indirect, or simple bystander). Thus, given the appropriate agents, intervention is theoretically feasible at all stages of progression in the neoplastic cutaneous melanocyte.

RATIONALE FOR USE OF INTERFERONS IN MELANOMA

The rationale for the use of interferons in melanoma is based on many different lines of evidence. The simplest effects of interferon, summarized in Table 1, are the direct effects. In fact, direct tumor stem cell inhibition has been correlated with response or lack of response to a number of antineoplastic agents.[10-12] The interferons have been shown to mediate additive or synergistic effects in multiple melanoma cell lines, as illustrated in Figure 1.

Table 1. Direct Effects of Interferon on Tumor

- Antiviral state and enzyme induction (2′–5′ A synthetase endonuclease, kinase)
- Inhibition of proliferation, phase-specific in some cells
- Down regulation of oncogene(s) associated with inhibition of proliferation
- Dependence upon binding to cell surface receptor of high affinity
- Receptor for alpha/beta differs from that for gamma
- Diverse dose-dependent effects—antiviral, antiproliferative, immune
- Combinations of alpha/beta and gamma variable—synergistic, additive, or antagonistic, according to cell studied

However real the direct in vitro inhibition of melanoma may be, it may be difficult to achieve similar effects in vivo given the requirement of continuous exposure to interferon at concentrations that are only transiently achievable pharmacologically in patients. However, with the synergism observed in certain tumor cells, meaningful direct antitumor effects may be achieved with combinations of interferons or interferon and other lymphokines. Phase-specific

Inhibition of in vitro growth of three human melanoma cell lines exposed to interferon alfa-2b (▨) or interferon gamma (▧) alone, at 100 U/mL and 10,000 U/mL, or to 50 or 5,000 U/mL of each (▩) for 48 hours.

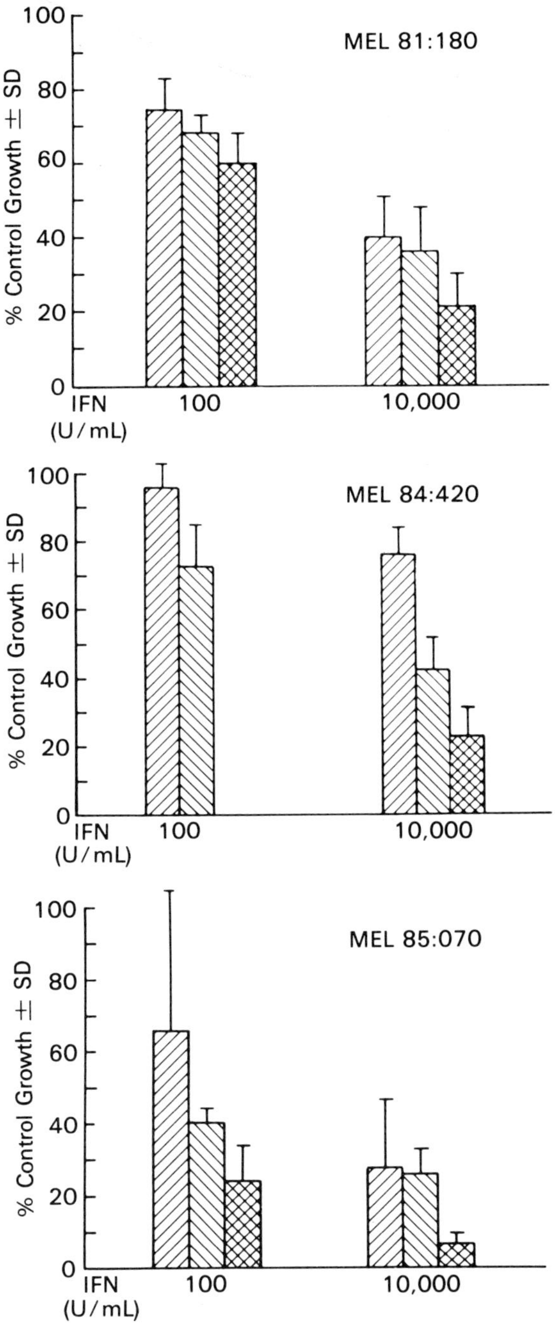

Figure 1. Subconfluent cultures of three human melanoma cell lines established in the author's laboratory show similar growth inhibition, with dose-dependent effects always greater for the combination of 5,000 U/mL of each ($p<0.01$ by t-test).

cell cycle effects first demonstrated in melanoma cells have now been analyzed at the level of oncogene expression. Interferon alpha inhibits the platelet-derived growth factor–induced nuclear competence family, including c-fos and c-myc, within minutes to hours of exposure to the growth factor. Consequently, interferon-treated cells fail to enter the S phase in the presence of the growth factor.[13] Interferon alpha has also been shown to inhibit transformation in 3T3 cells and LTK^- cells by multiple viral and cellular oncogenes (*v*-Ha-ras, *c*-Ha-ras, and *c*-Ki-ras) as well as the herpesvirus tk gene.[14,15]

The appearance of lymphoid host infiltrate in both the primary melanoma and the dysplastic nevi precursor but not in advanced metastatic lesions of melanoma suggests that the early disease process is perceived differently from the advanced disease. One possible explanation for this observation is the loss of immunogenic determinants in advanced disease. Alternatively, immunosuppression-inducing determinants may arise in the metastatic tumor cell.

Recently, primary melanomas have been shown to lose the expression of class I major histocompatibility complex (MHC) antigens as depth increases and prognosis worsens.[16-19] In fact, diminished expression of class I MHC gene products without gene deletions or rearrangements has been associated with increased tumorigenicity of human adenovirus-12–transformed cells, which can be inhibited by treatment of the transformed cells with interferon alpha.[20,21] The augmented expression of products of the MHC in tumor cells may facilitate recognition for induction of immune response, effector function of cellular elements, or antibody. In the case of class II antigens of the MHC, these are essential to antigen presentation (Table 2).

However, the role of class II products in melanoma cells is complex. Although MHC class II antigens are required for the induction of cellular immune response to primary melanoma cells, their presence in metastatic melanoma cells appears to be associated with the capacity of the metastatic cells to suppress proliferative-cytotoxic host immune response.[22,23]

Class II antigen induction by interferon may be important in a wide range of immunocytes, vascular endothelial cells, and the cells of a number of different tumors. The regulation of class II MHC antigen expression by interferon has been carefully studied and is classically a property of interferon gamma. Even when cells are resistant to the antiproliferative effects of interferon gamma and fail to modulate class I MHC product and 100 Kd as well as 240 Kd tumor-associated antigen expression, they continue to respond with increased expression of class II MHC products.[24,25] Human melanoma has been studied at a clonal level where phenotypic variation at baseline (untreated) is further complicated by variable interferon responsiveness of the cloned tumor cells derived from early melanoma cultures.[26] The hierarchy in DR>DP>DQ product expression noted in fresh and noncloned cultures of melanoma has been demonstrated in these clones as well. With the alpha/beta interferons (which induce predominantly class I MHC antigen expression without class II products in tumor cells), and with different ambient levels of gamma interferon (which has selectively greater effects upon class II [DR, DP, DQ] antigens), a gamut of afferent and efferent immune effects may be anticipated in the host.

The immunomodulating effects of interferon upon the host are of perhaps greatest interest to immunologists, for there has been long-standing evidence that the anticancer activity of interferon depends upon the host. Interferon is active in vivo against tumors resistant to the antiproliferative activity of interferon.[27] The subject of interferon and T, natural killer (NK), and macrophage effectors has been reviewed extensively and is not yet specifically pertinent to findings related to melanoma treatment in

Table 2. Augmentation of Cell Surface Antigens by Interferon

- Major histocompatibility complex (MHC)
  - Class I—all interferons
  - Class II—especially gamma
    - Cell-cell interactions in immune system
    - Antigen presentation
- Tumor-associated, tumor-restricted, (altered MHC) variable influence
  - Role of antigen shedding uncertain

Table 3. Modulation of Host Response Mechanisms by Interferon

- T cell
  - Suppressor T—inhibition
  - Helper or cytotoxic—activation
- B cell
  - Kinetic determinants—Ig augmented when interferon prior to antigen
- Natural killer cell activation
- Macrophage activation

vivo.[28,29] The parameters of host response (Table 3) critical in the antitumor response remain unknown. It is clear, however, that effects of interferon on all potential effectors are time-, dose-, and schedule-dependent and may differ according to the nature and stage of the disease being treated.

The analysis of published trials of interferon alpha has most commonly focused on NK cell function. Experimental designs have varied widely from single-dose to multiple-dose studies using schedules ranging from twice weekly to multiple daily intravenous (IV) or intramuscular (IM) administration.[30-40] Original clinical studies using partially purified leukocyte interferon alfa-2a revealed augmented NK activity 24 hours after initial daily IM treatment with 1.5 to 6 MU and sustained elevations of NK activity for up to 12 months.[33-35] The subsequent American Cancer Society–sponsored US multi-institutional trial conducted in more homogeneous (melanoma) patient populations showed a later peak of activation with IM doses of 1 to 9 MU/day and depression of NK activity at 1 day.[36] Further US trials in a more heterogeneous patient population suggested that sustained activation of NK function occurred primarily in patients with low baseline NK activity.[37]

Studies using more highly purified lymphoblastoid and recombinant DNA–synthesized interferon alfa-2's have recently been conducted. Single-dose studies showed suppression of NK activity 12 hours postadministration.[38] Results of more detailed crossover studies have suggested a relatively low optimal dose of 3 MU of IM recombinant interferon alfa-2's. This effect, however, could be detected only after overnight culture of lymphocytes in interferon-free medium and was expressed in terms of a log-transformed lytic unit index. Direct assay of freshly obtained blood lymphocytes revealed no such activation.[39,40] This finding suggests that certain control mechanisms occurring in vivo may be abrogated by overnight "resting" in vitro.

The heterogeneous patient populations involved in most studies have made clinical correlations of antitumor response difficult or impossible except in rare instances.[33-35,41,42] The dissection of multiple host parameters in homogeneous populations of patients is perhaps possible only now with the use of phenotypic and functional assays to determine the role of separate effector mechanisms against *autologous* tumor in vivo. The recently elucidated role of adherent monocytic suppressor cells in the regulation of NK function during in vivo treatment with interferon alpha points to the need for separate attention to T-T, T-B, NK-B, and macrophage-T, macrophage-B, and macrophage-NK interactions in the composite analysis of their role in cancer treatment.[43] The role of interferon must presently be ascertained in-

Table 4. Results of Early Clinical Trials With Leukocyte/Lymphoblast Partially Purified Interferon

Study	Treatment Regimen (IM)	Number of Patients		Responses		
		Entered	Evaluable	Complete	Partial	None
Retsas et al,[44] 1983	0.5 MU/m^2/day	17	17	1	1	15
Krown et al,[45] 1984	1 MU/day x 42	16	16	0	1	15
	3 MU/day x 42	14	14	0	0	14
	9 MU/day x 42	14	14	0	0	14
Goldberg et al,[46] 1984	15 MU/m^2 tiw 2/3 wks x 12 wks	21	17	1	1	15
	0.5 MU/m^2/wk x 12 wks	12	11	0	0	11
	0.5 MU/m^2/day x 6 wks	11	8	0	0	8

Table 5. Preliminary Reports of Systemically Administered Interferon Alfa-2b in Metastatic Melanoma

Study	Treatment Regimen	Number of Patients	Response		
			Complete	Partial	None
Bretaudeau, Pouillart,[57] 1984	10 MU/day, IV	19	0	6	13
Hawkins et al,[54] 1984	30 MU/m²/day, 5/21 days, IV	29	1	1	27
Robinson et al,[56] 1984	30 MU/m²/day, 5/21 days, IV	31	0	1	30
	30 MU/m²/day, tiw, SC	32	2	4	26
Total		111	3	12	96

dependently of any real conception of its mechanism of action. Subsequent analysis may then determine its mechanism and optimal use.

CLINICAL EXPERIENCE WITH INTERFERON

Results of empirical clinical trials using natural leukocyte and lymphoblastoid interferon have been disappointing. In 96 evaluable patients, only two complete and three partial responses were achieved. Median dosages of 1 to 3 MU/day were used in these early trials (Table 4).[44-46] One subgroup treated with a maximum of 15 MU/m² showed an 11.8% objective response rate (2/17). Treatment duration ranged from 4 to 6 weeks. The only schedule sustained for 12 weeks was an interrupted schedule given for 2 of 3 weeks.

Cimetidine, an H_2-receptor blocker with T-cell immunoregulatory activity, now appears to have little adjunctive activity when given with systemic interferon alpha. This observation contrasts with original findings obtained with intralesional interferon alpha in patients with cutaneous metastases.[47-55]

Experience with recombinant DNA-synthesized interferon alfa-2b and interferon alfa-2a has now been reported from several institutions. Preliminary data are available from several other centers (Table 5).[54,56,57] These trials, which employed diverse routes, doses, and schedules of administration, resulted in remarkably consistent findings. First, intermittent administration for 5 days every 3 weeks appeared less active than the thrice-weekly schedule. If the low-dose schedules of intermittent treatment are eliminated, a 23.5% response rate (12/51) was achieved, based on reports in the abstract literature.

More fully detailed trials (Table 6),[32,58-61] yield a response rate of 19.6% in 102 evaluable patients. Factors associated with response have been best examined systematically at the Mayo Clinic, where Creagan and associates observed 21 responses among 96 patients, and logistic regression enabled testing of prospectively identified clinical parameters, including performance status, prior chemotherapy, prior radiotherapy, age >56 years, male sex, dosage (12.5 MU *v* 50 MU/m²), and addition of cimetidine. None of these factors was found to correlate with treatment outcome. The single factor that proved to be a covariate of response in these studies was the presence of visceral-dominant metastases, which was identified as an adverse prognostic

Table 6. Published Studies of Systemically Administered Single-Agent Interferon Alfa-2's in Metastatic Melanoma

Study	Treatment Regimen	Number of Patients		Response		
		Entered	Evaluable	Complete	Partial	None
Creagan et al,[60] 1984	12 MU/m²/day, tiw x 12 wks, IM	30	30	1	5	24
Creagan et al,[61] 1984	50 MU/m²/day, tiw x 12 wks, IM	31	31	3	4	24
Kirkwood et al,[32] 1985	10–100 MU/day, x 5 days/wk, IV	16	16	2	0	14
	3–100 MU/day, IM	7	7	1	2	4
Hersey et al,[59] 1985	50 MU/m²/day, tiw, IM	20	18	1	1	16
Total		104	102	8	12	82

factor. It is notable that more than one fourth of the responses in this study occurred *after* the first month of treatment.

A recently published trial conducted in Australia using interferon alfa-2a involved 20 patients. Two patients were considered inevaluable and withdrawn at 2 to 4 weeks. One of these patients, however, had no evidence of tumor at operation for presumed (radiographically) progressive bony disease. Two complete responses were documented at 4 and 10 weeks of treatment among the remaining 18 patients evaluated. Treatment was stopped at ≤ 5 weeks in nine patients, and five other patients died within 8 weeks of the start of the study. The authors conclude that response is negatively correlated with performance status but that treatment is not well tolerated in patients of performance status 2. Table 7 lists the common factors that influenced tumor response in trials with interferon alpha. Again, it is uncertain which systemic effects are desirable and associated with increased response rates.

Table 7. Factors Associated With Tumor Response in Clinical Studies of Interferon Alpha in Melanoma

- Patient selection for tolerance of treatment
  - Dosage, route
  - Time on treatment
- Tumor selection
  - Nonvisceral metastases—cutaneous, soft tissue, nodal, lung
  - Size—micrometastases in the adjuvant setting
- Continuous treatment
  - Regular schedule
  - Sufficient dosage to attain systemic effects
- End points assuring sufficient treatment for evaluability
  - Definitions of toxicity for dose reduction, discontinuation of treatment
  - Definitions of progression as for hormonal modality <1 month, 2–3 months, >3 months

Two of three objective complete responses seen by investigators at Yale are sustained at >36 months. One relapse has occurred at 36 months, with the brain as the only site of recurrent melanoma. Three patients treated at the Mayo Clinic remain in remission 25, 26, and 35 months after the start of treatment. Thus, of the 18% to 26% of patients who have responded, one third have achieved complete and enduring regressions. The three patients in whom complete remission was achieved at our institution include two men and one woman with histologically documented metastatic recurrence at cervical nodes, multiple cutaneous and suspected osseous sites, and retroperitoneal soft tissues. These patients required 4, 24, and 8 weeks to enter remission and remain alive in remission for more than 36 months since initial interferon treatment by the IV or IV and subcutaneous routes and 12 to 24 months since the last interferon treatment.

CURRENT AND FUTURE DIRECTIONS

Although activity against melanoma is apparent in the phase I-II trials reviewed here, further randomized tests of interferon in phase II investigations are necessary to establish its activity. Such trials will be virtually senseless if not accompanied by an examination of the mechanism of action and a systematic effort to improve the outcome of therapy.

Toxicity reduction is one essential issue in need of further study. It remains uncertain whether we can ameliorate toxicity with the use of either conventional antipyretics/analgesics of the nonsteroidal anti-inflammatory drug class, or steroids, without abrogating antitumor activity. Trials focusing upon certain in vitro activities would be simplest, but such studies carry the risk that the parameter being followed is unrelated to antineoplastic function in vivo.

Micrometastatic Disease

The prognostic precision reached in melanoma trials of interferon is now possible in the adjuvant setting of postsurgical patients predicted to be at high risk of relapse within 1 to 3 years (Table 8). In the absence of demonstrable

Table 8. Interferon Applications in the Surgical Adjuvant Setting

Study	Disease Stage	Dosage	Duration of Treatment
ECOG	Stage I (>4 mm) and Stage II	20 MU/m²/day 5/7 days/wk, IV	4 wks
		10 MU/m² tiw, IM	48 wks
NCCSG	Stage II	12.5 MU/m² tiw, IM	12 wks

tumor masses, these patients have a defined microscopic burden of tumor that is perhaps the ideal proving ground for immunologic therapies. Optimal tumor antigenicity, expression of MHC products, and access to the agent and/or host response are to be anticipated in the adjuvant setting as compared to later stages of advanced disease.

Combination Therapy

The use of interferon in combination with other modalities is in part foreshadowed by the adjuvant postsurgical setting. In this volume, Torrisi reviews combinations of interferon and radiotherapy. The logic behind the use of interferon-chemotherapy combinations (Table 9) is similar. We have compared the effect of interferon alpha and dacarbazine, each given in a full dosage of 20 MU/m²/day IV for 5 of 7 days each week for 2 weeks or 10 MU/m²/day tiw, and 200 mg/m²/day IV for 5 days every 21 days, with the single agents given separately. Preliminary data show toxicity of this combination to be tolerable and no greater than that of the single agents. The evaluation of response is premature, with only 57 patients entered in the study to date.

A nonrandomized study in progress in Australia—with an encouraging overall response rate and a high complete response rate—suggests that the use of interferon alpha with dacarbazine has potential therapeutic rewards. Interferon alpha and 1,3-bis-(2 chloroethyl) 1 nitrosourea have been administered together in trials conducted at the Mayo Clinic (Creagan, personal communication); these feasibility studies are of particular importance given the use of nitrosoureas as reference drugs in melanoma over the years.

The most intriguing and potentially rational use of the interferons may, however, be in conjunction with other biologicals. The possibilities listed in Table 9 are only the most immediate and presently active considerations. The synergism of alpha or beta interferons with gamma interferons demonstrated in vitro may now be tested in vivo: Arming functions of interferons for multiple effector cells listed in Table 3 that may be targeted by means of tumor-restricted antibodies offer a unique means to reduce toxicity while improving the competence of the host to respond against the tumor. The potential of interferons to augment expression of tumor-restricted and MHC antigens that are expressed weakly or aberrantly in human melanoma cells further strengthens the rationale for the use of interferons in this disease. It will be essential to study the in vivo modulation of host response and the expression of tumor and normal cell surface markers against which the host response is directed to answer the critical questions about the role that immunity plays in cancer biology—as well as the role of interferons as immunomodulators.

Table 9. Interferon Combinations Currently Being Investigated in Melanoma

Interferon-Antibody	Alpha Interferon + R24 Anti-Melanoma Antibody
Interferon-H_2 Antagonist	Alpha Interferon + Cimetidine
Interferon I-Interferon II	Alpha Interferon + Gamma Interferon
	Beta Interferon + Gamma Interferon
Interferon-Chemotherapy	Alpha Interferon + BCNU
	Alpha Interferon + Dacarbazine Phase II—Australian Phase III—US Multi-institutional
	Beta Interferon + Dacarbazine and cimetidine—Canadian-cross

In summary, the current challenge with interferons is to learn how these mediators and modulators of host response operate. By understanding the in vivo role of each of the direct and indirect actions of interferons in melanoma, we can hope to improve the efficacy of interferon as a therapeutic agent, both alone and in combination with other biologicals or standard drugs.

ACKNOWLEDGEMENTS

The authors gratefully acknowledge the invaluable participation of Carol Ann Davis, RN, MSN, in the conduct and analysis of these clinical trials and the laboratory support of Graciela Hebert, Yoshihiro Nishida, and Nabonita Pall. They also thank Schering-Plough Corporation and Biogen Inc for support of their clinical investigations of the interferons in melanoma.

REFERENCES

1. Kirkwood JM, Ernstoff MS: Interferons in the treatment of human cancer. J Clin Oncol 2:336–352, 1984

2. Carey TE, Takahashi T, Resnick LA, et al: Cell surface antigens of human malignant melanoma: Mixed hemadsorption assay for humoral immunity to cultured autologous melanoma cells. Proc Natl Acad Sci USA 73:3278–3282, 1976

3. Shiku H, Takahashi T, Oettgen HF, et al: Cell surface antigens of human malignant melanoma. II. Serological typing with immune adherence assays and definition of two new surface antigens. J Exp Med 144:873–881, 1976

4. Kirkwood JM, Vlock DR: Augmentation of autologous antibody to human melanoma following acid dissociation and ultrafiltration of serum. Cancer Res 44:4177–4182, 1984

5. Real FX, Mattes MJ, Houghton AN, et al: Class I (unique) tumor antigens of human melanoma. J Exp Med 160:1219–1233, 1984

6. Balch CM, Murad TM, Soong S-J, et al: A multifactorial analysis of melanoma: Prognostic histopathological features comparing Clark's and Breslow's staging methods. Ann Surg 188:732–742, 1978

7. Balch CM, Soong S-J, Milton GW, et al: A comparison of prognostic factors and surgical results in 1786 patients with localized (stage I) melanoma treated in Alabama, USA and New South Wales, Australia. Ann Surg 196:677–684, 1982

8. Greene MH, Reimer RR, Clark WH Jr, et al: Precursor lesions in familial melanoma. Semin Oncol 5:85–87, 1978

9. Roush GC, Schymura MJ, Holford TR: Risk for cutaneous melanoma in recent Connecticut birth cohorts. Am J Public Health 75:679–682, 1985

10. Kirkwood JM, Marsh JC: *In vivo* drug sensitivity assay of clonogenic human melanoma cells, and correlation with treatment outcome. Cancer Res 43:3434–3440, 1983

11. Salmon SE, Durie BGM, Young L, et al: Effects of cloned human leukocyte interferons in the human tumor stem cell assay. J Clin Oncol 1:217–225, 1983

12. Meyskens FL Jr, Loescher L, Moon TE, et al: Relation of *in vitro* colony survival to clinical response in a prospective trial of single-agent chemotherapy for metastatic melanoma. J Clin Oncol 2:1223–1228, 1984

13. Einat M, Resnitzky D, Kimchi A: Inhibitory effects of interferon on the expression of genes regulated by platelet-derived growth factor. Proc Natl Acad Sci USA 82:7608–7612, 1985

14. Perucho M, Esteban M: Inhibitory effect of interferon on the genetic and oncogenic transformation by viral and cellular genes. J Virol 54:229–232, 1985

15. Czarniecki CW, Fennie CW, Powers DB, et al: Synergistic antiviral and antiproliferative activities of *Escherichia coli*-derived human alpha, beta, and gamma interferons. J Virol 49:490–496, 1984

16. Ruiter DJ, Bhan AK, Harrist TJ, et al: Major histocompatibility antigens and mononuclear inflammatory infiltrate in benign nevomelanocytic proliferations and malignant melanoma. J Immunol 129:2808–2815, 1982

17. Fossati G, Anichini A, Taramelli D, et al: Immune response to autologous human melanoma: Implications for class I and II MHC products. Biochim Biophys Acta Reviews in Cancer (in press)

18. Bröcker E-B, Suter L, Bruggen J, et al: Phenotypic dynamics of tumor progression in human malignant melanoma. Int J Cancer 36:29–35, 1985

19. Bröcker E-B, Suter L, Sorg C: HLA-DR antigen expression in primary melanomas of the skin. J Invest Dermatol 82:244–247, 1984

20. Hayashi H, Tanaka K, Jay F, et al: Modulation of the tumorigenicity of human adenovirus-12-transformed cells by interferon. Cell 43:263–267, 1985

21. Schrier PI, Bernards R, Vaessen RTMJ, et al: Expression of class I major histocompatibility antigens switched off by highly oncogenic adenovirus 12 in transformed rat cells. Nature 305:771–775, 1983

22. Taramelli D, Fossati G, Balsari A, et al: The inhibition of lymphocyte stimulation by autologous human metastatic melanoma cells correlates with the expression of HLA-DR antigens on the tumor cells. Int J Cancer 34:797–806, 1984

23. Fossati G, Taramelli D, Balsari A, et al: Primary but not metastatic human melanomas expressing DR antigens stimulate autologous lymphocytes. Int J Cancer 33:591–597, 1984

24. Ziai MR, Imberti L, Tongson A, et al: Differential modulation by recombinant immune interferon of the expression and shedding of HLA antigens and melanoma associated antigens by a melanoma cell line resistant to the antiproliferative activity of immune interferon. Cancer Res 45:5877–5882, 1985

25. Collins T, Korman AJ, Wake CT, et al: Immune interferon activates multiple class II major histocompatibility complex genes and the associated invariant chain gene in human endothelial cells and dermal fibroblasts. Proc Natl Acad Sci USA 81:4917–4921, 1984

26. Anichini A, Mortarini R, Fossati G, et al: Phenotypic profile of clones from early cultures of human metastatic melanomas, and its modulation by recombinant interferon gamma. Int J Cancer (in press)

27. Belardelli F, Gresser L, Maury C, et al: Antitumor effects of interferon in mice injected with interferon-sensitive and interferon-resistant Friend leukemia cells. I. Int J Cancer 30:813–820, 1982

28. Vogel S, Friedman R: Interferon and macrophages, in Vilcek J (ed): Interferon and the Immune System, vol 2. New York, Elsevier, 1984, pp 45–59

29. Herberman R: Interferon and cytotoxic effector cells, in Vilcek J (ed): Interferon and the Immune System, vol 2. New York, Elsevier, 1984, pp 61–84

30. Ernstoff MS, Fusi S, Kirkwood JM: Parameters of interferon action: II. Immunological effects of recombinant leukocyte interferon (IFN-alpha2) in phase I-II trials. J Biol Response Mod 2:540–547, 1983

31. Kirkwood JM, Ernstoff MS, Davis CA, et al: Immunological effects of interferon gamma (in preparation)

32. Kirkwood JM, Ernstoff MS, Davis CA, et al: Com-

parison of intramuscular and intravenous recombinant alpha-2 interferon in melanoma and other cancers. Ann Intern Med 103:32–36, 1985

33. Einhorn S, Blomgren H, Strander H: Interferon and spontaneous cytotoxicity in man. II. Studies in patients receiving exogenous leukocyte interferon. Acta Med Scand 204:477–483, 1978

34. Einhorn S, Blomgren H, Strander H: Interferon and spontaneous cytotoxicity in man. V. Enhancement of spontaneous cytotoxicity in patients receiving human leukocyte interferon. Int J Cancer 26:419–428, 1980

35. Einhorn S, Blomgren H, Johansson R, et al: Enhanced NK activity in patients treated by interferon alpha. Relation to chemical response, in Herberman RB (ed): NK Cells and Other Natural Effector Cells. New York, Academic Press, 1982, pp 1259–1263

36. Golub SH: NK cytotoxicity in interferon treated melanoma patients, in Herberman RB (ed): NK Cells and Other Natural Effector Cells. New York, Academic Press, 1982, pp 1265–1271

37. Lotzova E, Savary CA, Gutterman JU, et al: Modulation of natural killer cell-mediated cytotoxicity by partially purified and cloned interferon-alpha. Cancer Res 42:2480–2488, 1982

38. Laszlo J, Huang AT, Brenckman WD, et al: Phase I study of pharmacologic and immunological effects of human lymphoblastoid interferon given to patients with cancer. Cancer Res 43:4458–4466, 1983

39. Maluish AE, Ortaldo JR, Conlon JC, et al: Depression of natural killer cytotoxicity following in vivo administration of recombinant leukocyte interferon. J Immunol 131:503–507, 1983

40. Edwards BS, Merritt JA, Fuhlbrigge RC, et al: Low doses of interferon alpha result in more effective clinical natural killer cell activation. J Clin Invest 75:1908–1913, 1985

41. Neefe JR, Sullivan JE, Ayoob M, et al: Augmented immunity in cancer patients treated with alpha-interferon. Cancer Res 45:874–878, 1985

42. Hokland P, Olesen BK, Ernst P: Effect of recombinant alpha interferon on NK and ADCC function in lung cancer patients: Results from a phase II trial. J Interferon Res 4:561–569, 1984

43. Uchida A, Yanagawa E, Kokoschka EM, et al: *In vitro* modulation of human natural killer cell activity by interferon: Generation of adherent suppressor cells. Br J Cancer 50:483–492, 1984

44. Retsas S, Preistman TJ, Newton KA, et al: Evaluation of human lymphoblastoid interferon in advanced malignant melanoma. Cancer 51:273–276, 1983

45. Krown SE, Burk MW, Kirkwood JM, et al: Human leukocyte (alpha) interferon in metastatic malignant melanoma: The American Cancer Society Phase II trial. Cancer Treat Rep 68:723–726, 1984

46. Goldberg R, Silgals R, Ayoob M, et al: A phase II trial of lymphoblastoid interferon (IF) in malignant melanoma (MM). Proc Am Soc Clin Oncol 3:49, 1984 (abstr C-189)

47. Kirkwood JM, Ernstoff M: Melanoma: Therapeutic options with recombinant interferons. Semin Oncol 12:7–12, 1985 (suppl 5)

48. Borgstrom S, von Eyben FE, Flodgren P, et al: Human leukocyte interferon and cimetidine for metastatic melanoma. N Engl J Med 307:1080–1081, 1982

49. Flodgren P, Borgstrom S, Jonsson PE, et al: Metastatic malignant melanoma: Regression induced by combined treatment with interferon [HU IFN-Alpha (Le)] and cimetidine. Int J Cancer 32:657–665, 1983

50. Hill NO, Pardue A, Khan A, et al: Interferon and cimetidine for malignant melanoma. N Engl J Med 308:1286, 1983

51. Ernstoff MS, Davis CA, Kirkwood JM: Cimetidine (C) plus interferon alpha-2 (IFN) does not remit metastatic melanoma which has failed IFN alone. Proc Am Soc Clin Oncol 3:62, 1984 (abstr C-240)

52. Lipton A, Harvey HA, Simmonds MA, et al: Lack of enhanced activity of systemic interferon by cimetidine in malignant melanoma. Proc Am Soc Clin Oncol 3:56, 1984 (abstr C-215)

53. Slater DE, Krown SE, Pinsky CM, et al: Human leukocyte (alpha) interferon [HU IFN-alpha(Le)] and cimetidine in malignant melanoma. Proc Am Soc Clin Oncol 3:54, 1984 (abstr C-210)

54. Hawkins MJ, McCune CS, Speyer JL, et al: Recombinant $alpha_2$ interferon (IFN $alpha_2$) (SCH 30500) in patients with metastatic malignant melanoma (MMM): An ECOG pilot study. Proc Am Soc Clin Oncol 3:51, 1984 (abstr C-195)

55. Creagan ET, Ahmann DL, Green SJ, et al: Phase II study of recombinant leukocyte A interferon (IFN-rA) plus cimetidine in disseminated malignant melanoma. J Clin Oncol 3:977–981, 1985

56. Robinson WA, Kirkwood J, Harvey H, et al: Effective use of recombinant human alpha-2 interferon (IFN-$alpha_2$) in metastatic malignant melanoma: A comparison of two regimens. Proc Am Soc Clin Oncol 3:60, 1984 (abstr C-234)

57. Pouillart P, Bretaudeau B, Dorval T, et al: Clinical phase II study of recombinant DNA interferon (h.u. IFN alpha-2) in patients with metastatic malignant melanoma. Antiviral Res 1(3):92, 1984 (abstr D19, vol 4)

58. Creagan ET, Ahmann DL, Frytak S, et al: Phase II trials of recombinant leukocyte A interferon in disseminated malignant melanoma: Results in 96 patients. Cancer Treat Rep (in press)

59. Hersey P, Hasic E, MacDonald M, et al: Effects of recombinant leukocyte interferon (rIFN-alpha A) on tumour growth and immune responses in patients with metastatic melanoma. Br J Cancer 51:815–826, 1985

60. Creagan ET, Ahmann DL, Green SJ, et al: Phase II study of low-dose recombinant leukocyte A interferon in disseminated malignant melanoma. J Clin Oncol 2:1002–1005, 1984

61. Creagan ET, Ahmann DL, Green SJ, et al: Phase II study of recombinant leukocyte A interferon (rIFN-alpha A) in disseminated malignant melanoma. Cancer 54:2844–2849, 1984

Superficial Carcinoma of the Bladder: Natural History and the Role of Interferons

Frank M. Torti and Bert L. Lum

Superficial transitional cell carcinoma of the bladder is a chronic disease. Patients face a lifetime with the potential for further neoplastic manifestations—the recurrence of either superficial or deeply invasive tumor. To some extent, the likelihood of disease recurrence can be predicted. Further, certain clinical interventions can alter the probability of tumor recurrence. This paper focuses on those patient and tumor characteristics that predict for the propensity to develop recurrent disease, with emphasis on the potential of the interferons to both treat this disease and to modify its natural history.

THE PURPOSE of this paper is: (1) to outline the natural history and the indications for therapeutic intervention in superficial bladder cancer; (2) to detail the rationale for the use of interferon in bladder cancer; and (3) to summarize the preliminary data on the use of interferon in treating bladder cancer.

FACTORS PREDICTING RECURRENCE AND INVASION

The information currently available on the natural history of bladder cancer is inferential. There are virtually no data on untreated cancer, and much of our knowledge reflects experience in patients treated with endoscopic surgery, intravesical chemotherapy, or both.

Bladder cancer recurs after initial treatment in 40% to 85% of patients. Recurrence is most likely to occur within the first year but may occur after many years. In a group of 62 patients with carcinoma in situ (CIS), for example, Utz et al[1] reported a recurrence rate within the first year of 82%. Lerman et al[2] found an overall recurrence rate of bladder papillomas of 47% to 31% for unifocal lesions and 66% for multifocal lesions. Loening et al[3] reported that 85% of patients whose tumor recurred experienced recurrence within 1 year.

Although not generally emphasized, the word "recurrence" may have more than one biologic meaning. Animal models suggest that tumors implant in areas of previous trauma or surgery and that recurrence may, in fact, represent a form of local "metastasis." However, the predilection for subsequent tumor formation in the urothelium as a whole, even in areas that experience no trauma and have little opportunity for local dissemination, eg, the ureters and renal pelvis, is well known. This new occurrence of tumors is presumably attributable to the continuous exposure of the urothelium to tumorigenic stimuli, probably from the urine.

These biologic possibilities are not merely of theoretical interest but may relate to different etiologies for early and late recurrence of superficial bladder tumors. They may also be important in predicting the use and possible limitations of interferon and other intravesical treatments. For example, because the possibility of the development of tumor resistance with continuous or intermittent exposure of the same tumor cells to a drug is high, the optimal regimen of intravesical therapy may differ depending on whether tumor recurrence is related to intravesical dissemination or new tumor formation.

The factors predictive of tumor recurrence, regardless of the etiology, can be classified into a number of general categories, each of which will be discussed separately.

Grade and Stage

The histologic grade of the tumor has an important impact on the possibility of local recurrence. This is true in most studies, even when tumor stage (depth of invasion into the bladder wall) is considered. Broders[4] was the first to introduce uniform criteria for grading bladder cancer. His grading system was used by a number of investigators to show the influence of grade on overall prognosis. For example, in 1977, Barnes et al[5] reported an 85% survival rate for grade I tumors as compared with a 51% sur-

From Stanford University Medical Center, Stanford, California, The University of the Pacific, Stockton, California, and the Palo Alto VA Medical Center, Palo Alto, California.

Address reprint requests to Frank M. Torti, MD, Division of Medical Oncology, Stanford University Medical Center, Stanford, CA 94305.

vival rate for grade II neoplasms. Furthermore, although a number of investigators have shown that tumor stage is also of prognostic significance, Lutzeyer et al[6] demonstrated that grade, not stage, is important in identifying that subset of patients in whom the tumor will recur at a higher stage or grade—a poor prognostic group among patients with recurrent bladder cancer.

Multicentricity

Not surprisingly, patients with multiple bladder tumors at the time of diagnosis have a poorer prognosis than those with a single tumor at presentation. The influence of multicentricity is well documented. Lerman et al[2] found an overall recurrence rate of 31% in patients with a single tumor and 66% in those with multiple tumors.

Of greater importance than overall recurrence are those tumors that invade deeply into the bladder muscle when they recur—life-threatening neoplasms that require extensive surgery or irradiation for cure. In such cases, multicentricity of initial tumor presentation also confers important prognostic information. Lerman et al[2] showed that the probability of subsequent development of a muscle invasive tumor nearly trebled, from 4.6% to 13.6%, with multiple tumors on presentation. This observation, however, has not been confirmed in all studies. Williams et al[7] found no difference in survival between patients with single and multiple tumors, although the subsequent development of lamina propria invasion was higher in the group with multiple tumors.

CIS

The usual presenting symptoms of CIS are hematuria or symptoms of bladder irritability. The intensity and the nature of the symptoms of bladder irritation—frequency, dysuria, and urgency—separate this clinical syndrome from that of the papillary tumors, in which asymptomatic hematuria predominates at presentation. When these symptoms occur without hematuria, they often masquerade as urinary tract infections, making CIS an easily overlooked diagnosis.

CIS has three presentations which, regardless of whether they are different biologic entities, have important clinical and prognostic distinctions. The first and most common form of CIS, which we call type I CIS, is a small focus of in situ cancer surrounding the base of a papillary or sessile tumor. The occurrence of this focus of CIS has a profound effect on prognosis, perhaps overriding tumor grade and stage, although this issue has never been formally addressed. Althausen et al[8] demonstrated that 7% of patients with a normal mucosa surrounding papillary cancer, 36% of those with adjacent atypia, and 83% of those with CIS surrounding the papillary tumor eventually developed invasive cancer.

The second, or type II, presentation of CIS is characterized by atypia or in situ cancer distant from the papillary tumor. According to Soloway et al,[9] careful histologic examination of the bladder mucosa at the time of resection of superficial tumors revealed a 33% incidence of histologic abnormalities, 5% of which represented in situ cancer. In a number of these patients, biopsies were obtained from presumably normal urothelium, indicating the need for careful staging of the entire bladder at the time of cystoscopic resection. Even more striking was the restaging of the urothelium 1 year later. At that time, 46% of the patients showed atypia, 14% CIS, and 16% invasive cancer.

In the third, or type III, presentation of CIS, there is extensive involvement of the urothelium with the typical raised, erythematous changes that have become synonymous with the clinical syndrome often described simply as CIS. Irritative symptomology is frequently present in these patients, and as many as 50% to 80% will develop cancer, leading many investigators to

Table 1. Relationship of Carcinoma in Situ of the Bladder to the Incidence of Invasive Carcinoma*

Author	No. Patients	Invasion No. (%)	Follow-up Time (Yrs)
Melamed et al[19]	25	9 (36)	<5
Koss[20]	13	7 (54)	1–6
Utz et al[1]: Diffuse	62	37 (60)	<5
Barlebo[21]	10	0 (0)	6
Riddle et al[22]: Diffuse	23	18 (78)	1–11
Focal	13	1 (8)	1–16
Althausen et al[23]	12	10 (83)	1.5
Farrow et al[24]	58	8 (14)	<5

* Reprinted with permission from Torti and Lum.[25]

recommend prophylactic cystectomy. Table 1 summarizes the studies in which the association of CIS and eventual development of invasive carcinoma has been reported. It must be remembered that these studies are quite heterogeneous with regard to both treatment and prior patient history of urothelial disease. Nonetheless, the high percentage of patients with invasive disease in many of these series is noteworthy.

INTERFERON IN BLADDER CANCER

Interferons are cellular proteins whose production is augmented in response to a variety of stimuli. Viral infection, bacterial endotoxins, and a variety of other stimuli elicit interferon production, which is mediated through the increased transcription of the interferon genes of macrophages, lymphocytes, and other host cells. In addition to the classic action of interferon, namely, rendering cells resistant to infections by viruses, a number of other actions have been described, including the inhibition of cell growth and the maturation or differentiation of certain cells. cGMP and cAMP levels increase in certain cell lines; polymorphonuclear leukocytes are stimulated to increased phagocytosis; and the cytotoxic potential of natural killer (NK) cells and macrophages is increased.

The close association between bladder cancer and modulation of the immune system has been known for years. Reactivity to surface antigens, such as the ABO blood group antigens and the T-group antigens, is often lost with the development of a bladder neoplasm.[10-12] This observation, combined with the accessibility of the bladder mucosa to direct, topical treatment, has permitted and justified an immunotherapeutic approach to bladder cancer.

One such approach, bacillus Calmette Guerin (BCG) treatment, has been somewhat successful in the treatment of bladder cancer. BCG generates a vigorous, local inflammatory reaction in virtually all patients that involves both the mucosa and the submucosa.[13] Although the antitumor activity of BCG remains uncertain, evidence suggests that it may be linked to interferon production. In a normal host, this inflammatory response should elicit the activation of cytotoxic lymphocytes, macrophages, and other elements of the immune response. In fact, both animal and human studies demonstrate that BCG treatment stimulates circulating levels of interferon.[14] Whether this increased level of circulating interferon leads to any of the cytotoxic, cytostatic, or immunomodulatory activities of BCG remains uncertain.

Literature reports suggesting the value of intravesical interferon in treating bladder cancer led to the Stanford-NCOG trial of intravesical interferon alfa-2b (Intron® A) in superficial bladder cancer. Ikic et al[15] evaluated the use of intralesional injections of a nonrecombinant preparation of interferon. They treated eight patients, two of whom received concomitant intramuscular treatment. Four of the patients achieved a complete response, and two additional patients had a partial response. The duration of remission ranged from 3 to 24 months. Subsequently, Scorticatti et al[16] administered 1 million units of alpha interferon intramuscularly every other day for a 6-month period. All eight patients treated achieved a partial response.

Kemeny et al[17] tested the ability of poly I:C, an interferon inducer, to prevent recurrent tumor formation after endoscopic resection. Although no difference in recurrence rate was noted in the 32 patients studied, a difference in survival favoring the poly I:C group was observed. The median survival at the time of the report was 170+ months for the poly I:C group as compared with 76+ months for the control group, treated only with resection. Among the patients with CIS, all nine in the poly I:C group remained disease-free, whereas four of six CIS patients in the control group died of their disease. Maintenance of remission in the poly I:C group was associated with a twofold to eightfold elevation in interferon serum levels.

Torti et al[18] studied intravesical interferon alfa-2b in a phase I-II study that included patients with recurrent papillary tumors, CIS, or both. Interferon was administered intravesically each week for 8 weeks. Retention time was 2 hours with each administration. The interferon dose ranged from 50 to 200 million units. Patients were reevaluated by repeat cystoscopy with multiple bladder biopsies and urinary cytology 3 months after the start of treatment (approximately 30 days after the last interferon instillation). Prostatic urethral biopsies and upper tract cytologies were also performed in selected patients. Four of the eight patients with CIS achieved a complete response. These responses were achieved with virtually no local or systemic toxicity.

Although preliminary, these results suggest that the interferons may play a role in the treatment of superficial bladder cancer. Tumor response has been observed with intralesional administration and systemic therapy as well as with intravesical treatment. Further trials are needed to better define the optimal interferon dose and treatment schedule as well as to compare this agent with other intravesical treatments.

REFERENCES

1. Utz DC, Hanash KA, Farrow GM: The plight of the patient with carcinoma in situ of the bladder. J Urol 103:160–164, 1970

2. Lerman RI, Hunter RVP, Whitmore WF: Papilloma of the urinary bladder. Cancer 25:333–342, 1970

3. Loening S, Narayana A, Yoder L, et al: Factors influencing the recurrence rate of bladder cancer. J Urol 123:29–31, 1980

4. Broders AC: Epithelioma of the genitourinary organs. Ann Surg 75:574–604, 1922

5. Barnes RW, Dick AL, Hadley HL, et al: Survival following transurethral resection of bladder carcinoma. Cancer Res 37:2895–2897, 1977

6. Lutzeyer W, Rubben H, Dahm H: Prognostic parameters in superficial bladder cancer: An analysis of 315 cases. J Urol 127:250–252, 1982

7. Williams JC, Hammonds JC, Saunders N: T_1 bladder tumors. Br J Urol 49:663–668, 1977

8. Althausen AF, Prout GR, Daly JJ: Non-invasive papillary carcinoma of the bladder associated with carcinoma in situ. J Urol 116:575–580, 1976

9. Soloway MS, Murphy W, Rao MK: Serial multiple site biopsies in patients with bladder cancer. J Urol 120:57–59, 1978

10. Kovarik S, Davidsohn I, Stejskal R: ABO antigens in cancer: Detection with the mixed cell agglutination reaction. Arch Pathol 86:12–21, 1968

11. Sadoughi N, Mlsna J, Guinan P, et al: Prognostic value of cell surface antigens using immunoperoxidase methods in bladder carcinoma. Urol 20:143–146, 1982

12. Coon JS, Weinstein RS, Summers JL: Blood group precursor T-antigen expression in human bladder carcinoma. Am J Clin Pathol 77:692–699, 1982

13. Bloomberg SD, Brosman SA, Hausman MD, et al: The effects of BCG on the dog bladder. Invest Urol 12(6):427, 1975

14. Catalona WJ, Shapiro A, Ratliff TL, et al: Interferon induction during intravesical bacillus Calmette Guerin (BCG) therapy. XIX International Congress of the Societe Internationale d'Urologie, San Francisco, September 1982

15. Ikic D, Maricic Z, Oresic V, et al: Application of human leucocyte interferon in patients with urinary bladder papillomatosis, breast cancer, and melanoma. Lancet 1:1022, 1981

16. Scorticatti CH, LaPena NC, Bellora OG, et al: Systemic IFN-alpha treatment of multiple papilloma grade I or II patients: pilot study. J Interferon Res 2:339–343, 1982

17. Kemeny N, Yagoda A, Wang Y, et al: Randomized trial of standard therapy with or without poly I:C in patients with superficial bladder cancer. Cancer 48:2154–2157, 1981

18. Torti FM, Shortliffe LD, Williams RD, et al: Superficial bladder cancers are responsive to alpha-2 interferon administered intravesically. Proc Am Soc Clin Oncol 3:160, 1984

19. Melamed MR, Vousta NG, Grabstald H: Natural history and clinical behavior of in situ carcinoma of the human urinary bladder. Cancer 17:1533–1545, 1964

20. Koss LG, Melamed MR, Kelly RE: Further cytologic and histologic studies of bladder lesions in workers exposed to para-aminodiphenyl: Progress report. J Nat Cancer Inst 43:233, 1969

21. Barlebo H, Sorenson BL, Ohlson A: Carcinoma in situ of the urinary bladder. Scand J Urol Nephrol 6:213, 1972

22. Riddle PR, Chisholm GD, Trott PA: Flat carcinoma in situ of the bladder. Br J Urol 47:829–833, 1976

23. Althausen AF, Prout GR, Daly JJ: Non-invasive papillary carcinoma of the bladder associated with carcinoma in situ. J Urol 116:575–580, 1976

24. Farrow GM, Utz DC, Rife CC, et al: Clinical observations on sixty-nine cases of in situ carcinoma of the urinary bladder. Cancer Res 37:2794–2798, 1977

25. Torti FM, Lum BL: Therapeutic approaches, including interferon, to cancer in situ of the bladder. Cancer Treat Rev 12:45–59, 1985

Intraperitoneal Recombinant α-Interferon for "Salvage" Immunotherapy in Stage III Epithelial Ovarian Cancer: A Gynecologic Oncology Group Study[1,2]

Jonathan S. Berek,[3] Neville F. Hacker, Alan Lichtenstein, Tyler Jung, Celsa Spina, Reba M. Knox, Jeanine Brady, Teri Greene, Lupe M. Ettinger, Leo D. Lagasse, Eric M. Bonnem, Robert J. Spiegel, and Jacob Zighelboim

Fourteen patients with persistent epithelial ovarian cancer documented at second look laparotomy after combination chemotherapy were treated with 146 cycles of α-recombinant interferon (rIFN-α_2) administered i.p. The initial dose was 5 × 10^6 units which was escalated weekly to 50 × 10^6 units over 4 weeks and then continued weekly for a total of 16 weeks. Eleven patients underwent surgical reevaluation after therapy which confirmed four pathological complete responses (36%), one partial response (9%), and disease progression in six patients (55%). Five of seven patients (71%) with residual tumor <5 mm had a surgically documented response, whereas there was no response in the four patients whose tumors were ≥5 mm. Three patients were evaluable for clinical response only: one patient who refused surgery had a complete clinical response with total resolution of ascites; one had stable disease; and one had disease progression. Fever ≥38°C was seen in 58%, fever ≥39.0°C was seen in 18%, vomiting in 37%, abdominal pain was reported in 22%, and one patient had infectious peritonitis. Peripheral white blood cell counts and i.p. washings were obtained pretreatment and on days 1, 3, and 7 after treatment. While there was no consistent alteration in peripheral white blood cell counts, the numbers of i.p. monocytes and lymphocytes showed a significant boost on day 1 after each dose of rIFN-α_2. Natural killer lymphocyte cytotoxicity was elevated in the i.p. cavity fluid obtained from most patients on day 1 after treatment, while blood natural killer lymphocyte cytotoxicity values showed considerable variability. Pharmacokinetic studies show that i.p. levels of rIFN-α_2 were 30–1000 times blood levels. rIFN-α_2 i.p. may act by increasing concentrations of drug and augmenting regional host cells in patients with minimal residual ovarian cancer.

INTRODUCTION

IFNs* are a diverse group of locally active, naturally occurring, regulatory glycoproteins which are currently undergoing extensive clinical testing as antineoplastic agents.[1-9] Their biological activities are diverse, and in addition to their ability to modify immunoregulatory systems[1,2] they possess direct antineoplastic activity. These agents alter tumor cell function and structure and induce cellular inhibition of replication of many viruses.[1]

Therapeutic responses have been observed in a variety of tumor systems.[1-5,7,8] Human α-interferon, a specific antigenic type produced mainly by leukocytes,[2] is now produced in highly purified, large quantities because genetic recombinant DNA technology has permitted the production of specifically cloned products.[8]

In our experience patients treated with combination chemotherapy for epithelial ovarian cancer and in clinical remission have a 60–70% rate of persistent disease at second look laparotomy.[10] Therefore there is a need for improved primary or secondary therapies in order to improve survival and cure rates.

---

[1]This report is reprinted with permission from a prior publication by J. S. Berek et al. *Cancer Research* 1985; 45:4447–4453.

[2]Supported by grants from the Schering Corporation, the Concern Foundation, and The National Cancer Institute (Grant CA 12800, NIH); a USPHS CRC Grant RR865; and Gynecologic Oncology Group Grant CA 13630-13.

[3]To whom requests for reprints should be addressed, at Division of Gynecologic Oncology, Department of Obstetrics and Gynecology, UCLA School of Medicine, Los Angeles, CA 90024.

*The abbreviations used are: IFNs, interferons; rIFN-α_2, α-recombinant interferon; NK, natural killer lymphocyte cytotoxicity; MRD, minimal residual disease; BRM, biological response modifier.

Division of Gynecologic Oncology, the Departments of Obstetrics and Gynecology [J. S. B., N. F. H., T. J., R. M. K., T. G., L. M. E., L. D. L.], Medicine, and Microbiology and Immunology [A. L., C. S., J. Z.], the UCLA School of Medicine, and Jonsson Comprehensive Cancer Center [J. S. B., N. F. H., L. D. L.], Los Angeles, California 90024; and the Schering Corporation [J. B., E. M. B., R. J. S.], Kenilworth, New Jersey 07033; and the Gynecologic Oncology Group [J. S. B., N. F. H., L. M. E., L. D. L.], Philadelphia, Pennsylvania 19107

One approach which has been suggested is to treat the residual disease with the i.p. administration of antitumor agents.[11-13] Complete and partial responses have been surgically documented in response to the i.p. administration of *Corynebacterium parvum* as second line therapy in epithelial ovarian cancer patients.[11,12] These responses have been documented only in patients with MRD (*i.e.,* <5 mm maximum diameter of the residual tumor) at second look operations. However, since this BRM is relatively toxic when administered i.p., BRMs which induce a less intense peritonitis might be more practical and effective.[13,14] The i.p. instillation of BRMs for ovarian cancer has clinical appeal because of the potential for increasing the drug concentration at the tumor site and decreasing systemic toxicity.[11-15]

This report is a trial of the i.p. administration of recombinant (rIFN-α_2) in patients with persistent epithelial ovarian cancer documented at second look laparotomy. Evaluation of efficacy, toxicity, pharmacokinetics, and host cell parameters are presented.

MATERIALS AND METHODS

Patients. A total of 14 patients with persistent epithelial ovarian cancer were treated with 146 cycles of i.p. rIFN-α_2. All patients were evaluable for clinical response and toxicity. Eleven patients were surgically reevaluated after therapy. Serial rIFN-α_2 levels, studies of host cell populations, and lymphocyte cytotoxicity assays were performed on peritoneal washings and peripheral blood.

Patients ranged in age from 42 to 66 years with a mean age of 53.4 years. All patients were classified as International Federation of Gynecology and Obstetrics stage III. No patient had documented extraperitoneal disease at the initiation of immunotherapy.

Residual tumor prior to rIFN-α_2 treatments ranged from microscopic disease (positive cytology only) to a 4- × 4-cm palpable pelvic mass. Six patients (43%) had only positive peritoneal cytology (classes IV and V), two patients (14%) had measurable disease <5 mm in diameter, one patient (7%) had disease 5 to 15 mm in diameter, and five patients (36%) had disease >15 mm. Papillary serous cystadenocarcinoma was the histological type in 11 of the 14 patients. Two patients had grade I tumors, six had grade II lesions, and six had grade III lesions.

Cytology of peritoneal fluids were graded as follows: class I or II, negative; class III, equivocal or suspicious; and class IV or V, positive for frankly malignant cells.

Prior to i.p. rIFN-α_2 therapy each patient had undergone one to three exploratory laparotomies to resect tumor, including a total abdominal hysterectomy, bilateral salpingooophorectomy, as well as 5 to 13 (median, 9) cycles of combination chemotherapy with *cis*-platinum, doxorubicin, and cyclophosphamide. Two patients previously had received external pelvic radiation therapy. Immediately prior to entry onto this study, a second look minilaparotomy was performed at which time two Tenckhoff catheters were implanted using standard techniques:[11] the tip of one catheter was directed toward the pelvis; and the tip of the second catheter was directed cephalad up the right paracolic gutter. An operation to evaluate response to rIFN-α_2 was performed 1 to 6 weeks following the final course of rIFN-α_2 as described previously.[10,16] The protocol was approved by the Human Subject Protection Committee of the University of California, UCLA.

Dialysis fluid was instilled into the peritoneal cavity (Dyalasate with 1.5% dextrose) after being warmed to 37°C and was supplemented with sodium heparin (500 units/liter; Panheparin; Abbott Laboratories).

i.p. Therapy. After catheter placement several peritoneal lavages were performed using 1 to 2 liters of dialysis fluid until peritoneal rinses were free of blood. Three consecutive blood free peritoneal lavages were required before the first rIFN-α_2 treatment. Catheters were flushed every other day with 10 ml of heparinized saline except for treatment days in which only saline solution was used.

Once rIFN-α_2 treatment began peritoneal lavages were performed on days 2 and 7. Aliquots obtained prior to each lavage were examined cytologically for malignant cells, and total WBC differential counts and immunological assays of peritoneal host cells were performed.

Interferon Administration. Human rIFN-α_2 (SCh 30500, Schering Corporation, Kenilworth,

NJ) was administered i.p. in 250 ml normal saline after 1750 ml of dialysis solution were instilled i.p. via Tenckhoff catheters.

Ten patients in the first dose schedule of the study received an escalating weekly dosage of rIFN-α_2. The dosage of rIFN-α_2 was initially 5 $\times 10^6$ units, which was escalated to 10 $\times 10^6$ and then 20 $\times 10^6$ units and then followed by five consecutive courses at 50 $\times 10^6$ units. The second dose schedule initially called for patients to be infused with rIFN-α_2 three times a week (every other day) at 50 $\times 10^6$ units. This regimen was to be followed every other week for 16 weeks. However, because of toxicity the second dosage schedule was modified to 50 $\times 10^6$ units a week for 8 more weeks.

Patients were premedicated with 25 mg diphenhydramine hydrochloride and 650 mg acetaminophen p.o. The former was discontinued during the second dose schedule because no major allergic reactions from rIFN-α_2 were observed and the patients complained of somnolence. Acetaminophen was given every 4 h for the duration of the hospital visit (usually 24 h) and was then taken by patients upon discharge as needed.

When 24 h had elapsed after rIFN-α_2 treatment, 2 liters of warmed dialysis fluid were instilled into the peritoneal cavity and recovered for cytological and immunological assays. The exposed ends of the Tenckhoff catheters were resealed aseptically.

Response Criteria. Response was defined as follows: complete response, no evidence of disease at the completion of therapy, including the absence of malignant cells in the peritoneal fluid cytological evaluation in those patients whose cytologies had been positive; partial response, the presence of a positive cytology only at the completion of therapy in those patients who had had macroscopic disease, or the regression of macroscopic disease by at least 50% in tumor dimension; stable disease, no change in the positive cytology and/or the tumor dimension; progressive disease, evidence of tumor growth during or at the completion of treatment.

Toxicity. Toxicity was monitored and graded according to the criteria outlined by the Gynecologic Oncology Group[15] and modified to adapt to the expected effects of rIFN-α_2. rIFN-α_2 routinely causes fevers which at times are above 39°C and this was not considered a toxicity requiring dose reduction. For rIFN-α_2 dose-limiting toxicity is usually a cumulative one based on the patients' general condition and symptoms, *e.g.*, fatigue and malaise, rather than objective laboratory parameters.[1,2]

Toxicities which may be encountered by the patients receiving rIFN-α_2 include: (*a*) fatigue and malaise. If a subject experienced fatigue to the extent that she was unable to ambulate, the rIFN-α_2 was held. One to 2 weeks after the patient was again ambulatory, the rIFN-α_2 was resumed on the regular schedule at the last maximum tolerated dosage, or reduced by 25%, whichever dose was higher; (*b*) weight loss. The guidelines listed below were followed for weight loss believed to be solely induced by the rIFN-α_2 (for $\geq$15 pounds reduce dosage by 50%; for $\geq$20 pounds, hold treatment); (*c*) abdominal pain if the pain was intermittent over a time period of <24 h and required no analgesics, it was considered mild (grade I), if it lasted >24 h and necessitated p.o. analgesics which relieved the pain it was grade II, and severe (grade III) pain included that which was continuous weekly and not responsive to p.o. analgesics; (*d*) chills: grade I, those that lasted $\leq$10 min at a time and did not restrict patient activity in any way; grade II, those that lasted >10 but <30 min at a time and did not confine the patient to bed; and grade III, rigorous shivering that required the patient to stay in bed and that lasted continuously for a period of >30 min; (*e*) headache: grade I, those lasting <24 h relieved by p.o. analgesics; grade II, those that lasted >24 h and <48 h and are temporarily relieved by p.o. analgesics; and grade III, those lasting >48 h and temporarily relieved by p.o. analgesics; (*f*) temporary anorexia: grade I, $\leq$24 h; grade II, >24 h and <72 h; and grade III, $\geq$72 h; (*g*) pruritis: grade I, $\leq$24 h; grade II, >24 h and $\leq$48 h; and grade III, >48 h.

Blood Lymphocyte Analysis. Ten ml of blood were drawn before treatment for base-line analysis and one to three times/week during treatment. Samples were assayed for differential WBC, lymphocyte populations, and cytotoxic activity.

Peritoneal Cell Analysis. Peritoneal lavage fluid specimens were obtained two to three times/week during rIFN-α_2 treatment. An aliquot of 50 ml of fluid was examined cytologically for malignant cells. The remaining dialysis fluid was centrifuged at approximately 700 rpm for 5 min and resuspended with minimal essential media. Total WBC/ml were counted, Cytoprep slides were made, and differential cell counts/ml were performed.

Separation of peritoneal cells was performed with a Ficoll:Hypaque density gradient as described previously.[18] Specimens which had high concentrations of macrophages were treated with GAF iron fillings and removed with a magnet.[19] Differential WBC were performed. Lymphocyte populations were isolated and a specimen was assayed by the UCLA Clinical Immunological Research Laboratory for lymphocyte cytotoxicity.

Natural Killer Cell Activity. A constant number of ^{51}Cr-labeled target cells (1×10^4) was mixed with varying numbers of lymphocyte effector cells at an effector:target ratio of 25:1. Cultures were incubated in V-well microtiter plates for 3 h at 27°C. Supernatant was collected and ^{51}Cr release was assayed by γ-emission according to the method of Jondal *et al.*[20] The percentage of lysis was calculated as

$$\%\text{ of lysis} = \frac{[\text{cpm of target + effector}] - [\text{cpm of target alone}]}{[\text{cpm of target + detergent (Triton X)}] - [\text{cpm of target alone}]} \times 100$$

Addition of detergent to targets evaluated maximal release (always greater than 85% of incorporated cpm) while culture of targets alone served as background release (always less than 20% of incorporated cpm). The myeloid line K562 served as the target cell of the NK assay.

Neutralizing Antibodies. Frozen serum samples from each patient were obtained before and after treatment and were sent to the Schering Corporation Clinical Laboratories to assay for generation of antibodies specific for the rIFN-α_2. The procedure for detection of anti-IFN-α_2 antibody in human sera is a radioimmunological technique to screen for antibodies as described previously.[21]

Pharmacokinetics. From each patient 10 ml of blood were drawn prior to rIFN-α_2 (50×10^6) and 24 h afterward. Additionally five patients were studied after the administration of a rIFN-α_2 treatment at time 0 (pretreatment = base line), 4, 8, 12, 20, and 24 h from initiation of the i.p. infusion. Blood samples were centrifuged and subsequent frozen serum specimens were sent to the Schering Corporation Clinical Laboratories to determine rIFN-α_2 levels. The method for measuring rIFN-α_2 levels utilized a human foreskin diploid cell line, the murine EMC virus, and a crystal violet stain to visually detect cytopathic effects as described.[22]

Approximately 50 ml of dialysis fluid were obtained from peritoneal lavages at pretreatment (time = 0) and at 4 and 24 h following 50 million units of rIFN-α_2 infused at time 0. Additional peritoneal fluid samples (48 and 72 h) were obtained by peritoneal lavages consisting of approximately 1 liter of dialysis fluid. Specimens were frozen immediately and sent to the Schering Corporation Clinical Laboratories to determine rIFN-α_2 levels.

RESULTS

Response

Four of 11 surgically evaluated patients demonstrated complete responses to rIFN-α_2 treatment. Tumor disappearance was documented by a negative reassessment laparotomy and at least six consecutive negative (class I or II) peritoneal cytological washings at the completion of rIFN-α_2 therapy. Three of the complete responders entered the program with microscopic disease as documented by positive cytology only, and the other had 5–10 residual tumor nodules, approximately 1–2 mm in diameter in the pelvic peritoneum. All four patients remain alive without recurrence from 5 to 14 months posttreatment.

An additional patient had a partial response. This patient began the study with 6–10 peritoneal tumor nodules of 2–3 mm tumors in the pelvic cul-de-sac. Upon reassessment laparotomy the patient had no macroscopic evidence of disease, but a specimen for cytological evaluation obtained from the upper abdomen was positive for persistent malignant cells. Surgi-

Table 1. Surgically Documented Response by Residual Disease

Maximum Diameter	No. of Patients	Response Complete	Response Partial	%
Cytology positive	5[a]	3	0	60
<5 mm	2[a]	1	1	100
>5 mm	4	0	0	0
Total	11	4	1	45

[a] Five of seven (71%) of patients with <5 mm disease responded to therapy.

cally documented responses by residual disease are listed in Table 1.

Six surgically evaluated patients had disease progression during treatment. Four of these patients entered treatment with intraabdominal tumor nodules >1.5 cm in diameter, and two patients had only microscopic disease following optimal debulking. Of the two patients who entered with microscopic disease and progressed, one developed a 2- × 2-cm retroperitoneal tumor nodule which was removed. After whole abdominal radiation treatment she remained clinically free of disease for 12 months before abdominal recurrence. The other patient with microscopic disease was found to be free of disease by laparoscopy following her first eight cycles of treatment, but progressive abdominal disease was documented at the completion of the protocol by laparotomy where 1–2 mm studding on the small bowel mesentery was documented.

Aliquots of peritoneal fluid were obtained weekly during the course of therapy and examined cytologically for malignant cells (Chart 1). The six patients who were clinically free of disease and evaluated surgically at the completion of therapy retained evidence of malignant cells throughout treatment (class IV or V cytology), whereas those four patients who had surgically documented complete responses developed negative cytology by week 8 of treatment. This corresponds to the week after the patients had received their fourth treatment cycle at the maximum dose of 50 × 10^6 units/week.

Of the three patients who were only clinically evaluable, one had a complete resolution of ascites during treatment and remains clinically free of disease 16 months posttreatment. One patient had stable disease during treatment and remains stable after 4 months with 2 cm disease palpable in the recto-vaginal septum. The third had a 3–4-cm mass palpable in the rectovaginal septum progress to 5–6-cm disease after eight treatments.

Toxicity

Objective and subjective systemic reactions were monitored throughout the study in all patients (Table 2). Of the 146 courses monitored for subjective side effects, fatigue was noted in 65%, chills in 53%, temporary anorexia in 39%, headaches in 38%, nausea and/or vomiting in 37%, diarrhea in 27%, abdominal pain in 22%, and total body pruritis in 12%. Other common complaints included "abnormal" taste, "dry" mouth, back pain, and muscle aches, all of which were mild to moderate.

Vital signs were monitored during the first 24 h after treatment in 132 courses. Fever (≥38°C) was documented in 77 courses (58%). The degree of fever is listed in Table 2. Response could not be correlated with the fever because both nonresponding and responding patients had systemic temperature evaluations. A slight increase in pulse without tachycardia was mea-

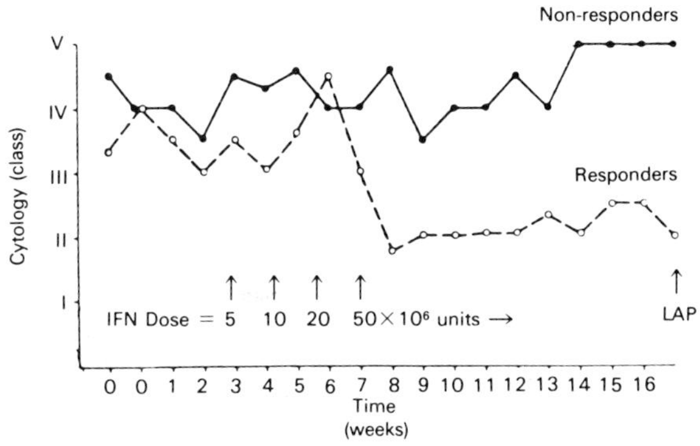

Chart 1. Plot of mean of the cytological classes of peritoneal washings by grade for responders and nonresponders in a group of 11 surgically evaluable patients treated with i.p. rIFN-α_2. Cytological grades I and II are negative, grade III is equivocal, and grades IV and V are frankly positive for malignant cells. Following two baseline (time = 0) cytological assays, specimens were obtained weekly while on treatment. The maximum dose of 50 × 10^6 units rIFN-α_2 was reached by week 4 and repeated weekly thereafter. *LAP*, laparotomy.

Table 2. Toxicity of Patients Receiving i.p. rIFN-α_2

Grade of Toxicity	Fever[a]	Abdominal Pain	Malaise	Headache	Chills	Nausea and Vomiting	Diarrhea	Pruritis	Temporary Anorexia	Anemia[b] Day 1	Anemia[b] Day 7	Leukopenia[b] Day 1	Leukopenia[b] Day 7
I. Mild	≥38°C: 40	11	30	19	36	21	19	6	31	31	34	26	9
II. Moderate	≥39°C: 17	10	33	16	16	16	8	6	7	22	24	9	4
III. Severe	≥40°C: 1	1	2	3	1				1	5	4	1	
Total	58	22	65	38	53	37	27	12	39	58	62	36	13

(Column group heading: % of Patients with Side Effects)

[a] Fever assessed in 132 of 146 cycles.
[b] Anemia and leukopenia assessed in 140 of 146 cycles.

sured in some patients during this first 24-h period; however, in all cases pulse rates returned to normal values within 24 h. Respiration and blood pressure remained normal during treatment.

Hematological analysis in 140 courses was performed pretreatment and 24 h and 7 days after treatment. Base-line (pretreatment = time 0) blood hemoglobin levels showed only 5% anemia, but by day 1, 31% had grade I anemia, 22% had grade II anemia, and 5% had grade III anemia. By day 7, 34% had grade I toxicity, 24% had grade II toxicity, and 4% had grade III toxicity. With base-line (pretreatment = time 0) values of leukopenia in only 1% of patients, leukopenia was noted in 36% of cases on day 1 and 13% of cases on day 7. In 90% of the courses the total WBC on day 1 was less than pretreatment value, but only 36% were <3000/ml (10% grade III), and those values returned to normal by day 3 in most cases. Additionally in 88% of these courses the WBC on day 7 was greater than the WBC on day 1, with only 13% having WBC <3000/ml on day 7. The mean base-line WBC for the 14 treated patients was 5350/ml. This level decreased slightly during treatment with mean values of 4400 on day 1 and 4900/ml on day 7. WBC for responders and nonresponders were not significantly different.

Blood chemistry tests performed every week of treatment revealed no elevation of liver enzymes, renal function tests, or other abnormalities.

The dose limiting toxicity occurred in the second dose schedule phase of the study during which patients received 50 × 10^6 units rIFN-α_2 three times every other week, but after two cycles persistent moderate toxicity (fatigue, abdominal pain, and headaches) required that the treatment schedule be modified so that the rIFN-α_2 was given weekly thereafter.

In an additional two patients Tenckhoff catheters were inserted with the intention of treating the patients with i.p. rIFN-α_2. One patient developed a clotted catheter and decided not to continue the study, and the catheter was removed prior to any rIFN-α_2 treatment. Another

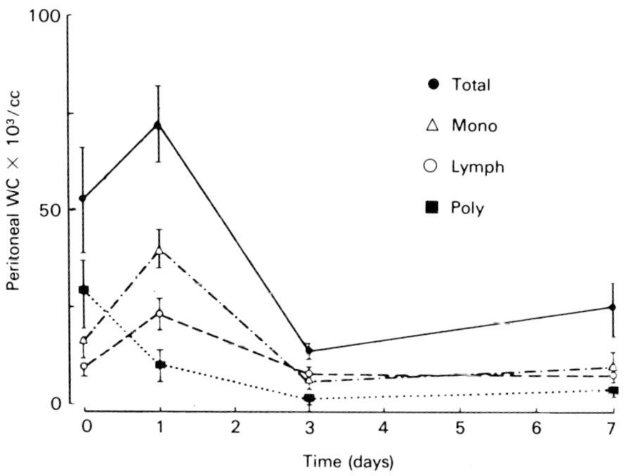

Chart 2. Fluid WBC of patients treated with i.p. rIFN-α_2 are presented. After three baseline values (pretreatment = time 0), specimens were obtained on days 1, 3, and 7 after most weekly treatments. Day 7 also represents the time immediately prior to the subsequent treatment. Values represent the mean integrated sum of all treatment cycles (*bars,* SD) showing a rapid rise in total WBC, lymphocytes, and mononuclear cells by day 1 after treatment, and a gradual return to below baseline by day 7. Total WBC are plotted, as well as polymorphonuclear leukocytes (*Poly*), lymphocytes, and monocytes.

patient had a catheter placed at the time of laparotomy but developed a postoperation thrombophlebitis and was thus excluded from the protocol.

Immunological Results

Peripheral Blood. Differential counts revealed that lymphocytes decreased each cycle for a mean base-line value of 1530/ml to 550/ml on day 1 and then rapidly returned to near base-line levels of 1300/ml by day 7. Blood monocytes and polymorphonuclear leukocytes remained relatively constant throughout treatment.

Peritoneal Fluid. The mean base-line peritoneal WBC for treated patients was 48,100/ml. A consistent increase was seen in the WBC by day 1 in all patients (83,100/ml), a mean value which returned to levels slightly below base line by day 7, *i.e.,* 22,000/ml (Chart 2). The absolute numbers of peritoneal monocytes and lymphocytes increased on day 1 of each cycle after treatment and returned to base-line values by day 7. Monocyte numbers increased from a mean base-line value of 16,300/ml to 52,600/ml

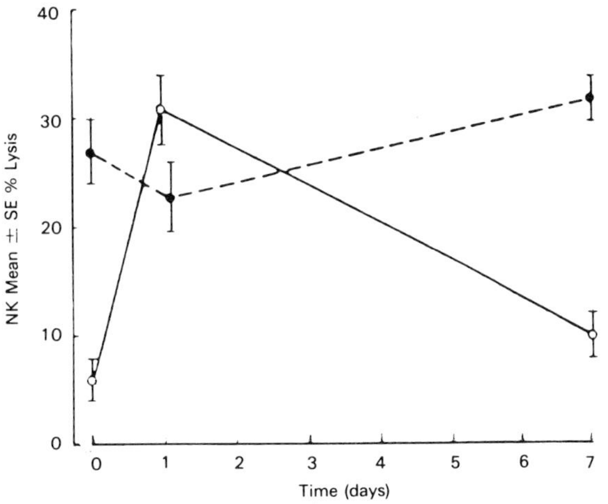

Chart 3. NK. *Points,* the mean percentage of specific lysis of each patient; *bars,* SE. The peripheral blood lymphocytes (- - -) and the peritoneal cavity lymphocytes (—) are presented. Time zero = baseline levels prior to initial treatment, and day 1 is the mean of NK 24 h after i.p. administration of rIFN-α_2. Specimens taken 7 days after treatment are also those taken immediately prior to subsequent treatment.

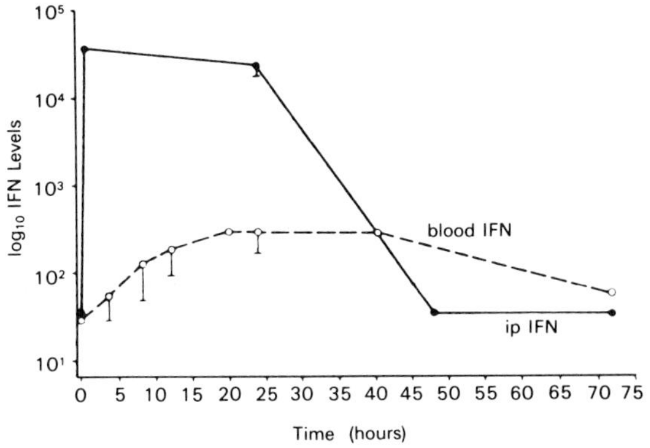

Chart 4. Mean values of blood (- - -) and i.p. fluid (——) rIFN-α_2 levels following the i.p. administration of 50 × 10^6 rIFN-α_2; *bars,* SE.

on day 1, while lymphocytes increased from a mean base-line value of 12,300/ml to 26,500/ml on day 1 and returned to 6,600/ml by day 7. By contrast polymorphonuclear leukocyte levels dropped from a base line of 19,500/ml to 4,000/ml on day 1 and rose to 7,700/ml on day 7. There were no significant differences in WBC counts and differential populations between responders and nonresponders. Some increase in total cell counts were observed by the seventh and eighth weeks of therapy.

NK

Evaluation of NK (effector:target ratio, 25:1) in blood and peritoneal fluid is presented (mean ± SE) in Chart 3. The NK base line in the blood was 27 ± 3, which was 24 ± 3 by day 1, and rose slightly to 32 ± 2 by day 7. In contrast the i.p. NK values were markedly boosted from a base line of 6 ± 2 to 31 ± 4 on day 1 and fell to 10 ± 2 by day 7. Over the successive treatment weeks alterations in NK were relatively homogeneous with no major variation over time; *i.e.,* there was no cumulative boost or depression in the NK over 8 to 16 weeks. Boosting of NK did not uniformly relate to response; *i.e.,* while all patients who had a documented response had significant elevation of i.p. NK on day 1, five of the eight patients who did not have a response also demonstrated some NK elevation.

Neutralizing Antibodies

Multiple serum samples obtained prior to treatment and on days 1 and 7 after treatment were tested for neutralizing antibodies specific to the human rIFN-α_2. No antibodies were detected at any time.

IFN Pharmacokinetics

Serum. Serum rIFN-α_2 levels rose from pretreatment base line of $\leq$38 units/ml to levels of 75–300 units/ml 8 h after treatment (Chart 4). By 24 h serum rIFN-α_2 levels consistently ranged from 150 to 600 units/ml. Serum samples taken from day 2 through day 7 were scarce due to the logistics of patient travel to and from the hospital on "off" days; however, from the small number of samples that we were able to obtain, it appears that rIFN-α_2 levels remained high or above base-line values up to day 6. Serum levels returned to base line by day 7.

Peritoneal Fluid. Peritoneal fluid rIFN-α_2 levels rose from a pretreatment level of $\leq$38 units/ml up to approximately 38,400 units/ml during the first 24 h of treatment at interferon dosage of 50×10^6 units of rIFN-α_2 (Chart 4). Thereafter coinciding with removal of dialysis fluid at the 24-h mark, levels of rIFN-α_2 in the peritoneal cavity returned to base line. Measurements of rIFN-α_2 levels in lavages at day 2 (48 h), day 3 (72 h), and day 7 (168 h) were equal to base-line levels of $\leq$38 units/ml.

DISCUSSION

This is the first report demonstrating efficacy for the i.p. administration of rIFN-α_2 in patients with persistent MRD epithelial ovarian cancer detected at second look laparotomy. The documentation of complete responses in 4 of the 11 surgically evaluated patients suggests that this biological response modifier may prove useful in the treatment of MRD ovarian cancer. Responses appeared to occur after four to six cycles of 50×10^6 units of rIFN-α_2, as indicated by the results obtained with serial peritoneal fluid cytologies performed on these patients. The toxicity of the i.p. rIFN-α_2 was moderate; the principal problem related to the use of the i.p. catheters.

In this study the rIFN-α_2 pharmacokinetic data suggest that very high i.p. concentrations of the agent are present for at least 24 h, at which time dialysis solution is withdrawn for study. However, a low level of rIFN-α_2 is detectable 48 and 72 h after treatment. Peripheral blood levels remained elevated for 5 to 6 days. These data might help to explain the biological efficacy of rIFN-α_2. Also the serum levels of rIFN-α_2 are quite high in comparison to the usual levels achieved with standard i.m. or s.c. administration, which usually ranges approximately 200 to 300 units/ml.[1-8] Thus the peritoneal cavity may be acting as a reservoir, leading to both constant surface exposure and to a persistent serum level. This feature has implications for cell cycle studies as indicated by *in vitro* data which demonstrate that constant exposure to rIFN-α_2 produces more marked cytotoxic and cytostatic effect than does pulse exposure.[3,4] This antitumor activity might result from exposure of the ovarian cancer cells to high concentrations of rIFN-α_2.

It is of interest that only patients with MRD (<5 mm maximum tumor diameter) achieved a surgically documented response and that patients with larger disease did not respond. Indeed five of seven surgically evaluated patients (71%) with MRD had a response. As such, future trials of this agent should probably be confined to patients with MRD. These data are similar to our previous experience using i.p. immunotherapy,[11,12] chemotherapy,[13] and whole abdominal radiation therapy[23] and with data obtained using a murine ovarian cancer model.[14,24-26] Therefore it would appear that the tumor burden prior to the initiation of therapy is critical in these patients; thus surgical resection of tumor might be important if larger tumors are present at the time of exploratory surgery.[27]

The only previous studies of the use of systemically administered IFNs for the treatment of ovarian cancer have been carried out in Scandinavia[2,9] and the United States.[28] The first group of authors reported partial clinical responses in 2 of 18 previously treated patients, 3 patients with "minimal" responses, and 3 patients who had stable disease for up to 1 year. The second group of authors[27] reported no responses, while 4 of their 13 patients had stable disease (median, 6 months).

In our experience ovarian cancer often remains confined to the peritoneal cavity, even after clinical recurrence.[10] Intracavitary therapies are appealing because of their potential for increasing the concentration of the agent and bringing the agent into direct contact with the residual tumor.[6,11-15] Historically, BRMs have been most effective in patients in whom the agent has been administered intralesionally or intracavitarilly.[6,11-15,24,25] Also the presence of tumor cytotoxic chemotherapy appears to be immunosuppressive in patients with ovarian cancer.[19]

BRMS have generally been unsuccessful in the treatment of ovarian cancer.[13] However, some studies have suggested that combinations of systemically administered *Bacillus* Calmette-*Guérin*[18] and *C. parvum*[30] administered concomitantly with cytotoxic chemotherapy induce a higher proportion of clinically documented complete responses than the use of combination chemotherapy alone. The i.p. administration of *C. parvum* in patients with MRD documented at second look has produced surgically documented responses.[11,12]

NK and antibody dependent cell mediated cytotoxicity may be partially responsible for tumor control and/or proliferation in the peritoneal cavity.[11,12,19,31] These effector cells have been shown to be deficient in the peritoneal cavities of women with ovarian cancer previously treated with combination chemotherapy.[18] The i.p. administration of *C. parvum* has been reported to augment peritoneal cavity cytotoxic effector lymphocytes, both NK[12,31] and antibody-dependent cell mediated cytotoxicity,[11,12] in responding patients. Since rIFN-α_2 has been shown to be a potent stimulator of NK,[6] its i.p. administration to patients with persistent epithelial disease thus seems rational. Our measurement of both blood and i.p. fluid NK in relationship to the rIFN-α_2 treatments shows that i.p. NK is significantly boosted after 1 day, while blood values showed considerable variability. No cumulative boosting or suppression is demonstrated. Also the values do not correlate with the objective response. The temporal dynamics of NK effectors relative to the rIFN-α_2 pharmacokinetics are the subject of a separate report.* Although mononuclear cells were not tested for cytotoxicity in these patients, future studies will focus on these potentially important cells.

IFNαs have been shown to have an antiproliferative effect against ovarian cancer cells grown in human tumor stem cell assays.[32] Also there is evidence that IFNs may act synergistically with cytotoxic chemotherapeutic agents *in vitro*.[33-36] These data suggest that the exposure of cancer cells to rIFN-α_2 prior to or concomitant with cytotoxic agent(s) can increase cell kill. Therefore i.p. rIFN-α_2 may be potentially useful in addition to cytotoxic chemotherapy in patients with ovarian cancer. Indeed there is the potential for the use of rIFN-α_2 in the treatment of patients after primary cytoreductive surgery in combination with chemotherapy or in an adjuvant setting after a negative second look laparotomy.

ADDENDUM (STATUS OF PATIENTS AS OF APRIL 1986)

Of the 11 surgically evaluable patients, 4 patients who had complete responses to the IFN therapy are alive at 21, 24, 28, and 30 months, respectively (mean follow-up is 26 months). Three of these patients are free of disease, and 1 patient whose disease recurred at 12 months is alive at 21 months. The one patient who had a partial response to the rIFN-α_2 treatment is alive and free of disease at 22 months. Of the patients whose disease progressed, the mean survival time was 12 months (with a range of 4 to 17 months). All these patients have died. Of the 3 patients who were clinically evaluable, only the patient who had a complete response survived 23 months before succumbing to recurrent disease. The one with clinically stable disease survived 12 months, and the one who had progressive disease survived 8 months.

*C. Spina, A. Lichtenstein, J. S. Berek, and J. Zighelboim. Regional modulation of natural immunity by interferon therapy to patients with ovarian cancer, submitted for publication.

REFERENCES

1. Borden, E. C. Progress toward therapeutic application of interferons. Cancer (Phila.), *54:* 2770–2776, 1984.

2. Kirkwood, J. M., and Ernstoff, M. S. Interferons in the treatment of human cancer. J. Clin. Oncol., *2:* 336–352, 1984.

3. Grossberg, S. E. The interferons and their inducers:

molecular and therapeutic considerations. Part I. N. Engl. J. Med., *287:* 13–19, 1972.

4. Grossberg, S. E. The interferons and their inducers: molecular and therapeutic considerations. Part II. N. Engl. J. Med., *287:* 79–85, 1972.

5. Grossberg, S. E. The interferons and their inducers: molecular and therapeutic considerations. Part III. N. Engl. J. Med., *287:* 122–128, 1972.

6. Oldham, R. K. Biologicals and biological response modifiers: fourth modality of cancer treatment. Cancer Treat. Rep., *68:* 221–232, 1984.

7. Quesada, J. R., Reuben, J., Manning, J. T., Hersh, E. M., and Gutterman, J. U. Alpha interferon for induction of remission in hairy-cell leukemia. N. Engl. J. Med., *310:* 15–18, 1984.

8. Foon, F. A., Sherwin, S. A., Abrams, P. G., Longo, D. L., Fer, M. F., Stevenson, H. C., Ochs, J. J., Bottino, G. C., Schoenberger, C. S., Zeffren, J., Jaffe, E. S., and Oldham, R. K. Treatment of advanced non-Hodgkin's lymphoma with recombinant leukocyte a interferon. N. Engl. J. Med., *311:* 1148–1152, 1984.

9. Einhorn, N., Cantell, K., Einhorn, S., and Strander, H. S. Human leukocyte interferon therapy for advanced ovarian cancer. Am. J. Clin. Oncol., *5:* 167–172, 1982.

10. Berek, J. S., Hacker, N. F., Lagasse, L. D., Poth, T., Resnick, B., and Nieberg, R. K. Second-look laparotomy in stage III epithelial ovarian cancer: clinical variables associated with disease status. Obstet. Gynecol., *64:* 207–212, 1984.

11. Bast, R. C., Berek, J. S., Obrist, R., Griffiths, C. T., Berkowitz, R. S., Hacker, N. F., Parker, L., Lagasse, L. D., and Knapp, R. C. Intraperitoneal immunotherapy of human ovarian carcinoma with *Corynebacterium parvum.* Cancer Res., *43:* 1395–1401, 1983.

12. Berek, J. S., Knapp, R. C., Hacker, N. F., Lichtenstein, A., Jung, T., Spina, C., Obrist, R., Griffiths, C. T., Berkowitz, R. S., Parker, L., Zighelboim, J., and Bast, R. C. Intraperitoneal immunotherapy of epithelial ovarian carcinoma with *Corynebacterium parvum.* Am. J. Obstet. Gynecol., in press, 1985.

13. Berek, J. S., and Hacker, N. F. Immunotherapy of gynecologic cancer. *In:* G. Deppe (ed.), Chemotherapy of Gynecologic Cancer, pp. 363–374. New York: Alan R. Liss, Inc., 1984.

14. Berek, J. S., Cantrell, J. L., Lichtenstein, A. K., Hacker, N. F., Knox, R. M., Nieberg, R. K., Poth, T., Elashoff, R. M., Lagasse, L. D., and Zighelboim, J. Immunotherapy with biochemically dissociated fractions of *Propionibacterium acnes* in a murine ovarian cancer model. Cancer Res., *44:* 1871–1875, 1984.

15. Pretorius, R. G., Hacker, N. F., Berek, J. S., Ford, L. C., Hoeschele, J. D., Butler, T. A., and Lagasse, L. D. al. The pharmacokinetics of intraperitoneal cisplatinum in refractory ovarian cancer. Cancer Treat. Rep., *67:* 1085–1092, 1983.

16. Berek, J. S., Griffiths, C. T., and Leventhal, J. L. Second-look evaluation in ovarian cancer. Obstet. Gynecol., *58:* 192–198, 1981.

17. Blessing, J. A. Design, analysis, and interpretation of chemotherapy trials in gynecologic cancer. *In:* G. Deppe (ed.), Chemotherapy of Gynecologic Cancer, pp. 49–83. New York: Alan R. Liss, Inc., 1984.

18. Boyum, A. Separation of lymphocytes from blood and bone marrow. Scand. J. Clin. Lab. Invest., *21* (Suppl. 97): *77,* 1968.

19. Berek, J. S., Bast, R. C., Lichtenstein, A., Hacker, N. F., Spina, C., Lagasse, L. D., Knapp, R. C., and Zighelboim, J. Lymphocyte cytotoxicity in the peritoneal cavity and blood of patients with ovarian cancer. Obstet. Gynecol., *64:* 708–714, 1984.

20. Jondal, M., Spina, C., and Targan, S. Human spontaneous killer cells: selective cytotoxicity against tumor-derived target cells. Nature (Lond.), *272:* 62–64, 1978.

21. Protzman, W. P., Jacobs, S. L., Minnicozzi, M., Oden, E. M., and Kelsey, D. K. A radioimmunologic technique to screen for antibodies to alpha-2 interferon. J. Immunol. Methods, in press, 1985.

22. Rubinstein, S., Samilletti, P., and Pestka, S. A convenient assay for interferon. J. Virol., *37:* 755–758, 1981.

23. Hacker, N. F., Berek, J. S., Burnison, C. M., Heintz, A. P. M., Eisen, K. P. S., Juillard, G. J. F., Fu, Y. S., and Lagasse, L. D. Whole abdominal radiation as salvage therapy for epithelial ovarian cancer. Obstet. Gynecol., *65:* 60–66, 1985.

24. Knapp, R. C., and Berkowitz, R. S. *Corynebacterium parvum* as an immunotherapeutic agent in an ovarian cancer model. Am. J. Obstet. Gynecol., *128:* 782–786, 1977.

25. Bast, R. C., Knapp, R. C., Mitchell, A. K., Thorston, J. F., Tucker, R. W., and Schlossman, S. F. Immunotherapy of a murine ovarian carcinoma with *Corynebacterium parvum* and specific heteroantiserum. J. Immunol., *123:* 1945–1951, 1979.

26. Vanhaelen, C. P. J., and Fisher, R. I. Requirements for successful immunotherapy and chemo-immunotherapy of a murine model of ovarian cancer. Cancer Res., *41:* 980–983, 1981.

27. Berek, J. S., Hacker, N. F., Lagasse, L. D., Nieberg, R. K., and Elashoff, R. M. Survival of patients following secondary cytoreductive surgery in ovarian cancer. Obstet. Gynecol., *61:* 189–193, 1983.

28. Freedman, R., Wharton, J. T., and Rutledge, F. Human leukocyte interferon (IFNα) in patients with epithelial ovarian cancer (a preliminary report). Proc. Am. Assoc. Cancer Res., *22:* 372, 1981.

29. Alberts, D. S., Salmon, E. S., and Moon, T. E. Chemoimmunotherapy for advanced ovarian carcinoma with Adriamycin-cyclophosphamide $\pm$ BCG: early report of a Southwest oncology group study. Recent Results Cancer Res., *68:* 160–165, 1978.

30. Creasman, W. T., Gall, S. A., and Blessing, J. A. Chemoimmunotherapy in the management of primary stage III ovarian cancer: a Gynecologic Oncology Group study. Cancer Treat. Rep., *63:* 319–323, 1979.

31. Lichtenstein, A., Berek, J. S., Bast, R. C., Spina, C., Hacker, N. F., Knapp, R. C., and Zighelboim, J. Activation of peritoneal lymphocyte cytotoxicity in patients with ovarian cancer by intraperitoneal treatment with *Cornyebacterium parvum.* J. Biol. Resp. Modifiers, *3:* 1–8, 1984.

32. Willson, J. K. V., Bittner, G., and Border, E. C. Antiproliferative activity of interferons against ovarian cancer

cells grown in human tumor stem cell assay. J. Interferon Res., *4:* 441–447, 1984.

33. Welander, C., Gaines, J., Homesley, H., and Rudnick, S. *In vitro* synergistic effects of recombinant human interferon $alpha_2$ (rIFN-α_2) and doxorubicin on human tumor cell lines. Proc. Am. Soc. Clin. Oncol., *2:* 42, 1983.

34. Inoue, M., and Tan, Y. H. Enhancement of actinomycin D- and *cis*-diamminedichloroplatinum(II) induced killing of human fibroblasts by human β-interferon. Cancer Res., *43:* 5484–5488, 1983.

35. Tozawa, M., Kidowaki, T., Terufusa, T., Schmidt, H. J., Abu-Ghazaleh, S., Whisnant, J. K., and Di Saia, P. J. Combination therapy of interferon and cyclophosphamide on murine neuroblastoma. J. Jpn. Soc. Cancer Ther., *17:* 613, 1982.

36. Aapro, M. S., Salmon, S. E., and Alberts, D. S. Schedule dependent synergism of vinblastine and cloned leukocyte interferon α. Stem Cells, *1:* 303–304, 1981.

Rationale for and Conduct of a Phase I Clinical Trial With Interferon Alfa-2b Plus Doxorubicin

Daniel D. Von Hoff,* Giselle Sarosy,† Thomas D. Brown,‡ John G. Kuhn,* and Daniel L. Kisner*

A human tumor cloning system was utilized to screen for the antitumor activity of recombinant interferon alfa-2b (Intron® A) alone and in combination with standard antineoplastic agents. These in vitro studies confirmed synergistic effects of alfa-2b plus doxorubicin against primary human tumors. Based on those in vitro findings, a phase I study has been conducted by Sarosy and colleagues[1] that demonstrated that recombinant interferon alpha-2b and doxorubicin could be given together. Myelosuppression was the dose-limiting toxicity. Because responses were noted in the phase I trials with the combination, phase II trials of the combination are warranted. Additional phase I studies that should be pursued include recombinant interferon alpha-2b plus 5-fluorouracil, interferon plus cisplatinum, and interferon plus DTIC.

IT HAS been adequately documented in the literature as well as in this issue of *Seminars in Oncology* that the interferons have some antitumor activity as single agents in a variety of diseases, including hairy cell leukemia (HCL), the lymphomas, renal cell carcinoma, melanoma, and Kaposi's sarcoma. However, the interferons have not had a major impact on survival of patients with cancer, except in the case of those with HCL. Because of this limited single-agent activity, a number of attempts have been made to combine the interferons with standard antineoplastic agents. In this article, we review the preclinical rationale for combining recombinant interferon alfa-2b and doxorubicin, and discuss the results of a recently completed phase I trial employing this combination.[1]

PRECLINICAL RATIONALE FOR COMBINING INTERFERONS AND DOXORUBICIN

Activity in a Human Tumor Cloning System

Utilizing a capillary cloning system similar to a human tumor cloning system described by Hamburger and Salmon,[2] we screened recombinant interferon alfa-2b (Intron® A) for activity against human tumor colony-forming units.[2-5] Tables 1 and 2 detail the results of testing concentrations of 10, 100, and 1,000 ng/mL of recombinant interferon alfa-2b at both 1-hour and continuous exposure. As can be seen in these tables, a clear-cut dose-response effect occurs with either type of exposure. It is also clear that continuous exposure to recombinant interferon alfa-2b produces cytotoxicity in a greater percentage of patients' tumors. These preclinical data support high and constant exposures to recombinant interferon alfa-2b for maximum antitumor effect. The results of clinical trials comparing high and low doses of interferon lead to the same conclusion.[6]

In vitro studies utilizing a combination of recombinant interferon alfa-2b plus doxorubicin at one-tenth peak plasma level (0.04 μg/mL) were also performed. As part of this research, each agent was tested separately, at continuous exposure, as well (Table 3). All specimens were examined for the synergistic effects of recombinant interferon alfa-2b plus doxorubicin by utilizing the method of Momparler.[7] This method calculates synergism by taking the surviving fraction of agent A and multiplying it by the surviving fraction of agent B. If the two agents administered together have a surviving fraction less than that produced by A × B, synergism is present. As can be seen in Table 3, nine (69%) of 13 specimens plated demonstrated synergism.

**Cancer Therapy and Research Foundation of South Texas and the Section of Drug Development, University of Texas Health Science Center at San Antonio, Division of Oncology, Department of Medicine, 7703 Floyd Curl Drive, San Antonio, Texas.*

†Investigational Drug Branch, Landow Building, Room 4C17, National Institutes of Health, Bethesda, Maryland.

‡Brooke Army Medical Center, Beach Pavilion, Fort Sam Houston, Texas.

Address reprint requests to: Daniel D. Von Hoff, MD, University of Texas Health Science Center at San Antonio, Medicine/Oncology, 7703 Floyd Curl Drive, San Antonio, TX 78284.

This investigation was supported in part by a grant from the Schering Corporation and by the Public Health Service, National Research Service award CA 09434 from the National Cancer Institute (G.S.), as well as by the General Clinical Research Center, NIH, DHHS (grant R R-01346) and the Clinical and Support Services of the Audie L. Murphy Memorial Veterans Hospital, San Antonio, Texas.

Table 1. In Vitro Activity of Recombinant Interferon Alfa-2b (1-Hour Exposure)

	Number of Responses* / Number Evaluable		
Tumor Types	10 ng/mL	100 ng/mL	1,000 ng/mL
Breast	0/1	0/1	0/1
Cervix	0/1	1/1	0/1
Colon	0/2	0/2	0/2
Lung, non–small-cell	1/3	1/3	2/3
Lung, small-cell	0/1	0/1	0/1
Melanoma	1/3	1/3	2/3
Ovary	0/5	0/5	3/5
Sarcoma	0/1	0/1	0/1
Pancreas	0/1	0/1	1/1
Totals (%)	2/18(11%)	3/18(17%)	8/18(44%)

* ≤50% survival of tumor colony-forming units.

Table 2. In Vitro Activity of Recombinant Interferon Alfa-2b (Continuous Exposure)

	Number of Responses* / Number Evaluable		
Tumor Type	10 ng/mL	100 ng/mL	1,000 ng/mL
Breast	2/4	4/6	3/4
Cervix	1/1	1/1	1/1
Corpus uteri		1/1	
Colorectal	0/5	2/5	2/5
Kidney	1/1	2/2	1/1
Lung, non–small-cell	8/10	9/11	9/10
Lung, small-cell	0/1	0/1	0/1
Head and neck		1/1	
Melanoma	2/7	5/7	6/7
Neuroblastoma	0/1	1/1	0/1
Ovary	2/6	2/6	3/6
Pancreas	1/1	1/2	1/1
Mesothelioma	0/3	0/3	0/3
Sarcoma	1/2	3/3	2/2
Stomach	0/2	0/2	1/2
Unknown primary		1/1	
Totals (%)	18/44(41%)	33/53(62%)	29/44(66%)

* ≤50% survival of tumor colony-forming units.

The synergism was observed across a variety of tumor types. It is particularly noteworthy that it occurred in four of six breast cancer patients' tumors and in the tumor of the one pancreas cancer patient (see clinical data below). In a similar study by Welander and colleagues,[8] true synergism was noted in two of 13 tumors. These in vitro results in a human tumor cloning assay indicated that recombinant interferon alfa-2b plus doxorubicin might be worthy of a clinical trial.

Activity in Other Systems

Welander and colleagues[8] have also documented true synergism of recombinant interferon alfa-2b plus doxorubicin against several human tumor cell lines growing in vitro (particularly ovarian cancer cell lines). In studying the effect of recombinant interferon alfa-2b plus doxorubicin against Burkitt's lymphoma cell lines, Morris and Spiegel[9] have also documented true synergism. Aapro and colleagues[10] have demonstrated only additive effects of a recombi-

Table 3. Activity of Recombinant Interferon Alfa-2b (rIFNα₂) Plus Doxorubicin Against Human Tumor Colony-Forming Units

	Survival			
Tumor Type	rIFNα_2* (%)	Doxorubicin† (%)	rIFNα_2 + Doxorubicin (%)	Synergism‡
Breast	49	66	35	No
Breast	14	65	14	No
Breast	127	99	102	Yes
Breast	33	127	14	Yes
Breast	72	100	29	Yes
Breast	100	82	32	Yes
Lung	45	116	68	No
Kidney	43	72	20	Yes
Stomach	52	71	39	No
Sarcoma	28	65	13	Yes
Pancreas	60	95	27	Yes
Uterus	48	64	16	Yes
Unknown primary	23	81	17	Yes

* rIFNα_2 was tested at 100 ng/mL.
† Doxorubicin was tested at 0.04 µg/mL.
‡ Synergism was demonstrated in a total of nine (69%) of 13 tumors.

nant alpha interferon against myeloma, breast, and colon lines. Slater et al[11] could find no synergistic effect of the agents against L1210 leukemia. Finally, Balkwill and Moodie[12] found that human interferon alpha (of lymphoid origin) plus doxorubicin was synergistic against human breast cancer growing in nude mice. They noted that this effect could be due to lengthening of the phase of the cell cycle (interferon is known to alter the phase of the cell cycle, but it does not appear to have a major effect on the metabolism of doxorubicin).[13] The majority of the in vitro and in vivo data suggested the appropriateness of a clinical trial of an alpha interferon plus doxorubicin regimen.

PHASE I CLINICAL TRIAL OF RECOMBINANT INTERFERON ALFA-2b PLUS DOXORUBICIN

Sarosy and colleagues[1] have conducted a phase I clinical trial of recombinant interferon alfa-2b plus doxorubicin. In this trial, recombinant interferon alfa-2b was given at a fixed dose of 10×10^6 IU/m² subcutaneously (SC) three times a week (Monday, Wednesday, and Friday) during weeks 1 and 2; no interferon was given during week 3. Interferon administration resumed according to the same schedule during weeks 4 and 5, with no interferon being administered during week 6; this schedule was repeated for the duration of the trial. The doxorubicin was given intravenously (IV), slowly over a 2- to 10-minute period on the Friday of every third week (ie, weeks 1, 4, etc). The escalations of doxorubicin were to proceed from 20 to 40 mg/m².

A total of 14 patients were entered in the study. All but one patient had undergone and failed prior chemotherapy. Two of the patients had previously been administered doxorubicin. All patients had solid tumors (five renal, three non–small-cell lung, two melanoma, and one each of pancreas, colon, skin, and unknown primary).

The dose-limiting toxicity in this study was hematologic toxicity. At a dose of 40 mg/m² of doxorubicin, unacceptable granulocytopenia (granulocyte count <500) was noted in four of six patients; two of the four patients were hospitalized (one with fever and pneumonia and the other with fever with negative cultures). Four other patients were treated at 30 mg/m². All had experienced prior chemotherapy and three had undergone chemotherapy plus radiotherapy. One patient at that dose level developed myelosuppression (granulocyte and platelet counts of 930 and of 39,000, respectively).

Based on these data, the recommended dose in patients with no prior therapy and a good performance status was 10 × 10^6 IU of recombinant interferon alfa-2b three times a week plus 40 mg/m^2 of doxorubicin every 21 days. The recommended dose for patients with extensive prior therapy and/or a poor performance status was the same amount of interferon with the doxorubicin portion reduced to 30 mg/m^2.

Nonhematologic side effects included the usual interferon-associated flu-like syndrome (fever and malaise) in about 80% of patients. Nausea and vomiting were noted in 50% of patients; 58% of patients developed alopecia.

Of particular interest is that two patients developed partial responses (lasting 5 months in one patient, who had pancreatic cancer, and 4 months in the other, who had squamous-cell carcinoma metastatic to the skin).

Table 4 details the other clinical studies involving the use of recombinant interferon alfa-2b plus doxorubicin. Green and colleagues[14] performed a phase I trial that utilized recombinant interferon alfa-2b at a dose of 10 × 10^6 IV three times a week for 3 weeks (with a 2-week rest), and doxorubicin at a dose of 7.5 to 25 mg/m^2 once a week. In this study, granulocytopenia was dose-limiting at a doxorubicin dose of 25 mg/m^2.

Welander and colleagues[15] have already performed a phase II trial of recombinant interferon alfa-2b plus doxorubicin in patients with advanced solid tumors. They administered recombinant interferon alfa-2b in simultaneous intramuscular injections of 10 × 10^6 IU/m^2 and IV infusions of 10 × 10^6 IU/m^2 given over 30 minutes. This was followed by a 2-hour infusion of 20 mg/m^2 of doxorubicin. Treatments were given once a week for three weeks. They reported clinical responses in patients with several different types of tumors, including those of ovarian cancer, cervical cancer, sarcoma, and endometrial cancers.

Muss and colleagues[16] treated 17 patients with renal-cell carcinoma in a phase II trial. Patients were given recombinant interferon alfa-2b at 10 × 10^6 IU SC and IV (30-minute infusion) once a week; 30 minutes after completion of recombinant interferon alfa-2b infusion, doxorubicin was administered in a dose of 20 mg/m^2 IV over 2 hours. Toxicity in this study consisted mainly of fever or flu-like symptoms. There were no responses in 15 evaluable patients.

Of major interest is the fact that the weekly schedule of recombinant interferon alfa-2b administration resulted in minimal myelosuppression in the studies by Welander et al[15] and Muss and colleagues.[16] However, with the three-times-a-week SC administration, the dose-limiting toxicity was myelosuppression (whether the doxorubicin was given every 3 weeks or weekly).

IMPLICATIONS FOR FUTURE CLINICAL STUDIES

Based on available preclinical and clinical information, it is clear that the use of recombinant interferon alfa-2b is feasible and can, in fact, produce responses in patients with solid tumors. The optimal schedule for administration of interferon plus doxorubicin remains obscure. However, the study by Sarosy et al,[1] as well as that by Welander and colleagues,[15] demonstrates that responses can be seen with at least two different schedules of interferon plus

Table 4. Other Published Clinical Trials of Recombinant Interferon Alfa-2b ($rIFN\alpha_2$) Plus Doxorubicin

Dose and Schedule			
$rIFN\alpha_2$	Doxorubicin	Comment	Study
10 x 10^6 IU TIW for 3 weeks	25 mg/m^2 weekly	Myelosuppression	Green et al[14]
10 x 10^6 IU IM and IV weekly	20 mg/m^2 weekly	Systemic symptoms; minimal myelosuppression	Welander et al[15]
10 x 10^6 IU subcutaneous and IV weekly	20 mg/m^2 weekly	Systemic symptoms; minimal myelosuppression	Muss et al[16]

Abbreviations: TIW, three times weekly; IM, intramuscularly.

Table 5. Summary of Evidence of Synergism of Recombinant Interferon Alfa-2b (rIFNα_2) Plus Other Anticancer Agents Against Human Tumor Colony-Forming Units

		Percent Survival			
Tumor Type	Drug	rIFNα_2	Drug	Combination	Synergism
Colon	5-fluorouracil	85	56	32	Yes
Colon	5-fluorouracil	24	10	3	No
Colon	5-fluorouracil	50	6	6	No
Lung	5-fluorouracil	143	194	101	Yes
Head and neck	5-fluorouracil	31	26	18	No
Melanoma	DTIC	4	10	36	No
Melanoma	DTIC	41	73	26	Yes
Melanoma	DTIC	27	72	4	Yes
Lung	Melphalan	7	74	10	No
Lung	Melphalan	42	121	39	Yes
Ovary	Cisplatinum	68	92	54	Yes
Cervix	Cisplatinum	24	131	13	Yes
Ovary	Cyclophosphamide	35	21	3	Yes
Kidney	Vinblastine	27	93	5	Yes

doxorubicin administration. There is certainly sufficient evidence of activity to proceed with phase II studies of recombinant interferon alfa-2b plus doxorubicin employing either of those two schedules.

ADDITIONAL COMBINATIONS WORTHY OF EXPLORATION

We have examined, in a preliminary manner, the activity of recombinant interferon alfa-2b plus other agents utilizing the human tumor cloning assay (Table 5). Although the number of tumors tested is small, it can be seen that there is synergism between recombinant interferon alfa-2b and all the agents examined, including 5-fluorouracil, DTIC, melphalan, cisplatinum, cyclophosphamide, and vinblastine. Overall, nine (64%) of the 14 tumors tested showed evidence of synergy between recombinant interferon alfa-2b and the particular antineoplastic agent used. In vitro and in vivo studies in other systems have also documented synergism.[10,11,17-20] Clinical trials utilizing a combination such as recombinant interferon alfa-2b plus DTIC in patients with metastatic malignant melanomas are definitely indicated.

REFERENCES

1. Sarosy GA, Brown TD, Von Hoff DD, et al: Phase I study of alpha-2 interferon (Intron) plus doxorubicin in patients with solid tumors. Cancer Res (in press)

2. Hamburger AW, Salmon SE: Primary bioassay of human tumor stem cells. Science 197:461–463, 1977

3. Von Hoff DD, Casper J, Bradley E, et al: Direct cloning of human neuroblastoma cells in soft agar culture. Cancer Res 40:3591–3597, 1980

4. Von Hoff DD, Clark GM, Stogdill BJ, et al: Prospective clinical trial of a human tumor cloning system. Cancer Res 43:1926–1931, 1983

5. Von Hoff DD: Plating efficiencies of human tumors in capillaries versus petri dishes, in Salmon SE, Trent JM (eds): Human Tumor Cloning. Orlando, Fla, Grune & Stratton, 1984, pp 153–161

6. Kirkwood JM, Harris JF, Vera R, et al: A randomized study of low and high doses of leukocyte α-interferon in metastatic renal cell carcinoma: The American Cancer Society collaborative trial. Cancer Res 45:863–871, 1985

7. Momparler RL: In vitro systems for evaluation of combination chemotherapy. Pharmacol Ther 8:21–35, 1980

8. Welander CE, Morgan TM, Homesley HD, et al: Combined recombinant human interferon alpha$_2$ and cytotoxic agents studied in a clonogenic assay. Int J Cancer 35:721–729, 1985

9. Morris L, Spiegel R: In vitro synergistic effect of recombinant human interferon alpha 2 (rIFN-α_2) and adriamycin (ADR) in a human Burkitt's lymphoma cell line. Proc Am Assoc Cancer Res 25:318, 1984 (abstr)

10. Aapro MS, Alberts DS, Salmon SE: Interaction of

human leukocyte interferon with vinca alkaloids and other chemotherapeutic agents against human tumors in clonogenic assay. Cancer Chemother Pharmacol 10:161–166, 1983

11. Slater LM, Wetzel MN, Cesario T: Combined interferon-antimetabolite therapy of murine L-1210 leukemia. Cancer 48:5–9, 1981

12. Balkwill FR, Moodie EM: Positive interactions between human interferon and cyclophosphamide or adriamycin in a human tumor model system. Cancer Res 44:904–908, 1984

13. Balkwill FR, Mowshowitz S, Seilman SS, et al: Positive interactions between interferon and chemotherapy due to direct tumor action rather than effects on host drug-metabolising enzymes. Cancer Res 44:5249–5255, 1984

14. Green MD, Speyer JL, Wernz JD, et al: A phase I study of the concurrent administration of alpha-2-interferon and doxorubicin. Clin Res 33:767A, 1985(abstr)

15. Welander CE, Muss HB, Homesley HD, et al: Phase II trial of combined human interferon alpha$_2$ (rIFNα_2) and doxorubicin in advanced solid tumors. Proc Am Soc Clin Oncol 4:220, 1985 (abstr)

16. Muss HB, Welander C, Caponera M, et al: Interferon and doxorubicin in renal cell carcinoma. Cancer Treat Rep 69:721–722, 1985

17. Namba M, Miyoshi T, Kanamori T: Combined effects of 5-fluorouracil and interferon on proliferation of human neoplastic cells in culture. Gann 73:819–824, 1982

18. Gresser I, Maury C, Tovey M: Efficacy of combined interferon cyclophosphamide therapy after diagnosis of lymphoma in AKR mice. Eur J Cancer 14:97–99, 1978

19. Charigos MA, Pearson JW: Cure of murine leukemia with drug and interferon treatment. J Natl Cancer Inst 51:1367–1368, 1973

20. Miyoshi T, Ogawa S, Kanamori T, et al: Interferon potential cytotoxic effects of 5-fluorouracil on cell proliferation of established human cell lines originating from neoplastic tissue. Cancer Lett 17:239–247, 1983

The Combined Use of Interferon and Radiotherapy in Cancer Management

John Torrisi, Christine Berg, Eric Bonnem*, and Anatoly Dritschilo

Preclinical studies have suggested combination therapy with interferon and radiation results in an enhanced cytotoxic effect. Both additive and synergistic effects have been reported in mammalian cells in tissue culture. A phase I trial was designed to determine patient tolerance to concomitant Schering interferon alfa-2b (Intron® A) and radiation therapy (RT). RT was delivered in standard fashion (five times a week in 180 rad fractions). Interferon was injected subcutaneously 2 hours prior to irradiation. Sixteen patients, divided into groups of three, received interferon at dose levels of 2 × 10^6 to 30 × 10^6 IU/m^2 given five or three times a week. Planned dose escalations were stopped at 5 × 10^6 IU/m^2 by patient tolerance. We observed a significant difference in tolerance to treatment between the patients receiving interferon three times a week and those receiving interferon five times a week. Eight of nine patients treated five times a week developed grade III-IV toxicity resulting in hospitalization and discontinuation of interferon; radiation was not discontinued. Only two of seven patients treated three times a week were hospitalized, with grade II toxicity (anorexia), but both were subsequently able to continue treatment with both interferon and radiation. We have identified a maximum tolerated dose and schedule of interferon (5 × 10^6 IU/m^2 three times a week) for use in future combined modality trials to assess the potential clinical effectiveness of interferon in combination with RT.

FUTURE improvements in the effectiveness of radiation therapy (RT) in the treatment of cancer may result from its combination with other treatment modalities. One area of interest has been the development of radiation sensitizers designed to shift the therapeutic ratio in favor of increased tumor destruction. Despite laboratory successes, little clinical progress has been achieved in the development of an optimal radiation sensitizer. Recent laboratory studies have shown that interferon has sensitizing properties when it is used in combination with ionizing radiation. Clinical trials using interferon and radiation are under development. In this article, we review the preclinical reports of interferon and radiation interactions, speculate on possible mechanisms, and report the results of a phase I clinical trial using Schering interferon alfa-2b in combination with RT.

IN VITRO STUDIES

The interest in the combined use of RT and interferon stems from several in vitro studies that demonstrated that interferon modifies the expression of radiation effects. Ortaldo and McCoy[1] demonstrated that mice given a single intraperitoneal injection of interferon one day after being administered a lethal dose of whole body irradiation had a survival rate significantly better than that of those exposed to radiation only. The researchers attributed the protective effect of interferon to the augmentation of immune function within the animals. Other studies, particularly those using tissue culture techniques, indicate that interferon has radiosensitizing properties. Dritschilo et al[2] demonstrated that radiation killing of mouse 3T3 cells was enhanced in the presence of mouse L-cell interferon. Exposure to interferon for 2 hours prior to radiation led to a potentiation of radiation cell killing, principally reflected in a reduction of the "shoulder" portion of the radiation survival curve. The effect was noted to be species specific; it was not reproducible using human interferon with mouse 3T3 cells. Split-dose experiments designed to test for changes in the repair of sublethal radiation injury failed to determine a difference between interferon-treated and untreated cells. The authors hypothesized that interferon potentiated the radiation effect by inhibiting the ability of cultured cells to accumulate sublethal radiation injury. Similar studies using the HeLa cell culture system appeared to confirm the above observations.[3] Gould et al[4] observed radiosensitization of human bronchogenic carcinoma cells when these were exposed to beta interferon, but not when they were exposed to alpha interferon.

*From the Department of Radiation Medicine, Georgetown University Medical Center, Washington, DC and the*Clinical Research Division, Schering Corporation, Kenilworth, New Jersey.*

Address reprint requests to Anatoly Dritschilo, MD, Department of Radiation Medicine, Georgetown University Medical Center, 3800 Reservoir Road, NW, Washington, DC 20007.

The antiproliferative effect of each interferon on the cell line was determined in the absence of ionizing radiation and was noted to parallel closely the degree of radiosensitization obtained in combined therapy. Comparison of the cell survival curves obtained using interferon and RT combined with that obtained using RT alone indicated that the major effect of interferon was a reduction in the shoulder of the survival curve. The slopes of the radiation survival curves, as reflected in the D_0 values, were similar in the two groups. The antineoplastic effects of the combined interferon and RT treatment was supraadditive—ie, greater than that yielded by adding the individual effects of the two agents—indicating that true radiosensitization had occurred.

Contrary results were obtained by Nederman and Benediktsson[5] in their study of human glioma cell cultures. Using growth retardation instead of cell death as an end point, they noted that the increased effect of combined interferon and RT could be explained by the sum of each therapy used alone. Radiosensitization could not be confirmed in their model system.

Table 1 summarizes the preclinical studies using interferon with radiation. Additional work in our laboratory (unpublished data) suggests a correlation between the response of cells to interferon alone and the supraadditive cytotoxicity observed with interferon plus radiation. We have observed three general characteristics of cytotoxic responses of cells in tissue culture to interferon alfa-2b alone (Figure 1): (1) *growth stimulation* for the normal human fibroblasts; (2) *minimal growth inhibition* for the glioblastoma cells; and (3) *marked growth inhibition* for the osteosarcoma cells. Other cell lines tested fall into these three categories. In general, it may be predicted that cells in category (3) will respond to radiation in the presence of interferon in a synergistic manner, whereas the cells in the other categories either undergo no enhanced cell killing or are affected only additively.

Use of an interferon inducer such as poly (ICLC)—a complex of polyinosinic acid-polycytidylic acid with poly-L-lysine and carboxymethylcellulose—offers the possibility of endogenously achieving high serum interferon levels in animals. Combined use of poly (ICLC) and RT has been studied in the treatment of Lewis lung carcinoma in C_{57} B1 mice.[6] Compared with the mice that received either the inducer or radiation alone, mice in the combined therapy group exhibited a supraadditive improvement in local control, which was determined by measuring the delay in tumor regrowth. Prolonged survival was also noted in the combined treatment group.

Table 1. Preclinical Studies Utilizing Combined Interferon and Radiation

System	Interferon Type	Results/Conclusions	Study
Murine Swiss 3T3 cells	Mouse L cell	Potentiation of radiation killing; reduction of the shoulder of the radiation survival curve	Dritschilo et al,[2] 1982
Human glioma cells (U-118, U-251)	Human alpha	Additive effect on growth delay	Nederman and Benediktsson,[5] 1982
HeLa cells	Human beta	Synergistic cytotoxic effect; reduction of the shoulder of the radiation survival curve	Namba et al,[3] 1984
Human bronchogenic carcinoma cells (A549)	Human alpha and beta	Sensitization of radiation killing by interferon beta, but not by interferon alpha; reduction of the shoulder of the radiation survival curve	Gould et al,[4] 1984
Lewis lung carcinoma in C_{57} B1 mice	Interferon inducer, poly (ICLC)	Improved tumor response and survival in vivo following combined interferon inducer and irradiation	Lvovsky et al,[6] 1985

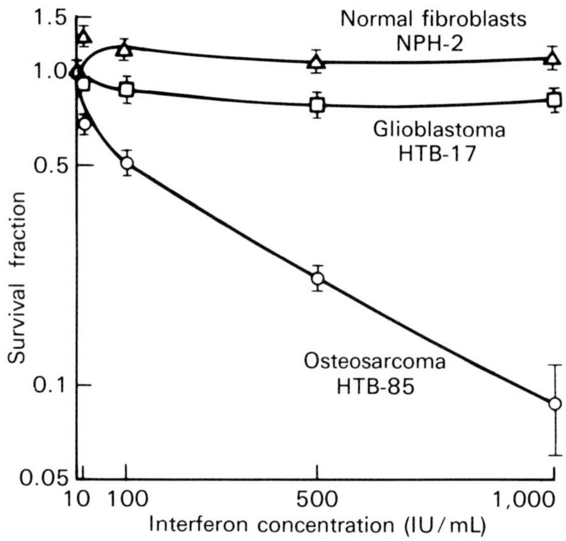

Figure 1. Response to interferon alfa-2b of normal human fibroblast (△), glioblastoma (□), and osteosarcoma (○) cell lines.

INTERFERON AND RADIATION: CLINICAL STUDIES

Interferon has not lived up to the expectation that it would be a "cure for all cancers." Initial clinical studies have shown antitumor effects in small, albeit consistent, percentages of patients with renal-cell carcinoma, melanomas, non-Hodgkin's lymphomas, Kaposi's sarcoma, and other tumors. Table 2 summarizes the reported clinical results of interferon and RT combined modality treatment. Mahaley et al[7,8] were able to use full-dose RT *sequentially* following interferon therapy in the treatment of anaplastic gliomas without provoking unexpected morbidity.

In this study nine patients underwent subtotal resection of anaplastic gliomas and within 3 weeks were started on postoperative therapy. Interferon was administered on 3 consecutive days a week for a total of 3 weeks at doses of 10, 20, and 30 $\times$ 10^6 IU/m^2/day during the first, second, and third weeks, respectively. An infusional pump was used to administer the interferon intravenously over a 4-hour period. Side effects experienced included chills, fever, headache, lethargy, and back pain. These were most pronounced during the first week of treatment. Leukopenia, granulocytopenia, and serum hepatic enzyme elevation were reported as mild. Lumbar cerebral spinal fluid determinations performed in six patients failed to detect interferon; however, the tumor bed of one patient contained an interferon concentration of 120 units/mL.

One week following completion of interferon administration, RT was initiated with delivery of 43 Gy to the whole brain followed by a 17.2-Gy boost to the tumor site. No further therapy

Table 2. Clinical Studies of Combined Interferon and Radiation

Diagnosis	Interferon Dose	Radiation Dose	Results/Comments	Study
Anaplastic glioma				
9 patients	10–30 MU/day, 3 days a week for 3 weeks	60.2 Gy	Sequential interferon and RT; no excess toxicity; no therapeutic benefit	Mahaley et al,[8] 1984
Kaposi's sarcoma (acquired immune deficiency syndrome)				
2 patients	36 MU/day	11–21 Gy	Concomitant interferon and RT; marked mucositis, requiring hospitalization for supportive care	Real et al,[9] 1985
Various malignancies				
16 patients	2–5 MU/m^2, 3 or 5 days a week	39.6–59.4 Gy	Concomitant interferon and RT; marked exacerbation of toxicity in patients receiving treatment 5 days a week	Torrisi et al,[11] 1986

4.6)/mm^3 and 302 (261 to 341)/mm^3, respectively, for those receiving treatment five times a week, and 2.7 (1.9 to 3.0)/mm^3 and 160 (143 to 185)/mm^3, respectively, for those receiving treatment three times a week.

Tumor response was determined by means of serial radiographic studies using standard perpendicular diameter measurements. Complete response, defined as the disappearance of all measurable disease as determined by observations separated by at least 4 weeks, was seen in one patient; partial responses were seen in five others. Stable disease was noted in eight patients. Two patients were declared inevaluable because they were unable to complete the radiotherapeutic course (one died during treatment; the other refused further therapy). Because this trial involved patients with advanced disease, it was not possible to determine if the clinical responses were different from those expected from RT alone.

On the basis of these findings, we define the administration of interferon alfa-2b five times a week to be a nontolerated dose schedule when such administration occurs in conjunction with RT. We believe that the tolerance exhibited by the patients receiving treatment three times a week and the ability to manage the toxicities associated with a dose of 5×10^6 IU/m^2 in these patients indicate that this dose and schedule can be safely utilized in phase II-III studies comparing combination therapy with radiation monotherapy.

COMMENT

The interferons are a diverse group of biologically active glycoproteins that have become available for clinical investigation only relatively recently. In vitro and in vivo studies of the combined use of interferon and RT offer the promise of a supraadditive effect (radiosensitization). Testing of tumor cell lines in vitro offers an opportunity to predict the potential synergistic result of combining interferon with RT. In such selected cases, it may be appropriate to conduct clinical trials in an effort to improve the therapeutic ratio. Normal tissue toxicity, however, also appears to be enhanced, and the long-term effects of the combination therapy remain to be established. At least one dose schedule of concomitant therapy has been established. Phase II and phase III studies are required to fully evaluate the effectiveness of the combined use of interferon and RT.

ACKNOWLEDGMENT

We would like to thank Ms Sandra Hawkins for her contribution to the preparation of this manuscript.

REFERENCES

1. Ortaldo JR, McCoy JL: Protective effects of interferon in mice previously exposed to lethal irradiation. Radiat Res 81:262–266, 1980

2. Dritschilo A, Mossman K, Gray M, et al: Potentiation of radiation injury by interferon. Am J Clin Oncol 5:79–82, 1982

3. Namba M, Yamamoto S, Tanaka H, et al: In vitro and in vivo studies on potentiation of cytotoxic effects of anticancer drugs or cobalt-60 gamma ray by interferon on human neoplastic cells. Cancer 54:2262–2267, 1984

4. Gould M, Kakria R, Olson S, et al: Radiosensitization of human bronchogenic carcinoma cells by interferon. J Interferon Res 4:123–128, 1984

5. Nederman T, Benediktsson G: Effects of interferon on growth rate and radiation sensitivity of cultured, human glioma cells. Acta—Radiol [Oncol] 21:231–234, 1982

6. Lvovsky E, Mossman K, Levy H, et al: Response of mouse tumor to interferon inducer and radiation. Int J Radiat Oncol Biol Phys 11:1721–1725, 1985

7. Mahaley M, Urso M, Whaley R, et al: Immunobiology of primary intracranial tumors. IX. Phase I study of human lymphoblastoid interferon. J Biol Response Mod 3:19–25, 1984

8. Mahaley M, Urso M, Whaley R, et al: Interferon as adjuvant therapy with initial radiotherapy of patients with anaplastic gliomas. J Neurosurg 61:1069–1071, 1984

9. Real F, Krown S, Nisce L, et al: Unexpected toxicity from radiation therapy in two patients with Kaposi's sarcoma receiving interferon. J Biol Response Mod 4:141–146, 1985

10. Maitson K, Holsti L, Niiranen A, et al: Human leukocyte interferon as part of a combined treatment for previously untreated small cell lung cancer. J Biol Response Mod 4:8–17, 1985

11. Torrisi J, Berg C, Harter K, et al: Phase I combined modality clinical trial of alpha-2-interferon and radiotherapy. Int J Radiat Oncol Biol Phys, Pergamon Press, Ltd. (in press)

Interferon Alfa-2b–Cyclophosphamide Combination Studies: In Vitro and Phase I-II Clinical Results

Brian G.M. Durie, Lawrence Clouse, Theodore Braich, Meredith Grimm,* and Aurelia B. Robertone

Since interferon alfa-2b (Intron® A) is useful as a single agent, it is important to determine if interferon can be combined with standard chemotherapy to improve both response and survival in patients with cancer. Using clonogenic assays, interferon was tested alone and in combination with cyclophosphamide (Cytoxan) or melphalan (Alkeran) using several dose and exposure schedules to evaluate cytotoxicity. In vitro, continuous-exposure interferon produced optimal cell kill. Maximum enhancement of cytotoxicity occurred with cyclophosphamide or melphalan pretreatment (1 hour) and/or simultaneous interferon treatment. Based upon these data, a phase I-II study was designed to determine the tolerance of cancer patients to a fixed dose of cyclophosphamide (150 mg/m^2 p.o. daily × 4 days [days 2 to 5]) combined with increasing doses of interferon. Interferon was administered subcutaneously on treatment cycle days 1 to 5, plus days 8, 10, 12, 15, 17, and 19 of the 21-day regimen. Three patients had partial responses: one breast cancer, one angiosarcoma, and one myeloma (mixed). All patients reported mild flu-like symptoms, fatigue, and anorexia. Leukopenia occurred in all patients; three required treatment interruption to allow recovery. Eight patients had a fall in hemoglobin (mean decrease 1.4 g/dL). The combination of cyclophosphamide and interferon was safe and deserves further trial in cancer treatment. However, using this combination schedule, interferon doses ≥5 × 10^6 IU were poorly tolerated and compromised administration of full-dose cyclophosphamide.

INTERFERONS are natural cellular proteins, which have a wide range of immunomodulatory and antiproliferative properties.[1-4] In addition to their antiviral effects, interferons (particularly alpha interferons) have significant antitumor effects both in vitro and in vivo in a wide variety of hematologic and solid tumors.[5-7] Therefore, a major clinical research objective is to determine how best to integrate alpha interferons into conventional chemotherapeutic strategies for treatment of malignancies in which alpha interferons have activity.[8-10]

Since alpha interferons have shown activity against lymphomas, breast cancer, leukemias, and multiple myeloma, for which cyclophosphamide (Cytoxan) is commonly used,[5,6,10] this study was designed to evaluate the combined administration of cyclophosphamide and interferon alfa-2b (Intron® A). The clinical protocol of the phase I-II study reported in this paper was based upon the preliminary in vitro evaluation of the interferon-cyclophosphamide combination. Although the potential synergism of the two agents was evaluated in vitro, the major clinical question was the toxicity of combined administration of the two agents and whether full doses of cyclophosphamide could be administered in addition to interferon alfa-2b.

MATERIALS AND METHODS

Experimental

The procedure for preparing and culturing single-cell suspensions of human tumor cells has been previously described in detail.[6] The human myeloma cell line RPMI 8226 was obtained from the American Type Culture Collection, Rockville, Maryland. The cells were harvested 24 to 48 hours after splitting the cultures and adding fresh medium. All dilutions of the alfa-2b interferon (obtained from the Schering Corporation, Kenilworth, New Jersey) were done in McCoy's 5A medium containing 10% heat-inactivated fetal bovine serum. The RPMI 8226 cell line was plated at a cell concentration of 8 × 10^4/plate in RPMI 1640 medium with 10% fetal calf serum. The alfa-2b interferon was incorporated into the medium at a final concentration ranging from 0.05 to 5 ng/mL, which is equivalent to 10 to 1,000 units/mL of interferon activity. The interferon was added to the mixture just prior to plating.

The plates were incubated at 37 °C in a humidified atmosphere of 7% CO_2. All plates were monitored for aggregation on the morning after

From the Department of Internal Medicine, Section of Hematology/Oncology, University of Arizona College of Medicine, Tucson, Arizona.

**Schering-Plough Pharmaceutical Research Division, Kenilworth, New Jersey.*

Address reprint requests to Brian G.M. Durie, MD, Department of Internal Medicine, University of Arizona Health Sciences Center, 1501 North Campbell Avenue, Tucson, AZ 85724.

plating and discarded if significant aggregation was present. Colony counts were carried out between days 14 and 17 using the Bausch and Lomb FAS II image analyzer, specially equipped and programmed for tumor colony counting.[11] At the time of counting, control plates were also compared with additional control plates fixed in 3% glutaraldehyde kept at 4 °C for the incubation period to prevent proliferation. Cell aggregates greater than 60 μm were counted as colonies.

Clinical

The clinical phase I-II study was sponsored by the Schering Corporation. Details of the drug treatment protocol are outlined in Table 1. The goal of the study was to administer cyclophosphamide at full dosage using a 3-week p.o. schedule. Alfa-2b interferon, administered subcutaneously (SC), was added to the cyclophosphamide schedule to identify the maximum tolerated dose of interferon that could be administered simultaneously with the 4 days of cyclophosphamide therapy and on a Monday-Wednesday-Friday schedule in between the 3-week pulses of cyclophosphamide. The starting dose of interferon was 3 million IU with escalation to 15 million IU (all SC).

As outlined in Table 2, 13 patients were entered into this phase I study. All patients with a confirmed pathologic diagnosis of cancer refractory to conventional therapy (or for which no conventional therapy is available) were eligible for this study. Following a discussion with the principal investigator, appropriate informed consent (as approved by the University of Arizona Human Subjects Committee) was obtained.

Detailed subjective and objective monitoring was carried out to evaluate the toxicity and efficacy of the treatment protocol.

RESULTS

In Vitro Studies

The major results of in vitro testing are summarized in Tables 3 through 5. Table 3 shows the dose response of the 8226 myeloma cell line to alfa-2b interferon, indicating substantial cytotoxicity with continuous exposure to 100 units/mL of interferon and complete elimination of colony growth with continuous exposure to 1,000 units/mL. Based on these data, continuous exposure of the cell line to lower interferon doses (in the range of 10 to 100 units/mL) were used in combination with cyclophosphamide and/or melphalan to evaluate potential synergism.

As shown in Table 4, a combination of 10 units/mL alfa-2b interferon plus 0.1 mg/mL cyclophosphamide clearly enhanced in vitro cell kill of the 8226 myeloma line. The cells were preincubated for 1 hour in 4-hydroperoxy cyclophosphamide prior to plating, with subsequent continuous exposure to the alfa-2b interferon. Only 8% of myeloma colonies survived when exposed to a combination of 50 units/mL alfa-2b interferon plus 0.1 mg/mL cyclophosphamide

Table 1. Cyclophosphamide–Alfa-2b Interferon Phase I–II Study: Treatment Protocol

Cyclophosphamide 150 mg/m²* p.o. QD x 4 (days 2–5)
Alfa-2b interferon 3→ 15 million IU† SC days 1–5 and days 8, 10, 12, 15, 17, and 19 of a 21-day cycle

* Fixed dose.
† Escalated as tolerated (see the text).

Table 2. Cyclophosphamide–Alfa-2b Interferon Phase I–II Study: Patient Profile

Male: 9, Female: 4 } 13
Age: 40–67 years (median 62)
Prior therapy: 11/13 (85%)

Table 3. Dose Response of 8226 Myeloma Cell Line to Alfa-2b Interferon

Interferon Dose (U/mL)	Dose Response (Number of Colonies)	Survival %
Control	425 ± 34	100
Continuous exposure		
10	567 ± 49	133
50	125 ± 29	29
100	27 ± 29	6
1,000	0	0

Table 4. Dose Response of 8226 Myeloma Cell Line to Alfa-2b Interferon Plus Cyclophosphamide

In Vitro Exposure	Response ± Cyclophosphamide (Number of Colonies)	Survival %
Control	425 ± 34	100
Alfa-2b interferon 10 U/mL (continuous)	567 ± 49	133
Cyclophosphamide 0.1 mg/mL (1 hour)	618 ± 115	145
Alfa-2b interferon 10 U/mL (continuous) + cyclophosphamide 0.1 mg/mL (1 hour)	364 ± 64	85*
Alfa-2b interferon 50 U/mL (continuous)	125 ± 44	29
Alfa-2b interferon 50 U/mL (continuous) + cyclophosphamide 0.1 mg/mL (1 hour)	34 ± 7	8*

* $p<0.01$.

Table 5. Dose Response of 8226 Myeloma Cell Line to Alfa-2b Interferon Plus Melphalan

In Vitro Exposure	Response ± Melphalan (Number of Colonies)	Survival %
Control	425 ± 34	100
Alfa-2b interferon 10 U/mL (continuous)	567 ± 49	133
Melphalan 0.1 mg/mL (1 hour)	726 ± 52	171
Alfa-2b interferon 10 U/mL (continuous) + melphalan 0.1 mg/mL (1 hour)	262 ± 66	62*
Alfa-2b interferon 50 U/mL (continuous)	125 ± 44	29
Alfa-2b interferon 50 U/mL (continuous) + melphalan 0.1 mg/mL (1 hour)	50 ± 14	13

* $p<0.01$.

(1-hour exposure). A similar enhancement of cell kill (13% survival) was noted with the combination of 50 units/mL alfa-2b interferon plus 0.1 mg/mL melphalan (Table 5; Figure 1). When 1 hour of pretreatment with alfa-2b interferon was used, there was less enhancement of cell kill. Therefore, the essential feature of greater cytotoxicity was continuous exposure to interferon during the culture period.

Conclusions drawn from these in vitro studies were that (1) combined exposure of cells to both melphalan and cyclophosphamide was important and (2) subsequent continuous exposure to interferon enhanced in vitro cell kill.

Clinical Phase I-II Study

The in vitro studies were the basis for the clinical phase I-II study. The goal was to maximize the amount of interferon that could be administered simultaneously with the cyclophosphamide, as well as the amount that could be administered between the 3-week pulses of oral cyclophosphamide (days 2 to 5).

The interferon was administered SC on days 1 through 5 plus days 8, 10, 12, 15, 17, 19, and

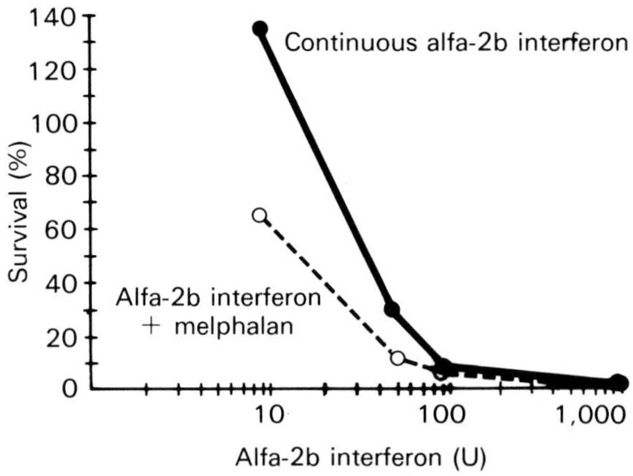

Figure 1. Survival of RPMI 8226 cell line following continuous exposure to 10–1,000 U/mL alfa-2b interferon alone and to 50 U/mL alfa-2b interferon plus 0.1 mg/mL melphalan.

21 of the 3-week cycle. The first three patients received 3×10^6 IU of interferon on all of these days. Patients 5 and 6 received 10×10^6 IU of interferon on days 1 through 5 and 3×10^6 IU on the remaining days of the cycle. Patients 7 through 9 received 10×10^6 IU of interferon on days 1 through 5 and then 5×10^6 IU of interferon on the other days between the cycles of cyclophosphamide. Patients 10 through 13 received 15×10^6 IU of interferon on days 1 through 5 and then 5×10^6 IU for the balance of the days between the cyclophosphamide cycles.

Patients with both hematologic and solid tumor malignancies were evaluated as part of the study (see Table 6). Although the determination of therapeutic response was not a major goal of this investigation, partial responses were seen in one patient with breast cancer (local disease of the chest wall) and one with angiosarcoma (retroperitoneal mass visualized on serial computed tomography). In addition, a mixed response to therapy occurred in one patient with refractory multiple myeloma. Therefore, responses were seen in three of the 13 patients evaluated, a response rate of 23%.

The major goal of this study was to evaluate tolerance of the treatment protocol. Toxicities that limited therapy are detailed in Table 7. Cumulative myelosuppression occurred with all alfa-2b interferon doses $>3 \times 10^6$ IU, necessitating a decrease in interferon dosage and/or a delay in the treatment cycle. Other major effects included neutropenia and cumulative decreases in the hemoglobin level. Eight patients had a significant fall in hemoglobin (mean decrease of 1.4 g/dL), and several required transfusion to correct this effect. Additionally, transient increases in liver transaminase levels (that returned to normal with discontinuation of treatment) were observed.

Table 6. Cyclophosphamide–Alfa-2b Interferon Phase I–II Study: Malignancies Represented

Myeloma (2)	Breast (1)
Lymphoma (2)	Lung (1)
Melanoma (2)	Kidney (1)
Sarcoma (2)	Esophagus (1)
Carcinoid (1)	

Table 7. Cyclophosphamide–Alfa-2b Interferon Phase I–II Study: Toxicity

Limiting Factors
Cumulative myelosuppression (white blood cells + hemoglobin) at $>3 \times 10^6$ IU interferon
Subjective toxicity (flu-like; ↓ performance status) at $\geq 10 \times 10^6$ IU interferon

Table 8. Cyclophosphamide–Alfa-2b Interferon Phase I–II Study: Conclusions

Full-dose cyclophosphamide plus 3×10^6 IU interferon is well tolerated
Interferon doses $\geq 5 \times 10^6$ IU lead to treatment-limiting toxicity
Cyclophosphamide-interferon is a clinically active combination

The true limiting toxicity of interferon was subjective in nature, the most prominent features being a flu-like syndrome, substantial decrease in the performance status, and weight loss (in patients receiving higher doses of interferon). Subjective toxicity was dose-limiting with alfa-2b interferon dosages $\geq 10 \times 10^6$ IU.

CONCLUSIONS

The conclusions of this study are summarized in Table 8. It was possible to administer full-dose cyclophosphamide therapy plus 3×10^6 IU interferon to all of the patients evaluated in this study. Individuals receiving higher dosages of interferon frequently required reduction to 3×10^6 IU in order to tolerate ongoing treatment without major difficulties. Interferon doses above this level led to treatment-limiting subjective and objective toxicity, which usually compromised the ability to administer full-dose cyclophosphamide and also necessitated a delay in the treatment schedules.

Interestingly, the cyclophosphamide-interferon schedule was clinically active in three patients. This may indicate that the interferon did not interfere with cyclophosphamide metabolism or efficacy.

It was concluded that the combination of cyclophosphamide and alfa-2b interferon is safe and deserves further evaluation in cancer treatment. However, using this particular combination schedule, interferon doses $\geq 5 \times 10^6$ IU were poorly tolerated and compromised the administration of full doses of cyclophosphamide. Therefore, in similar studies, caution will be required when interferon doses $>3 \times 10^6$ IU are employed.

REFERENCES

1. Isaacs A, Lindemann J: Virus interference. I. The interferon. Proc R Soc Lond (Biol) 147:258–267, 1957

2. Gresser I, Tovey MG, Bandu MT, et al: Role of interferon in the pathogenesis of virus disease in mice as demonstrated by the use of anti-interferon serum. I. Rapid evolution of EMC virus infection. J Exp Med 144:1305–1315, 1976

3. Gresser I: On the varied biologic effects of interferon. Cell Immunol 34:406–415, 1977

4. Linhorn S, Strander H: Is interferon tissue specific? Effect of human leukocyte and fibroblast interferons on the growth of lymphoblastoid and osteosarcoma cell lines. J Gen Virol 35:573–577, 1977

5. Kirkwood JM, Ernstoff MS: Interferons in the treatment of human cancer. J Clin Oncol 2(4):336–352, 1984

6. Salmon SE, Durie BGM, Young L, et al: Effects of cloned human leukocyte interferons in the human tumor stem cell assay. J Clin Oncol 1(3):217–225, 1983

7. Billiau A, Bloemmen J, Bogaerts M, et al: Interferon therapy in multiple myeloma: Failure of human fibroblast interferon administration to affect the course of light chain disease. Eur J Cancer Clin Oncol 17(6):875–882, 1981

8. Ahre A, Bjorkholm M, Mellstedt H, et al: Human leukocyte interferon and intermittent high-dose melphalan-prednisone administration in the treatment of multiple myeloma: A randomized clinical trial from the myeloma group of Central Sweden. Cancer Treat Rep 68(11):1331–1338, 1984

9. Creagan ET, Kovach JS, Long HJ, et al: Phase I study of recombinant leukocyte A human interferon combined with BCNU in selected patients with advanced cancer. J Clin Oncol 4(3):408–413, 1986

10. Costanzi JJ, Cooper MR, Scarffe JH, et al: Phase II study of recombinant alpha-2-interferon in resistant multiple myeloma. J Clin Oncol 3(5):654–659, 1985

11. Salmon SE, Young L, Lebowitz J, et al: Evaluation of the Omnicon Image analysis system for counting human tumor colonies, in Salmon SE, Trent JM (eds): Human Tumor Cloning. Orlando, Fla, Grune & Stratton, 1984, pp 163–171

Intron® A (Interferon Alfa-2b): Clinical Overview and Future Directions

Robert J. Spiegel

The clinical development of the recombinant alpha interferons represents a prototype for the clinical development of biological compounds. Their testing raises fundamental questions concerning phase I objectives and strategies for biologicals, eg, study design in an immune model *v* a cytotoxic model. However, with over 5,000 patients treated with these compounds, some general principles have emerged. There is a suggestion of dose-response relationships, and a clearer picture of schedule dependence. The extent of tumor burden and identification of sensitive subtypes of patients also appear to be critical factors in evaluating the true potential activity of biological compounds. The toxicity profile of the alpha interferons is unusual. Fever and flu-like symptoms occur almost universally in all doses and schedules, and are usually dose-limiting. Somnolence and other CNS effects occur in a small percentage of patients. Hematologic toxicity occurs but is minimal at lower doses and is noncumulative and rapidly reversible at all doses. Gastrointestinal toxicity is mild. No other unusual or unexpected toxicities have been reported, and early reports of cardiovascular toxicity have not been confirmed in large trials. The use of these pioneer recombinant DNA products raised concerns about the potential production of antibodies and serum-neutralizing factors. Reports with small patient numbers confirmed the occasional development of serum-neutralizing activity to some alpha interferons, which may coincide with a loss of detectable serum interferon and loss of clinical activity. A large study with interferon alfa-2b (Intron® A) has reported a low overall incidence of neutralizing activity (2.5%) and no association with loss of clinical activity. The significance of the neutralizing activity and the reasons for an apparently higher incidence of this phenomenon with other alpha interferon preparations remain to be determined. The full role of alpha interferon by itself or in combination with other available therapies will be resolved in coming years. Efficacy data available to date and phase I combination studies are reviewed.

ALTHOUGH interferon was first discovered by Isaacs and Lindemann in 1957, it was not until the early 1980s, when large quantities of highly purified interferon became available through recombinant DNA technology, that conventional phase I-II testing of interferon could begin. Earlier clinical studies had utilized interferon produced by viral induction of human peripheral blood leukocytes; that process resulted in products with low specific activity ($<1 \times 10^6$ IU/m^2) and less than 1% purity. The scarcity of this material precluded the evaluation of interferon in comprehensive phase I-II studies that could ask dose or schedule questions, and toxicity was frequently ascribed to impurities in the preparations rather than to interferon itself.

In 1979, Dr. Charles Weissman successfully isolated and cloned the gene for human alpha interferon. Using recombinant DNA technology, this gene has been introduced into *Escherichia coli* bacteria, and now can be utilized for the production of large quantities of highly purified human alpha interferon. This clone, developed by Schering Corporation, Kenilworth, NJ, is now designated interferon alfa-2b (Intron® A). Interferon alfa-2b is a 98% pure preparation of a single species of human alpha interferon with a specific activity of 2×10^8 IU/mg protein. The molecule consists of 165 amino acids and has a molecular weight of approximately 20,000 daltons.

Clinical trials with interferon alfa-2b were initiated in 1981, although comprehensive animal toxicology studies or preclinical testing in classic animal tumor models could not be done due to the species specificity of interferon. Since alpha interferon was a prototype biological response modifier, early studies involved an unusually wide variety of administration regimens in an attempt to capitalize on its many putative attributes, such as immune modulation, cell differentiation, radiation sensitization, chemotherapy synergism, and direct cytotoxicity. Various doses and schedules were tested by the intravenous (IV), intramuscular (IM), and subcutaneous (SC) routes. Phase I trials alone involved 165 individuals. In phase II and III trials, interferon alfa-2b has been administered to over 2,000 cancer patients with a broad spec-

Address reprint requests to Robert J. Spiegel, MD, Schering Corporation, 2000 Galloping Hill Road, Kenilworth, NJ 07033.

trum of malignancies. This review summarizes the safety and efficacy results obtained in these studies.

OVERVIEW OF INTERFERON ALFA-2b SAFETY AND TOXICITY

Safety and tolerance data have been obtained and analyzed for 867 patients who were treated systemically with interferon alfa-2b in phase I-II trials and represent more than 3,000 patient-months of exposure. The overall incidence of clinical adverse effects and laboratory abnormalities in this patient population is presented and analyzed for relationships to dose, duration of treatment, and patient age.

Of the 867 patients, 480 received only SC treatment, 312 received only IV treatment, and 75 received both SC and IV treatment. This represents 942 patient-courses of treatment (555 SC and 387 IV). Most patients receiving the SC dose were treated three times per week with self-administered injections. Prior pharmacokinetic studies demonstrated that SC and IM dosing give comparable T_{MAX} and AUC values.[1,2] Subcutaneous doses ranged from 2 to 50 MU/m^2 (MU = 1×10^6 IU), with the majority of patients receiving 2 to 10 MU/m^2 per dose. Intravenous doses ranged from 1 to 100 MU/m^2, with the majority of patients receiving >50 MU/m^2 per dose. Patients receiving interferon alfa-2b by other schedules and routes—eg, continuous IV infusion, intraperitoneal, or intravesicular dosing—are not included in this analysis. Table 1 shows the distribution of patients by duration of treatment: 481/867 (55%) of the patients were treated for at least 8 weeks, and 334/867 (39%) were treated for at least 12 weeks.

Table 1. Distribution of Patients by Treatment Duration

Treatment Duration (Weeks)	N	%
<4	190	22
4–8	196	23
8–12	147	17
12–24	141	17
24–36	96	11
36–48	59	7
48–72	34	4
72–96	3	<1
>96	1	<1

A variety of malignancies are included in this analysis. The major patient groups include multiple myeloma (97 patients), renal-cell carcinoma (75), hairy cell leukemia (92), malignant melanoma (86), and Kaposi's sarcoma (53). However, the patient entry and exclusion criteria for each study were similar. In general, patients eligible for entry into these clinical trials were 18 years of age or older, had histopathologically confirmed malignant disease, life expectancy ≥ 8 weeks, performance status $\leq$ECOG 2, no prior hormonal therapy or chemotherapy within 1 month of treatment, and no prior history of exposure to interferon. Written informed consent was obtained from all patients. Those excluded from entry into these studies were patients with a history of cardiac disease, CNS metastases, severe intercurrent infection, or previous malignancy. Impaired renal, hepatic, and/or hematologic functions were also criteria for exclusion.

Induction therapy usually consisted of daily dosing or three doses per week. Occasionally, an escalating dose schedule was used during induction. Therapy was then continued at the highest tolerated dose for the remainder of treatment. In most studies, stable or responding patients were permitted to continue treatment on a maintenance schedule until their disease progressed or until they were removed from the trial. Dose attenuation was permitted based on

Table 2. Best-Tolerated Doses and Administration Schedules for Intron® A

Indication	Schedule	Starting Dose/m^2
Hairy cell leukemia	SC TIW	2 MU/m^2
Multiple myeloma	SC TIW	2–10 MU/m^2
Kaposi's sarcoma	IV qd x 5, q2 wks*	50 MU/m^2
	SC TIW†	10–15 MU/m^2
Melanoma	SC TIW	10 MU/m^2
Lymphoma	SC TIW	2–10 MU/m^2
Renal-cell cancer	SC TIW	10 MU/m^2
Chronic myelogenous leukemia	SC qd*	4 MU/m^2
	SC TIW†	3–5 MU/m^2
Other miscellaneous solid cancers	SC TIW	5–10 MU/m^2

TIW = Three times weekly; qd = daily.
* Induction.
† Maintenance.

Table 3. Recommendations for Dose Adjustment*

		WHO Grade Severity	Toxicity	Recommended IFN Dose
Hematologic				
Granulocytes/mm³	Platelet/mm³			
>1,500	>75,000	0–1	None to mild	100%
	50–75,000	2	Moderate	75%
	<50,000	3–4	Severe	0
1,000–1,500	>75,000	2	Mild	75%
	50–75,000	2	Moderate	0
	<50,000	3–4	Severe	0
<1,000	Any	3–4	Severe	0
Hepatic Function				
SGOT/SGPT/alkaline phosphatase				
≤1.25 x upper limit of normal		0	None to mild	100%
1.26–2.5 x upper limit of normal		1	Mild	75%
2.6–5 x upper limit of normal		2	Moderate	50%
>5 x upper limit of normal		3–4	Severe	0
Nausea		1	Mild: nausea	100%
		2	Moderate: transient vomiting	100%
		3–4	Severe: vomiting requiring therapy or intractable	0
Diarrhea		1	Mild: transient stools 2/d	100%
		2	Moderate: diarrhea with >8 stools/d lasting >4 days	50%
		3–4	Severe: diarrhea with >8 stools/d	0
Anorexia			Mild	100%
			Moderate: anorexia, weight loss of 10% to 20%	50%
			Severe: weight loss >20%	0
Fever		1–2	Mild: 35–40°C	100%
		3–4	Severe: >40°C	0
Neurotoxicity		1	Mild: transient lethargy	100%
		2	Moderate: somnolent <50% of waking hours	100%
		3–4	Severe: somnolent >50% of waking hours	0
Cardiac		1	Mild: sinus tachycardia <120 at rest	100%
			Moderate: unifocal PVC, atrial arrhythmia	100%
			Severe: multifocal PVC, ventricular tachycardia	0
Hypotension			Mild: asymptomatic, fall ≤20 mm Hg diastolic	100%
			Moderate: symptomatic, fall ≤20 mm Hg diastolic	50%
			Severe: fall >20 mm Hg, whether or not symptomatic	0
Allergic/cutaneous		1	Edema, erythema of injection site	100%
		2	Injection site rash, vesiculation, pruritis	100%
		3–4	Bronchospasm, anaphylaxis, exfoliative dermatitis	0

* Occurrence of the noted side effects should be an indication to adjust the next one to three dose administrations as noted. Following a recommendation to withhold a dose altogether, treatment should be reinitiated at 50% of the last dose. If patients tolerate reduced dosing well, an attempt may be made to reinstitute full dosing.

toxicity. Best-tolerated doses utilized in each major study and guidelines for dose modification appear in Tables 2 and 3.

Adverse experiences were graded according to the World Health Organization (WHO) recommendations for grading of acute and subacute toxicity.[3] WHO grades correspond to the following general descriptions of severity: 0, no toxicity; 1, mild; 2, moderate; 3, severe; and 4, very severe or life-threatening. Only adverse experiences that were considered by investigators to be possibly or probably related to interferon treatment are tabulated in this analysis.

Serum was collected for the determination of neutralizing activity to interferon. The methodology used is highly sensitive, with the ability to detect serum with neutralizing activity against 50 units of interferon/mL.[4-6] Samples were collected pretreatment, during treatment, and after therapy had been discontinued.

TOXICITY RESULTS

Virtually all patients experienced toxicity at some time during therapy. However, this involved primarily flu-like symptoms, ie, fever, chills, and malaise. These symptoms, as well as the other more common side effects, were dose-related and rapidly reversible upon treatment discontinuation or dose modification. Overall, 93/867 (11%) patients discontinued treatment because of adverse experiences. However, in studies in which patients received doses of <5 MU, the discontinuation rate for adverse experiences was less than 3%. In addition to flu-like symptoms, frequent toxicities included transient leukopenia and asymptomatic increases in hepatic transaminases. Central nervous system toxicity consisting of somnolence and confusion occurred in up to one third of patients; it was more prevalent in the elderly and was generally mild. Cardiovascular toxicity consisted primarily of asymptomatic hypotension and tachycardia. Direct cardiotoxicity or true arrhythmogenic activity was not seen. Cardiovascular side effects were also more prevalent in older patients. There was no appreciable evidence of renal toxicity.

There was no evidence of cumulative toxicity in any organ system; in fact, during long-term treatment, patients developed increasing tolerance to some symptoms. A listing of toxicities is shown in Table 4.

Flu-like symptoms occurred in almost all patients (98%) but were grade III in only 41% and grade IV in only 2%. In doses <5 MU, grade III flu-like toxicity occurred in only 16% of patients and no grade IV toxicity occurred. Fever (80%), fatigue (73%), rigors (61%), and anorexia (50%) were the predominant adverse experiences in this category. The severity of symptoms tended to increase with higher doses, particularly for IV administration. A decreased incidence over time was evident. Only 20/867 (2%) of patients had very severe (Grade IV) flu-like symptoms, primarily fatigue and fever. Symptoms were usually controlled by the administration of acetaminophen or by dose reduction, and were rapidly reversible within 1 to 2 days of treatment discontinuation.

Gastrointestinal disorders. Nausea and vom-

Table 4. Incidence (%) of Adverse Experiences

	All Patients (N = 867)			Courses with Maximum Dose <10 MU (N = 282)	
Adverse Effect	Any Severity	Grade III	Grade IV	Any Severity	Grade III or IV
Flu-like symptoms	98	41	2	94	26
Nausea/vomiting	50	6	<1	28	2
Other GI	27	2	<1	20	0
Central nervous system	34	8	1	29	6
Cardiovascular	14	2	<1	6	0
Skin	12	<1	0	12	0
Respiratory	7	2	<1	5	1
Alopecia	4	<1	0	2	0
Weight loss	4	1	0	1	<1

iting occurred in 50% of patients, and were grade III or IV in 7%. With SC administration, the incidence was 28% during cycles in which the maximum dose was <10 MU, and 21% when doses were <5 MU. At this latter dose, grade III or IV toxicity occurred in only 1% of patients. However, at SC doses larger than 10 MU, the incidence of gastrointestinal (GI) toxicity rose to 45%. With IV dosing, nausea and vomiting occurred in 20% of patients at doses <10 MU and in 50% of patients at higher doses. Over time, tachyphylaxis developed to all GI effects at all doses.

Gastrointestinal disorders other than nausea and vomiting occurred in 27% of patients, but were grade III or IV in only 2%. Diarrhea was the predominant symptom, occurring in 24% of patients; abdominal pain occurred in 2%.

Central and peripheral nervous system disorders occurred in 34% of patients, but were grade III or IV in only 8%. Somnolence (14%) and confusion (12%) were the major adverse effects in this category. Notably, these disorders were often associated with flu-like symptoms and may not be truly independent toxicities.

The incidence of central and peripheral nervous system effects appeared to be dose-related. At doses <5 MU, the overall incidence of any CNS effects was 27% (these were grade III in only 3% of patients and grade IV in none). At all doses, the incidence and severity of CNS effects decreased over time, and tolerance appeared to develop.

The incidence of CNS symptoms was related to age (Table 5). In persons aged 40 or younger, the incidence of nervous system disorders was 25%, compared with 43% in those over 60. Although CNS effects were reversible, in some cases they did not fully resolve until 1 to 2 weeks after treatment was discontinued.

Cardiovascular disorders occurred in 14% of patients, but were grade III in only 2% and grade IV in 1%. These toxicities were primarily hypotension (8%) and tachycardia (3%). The incidence of cardiovascular disorders was higher at doses >20 MU than at lower doses in patients receiving IV treatment. With SC treatment at doses <5 MU, the incidence of cardiovascular toxicities was only 5%, with a single grade III incidence of deep vein thrombosis. At SC doses of 20 to 50 MU, 13 (11%) of 119 patients had cardiovascular toxicities. Table 5 shows the incidence of cardiovascular disorders by age group. A lower proportion of patients younger than 40 (8%) had cardiovascular disorders than did those aged 40 to 60 (13%) or those over 60 (22%). Notably, 13 (52%) of 25 of the grade III or IV adverse experiences occurred within the first 5 days of treatment, and most resolved while the patient remained on treatment. There was no evidence of direct arrhythmogenicity or cardiotoxicity in this group of patients, and no cumulative effect was evident.

Table 5. Relationship of Cardiovascular and CNS Side Effects to Age

Age	Incidence of Side Effects (Any Severity) to Age: Cardiovascular	CNS
<40	8%	25%
40–60	13%	34%
>60	22%	43%

Skin disorders occurred in 12% of patients, but were grade III or IV in less than 1%. Transient rashes and pruritus were the predominant experiences in this category. Dry skin and nonspecific dermatitis also occurred. The rashes were intermittent, did not progress to more serious manifestations, and did not require dose adjustment or treatment discontinuation. Skin testing in affected patients failed to yield evidence of true hypersensitivity reactions.

Renal function abnormalities did not occur. The lack of substantial changes in measured BUN and creatinine values—even at the highest doses and for extended treatment periods—indicates that interferon alfa-2b treatment had minimal effect on renal function. Adverse experiences involving the urinary system occurred in 20 patients, but were grade III or IV in only two patients. Many of these patients had underlying conditions, such as multiple myeloma, that predispose to renal decompensation over long periods of observation.

Hepatic function abnormalities were limited to transient elevations in hepatic transaminases; increased SGOT and SGPT values occurred in 11% and 10%, respectively, of the overall population. Increases appeared to be related to dose, particularly with SC administration. Only 2% to 5% of patients treated with SC doses smaller than 5 MU developed transaminase elevations, while the incidence was 10% to 13% at a dose of 50 to 75 MU. In the IV treatment group, a dose relationship was also evident. Alkaline phosphatase and lactate dehydrogenase (LDH) were less consistently affected by treatment than were transaminase levels, and no dose relationship was seen.

No clinical evidence of treatment-related hepatic dysfunction was seen, and no cumulative toxicity was evident in the 334 patients who were treated longer than 12 weeks. In fact, a lower proportion of patients had substantial changes in SGOT and SGPT values after 12 weeks of treatment than in their first 12 weeks. Few patients discontinued treatment because of increases in hepatic enzyme levels; such increases were usually managed by dose reduction. Elevated transaminase levels usually returned to normal within 4 to 7 days after discontinuing therapy.

Hematologic toxicity was manifested primarily as changes in total WBC count and granulocyte count. Changes from WHO grade 0, I, or II at baseline to grade III or IV occurred in 18% and 20%, respectively, of patients with solid tumors, and in 35% and 55%, respectively, of patients with leukemia or multiple myeloma. Granulocytopenia was clearly dose-related. Despite the considerable proportion of patients with laboratory evidence of leukopenia, infection occurred in only 7% of patients and was rarely severe. Hemoglobin levels and platelet counts were minimally affected by treatment, and no dose effect was apparent. There was no evidence of cumulative hematologic toxicity, and WBC and platelet counts usually recovered within 2 to 3 days after discontinuing therapy. It has been suggested that some of the granulocytopenia observed during interferon treatment might represent bone marrow sequestration and delayed release rather than myelotoxicity.[7]

SERUM-NEUTRALIZING ACTIVITY

The species specificity of the interferons led early investigators to believe that the interferons would not be immunogenic in homologous systems. However, in 1981, Vallbracht et al[8] reported that some patients treated with human fibroblast interferon had developed detectable levels of IgG antibodies that could neutralize human beta interferon. Subsequently, Trown et al[9] described a patient in whom IgG antibodies to human leukocyte (alpha) interferon developed following treatment with Cantell purified alpha interferon.

Early results with the most widely utilized recombinant alpha interferon preparations, alfa-2a (Roche) and alfa-2b (Schering), suggested that these two molecules might have quite different immunogenic properties. In studies using the alfa-2a preparation, serum neutralizing factors were detected in 3 of 16, 1 of 13, 2 of 12, and 16 of 41 patients in pharmacokinetic, Kaposi's sarcoma, multiple myeloma, and hypernephroma studies, respectively.[10-13] In contrast, phase I-II studies conducted with the alfa-2b preparation reported no development of serum-neutralizing factors.[14-17]

The lower immunogenic potential of interferon alfa-2b has since been borne out in large studies. Jones and Itri,[18] summarizing a large clinical experience, reported that 153 (27.4%) of 559 evaluable patients developed neutralizing antibodies during the course of treatment with interferon alfa-2a. Thirty-eight patients also developed neutralizing antibodies to human alpha interferon. Certain patient subsets seemed to have a particularly high rate of development of antibodies (eg, renal-cell carcinoma, 45.9%, and Kaposi's sarcoma, 36.6%). Notably, other reports have suggested that the development of these antibodies coincided with the loss of clinical effect and a decrease in detectable serum levels of interferon.[13,19]

In contrast, in recent studies employing interferon alfa-2b, only ten (2.4%) of 423 systemically treated cancer patients developed neutralizing antibodies.[4] In many of these cases, the antibody disappeared spontaneously. Additionally, in all but one patient, the titers were extremely low and did not show increases with continued dosing. In two of the ten patients, clinical response to the interferon continued despite the development of antibodies.

At the present time, the difference in antigenic potential between interferon alfa-2a and interferon alfa-2b appears to be real; however, the clinical significance of this is not yet known.

OVERVIEW OF EFFICACY

Phase II Studies

In ongoing phase II-III studies, interferon alfa-2b has been administered to more than 2,000 patients with a wide range of tumor types. These trials are helping to delineate those malignancies that are sensitive to interferon, as well as optimal doses and schedules. Generally, where activity has been reported with natural interferons, confirmatory activity has also been found with interferon alfa-2b. Table 6 provides an overview of the activity of this agent against a variety of tumor types.

Phase II studies with interferon alfa-2b, as well as other interferon products, have been largely negative in most adult solid tumors. It should be noted that most of these trials have been conducted in patients with advanced disease; therefore, they may reflect inactivity against large bulky tumors rather than absolute inactivity against particular tumor types. Also, preliminary results indicate that interferon exhibits schedule dependency and perhaps also dose dependency: Continuous dosing in daily or three-times-per-week schedules appears to be superior to more intermittent dosing. For these reasons—as well as the potential for interferon to work synergistically with other forms of therapy—low response rates in some tumor types might belie the role of interferon or other biologicals. In the following section, the clinical experience with interferon alfa-2b in those malignancies that have been studied most extensively is briefly reviewed.

Table 6. Activity of Alpha Interferon Against Various Malignancies in Phase II Studies

Active	Hairy cell leukemia
	Chronic myelogenous leukemia
	Non-Hodgkin's lymphoma
	Mycosis fungoides
	Cutaneous T-cell lymphomas
	Kaposi's sarcoma
	Multiple myeloma
	Malignant melanoma
	Renal-cell cancer
	Bladder cancer (intravesical)
	Ovarian cancer (intraperitoneal)
Inactive	Breast cancer
	Colon cancer
	Non–small-cell lung cancer
	Prostate cancer
	Acute myelogenous leukemia
Further study required	Chronic lymphocytic leukemia
	Acute lymphocytic leukemia
	Preleukemia
	Hodgkin's disease
	Osteogenic sarcoma
	Astrocytoma

Malignancies of B-Cell Origin: Hairy Cell Leukemia, Lymphoma, and Multiple Myeloma

In this subset of hematologic malignancies, interferon has demonstrated important and in some cases remarkable activity. As detailed elsewhere in this volume and in other published reports, interferon alfa-2b administered at low doses (2 MU/m^2 SC three times per week) has produced objective responses in approximately 75% of patients with hairy cell leukemia (HCL), and meaningful hematologic responses in almost 90% of patients.[20-23] Comparable responses have also been reported with interferon alfa-2b in nonsplenectomized patients.[24] The ability of interferon to actually reduce, or in some cases eliminate, the presence of hairy cells in the bone marrow suggests that—through direct or indirect mechanisms of action—this agent is producing cytoreductive effects against the malignant clone. The long time required to achieve optimal response (in many cases greater than 6 months) indicates that mechanisms other than direct cytotoxicity may be involved. In fact, some in vitro studies suggest that interferon may produce changes in hairy cells by inducing differentiation.[25]

High activity, with response rates of 40% to 50%, has also been demonstrated with single-agent, low-dose interferon alfa-2b in the low-grade lymphomas, similar to reports with other alpha interferons.[26-28] Interestingly, a study by Wagstaff and Crowther[29] has shown that a low dose of interferon alfa-2b (2 MU/m^2 SC three times per week) can produce response rates comparable to higher dosing schedules in good-prognosis non-Hodgkin's lymphomas. Studies are now under way in NCI Cooperative Groups to determine alpha interferon's role as part of combination induction therapy or as a single agent in consolidation/maintenance phases of lymphoma treatment.

A number of studies have demonstrated the activity of the alpha interferons in multiple myeloma. Although the overall response rate in patients with resistant disease is low (15% to 25%), some subsets of patients (eg, relapsers with minimal prior therapy) might do particularly well; some patients have achieved complete or partial responses of long duration. Costanzi et al[30] reported an overall response rate of 18%. Responses were seen in five of 19 patients who were relapsing after previously responding to conventional chemotherapy, and in two of five patients who had been previously treated with only alkylating agents. In contrast, only three of 25 patients who had failed multiple-drug therapies responded to interferon alfa-2b as third- or fourth-line therapy. Some of the responders have now been maintained in remission for over 3 years, and one has achieved a complete response with bone healing.

Interferon has activity against all subtypes of myeloma, ie, IgG, IgA, IgM, and kappa and lambda forms, and the low response rate demonstrated overall in phase II studies may underestimate the real potential for interferon alfa-2b in multiple myeloma.[30] A pilot study described by Cooper et al[31] has shown the feasibility of combining interferon with full doses of melphalan and prednisone as first-line therapy. The efficacy of this combination as compared to melphalan and prednisone alone is currently the subject of a large phase III trial being conducted by the Cancer and Leukemia Group B (CALGB).

Other Leukemias and Lymphomas

Chronic myelogenous leukemia (CML) also appears to have marked sensitivity to alpha interferon. In two studies reported to date, patients have achieved significant improvement in their peripheral blood counts and prolonged therapy appears to be capable of reducing or eliminating Philadelphia chromosome positive cells from the bone marrow. The initial report of alpha interferon's activity in this disease was by Talpaz et al[32] using nonrecombinant alpha interferon. These findings have been confirmed and extended by Talpaz with interferon alfa-2a. Similar results have since been reported with interferon alfa-2b by Niederle et al.[33,34] As is the case with HCL, achievement of an optimum response in CML requires more than 6 months. This again indicates that interferon may be working through mechanisms other than direct cytotoxicity.

Aside from interferon's utility as a single agent in this setting, Bersagel in this volume reports that when it is administered between cycles of alkylating agent treatment, interferon may be able to prolong the doubling time of the malignant clone of CML. Long-term large-scale studies will be necessary to demonstrate whether either this strategy or single-agent interferon is capable of actually prolonging survival and delaying or eliminating transformation to the acute blastic phase of CML.

In chronic lymphocytic leukemia, alpha interferons have not shown activity to date. However, in acute lymphoblastic leukemia (ALL), interferon's activity may be significant. A phase II study administering interferon as a single agent to children in acute relapse suggested that interferon might have some activity in ALL.[35] A study now being conducted by the Pediatric Oncology Group will assess interferon's potential, in combination with chemotherapy, in the treatment of ALL patients with first bone marrow relapse.

Interferon's activity in hematologic malignancies does not appear to be limited to those cells that are of B-cell origin or to CML. The cutaneous T-cell lymphomas (CTCLs) have also demonstrated marked sensitivity, with response rates approaching 50%.[36] It is unclear what features of the cell types mentioned above might predict for interferon's sensitivity. Nevertheless, the wide-ranging activity of alpha interferon in a variety of hematologic malignancies is clear.

AIDS-Related Kaposi's Sarcoma

Shortly after its initial appearance, acquired immune deficiency syndrome (AIDS)–related Kaposi's sarcoma was identified as a potentially important area for therapeutic intervention with biological response modifiers. Numerous studies have now confirmed that both interferon and other natural and recombinant interferon products have high activity in this disease although none of these agents has consistently demonstrated improvement of the underlying immunologic disorders. Overall response rates of 40% to 50% have been reported by a number of investigators, and these rates are considerably higher in patients with early-stage disease.[37] Moreover, these responses seem to be of long duration, in contrast to results obtained with chemotherapy. The results obtained with interferon in this disease setting are described by Abrams elsewhere in this volume.

Further studies are now under way with interferon alfa-2b in the setting of early HTLV-III infection. Since in vitro interferon seems to have real activity against retrovirus replication, it will be important to determine clinically whether interferon is more effective when applied earlier in the course of this infection.

Solid Tumors: Systemic Interferon Trials

In most phase II trials in which interferon was administered to patients with advanced solid tumors, the results have been disappointing. Despite some preclinical research suggesting that alpha interferons have activity against breast and colon cancer, phase II studies conducted in these diseases were negative.[38-42] Phase II studies in such other common adult malignancies as non–small-cell lung cancer and prostate cancer have also been negative. In these settings, interferon administered as a single agent appears unable to eradicate bulky disease that is resistant to prior therapies. Whether interferon might yet have a role in these diseases when combined with other chemotherapy, applied in the adjuvant setting, or administered with local-regional application remains to be tested.

Some solid tumors, namely malignant melanoma and renal-cell carcinoma, have shown sensitivity to interferon even in the phase II setting. In both those cases the overall response rates appear to be low, in the 20% to 25% range. However, the activity does appear to be real and is encouraging for future trials. In clinical trials of interferon alfa-2b in melanoma, efficacy appeared to be schedule-dependent. Although the numbers are small, the results suggest that more continuous dosing schedules produce higher response rates than do intermittent or interrupted schedules.[43]

The phase II trials in melanoma also highlight the importance of tumor burden. Patients who had large tumors at entry (>1.5 cm) had considerably less chance of obtaining a complete or partial response (3/40) than did patients whose tumor burden was small (<1.5 cm) at entry (8/26).

Notably, during the phase II melanoma trials, some patients were able to achieve complete responses of long duration. Two of the patients in the original phase I-II studies are now enjoying sustained complete remissions more than 3 years after study entry. This unusual finding—that some patients can achieve complete responses of very long duration—has been previously reported.[44] To pursue the potential of interferon in this disease setting and perhaps maximize its ability to be effective in a minimal tumor burden situation, the Eastern Cooperative Oncology Group (ECOG) is now performing a randomized trial of interferon alfa-2b in the adjuvant setting in high-risk patients after initial surgery.

The other solid tumor that has shown low but real response to interferon is renal-cell carcinoma. Response rates have ranged from 10% to 25%. The difference in results seems to reflect primarily patient selection. When patients are selected for good prognostic factors, the response rate falls in the 20% to 25% response range.[45] A number of studies have begun to look at the potential for utilizing interferon with other agents for combination therapy of renal-cell carcinoma; the rationale for adjuvant therapy with interferon is also being explored.

Solid Tumors: Local-Regional Treatment With Alpha Interferon

It is unclear whether interferon's effect in in vivo tumor systems is dose-dependent. However, clinically, SC administration will achieve peak serum levels of only 200 to 300 IU/mL, and an IV bolus administration will achieve peak levels of only 500 to 700 IU/mL, which will be sustained only briefly.[1,2] In contrast, intraperitoneal and intravesical administration have been shown to produce sustained levels as high as 30,000 IU/mL, and these levels can be achieved with little or no systemic toxicity. Both of these administration routes have produced promising results in preliminary clinical trials.

Berek et al[46] found that intraperitoneal administration of interferon alfa-2b resulted in complete responses in five of 11 women with ovarian cancer when administered after positive second-look laparotomy. This trial clearly demonstrates the effect of tumor burden on response: Responses only occurred in women with residual disease <5 mm, and complete responses were achieved in three of five women with only positive cytology at entry. In contrast, none of the patients with larger bulky disease achieved a response. Berek's paper in this supplement provides the details and updated results of this trial.

A similar form of local-regional therapy has produced promising results in superficial bladder cancer.[47,48] Responses have been seen in patients with both carcinoma in situ and papillary transitional cell histologies. This subject is reviewed by Torti et al in this publication.

Combination Studies: Interferon and Chemotherapy

Interferon has demonstrated synergy with many common antineoplastic drugs in a variety of preclinical models. In the human tumor stem cell assay, synergy has occurred when interferon has been used in combination with doxorubicin, cyclophosphamide, vinblastine, and cisplatin.[49-51] In mouse models, significant improvements in life span and, in some cases, complete eradication of implanted tumors have been seen following administration of interferon together with various chemotherapeutic agents.[52-54] A number of phase I trials have been conducted to determine the tolerance of interferon administered together with conventional chemotherapy. Studies testing interferon with doxorubicin, cyclophosphamide, and 5-fluorouracil have been completed and demonstrate acceptable tolerance.[51,55-57] Interferon has also been given safely in combination with high-dose steroids and with melphalan and prednisone.[31] This area will certainly be one of future study.

It should be noted that the actual mechanism of these interactions remains unknown, and some preclinical studies have produced contradictory results.[53] Interferon may work either synergistically with chemotherapeutic drugs through a variety of potential mechanisms (eg, enhanced cellular uptake of drug, cell cycling effects, interference with cellular repair mechanisms) or in a complimentary fashion through entirely different mechanisms than those exerted by the cytotoxics.

FUTURE DIRECTIONS

The potential role of alpha interferon in antineoplastic therapy has only just begun to be explored. A number of general study designs appear to be emerging for an expanded role of interferon alfa-2b in cancer treatment. In certain hematologic malignancies (eg, HCL, CML) interferon alfa-2b appears to offer a unique form of therapy; in some cases it is producing unprecedented responses in diseases for which no prior therapy was successful, or at least not successful in specifically eliminating the malignant clone. In other hematologic malignancies (eg, non-Hodgkin's lymphomas, mycosis fungoides, cutaneous T-cell lymphomas), interferon shows a potential high response rate that needs to be explored further in long-term studies. In still other hematologic malignancies (eg, CLL, ALL), interferon's real role needs further testing.

With a few exceptions, interferon has not produced dramatic response rates in the common solid tumors when given as a single agent to patients with advanced refractory disease. Interferon's larger potential role might be after primary tumor reduction with other modalities (surgery, radiation, or chemotherapy), a time when the tumor burden is minimal and when patients may be expected to survive long enough for the maximal effect of interferon to be operative. Clinical trials now under way for lymphoma, for example, are testing the role of interferon in maintenance therapy. Other hematologic malignancies might also be candidates for this type of approach. Additionally, there is a theoretical rationale for extended studies in the adjuvant setting in certain solid tumors.

One of the most intriguing future areas for

investigation involves the local-regional use of interferon. Intraperitoneal and intravesicular therapy have produced promising results in ovarian cancer and superficial bladder cancer. Other areas that remain to be explored include intrapleural trials and perhaps limb perfusion.

Combination trials with interferon represent another important area for future study. More needs to be understood about mechanisms of action and optimal sequencing to place the clinical combination trials on firmer scientific ground. In addition to testing combinations of interferon with conventional chemotherapy, there is great interest in administering interferon with other biological response modifiers; testing of these concepts is just beginning.

Finally, it should be acknowledged that we remain at a very early stage in our understanding of interferon. As with any form of cancer therapy, the better we can understand mechanisms of action of this agent, the more effectively it can be utilized. Clinical results to date suggest that, although interferon is unlikely to be a direct cytotoxic agent in most malignant disease settings, it does appear to exert its effect through direct effects on tumor cells. Clinical studies have not demonstrated that interferon is truly working through immune stimulation, although this remains possible. Further studies are necessary to determine what mechanisms of action are operational. It would also be optimal if in vitro modeling could be designed to better predict those tumor types or specific patients most likely to respond to interferon therapy.

REFERENCES

1. Spiegel RJ: Intron-A (interferon alfa-2b): Clinical overview. Cancer Treat Rev 12 (suppl B):5–16, 1985
2. Shah I, Band J, Samson M, et al: Pharmacokinetics and tolerance of intravenous and intramuscular recombinant alpha-2 interferon in patients with malignancies. Am J Hematol 17:363–371, 1984
3. Miller AB, Hoogstraten B, Staquet M, et al: Reporting results of cancer treatment. Cancer 47:207–214, 1981
4. Spiegel RJ, Spicehandler JR, Jacobs SL, et al: Low incidence of serum neutralizing factors in patients receiving recombinant ALFA-2b interferon (Intron-A). Am J Med 80:223–228, 1986
5. Protzman WP, Jacobs SL, Minnicozzi M, et al: A radioimmunologic technique to screen for antibodies to alpha-2 interferon. J Immunol Methods 75:317–323, 1984
6. Yeh TJ, McBride PJ, Overall JC, et al: Automated, quantitative cytopathic effect reduction assay for interferon. J Clin Microbiol 16:413, 1982
7. Ernstoff MS, Kirkwood JM: Changes in the bone marrow of cancer patients treated with recombinant interferon alpha-2. Am J Med 76:593–596, 1984
8. Vallbracht A, Treuner J, Flehmig B, et al: Interferon-neutralizing antibodies in patients treated with human fibroblast interferon. Nature 299:496–497, 1981
9. Trown PW, Kramer MJ, Dennin RA, et al: Antibodies to human leukocyte interferon in cancer patients. Lancet 1:81–84, 1983
10. Gutterman JU, Seymour F, Quesada J, et al: Recombinant leukocyte A interferon: Pharmacokinetics, single-dose tolerance and biologic effects in cancer patients. Ann Intern Med 96:549–556, 1982
11. Krown SE, Real FX, Cunningham-Rundles S, et al: Preliminary observations on the effect of recombinant leukocyte A interferon in homosexual men with Kaposi's sarcoma. N Engl J Med 308:1071–1076, 1983
12. Quesada JR, Hawkins M, Horning S, et al: Collaborative phase I-II study of recombinant DNA-produced leukocyte interferon (clone A) in metastatic breast cancer, malignant lymphoma, and multiple myeloma. Am J Med 77:427–432, 1984
13. Quesada JR, Rios A, Swanson D, et al: Antitumor activity of recombinant-derived interferon alpha in metastatic renal cell carcinoma. J Clin Oncol 3:1522–1528, 1985
14. Muss HB, Kempf RA, Martino S, et al: A phase II study of recombinant alpha interferon in patients with recurrent or metastatic breast cancer. J Clin Oncol 2:1012–1016, 1984
15. Shah I, Band J, Rudnick S: Pharmacokinetics and tolerance of intravenous recombinant alpha-2 interferon (alpha-2 IFN) in patients with lymphoproliferative malignancies. Clin Res 30:732A, 1982 (abstr)
16. Edelstein MB, Schellekens H, Laurent T, et al: A phase I clinical tolerance study of rDNA alpha-2 human interferon in patients with non-reticuloendothelial system malignancies. Eur J Cancer 19:891–894, 1983
17. Bretaudeau B, Palangie T, Giralt E, et al: Phase I trial of tolerance to increasing doses of recombinant DNA human alpha-2 interferon in patients with advanced cancer. Cancer 71:40–49, 1984
18. Jones GJ, Itri LM: Safety and tolerance of recombinant alfa-2b (Roferon-A) in cancer patients. Cancer 57:1709–1715, 1986
19. Quesada JR, Gutterman JU: Clinical study of recombinant DNA-produced leukocyte interferon (clone A) in an intermittent schedule in cancer patients. J Natl Cancer Inst 70:1041–1046, 1983
20. Ratain MJ, Golomb H, Vardiman J, et al: Treatment of hairy cell leukemia with recombinant alpha-2 interferon. Blood 65:644–648, 1985
21. Thompson JA, Brady J, Kidd P, et al: Recombinant alpha-2 interferon in the treatment of hairy cell leukemia. Cancer Treat Rep 69:791–793, 1985

22. Golomb HM, Jacobs A, Fefer A, et al: Alpha-2 interferon therapy of hairy cell leukemia: A multi-centered study of 64 patients. J Clin Oncol 4:900–905, 1986

23. Jacobs AD, Champlin RE, Golde DW: Recombinant alpha-2 interferon for hairy cell leukemia. Blood 65:1017–1020, 1985

24. Ehman WC, Silber R: Recombinant alpha-2 interferon is an effective agent in the treatment of hairy cell leukemia without prior splenectomy. Am J Med 80:1111–1114, 1986

25. Samuels BL, Brownstein BH, Golomb HM: In vitro induction of proteins by alpha-2 interferon in hairy cell leukemia. Cancer Res (in press)

26. Foon KA, Sherwin SA, Abrams PG, et al: Treatment of advanced non-Hodgkin's lymphoma with recombinant leukocyte A interferon. N Engl J Med 311:1148–1152, 1984

27. Leavitt RD, Ratanatharathorn V, Ozer H, et al: A phase II study of recombinant alpha-2 interferon in patients with malignant lymphoma with unfavorable histology. Proc Am Soc Clin Oncol 2:54, 1983

28. Leavitt RD, Kaplan RS, Bonnem EB, et al: High and low dose treatment for high and low grade non-Hodgkin's lymphoma. Proceedings of the Second International Conference on Malignant Lymphoma. Lugano, Switzerland, June 13–15, 1984

29. Wagstaff J, Crowther D: Human alpha-2 interferon (SCH 30500) in the non-Hodgkin's lymphomas (NHL): A report of 2 phase II studies. Br J Cancer 50:244, 1984

30. Costanzi JJ, Cooper MR, Scarffe JH, et al: Phase II study of recombinant alpha-2 interferon in resistant multiple myeloma. J Clin Oncol 3:654–659, 1985

31. Cooper MR, Fefer A, Thompson J, et al: Alpha-2 interferon/melphalan/prednisone in previously untreated patients with multiple myeloma—A phase I/II trial. Cancer Treat Rep 70:473–476, 1986

32. Talpaz M, Kanterjian HM, McCredie K, et al: Hematologic remission and cytogenetic improvement induced by recombinant human interferon alpha-2 in chronic myelogenous leukemia. N Engl J Med 314:1065–1069, 1986

33. Niederle N, Doberaver C, Kloke O, et al: Treatment of chronic myelogenous leukemia with recombinant interferon alpha (IFN-alpha 2b). Proc Am Soc Clin Oncol 5:236, 1986

34. Niederle N, Kloke O, Doberaver C, et al: α^2 interferon: erste behandlungsergebnisse bei der chronischen myeloischen leukämie. Dtsch Med Wochenschr 111:767–772, 1986

35. Ochs J, Abramowitch M, Rudnick S, et al: Phase I/II study of recombinant alpha-2 interferon against advanced leukemia and lymphoma in children. J Clin Oncol 4:883–887, 1986

36. Bunn PA, Foon KA, Idhe DC, et al: Recombinant leukocyte A interferon: An active agent in advanced cutaneous T-cell lymphomas. Ann Intern Med 101:484–487, 1984

37. Volberding PA, Mitsuyasu RT, Golando JP, et al: Treatment of Kaposi's sarcoma with alfa-2b interferon (Intron-A). Cancer (in press)

38. Silgals RM, Ahlgren JD, Neefe JR: A phase II trial of high dose intravenous interferon alpha-2 in advanced colorectal cancer. Cancer 54:2257–2261, 1984

39. Muss HB, Kempf RA, Martino S, et al: A phase II study of recombinant alpha interferon in patients with recurrent or metastatic breast cancer. J Clin Oncol 2:1012–1016, 1984

40. Balkwill FR, Bodmer J, Rubens RD: Recombinant DNA human interferon alpha-2 (IFN) in advanced breast cancer (ABC). Br J Cancer 49:390, 1984

41. Wasserman J, Lundell G, Blomgren H, et al: Treatment of patients with disseminated colorectal cancer with recombinant human alpha-2 interferon: Studies on the immune system. Int J Cancer 33:251–256, 1984

42. Niederle N, Kurschel E, Schmidt CG: Biologic effects of recombinant leukocyte alpha-2 interferon in metastatic carcinomas. Dtsch Med Wochenschr 109:779–782, 1984

43. Robinson WA, Kirkwood J, Harvey H, et al: Effective use of recombinant human alpha-2 interferon (IFN alpha-2) in metastatic malignant melanoma: A comparison of two regimens. Proc Am Soc Clin Oncol 3:60, 1984

44. Kerr R, Ayoub M, Goldberg R, et al: Treatment of metastatic malignant melanoma (MMM) with human leukocyte interferon (IFN). Proc Am Soc Clin Oncol 4:231, 1985

45. Muss HB, Costanzi JJ, Leavitt R, et al: Recombinant alfa interferon in renal cell carcinoma: A randomized trial of two routes of administration. J Clin Oncol (in press)

46. Berek JS, Hacker NF, Lichtenstein A, et al: Intraperitoneal recombinant alpha interferon for "salvage" immunotherapy in stage III epithelial ovarian cancer: A gynecologic oncology group study. Cancer Res 45:444–453, 1985

47. Torti FM, Shortliffe LD, Williams RD, et al: Superficial bladder cancers are responsive to alpha-2 interferon administered intravesically. Proc Am Soc Clin Oncol 3:160, 1984

48. Freiha FS, Hanningan JF, Higgins M, et al: Intravesical interferon therapy for carcinoma in-situ and transitional cell carcinoma of the bladder. J Urol 131:171A, 1984

49. Aapro MS, Alberts DS, Salmon SE, et al: Interaction of human leukocyte interferon with vinca alkaloids and other chemotherapeutic agents against human tumors in clonogenic assay. Can Chemo Pharm 10:161–166, 1985

50. Welander CE, Morgan TM, Homesley MD, et al: Combined recombinant human interferon alpha-2 and cytotoxic agents studies in a clonogenic assay. Int J Cancer 35:721–729, 1985

51. Green MD, Speyer J, Wernz J, et al: Doxorubicin and interferon: rationale and clinical experience. Can Treat Rev 12:61–67, 1985

52. Balkwill FR, Moodie EM: Positive interaction between human interferon and cyclophosphamide or Adriamycin in a human tumor model system. Cancer Res 44:904–908, 1984

53. Balkwill FR: Antitumor effects of interferon in animals. Interferon 4:23–45, 1985

54. Carmichael J, Wolf CR, Balkwill FR, et al: Potentiation of cisplatinum activity by interferon in non-small cell lung cancer xenografts. Br J Cancer 52:427–428, 1985

55. Sarosy GA, Brown TD, Von Hoff DD, et al: Phase I study of alpha-2 interferon (Intron) plus doxorubicin in patients with solid tumors. Cancer Res (in press)

56. Muss HB, Welander C, Caponera M, et al: Interferon

and doxorubicin in renal cell carcinoma. Cancer Treat Rep 69:721–722, 1985

57. Clouse L, Braich T, Grimm M, et al: A phase I trial of oral cyclophosphamide (CTX) and subcutaneous recombinant alpha-2b interferon (IFN) in patients with malignant disease. Proc Am Soc Clin Oncol 5:228, 1986

VOL XIII, NO 3, SUPPL 3 SEPTEMBER 1986

Seminars in Oncology

New Developments in the Treatment of Lung Cancer

Proceedings of a Symposium held March 1986 in St Thomas, United States Virgin Islands

Contributors

Lawrence H. Einhorn • William K. Evans • Ronald Feld
Nevin Murray • J. Pater • W. Shelley • A. Willan
David Osoba • M. Levitt • P. Coy • I. Hodson • D.G. Payne
A.S. MacDonald • Frances A. Shepherd • Gerrit DeBoer • A. Shah
E. Brown • E. Kostashuk • E. Laukkanen • J. Goldie • P. Band
J. Van den Hoek • K. Murphy • T. Sparling • M. Noble
Joseph D. McCracken • Lalitha M. Janaki • Sarah B. Taylor • P.G. Shankar Giri
Gary B. Weiss • William Gordon, Jr • Ralph B. Vance • John Crowley
David H. Johnson • Kenneth R. Hande • Lester L. Porter • John D. Hainsworth
Steven N. Wolff • F. Anthony Greco • Robert L. Comis • Paul A. Bunn, Jr
Joseph Aisner • Margaret Whitacre • Jeffrey Abrams • Kathleen Propert
Don V. Jackson, Jr • L. Douglas Case • Terry L. Evans • Philip Bonomi
T. Splinter • T. Kok • S. Kho • H. Lameris • F. ten Kate • O. Dalesio
B. Dolman • F. Palmen • J. Bouvy • J. Burghouts • F. Simonis • P. Harper
E. Rankin • I. van Reijswoud • J. van Hoogenhuijze • Jean Klastersky
Kendrith Rowland • Samuel G. Taylor, IV • Salitha Reddy • Myung-Sook Lee
L. Penfield Faber • William Warren • J.J. Rusthoven • K.A. Turnbull

GRUNE & STRATTON
Harcourt Brace Jovanovich, Inc.

Seminars in Oncology

New Developments in the Treatment of Lung Cancer

Proceedings of a symposium held March 1986 in St Thomas, US Virgin Islands. The meeting was sponsored under educational grants from Bristol-Myers Oncology Division and Bristol-Myers International Group.

VOL XIII, NO 3, SUPPL 3 **SEPTEMBER 1986**

Table of Contents

SMALL-CELL LUNG CANCER

Cisplatin Plus VP-16 in Small-Cell Lung Cancer .... *Lawrence H. Einhorn* 3

Initial Therapy With Cisplatin Plus VP-16 in Small-Cell Lung Cancer .... *Lawrence H. Einhorn* 5

The Use of VP-16 Plus Cisplatin During Induction Chemotherapy for Small-Cell Lung Cancer *W.K. Evans, R. Feld, N. Murray, J. Pater, W. Shelley, A. Willan, D. Osoba, M. Levitt, P. Coy, I. Hodson, D.G. Payne, and A.S. MacDonald* 10

First-Line Therapy With VP-16 and Cisplatin for Small-Cell Lung Cancer *William K. Evans, Frances A. Shepherd, Ronald Feld, David Osoba, and Gerrit DeBoer* 17

Alternating Chemotherapy and Thoracic Radiotherapy With Concurrent Cisplatin-Etoposide for Limited-Stage Small-Cell Carcinoma of the Lung .... *N. Murray, A. Shah, E. Brown, E. Kostashuk, E. Laukkanen, J. Goldie, P. Band, J. Van den Hoek, K. Murphy, T. Sparling, and M. Noble* 24

Concurrent Chemotherapy and Radiotherapy for Limited Small-Cell Carcinoma of the Lung: A Southwest Oncology Group Study .... *Joseph D. McCracken, Lalitha M. Janaki, Sarah B. Taylor, P.G. Shankar Giri, Gary B. Weiss, William Gordon, Jr, Ralph B. Vance, and John Crowley* 31

High-Dose Pilot Studies in Extensive-Stage Small-Cell Lung Cancer .... *David H. Johnson, Kenneth R. Hande, Lester L. Porter, John D. Hainsworth, Steven N. Wolff, and F. Anthony Greco* 37

Clinical Trials of Cyclophosphamide, Etoposide, and Vincristine in the Treatment of Small-Cell Lung Cancer .... *Robert L. Comis* 40

Cyclophosphamide, Doxorubicin, and Etoposide as First-Line Therapy in the Treatment of Small-Cell Lung Cancer .... *Paul A. Bunn, Jr, F. Anthony Greco, and Lawrence Einhorn* 45

(*Continued on following page*)

Doxorubicin, Cyclophosphamide, Etoposide and Platinum, Doxorubicin, Cyclophosphamide, and Etoposide for Small-Cell Lung Cancer .... *Joseph Aisner, Margaret Whitacre, Jeffrey Abrams, and Kathleen Propert* 54

Small-Cell Lung Cancer: A 10-Year Perspective .... *Don V. Jackson, Jr and L. Douglas Case* 63

Oral Etoposide in Small-Cell Lung Cancer .... *Robert L. Comis* 75

Outpatient Administration of VP-16 and Cisplatin .... *Terry L. Evans* 79

St Thomas Consensus on the Treatment of Small-Cell Lung Cancer 83

NON–SMALL-CELL LUNG CANCER

Brief Overview of Combination Chemotherapy in Non–Small-Cell Lung Cancer .... *Philip Bonomi* 89

Rationale for Chemotherapy for Patients With Advanced Non–Small-Cell Lung Cancer *F. Anthony Greco* 92

A Multicenter Phase II Trial of Cisplatin and Oral Etoposide (VP-16) in Inoperable Non–Small-Cell Lung Cancer .... *Ted Splinter, Tjebbe Kok, Siangh Kho, Han Lameris, Fiebo ten Kate, Otilia Dalesio, Bram Dolman, Fernand Palmen, Jaap Bouvy, Jos Burghouts, Frank Simonis, Peter Harper, Elaine Rankin, Ineke van Reijswoud, and Jan van Hoogenhuijze* 97

Therapy With Cisplatin and Etoposide for Non–Small-Cell Lung Cancer .... *Jean Klastersky* 104

Phase II Trial of Etoposide, Cisplatin, Continuous Infusion 5-Fluorouracil, and Simultaneous Split-Course Radiation Therapy in Stage III Non–Small-Cell Bronchogenic Carcinoma *Philip Bonomi, Kendrith Rowland, Samuel G. Taylor, IV, Salitha Reddy, Myung-Sook Lee, L. Penfield Faber, and William Warren* 115

Combined Chemotherapy and Radiation Therapy for Non–Small-Cell Lung Carcinoma *David Osoba, J.J. Rusthoven, W.K. Evans, and K.A. Turnbull* 121

Seminars in Oncology

Seminars in Oncology (ISSN 0093–7754) is published quarterly by Grune & Stratton, Inc., 6277 Sea Harbor Dr, Orlando, FL 32821. Months of issue are March, June, September, and December. Second class postage paid at Duluth, MN, and at additional mailing offices.

POSTMASTER: Send change of address to *Seminars in Oncology*, c/o Grune & Stratton, Inc., PO Box 6280, Duluth, MN 55806.

Editorial correspondence should be addressed to John W. Yarbro, MD, PhD, School of Medicine, University of Missouri at Columbia, Columbia, MO 65201.

Business correspondence (subscriptions, change of address) should be addressed to the Publisher, Grune & Stratton, Inc., PO Box 6280, Duluth, MN 55806.

Change of address notices, including both the old and new addresses of the subscriber, should be sent to the Publisher at least one month in advance.

Customer Service: (218) 723-9830.

Subscription rates: one volume of four issues, $58.00 in the United States and Canada; elsewhere, $83.00. Libraries and institutions: $75.00 in the United States and Canada; elsewhere, $83.00. Single copies, $19.50 in the United States and Canada; elsewhere, $22.50. Students, fellows, interns, and residents in the United States, Canada, and Australia may subscribe at a discount rate of $34.00 per year (a letter giving qualifying data must accompany order). Subscriptions are accepted on a calendar year basis. Prices are subject to change. Current prices are in effect for back volumes and back issues. Single issues, both current and back, exist in limited quantities and are offered for sale subject to availability. Journal orders are payable in advance. *Checks* should be sent to Grune & Stratton, Inc., PO Box 6209, Duluth, MN 55806.

Advertising representative: Cunningham Associates, PO Box 308, Park Ridge, NJ 07656, telephone (201) 767-4170.

Agents for Great Britain: Grune & Stratton Limited, 24–28 Oval Rd, London NW1 7DX, England. Agents for Australia and New Zealand: Grune & Stratton Australia, PO Box 300, North Ryde, NSW 2113, Australia. Publication of an advertisement in *Seminars in Oncology* does not imply endorsement of its claims by the Editor(s) or Publisher of the journal.

G&S

Orlando, FL

Harcourt Brace Jovanovich, Inc.

Seminars in Oncology

Seminars in Oncology

New Developments in the Treatment of Lung Cancer
Proceedings of a Symposium
March 1986
St Thomas, US Virgin Islands

Supported by educational grants from
Bristol-Myers Oncology Division, Evansville, Indiana
Bristol-Myers International Group, New York, New York

Dosages, indications, and methods of use for products that are referred to in the supplemenmt by the authors are not necessarily the same as indicated in the package insert for the product and may reflect the clinical experience of the authors or may be derived from the professional literature or other clinical sources. Because of differences between in vitro and in vivo systems and between laboratory animal models and clinical data in humans, in vitro and animal data may not necessarily correlate with clinical results.

SMALL-CELL LUNG CANCER

Seminars in Oncology

Vol 13, No 3, Suppl 3 **September 1986**

Cisplatin Plus VP-16 in Small-Cell Lung Cancer

By Lawrence H. Einhorn

LUNG CANCER is the most common cause of death from cancer in the United States. In 1985, there were approximately 145,000 newly diagnosed cases. Approximately 25% of these were small-cell lung carcinoma (SCLC). SCLC differs both biologically and clinically from the other histologic forms of lung cancer. Its unique response to chemotherapy, compared with that of non–small-cell lung cancer, is well established and has led to improved survival and a small but definite cure rate.[1,2]

During the past decade, combination chemotherapy has become standard therapy in both extensive and limited SCLC. Although many combination regimens give similar results, perhaps the most commonly used regimen has been cyclophosphamide plus doxorobicin (Adriamycin) plus vincristine (CAV). The CAV regimen, combined with prophylactic CNS irradiation and chest radiotherapy was begun in 1974 at Indiana University.[1] With a minimal follow-up of 5 years, 18 of 123 patients (15%) with limited SCLC are alive and continuously disease free and presumably cured of their cancer.

Second-line chemotherapy after failure with CAV has been largely unsuccessful, with only modest response rates of brief duration, and a median survival of only 2 to 3 months after progression on CAV. Etoposide (VP-16) has a high objective response rate (44%) in patients with no prior chemotherapy or prior single-agent cyclophosphamide.[3] However, the results with single-agent VP-16 after failure on CAV have been disappointing. A large multi-institutional study evaluated VP-16 80 mg/m^2 $\times$ 5 every 3 weeks, and only 11 of 116 (9%) patients achieved an objective response.[4] Furthermore, three additional studies, utilizing doses of 125 to 140 mg/m^2 on days 1, 3, and 5 had similar negative results, with only one of 62 objective responses.[5–7]

Single-agent cisplatin has also been evaluated in heavily pretreated SCLC patients, and overall, 15 of 116 (13%) patients had an objective response (cumulative data from eight separate trials). Furthermore, single-agent carboplatin (CBDCA), a cisplatin analog, has been used as *initial* chemotherapy (300 to 400 mg/m^2 every 4 weeks) and 18 of 30 patients (60%) achieved an objective response, including three (10%) complete remissions.[8] Thus, platinum compounds are as active, if not more active, than VP-16, both as initial therapy and for refractory disease.

Cisplatin plus VP-16 is a highly synergistic combination in many animal models.[9] This prediction for human synergism has been realized in germ cell neoplasms not cured with cisplatin plus vinblastine plus bleomycin (PVB). In our experience, giving the identical PVB drugs after relapse has never resulted in a >1-year disease-free survival. Although VP-16 has single-agent activity in refractory testis cancer, the responses are only brief partial remissions. However, the combination of cisplatin plus VP-16 has resulted in a 25% cure rate as salvage therapy for patients not curable with PVB.[10]

The results of cisplatin plus VP-16 combination chemotherapy in refractory SCLC represents one of the most remarkable examples of clinical synergism in human oncology. Despite

---

From the Department of Medicine, Indiana University Medical Center, Indianapolis.

Dr Einhorn is an American Cancer Society Clinical Professor of Oncology.

Supported in part by PHS Grant No. 1 R35 CA 39844–01 awarded by the National Cancer Institute, DHHS.

Address reprint requests to Lawrence H. Einhorn, MD, 926 W Michigan, University Hospital N–582, Indianapolis, IN 46223.

0093–7754/86/1303–3001$05.00/0

unimpressive single-agent activity in CAV failures, there is a reproducible 50% objective response rate in numerous published studies.[11–16]

Although cisplatin plus VP-16 has become standard salvage therapy for CAV failures, it has had, at best, only a modest effect upon palliation of symptomatology and overall survival. However, now there is a regimen available that is non–cross-resistant with CAV and is competitive with CAV as first-line therapy. Thus, for the first time since the introduction of combination chemotherapy in the early 1970s, we may be at the threshold of another quantum leap forward in the management of SCLC by successfully incorporating a platinum compound and an epipodophyllotoxin derivative (VP-16 or VM-26) as an integral component of the therapeutic strategy. VM-26 has only rarely been tested in SCLC, but may be as active, if not more active, than VP-16, if the studies from Finsen Institute in Copenhagen can be confirmed. They studied VM-26 in refractory disease and demonstrated a 15% response rate, with six of 40 patients responding to single-agent VM-26, including five of 20 who had received no prior VP-16.[17] They then evaluated single agent VM-26 as initial therapy (60 mg/m^2 days 1 to 5 every 3 weeks), and 30 of 33 patients (90%) responded, including seven (21%) complete remissions.[18] Toxicity was mild, with only 30% developing leukocyte counts $<2,000/\mu L$.

In conclusion, the present and future strategies for SCLC can include the following: (1) Initial induction therapy with cisplatin plus VP-16. This regimen might be especially attractive in limited disease when combined with chest radiotherapy. (2) Late consolidation with cisplatin plus VP-16, after achieving a partial or complete remission with CAV. (3) Alternating chemotherapy (CAV courses 1, 3, and 5 and cisplatin plus VP-16 courses 2, 4, and 6) in a Goldie-Coldman schema. (4) The combination of CBDCA (or cisplatin) plus VM-26 is another attractive possibility.

REFERENCES

1. Einhorn LH, Bond WH, Hornback H, et al: Long term results in combined modality treatment of small cell carcinoma of the lung. Semin Oncol 5:309–313, 1978

2. Hande KR, DesPrez RM: Current perspectives in small cell lung cancer. Chest 85:669–677, 1984

3. Issell BF, Crooke ST: Etoposide (VP-16-213). Cancer Treat Rev 6:107–124, 1979

4. Issell BF, Einhorn LH, Comis RL, et al: Multicenter phase II trial of etoposide in refractory small cell lung cancer. Cancer Treat Rep 69:127–128, 1985

5. Antman K, Pomfret E, Karp G, et al: Phase II trial of etoposide in previously treated small cell carcinoma of the lung. Cancer Treat Rep 68:1413–1414, 1984

6. Asbury RF, Rubins J, Bennett JM: Etoposide in small cell lung cancer resistant to prior chemotherapy. Cancer Treat Rep 67:951–952, 1983

7. Evans WK, Feld R, Osoba D, et al: VP-16 alone and in combination with cisplatin in previously treated patients with small cell lung cancer. Cancer 53:1461–1466, 1984

8. Smith IE, Harland SJ, Robinson BA, et al: Carboplatin: A very active new cisplatin analog in the treatment of small cell lung cancer. Cancer Treat Rep 69:43–46, 1985

9. Schabel FM, Trader MW, Laster WK, et al: Cis-dichlorodiammineplatinum (II): Combination chemotherapy and cross-resistance studies with tumors of mice. Cancer Treat Rep 63:1459–1473, 1979

10. Hainsworth JD, Williams SD, Einhorn LH, et al: Successful treatment of resistant germinal neoplasms with VP-16 and cisplatin: Results of a Southeastern Cancer Study Group Trial. J Clin Oncol 3:666–671, 1985

11. Einhorn LH, Williams SD, Loehrer PJ: Platinum + VP-16 chemotherapy for refractory small cell lung cancer. Proc Am Assoc Cancer Res 25:174, 1984 (abstr)

12. Sierocki JS, Hilaris BS, Hopfan S, et al: Cis-dichlorodiammeplatinum and VP-16-213: An active regimen for small cell cancer of the lung. Cancer Treat Rep 63:1593–1597, 1979

13. Lopez JA, Mann J, Grapski R, et al: Salvage chemotherapy of refractory small cell lung cancer with VP-16 and cisplatinum. Proc Am Soc Clin Oncol 1:151, 1982 (abstr)

14. Tinsley R, Comis R, Difino S, et al: Potential clinical synergy observed in the treatment of small cell lung cancer with cisplatin plus VP-16. Proc Am Soc Clin Oncol 2:183, 1983 (abstr)

15. Porter L, Johnson D, Hainsworth J, et al: Recurrent small cell lung carcinoma treated with VP-16 and cisplatinum. Proc Am Soc Clin Oncol 3:215, 1984 (abstr)

16. Evans WK, Osoba D, Feld R, et al: Etoposide (VP-16) and cisplatin: An effective treatment for relapse in small cell lung cancer. J Clin Oncol 3:65–71, 1985

17. Pedersen AG, Bork E, Osterlind K, et al: Phase II study of teniposide in small cell carcinoma of the lung. Cancer Treat Rep 68:1289–1291, 1984

18. Bork E, Hansen M, Dombernowsky P, et al: VM-26: The most active single agent in small cell lung cancer? Proceedings of the Second International Lung Cancer Congress, Toronto, 1985, p 400

Initial Therapy With Cisplatin Plus VP-16 in Small-Cell Lung Cancer

By Lawrence H. Einhorn

Cisplatin plus VP-16 has become a widely used salvage regimen for CAV (cyclophosphomide, doxorubicin [Adriamycin], and vincristine) failures. However, the major value of this two-drug combination will probably be as an integral part of the initial therapeutic strategy. Cisplatin plus VP-16 has been used as induction therapy in four separate published studies involving 238 patients. The response rates ranged from 71% to 94% and complete remission (CR) rates varied from 30% to 53%. Cisplatin plus VP-16 has also been alternated with CAV in several phase II studies with encouraging results. A Southeastern Cancer Study Group (SECSG) protocol in extensive disease is currently testing this hypothesis in a random prospective study. A recently completed SECSG protocol in limited small-cell lung cancer tested the concept of late intensification with two courses of cisplatin plus VP-16 following six courses of CAV, *v* six courses of CAV alone. Presently, there is a statistically significant survival advantage for cisplatin plus VP-16.

SMALL-CELL LUNG CANCER (SCLC) accounts for approximately 25% of all cases of lung cancer. In 1985, there were an estimated 36,000 newly diagnosed cases of SCLC.

SCLC differs from non–small-cell lung cancer by virtue of early hematogenous dissemination, paraneoplastic syndromes, such as inappropriate antidiuretic hormone secretion (SIADH) and ectopic ACTH production, and especially important, chemosensitivity. It has been recognized for the past 10 to 15 years that all patients with SCLC require chemotherapy as an integral part of therapeutic strategy, even if disease is limited to the chest.

In the 1970s, the most common combination chemotherapy regimens included cyclophosphamide plus doxorubicin (Adriamycin [Adria Laboratories, Columbus, Ohio]) plus vincristine (CAV). Many patients with limited-extent disease concomitantly received chest irradiation with or without prophylactic cranial irradiation. Patients with extensive disease had a very high objective response rate (50% to 90%), which included 10% to 20% complete remissions (CR). These patients were afforded significant palliation and prolongation of survival, with median survival time of 9 months, compared with 2 months with supportive care alone. However, only 1% to 2% of these patients were alive and disease free at 3+ years. Patients with limited SCLC fared better, with 40% to 70% CR, 12- to 18- month median survival time, and 15% to 20% of patients continuously disease free at 3+ years. Similar results have been achieved with cyclophosphamide plus methotrexate plus CCNU, with or without vincristine.

Second-line, or salvage therapy, after failure on CAV on similar first-line regimens had been largely unsuccessful until the development of recent programs using cisplatin plus VP-16.[1–5] Most of these studies demonstrated a 40% to 50% objective response rate with perhaps modest prolongation of survival, and rare long-term remissions. The major importance of these salvage regimen studies was the demonstration that for the first time, a new regimen that was non–cross-resistant with CAV has been developed, and that the major utility of this program might well be as initial therapy rather than reserving its usage for refractory disease. Several therapeutic strategies are possible: (1) cisplatin plus VP-16 as initial therapy, either alone, or combined with thoracic irradiation; (2) CAV alternating with cisplatin plus VP-16 (Goldie-Coldman hypothesis); or (3) late intensification with cisplatin plus VP-16 after partial remission (PR) or CR with CAV. The concept of late intensification will be discussed in a separate chapter.

CISPLATIN PLUS VP-16 AS INITIAL CHEMOTHERAPY

Sierocki et al at Memorial Sloan-Kettering Cancer Center first used cisplatin plus VP-16 as

---

From the Department of Medicine, Indiana University Medical Center, Indianapolis.

Dr Einhorn is an American Cancer Society Clinical Professor of Oncology.

Supported in part by PHS Grant No. 1 R35 CA 39844-01 awarded by the National Cancer Institute, DHHS.

Address reprint requests to Lawerence H. Einhorn, MD, 926 W Michigan, University Hospital N-582, Indianapolis, IN 46223.

0093–7754/86/1303–3007$05.00/0

initial therapy in SCLC.[6] They treated 38 patients from April 1977 to March 1978 with cisplatin (60 mg/m^2) on days 1 and 22 plus VP-16 (120 mg/m^2) days 4, 6, 8, 25, 27, and 29. Following two courses of cisplatin plus VP-16, all patients then received four courses of CAV followed by two courses of cisplatin plus VP-16 and another four courses of CAV. The total duration of therapy was 18 months. All patients received prophylactic cranial irradiation. The therapeutic results are depicted in Table 1. The objective response rates were completely a reflection of the initial two courses of cisplatin plus VP-16. No further responses or improvement of partial response to CR was seen with subsequent CAV. At the initiation of this study, there were not yet any significant positive single-agent data for cisplatin in SCLC, nor were there any published data on potential dramatic synergy with the two-drug combination in preclinical or clinical studies. The Memorial group was probably also the first group to evaluate cisplatin plus VP-16 as salvage therapy in SCLC. Of six patients who failed to respond to first-line combination chemotherapy, one CR and four PRs were achieved.[7]

Toxicity included nausea, vomiting, and alopecia. Five of 38 patients experienced leukocyte counts < 2,000/μL and 11 patients had platelets < 100,000/μL (including eight with platelets < 50,000). The average hemoglobin decrease during chemotherapy was 4 g/dL. Two patients had creatinine rises to >2 mg/dL.

Evans et al treated 31 patients (11 with limited and 20 with extensive disease) with cisplatin plus VP-16 as initial therapy in SCLC.[8] These patients were entered in the study from March 1981 to February 1984. This was clearly a patient population with adverse prognostic characteristics, as in the majority of cases a doxorubicin-containing regimen was contraindicated because of severe cardiac or hepatic metastases.

Table 1. Memorial: Cisplatin Plus VP-16*

Extent	No. Patients	CR (%)	PR (%)	Median Survival Time (mo)
Limited	21	52	48	22
Extensive	17	41	47	9

Note. Four patients with limited disease remain disease free at 3+ years.

*Experience at Memorial Sloan-Kettering Cancer Center.[6]

Patients were candidates for this study if they had documented CNS metastases, serum bilirubin >3.0/dL or serious cardiac disease. The dosages administered were cisplatin (25 mg/m^2) for three consecutive days plus VP-16 (100 mg/m^2) for the same three consecutive days, with a total of six courses administered every 3 to 4 weeks. Responding patients with limited disease were treated with 2,500 rad to the primary site after completion of six courses of cisplatin plus VP-16. Of the 28 evaluable patients, 12 (43%) achieved a CR and 12 (43%) had a PR. The median duration of response was 39 weeks for patients with limited disease and 26 weeks for those with extensive disease. The median survival time for limited-disease patients was 63 weeks; seven of 11 limited-disease patients achieved a CR and two a PR. The median survival time for extensive disease was 39 weeks, with five of 17 (29%) CRs and ten (59%) PRs. All patients achieving a CR did so before receiving irradiation to the primary site.

Three patients were treated with CAV following relapse or failure to respond to cisplatin plus VP-16. One patient achieved a CR and one a PR.

Toxicity consisted primarily of nausea, vomiting, alopecia, myelosuppression, and nephrotoxicity. Most patients were treated on an outpatient basis. Nineteen percent required a dosage reduction for myelosuppression, and 23% also required a delay in treatment because of low granulocyte counts. Twenty-nine percent of the patients had at least one nadir granulocyte count < 1,500μL and 18% < 1,000/μL. There were four (13%) febrile granulocytopenic episodes and one drug-related mortality due to sepsis. Forty percent had platelet counts < 90,000, but there were no episodes < 25,000/μL and no thrombocytopenic bleeding. Two thirds of the patients developed anemia with hemoglobins below 10.0 g/L. The anemia was a cumulative effect with succeeding courses of chemotherapy. Two patients required discontinuation of cisplatin because of rising serum creatinines (maximum 4.0 mg/mL).

Other recent studies have confirmed the high objective response rate of cisplatin plus VP-16 as initial chemotherapy in SCLC. Kim and McDonald observed 21 of 24 responses (88%) with cisplatin (75 mg/m^2) day 1 plus VP-16 (125 mg/m^2) days 1, 3, and 5.[9] Woods and Levi treated 148 patients with cisplatin (80 mg/m^2) plus VP-16 (60 mg/m^2) days 1 to 3 every days for four courses.[10] Radiotherapy (3,900 rad) was also administered to the chest and prophylactically to the brain during the first 6 weeks of chemotherapy. The response rate was similar to the previous studies, with 48% CRs and 36% PRs in 50 patients with limited disease and 21% CRs and 43% PRs in 98 patients with extensive disease. An interesting aspect of this study was a randomization, after completion of cisplatin plus VP-16 plus radiotherapy, to receive ten courses of maintenance CAV *v* no further therapy. No patients improved their remission status while receiving CAV, and there was no significant difference in survival duration between the maintenance and no-maintenance groups (median overall survival, 50 weeks). Thus, this study and other studies suggest that: (1) cisplatin plus VP-16 is competitive with, if not superior to, CAV as initial therapy; (2) cisplatin plus VP-16 can be safely combined with thoracic irradiation. Whether the results of this type of combined modality therapy are less toxic or more therapeutic than CAV plus radiotherapy is still unresolved; and, (3) although cisplatin plus VP-16 has no cross-resistance with CAV, as it demonstrates a 40% to 50% objective response rate in CAV failures, the converse may not be the case; ie, when cisplatin plus VP-16 is used as first-line therapy, CAV may be an ineffective regimen when used as second-line therapy.

CISPLATIN PLUS VP-16 ALTERNATING WITH CAV

Murray et al evaluated an alternating regimen in 67 patients with limited SCLC.[11] CAV was alternated with cisplatin (60 mg/m^2) day 1 plus VP-16 (120 mg/m^2) days 1, 2, and 3 at 3-week intervals for a total of six courses. Thoracic radiotherapy (3,000 rad) was administered concurrently with the first cisplatin plus VP-16 course. There were 70% CRs and 24% PRs; the median survival was 82 weeks, and the projected 2-year survival was 35%. These survival results were superior to those in the historical control group receiving CAV plus thoracic irradiation (P = .01).

An interesting variation on the same theme has recently been published by the Memorial Sloan-Kettering Cancer Center group.[12] This study was a follow-up to their previous study using two courses of cisplatin plus VP-16 as initial therapy.[6] Forty-four patients with SCLC were treated with an induction program of CAV rapidly alternating (every 2 weeks) with cisplatin plus VP-16. The investigators felt the treatment interval between two mutually non–cross-resistant drug regimens may be critical to the emergence of a doubly resistant tumor cell population. Furthermore, in an attempt to eradicate residual tumor following chemotherapy induction, high-dose radiotherapy (250 rads on four days a week for a total of 18 fractions) to the primary disease complex and mediastinum was given to patients with limited disease following four courses of chemotherapy. Cyclophosphamide (500 mg/m^2) plus vincristine (1.4 mg/m^2) was administered on days 1 and 15 of radiotherapy. Chemotherapy cycles 1 and 3 consisted of cyclophosphamide (1,200 mg/m^2), doxorubicin (50 mg/m^2), and vincristine (1.4 mg/m^2), and cycles 2 and 4 consisted of cisplatin (60 mg/m^2) day 1 plus VP-16 (120 mg/m^2) days 4, 6, and 8. Each cycle was given as soon as the WBC count returned to >3,000/μL and platelets over 100,000/μL. It was found that CAV could be alternated with cisplatin plus VP-16 at 2-week intervals in 80% of patients.

Patients with limited disease not in CR (after four courses of chemotherapy plus thoracic irradiation) and all patients with extensive disease received maintenance chemotherapy for a total of 12 months with CCNU (100 mg/m^2) day 1 plus methotrexate (30 mg/m^2) intravenously days 1, 8, 15, and 22, and procarbazine (100 mg/m^2) days 1 to 14. Cyclophosphamide (1,000 mg/m^2) plus doxorubicin (30 mg/m^2) plus vincristine (1.4 mg/m^2) were administered on day 43, and cisplatin (50 mg/m^2) on day 71, plus VP-16 (120 mg/m^2) days 74, 76, and 78. The entire sequence was recycled on day 99.

Twenty-four patients with limited disease and 20 with extensive disease were entered in this study. Following the four courses of chemotherapy induction, CR was achieved in 16 (67%) limited- and 13 (65%) extensive-stage patients. Thirteen of the 15 remaining patients had PRs. Following thoracic irradiation, four of the eight PRs in the limited category converted to CR. The median duration of response in limited-disease patients was 12.7 months (range, 4 to 70+

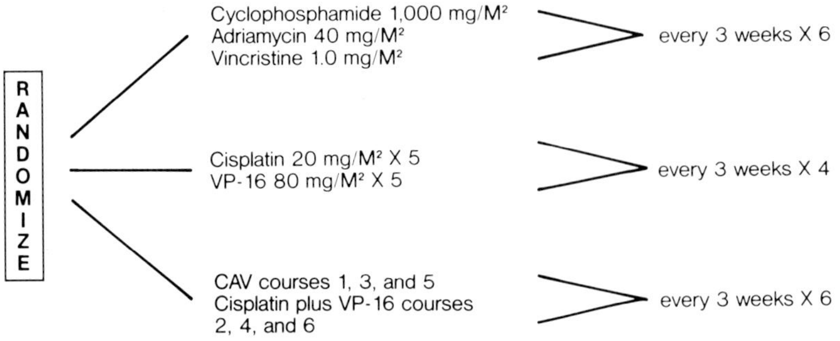

Fig 1. Protocol for SECSG LUN 302 trial—Extensive SCLC.

months) and 10.1 months in extensive disease (range, 2 to 63+ months). Analysis of survival with a minimal follow-up of 5 years revealed a median survival of 18.5 months for limited-disease patients and 12.2 months for those with extensive disease. Five patients (four with limited disease and one with extensive disease) remain continuously disease free and presumably cured of their neoplasm.

NEW STUDIES

A recently activated random prospective study by the Southeastern Cancer Study Group (SECSG) promises to answer the important questions about the role of cisplatin plus VP-16 in extensive SCLC. In this three-arm study, patients with extensive SCLC are randomized to six courses of CAV *v* four courses of cisplatin plus VP-16 *v* CAV courses 1, 3, and 5 alternating with cisplatin plus VP-16 for courses 2, 4, and 6 (Goldie-Coldman hypothesis). The schema for this study is depicted in Fig 1. This study will directly compare four courses of cisplatin plus VP-16 with six courses of CAV as initial therapy, and also will confirm or refute the concept of alternating non–cross-resistant regimens. SCLC remains the best solid tumor to test the Goldie-Coldman hypothesis, as there are two competitive regimens (CAV and cisplatin plus VP-16) as initial therapy, and cisplatin plus VP-16 is clearly a non–cross-resistant regimen with CAV. However, there is still controversy as to whether CAV is non–cross-resistant with cisplatin plus VP-16.[6,8,10]

Another important research question is the precise role of cisplatin plus VP-16 as initial therapy in limited SCLC, combined with thoracic irradiation. Most investigators feel that there is modest, but definite survival advantage (especially the potential for long-term disease-free survival) with chemoradiotherapy as opposed to chemotherapy alone in limited SCLC.

SUMMARY

There is little, if any, controversy about the ability of cisplatin plus VP-16 to achieve a 40% to 50% objective response rate in refractory SCLC. This represents the first truly new and innovative chemotherapy regimen in SCLC in the last 10 years. What is controversial, however, is how to best use this relatively new therapeutic regimen as an integral component of first-line chemotherapy. Some potential strategies and questions are listed below:

1. Can "late intensification" with cisplatin plus VP-16 improve the survival after an initial remission with CAV? A recently completed SECSG protocol (LUN 343) in limited disease is presently demonstrating a statistically significant survival advantage for two courses of cisplatin plus VP-16 (after six courses of CAV) *v* no late intensification.

2. Is cisplatin plus VP-16 as effective as CAV and other front-line regimens in SCLC? There

Table 2. Cisplatin Plus VP-16 as Initial Therapy

Reference	No. Patients	Cisplatin	VP-16	CR (%)	PR (%)
Sierocki[6]	38	60/m² d 1, 22	120/m² d 4, 6, 8, 25, 27, 29	18 (47)	18 (47)
Evans[8]	28	25/m² × 3	100/m² × 3	12 (43)	12 (43)
Kim[9]	24	75/m²	125/m² d 1, 3, 5	21 of 24 (88)	
Woods[10]	148	80/m²	60/m² × 3	78 (53)	55 (37)
				45 (30)	60 (41)

are several studies[6,8–10] indicating competitive, if not superior response rate and survival data compared with CAV or other regimens (nonrandomized studies). The current SECSG protocol for extensive disease will prospectively evaluate the role of four courses of cisplatin plus VP-16 *v* six courses of CAV.

3. What are the toxicity and therapeutic value of cisplatin plus VP-16 plus thoracic irradiation in patients with limited SCLC? Data from Murray et al[11] and Natale et al[12] demonstrate the safety and impressive therapeutic results with cisplatin plus VP-16 plus radiotherapy. The true value, compared with CAV plus chest radiotherapy, should be tested in a random prospective study in patients with limited-stage SCLC.

4. What is the proper dosage of cisplatin plus VP-16 when used as initial chemotherapy? It is very probable that the higher dosages used in salvage regimens[1–5] may not be necessary to achieve high response rates. Table 2 summarizes various regimens. The cisplatin doses have ranged from 60 to 80 mg/m^2 (compared with 20 mg/m^2 × 5 in most salvage regimens), and the VP-16, 180 to 375 mg/m^2 (as opposed to 80 to 100 mg/m^2 × 5 for refractory disease). The four studies listed in Table 2 had excellent response rates (71% to 94%, including 30% to 53% CRs) with the lower doses of cisplatin plus VP-16.

5. Is there value in alternating CAV with cisplatin plus VP-16? There are two nonrandomized studies[11,12] that imply therapeutic superiority using the Goldie-Coldman hypothesis. However, the true value of this principle of alternating two non–cross-resistant regimens such as CAV and cisplatin plus VP-16 will best be determined by the present SECSG protocol in extensive SCLC (Fig 1).

REFERENCES

1. Einhorn LH, Williams SD, Loehrer PJ: Platinum + VP-16 chemotherapy for refractory small cell lung cancer. Proc Am Assoc Cancer Res 25:174, 1984 (abstr)
2. Lopez JA, Mann J, Grapski R, et al: Salvage chemotherapy of refractory small cell lung cancer with VP-16 and cisplatinum. Proc Am Soc Clin Oncol 1:151, 1982 (abstr)
3. Tinsley R, Comis R, Difino S, et al: Potential clinical synergy observed in the treatment of small cell lung cancer with cisplatin plus VP-16. Proc Am Soc Clin Oncol 2:183, 1983 (abstr)
4. Porter L, Johnson S, Hainsworth J, et al: Recurrent small cell lung carcinoma treated with VP-16 and cisplatinum. Proc Am Soc Clin Oncol 3:215, 1984 (abstr)
5. Evans WK, Osoba D, Feld R, et al: Etoposide (VP-16) and cisplatin: An effective treatment for relapse in small cell lung cancer. J Clin Oncol 3:65–71, 1985
6. Sierocki JS, Hilaris BS, Hopfan S, et al: Cis-dichlorodiammineplatinum and VP-16–213: An active regimen for small cell cancer of the lung. Cancer Treat Rep 63:1593–1597, 1979
7. Sierocki JS, Golby RS, Wittes RE: Combination chemotherapy for small cell carcinoma of the lung. Proc Am Assoc Cancer Res 19:352, 1978 (abstr)
8. Evans WK, Shepherd FA, Feld R, et al: VP-16 and cisplatin as first-line therapy for small-cell lung cancer. J Clin Oncol 3:1471–1477, 1985
9. Kim RN, McDonald DB: The combination of VP-16-213 and cisplatin in the treatment of small cell carcinoma of the lung. Proc Am Soc Clin Oncol 1:141, 1982 (abstr)
10. Woods RL, Levi JA: Chemotherapy for small cell lung cancer: A randomized study of maintennce therapy with cyclophosphamide, Adriamycin, and vincristine (CAV) after remission induction with cisplatinum, VP-16, and radiotherapy. Proc Am Soc Clin Oncol 3:214, 1984 (abstr)
11. Murray N, Hadzic E, Shah A, et al: Alternating chemotherapy and thoracic irradiation with concurrent cisplatin for limited stage small cell carcinoma of the lung. Proc Am Soc Clin Oncol 3:214, 1984 (abstr)
12. Natale RB, Shank B, Hilaris BS, et al: Combination cyclophosphamide, Adriamycin, and vincristine rapidly alternating with combination cisplatin and VP-16 in treatment of small cell lung cancer. Am J Med 79:303–308, 1985

The Use of VP-16 Plus Cisplatin During Induction Chemotherapy for Small-Cell Lung Cancer

By W.K. Evans, R. Feld, N. Murray, J. Pater, W. Shelley, A. Willan, D. Osoba, M. Levitt, P. Coy, I. Hodson, D.G. Payne, and A.S. MacDonald

In an attempt to circumvent innate or acquired tumor-cell resistance to chemotherapy, patients with small-cell lung cancer (SCLC) were treated with induction therapy that incorporated two active and potentially non–cross-resistant chemotherapy regimens on two National Cancer Institute of Canada (NCI-C) trials. Patients with limited disease (LD) SCLC were treated with cyclophosphamide, doxorubicin (Adriamycin [Adria Laboratories, Columbus, Ohio]) and vincristine (CAV) and VP-16 plus cisplatin in two different sequences. One arm was randomized to receive CAV alternating with VP-16 plus cisplatin for a total of six treatment cycles, and the other arm received three courses of CAV followed by three courses of VP-16 plus cisplatin. Both treatment strategies produced similar response rates and survival curves, and each treatment group has a projected 2-year survival of 20%. Patients with extensive disease (ED) were treated with either six cycles of CAV (standard regimen) or CAV alternating with VP-16 plus cisplatin for a total of six treatment cycles. In this study, the alternating regimen produced a higher complete response (CR) rate (40% *v* 27%) and overall response rate (61% *v* 39%; *P* < .01). The progression-free survival was also superior for the alternating arm (*P* = .001), as was overall survival (*P* < .05). The frequency of thrombocytopenia and severe gastrointestinal toxicity was slightly greater in the alternating arm, but the frequency of neutropenia and infection was less. The alternation of CAV and VP-16 plus cisplatin during induction therapy is an effective treatment strategy in the management of SCLC and superior to CAV alone in extensive SCLC.

SMALL-CELL LUNG CANCER (SCLC) is characterized clinically by rapid cell growth and early dissemination.[1] Over 40% of patients present with evidence of distant metastases, and it is assumed that the remainder have occult spread. In contrast to the other major types of lung cancer, SCLC is sensitive to both chemotherapy and radiation therapy. This has led to significant improvements in the overall survival of patients with this disease, although treatment results appear to have plateaued.[2] Despite the fact that the majority of patients initially respond to cytotoxic chemotherapy, mot ultimately die of their disease due to the development of chemotherapy-resistant disease. Whether the development of drug resistance represents the expansion of drug-resistant clones of cells present at diagnosis or a change within cells exposed to cytotoxic therapy that renders them resistant to treatment remains to be determined.

Studies on the biology of cancer clearly demonstrate that cell populations within neoplasms are heterogeneous with respect to such properties as antigenicity, growth rate, karyotype, chemotherapeutic sensitivity, and metastatic potential.[3,4] Based on animal models, it is postulated that the greater the metastatic capacity of a tumor, the greater will be the tendency for the cells of the tumor to undergo spontaneous mutation and to give rise to cells with diverse phenotypic expression, including survival mechanisms for overcoming therapeutic insults.[5] In 1979, Goldie and Coldman presented a mathematical model relating the potential for chemotherapeutic cure of a malignant tumor to the spontaneous mutation rate toward phenotypic drug resistance.[6] In this model, it was proposed that stable drug-resistant phenotypes arise spontaneously in malignant tumors with a definite frequency, independent of the selecting agent. Therefore, the probability of developing drug-resistant mutant clones in a tumor would, according to the model, be directly related to the number of cell divisions that had occurred. It would therefore logically follow that the larger the tumor mass or the longer the delay in initiating therapy, the greater the likelihood that the tumor would contain a subpopulation of resistant cells.

In SCLC, spontaneous rapid mutation to drug resistance may provide one explanation for the

From the National Cancer Institute of Canada Clinical Trials Group, Kingston, Ontario.
Supported by the National Cancer Institute of Canada.
Address reprint requests to W.K. Evans, MD, Ottawa Regional Cancer Centre, 190 Melrose Ave, Ottawa, Ontario, Canada K1Y 4K7.

0093-7754/86/1303-3008$05.00/0

failure of current best therapy to eradicate the tumor. SCLC is generally very responsive to initial chemotherapy, indicating that sensitive subpopulations of cells are commonly present. At the time of relapse, the tumor usually fails to respond to the initial chemotherapy, implying that resistant subpopulations have developed. The frequency of response to second-line chemotherapy has generally been low, and survival following relapse has been short.[1] Presumably, the recurrent tumor is predominantly made up of drug-resistant cells.

It is well recognized that SCLC patients with relatively small tumor burdens (limited disease [LD]) have higher response rates and longer survival that those with large tumor burdens (extensive disease [ED]). Within the category of LD, patients with small primaries and no nodal involvement T_1N_0 have a 5-year survival of approximately 60% when treated with surgery and chemotherapy, compared with 30% for T_1N_1 and 9.0% for T_2N_1.[7] These observations, which link the curability of SCLC to total tumor mass, are best explained by the Goldie-Coldman model, which predicts that larger tumor volumes would more commonly contain drug-resistant subpopulations.

In SCLC, responses to multi-agent chemotherapy occur more frequently and are of longer duration than with single-agent therapy.[8] The better treatment effect of two or more agents given concurrently is also predicted by the model. Tumor cell subpopulations resistant to one agent may be sensitive to another, and, therefore, a greater proportion of tumor cells might be killed by a combination than when one drug is used alone.

There are several important implications of the Goldie-Coldman model for the treatment of SCLC. The model predicts that the period in which the tumor would be most susceptible to a chemotherapeutic cure is short and decreases rapidly with each cell division. Therefore, treatment should be administered early in the natural history of the tumor. In practice, however, the majority of SCLC patients present with far-advanced disease, and the possibility of administering drugs early, before mutations have occurred, is probably beyond the realm of possibility.

The second implication of the model is that a large number of active agents with differing mechanisms of action should be applied in the treatment of the malignancy. The number of drugs that can be administered simultaneously in combination is limited by additive toxicities, most commonly myelosuppression. Among the most active single agents are cyclophosphamide, doxorubicin (Adriamycin), CCNU (lomustine), methotrexate, vincristine, procarbazine, VP-16, and hexamethylmelamine.[9] A number of useful combination regimens have been developed using these agents.

One of the most commonly used combinations for SCLC is cyclophosphamide, doxorubicin, and vincristine (CAV). In two previous studies by the Toronto Lung Cancer Study Group, responses occurred in approximately 85% of LD patients and in 65% to 75% of ED patients receiving this combination.[10,11] The median survival time (MST) of LD patients was approximately 48 weeks, while that for patients with ED was 35 weeks. Approximately 10% of patients survived beyond two years (20% with LD and 3% with ED). These results with the CAV regimen are generally as good as most induction regimens, and in addition, therapy is well tolerated and suitable for outpatient administration.

The Goldie-Coldman model predicts that for those tumors for which two different active combinations are available, the highest probability of cure would occur if the combinations were administered as alternating courses as opposed to the sequential administration of several courses of the same combination.

Sierocki et al were the first to describe the clinical activity of the combination of VP-16 plus cisplatin in CAV-refractory patients.[12] We subsequently confirmed that VP-16 plus cisplatin was active against SCLC that had failed to respond or relapsed after CAV induction chemotherapy.[13] Of 78 evaluable patients, (LD, 24; ED, 54), six (8%) achieved a complete response (CR), while 37 (47%) had a partial response (PR). The median duration of response was 22 weeks (range, 4 to 50 weeks) for patients with LD and 18 weeks (range, 4 to 49 weeks) for those with ED. The MSTs of LD patients who had either CR or PR were 59 and 34 weeks, respectively, whereas the comparable figures for responding ED patients were 45 and 23 weeks, respectively.

Table 1. VP-16 and Cisplatin for Nonresponding or Relapsed SCLC

Reference	Dose and Schedule		Prior Chemotherapy	Disease Extent		No. Evaluable/ No. Treated	Response Rate (%)		MDR (wk)	MST (wk)
	VP-16	Cisplatin		LD	ED		CR	PR		
Evans[13]	100 mg/m^2 d 1–3	25 mg/m^2 d 1–3	CAV	25	53	77/78	LD 16	52	22	35
							ED 4	42	18	21
Porter[17]	200 mg/m^2 d 1–3	40 mg/m^2 d 1–3	15/29 prior VP-16	NS	NS	26/29	7	45	12	16
Figoli[18]	75 mg/m^2 d 1	20 mg/m^2 d 1–5	Multiple agents, 19 pts had 7 prior drugs	6	23	25/29	8	38	NS	56 (from original diagnosis
Einhorn[16]	100 mg/m^2 d 1–5	20 mg/m^2 d 1–5	CAV, 3 pts also had CCNU + MTX	9	23	32/32	9	72	19	21
Tinsley[19]	100 mg/m^2 d 1–5	20 mg/m^2 d 1–5	NS	7	8	15/15	0	47	NS	NS
Batist[20]	80 mg/m^2 d 1–3	75 mg/m^2 d 1	6 prior agents	5	13	18/18	0	11	NS	NS

Abbreviations: MDR, median duration of response; NS, not stated; pts, patients; MTX, methotrexate.

Numerous other investigators have found similar antitumor activity using VP-16 plus cisplatin in nonresponding or relapsed patients (Table 1).[13-20] Only Batist et al have reported a low response rate (11%), but the patients in this study had all had multiple drugs prior to VP-16 plus cisplatin and the dose of VP-16 was the lowest used in any of the reported series.[20]

The activity of VP-16 plus cisplatin as second-line therapy following CAV suggested that this combination might be non–cross-resistant with the CAV regimen and, therefore, it seemed reasonable to consider the use of VP-16 plus cisplatin as part of an aggressive induction regimen for SCLC.

In 1982, the National Cancer Institute of Canada (NCI-C) commenced two prospective randomized trials incorporating CAV and VP-16 plus cisplatin in the induction therapy. The study in limited disease (BR3) evaluated two different sequences of administration of the CAV and VP-16 plus cisplatin regimens (Table 2). One arm was randomized to receive CAV alternating with VP-16 plus cisplatin. The second arm received three courses of CAV followed by three courses of VP-16 plus cisplatin. Patients received prophylactic cranial irradiation (PCI) between the third and fourth courses of chemotherapy, and at the completion of the chemotherapy, patients received locoregional radiotherapy. No maintenance chemotherapy was given.

Chemotherapy consisted of cyclophosphamide (1,000 mg/m^2), doxorubicin (50 mg/m^2), and vincristine (2 mg) on day 1 or VP-16 (100 mg/m^2) days 1 to 3 and cisplatin (25 mg/m^2) days 1 to 3. Each of these regimens was repeated at approximately 3-week intervals and generally administered on an outpatient basis. Dose adjustments were made for low counts or abnormal renal function. PCI was administered as 2,000 rad to the entire brain in five fractions over 1 week. Thoracic irradiation was given to cover the prechemotherapy extent of disease, and patients in this study were randomized to receive either 2,500 rad in ten fractions in 2 weeks or 3,750 rad in 15 fractions in 3 weeks, with partial shielding of the thoracic spinal cord. Response and toxicity were evaluated using standard cooperative group criteria.

A preliminary analysis of 301 eligible randomized patients was recently reported at the Fourth World Conference on Lung Cancer.[21] One hundred fifty-two patients were randomized to the alternating arm and 145 to the sequential arm. The characteristics of the patients in the two arms were similar. The mean age was 61 years (range, 35 to 80). The Eastern Cooperative Oncology Group (ECOG) performance status of the patients was generally good, with 22% ECOG 0 and 65% ECOG 1.

The overall response rate was 76% (45% CR and 31% PR) after six courses of chemotherapy. The CR rate for alternating was 48% and for sequential was 42%, but this difference was not significant. The projected overall MST was 54 weeks (sequential, 60 weeks, and alternating, 59 weeks) and the projected 2-year survival was 19%, with no difference between the two arms. Patients tolerated the treatment well, although 62% had at least one episode of neutropenia (granulocytes $< 0.5 \times 10^9$/L) and 16% had thrombocytopenia of $< 50 \times 10^9$/L. Most of the neutropenic episodes occurred on the CAV regimen ($P < .0001$), whereas thrombocytopenia occurred most commonly when patients were receiving VP-16 plus cisplatin ($P < .0001$).

Table 2. Schema for NCI-C Study of CAV and VP-16 Plus Cisplatin in Limited SCLC (BR 3) Sequential *v* Alternating

Sequential		
Cyclophosphamide	1,000 mg/m^2	Every 3 wk for 3 cycles
Doxorubicin	50 mg/m^2	
Vincristine	2 mg	
followed by		
VP-16	100 mg/m^2	IV daily × 3 every 3 wk for 3 cycles
Cisplatin	25 mg/m^2	
Alternating		
CAV Alternating with VP-16 plus cisplatin every 3 wks for 6 cycles		

Table 3. Schema for NCI-C Study of CAV and VP-16 Plus Cisplatin in Extensive SCLC (BR 4) Standard *v* Alternating

Standard		
Cyclophosphamide	1,000 mg/m^2	IV Every 3 wk for 6 cycles
Doxorubicin	50 mg/m^2	
Vincristine	2 mg	
Alternating		
CAV alternating with VP-16 plus cisplatin every 3 wk for 6 cycles		
VP-16	100 mg/m^2	IV daily × 3
Cisplatin	25 mg/m^2	

Infections occurred in 7% of patients and proved fatal in two cases. There were only two cases of severe, but reversible renal failure, even though treatment was administered almost uniformly on an outpatient basis. To date, no unusual toxicities secondary to the cranial or thoracic irradiation have been observed.

The two treatment strategies incorporating CAV and VP-16 plus cisplatin into induction therapy have produced survival curves comparable to the best current protocols, and there is a projected 2-year survival of approximately 20%. However, the study did not demonstrate any significant difference between the alternating and sequential approaches.

On the other hand, ED patients were treated on a second NCI-C trial (BR4) in which they were randomized to receive either six courses of CAV alone ("standard") or CAV alternating with VP-16 plus cisplatin for a total of six treatment cycles (Table 3). Extensive disease was defined as disease spread beyond the primary site, mediastinum, and ipsilateral supraclavicular nodes. Patients with malignant pleural effusions were classified as ED and included in the study if they had other measurable or evaluable disease. Patients with CNS metastases were excluded, as were those with a performance status > ECOG 3 (Table 4). The doses of drugs in the CAV and VP-16 plus cisplatin regimens were similar to those used in BR3. Responding patients were treated with PCI following the third course of treatment in a dose of 2,000 rad in five fractions. A preliminary analysis of patients entered in this study has also been recently presented.[22] Of the 243 patients who have been randomized in the study, 230 had completed six courses of chemotherapy at the time of the analysis. A good balance for most known prognostic factors was achieved by the randomization process. However, the performance status of those in the alternating arm was slightly better than those in the standard arm. Fifty-three percent of the patients in the standard arm had an ECOG performance status of 0 to 1 compared with 66% of those in the alternating arm. In addition, there were slightly more patients in the alternating arm[19] with locoregional disease than in the standard arm.[16] In the majority of these cases, the locoregional disease was a pleural effusion.

The response rate after six cycles of chemotherapy in the alternating arm (61%) was significantly better than in the standard arm (39%)

Table 4. NCI-C Trial BR4: Ineligibility Criteria

CNS metastasis
Prior chemotherapy or radiotherapy
ECOG 4
Prior malignant tumor (except nonmelanoma skin tumor)
Inadequate marrow function (WBC < 3,000/μL, granulocytes < 1,500/μL, platelet count < 75,000/μL)
Bilirubin > 2 mg/dL
Serum creatinine > 1.5 g/dL, BUN > 30 mg/dL, creatinine clearance < 50 mL/min
Serious cardiac disease (myocardial infarction within 3 months of diagnosis, CHF, or arrhythmia requiring treatment)
Age > 80 yr

Table 5. NCI-C-Trial BR4: Analysis of Toxicity*

	Regimen	
	Standard	Alternating
Toxic deaths	3	4
Neutropenia < 0.500	70	58
Thrombocytopenia < 50,000	3	9
Hemorrhage	0	1
Infection	19	10
GI—severe	17	21
Renal	0	4
Total	112	107

*In 229 evaluable patients.

($P < .01$). When the best response to chemotherapy at any time during treatment was compared between the two treatment regimens, the percentage of patients with CR was higher in the alternating arm (40% *v* 27%). CR was also analyzed following the completion of six courses of chemotherapy. Again, the response rate was significantly better in the alternating arm ($P <$ .005). A statistically significant advantage for the alternating arm was also seen in progression-free survival ($P = .001$). Finally, when the overall survival of the two groups was compared, there was an advantage in favor of the alternating arm, but it was less impressive ($P < .05$). The absolute difference in MST was approximately 2 months.

The frequency of thrombocytopenia and severe gastrointestinal toxicity was slightly greater in the alternating arm, but the frequency of neutropenia and infection was less (Table 5). Renal injury was only observed on the alternating arm, but only four of 112 cases were identified with renal toxicity. The most common cause of death in this study was progressive cancer; however, there were seven treatment-related deaths, including two patients in the standard arm and three in the alternating arm who succumbed to sepsis during periods of neutropenia.

From the preliminary analysis of this study, it appears that the alternation of CAV and VP-16 plus cisplatin is a more effective treatment strategy in patients with extensive SCLC. Whether the improvement in progression-free survival and the marginal improvement in overall survival were due to the strategy of alternating VP-16 plus cisplatin and CAV regimens or to the fact that VP-16 plus cisplatin is itself a highly active drug combination in this disease is not yet known.

Although we have observed that VP-16 plus cisplatin can induce responses in patients relapsing after CAV chemotherapy, the activity of CAV after failure of VP-16 plus cisplatin is less well defined. In our experience with VP-16 plus cisplatin as first-line therapy, we have had the opportunity to treat 12 patients with CAV at the time of relapse. Two patients had CRs and one had a PR. Five other patients have been treated with the anthraquinone mitoxantrone at the time of relapse. One achieved a PR, one had stable disease, and the other three progressed on treatment. Scher observed no major responses to CAV chemotherapy in 18 patients when it was administered after incomplete response or progression following three courses of VP-16 plus cisplatin.[23]

Although the amount of data is limited at the present time, it would appear that true bidirectional non–cross-resistance does not exist between CAV and VP-16 plus cisplatin. Nonetheless, it is clear that induction regimens that include CAV and VP-16 plus cisplatin yield results as good as any previously reported. In ED patients, the strategy of alternating VP-16 plus cisplatin with CAV has yielded modestly superior results compared with the administration of CAV alone. Whether these results are due to the strategy of early administration of two active chemotherapy regimens or to the high level of antitumor activity with VP-16 plus cisplatin alone will require further study in a randomized clinical trial.

ACKNOWLEDGMENT

The authors wish to express their gratitude to the many physicians who entered and managed patients in these studies and to the clinical trials secretaries who collected the data at the participating centers. We also thank Chris Allen for her careful preparation of the manuscript.

REFERENCES

1. Hansen HH, Dombernowsky P, Hirsch FR: Staging procedures and prognostic features in small cell anaplastic bronchogenic carcinoma. Semin Oncol 5:280–287, 1978

2. Morstyn G, Ihde DC, Lichter AS, et al: Small cell lung cancer 1973–1983: Early progress and recent obstacles. Int J Radiat Oncol 10:515–539, 1984

3. Fidler IJ, Hart IR: Biological diversity in metastatic neoplasms: Origins and implications. Science 217:998–1003, 1982

4. Heppner G: Tumor heterogeneity. Cancer Res 214:2259–2265, 1984

5. Fidler IJ, Poste G: The cellular heterogeneity of malignant neoplasms: Implications. Semin Oncol 12:207–221, 1985

6. Goldie JH, Coldman AJ: A mathematical model for relating the drug sensitivity of tumours to their spontaneous mutation rate. Cancer Treat Rep 63:1727–1733, 1979

7. Shields TW, Higgins GA, Matthews MJ, et al: Surgical resection in the management of small cell carcinoma of the lung. J Thorac Cardiovasc Surg 84:481–488, 1982

8. Greco FA, Einhorn LH, Richardson RL, et al: Small cell lung cancer: Progress and perspectives. Semin Oncol 5:323–335, 1978

9. Weiss RB: Small cell carcinoma of the lung: Therapeutic management. Ann Int Med 88:522–531, 1978

10. Feld R, Pringle JF, Evans WK, et al: Combined modality treatment of small cell carcinoma of the lung. Arch Int Med 242:469–473, 1981

11. Feld R, Evans WK, DeBoer G, et al: Combined modality induction therapy without maintenance chemotherapy for small cell carcinoma of the lung. J Clin Oncol 2:294–304, 1984

12. Sierocki JS, Golberg RB, Wittes RE: Combination chemotherapy for small cell carcinoma of the lung. Proc Am Assoc Cancer Res 19:352, 1978 (abstr)

13. Evans WK, Osoba D, Feld R, et al: Etoposide (VP-16) and cisplatin: An effective treatment for relapse in small cell lung cancer. J Clin Oncol 3:65–71, 1985

14. Kim PN, McDonald DB: The combination of VP-16-213 and cisplatinum in the treatment of small cell carcinoma of lung. Proc Am Soc Clin Oncol 141, 1982 (abstr C-547)

15. Lopez JA, Mann J, Grapski R: Salvage chemotherapy for refractory small cell lung cancer with VP-16 and cisplatinum. Proc Am Soc Clin Oncol 151, 1982 (abstr C-586)

16. Einhorn LH, Williams SD, Loehrer PG: Platinum + VP-16 chemotherapy for refractory small cell lung cancer. Proc Am Assoc Cancer Res 174, 1984 (abstr 689)

17. Porter L, Johnson D, Hainsworth JL: Recurrent small cell lung carcinoma treated with VP-16 and cisplatinum. Cancer Treat Rep 69:479–481, 1985

18. Figoli F, Veronesi A, Frustacis S, et al: Cisplatin and etoposide as second line therapy in patients with small cell lung cancer. Proc IVth World Conference on Lung Cancer p 8, 1985 (abstr 501)

19. Tinsley R, Comis R, Difimo S, et al: Potential clinical surgery observed in the treatment of small cell lung cancer with cisplatin and VP-16–213. Proc Am Soc Clin Oncol 198, 1983 (abstr C-772)

20. Batist G, Ihde DC, Cowan K, et al: Phase II trial of cisplatin and VP-16 in previously treated small cell lung cancer. Proc Am Assoc Cancer Res 175, 1984 (abstr 694)

21. Feld R, Evans WK, Coy P, et al: Canadian multicentre randomized trials comparing sequential and alternating administration of two non-cross resistant chemotherapy combinations in patients with limited small cell carcinoma of the lung. Proc IVth World Conference on Lung Cancer p 77, 1985 (abstr 542)

22. Evans WK, Murray N, Feld R, et al: Canadian multicentre randomized trial comparing standard and alternating combination chemotherapy in extensive small cell lung cancer. Proc IVth World Conference on Lung Cancer p 77, 1985 (abstr 560)

23. Scher H, Casper E, Gralla R: Intensive induction chemotherapy with cisplatin plus etoposide with radiotherapy for small cell lung cancer. Proc IVth World Conference on Lung Cancer: 95, 1985 (abstr 483)

First-Line Therapy With VP-16 and Cisplatin for Small-Cell Lung Cancer

By William K. Evans, Frances A. Shepherd, Ronald Feld, David Osoba, and Gerrit DeBoer

VP-16 and cisplatin were used as first-line therapy in 31 patients with small-cell lung cancer (SCLC) in whom chemotherapy regimens that contained doxorubicin (Adriamycin [Adria Laboratories, Columbus, Ohio]) were contraindicated because of severe cardiac or hepatic disease. Eight patients who had cerebral metastases at presentation were also included in the study. There were 11 patients with limited disease (LD) and 20 with extensive disease (ED). Of the 28 evaluable patients, 12 (43%) had a complete response (CR) and 12 (43%) had a partial response (PR). Four patients (14%) failed to respond. The median duration of response (MDR) for LD patients was 39 weeks and for ED patients was 26 weeks. Patients with LD who responded (CR and PR) had a median survival time (MST) of 70 weeks (range, 28 to 232+ weeks), whereas ED patients who responded had an MST of 43 weeks (range, 17 to 68 weeks). Gastrointestinal toxicity was mild, but leukopenia and thrombocytopenia were common. Mild degrees of reversible nephrotoxicity occurred in 15 patients, but required discontinuation of cisplatin in only two. The results of this study are compared with several other recently published reports of VP-16 and cisplatin used as first-line therapy in SCLC.

THE EPIPODOPHYLLOTOXIN VP-16 is probably the single most active agent against small-cell lung cancer (SCLC).[1–4] In phase II clinical trials, response rates from 20% to 60% have been reported in previously untreated patients. On the other hand, VP-16 shows only marginal activity in patients who have had prior chemotherapy.[5–9] Cisplatin appears to have only modest activity as a single agent in SCLC,[10,11] but, in combination with VP-16, marked synergism has been observed in some animal tumor systems.[12,13]

In our early experience with these agents at the University of Toronto, we saw very little antitumor activity when VP-16 was used alone in SCLC patients who had failed therapy with cyclophosphamide, doxorubicin (Adriamycin), and vincristine (CAV).[5] In fact, only one of 18 evaluable patients treated had a partial response (PR) to VP-16 alone. However, the patient who did have a PR achieved a complete response (CR) when cisplatin was combined with VP-16. Subsequently, in a series of 78 patients who failed to respond to CAV or relapsed following it, we observed a 55% response rate.[14] The median duration of response (MDR) to VP-16 and cisplatin in these patients was 22 weeks (range, 4 to 50 weeks) for limited-disease (LD) patients and 18 weeks (range, 4 to 49 weeks) for those with extensive disease (ED). These observations, coupled with the report of Sierocki et al on the activity of the VP-16 and cisplatin combination in refractory SCLC,[15] led us to evaluate this combination as first-line therapy in individuals who were not candidates for CAV by virtue of poor cardiac or hepatic function. Patients with treated cerebral metastases were also treated on this study because of their known poor prognosis. We have recently reported the results of this study in detail elsewhere.[16]

PATIENTS AND METHODS

Patients were accrued to the study from the Toronto General Hospital; and The Ontario Cancer Institute, incorporating the Princess Margaret Hospital; and the Toronto-Bayview Regional Cancer Centre of the Ontario Cancer Foundation. All patients had histologically or cytologically proven SCLC and none had received previous chemotherapy or radiotherapy other than as treatment for symptomatic cerebral metastases.

Prior to treatment with VP-16 and cisplatin, all patients had a careful history and physical examination, assessment of performance status using the Eastern Cooperative Oncology Group (ECOG) scale, biochemical tests of renal and hepatic function, a chest radiograph, radionuclide brain, bone and liver scans, and a bone marrow aspiration and biopsy.

Suitable study candidates included patients with documented CNS metastases at presentation, clinical evidence of jaundice or a serum bilirubin >50 μmol/L (3.0 mg/100 mL), or serious cardiac disease. This included patients who had congestive heart failure secondary to myocardial infarction or valvular heart disease who required digoxin and/or diuretics.

Patients had to have a performance status of 0 to 3 (ECOG scale), a granulocyte count $>1.5 \times 10^9$ cells/L, a platelet

From the Department of Medicine, University of Toronto, and the Department of Biostatistics, The Ontario Cancer Institute.

Address reprint requests to W.K. Evans, MD, The Ontario Cancer Foundation, Ottawa Regional Cancer Centre, 190 Melrose Ave, Ottawa, Ontario, Canada K1Y 4K7.

0093–7754/86/1303–3006$05.00/0

count >125 × 10^9 cells/L, and a serum creatinine <130 μmol/L (2 mg/100 mL).

Chemotherapy Administration

Prior to each course of chemotherapy, all patients were premedicated with a combination of antiemetics that usually consisted of the following: dexamethasone 10 mg intravenously (IV); metoclopramide, 10 mg IV or orally; prochlorperazine, 10 mg orally or intramuscularly (IM). Following chemotherapy, prochlorperazine was continued every six hours for at least four doses following the last chemotherapy injection (Table 1). If this regimen was not optimally effective, dexamethasone 1 to 2 mg was also administered every six hours orally. VP-16 was diluted in normal saline to a concentration of 0.4 mg/mL and administered IV over a minimum of 30 minutes. The dose of VP-16 was 100 mg/m^2 IV on days 1, 2, and 3, and cisplatin was administered in a dose of 25 mg/m^2 by slow IV push at the end of the VP-16 infusion on days 1 to 3 also. Treatment cycles were repeated at 3- to 4-week intervals depending on treatment-day blood counts.

Pulse rate and BP were monitored at 15 minute intervals during the VP-16 infusion. No special efforts were made to hydrate patients, although they were encouraged to increase their fluid intake during treatment and they generally received in excess of 500 mL of normal saline on each treatment day with the VP-16 infusion. Mannitol and diuretics were not administered. Adjustments in drug dosage were made according to nadir and treatment-day blood counts. A 25% reduction in the dosage of both drugs was made if the nadir granulocyte count was <0.5 × 10^9/L or the nadir platelet count was <75 × 10^9/L. A similar reduction was made if the pretreatment granulocyte count was between 1.5 and 2.0 × 10^9/L or the pretreatment platelet count was between 100 and 125 × 10^9/L. If the pretreatment granulocyte count or platelet count fell below those levels that required a 25% dosage reduction, treatment was delayed for 1 week until the blood counts recovered. An arbitrary 25% dosage reduction was made for patients 70 years of age or older.

Patients who had no evidence of tumor spread beyond the mediastinum and/or ipsilateral supraclavicular nodes (LD) were treated with six cycles of chemotherapy followed by irradiation to the primary site (2,500 rad in ten fractions). Responding LD patients were also administered prophylactic cranial irradiation (PCI) in a dose of 2,000 rad in five fractions between the third and fourth treatment cycle. Responding ED patients also received PCI, but locoregional radiotherapy was used only for persistent local symptoms after six chemotherapy cycles. No maintenance chemotherapy was administered.

If disease progression occurred on VP-16 and cisplatin, patients were treated with CAV, if possible, or the anthraquinone, mitoxantrone. If neither approach was appropriate or possible, patients were treated at the investigator's discretion.

RESPONSE CRITERIA

Response to therapy was assessed at each treatment cycle by clinical examination of the patient, CBC, renal and liver function tests, chest radiograph, and repeat examination by radioisotope or computerized tomography (CT) scan as clinically indicated. A CR was defined as complete disappearance of all clinically and radiologically evident disease. Bronchoscopy was not used routinely to document the completeness of response to therapy. PR was defined as a decrease of at least 50% in the product of two perpendicular diameters of measurable lesions for at least 4 weeks. The term "stable" (STAB) was used to define the situation in which there was <50% decrease in measurable disease, improvement in the appearance of radionuclide scans or other evaluable, but nonmeasurable disease, or <25% increase in tumor size over a 12-week period. Those patients who met the criteria for stable disease, but had their treatment changed to another regimen before 12 weeks were classified as no response (NR) and grouped with the progressive disease (PD) patients. Progression was defined as an increase of >25% in the product of perpendicular diameters of measurable disease, or the development of new lesions.

Response duration was measured from the

Table 1. Chemotherapy Administration

VP-16 100 mg/m^2 d 1, 2, 3	Diluted to concentration of 0.4 mg/mL and administered over 30 min to 1 h
Cisplatin 25 mg/m^2 d 1, 2, 3	Administered slow IV push at end of VP-16 infusion
Repeat treatment cycles every 3 to 4 wk for six cycles	
	Antiemetic Schedule
Dexamethasone 10 mg IV Metoclopramide 10 mg IV (or orally)	Immediately prior to chemotherapy
Prochlorperazine	10 mg orally prior to chemotherapy and every 6h orally (or IM) for at least 3 d

date of first treatment to the date of disease progression or last follow-up. Survival time was measured from the time of first treatment with VP-16 and cisplatin to the date of last follow-up. Toxicity was graded according to ECOG toxicity criteria.[17]

Thirty-one patients have been treated on this study protocol. Twenty-four were men, seven were women, and their median age was 61 years (range, 29 to 77). Fifty percent of the patients had an ECOG performance status of 0 or 1, 43% were 2, and 6% (two patients) were 3. Eleven patients had LD confined to the primary site in the lung, with extension limited to the mediastinum and/or ipsilateral supraclavicular fossa. Of the 20 patients with extensive disease, 11 had liver involvement, eight had brain metastases, seven had bone metastases, and three had bone marrow involvement. In addition, two patients had adrenal metastases and one had a cytology-positive pleural effusion. One patient presented with superior vena cava obstruction. Sixty-five percent of patients had ischemic or valvular heart disease significant enough to preclude the safe use of doxorubicin, and 9% had a bilirubin level >50 μmol/L. Twenty-six percent of the patients had brain metastases at presentation. Twenty-eight of the 31 patients were evaluable for response. One patient was inevaluable because there was no obvious lesion on chest radiograph, but this patient had the syndrome of inappropriate antidiuretic hormone secretion (SIADH), which resolved with treatment. Two early deaths occurred in the study at 11 and 20 days from the first treatment. One of these deaths was treatment-related, but the other was the result of severe bleeding from a duodenal ulcer and appeared to be unrelated to the chemotherapy treatment.

Of the 28 evaluable patients, there were 11 with LD and 17 with ED. Seven of the LD patients (64%) achieved a CR and two (18%) had a PR. Two patients progressed on treatment. All patients achieving a CR did so before receiving irradiation to the primary site. The MDR for those patients achieving either a CR or PR was 39 weeks (range, 12 to 232+). The median survival time (MST) for the whole group of LD patients was 63 weeks. The MST for responding patients was 70 weeks, and for those patients who failed to respond, it was only 15 weeks.

Five of the 17 ED patients (29%) achieved a CR; an additional ten patients (59%) achieved a PR. Two patients progressed on treatment. The median duration of response was 26 weeks (range, 13 to 42 weeks). The MST for the whole group of extensive disease patients was 39 weeks compared with 68 weeks for those achieving CR and 40 weeks for those achieving PR. For those who had no response or whose disease progressed on treatment, the MST only 17 weeks.

The median number of treatment cycles to a PR was two and to a CR, three. Seventy-five percent of patients achieving a CR had a performance status of 0 or 1, whereas three of the four patients with no response or PD had a performance status of 2 or 3.

Ten patients failing VP-16 and cisplatin were treated with alternate treatment regimens. Three received CAV, and one patient achieved a CR, one a PR, and one progressed. Two patients were treated with VP-16, vincristine, and cyclophosphamide when cisplatin-induced nephrotoxicity precluded further safe use of cisplatin in one case and local recurrence occurred in a second case. The latter patient achieved a CR and the former had STAB disease. Five patients were treated with mitoxantrone at the time of relapse; one achieved a PR, one had stable disease, and the other three progressed on treatment. Two deaths unrelated to cancer occurred during this study and both were due to cardiac disease. One occurred in a patient with LD who had achieved a CR of 17 weeks' duration, and the other occurred in a patient with ED who had achieved a PR.

TOXICITY

Most patients were treated as outpatients throughout the treatment program. Only 16% of patients required hospital admission at some point to manage either treatment-related toxicities or to receive their chemotherapy.

Nineteen percent of patients required dosage reduction because of myelosuppression at some point during their treatment. Twenty-three percent of patients also required a delay in treatment because of low pretreatment granulocyte counts. Twenty-nine percent of patients had at least one granulocyte count below 1.5×10^9/L and 18% had a nadir granulocyte count below 1.0×10^9/L. Three patients (11%) had <500 granulocytes at some point in their treatment course. There were four febrile episodes associated with drug-induced neutropenia. Three of these resolved with broad-spectrum antibiotics, but one patient died because of severe neutropenia and sepsis.

Thrombocytopenia was common. Forty percent of patients had platelet counts $<90 \times 10^9/L$ at some point during treatment. There were no bleeding episodes associated with thrombocytopenia and no patient had a platelet count $<25 \times 10^9/L$. Anemia of 100 g/L or less occurred in 64% of patients. The frequency of anemia increased with successive treatment cycles and 32% of the patients required one or more blood transfusions. It was encouraging to note that 28% of the patients had no gastrointestinal toxicity during their chemotherapy treatment. The majority of patients did experience mild nausea and vomiting despite the antiemetic program; however, only one patient was hospitalized because of dehydration secondary to vomiting, and one other patient required a delay in one of his treatment cycles because of persistent nausea. Diarrhea was not observed.

Mild increases in serum creatinine level above baseline were seen in over half the patients. The mean increase was 1.6 times baseline, but increases ranged from 1.1 to 3.4 times baseline. The serum creatinine generally decreased with a reduction in the dose of cisplatin, but two patients required discontinuation of the drug because of increasing creatinine values. Neither of these patients developed clinically significant renal failure. Symptomatic hypomagnesemia developed in two patients and required magnesium supplementation. Hypotension during the VP-16 infusion was not observed. Alopecia occurred in all patients and was usually moderate to severe.

DISCUSSION

The combination of VP-16 and cisplatin has been shown to be synergistic against P-388 and L-1210 leukemia in mice[12,13] and to have an additive effect in an in vitro assay system using a human lymphoma cell line.[18] Studies using this combination in patients with refractory SCLC have generally demonstrated high objective response rates.[14,15,19–23] In one study, however, the response rate was only 11%, but all patients had been extensively pretreated with at least six other chemotherapeutic agents.[24]

In the present study, 43% of evaluable patients achieved a CR and an additional 43% had a PR. In LD patients, the median duration of response was 39 weeks and for extensive-disease patients it was 26 weeks. The MST for responding LD patients was 70 weeks, and for ED patients it was 43 weeks. These results are quite comparable with those reported for standard induction chemotherapy regimens such as CAV.[25] Considering the fact that the patients in this study had poor prognostic features such as extensive liver disease and brain metastases, as well as serious cardiac disease, these results are quite impressive.

Similarly encouraging results have been reported by several other centers. Table 2 shows the response rates to first-line VP-16 and cisplatin administered in a variety of dosage schedules. Sierocki et al first reported that this combination is active as an induction regimen in previously untreated SCLC.[26] They administer two cycles of VP-16 (120 mg/m^2) on days 4, 6, and 8 and cisplatin (60 mg/m^2) on day 1, 3 weeks apart, followed by four cycles of CAV chemotherapy and PCI. They noted that response to VP-16 and cisplatin was rapid and invariably maximal by the end of two induction cycles. Ninety-five percent of patients responded (LD, 52% CR; 48% PR; ED, 41% CR; 37% PR). The MDR for PRs with LD was only 4.5 months, but the MDR for those achieving CR had not been reached at the time of reporting. The MST for ED patients was approximately 9 months, whereas the MST for LD patients was in excess of 14 months. Long-term follow-up results on these patients have not yet been reported. Kim and McDonald treated patients with VP-16 (125 mg/m^2) on days 1, 3, and 5 and cisplatin (75 mg/m^2) on day 1. Twenty-one of 24 evaluable patients (88%) demonstrated a major response.[19] Woods and Levi administered VP-16 (80 mg/m^2) on days 1, 2, and 3 and cisplatin 80 mg/m^2 on day 1 every 3 weeks with split-course radiotherapy between the first and third chemotherapy cycles.[27] Fifty-three percent of patients achieved a CR and 37% a PR on this program.

Stoller et al reported that eight of nine patients had a major response to VP-16 (200 mg/m^2) days 1 and 2 and cisplatin (100 mg/m^2) day 1,

Table 2. Studies of Cisplatin Plus VP-16 as First-Line Therapy for SCLC

Reference/Yr	Dosage (mg/m²) Cisplatin	VP-16	No. of Evaluable Patients	PR (%)	CR (%)
Evans, 1985[16]	25 d 1, 2, 3	100 d 1, 2, 3	LD 11	2 (18)	7 (64)
			ED 17	10 (59)	5 (29)
Sierocki, 1979[26]	60 d 1	120 d 4, 6, 8	LD 21	10 (48)	11 (52)
			ED 17	8 (47)	7 (41)
Kim, 1982[19]	75 d 1	125 d 1, 3, 5	LD 11	6 (55)	4 (36)
			ED 13	9 (69)	2 (15)
Stoller, 1983[28]	100 d 1	200 d 1, 2	9	8 "Responded" (89)	
Tinsley, 1983[29]	20 d 1–5	100 d 1–5	ED 8	4 (50)	
Salvati, 1985[30]	60 d 1	120 d 2, 3, 4	LD 18	9 (50)	7 (39)
Wilke, 1985[31]	50 d 1–7	170 d 3, 4, 5	24	5 (21)	18 (75)
Boni, 1985[32]	60 d 1	120 d 4, 6, 8	LD 12	4 (33)	8 (67)
			ED 10	4 (40)	5 (50)
Scher, 1985[33]	125 d 1	120 d 4, 6, 8	37	11 (30)	20 (54)
		Total	208	90 (43)	94 (45)

repeated every 3 weeks for two cycles and followed by CAV chemotherapy ×4. One of the eight responding patients had a tumor lysis syndrome following the first course of VP-16 and cisplatin.[28] Tinsley et al obtained four PRs in eight patients when VP-16 (100 mg/m²) was administered days 1 to 5 and cisplatin (20 mg/m²) was administered days 1 to 5.[29] Unfortunately, three drug-related deaths occurred in this study. Salvati et al gave a single course of VP-16 (120 mg/m²) days 2, 3 and 4 and cisplatin (60 mg/m²) day 1 followed 4 weeks later by cyclophosphamide (600 mg/m²) and doxorubicin (50 mg/m²).[30] Of 18 evaluable patients, seven achieved a CR and nine a PR for an overall response rate of 89%. The MST of these patients was 52 weeks with a range of 28 to 104+ weeks. Wilke et al split the cisplatin dose and gave 50 mg/m² on day 1 and day 7 with VP-16 170 mg/m² days 3, 4, and 5.[31] Of 24 evaluable patients, 18 achieved a CR and five a PR.

Boni et al administered cisplatin (60 mg/m²) day 1 and VP-16 (120 mg/m²) days 4, 6, and 8 every 21 days to 24 previously untreated patients.[32] Radiotherapy to the primary site and brain was administered to all LD patients achieving a CR. Those achieving a PR were given chest radiotherapy alone. Chemotherapy was continued at 50% doses during radiotherapy. After three cycles of chemotherapy, response was assessed clinically and bronchoscopically. Ninety-five percent of the 22 evaluable patients responded: 100% of LD patients (eight CR, four PR) and 90% of ED patients (five CR, four PR). The MST of LD patients was 60 weeks and 41 weeks for ED. Thrombocytopenia (platelets <50,000 cells/μL) occurred in 13% of patients and three patients withdrew from further therapy at 13 and 14 weeks because of neurological toxicity. Finally, Scher et al attempted to escalate the dose of VP-16 starting at 120 mg/m² days 4, 6, and 8 with cisplatin (125 mg/m²) day 1.[33] On subsequent treatments, the VP-16 was escalated to 180 mg/m² and then to 240 mg/m² if blood counts permitted. There were 37 evaluable patients in this study; 54% achieved a CR and 30% a PR. The MST for LD patients was 18 months and 8 months for extensive disease. Scher noted that the response rate was not increased at higher doses of VP-16. A second important observation was that no major responses were seen when CAV was administered after incomplete response or progression on VP-16 and cisplatin.

We observed relatively few serious toxicities during the treatment of our patients with VP-16 and cisplatin. Thrombocytopenia (platelet count <90,000/μL) occurred in 40% of patients at some point during treatment. However, there were no bleeding episodes, and there was no requirement for platelet transfusions. This high frequency of thrombocytopenia, however, has been observed by others using this drug combination and may represent a synergistic toxic effect on megakaryocytes. Neutropenia was also common, but only three patients had granulocyte counts $<0.5 \times 10^9/L$. There was one death from sepsis in our series, and other investigators have also reported serious myelosuppression complicated by sepsis and death. This appears to be more common when VP-16 and cisplatin are used as second-line therapy.[21,22] Anemia occurred in over 60% of the patients on treatment. As treatment continued, the degree of anemia worsened and blood transfusions were required in half of our patients.

Some degree of renal dysfunction was seen in over half the patients in this study. This is higher than the observed frequency of renal dysfunction we observed in 78 previously treated patients reported.[14] The increased frequency of renal dysfunction in this series may, in part, be due to the greater number of treatment cycles given to these patients as opposed to those with prior chemotherapy and to a lower frequency of dose reductions for myelosuppression because of greater bone marrow reserve. In addition, because many of these patients had serious cardiac disease, the amount of fluid given with each treatment cycle was generally conservative. We would favor a somewhat more vigorous effort to hydrate patients in future studies. The use of platinum analogues with less nephrotoxicity may help to circumvent this problem.[34,35]

The data emerging on VP-16 and cisplatin as first-line therapy in SCLC clearly indicate that this regimen is highly active with response rates comparable to the traditionally best regimens. Durations of response and survival also appear comparable. There is no evidence that doses of VP-16 or cisplatin higher than those used in the current study produce better overall results, although it is clear that more intensive regimens produce greater degrees of toxicity. The high frequency of response in patients refractory to, or relapsing after, induction chemotherapy consisting of cyclophosphamide, doxorubicin, and vincristine suggested that the VP-16 and cisplatin combination might well be the long sought after non–cross-resistant chemotherapy regimen. On the other hand, the infrequency of response to CAV following VP-16 and cisplatin reported by Scher suggests that the non–cross-resistance may not be bidirectional. Whether the combination of VP-16 and cisplatin is superior to CAV as an induction chemotherapy regimen will need to be addressed in a prospective randomized trial. Clearly, however, the activity of the VP-16–cisplatin combination as first-line therapy justifies its use in those patients in whom there is a contraindication to other commonly used regimens.

ACKNOWLEDGMENT

The authors wish to thank Else Johansen, Lesley Steward, and Kathy Turnbull for their assistance in data collection and Chris Allen for her careful preparation of the manuscript.

REFERENCES

1. Arnold AM: General review. Podophyllotoxin derivative VP-16-213. Cancer Chemother Pharmacol 3:71–80, 1979

2. Cavalli F, Sonntag RW, Jungi F, et al: VP-16-213 monotherapy for remission induction of small cell lung cancer: A randomized trial using three dosage schedules. Cancer Treat Rep 62:473–475, 1978

3. Hansen M, Hirsch F, Dombernowsky P, et al: Treatment of small cell anaplastic carcinoma of the lung with the oral solution of VP-16-213 (NSC 141 540, 4'-Demethyl epipodophyllotoxin 9-4, 6-0-ethylidene-beta-D-glucopyranoside). Cancer 40:633–637, 1977

4. Tucker RD, Ferguson A, Van Wyck C, et al: Chemotherapy of small cell carcinoma of the lung with VP-16-213. Cancer 41:1710–1714, 1978

5. Evans WK, Osoba D, Feld R, et al: VP-16 alone and in combination with cisplatin for relapse in small cell lung cancer. Cancer 53:1461–1466, 1984

6. Cohen NH, Broder LE, Fossieck BE, et al: Phase II clinical trial of weekly administration of VP-16-213 in small cell bronchogenic carcinoma. Cancer Treat Rep 61:489–490, 1977

7. Tempero M, Kessinger A, Lemon HM: VP-16-213 therapy in patients with small cell carcinoma of the lung after failure on combination chemotherapy. Cancer Clin Trials 4:155–157, 1981

8. Dally MB, Harper P, Smyth JF, et al: Epipodophyllotoxin (VP-16-213) on small cell carcinoma of the bronchus resistant to initial combined chemotherapy. Br J Dis Chest 74:312, 1980

9. Karp G, Antman K, Canellos G: VP-16-213: A phase II trial using a weekly schedule. Cancer Clin Trials 4:465–468, 1981

10. Rossof AH, Bearden JD III, Coltman CA Jr: Phase II evaluation of cis-diamminedichloroplatinum (II) in lung cancer. Cancer Treat Rep 60:1979–1980, 1976

11. Dombernowsky P, Sorenson S, Aisner J, et al: Cisdichlorodiammineplatinum (II) in small cell anaplastic bronchogenic carcinoma: A phase II study. Cancer Treat Rep 63:543–545, 1979

12. Von Hoff DD, Elson D: Clinical results with cisplatin in lung cancer, in Prestayko AW, Crooke S, Carter SK (eds): Cisplatin, Current Status and New Developments, vol 1. Orlando, Fla, Academic, 1980, pp 445–458

13. Schabel FM, Trader MW, Laster WK, et al: Cisdichlorodiammineplatinum (II): Combination chemotherapy and cross-resistance studies with tumours of mice. Cancer Treat Rep 63:1459–1473, 1979

14. Evans WK, Osoba D, Feld R, et al: VP-16 and cisplatin: An effective treatment for relapse in small cell lung cancer. J Clin Oncol 3:65–71, 1985

15. Sierocki JS, Golbey RB, Wittes RE: Combination chemotherapy for small cell carcinoma of the lung. Proc Am Assoc Cancer Res 19:352, 1978 (abstr)

16. Evans WK, Shepherd FA, Feld R, et al: VP-16 and cisplatin as first-line therapy for small cell lung cancer. J Clin Oncol 3:1471–1477, 1985

17. Oken MM, Creech RH, Tormey DC, et al: Toxicity and response criteria of the Eastern Cooperative Oncology Group. Am J Clin Oncol 5:649–655, 1982

18. Drewinko B, Green C, Loo TL: Combination chemotherapy in vitro with cis-dichlorodiammineplatinum (II). Cancer Treat Rep 60:1619–1625, 1976

19. Kim P-N, McDonald DB: The combination of VP-16-213 and cis-platinum in the treatment of small cell carcinoma of lung. Proc Am Soc Clin Oncol 1:141, 1982 (abstr)

20. Lopez JA, Mann J, Grapski R, et al: Salvage chemotherapy for refractory small cell lung cancer (SCLC) with VP-16 and cis-platinum (DDP). Proc Am Soc Clin Oncol 1:151, 1982 (abstr)

21. Porter L, Johnson D, Hainsworth J, et al: Recurrent small cell lung carcinoma treated with VP-16 and cisplatinum. Proc Am Soc Clin Oncol 3: 215, 1984 (abstr)

22. Einhorn LH, Williams SD, Loehrer PJ: Platinum + VP-16 chemotherapy for refractory small cell lung cancer. Proc Am Assoc Cancer Res 25:1774, 1984 (abstr)

23. Figoli F, Veronesi A, Fristaci S, et al: Cis-platin and etoposide as second line therapy in patients with small cell lung cancer. Proc IVth World Conference on Lung Cancer p 8, 1985 (abstr 501)

24. Batist G, Ihde D, Cowan K, et al: Phase II trial of cisplatin and VP-16 in previously treated small cell lung cancer. Proc Am Assoc Cancer Res 25:775, 1984 (abstr)

25. Bunn PA, Cohen MH, Ihde DC, et al: Commentary: Advances in small cell bronchogenic carcinoma. Cancer Treat Rep 61:333–340, 1977

26. Sierocki JS, Hilaris BS, Hopfan S, et al: Cis-diamminedichloroplatinum (II) and VP-16-213: An active induction regimen for small cell carcinoma of the lung. Cancer Treat Rep 63:1593–1597, 1979

27. Woods RL, Levi JA: Chemotherapy for small cell lung cancer (SCLC): A randomized study of maintenance therapy with cyclophosphamide, Adriamycin and vincristine (CAV) after remission induction with cisplatinum (Cis, DDP), VP-16-213 and radiotherapy. Proc Am Soc Clin Oncol 3:214, 1984 (abstr C836)

28. Stoller RG, Jacobs SA, Earle MF, et al: Combination cisplatinum (CDDP/VP-16) as initial therapy in small cell lung carcinoma. Proc Am Soc Clin Oncol 2:197, 1983 (abstr C769)

29. Tinsley R, Comis R, DiFimo S, et al: Potential clinical synergy observed in the treatment of small cell lung cancer with cisplatin and VP-16-213. Proc Am Soc Clin Oncol 2:198, 1983 (abstr C772)

30. Salvati F, Mugnaini L, Cruciani AR: Cisplatin and etoposide followed by Adriamycin and cytoxan for treatment of SCLC limited disease. Proc IVth World Conference on Lung Cancer p 7, 1985 (abstr 523)

31. Wilke H, Achterrath W, Gunzer U, et al: High remission rates in the treatment of small cell lung cancer with etoposide and splitted doses of cisplatin. Proc IVth World Conference on Lung Cancer: 8, 1985 (abstr 480)

32. Boni C, Bisagni G, Ceci G, et al: Cisplatinum plus VP-16 chemotherapy as front-line treatment in small cell lung cancer. Proc Am Soc Clin Oncol 4:196, 1985 (abstr C765)

33. Scher H, Casper E, Gralla R, et al: Intensive induction chemotherapy with cisplatin + etoposide with radiotherapy for small cell lung cancer. Proc IVth World Conference on Lung Cancer: 95, 1985 (abstr 483)

34. Evans BD, Weston C, Smith IE. Carboplatin (JM8) and VP-16 combination chemotherapy for untreated small cell lung carcinoma (SCLC): A Phase II study. Proc Am Soc Clin Oncol 4:188, 1985 (abstr C734)

35. Takita H, Madajewicz S, Plager J, et al: Phase II study of Iproplatin (CHIP) and etoposide in small cell lung carcinoma. Proc Am Soc Clin Oncol 4:193, 1985 (abstr C755)

Alternating Chemotherapy and Thoracic Radiotherapy With Concurrent Cisplatin-Etoposide for Limited-Stage Small-Cell Carcinoma of the Lung

By N. Murray, A. Shah, E. Brown, E. Kostashuk, E. Laukkanen, J. Goldie, P. Band, J. Van den Hoek, K. Murphy, T. Sparling, and M. Noble

Seventy patients with limited-stage small-cell lung cancer (SCLC) were given six courses of chemotherapy alternating two drug combinations: a combination of cyclophosphamide, doxorubicin (Adriamycin [Adria Laboratories, Columbus OH]) and vincristine (CAV) was alternated with cisplatin and etoposide at 3-week intervals. Thoracic radiotherapy was administered concurrently with the first cisplatin-etoposide chemotherapy. Prophylactic cranial irradiation (PCI) was administered after the completion of all chemotherapy. No maintenance treatment was used. Seventy-six percent of patients achieved a complete clinical response. The median survival was 78 weeks and the 2-year survival rate was 32% with an average follow-up of 3 1/2 years. Seventeen percent are currently alive and disease free. Cisplatin and etoposide can be administered concurrently with thoracic irradiation with acceptable toxicity. Our results justify further clinical research using alternating chemotherapy and concurrent thoracic irradiation and cisplatin-etoposide chemotherapy.

THE PRODUCTION of a complete or "nearly" complete remission of a rapidly growing small-cell lung cancer (SCLC) is a dramatic phenomenon that unavoidably encourages an oncologist to believe that the cure of this neoplasm should be feasible in many patients. Few things generate more despair and discouragement than the relentless recurrence of the tumor that usually has become impervious to meaningful control by the original or alternative treatments. Minimal progress has occurred in the treatment of SCLC in this decade.[1] A large amount of currently available data indicates that the development of drug-resistant cells within tumors is a critical factor in determining curability by chemotherapeutic agents.[2,3] Although resistance due to altered cell kinetics and pharmacologic sanctuaries is possible, evidence strongly implies a genetic origin for most of these drug-resistant phenotypes.[4] The high relapse rates observed, despite aggressive chemotherapy for limited-stage SCLC, indicate that most patients harbor chemotherapy-resistant tumor stem cells.

One obvious way to remedy this problem is to give improved chemotherapy. Although alternating non–cross-resistant chemotherapy has improved the results of treatment for Hodgkin's disease,[5,6] results of clinical research in SCLC have been controversial.[7] The difficulty with the interpretation of these results lies in the data proving that combinations used are symmetrically effective and non–cross-resistant. Our own group has experienced frustration in this regard.[8] The theoretical conditions under which alternating chemotherapy may offer an advantage are precisely described.[9] There is convincing evidence that the etoposide-cisplatin regimen is highly effective[10,11] and at least partially non–cross-resistant with cyclophosphamide, doxorubicin, and vincristine (CAV).[12,13] Recently, a large randomized trial, conducted under the auspices of the National Cancer Institute of Canada, that treated extensive-stage SCLC patients has shown better response rates, progression-free survival, and overall survival for CAV and etoposide-cisplatin alternation as compared with sequential CAV with etoposide-cisplatin salvage chemotherapy.[14] A parallel multicenter Canadian trial for limited-stage SCLC did not observe any difference for an early *v* a delayed alternation of CAV and etoposide-cisplatin.[15] These data plus encouraging results from Memorial Sloan-Kettering Cancer Center,[16] have convinced us that alternating CAV and etoposide-cisplatin chemotherapy is state-of-the-art drug treatment for this disease.

Another issue critical to evolving a strategy for eliminating all chemotherapy-resistant cells in limited-stage SCLC is the timing of thoracic irradiation relative to chemotherapy. Although not all randomized trials have been positive, it is

---

From the Lung Tumour Group, Cancer Control Agency of British Columbia, and the Department of Medicine, University of British Columbia, Vancouver, Canada.

Address reprint requests to Nevin Murray, MD, Cancer Control Agency of BC, 600 W 10th Ave, Vancouver, BC, V5Z 4E6, Canada.

0093-7754/86/1303-3010$05.00/0

now widely accepted that locoregional irradiation plus chemotherapy is better than chemotherapy alone for long-term survival of patients with limited-stage disease.[17–20] We hypothesize that early thoracic irradiation is better than radiotherapy administered late in the treatment program to consolidate a chemotherapy response. The event that leads to treatment failure in SCLC is a very succinct one. It occurs when the first fully chemotherapy-resistant clonigenic tumor stem cell escapes from the primary tumor and mediastinal node complex to seed the periphery. This event will have occurred in some patients prior to initiation of therapy, and they are incurable by definition, regardless of whether or what kind of regional radiotherapy is offered. For the remainder, the drug-resistant cells reside in the major repository of tumor stem cells in the regional disease. The probability of these resistant stem cells disseminating is a function of their number and time. Even though the patient will appear to be doing well clinically with chemotherapy alone, the drug-resistant cells in the regional disease will be multiplying and seeding hematogenously in a continuous fashion. We believe that the probability of destroying chemotherapy-resistant stem cells is best when thoracic irradiation is administered early, when their number is smallest and chance for spread is least.

We report here the results of a pilot study incorporating these principles in a combined modality regimen attempting to improve the results for our patients with limited-stage SCLC.

MATERIALS AND METHODS

Patient Eligibility

All patients with histologic or cytologic proof of SCLC seen at the University of British Columbia teaching hospitals by the Lung Tumour Group of the Cancer Control Agency of British Columbia (CCABC) between May 1981 and September 1983 were considered for this pilot study. Patients were eligible if they had undergone no prior treatment with chemotherapy or radiotherapy, were ambulatory, had adequate renal (creatinine <1.5 mg/100 mL), hepatic (bilirubin <2 mg/100 mL) and bone marrow function (granulocytes $>2{,}000/\mu L$ and platelet count $>150{,}000/\mu L$), and were free of congestive heart failure or recent (<3 months) myocardial infarction. Patients with prior malignancy within the previous 5 years, excepting nonmelanoma skin cancers, were excluded.

All patients had a complete history, physical examination, pathology review by CCABC reference pathologist, chest radiography, complete blood count (CBC), serum chemistries, unilateral bone marrow aspiration and biopsy, radionuclide bone scan, brain scan (radionuclide or computed tomography [CT]) and liver image (radionuclide scan, ultrasound, or CT scan). Limited-stage disease included tumor restricted to the ipsilateral lung parenchyma, mediastinum, and ipsilateral supraclavicular fossa. All other patients with clinical evidence of disease spread beyond the extent defined for limited disease or cytology-positive pleural effusions were considered to have extensive-stage disease and were excluded from the study.

Treatment

The treatment schema is illustrated in Fig 1. Cyclophosphamide (750 mg/m^2), doxorubicin (60 mg/m^2), and vincristine (2 mg) (CAV) by bolus intravenous (IV) injection were alternated with etoposide (120 mg/m^2) for three successive days and cisplatin (60 mg/m^2) on one day only. Etoposide was diluted in normal saline to a concentration of 0.4 mg/mL and infused IV over 30 minutes. Cisplatin was diluted in 1 L of normal saline and administered over a two-hour period. The interval between chemotherapy treatments was 3 weeks,

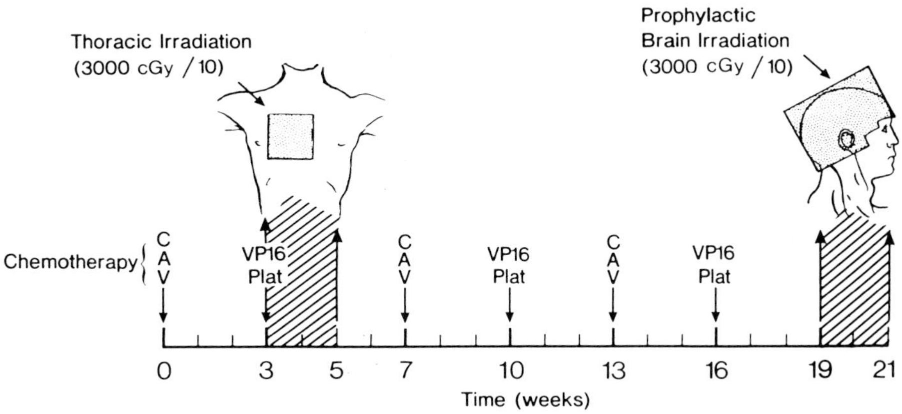

Fig 1. Treatment schema (XRT, x-ray therapy).

and three cycles of each combination were administered. The interval between the second and third chemotherapy was 4 weeks to allow for recovery from any side effects from the concurrent thoracic irradiation. Nadir blood counts were not considered for dose modifications. Drug dosage modifications were made according to treatment day counts (Table 1).

Thoracic radiotherapy consisted of 3,000 cGy in ten fractions over 2 weeks, beginning concurrently with the first cycle of etoposide-cisplatin chemotherapy. Treatment ports included the prechemotherapy intrathoracic disease and the mediastinal nodes. The supraclavicular fossae were not routinely included unless they were originally involved. Thoracic irradiation was not interrupted because of reduced blood counts unless the patient was clinically infected. Severely granulocytopenic patients ($<500/\mu L$) were given prophylactic trimethoprim-sulfamethoxazole.

Prophylactic cranial irradiation (PCI) consisted of 3,000 cGy in ten fractions over 2 weeks administered 3 weeks following the final (sixth) cycle of chemotherapy to all patients without progressive disease. A CT scan of the brain was routinely repeated before PCI. No maintenance chemotherapy was used.

Response Criteria

A complete response was defined as the disappearance of all known cancer. The assessment was based primarily on the chest radiograph, since CT scans of the chest and repeat bronchoscopies were not routinely performed. A partial response was defined as a >50% decrease of the product of the two greatest perpendicular diameters of the tumor mass lasting for the entire induction regimen with no evidence of progression at a metastatic site. Progressive disease was defined as a >25% increase in the cross-sectional area of any lesion or the occurrence of a metastatic lesion at any time before the treatment was finished (completion of PCI).

Measurements of Survival and Time to Progression

Survival was measured from the time of first therapy until death, and time to progression was measured from the beginning of therapy to the date of disease progression.

Statistical Methods

Actuarial survival curves were calculated by the Kaplan and Meier method,[21] and comparisons of survival were done with the log rank test.[22]

RESULTS

Patient Characteristics

Seventy-seven patients were registered in the study. Three of these were ineligible on pathology review because they had large-cell carcinoma (two patients) or carcinoid tumor (one patient). Four cases underwent surgery, and all evident disease was resected. The remaining 70 patients are fully evaluable. At the time of this analysis, time in the study ranged from 27 to 56 months with a median study time of 43 months.

There were 44 males and 26 females with an age range of 39 to 81 years with a median of 61 years. The Eastern Cooperative Oncology Group (ECOG) performance status was 0 in seven (10%), 1 in 40 (57%), 2 in 18 (26%), and 3 in five (7%). Forty-seven patients had oat-cell–type SCLC and 23 had intermediate-cell–type disease. Five patients (7%) had supraclavicular lymphadenopathy.

Table 1. Adjustment of Drug Dose of Cyclophosphamide, Doxorubicin, and Etoposide for Hematologic Toxicity

Granulocytes/μL	Platelets/μL	Drug Dose
>2,000	>125,000	Full
1,500–1,999	75,000–124,000	Decrease 25%
<1,500	<75,000	Delay 1 wk

Response Rates and Duration of Response

The response rates by cell type are displayed in Table 2. Overall, the complete remission rate by chest radiograph assessment was 76%. The response status according to cell type was remarkably similar. Only five patients (7%) developed progressive disease during the entire treatment regimen. Two asymptomatic patients (3%) had metastatic disease discovered on routine pre-PCI CT brain scans. Other sites of early progression included cervical nodes, lymphangitic lung disease, and carcinomatous meningitis.

The median time to progression was 60 weeks. Twenty-six percent of patients were progression free at 2 years (Fig 2).

Survival

The actuarial median survival time for all 70 patients (Fig 2) was 78 weeks. The 2-year survival rate was 32%, and currently 12 patients (17%) are alive and clinically free of SCLC. The median survival for oat-cell type was 71 weeks, and for intermediate-cell type, 88 weeks; the

Table 2. Response Rates

		Response (%)		
Cell Type	No.	CR	PR	Progression
Oat cell	47	77	15	8
Intermediate	23	74	21	5
Total	70	76	17	7

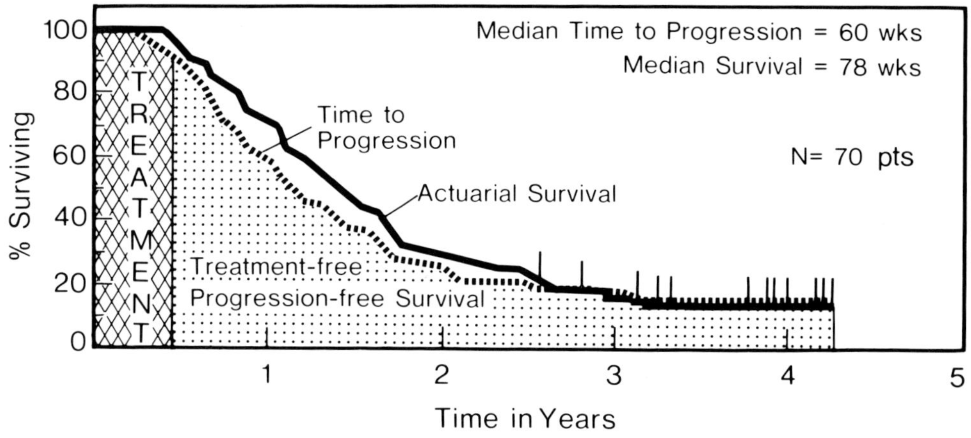

Fig 2. Actuarial survival (solid line) and progression-free survival (broken line).

respective 2-year survival rates were 24% and 40% ($P > .05$).

Toxicity

Treatment toxicity is summarized in Table 3. One patient died of interstitial pneumonitis 2 months after completing the entire regimen. Although most patients developed the expected radiation fibrosis within the treatment ports, no unusual lung toxicity was observed other than the case described earlier. Five patients had six episodes of neutropenia with fever, but no patient died of sepsis. There was no thrombocytopenic bleeding, but 22% of patients required supportive RBC transfusions. One patient has developed pancytopenia with a hypercellular bone marrow without excess blasts after 4 years of SCLC-free follow-up. There was a single case of hemorrhagic cystitis from cyclophosphamide. Although most patients developed some degree of esophagitis during the concurrent etoposide-cisplatin therapy and thoracic irradiation, only three patients (4%) required hospitalization for supportive care, and no strictures were observed. Recall radiation reactions after doxorubicin were not problematic for the skin or esophagus. Skin reactions were generally minor. No patient developed a serum creatinine above 2 mg/100 mL. None of the long-term survivors have become demented clinically, but detailed radiographic and neuropsychologic assessments are underway and will be the subject of a separate report.

Table 3. Treatment-Related Toxicity

	No. (N = 70)	Percent
Mortality	1	2
Morbidity		
Systemic infections*	5	7
Anemia†	15	22
Preleukemia	1	2
Hemorrhagic cystitis	1	2
Esophagitis‡		
Asymptomatic	11	16
Mild dysphagia/normal diet	18	26
Moderate dysphagia/soft diet	23	33
Severe dysphagia/fluids only	15	21
Hospitalized for supportive care	3	4
Strictures	0	0
Skin reactions‡		
None	35	50
Erythema	34	48
Dry desquamation	1	2

*Proved or suspected, and severe enough to require hospitalization.

†Requiring RBC transfusions.

‡Thoracic irradiation and etoposide-cisplatin.

Regimen Feasibility and Drug Delivery

For the 70 patients in the study, 420 chemotherapy courses were planned and 393 (94%) were actually administered. Ninety-six percent received four or more, and 82% had all six cycles. When chemotherapy was given, the percentages of full protocol doses actually administered were: cyclophosphamide 92%, doxorubicin 93%, vincristine 92%, etoposide 97%, and cisplatin 99%.

The treatment schema (Fig 1) calls for all six chemotherapy courses and thoracic irradiation to be administered in 16 weeks. The actual average time to chemotherapy completion for those patients receiving all six drug courses was 17.4

weeks, with 80% completing treatment at 18 weeks.

Failure Patterns and Causes of Death

Twelve of 70 patients are currently alive and free of SCCL. Four patients died of other unrelated causes (two cerebrovascular accidents and two myocardial infarctions) with no clinical evidence of SCLC. One patient died of a second primary lung cancer (squamous cell) after 3 years of SCLC remission. There was one toxic death. The remaining 52 patients are evaluable for relapse analysis, and this is summarized in Table 4. Twenty of 52 relapses occurred locally within the limited-stage definition. Sixteen were in the radiation treatment ports and four were outside (supraclavicular nodes in three and chest wall in one). Eight of 17 systemic relapses occurred beyond 18 months of follow-up. Although brain relapses occurred in 11 patients (22%), four patients did so not having received PCI (two before PCI was prescribed and two having refused PCI). Both local and systemic relapse occurred simultaneously in four cases (8%).

The average time from initiation of therapy to progression for the different sites was: local, 57 weeks; systemic, 64 weeks; brain (excluding the four cases not having PCI), 56 weeks; and local plus systemic, 68 weeks. The average time from progression to death was: local, 24 weeks; systemic, 13 weeks; brain, 13 weeks; and local plus systemic, 8 weeks.

Patients receiving the original chemotherapeutic agents at relapse did not derive any meaningful benefit (19 attempts).

DISCUSSION

Chemotherapy alone infrequently cures macroscopic quantities of SCLC. The fact that the cure rate for extensive-stage disease is only 1% and the proportion of long-term survivors for most mature studies using only chemotherapy for limited-stage disease is usually around 5% suggests that the large majority of patients with this cancer have drug-resistant tumor stem cells at diagnosis. For limited-stage cases in which macroscopic disease can be treated with potentially non-cross-resistant radiation therapy, the chance for extermination of the drug-resistant clonogenic cells persists as long as these cells remain within the radiotherapy field. A large Canadian multicenter trial for limited-stage disease using CAV and etoposide-cisplatin chemotherapy and consolidative chest irradiation resulted in a median survival of 60 weeks and a 2-year survival rate of 19%.[15] In our introductory remarks, we explained why early chest irradiation should be superior to late or consolidative irradiation. The encouraging 78-week median survival and 32% 2-year survival observed in this present study support this hypothesis. The concept is additionally supported by mathematical modeling[23] and the favorable results of other "front-end loaded" regimens.[24,27]

Our regimen includes the delivery of thoracic irradiation concurrently with etoposide-cisplatin chemotherapy after one cycle of CAV. The potential advantages of this plan include (1) thoracic radiation is given early; (2) the initial cycle of CAV usually markedly reduces the tumor size, improving the patient's general condition for the vigorous combined therapy; (3) the reoxygenation of the tumor by a chemotherapy response may make it more vulnerable to radiation[25]; (4) cisplatin administered concurrently with radiation may have radiosensitizing properties[26]; (5) the early delivery of radiation promptly opens obstructed bronchi, decreasing the probability of infection, particularly during later granulocyte nadirs caused by chemotherapy; and (6) the concurrent use of chemotherapy and irradiation allows the cadence of chemotherapy to continue without an interruption that allows tumor cells to regrow in unirradiated sites, as is unavoidable when the "sandwich" technique is used.

An analysis of treatment factors contributing to long-term survival in SCLC[27] concluded that both early and concurrent thoracic irradiation are advantageous. Toxicity, particularly to lung,

Table 4. Relapse Sites *v* Time (mo)

	Number (%)				
Relapse Site	0–6	6–12	12–18	18+	Total
Local	1 (2)	4 (8)	11 (22)	4 (8)	20 (38)
Systemic	2 (4)	6 (11)	1 (2)	8 (15)	17 (32)
Brain	2 (4)	5 (10)	2 (4)	2 (4)	11 (22)
Local and systemic	2 (4)	0 (0)	2 (4)	0 (0)	4 (8)
Total	7 (14)	15 (29)	16 (32)	14 (27)	52 (100)

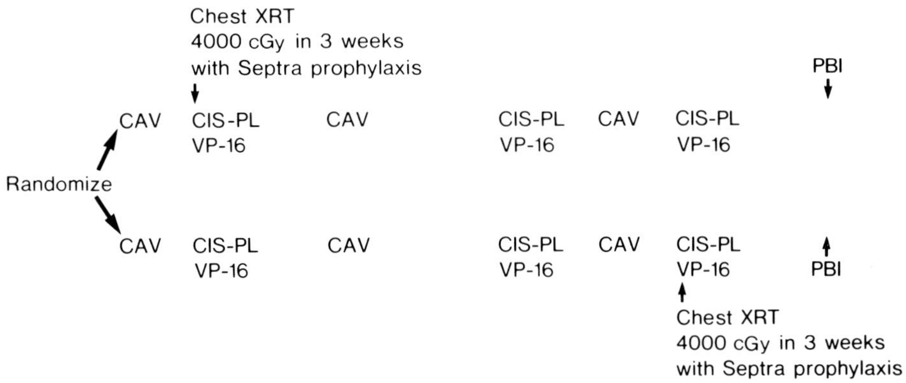

Fig 3. Schema for the National Cancer Institute of Canada trial of early *v* late thoracic irradiation for limited-stage SCLC (BR 6).

heart, esophagus, and skin from doxorubicin[27–29] and nitrosourea-radiation interactions[30] can be daunting. Data from the present study show that etoposide-cisplatin chemotherapy can be administered concurrently with radiation with acceptable toxicity. The good compliance and dose delivery data for this regimen verify its feasibility.

The timing of thoracic radiotherapy is a critical issue that is amenable to clinical trial analysis. The schema of the most recent protocol for limited-stage SCLC being conducted under the auspices of the National Cancer Institute of Canada Clinical Trials Group (Kingston, Ontario) is outlined in Fig 3. The trial builds on the results of previous SCLC studies by this group,[14, 15] and additionally tests the hypothesis suggested by the present study. Only one question is asked in the randomized trial: Is there a difference in outcome for patients treated with early *v* late thoracic irradiation administered concurrently with etoposide-cisplatin chemotherapy? This question of timing must be answered before other important issues (treatment volumes, optimal dose fractionations, radiosensitizers, and surgical options) can be addressed. We hypothesize that although consolidative radiotherapy may have some intuitive and practical appeal, it is a fundamentally flawed concept, and early thoracic irradiation will be proved a superior approach.

A summary of the second workshop on SCLC has indicated that "there is a tendency to shorten the duration of treatment and limit it to a period of 6 to 12 months."[1] Since limited-stage median survival times commonly range from 13 to 15 months and only 10% to 15% of patients are cured, it follows that the majority of patients are either on treatment or suffering from recurrent disease most of the time.[1] Our study demonstrates that a short treatment program lasting only 21 weeks can generate good results with a 19.5-month median survival and a long-term survival rate in the 15% to 20% range. Moreover, our short regimen decreases morbidity and results in longer good-quality survival, during which patient is free of acute treatment side effects and progressive cancer (average, 10 months; Fig 2). We are optimistic that similar results will be generated in the ongoing multicenter Canadian trial (Fig 3).

ACKNOWLEDGMENT

We thank Dr Chris Coppin and Dr Joe Connors for reviewing the manuscript, Dr Gedy Gedauskas and Ruth Page for their data contributions, and Lorraine Cho for typing the manuscript.

REFERENCES

1. Hansen HH, Smyth JF: The second workshop on small cell carcinoma of the lung, Gleneagles, Scotland. September 1984. Lung Cancer 1:9–13, 1985

2 Goldie JH, Coldman AJ: Genetic origin of drug resistance in neoplasms. Cancer Res 44:3643–3653, 1984

3. De Vita VT Jr: The relationship between tumour mass and resistance to chemotherapy. Cancer 51:1209–1220, 1983

4. Ling V: Genetic basis of drug resistance in mammalian cells, in Bruchovsky N, Goldie JH (eds): Drug and Hormone

Resistance in Neoplasia, vol 1. Boca Raton, Fla CRC, 1982, pp 1–19

5. Santoro A, Bonadonna G, Bonfant V, et al: Alternating drug combinations in the treatment of advanced Hodgkin's disease. N Engl J Med 306:770–775, 1982

6. Klimo P, Connors JM: MOPP/ABV hybrid program: Combination chemotherapy based on early introduction of seven effective drugs for advanced Hodgkin's disease. J Clin Oncol 3:1174–1182, 1985

7. Elliott JA, Osterlind K, Hansen HH: Cyclic alternating noncross-resistant chemotherapy of small cell anaplastic carcinoma of the lung. Cancer Treat Rev 103–113, 1984

8. Murray N, Shah A, Wilson K, et al: Cyclic alternating chemotherapy for small cell carcinoma of the lung. Cancer Treat Rep 69:1241–1242, 1985

9. Goldie JH, Coldman AJ, Gudauskas G: Rationale for the use of alternating noncross-resistant chemotherapy. Cancer Treat Rep 66:439–449, 1982

10. Sierocki JS, Hilaris BS, Hopfan S, et al: Cisdiamminedichloroplatinum and VP-16-315: An active induction regimen for small cell carcinoma of the lung. Cancer Treat Rep 63:1593–1597, 1979

11. Evans WK, Shepherd FA, Feld R, et al: VP-16 and cisplatin as first-line therapy for small cell lung cancer. J Clin Oncol 3:1471–1477, 1985

12. Evans WK, Osoba D, Feld R, et al: VP-16 and cisplatin: An effective treatment for relapse in small cell cancer. J Clin Oncol 3:65–71, 1985

13. Porter LL, Johnson DH, Hainsworth JD, et al: Cisplatin and etoposide combination chemotherapy for refractory small cell carcinoma of the lung. Cancer Treat Rep 69:479–481, 1985

14. Evans WK, Murray N, Feld R, et al: Canadian multicentre randomized trial comparing standard and alternating chemotherapy in extensive stage small cell lung cancer. Proc IV World Conference on Lung Cancer, Toronto, August 1985, p 77 (abstr 560)

15. Feld R, Evans WK, Coy P, et al: Canadian multicentre trial comparing sequential and alternating noncross-resistant chemotherapy in patients with limited small cell lung cancer. Proc IV World Conference on Lung Cancer, Toronto, Ontario, August 1985, p 77 (abstr 542)

16. Natale RB, Shank B, Hilaris BS, et al: Combination cyclophosphamide, Adriamycin and vincristine rapidly alternating with combination cisplatin and VP-16 in treatment of small cell lung cancer. Am J Med 79:303–308, 1985

17. Bleehen NM, Cox JD: Radiotherapy for lung cancer. Int J Rad Oncol Biol Phys 11:1001–1007, 1985

18. Lichter AS, Bunn PA, Ihde DC, et al: The role of radiation therapy in the treatment of small cell lung cancer. Cancer 55:2163–2175, 1985

19. Perez CA, Einhorn L, Oldham RK, et al: Randomized trial of radiotherapy to the thorax in limited small cell carcinoma of the lung treated with multiagent chemotherapy and elective brain irradiation: A preliminary report. J Clin Oncol 2:1200–1208, 1984

20. Bunn P, Ihde D, Lichter A, et al: Randomized trial of combination chemotherapy with or without chest radiotherapy in limited stage small cell lung cancer. Proc IV World Conference on Lung Cancer, Toronto, August 1985, p 87 (abstr 365)

21. Kaplan EL, Meier P: Non-parametric estimation from incomplete observations. J Am Stat Assoc 457–481, 1958

22. Peto R, Pike MC, Armitage P, et al: Design and analysis of randomized clinical trials requiring prolonged observation of each patient: II analysis and examples. Br J Cancer 35:11–39, 1977

23. Goldie JH, Coldman AJ: Clinical implications of the phenomenon of drug resistance, in Bruchovsky N, Goldie JH (eds): Drug and Hormone Resistance in Neoplasia, vol 2. Boca Raton, Fl, CRC, 1983, pp 111–127

24. Arriagada R, LeChevalier T, Tubiana M, et al: Alternating radiotherapy and chemotherapy schedules in small cell lung cancer, limited disease. Int J Radiat Oncol Biol Phys 11:1461–1467, 1985

25. Tomlinson RH, Gray LH: The histological structure of some human lung cancers and the possible implications for radiotherapy. Br J Cancer 9:539–549, 1955

26. Douple FB, Richmond RC: A review of platinum complex biochemistry suggests a rationale for combined platinum-radiotherapy. Int J Radiat Oncol Biol Phys 5:1335–1339, 1979

27. Catane R, Lichter A, Lee YT, et al: Small cell lung cancer: Analysis of treatment factors contributing to prolonged survival. Cancer 48:1936–1943, 1981

28. Greco FA, Brereton HD, Kent H, et al: Adriamycin and enhanced radiation reaction in normal esophagus and skin. Ann Intern Med 85:294–298, 1976

29. Merrill J, Greco FA, Zimbler H: Adriamycin and radiation synergistic cardiotoxicity. Ann Int Med 82:122–123, 1975

30. Ihde D, Brooks B, Sieffer, et al: Pulmonary toxicity with combined modality therapy for limited stage small cell lung cancer. Proc IV World Conference on Lung Cancer. Toronto, Ontario, 1985, p 142 (abstr 112)

Concurrent Chemotherapy and Radiotherapy for Limited Small-Cell Carcinoma of the Lung: A Southwest Oncology Group Study

By Joseph D. McCracken, Lalitha M. Janaki, Sarah B. Taylor, P.G. Shankar Giri, Gary B. Weiss, William Gordon, Jr, Ralph B. Vance, and John Crowley

This pilot study in limited-stage small-cell carcinoma of the lung using concurrent cisplatin (Platinol) and etoposide (VePesid) chemotherapy with radiotherapy has yielded a high complete response rate in 23 of 40 patients evaluable for response. Five of these responders have survived greater than 2 years off all therapy with a stable, high performance status. Median survival of all patients is 18 months. Toxicity has been acceptable, the most common being neutropenia. Radiation toxicities include 17 of 40 patients experiencing mild to moderate esophagitis, with one severe toxicity; and three of 40 patients developing mild to moderate radiation pneumonitis. The high complete remission observed with this program and the long tumor-free interval seen off maintenance therapy deserve further exploration. Toxicities appear only moderately greater than with other programs currently utilized.

ETOPOSIDE (VePesid, Bristol-Myers Oncology Division, Evansville, Ind) and cisplatin (Platinol, Bristol-Myers Oncology Division, Evansville, Ind) have shown considerable activity as "salvage drugs"[1] and now are being explored up front as initial therapy in small-cell lung carcinoma (SCLC).[2] Preclinical studies in laboratory animals suggested a synergism between etoposide and cisplatin. Schabel[3] and associates reported marked synergism for the combination in mice bearing P388 murine leukemia. Similarly, Burchenal et al[4] reported that etoposide and a platinum analog were synergistic in curing L1210 leukemia in mice.

The use of these drugs in combination has not been associated with serious myelosuppression as a side effect.[5–10] In addition, cisplatin has radiosensitizing properties[11–15] and is attractive for use as a combined modality agent with radiation therapy.

This Southwest Oncology Group (SWOG) pilot study has demonstrated that these two agents can be successfully given with simultaneous radiotherapy with a complete response rate of 57%. Toxicities have been acceptable and responders have associated long-term high performance status survival. An additional study in progress at the National Cancer Institute (NCI)[16] suggests an advantage for simultaneous cyclophosphamide, methotrexate, and CCNU (lomustine) (CMC) plus chest radiation over CMC alone.

The concept of administering simultaneous radiotherapy with chemotherapy allows for shorter overall treatment time and less long-term patient morbidity. With new techniques in consolidation therapies, a potential advance in the long-term survival of limited-disease patients appears possible.

PLATEAU OF SURVIVAL WITH "TRADITIONAL" THERAPIES

SWOG has conducted three studies in limited SCLC. In the first two studies, SWOG 7115[17] and SWOG 7628,[18] induction chemotherapy was administered for 6 weeks, followed by radiation therapy to the primary disease in the chest. Prophylactic radiation therapy was also given to the whole brain. Median survival in these two studies was 48 and 46 weeks, respectively. The recently completed study, SWOG 7924,[19] randomized complete responders (CRs) with chemotherapy to receive either radiation therapy to the chest primary or no radiation therapy with "consolidation chemotherapy." Although the data are immature at present, it appears that patients receiving radiation therapy have improved survival over those patients receiving no radiation therapy. Survival is superior in patients achieving CR in this study over those

From the Brooke Army Medical Center, San Antonio; the University of Texas, Galveston; the University of Kansas Medical Center, Kansas City; the University of Mississippi Medical Center, Jackson; and the Southwest Oncology Group Statistical Center, Seattle.

Supported in part by the following PHS Cooperative Agrement grant numbers awarded by the National Cancer Institute, DHHS: CA-22411, CA-03096, CA-12644, CA-22433, CA-16385, CA-37429 and CA-32102.

Address reprint requests to Southwest Oncology Group(SWOG-8269), Operations Office, 5430 Fredericksburg Rd, Suite 618 San Antonio, TX 78229.

0093–7754/86/1303–3009$05.00/0

patients not achieving CR: 74 weeks for responders; 53 weeks for partial responders (PRs); 23 weeks for nonresponders. Overall, there is no significant improvement in the median survival of these three successive studies.

Attempts at improving survival with cyclic and non–cross-resistant combinations using the Goldie-Coldman hypothesis have also been disappointing in producing improved survivals.[20–24] It would thus appear evident that no major breakthroughs appear imminent in the common technique of using chemotherapy followed by radiotherapy to the chest primary.

RATIONALE FOR THE USE OF RADIATION THERAPY IN LIMITED SMALL-CELL CARCINOMA

Relapse at the primary site has been a problem with patients receiving <4,500 rad of radiotherapy. In SWOG 7628, a preamendment version of the protocol used 3,000 rad to the chest primary.[25] An increased number of local failures in the chest were noted in this regimen compared with those in postamendment patients who received 4,500 rad. In SWOG 7828, a program using combination chemotherapy alone in extensive small-cell carcinoma without radiotherapy to the chest, 67% of the patients who experienced CR relapsed in the chest only, without evidence of distant metastases.[26] This represented a dramatic change from the SWOG 7415 study in which only seven of 27 CRs with extensive disease had failure in the chest (19%). On SWOG 7415,[17] patients received 4,500 rad of radiotherapy to the chest. A recent review[27] of patients who survived 2 years or more with SCLC revealed that: (1) local therapy (either surgery or radiation therapy) was an important part of therapy for long-term survival; (2) local tumor control of the lung was superior in the patients treated with surgery or high-dose irradiation (>4,800 rad) compared with patients treated with low-dose irradiation (<3,500 rad); and (3) 33% of patients who were without evident disease at 2 years eventually relapsed, implying that even 2-year follow-up is inadequate to fully assess treatment efficacy. From these data, it is clear that local control remains a major problem with programs using combination chemotherapy only, with or without sequential radiation therapy.

CLINICAL EFFECTIVENESS OF RADIATION THERAPY WITH SIMULTANEOUS CHEMOTHERAPY

Cisplatin in combination with fluorouracil has demonstrated significant synergy with radiation therapy administerd simultaneously in head and neck[28–33] and esophageal cancers.[34] Cisplatin has attractiveness as an agent to use with radiation as it appears to have only weak radiosensitizing properties,[11–15] rather than the strong radiosensitizing properties of doxorubicin (Adriamycin [Adria Laboratories, Columbus, OH]).

Catene[35] reported on seven regimens used at the NCI, three of which used concurrent chemotherapy and radiation therapy (Table 1). The chemotherapy agents used were doxorubicin, cyclophosphamide, and vincristine (CAV). One program used 4,500 rad with small daily fractions administered over 62 days, with 9 weeks of concurrent chemotherapy-radiotherapy. A 71% CR rate was achieved with only one relapse within the field of radiation. However, seven of 14 patients (50%) experienced death from toxic-

Table 1. NCI Experience With Concurrent Radiation Therapy and Chemotherapy in Limited SCLC

Chemotherapy for All Studies	No. of Patients	Radiation Therapy Total Dose (Rad)	Radiation Therapy Period (Days)	No. of Weeks of Concurrent Radiation Therapy and Chemotherapy	No. of CR (%)	No. of Deaths From Toxicity (%)	No. of CR Who Relapsed Within Field of RT	2-Year Survival (%)
CAV								
Cyclo 1,500 mg/m² IV day 1	10	3,000	20	3	8 (80)	1 (10)	2	5 (50)
Dox 40 mg/m² IV day 1	12	3,000	42	6	8 (67)	3 (25)	3	4 (33)
VCR 2 mg IV day 1								
Plus thoracic RT	14	4,500	62	9	10 (71)	7 (50)	1	4 (29)
Repeat CAV every 3 weeks								
Repeat RT as indicated in protocol*								

*Refer to column entitled "No. of Weeks of Concurrent Radiation Therapy and Chemotherapy" for additional information.

Abbreviations: Cyclo, Cytoxan (cyclophosphamide); Dox, doxorubicin; VCR, vincristine; RT, radiation therapy.

ity of the treatment. In their programs using 3,000 rad of radiotherapy, although deaths from toxicity were fewer, local failures were no better than other studies using sequential chemotherapy plus radiotherapy. The radiation toxicity was probably greatly enhanced by the use of doxorubicin therapy, which is a potent radiation sensitizer.

The substitution of cisplatin for doxorubicin and the addition of doxorubicin to cisplatin appeared quite attractive to use in the combined modality setting with simultaneous use of radiation therapy for the treatment of SCLC.

For these reasons, a pilot study was performed by SWOG to explore the response rate with concurrent use of radiation therapy plus chemotherapy using cisplatin, etoposide, and vincristine in limited SCLC and to observe the toxicities of this combined modality program.

MATERIALS AND METHODS

The treatment program/schema (Table 2) used cisplatin (50 mg/m^2, IV) days 1, 8, 29, 36, 57, and 64; VP-16 (50 mg/m^2, IV), days 1 through 5, 29 through 33, and 57 through 61; vincristine (1.4 mg/m^2, IV), days 15, 22, 43, and 50 (maximum dose, 2 mg). Treatment was given if on the day of therapy, WBC was >3,000 μL and platelet count >100,000 μL. Concurrent radiation therapy to the primary tumor was given at 180 rad per day for 25 treatments to a total dose of 4,500 rad beginning day 1 of the study. Therapy to the whole lung was limited to a maximum dose of 2,000 rad. Three thousand rad of prophylactic brain radiotherapy were administered to all patients. On day 85 of the study, consolidation chemotherapy was begun, consisting of vincristine (1 mg, IV), days 1, 8, 15, 22, 29, and 35; methotrexate (60 mg/m^2, IV), days 1 and 43; VP-16 (50 mg/m^2, IV), days 1 through 5 and 43 through 47; doxorubicin (60 mg/m^2, IV), days 22 and 64, cyclophosphamide (1,000 mg/m^2, IV), days 22 and 64. After 12 weeks of consolidation chemotherapy, patients with a CR had all therapy discontinued and were observed.

Table 3. Response

	No.	%
CR	23	57
PR	10	25
Mixed response	0	0
Stable/no response	1	2
Increasing disease	1	2
Early death	2	5
No evaluation, assumed no response	3	7
Total	40	100

RESULTS

Forty-one patients have been registered at four different SWOG institutions. Forty patients were judged evaluable, with one patient ineligible for study. Responses (Table 3) include 23 CRs, ten PRs, and two progressive disease.

Five CRs are >2 years from treatment start and off all therapy with a stable good-performance status. Median survival of all patients is 18 months (Fig 1). Seventeen patients have expired. Ten patients have died from relapse or progressive disease. Seven patients died of non-neoplastic causes (Table 4); two from myocardial infarction after completion of therapy (both in remission), one from organic mental syndrome in PR off therapy, one from pulmonary edema in CR off therapy, one from pneumonia in CR off therapy, and one from myocardial infarction during therapy. Six of the patients died of non-neoplastic disease while in remission.

Only two patients have relapsed just in the

Table 2. Concurrent Chemotherapy With Cisplatin, Etoposide, and Vincristine and Radiation Therapy for SCLC: Treatment Regimen

Regimen	Days of Administration
Chemotherapy	
Cisplatin* 50 mg/m^2 IV	1, 8, 29, 36, 57, 64, 71
Etoposide† 50 mg/m^2 IV	1–5, 29–33, 57–61
Vincristine 1.4 mg/m^2 IV (maximum dose, 2 mg)	15, 22, 43, 50
RT: (thoracic) 180 rad/d × 25; (whole brain) 3,000 rad over 2 wk, 5 treatments/wk	1–25 (thoracic RT), 57–71 (whole brain RT)
Consolidation chemotherapy (cycle begins day 85)	
Vincristine 1 mg IV	1, 8, 15, 22, 29, 36
Methotrexate 60 mg/m^2 IV	1, 43
Etoposide 50 mg/m^2 IV	1–5, 43–47
Doxorubicin 60 mg/m^2 IV	22, 64
Cyclophosphamide 1,000 mg/m^2 IV	22, 64

*Cisplatin for injection.

†Etoposide injection.

Abbreviation: RT, radiation therapy.

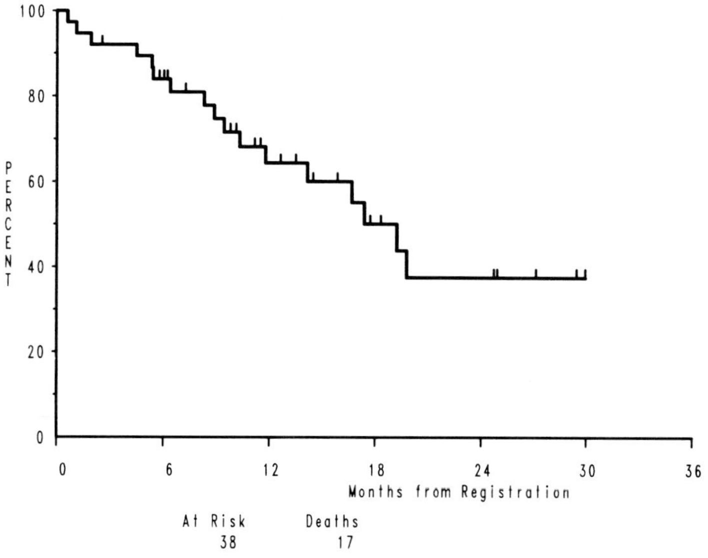

Fig 1. Concurrent chemotherapy for limited small-cell carcinoma of the lung (a Southwest Oncology Group Study: SWOG pilot protocol 8269 survival distribution; all eligible patients with follow-up).

primary tumor site in the field of radiotherapy. Two other patients had relapse in radiotherapy port: one with the onset of bone metastases, the other with adrenal metastases. One patient relapsed in the CNS. One patient relapsed during induction therapy outside the port of primary treatment in the chest, and one patient relapsed with spinal cord metastases. All other relapses have been at multiple organ sites, with bone being the most common.

Toxicity (Table 5) has been acceptable, with the most common being neutropenia with 14 severe and five life-threatening toxicities observed in 32 of the 40 evaluable patients. Radiation toxicities have been acceptable. One patient developed severe radiation-induced esophagitis, eight developed moderate symptoms, and nine developed mild symptoms. Three patients developed mild to moderate radiation pneumonitis that resolved with standard treatment. Two patients in remission are reported as having a grade 3 performance status because of chronic obstructive pulmonary disease, one on biopsy felt to be chronic radiation pneumonitis. Six patients required a significant radiation therapy delay of >1 week because of toxicities. Ten patients did not complete the entire treatment program and refused further therapy. Complete summary of the toxicities is outlined in Table 5.

Table 4. Deaths

No.	Cause
10	Progressive disease
2	Myocardial infarction after completion of therapy, both in remission
1	Organic mental syndrome in PR; off therapy
1	Pulmonary edema in CR; off therapy
1	Pneumonia in CR; off therapy
1	Myocardial infarction during therapy
1	Generalized debilitation, no tumor at autopsy

Abbreviation: CR, complete response.

SUMMARY

The high CR rate observed with combined cisplatin and etoposide and simultaneous chest irradiation, improved median survival over prior SWOG studies,[17–19] and the long tumor-free intervals seen off maintenance therapy deserve further exploration. Toxicities appear only moderately greater than other programs currently used. Seventy-five percent of patients treated

Table 5. Toxicity

	0	1	2	3	4	5
Anemia	17	7	8	0	0	0
Diarrhea	30	0	1	0	1	0
Leukopenia	0	2	11	14	5	0
Mucositis/ulcers/stomatitis	31	0	1	0	0	0
Nausea/vomiting/anorexia	10	9	6	7	0	0
Peripheral neuropathy	20	4	8	0	0	0
Renal—other (specify)	29	2	1	0	0	0
Thrombocytopenia	21	6	3	2	0	0
XRT esophagitis	14	9	8	1	0	0
XRT pneumonitis	29	2	1	0	0	0
Maximum degree any toxicity						
Number	0	1	9	17	5	0

Abbreviation: XRT, x-ray therapy.

0, none; 1, mild; 2, moderate; 3, severe; 4, life-threatening; 5, fatal.

completed the entire program, and five patients are >2 years from treatment start with a good-performance–status quality survival. The short overall duration of the treatment program (24 weeks) eliminates the long-term debilitation commonly seen in survivors of standard treatment programs.[36,37]

The short duration of the initial combined chemotherapy/radiotherapy program allows for new experimentation with techniques of consolidation/intensification that have appeared to have major impact on long-range survival and cure in leukemia and lymphomas. The minimal cumulative myelosuppressive effects of this initial program would allow for experimentation of such aggressive consolidation techniques as high-dose conventional chemotherapy, hemibody irradiation, or autologous bone marrow transplantation with high-dose chemotherapy.

There is also reemergence of the role of surgery in limited SCLC. A recent analysis[38] of long-term survivors in SWOG 7628 indicated those patients who underwent surgical removal of their tumor had improved survival over patients of similar stage who had not undergone surgical removal. As local relapse has occurred in 10% of patients to date on this treatment program, there remain several pertinent questions to be answered in future years as to the role of additional surgical excision of the primary tumor area after such induction therapy. An alternate approach would be to remove the primary tumor and follow this with involved field radiotherapy plus cisplatin and etoposide.

Difficulties in administering cisplatin are its problems with nausea, vomiting, and renal toxicities, which may continue, despite antiemetic coverage and IV hydration. These toxicities were the major cause of patients refusing further therapy. The newer platinum analogs may very well negate this problem and create better patient acceptance of such a treatment program. Unfortunately, the toxicities of the newer analogs appear to be bone marrow suppression,[39] and careful phase I-II type studies will need to be performed to explore their potential as agents in this disease.

This pilot study has now been activated as a group-wide study in SWOG to confirm these data as a base for future studies using concurrent chemotherapy and radiotherapy in limited SCLC.

REFERENCES

1. Evans WK, Osoba D, Feld R, et al: Etoposide (VP-16) and cisplatin: An effective treatment for relapse in small cell lung cancer. J Clin Oncol 3:65–71, 1985

2. Sierocki JS, Hilaris BS, Hopfan S, et al: Cisdichlorodiammine-platinum-II and VP-16-213: An active induction regimen for small cell carcinoma of the lung. Cancer Treat Rep 63:5093–5097, 1979

3. Schabel FM Jr, Trader MW, Laster WR Jr, et al: Cis-dichlorodiammineplatinum (II): Combination chemotherapy and cross-resistance studies with tumors of mice. Cancer Treat Rep 63:1459–1473, 1979

4. Burchenal JH, Lokys L, Turkevich J, et al: Rationale of combination chemotherapy, in Prestayko AW, Crooke ST, Carter SK (eds): Cisplatin: Current Status and New Developments. Orlando, Fla, Academic, 1980, pp 113–123

5. Lopez JA, Mann J, Grapski RT, et al: Etoposide and cisplatin salvage chemotherapy for small cell lung cancer. Cancer Treat Rep 69:369–371, 1985

6. Evans WK, Osoba D, Feld R, et al: Etoposide (VP-16) and cisplatin: An effective treatment for relapse in small cell lung cancer. J Clin Oncol 3:65–71, 1985

7. Figoli F, Crivellari D, Gagligioni E, et al: Cis-platinum and etoposide (D-V) as second line chemotherapy in patients (pts) with extended small cell lung cancer (SCLC). Cancer Chemother Pharmacol 14:25, 1985 (suppl)

8. Porter L, Johnson D, Hainsworth J, et al: Cisplatin and etoposide combination chemotherapy for refractory small cell carcinoma of the lung. Cancer Treat Rep 69:479–481, 1985

9. Einhorn LH, Williams SD, Loehrer PJ: Platinum (P) + VP-16 chemotherapy for refractory small cell lung cancer (RSCLC). Proc Am Assoc Cancer Res 25:174, 1984

10. Batist G, Ihde DC, Cowan K, et al: Phase II trial of cisplatin and VP-16 in previously treated small cell lung cancer (SCLC). Proc Am Assoc Cancer Res 25:175, 1984

11. Schaake-Koning C, Bartelink H, Hora Adema B, et al: Radiotherapy enhanced by cis-diamminedichloro-platinum (II) (C-DDP), in Inoperable Non-Small Cell Lung Cancer (NSCLC): A Dose Finding Study. Presented at the Third Annual Meeting of the European Society for Therapeutic Radiology and Oncology, September 9–15, Jerusalem, Israel, 1984, p 60

12. Sand J, Rosenthal CJ, Rotman M, et al: Lack of toxicity of cis platin administered as radiosensitizer by long term continuous infusion. Pro Am Soc Clin Oncol 3:44, 1984 (abstr C-172)

13. Leipzig B: Cisplatin sensitization to radiotherapy of squamous cell carcinomas of the head and neck. Am J Surg 146:462–465, 1983

14. Pinedo HM, Karim ABMF, Van Vliet WH, et al: Daily cis-dichlorodiammineplatinum (II) as a radio-enhancer: A preliminary toxicity report. J Cancer Res Clin Oncol 105:79–82, 1983

15. Leipzig B, Wetmore SJ, Putzeys R, et al: Cisplatin potentiation of radiotherapy: Long term follow-up. Arch Otolaryngol 111:114–118, 1985

16. Bunn P, Cohen M, Lichter A, et al: A randomized trial

of chemotherapy vs chemotherapy plus radiotherapy in limited small cell lung cancer. Proc Am Soc Clin Oncol 2:200, 1983 (abstr)

17. Livingston RB, Moore TN, Heilbrun L, et al: Small cell carcinoma of the lung: Combined chemotherapy and radiation. Ann Intern Med 88:194–199, 1978

18. McCracken JD, Chen T, White J, et al: Combination chemotherapy, radiotherapy and BCG immunotherapy in limited small cell carcinoma of the lung. Cancer 49:2252–2258, 1982

19. Mira JG, Keys MS, Chen T: Influence of chest radiotherapy and response remission duration and survival in chemotherapy responders on localized small cell lung carcinoma: The Southwest Oncology Group Study. Proc Am Soc Clin Oncol 3:212, 1984 (abstr)

20. Timothy AR, Calman FMB, Bateman NT, et al: Single-dose etoposide in combination with vincristine and doxorubicin in the treatment of small cell lung cancer (SCLC). Semin Oncol 12:45–47, 1985 (suppl 2)

21. Reddy SK, Takita H, Lane WW, et al: Cyclic alternating chemotherapy for small cell lung cancer. Cancer Chemother Pharmacol 12:190–193, 1984

22. Rudolph A, Einhorn L, Wampler G, et al: The substitution of etoposide for vincristine in established therapy for small cell carcinoma of the lung. Proceedings of the 13th International Congress of Chemotherapy, Vienna, 1983

23. Issell B, Rudolph A, Lawson R, et al: The substitution of etoposide for doxorubicin in small cell lung cancer combination chemotherapy. Proceedings of the 13th International Congress of Chemotherapy, Vienna, 1983

24. Feld R, Evans WK, Coy P, et al: Canadian multicenter randomized trial comparing sequential alternating administration of two noncrossresistant chemotherapy combinations in patients with limited small cell carcinoma of the lung. Proc Am Soc Clin Oncol 4:177, 1985 (abstr)

25. White JD, McCracken JD, Chen T: Radiation therapy limited oat cell carcinoma of the lung. Proc Am Soc Clin Oncol: 339, 1980 (abstr C-80)

26. Mira JG, Livingston RB, Moore TN, et al: Influence of chest radiotherapy in frequency and patterns of chest relapse in disseminated small cell lung carcinoma. Cancer 15:1226–1272, 1982

27. Peschel RE, Capp DS, Carter D, et al: Long term survivor with small cell carcinoma of the lung. Int J Radiat Oncol Biol Phys 7:1545–1548, 1981

28. Adelstein DJ, Sharan VM, Earle AS, et al: Combined modality therapy (CMT) with simultaneous 5-fluorouracil (5FU), cis-platinum (DDP) and radiation therapy (RT) in the treatment of squamous cell cancer of the head and neck. Proc Am Soc Clin Oncol 4:131, 1985 (abstr)

29. Al-Sarraf M, Kinzie J, Marcial V, et al: Combination of cis-platinum and radiotherapy in patients with advanced head and neck cancer: Radiation Therapy Oncology Group Progress Report. Proc Am Soc Clin Oncol 3:180, 1984 (abstr)

30. Coughlin CT, Richmond RC: Platinum based combined modality approach for locally advanced head and neck carcinoma. Int J Radiat Oncol Biol Phys 11:915–191, 1985

31. Creagan ET, Fountain KS, Frytak S, et al: Concomitant radiation therapy and cis-diamminedichloroplatinum (II) in patients with advanced head and neck cancer. Med Pediatr Oncol 9:119–120, 1981

32. Green MD, Cooper JS, Cohen N, et al: A pilot study of the concomitant use of cis-platinum chemotherapy and radiation therapy in patients with advanced head and neck cancer. Dev Oncol 17:348, 1984 (abstr)

33. Haselow RE, Adams GS, Oken MM, et al: Cisplatinum (DDP) with radiation therapy (RT) for locally advanced unresectable head and neck cancer. Proc Am Soc Clin Oncol 2:160, 1983 (abstr)

34. Leichman L, Seydel HG, Steiger Z: Preoperative adjuvant therapy for squamous cell cancer of the esophagus: SWOG and RTOG clinical trials. Proc Am Soc Clin Oncol 3:147, 1984 (abstr)

35. Catane R, Lichter A, Lee Y, et al: Small cell lung cancer analysis of treatment factors contributing to prolonged survival. Cancer 48:1936–1943, 1981

36. Volk SA, Mansour RP, Gandara DR, et al: Morbidity and long term survivors of small cell carcinoma of the lung. Proc Am Soc Clin Oncol 2:185, 1983 (abstr)

37. Johnson BE, Ihde DC, Lichter AS, et al: Five to ten year follow-up of small cell lung cancer patients disease free at thirty months: Chronic toxicities and late relapses. Proc Am Soc Clin Oncol 3:218, 1984 (abstr)

38. Friess G, McCracken JD, Troxell L, et al: Effect of initial resection of small cell carcinoma of the lung: A review of Southwest Oncology Group Study 7628. J Clin Oncol 3:964, 1985

39. Creekmore SP, Micetich KC, Vogelzang N, et al: Low toxicity in significant tumor responses in phase II trials of carboplatin (CVDCA) in head & neck, nonsmall cell lung, urothelial and ovarian cancers. Proc Am Soc Clin Oncol 4:144, 1985 (abstr)

High-Dose Pilot Studies in Extensive-Stage Small-Cell Lung Cancer

By David H. Johnson, Kenneth R. Hande, Lester L. Porter, John D. Hainsworth, Steven N. Wolff, and F. Anthony Greco

Small-cell lung cancer is rarely cured with standard chemotherapy, despite initial good responses. The concept of high-dose induction therapy for extensive-stage patients has been explained in a series of pilot studies. The rationale of this approach and the most recent preliminary results will be presented.

FOR THE PAST FEW YEARS, we have been interested in the concept of high-dose induction therapy for patients with extensive-stage small-cell lung cancer (SCLC). We have now completed a series of three pilot studies using a similar design. The first study explored the use of high-dose etoposide as a single agent. The second study used the same dose of etoposide and added high-dose cyclophosphamide. The third study retained the first two agents and added relatively high-dose cisplatin.

The rationale for embarking on these high-dose induction therapy studies came in part from a recognition of the shortcomings of standard chemotherapy for patients with SCLC. Although the overall response is excellent to standard chemotherapy, resistant tumor becomes a problem for the large majority of patients. We decided to address the problem of drug resistance with high-dose chemotherapy. There are certainly several examples in clinical oncology where dose is an important feature of successful therapy and in many animal tumor models dose and dose rate are critical to tumor cell kill. Many chemoresponsive neoplasms, including SCLC, demonstrate a dose-reponse relationship.[1] The importance of dose was succinctly stated by Dr Frank Schabel, Jr, "The dependence upon maximum dosing for greatest tumor cell kill and optimal therapeutic effect is probably the most consistent principle in cancer chemotherapy that we observe with essentially all drugs and certainly with all murine tumor models, and we believe clinical protocol planning would be well guided in using it."[2]

It is likely that a substantial population of SCLC cells is resistant or relatively resistant to many chemotherapeutic agents even before the initiation of treatment. There are several implications of the Goldie-Coldman hypothesis that are probably relevant in SCLC. Combination chemotherapy will be required to minimize the ultimate impact of the relatively resistant neoplastic cells, and ideally all active agents should be used concurrently. Toxicity to normal cells is the major limitation to dose escalation or frequent administration of various drugs. The necessary reduction in doses, as used in standard chemotherapy, likely leads to a reduction in the fractional cell kill and subsequently increased mutation to resistance. Therefore, standard chemotherapy may actually increase the drug-resistant population, which later progresses and kills the patient. This problem may possibly be overcome by using the maximum effective therapy early. The drugs must be active, administered at the highest possible dose, and have additive or synergistic effects with one another.

We have been impressed by the activity of etoposide and cisplatin in patients with progressive tumor resistant to cyclophosphamide, doxorubicin, and vincristine. Several groups have shown that etoposide and cisplatin are probably synergistic and can produce about a 40% response rate in these resistant patients.[3] As single agents in this setting, the response rate to either drug is 10% to 13%. Additionally, etoposide and cisplatin are very active in previously untreated patients. The synergism of these drugs is probably best demonstrated in the clinic for patients with resistant, progressive germ-cell neoplasms. Even those patients who have progressive resistant disease following vinblastine, bleomycin, and cisplatin have about a 20% cure rate following etoposide and cisplatin.[4] Neither drug as a single agent has been curative in this setting. There are also considerable in vitro and animal model data supporting the synergism and/or potentiation of the combination of etopo-

From the Division of Oncology, Vanderbilt University Medical Center, Nashville.

Address reprint requests to F. Anthony Greco, MD, Division of Oncology Vanderbilt University Medical Center, Nashville, TN 37232.

0093–7754/86/1303–3011$05.00/0

side, cisplatin, and cyclophosphamide. In addition, high-dose cyclophosphamide given alone to limited-stage patients is a very active agent capable of producing a complete response (CR) rate of near 40%.[5]

The results of our first two pilot studies with extensive-stage SCLC patients have been published.[6,7] The first study of high-dose etoposide as a single agent produced a CR rate of 30%. In the second study, high-dose cyclophosphamide was added to high-dose etoposide. The CR rate for this second study was also 30%. Furthermore, there was no significant increase in myelotoxicity compared with high-dose etoposide alone, suggesting subadditive toxicity. We are now completing our third study. Relatively high-dose cisplatin has been added to high-dose etoposide and high-dose cyclophosphamide. The preliminary results of this study will be briefly described here.

METHODS

Eighteen previously untreated patients (13 men and five women) have thus far entered this trial. Patient characteristics and metastatic sites are outlined in Table 1. The goal was to choose only patients who were ambulatory, but one patient with a performance status of 40% was included in this trial. Patients with severe cardiac disease (ejection fraction <45%) were excluded. The staging evaluation included physical examination; bronchoscopy; chest radiograph; CT scans of chest, brain, and abdomen; bone scan; and bone marrow aspiration and biopsy. The patients had widespread evidence of metastases and most patients had two or more sites of metastatic disease.

Induction therapy consisted of two cycles of high-dose etoposide (400 $mg/m^2/d \times 3$ d), high-dose cyclophosphamide (50 mg/kg/d × 2 d), and cisplatin (40 $mg/m^2/d \times$ 3 d), administered intravenously (IV) at 3- to 4-week intervals, depending on bone marrow recovery. Patients were hospitalized during their treatment until peripheral blood counts returned (>500/μL polys, >60,000/μL platelets) and there were no signs of fever or infection. Patients subsequently received four cycles of cyclophosphamide, doxorubicin, and vincristine administered IV in standard doses every 3 weeks. No additional chemotherapy was administered until relapse or progression was documented. Patients in CR received prophylactic whole brain radiotherapy. Responses were assessed after the two courses of high-dose induction therapy and following completion of all chemotherapy. Evaluation of response included bronchoscopy with biopsies and washings; CT scans of the chest, as well as CT scans of the brain or abdomen; and bone marrow biopsy and aspiration in those who had involvement before treatment.

Table 1. Patient Characteristics and Metastatic Sites

Patient characteristics	
	Number: 18
	Sex: 13 males, 5 females
	Age: 55.5 years (48-66)
	Performance status: 80% (40%-100%)
Metastatic sites	
	Liver: 6
	Bone marrow: 9
	Bone: 3
	CNS: 6
	Adrenal: 4
	Other: 10

RESULTS

Following the two courses of high-dose induction therapy, 16 of 18 patients achieved an objective response (12 CR, 4 partial response [PR]). Two patients who had PR improved to CR after receiving cyclophosphamide, doxorubicin, and vincristine. The overall response rate after completion of all chemotherapy was 93%. At the completion of the two high doses of chemotherapy, 12 of 18 patients (67%) had a CR (confidence interval ±23%). However, the duration of responses was relatively short (6+ months, ranging from 2 to 12 months). Median survival of these patients is about 8 months (2 to 17+ months) and five patients currently remain free of disease (4+ to 7+ months).

Toxicity of the first two courses of induction therapy are listed in Table 2 in the third column. This table also compares these toxicities with our previous two trials of high-dose etoposide alone and high-dose cyclophosphamide plus high-dose etoposide. All 33 courses of induction therapy with high-dose etoposide, cyclophosphamide, and cisplatin were associated with leukopenia (<200/μL) and thrombocytopenia (<32,000/μL). In addition, 30 of 33 courses (91%) were associated with fever >38.5 °C. Thirteen of these (39%) were associated with documented infections. Two deaths were related to treatment. One of these treatment-related deaths occurred in the patient with a pretreatment performance status of 40%. In general, these toxicities were not significantly different from our two previous trials. Mild to moderate mucositis represented the most important nonhematologic toxicity seen in 20 of 33 courses (61%). This was significant compared with ten of 31 courses (32%) seen in our previous study with high-dose etoposide and high-dose cyclophosphamide.

DISCUSSION

Combination high-dose induction chemotherapy with etoposide, cyclophosphamide, and cis-

Table 2. Toxicities of High-Dose Etoposide-Containing Regimens

	HDE	HCDE	HDCEP
No. of courses	26	31	33
WBC nadir	600/μL	100/μL	100/μL
	(80–2,100)	(0–400)	(0–200)
Days WBC < 1,000/μL	8	9	10
	(7–10)	(5-14)	(7-13)
Platelet nadir	23,000/μL	14,000/μL	16,000/μL
	(6.5–136k)	(6.0–77k)	(2.0–32k)
Days platelets < 20k	1	2	4
	(0–10)	(0–10)	(0–15)
Fever > 38.5 °C	11 (42%)	24 (77%)	30 (91%)
Infections	5 (19%)	8 (26%)	13 (39%)
Hemorrhage	0 (0%)	1 (3%)	3 (9%)
Deaths	3/13 (23%)	1/17 (6%)	2/18 (11%)

Abbreviations: HDE, high-dose etoposide; HDCE, high-dose cyclophosphamide and etoposide; HDCEP, high-dose cyclophosphamide, etoposide, and cisplatin; K, thousand.

platin produced a high CR rate (67%) in patients with extensive-stage SCLC. The CR rate appears to be the highest reported in this group of patients, and compares to the 20% to 30% from many series with standard therapy.[3] The tumor-cell kill is superior to standard chemotherapy. Unfortunately, the CRs reported here are of short duration, suggesting that patients still have a relatively large tumor burden and soon develop progressive disease. It is likely that an even greater amount of tumor-cell kill will be required in these particular patients to substantially improve overall survival.

Clinical progress in cancer chemotherapy has been characterized in the past by increasing PR rates leading eventually to an increase in the CR rates followed by strategies to increase the duration of CR until at least a portion of the patients experience long-term disease-free survival. Modification of the high-dose regimen as reported here may improve the remission duration. It is tempting to speculate that high-dose induction therapy, as used in this study, might be much more effective in the treatment of patients with limited-stage SCLC. Such patients probably have one or two logs fewer tumor cells at the beginning of therapy than do extensive-stage patients. This difference may mean that an improvement in survival may result from therapy with high-dose induction therapy of the variety described here. We are currently testing this concept in a prospective randomized trial comparing two cycles of high-dose etoposide, cyclophosphamide, and cisplatin, followed by thoracic radiotherapy *v* standard chemotherapy with cyclophosphamide, doxorubicin, and vincristine for six cycles plus thoracic radiotherapy. Although the high-dose induction therapy may produce a greater degree of tumor-cell kill, further study will be required to determine if this approach significantly improves survival compared with standard therapy.

REFERENCES

1. Frei E, Canellos GP: Dose: A critical factor in cancer chemotherapy. Am J Med 69: 585–591, 1980

2. Schabel FM, Griswald DP, Corbett TH, et al: Testing therapeutic hypotheses in mice and men: Observations on the therapeutic activity against solid tumors of mice treated with anticancer drugs that have demonstrated a potential clinical utility for treatment of advanced solid tumor of man, in DeVita VT, Busch H (eds): Methods in Cancer Research, vol 17, Cancer Drug Development (part B). Orlando, Fla, Academic, 1979, pp 3–51

3. Johnson DH, Greco FA: Small cell carcinoma of the lung. CRC Crit Rev Oncol/Hematol 4:303–336, 1986

4. Hainsworth JD, Williams SD, Einhorn LH, et al: Sucessful treatment of resistant germinal neoplasms with VP-16 and cisplatin. J Clin Oncol 3:666–671, 1985

5. Souhami RL, Harper PG, Linch D, et al: High-dose cyclophosphamide with autologous bone marrow transplantation as initial treatment of small cell carcinoma of the lung. Cancer Chemother Pharmacol 8:31–35, 1982

6. Wolff SN, Johnson DH, Hande KR, et al: High-dose etoposide as single-agent chemotherapy for small cell carcinoma of the lung. Cancer Treat Rep 67:957–958, 1983

7. Johnson DH, Wolff SN, Hainsworth JD, et al: Extensive-stage small cell caricnoma: Intensive induction chemotherapy with high dose cyclophosphamide and etoposide. J Clin Oncol 3:170–175, 1985

Clinical Trials of Cyclophosphamide, Etoposide, and Vincristine in the Treatment of Small-Cell Lung Cancer

By Robert L. Comis

Etoposide is one of the most active drugs used in the treatment of small-cell lung cancer (SCLC). Recently, studies were completed that evaluated the substitution of etoposide for doxorubicin (Adriamycin) used in combination with cyclophosphamide and vincristine. This study has shown that equivalent antitumor activity, as measured by objective response, can be obtained with the combination of cyclophosphamide, etoposide, and vincristine (CEV) as compared with the CAV combination. A longer response duration and median survival are seen in extensive-disease patients treated with the CEV combination. As expected, no cardiotoxicity is associated with CEV therapy, and interestingly, there is no potentiating neurotoxicity with CEV. A study recently completed has shown that CEV can be effectively combined with intensive radiation therapy to the chest administered simultaneously. CEV appears to be an effective alternative to CAV, and it can be readily combined with aggressive radiation therapy.

ETOPOSIDE is one of the most important drugs for the treatment of small-cell carcinoma of the lungs (SCLC). A variety of studies indicate that the agent has important schedule-dependent properties and that the resistance conferred by previous exposure to other therapeutic agents induces resistance to etoposide. The single-agent response rate for etoposide in SCLC is dependent on the intensity of previous chemotherapy (Table 1). In addition, it appears that multiple-day exposure is superior to single-day intermittent therapy.[1] The activity of the drug, the ability of previous combination chemotherapy exposure to induce resistance, and the schedule dependency of the agent imply that etoposide, used at an optimal dose and schedule, would be best employed in front-line chemotherapy programs.

One of the most extensively used combination chemotherapy programs in SCLC is cyclophosphamide/doxorubicin (Adriamycin [Adria Laboratories, Columbus, Ohio])/vincristine (CAV). Results of studies using this regimen have shown that the complete remission rates for patients with limited and extensive disease are approximately 40% and 15%, respectively.[2] Large studies have also shown that chest radiation therapy combined with CAV is superior to CAV chemotherapy alone.[3] Doxorubicin has been shown to be a radiopotentiator both experimentally and clinically. Doxorubicin potentiates both the mucosal and cardiac toxicities of chest radiotherapy.

The former considerations led to chemotherapy-oriented studies in which etoposide was substituted for doxorubicin (ie, CAV *v* CEV [cyclophosphamide, etoposide, vincristine]), as well as to studies that substituted etoposide for doxorubicin during intensive radiotherapy to avoid the potentiating interaction between doxorubicin and radiotherapy.

CAV *v* CEV *v* CV

One study directly compared etoposide *v* doxorubicin in combination with cyclophosphamide and vincristine. Patients were randomly assigned to one of three treatment groups—CEV *v* CAV *v* CV (cyclophosphamide and vincristine)—as outlined in Table 2. Prior to randomization, patients were stratified according to sex, disease extent, and performance status. The CV arm included high-dose cyclophosphamide with an escalation, according to the degree of hematologic toxicity encountered. Disease extent, objective response, and survival were defined by currently accepted criteria. Patients with limited disease who had not achieved a complete remission after four courses of chemotherapy were given radiotherapy to residual intrathoracic tumor (3,000 cGy in 2 weeks).

A total of 353 patients were entered into the study. A breakdown by treatment group of the pretreatment stratification variables is shown in Table 3. Analysis of objective response, response duration, and survival included all patients assigned to a given treatment arm, whether or not they were considered evaluable. A three-way comparison of complete response rates revealed

---

From the Fox Chase Cancer Center, Philadelphia.

Address reprint requests to Robert L. Comis, MD, Medical Director, Fox Chase Cancer Center, 7701 Burholme Ave, Philadelphia, PA 19111.

0093-7754/86/1303-3002$05.00/0

Table 1. Response to Single-Agent Etoposide Based on Previous Chemotherapy

	No. of Studies	No. of Patients	Response* No. (%)
No. previous chemotherapy	7	106	54 (51)
Previous chemotherapy			
Before 1980	4	61	26 (43)
After 1980	6	132	12 (11)
Overall	17	299	92 (31)

*Complete plus partial response.

no statistically significant difference for limited- (31% to 42%) or extensive-disease patients (7% to 13%); nor were there significant differences according to other prognostic factors.

Response duration, as measured from day 1 of treatment to first evidence of disease progression, ranged from 27 to 34 weeks: the three-drug regimens were significantly superior statistically to the two-drug program. A three-way comparison of response duration in extensive-disease patients (Table 4) showed a highly significant difference in favor of the three-drug programs; medians were 23, 30, and 32 weeks for CV, CAV, and CEV, respectively (P = .004). Survival in extensive-disease patients was also superior with the three-drug combinations. Moreover, in the extensive-disease patients, response duration and survival were superior with CEV as compared with either CAV or CV (Table 5).

Interestingly, the nadirs of leukopenia and granulocytopenia were substantially increased in patients who received the two-drug program

Table 2. Treatment Plan

Drug Program	Dose (mg/m^2)	Route	Schedule
CEV			
Cyclophosphamide	1,000	IV	Day 1
Etoposide	50	IV	Day 1
Etoposide	100	PO	Days 2-5
Vincristine*	1.4	IV	Day 1
CAV			
Cyclophosphamide	1,000	IV	Day 1
Doxorubicin	50	IV	Day 1
Vincristine*	1.4	IV	Day 1
CV			
Cyclophosphamide	2,000	IV	Day 1
Vincristine*	1.4	IV	Day 1

Abbreviations: IV, intravenous; PO, oral.
*Maximum total dose per injection: 2 mg.

Table 3. Demographic Summary

	No. of Patients (%)		
	CEV	CAV	CV
Total patients	115	101	86
Extent of disease			
Limited	36 (31)	35 (35)	26 (30)
Extensive	79 (69)	66 (65)	60 (70)
Sex			
Male	83 (72)	83 (82)	61 (71)
Female	32 (28)	18 (18)	25 (29)
Performance status			
0	19 (17)	24 (24)	9 (10)
1	62 (54)	52 (51)	49 (57)
2	20 (17)	18 (18)	16 (19)
3	11 (10)	7 (7)	9 (10)
4	3 (3)	0	3 (3)

compared with the three-drug programs, yielding P values of .001 and .025, respectively. These data imply that the addition of etoposide or doxorubicin to CV adds activity that is unrelated to the intensity of the pharmacologic effect as measured by leukopenia.

The analysis of nonhematologic toxicities in this three-way comparison is of particular importance. Reports from uncontrolled trials had indicated that etoposide may accentuate the neurotoxicity of vincristine.[3] In this controlled study, the incidence of neurotoxicity was similar for CEV (31%), CAV (36%), and CV (26%)[4] (P = .334). Cardiotoxicity was rare and only seen in patients who received doxorubicin. Three patients developed decreased ejection fractions as measured by radionuclide ventriculogram; two of the three patients had symptomatic congestive heart failure (their cumulative doses ranged from 300 to 402 mg/m^2). As expected, hemorrhagic cystitis was more common in the high-dose cyclophosphamide-treated group (CV: 16%) than in the three-drug groups (1%) (P = .001).

CAV *v* CEV

Because of early evidence of superiority of the three-drug programs (CEV and CAV), randomization to CV was prematurely discontinued. By the end of the study, more than 170 patients had been randomized to one of the three-drug programs. Within these two groups no statistically significant differences relative to disease extent, sex, age, or performance status were apparent.

Table 4. Response Duration by Extent of Disease

	CEV	CAV	CV	Total	*P* Values	
					Mantel-Cox	Gehan-Breslow
Extensive disease					.002*	.004*
No. of responders	38	29	24	91		
Duration (wk)						
Median	32	30	23	28		
Range	11–179+	9–217+	9–40	9–217+		
Limited disease					.739	.830
No. of responders	22	23	13	58		
Duration (wk)						
Median	42	41	45	42		
Range	9–158	9–144+	16–166+	9–166+		

*CEV *v* CV: Mantel-Cox $P = .001$; Gehan-Breslow $P = .001$. CAV *v* CV: Mantel-Cox $P = .011$; Gehan-Breslow $P = .065$.

Complete, partial, and overall response rates were not significantly different between the two treatment groups. Although the complete response rate in extensive-disease patients for CEV was more than twice that for CAV (14% *v* 6%), this was not statistically significant ($P = .133$) within the treated sample size.

Response duration in extensive-disease patients was superior for CEV compared with CAV (33 *v* 25 weeks; $P = .02$). Survival was also superior for the CEV regimen (Table 6) ($P = .012$).

In summary, this study, which is the largest comparative trial addressing the value of using etoposide in an "up-front" regimen, indicates that (1) three-drug programs (CEV and CAV) appear to be more effective than the two-drug program (CV), given to at least equivalent toxicity; (2) CEV appears to be associated with equivalent objective response, yet better response duration and survival than CAV; (3) neurotoxicity is not augmented by the interaction of etoposide and vincristine; and (4) as expected, cardiotoxicity is a more significant problem with doxorubicin-containing regimens.

CEV COMBINED WITH RADIOTHERAPY

A study of patients with limited-disease SCLC was designed in the spring of 1980.[5] At that time, the preliminary data from the CEV *v* CAV *v* CV study indicated the following: CEV response was at least comparable to CAV; there was a radiation dose-response effect in SCLC[6]; simultaneous chemotherapy combined with high-dose radiotherapy might be superior to sandwich radiation therapy.[7] In addition, results of small trials indicated that combination chemotherapy alone might be equivalent to combined modality approaches.[8] Thus, the design of our study was to determine whether a regimen of aggressive radiotherapy given simultaneously with effective chemotherapy (arm I) was superior to the same approach after three cycles of cytoreductive chemotherapy (arm II), or to chemotherapy

Table 5. Survival by Treatment Group

	CEV	CAV	CV	*P* Values	
				Mantel-Cox	Gehan-Breslow
Total patients	115	101	86		
Survival*				.235	.076
Median	44	36	33		
Range	1–179+	1–231+	0–217+		
Alive at last follow-up, No. (%)†	12 (10)	12 (12)	9 (10)		
2-yr survivors, No. (%)‡	10 (9)	6 (6)	4 (5)		
2-yr survivors, free of disease, No. (%)§	4 (3)	2 (2)	1 (1)		

*CEV *v* CV: Mantel-Cox $P = .085$, Gehan-Breslow $P = .025$. CAV *v* CV: Mantel-Cox $P = .445$, Gehan-Breslow $P = .308$.

†$P = .932$.

‡$P = .493$.

§$P = .538$.

Table 6. Response Duration in Extensive-Disease Patients at Final Evaluation

	CEV	CAV	Total	*P* Value
Total patients (no.)	94	83	177	
Survival (wk)				.012
Median	39	33	36	
Range	1–179+	0–217	0–217	

Table 7. CALGB Study: Chemotherapy Regimen

Drug	Dosage
Cyclophosphamide	1.0 g/m² × 1
Etoposide	80 mg/m²/d × 3
Vincristine	2 mg
Adriamycin* (doxorubicin)	45 mg/m²

*CAV alternates with CEV after week 15.

alone (arm III). The design of the study and the CEV program are outlined in Fig 1 and Table 7. Radiation therapy to the chest was delivered at a dose of 5,000 cGy in 5 weeks.

CEV was chosen due to the preliminary activity data and also because less cardiopulmonary toxicity could be anticipated with CEV (as compared with CAV) delivered at an acceptably intensive dose and schedule, combined with radiation therapy. The crossover to CAV was based on the desire of many investigators to employ doxorubicin at some time during the treatment period.

The Cancer and Acute Leukemia Group B (CALGB) primary investigators responsible for the design of this study were Drs Michael Perry (principal investigator), Walter Eaton (radiotherapy), Charles Faulkner (pathology), James Ware (biostatistician), and myself.

Between January 1981 and June 1984, 426 patients were randomly assigned to one of the three treatment arms. Twenty-seven patients (6%) were excluded for a variety of reasons, leaving 399 patients for analysis. There were no statistically significant differences in any major patient-related characteristic, including performance status, sex, or age.

There was a highly significant difference in complete response rate with chemotherapy alone as compared with the combined modality programs (35% *v* 48% to 57%, $P = .0017$). The results of the trial also established the activity of CEV as an induction program for limited SCLC. The complete response rate of 35% for CEV is consistent with the complete response rate of 42% seen in the 36 limited-disease patients treated in the study of CEV *v* CAV *v* CV. Although patients were crossed over to CAV at 15 weeks in the CALGB trial, most of them had obtained a complete remission or progressed by that time. Since current studies do not support a profound effect of fixed alternating chemotherapy, it is unlikely that the late crossover to CAV substantially altered the response rate.

Failure-free and overall survival computed from the day of entry into the study were superior for the combined modality programs as well. In addition, 2-year disease-free survivals for regimens I, II, and III were 15%, 23%, and 6%, respectively, which is a highly significant difference ($P < .0001$). This survival advantage was paralleled by a striking difference in chest relapse rate. In the chemotherapy-alone arm (arm III), the relapse rate was approximately 60%, whereas chest relapse was seen in only 30% to 40% of patients treated with combined modality therapy. It is also interesting that the arm that included three cycles of cytoreductive chemotherapy prior to simultaneous chemotherapy and radiation therapy (arm II) was superior to the simultaneous program (arm I), which began on day 1 in all parameters. This result cannot be explained on the basis of attenuated dose, schedule, or total drug administered to patients in arm I.

As expected, the combined modality programs were associated with more severe and life-threatening myelosuppression than the chemotherapy-alone programs. No life-threatening cardiac or mucosal toxicity was encountered. The incidence of severe cardiac toxicity was 1% in both combined modality arms and 0% in the chemothera-

Fig 1. Schema of three-arm study on the treatment of patients with limited-disease small-cell lung cancer, conducted by Cancer and Leukemia Group B. All three groups received CNS radiotherapy.

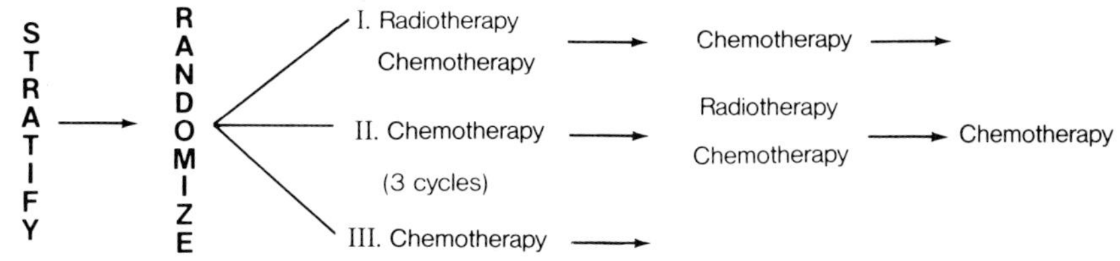

py-alone arm. The incidence of severe mucosal toxicity was 8% to 10% in the combined modality groups and 0% in the chemotherapy group.

DISCUSSION

The two studies cited above are the only studies that have extensively evaluated the role of etoposide substituted for doxorubicin in the primary treatment of SCLC. As mentioned, it was anticipated that certain toxicity advantages would accrue from such substitution studies. The obvious advantage relative to cardiotoxicity was substantiated by the study comparing CAV, CEV, and CV. In addition, the possible problem of potentiating neurotoxicity by using both etoposide and vincristine was addressed by the study design. The results of this controlled randomized trial did not substantiate this potential problem. For those involved in the design of this substitutive trial, the toxicity advantages for etoposide were expected.

The potential therapeutic benefit of an etoposide/doxorubicin substitution was less apparent. The rigorous analysis of results with CAV *v* CEV *v* CV, which is alluded to here and will be published in detail in the future, indicates that use of etoposide is associated with a detectable advantage in response duration and survival for extensive-disease patients. This effect is consonant with results of randomized studies, which show an advantage to adding etoposide to CAV for the treatment of extensive-disease patients.[9]

The results of the CALGB study indicate that CEV is associated with a complete response rate of 35% in limited-disease patients. More importantly, the results show that CEV can be combined effectively with intensive radiation therapy with acceptable toxicity and definite therapeutic benefit. Few studies have effectively combined intensive radiation therapy programs with doxorubicin-containing combination chemotherapy programs with minimal mucosal and/or cardiac toxicity.

In conclusion, it appears that etoposide may be of some benefit in increasing response duration and survival in extensive-disease patients in whom etoposide is substituted for doxorubicin. The CEV combination is also associated with less potential for cardiac toxicity, and an apparent increased ability to deliver full doses with simultaneous radiation therapy. Although the results of these trials do not represent dramatic therapeutic advances in the treatment of SCLC, they do represent potentially important informational building blocks for the development of future programs.

REFERENCES

1. Cavalli F, Sonntag RW, Jungi F, et al: VP-16-213 monotherapy for remission induction of small cell lung cancer: A randomized trial using three dosage schedules. Cancer Treat Rep 62:473–475, 1978

2. Livingston RB, Moore TN, Heilbrun L, et al: Small cell carcinoma of the lung: Combined chemotherapy and radiation: A Southwest Oncology Group Study. Ann Intern Med 88:194–199, 1978

3. Perez CA, Einhorn L, Oldham RK, et al: Randomized trial of radiotherapy to the thorax in limited small-cell carcinoma of the lung treated with multiagent chemotherapy and elective brain irradiation: A preliminary report. J Clin Oncol 2:1200–1208, 1984

4. Thant M, Hawley RJ, Smith MT, et al: Possible enhancement of vincristine neuropathy by VP-16. Cancer 49:859–864, 1982

5. Perry MC, Eaton WL, Chahinian P, et al: Chemotherapy (CT) with or without radiation therapy (RT) in limited small cell cancer of the lung (SCCL). Proc Am Soc Clin Oncol 5:173, 1986 (abstr 678)

6. Choi H, Carey RW: Small cell anaplastic carcinoma of the lung. Cancer 37:2651–2657, 1976

7. Catane R, Lichter A, Lee YJ, et al: Small cell lung cancer. Analysis of treatment factors contributing to prolonged survival. Cancer 48:1936–1943, 1981

8. Stevens E, Einhorn L, Rohn R: Treatment of limited small cell lung cancer. Proc Am Assoc Cancer Res 20:435, 1979 (abstr)

9. Jackson DV, Zekan PJ, Caldwell RD, et al: VP-16-213 in combination chemotherapy with chest irradiation for small-cell lung cancer: A randomized trial of the Piedmont Oncology Association. Clin Oncol 2:1343–1351, 1984

Cyclophosphamide, Doxorubicin, and Etoposide as First-Line Therapy in the Treatment of Small-Cell Lung Cancer

By Paul A. Bunn, Jr, F. Anthony Greco, and Lawrence Einhorn

The discovery that etopside is one of the most active drugs in small-cell lung cancer (SCLC) led to its incorporation into a number of first-line combination chemotherapy regimens. The cyclophosphamide/doxorubicin/etoposide (CAE) regimen was shown to be as active or more active than other standard regimens in nonrandomized studies. In a randomized study presented in this report, the CAE regimen was significantly superior to the cyclophosphamide/doxorubicin/vincristine (CAV) regimen for response duration and survival in extensive-stage patients. In limited-stage patients the results were slightly better with CAE. In addition, CAE lacked the neurotoxicity of CAV.

SMALL-CELL LUNG CANCER (SCLC) is one of the most common (approximately 38,000 cases per year) and lethal (approximately 34,000 deaths per year) cancers occurring in the United States.[1,2] Its propensity for early spread, rapid growth, and sensitivity to drugs has led to the establishment of combination chemotherapy as the cornerstone of treatment.[2] Studies during the early 1970s demonstrated that drug combinations were superior to single agents. Chemotherapy regimens containing relatively high drug doses (sufficient to frequently produce granulocyte nadirs of $\leq 1,000/\mu L$) were shown to be superior to regimens producing little myelosuppression.[3]

Etoposide (VP-16–213, VePesid) was discovered to be one of the most active single agents (and perhaps the most active agent)[4] after at least eight drugs (cyclophosphamide, nitrogen mustard, doxorubicin, vincristine, methotrexate, nitrosoureas, procarbazine, hexamethylmelamine) had been proven to be efficacious and after several three- and four-drug regimens had shown considerable activity. Only recently has etoposide been incorporated into several combinations, which were designed to use the most active agents with differing mechanisms of action and to avoid some of the toxicities and problems of established regimens. Prior to the recognition of etoposide's activity, the three-drug CAV (cyclophosphamide/doxorubicin/vincristine)[5,7] and CMC (cyclophosphamide/methotrexate/CCNU [lomustine]) three regimens were shown to be highly active combinations by many groups. However, many SCLC patients are elderly and suffer from varying degrees of neuropathy and pulmonary and heart disease: CMC regimen causes significant myelosuppression (often requiring weeks of hospitalization) and frequently pulmonary toxicity[3,8]; the CAV regimen has neurologic and cardiac toxicities. The discovery of etoposide led to the study of regimens without these potential toxicities. In this discussion, we will review multicenter results with CAE (cyclophosphamide/doxorubicin/etoposide)-based combinations. These studies show that CAE is as effective as other regimens for SCLC patients, that it virtually eliminates the neurotoxicity of CAV, and that it may be the most effective regimen in extensive-stage SCLC patients with response and survival advantages over CAV. The four-drug CAEV (cyclophosphamide/doxorubicin/etoposide/vincristine) regimen is superior to CAV in extensive-stage patients; however, it does not appear to be superior to CAE in patients with limited-stage disease; it is unclear whether CAE or CAEV is superior in extensive-stage disease.

NONRANDOMIZED STUDIES OF CAE IN LIMITED-STAGE SCLC PATIENTS

Published trials utilizing CAE in limited-stage SCLC are reviewed in Table 1. The partial response and complete response rates as well as survival in these studies are equivalent to the best published results from studies using other combinations. Results listed from Aisner are compiled from three separate studies conducted at the University of Maryland.[9–11] One showed no benefit from adding the immunostimulant methanol

From the Division of Medical Oncology, University of Colorado Health Sciences Center, Denver; Division of Medical Oncology, Vanderbilt University School of Medicine, Nashville, Tenn; and the Division of Medical Oncology, University of Indiana School of Medicine, Indianapolis.

Address reprint requests to Paul A. Bunn, Jr, MD, Head, Division of Medical Oncology, University of Colorado Health Sciences Center, 4200 E Ninth Ave, Campus Box B171, Denver, CO 80262.

0093–7754/86/1303–3003$05.00/0

Table 1. Results With CAE in Limited-Stage SCLC

Author	C	A	mg/m² E Schedule (d)	CRT	PCI	No. of Patients	PR No. (%)	CR No. (%)	CR + PR No. (%)	Median Survival (mo)
Aisner et al[9-11]*	1,000	45	50 (1-5) 100 (1-5)	—	±	43	4	28	(91)	14.0
DeMarinis et al[14]	1,000	50	80 (1, 3, 5)	±	±	8	0	6	(75)	12.0†
Hoth et al[30]	400	40	100 (1, 3, 5)	—	—	23	8	10	(78)	7.8†
Klastersky et al[31]	1,000	45	80 (1-3)	+	±	34	21	7	(82)	14.0
Vogl et al[12]	700	40	150-200 (1-5)	—	±	8	42	4	(75)	6.5†
Total						116	42(36)	55(47)	97/116(84)	6.5±14

Abbreviations: C, cyclophosphamide; A, doxorubicin; E, etoposide; CRT, chest radiotherapy; PCI, prophylactic cranial irradiation; PR, partial response; CR, complete response.

*Compiled from three studies. In one study,[10] CAE was alternated with COMP (CCNU/vincristine/methotrexate/procarbazine) in one arm of a randomized study. There was no advantage over CAE, and data on these patients are excluded. There were no differences in another study[11] comparing the 50-mg (day 1 to 5) bolus schedule with the 100 mg/m² intravenous 5-day continuous infusion schedule. In the third study, MER did not improve results over CAE alone.[9]

†CAE given in cycles 1 + 2; methotrexate (100 mg/kg) on day 1 with CAE on day 8 given in cycles 3 to 8.

extractable residue of BCG (MER) to the CAE regimen[9]; a second, that switching to the non-cross-resistant COMP regimen (CCNU/vincristine/methotrexate/procarbazine) at the time of maximal response did not improve results over CAE alone[10]; and a third, that the continuous five-day infusion schedule of etoposide did not improve results over intermittent bolus infusion of three days.[11] Comparison of all trials in Table 1 suggests that the schedule of etoposide administration did not have a major influence on results and, consequently, the more convenient, one- to three-day schedule may be preferred. Most of the studies used total etoposide doses of 240 to 250 mg/m²/course. The study of Vogl et al[12] with higher etoposide doses did not appear to improve results. The lowest response rates were seen with cyclophosphamide doses of <1,000 mg/m².

Not surprisingly, the results in extensive-stage patients (Table 2) are worse than those with limited-stage disease, but are equivalent to the best results from studies of other combinations. Once again, the etoposide dose and schedule did not have an apparent influence on response rate or survival. The two studies with the shortest median survival gave the lowest dose of cyclophosphamide. However, the Abeloff[13] study with extremely high doses of all three drugs did not appear to improve results over the doses employed by Aisner et al.[9-11,14]

Table 2. Results With CAE in Extensive-Stage SCLC

Author	C	A	mg/m² E Schedule (d)	CRT	PCI	No. of Patients	PR No. (%)	CR No. (%)	CR + PR No. (%)	Median Survival (mo)
Aisner et al[9-11]*	1,000	45	50 (1-5) 100 (1-5)	—	±	67	28	31	(88)	10.0
Abeloff et al[13]†	2,400	60	125 (1, 3, 5)	—	CR	15	10	3	(87)	9.9
DeMarinis et al[14]	1,000	50	80 (1, 3, 5)	±	±	13	NR	NR	(20)	8.0†
Klastersky et al[31]	1,000	45	80 (1, 3, 5)	±	±	27	16	2	(66)	8.3
Matelski et al[32]	500	50	50 (1-5)	—	—	24	10	1	(46)	7.9
Vogl et al[12]	700	40	150-200 (1-5)	NR	NR	8	3	3	(63)	6.0
Total						154	67/141(48)	40/141(28)	107/141(76)	6.0-10.0

Abbreviations: C, cyclophosphamide; A, doxorubicin; E, etoposide; CRT, chest radiotherapy; PCI, prophylactic cranial irradiation; PR, partial response; CR, complete response; NR, not reported.

*Compiled from three studies. In one study,[10] CAE was alternated with COMP (in one arm of a randomized study). There was no advantage over CAE, and data on these patients are excluded. There were no differences in another study[11] comparing the 50-mg (day 1 to 5) bolus schedule with the 100 mg/m² intravenous 5-day continuous infusion schedule. In the third study, MER did not improve results over CAE alone.[9]

†CAE was given for two cycles, then BOMP for two cycles, then alternate. BOMP = BCNU (60 mg/m² IV day 1) + vincristine (1.4 mg/m², day 1) + methotrexate (30 mg/m² IV, day 1) + procarbazine (100 mg/m² orally, days 1 to 10).

Table 3. Results with CAEV in Limited-Stage SCLC

Author	C (mg/m²)	Schedule (d)	A (mg/m²)	Schedule (d)	E (mg/m²)	Schedule (d)	V (mg/m²)	Schedule (d)	CRT	PCI	Patients (No.)	PR (No.)	CR (No.)	CR + PR (%)	Median Survival (mo)
Zekan,[15] Jackson[19]*	1,000		50		60	(1–5)	1.5		+	+	35	11	19	(86)	15.0
Evans et al[17]†	1,000		50		125	(1–3)	2.0		±	+	13	NR	12	NR	20.0
Rome et al[18]‡	1,000		40		125	(21, 23, 25)	1.4		±	±	7	0	5	(71)	14.0
Goodman et al[19]	200	(3–6)	40		150	(1, 8)	1.0	(1, 8)	+	+	33	4	25	(88)	21.3
von Eyben et al[20]	1,000		50		80	(2, 4, 6)	1.0		–	–	2	0	2	(100)	11.0†
Gracia and Jimenez[21]§	800		50		100	(14–18)	1.4	(1, 8, 15, 22)	–	–	19	5	9	(73)	16.5 CR 12.2 PR
Eagan et al[22]§	150	(1–3)	15	(1–3)	50	(1–3)	1.4		+	+	31	17	9	(84)	15.5
Total											140	37/127(29)	81/140(58)	(84)	11.0 ± 21.0

Abbreviations: C, cyclophosphamide; A, doxorubicin; E, etoposide; V, vincristine; CRT, chest radiotherapy; PCI, prophylactic cranial irradiation; PR, partial response; CR, complete response; NR, not reported.

*Doses listed are the induction doses given for the first three cycles. During maintenance (cycles 3 to 6), the cyclophosphamide dose was reduced by 25% and the etoposide dose was 250 mg/m² intravenous day 1.

†Methotrexate 3,000 mg/m² intravenous day 15 with leucovorin rescue was given on alternate cycles.

‡6-week cycles.

§4-week cycles.

Table 4. Results With CAEV in Extensive-Stage SCLC

Author	mg/m² C	Schedule (d)	A	E	Schedule (d)	V	Schedule (d)	CRT	PCI	Patients (No.)	PR (No.)	CR (No.)	CR + PR (%)	Median Survival (mo)
Zekan et al,[15] Jackson et al[16]*	1,000		50	60	(1–5)	1.5		+	+	61	30	21	(84)	9.4
Evans et al[17]†	1,000		50	125	(1–3)	2.0		±	±	13	NR	3	NR	8.5
Rome et al[18]‡	1,000		40	125	(21, 23, 25)	1.4		±	±	11	5	1	(55)	6.0
Lowenbraun et al[23]	1,000		40	100	(1–3)	1.0		—	±	108	65	15	(74)	9.8
Valdivieso et al[24]§	750–1,000		50–60	75–100	(3–5)	1.5	(1, 8)	—	+	48	23	25	(100)	14.5 CR 8.5 PR
Brower et al[25]‖	1,000		50	125		1.4		—	±	48	31	11	(88)	11.8
Dillman et al[26]¶	800		50	200		1.4		TBI	+	19	11	4	(79)	9.3–10.2
Goodman et al[19]	200	(3–6)	40	150	(1, 8)	1.0	(1, 8)	+	+	32	14	11	(78)	8.3
von Eyben et al[20]	1,000		50	80	(2, 4, 6)	1.0		—	—	10	4	4	(80)	8.0
Gracia and Jimenez[21]#	800		50	100	(14–18)	1.4	(1, 8, 15)	—	—	5	4	1	(100)	12.5 CR 6.9 PR
Lowenbraun et al[27]	1,000		40	100	(1–3)	1.0		—	—	46	31	6	(80)	9.7
Total/No. (%)										401	218/388(56)	102/401(25)	(81)	6.0–12.0

Abbreviations: C, cyclophosphamide; A, doxorubicin; E, etoposide; V, vincristine; CRT, chest radiotherapy; PCI, prophylactic cranial irradiation; PR, partial response; CR, complete response; NR, not reported; TBI, total body irradiation.

*Doses listed are the induction doses given for the first three cycles. During maintenance (cycles 3 to 6) the cyclophosphamide dose was reduced by 25% and the etoposide dose was 250 mg/m² IV, day 1.

†Methotrexate (3,000 mg/m² IV, day 15) with leucovorin rescue was given on alternate cycles.

‡6-week cycles.

§Autologous bone marrow and laminar airflow used in some patients.

‖Induction cycles given first 6 weeks varied from 2 to 6. Maintenance cycles (3 to 6) had reductions in cyclophosphamide to 500 mg/m² and etoposide to 100 mg/m² on day 1.

¶After four induction cycles, six consolidation cycles of cyclophosphamide (750 mg/m² IV, day 1) + methotrexate (30 mg/m² IV day 1) + hexamethyamelamine (100 mg/m² orally, days 1 to 10) were given.

#4-week cycles.

NONRANDOMIZED TRIALS OF CAEV IN LIMITED-STAGE SCLC PATIENTS

Results have been reported from at least seven studies with 140 limited-stage SCLC patients adding vincristine to the CAE regimen (Table 3).[15–22] Overall, complete and partial response rates, as well as survival, do not appear to be different from results obtained with the three-drug CAE regimen, although the added toxicity from vincristine must be considered. Once again, it is not clear that the schedule of etoposide administration influenced the results. The trial done by the Piedmont Oncology Group, reviewed by Jackson[15,16] elsewhere in this publication, showed no significant differences in response rates or survival between the three-drug CAV regimen and the four-drug CAEV regimen.

RESULTS OF CAEV IN EXTENSIVE-STAGE SCLC PATIENTS

Rather uniform results were obtained with the CAEV regimen in extensive-stage SCLC patients as reported from 11 studies with 401 patients (Table 4).[15–21,23–27] There was no obvious association between etoposide schedule and response or survival. The longest median survival was reported by Brower et al.[25] This trial used the most aggressive drug schedule, with up to six cycles given in the first 12 weeks. However, three different schedule intensities were used, and there were no significant differences between schedules. Extensive neurotoxicity was reported among patients given vincristine in the most frequent schedule.[28] The other trials did not report similar degrees of neurotoxicity. Thus, the results of CAEV trials are no better than those obtained with CAE, plus there was the added toxicity of vincristine. The complete response rate, in fact, was slightly lower in the CAEV trials (25% *v* 28%).

There have been several major randomized trials designed to evaluate the role of etoposide in comparison with older regimens. The first trial sought to determine whether adding etoposide directly to the CAV regimen would improve results without adding toxicity[15,16] and is reviewed in a subsequent article in this journal by Dr Jackson. The second trial was designed to study the substitution of etoposide for doxorubicin and is discussed by Dr Comis in another article in this journal. A third trial was designed to determine whether etoposide could be substituted for vincristine with equivalent or superior results to CAV. The results of this trial are discussed here.

A RANDOMIZED COMPARISON OF CAV *v* CAE

Many SCLC patients are elderly and at risk for the toxic neurologic complications produced by vincristine. Since etoposide appears to be the most active single agent in SCLC and lacks neurotoxicity, a multi-institutional randomized trial was instituted to determine whether CAE

Table 5. Drug Doses and Schedules in a Randomized Trial of CAE *v* CAV

Drug	Dose (mg/m²)	Route	Schedule (d)
CAE			
Cyclophosphamide	100	IV	1
Doxorubicin	45	IV	1
Etoposide	50	IV	1–5
CAV			
Cyclophosphamide	1,200	IV	1
Doxorubicin	45	IV	1
Vincristine	1.4*	IV	1

Abbreviation: IV, intravenous.

*Maximum dose 2.0 mg.

Table 6. Patient Characteristics in a Randomized Trial of CAE *v* CAV

Patient Characteristic	CAE	CAV	*P* Value
Median age (yr)	60	62	NS
White/nonwhite (no. of patients)	147/22	145/29	NS
	122/47	119/55	NS
Performance status (no. of patients)			
0–1	109	106	NS
2	29	39	
3	29	23	
4	2	6	
Limited-stage disease (no. of patients)	39	41	NS
Extensive-stage disease (no. of patients)	130	133	NS
CNS	39	20	.064
Bone marrow	32	34	NS
Liver	45	51	NS
Bone	61	57	NS
PCI (no. of patients)	36	35	NS
Median no. cycles of Rx (range)	6 (1–20)	5 (1–20)	NS

Abbreviations: Rx, treatment; PCI, prophylactic cranial irradiation; NS, not significant.

Table 7. Treatment Results in a Randomized Study of CAE v CAV

	No. of Patients	PR No. (%)	CR No. (%)	CR + PR (%)	MDR (wk)	Median Survival (wk)	2-yr Survival No. (%)	2-yr DFS (No.)
Limited-stage SCLC								
CAE	39	15(38)	10(26)	64	46	48	3(8)	2
CAV	41	13(32)	10(24)	56	42	58	6(3)	4
Extensive-stage SCLC								
CAE	130	54(42)	16(12)	54	40*	39†	4(3)	0
CAV	133	47(35)	13(10)	45	31*	31†	2(2)	0

Abbreviations: PR, partial response; CR, complete response; MDR, median duration of response; 2-yr DFS, 2-year disease-free survival.

*$P = .002$ Mantel-Cox; $P = .037$ Gehan.

†$P = .030$ Mantel-Cox; $P = .068$ Gehan.

would provide equivalent or superior results compared with CAV. The drug doses and schedules for each arm of this trial are shown in Table 5.

The study design called for stratification of patients by stage of disease. The treatment groups were equally balanced with respect to established prognostic factors and amount of drugs and radiation received (Table 6). The preliminary results of this multi-institutional trial[29] (Rudolph A, personal communication, 1986) are provided by stage in Table 7 and Figs 1 and 2. In 80 limited-stage patients, there were no significant difference in partial (38% v 32%) or complete (26% v 24%) response rates. The median duration of response was slightly longer in the CAE group, whereas median survival was a little longer in the CAV group. However, none of these differences was significant (Fig 1A, Table 7). The proportion of 2-year survivors and 2-year disease-free survivors was low and equivalent in each group.

In 263 extensive-stage patients, the CAE regi-

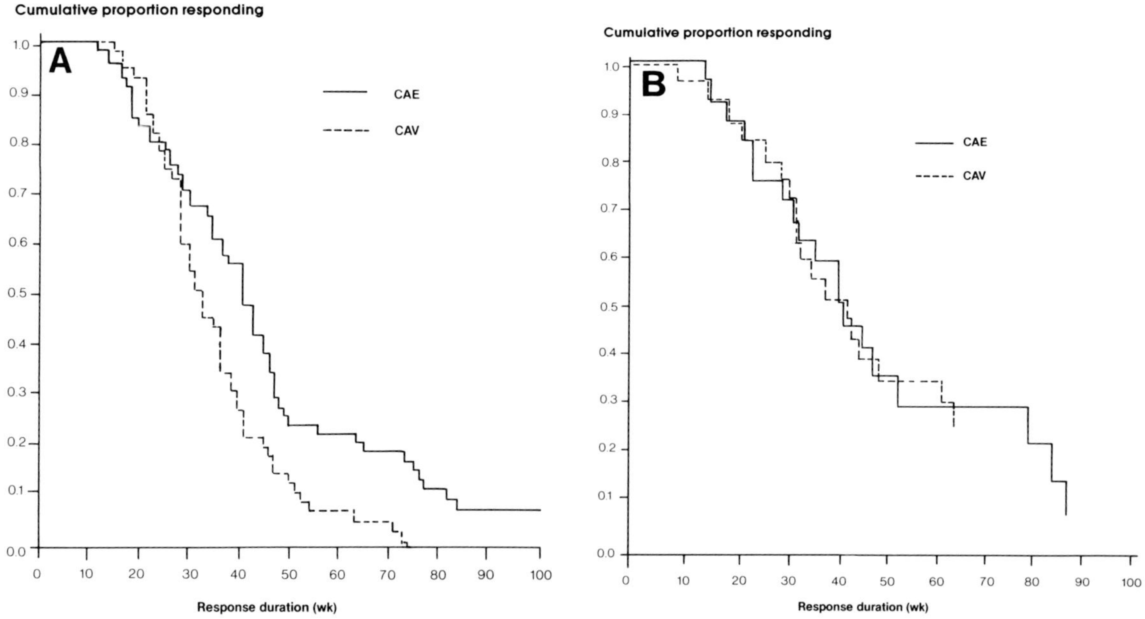

Fig 1. Response duration following CAE and CAV chemotherapy: (A) Actuarial response duration for limited-stage SCLC patients. For 25 patients responding to CAE, the median response duration was 46 weeks, with a 95% confidence interval of 36 to 53 weeks. For 23 responders to CAV, the median response duration was 42 weeks, with a 95% confidence interval of 36 to 50 weeks. (B) Actuarial response duration for extensive-stage SCLC patients. The medians were 40 and 31 weeks for CAE and CAV, respectively. The 95% confidence intervals were 34 to 44 and 28 to 34 weeks, respectively. These differences were statistically significant. CAV denoted by broken line; CAE denoted by solid line. (From Rudolph et al,[29] and Rudolph A, personal communication, 1986.)

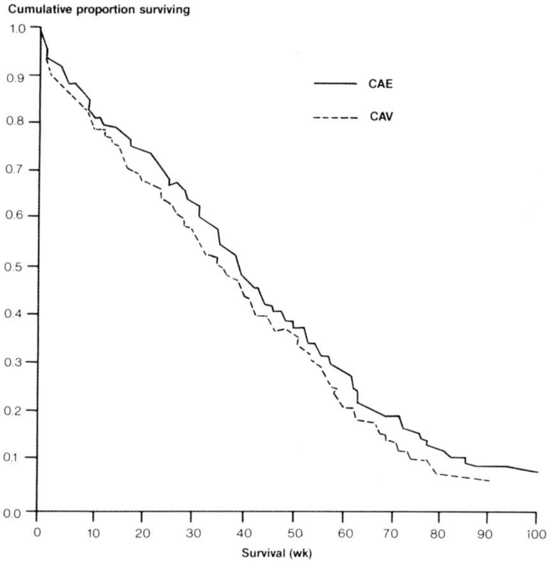

Fig 2. Actuarial survival for all patients by treatment group. Survival was better in the CAE group (median 40 *v* 37 weeks), but the differences were not statistically significant. For extensive-stage SCLC patients, survival was significantly better in CAE-treated patients. CAV denoted by broken line; CAE denoted by solid line. (From Rudolph et al,[29] and Rudolph A, personal communication, 1986.)

men produced a slightly higher partial (42% *v* 35%) and complete (12% *v* 10%) response rate. The differences in response duration and survival were more strikingly in favor of the CAE regimen with response durations of 40 *v* 31 weeks and median survival of 39 *v* 31 weeks, respectively (Fig 1B). These differences were statistically significant.

Both regimens were relatively well tolerated with one death occurring during induction. Hematologic toxicity was more severe in the CAE group; nonhematologic toxicities were comparable in the two groups with the exception of neurologic toxicity, which was significantly more severe in the CAV group. Myelosuppression was the most frequent toxicity in both groups, but was more severe in the CAE group (Table 8). The WBC count nadir was <1,000/μL in 53% of the CAE patients, but only 41% of the CAV patients (P = .04). The median WBC count nadir was 900/μL and 1,200/μL in the two groups, respectively. Granulocyte nadirs were also lower in the CAE group, although these differences were not significant. Thrombocytopenia was less severe than granulocytopenia in both groups and nadir counts were significantly lower with CAE. Platelet nadirs <25,000/μL occurred in 11% of CAE patients and 4% of CAV patients: the median nadirs were 100,000/μL and 149,000/μL, respectively. Anemia was also more severe in the CAE group with median hemoglobin count nadirs of 9.1 g/dL and 10.0 g/dL, respectively.

Despite the more striking myelosuppression in the CAE group, the frequency of antibiotic usage, the number of infections, and the deaths from toxicity and infection were similar in each group (Table 8). Documented infections occurred in 28% of the CAE-treated patients and 23% of the CAV patients, whereas sepsis developed in 6% and 5%, respectively. Antibiotics were given to 56% of the patients in the CAE group and 51% in the CAV group. The drug-related and possibly drug-related deaths are also summarized in Table 8. Of the 12 deaths in the CAE group, two occurred in limited-stage and ten in extensive-stage patients. Among the CAV-treated patients, there were no deaths in those with limited-stage disease and eight deaths in those with extensive-stage disease; and there were no significant differences between the CAE and CAV groups. Most of the drug-related deaths occurred during induction (first cycle) and these were related to infections in at least seven patients (four CAE, three CAV). After the

Table 8. Hematologic and Infectious Complications in a Randomized Trial of CAE *v* CAV

	CAE	CAV	*P* Value
WBC ≤ 1,000/μL	53%	41%	.038
Median WBC nadir (range)	0.9 (0.1–7.0) × 10^3/μL	1.2 (0.1–11.3) × 10^3/μL	.003
Platelet nadirs ≤ 25,000/μL	11%	4%	.034
Median platelet nadir (range)	100 (6–550) × 10^3/μL	149 (5–1,094) × 10^3/μL	.001
Antibiotics (no. of patients)	94 (56%)	88 (51%)	NS
Sepsis (no. of patients)	10 (6%)	8 (5%)	NS
Infection (no. of patients)	47 (28%)	40 (23%)	NS
Drug-related death (No. of patients)	12	8	NS

Abbreviation: NS, not significant.

Table 9. Nonhematologic Toxicities in a Randomized Trial of CAE *v* CAV

	CAE No. (%)	CAV No. (%)	*P* Value
Polyneuropathy	6 (4)	54 (31)	<.001
Constipation	3 (2)	14 (8)	<.007
Cardiotoxicity	7 (4)	3 (2)	NS
Nausea/vomiting	128 (76)	137 (79)	NS
Anorexia	49 (29)	43 (25)	NS
Alopecia	76 (45)	70 (40)	NS
Stomatitis	27 (16)	20 (11)	NS
Fatigue	32 (19)	33 (19)	NS

Abbreviation: NS, not significant.

first cycle of therapy, there were five deaths in the CAE group *v* one in the CAV group.

Polyneuropathy and constipation were the only nonhematologic toxicities that occurred with greater frequency in the CAV group (Table 9). These developed in 31% and 8%, respectively, of the CAV-treated patients *v* 4% and 2%, respectively, of the CAE group. Nausea and vomiting occurred in most patients and alopecia and anorexia in 24% to 45%. Cardiotoxicity was relatively uncommon, occurring in 4% and 2% of the CAE and CAV patients, respectively.

DISCUSSION AND CONCLUSIONS

The treatment of SCLC has improved markedly over the past two decades. In 1970, the median survival of all patients was about 4 months and less than 1% of patients survived 5 years. Current combination chemotherapy regimens produce median survivals of approximately 1 year with approximately 5% of patients surviving 2 to 5 years. The most effective drug combinations usually contain three active single agents given with sufficient intensity to produce WBC count nadirs of 1,000/μL or less in the majority of patients. Most of these regimens contain doxorubicin and/or vincristine, which may be less than ideal agents for elderly lung cancer patients with significant heart disease or peripheral neuropathies.

The more recent discovery that etoposide is perhaps the most active agent in SCLC has led to a number of trials in which doxorubicin and/or vincristine were replaced by etoposide or etoposide was added to existing regimens. These trials demonstrated that etoposide can replace doxorubicin or vincristine without loss of activity. The CAE regimen has been shown to be as active as any other regimen in SCLC. In comparison with CAV, the CAE regimen exhibited a significantly longer response duration and median survival in extensive-stage disease patients. The four-drug CAEV regimen is also superior to CAV in extensive-stage disease. There are no data to determine whether CAE or CAEV should be preferred in patients with extensive-stage SCLC. In limited-stage disease, however, CAE can be considered as effective as any other regimen without the toxicities associated with vincristine.

REFERENCES

1. Silverberg E: Cancer statistics, 1985. CA 35:19–35, 1985

2. Minna JD, Higgins GA, Glatstein EJ: Cancer of the lung, in Devita VT, Hellman S, Rosenberg S (eds): Principles and Practice of Oncology. Philadelphia, Lippincott, 1982, pp 396–474

3. Cohen MA, Creaven PH, Fossick BE Jr, et al: Intensive chemotherapy of small cell bronchogenic carcinoma. Cancer Treat Rep 61:349–354, 1977

4. O'Dwyer PJ, Leyland-Jones B, Alenso MT, et al: Etoposide (VP–16–213): Current status of an active anticancer drug. N Engl J Med 312:692–700, 1985

5. Greco FA, Richardson RL, Snell JD, et al: Small cell lung cancer: Complete remission and improved survival. Am J Med 66:625–630, 1979

6. Johnson RE, Brereton HD, Kent CH: "Total" therapy for small cell carcinoma of the lung. Ann Thorac Surg 25:510–515, 1978

7. Mandelbaum I, Williams SD, Hornback NB, et al: Combined therapy for small cell undifferentiated carcinoma of the lung. J Thorac Cardiovasc Surg 76:292–296, 1978

8. Brooks J, Seifter ES, Walsh TE, et al: Pulmonary toxicity with combined modality therapy for limited stage small cell lung cancer. J Clin Oncol 4:200–209, 1986

9. Aisner J, Wiernik PH: Chemotherapy versus chemoimmunotherapy for small cell undifferentiated carcinoma of the lung. Cancer 46:2543–2549, 1980

10. Aisner J, Whitacre M, Van Echo DA, et al: Combination chemotherapy for small cell carcinoma of the lung: Continuous versus alternating non-cross-resistant combination. Cancer Treat Rep 66:221–230, 1982

11. Aisner J, Whitacre M, Van Echo DA, et al: Doxorubicin, cyclophosphamide, and etoposide (ACE) by bolus or continuous infusion for small cell carcinoma of the lung (SCCL). Proc Am Soc Clin Oncol 2:196, 1983 (abstr)

12. Vogl S, Bonomi P, Chang A: Etoposide (VP–16) in very high doses in combination for small cell bronchogenic carcinoma (SCBC) with moderate doses of Adriamycin (A) and cyclophosphamide (C): Modest results. Proc Am Assoc Cancer Res 25:177, 1984 (abstr)

13. Abeloff MD, Ettinger DS, Order SE, et al: Intensive

induction chemotherapy in 54 patients with small cell carcinoma of the lung. Cancer Treat Rep 65:639–646, 1981

14. DeMarinis F, Maccone C, Migliorino MR, et al: Cisplatin, Adriamycin, etoposide (PAE) vs Cytoxan, Adriamycin, etoposide (CAE) in the chemotherapy (CT) of small cell lung cancer (SCLC). Cancer Chemother Pharmacol 14:S19, 1985 (suppl)

15. Zekan P, Jackson D, Muss H, et al: VP–16 enhancement of treatment results in extensive small cell cancer of the lung. A randomized trial of the Piedmont Oncology Association. Proc Am Soc Clin Oncol 4:192, 1985 (abstr)

16. Jackson DV Jr, Zekan PJ, Caldwell RD, et al: VP–16–213 in combination chemotherapy with chest irradiation for small cell lung cancer. A randomized trial of the Piedmont Oncology Association. J Clin Oncol 2:1343–1351, 1984

17. Evans T, Jacobs SA, Earle MF, et al: Up-front VP–16/platinum (CDDP) in small cell lung cancer (SCCL). Proc Am Soc Clin Oncol 4:189, 1985 (abstr)

18. Rome LS, Portlock CS, Kapp DS, et al: Cyclophosphamide, Adriamycin, vincristine (CAV) vs. cyclophosphamide, Adriamycin, vincristine alternating with VP–16 (etoposide) (CAV/E) in the treatment of small cell cancer (SCC) of the lung. Proc Am Soc Clin Oncol 4:191, 1985 (abstr)

19. Goodman GE, Miller TP, Manning MM, et al: Treatment of small cell lung cancer with VP–16, vincristine, doxorubicin (Adriamycin), cyclophosphamide (EVAC), and high dose chest radiotherapy. J Clin Oncol 1:483–488, 1983

20. Von Eyben FE, Arwidi A, Hellekant C, et al: Vincristine, Adriamycin, cyclophosphamide, and etoposide (VP–16–213) in small-cell anaplastic carcinoma of the lung. Cancer Chemother Pharmacol 7:195–197, 1982

21. Gracia JM, Jimenez A: Chemotherapy combination with cyclophosphamide (CTX), Adriamycin (ADM), vincristine (VCR), and VP16–213 in small cell carcinoma of the lung (SCCL). Cancer Chemother Pharmacol 7:199–201, 1982

22. Eagan RT, Lee RE, Frytak S, et al: An evaluation of low-dose cisplatin as part of combined modality therapy of limited small cell cancer. Cancer Clin Trials 4:267–271, 1981

23. Lowenbraun S, Birch R, Buchanan R, et al: Combination chemotherapy in small cell lung carcinoma: A randomized study of two intensive regimens. Cancer 54:2344–2355, 1984

24. Valdivieso M, Cabanillas F, Keating M, et al: Effects of intensive induction chemotherapy for extensive-disease small cell bronchogenic carcinoma in protected environment-prophylactic antibiotic units. Am J Med 76:405–412, 1984

25. Brower M, Ihde DC, Johnston-Early A, et al: Treatment of extensive stage small cell bronchogenic carcinoma: Effects of variation in intensity of induction chemotherapy. Am J Med 75:993–1000, 1983

26. Dillman RO, Teatle R, Seatgren S, et al: Extensive disease small cell carcinoma of the lung: Trial of non-cross resistant chemotherapy and consolidation radiotherapy. Cancer 49:2003–2008, 1982

27. Lowenbraun S, Buchanan R, Birch R, et al: Intensive chemotherapy in small cell lung carcinoma (SCLC). Proc Am Clin Oncol 22:504, 1981 (abstr)

28. Thant M, Hawley PJ, Smith MT, et al: Possible enhancement of vincristine neuropathy by VP16. Cancer 49:859–864, 1982 (abstr)

29. Rudolph A, Einhorn L, Wampler G, et al: The substitution of etoposide for vincristine in established therapy for small cell carcinoma of the lung. Proceedings of the 13th International Congress of Chemotherapy, Vienna, 1983

30. Hoth D, Lokey J, Baker J, et al: Limited small cell lung carcinoma: Treatment with chemotherapy alone. Proc Am Soc Clin Oncol 21:455, 1980 (abstr)

31. Klastersky J, Sculier JP, Dumont JP, et al: Combination Chemotherapy with Adriamycin, etoposide, and cyclophosphamide for small cell carcinoma of the lung. A study by the EORTC Lung Cancer Working Party (Belgium). Cancer 56:71–75, 1985

32. Matelski HW, Lokich JJ, Huberman MS, et al: Adriamycin, cyclophosphamide and etoposide (VP–16–213) in extensive-stage small cell lung cancer. Am J Clin Oncol 7:729–732, 1984

Doxorubicin, Cyclophosphamide, Etoposide and Platinum, Doxorubicin, Cyclophosphamide and Etoposide for Small-Cell Carcinoma of the Lung

By Joseph Aisner, Margaret Whitacre, Jeffrey Abrams, and Kathleen Propert

Small-cell lung cancer (SCLC) is a disseminated disease regardless of our ability to document all sites. Chemotherapy is thus the cornerstone of treatment. There are multiple active single agents, resulting in many combination chemotherapy regimens. Optimal combinations are probably derived from the use of synergistic drug interactions. A three drug combination of doxorubicin (Adriamycin), cyclophosphamide, and etoposide (ACE) has been used at the University of Maryland Cancer Center (UMCC) for more than a decade in sequential studies. Two hundred four patients, 143 men and 61 women, were treated on these studies. Eighty-five had limited disease (LD) and 119 had extensive disease (ED). The complete response (CR) frequencies were 65% and 43% for LD and ED, respectively, and the median survivals were 15 and 9.5 months, respectively. Twenty-two percent of the LD patients were alive at 2 years. To improve upon response or survival, and because of synergy, cisplatin was added to ACE (PACE). PACE chemotherapy was administered in two studies—study 1 at UMCC for both LD and ED, and study 2 by Cancer and Acute Leukemia Group B (CALGB) for ED only. Preliminary review suggests that CR frequencies for LD (53%, study 1) and ED (44%, study 1; 37%, study 2) were similar to prior studies, but median survivals (LD, 18+ months, study 1; ED, 15 months, study 1, 10.5 months, study 2) appears superior to previous studies. However, PACE is more toxic than ACE. Further studies of PACE are needed to assess if the additional toxicities are warranted.

SMALL-CELL LUNG CANCER (SCLC) has received considerable attention in the medical literature in recent years because of its unique histology, biologic behavior, and response to both chemotherapy and radiation therapy. Clinical manifestations of the high labelling index and short doubling times seen in in vitro studies include rapid and fulminant clinical course of the disease, abrupt onset of signs and symptoms, early dissemination of widespread metastases, and short median duration of survival without systemic treatment.[1–5] One of the most important advances in this disease occurred in the early 1970s when its systemic nature was completely appreciated. More than half of all patients present with disease outside the thorax, and a vast majority of all patients present with disease involving local and regional lymph nodes, rendering the disease technically unresectable.[6,7] In the past, surgical series among patients with disease confined to the chest showed early death with high early systemic failure (widespread metastases at autopsy) and no apparent cures.[8,9] The pattern of treatment failure, metastases, and widespread regional involvement has led to the general recognition that SCLC is a systemic disease process. Even though various radiation therapy series for limited disease produced an increase in the median duration of survival, still nearly all patients died of the disease and showed evidence of widespread metastases; this gave further support to the concept that localized forms of treatment were inadequate for overall disease control or potential cure.[10–12] Appreciation of the systemic nature of SCLC, therefore, led to the general acceptance of chemotherapy as the cornerstone of treatment for this disease.[13]

TREATMENT APPROACHES

The approach to treatment of SCLC has evolved over the past 15 years and is currently undergoing further refinement. Most importantly realized from the study of treatment programs in SCLC is that aggressive treatment approaches are necessary in order to achieve the highest possible cure rate.[13] Every study that has examined the issue of dose response of chemotherapy for SCLC has suggested a dose-response curve for these chemotherapeutic agents where dose and/or schedule are important factors. Another important factor in the understanding of a potential treatment approach is the necessity

From the Division of Medical Oncology, University of Maryland Cancer Center, University of Maryland School of Medicine Baltimore Veterans Administration Medical Center; and the Biostatistical Center, Cancer and Leukemia Group B, Harvard School of Public Health, Boston.

Address reprint requests to Joseph Aisner, MD, Division of Medical Oncology, Univerisity of Maryland Cancer Center, 22 S Greene, Baltimore, MD 21201.

0093–7754/86/1303–3005$05.00/0

for careful staging. Currently, the most useful staging system for the purpose of assessing treatment options is the limited/extensive disease staging categories.[7] Limited disease is defined as that disease confined to one hemithorax, plus or minus mediastinal or hilar nodes, plus or minus ipsilateral supraclavicular lymph nodes. Ipsilateral pleural effusion, whether cytologically positive or not, is now believed to represent limited disease. With the possible exception of an ipsilateral pleural effusion, extensive disease is any disease beyond the confines of the limited disease definition. In evaluating literature reports of treatment series, it is necessary to carefully assess the staging techniques used. Nearly every series that has carefully staged SCLC, and compared limited and extensive disease, has shown a significant difference in treatment outcome (response and survival) between the two stages. Thus, the more carefully staged the disease, the better both subgroups (limited and extensive disease) will apparently do. This is due to staging shifts (ie, the poorer-outcome limited-disease patients become the better-outcome extensive-disease patients, thereby improving both groups) and is not necessarily a treatment outcome attributable to the treatment approach and/or treatment modality. Thus, interinstitutional differences may be seen solely on the basis of staging rigor. At the University of Maryland Cancer Center, the same vigorous staging criteria have been applied for nearly a decade, with a resultant stability in treatment outcome.[14–16] Newer technologies, such as computed tomographic scanning and biomarkers, however, have simplified staging and offered new prognostic factors.[17]

Based on the outcome of staging evaluations, treatment applications may differ according to treatment modalities applied for regional (limited) or extensive disease. Patients with extrathoracic disease, except for intracranial involvement, are unlikely to benefit from the application of irradiation to all areas of bulk disease. Irradiation to liver, bone marrow, adrenal glands, and other organs is likely to be time consuming and cause delays in chemotherapy or reduction in chemotherapy doses, or both. Thus, the approach to extensive disease is the use of aggressive combination chemotherapy alone, with cranial irradiation as indicated. For limited disease, however, there is incomplete agreement concerning the role of chest irradiation in controlling areas of bulk disease within the chest.[12,18–25] Multiple studies, including prospectively randomized controlled studies, have addressed these issues[18–25] and led us to conclude that when chest irradiation is administered between courses of combination chemotherapy, there is no demonstrable effect on survival; there is, however, improved local control. Thus there is an increased distal failure rate. When chest irradiation is given concomitantly with combination chemotherapy, there is a small but consistent survival advantage of about 5% to 10% in favor of the combined modality treatment. In most studies, however, in order to administer concurrent therapies, the dose of chemotherapy is modified to permit chest irradiation, and the dose of chest irradiation is accommodated for chemotherapy. One study applied both treatment modalities maximally with the suggestion that enhanced disease control might be obtained.[25] There was, however, an unacceptable toxicity, with death due to esophageal and pulmonary fibrosis induced by the chemotherapy-radiotherapy interactions. Newer approaches to radiation treatment planning, however, may allow for more aggressive application of both modalities, with more acceptable levels of toxicity.

If one were to evaluate patterns of treatment failure for both aggressive chemotherapy and combined modality therapy, it would become evident that most treatment failure occurs with distant metastases regardless of treatment modality application.[26] For patients given chemotherapy alone, nearly two thirds fail systemically, or both locally and systemically, whereas for patients given combined modality treatment, 75% or more have treatment failure at distant sites. Thus, in order to achieve better control of SCLC and improve the number of people achieving long-term survival, better systemic therapy is currently needed. As better systemic therapy is achieved, it is highly probable that the issues of local control and control of bulk tumor will be highly critical in achieving long-term disease-free survival.

SINGLE-AGENT CHEMOTHERAPY

Coincident with the recognition of SCLC as a distinct entity, was the recognition of antitumor

Table 1. Activity of Single Agents in SCLC

Drug	Approximate Response (%)*
Teniposide (VM-26)	65
Carboplatin (CBDCA)	50
Etoposide (VP-16)	45
Cyclophosphamide	40
Vincristine	35
Mechlorethamine	35
Methotrexate	30
Doxorubicin	30
Vindesine	25
Carmustine (BCNU)	25
MeCCNU	25
Lomustine	15
Hexamethylmelamine	30†
Procarbazine	25†

*Data derived from compilation of this list do not consider dose and schedule.

†Recent phase II studies failed to confirm activity.

Table 3. ACE Combination Chemotherapy*

Drug	Dosage and Schedule	
Doxorubicin	45 mg/m^2	IV day 1
Cyclophosphamide	1,000 mg/m^2	IV day 1
Etoposide	50 mg/m^2	IV days 1-5
Each course	21 days	Courses 1-3
	28 days	Course 4-8

*CAE regimen: Courses were given every 21 days or as tolerated. Initial doxorubicin doses were modified for hepatic function. Doxorubicin was given as a full dose if bilirubin was ≤1.5 mg/dL and serum SGOT was <60 IU. The dose was reduced to 50% if bilirubin was between 1.5 and 3.0 mg/dL, or SGOT was between 60 and 180 IU. The dose was reduced to 25% if bilirubin was >3.1 mg/dL, or SGOT was >180 IU. Doxorubicin was continued until total cumulative dose of 540 mg/m^2. All chemotherapy doses were adjusted after three courses for myelotoxicity.

Abbreviation: IV, intravenous.

activity of many single agents with dramatic short-term objective tumor regressions. Table 1 shows the approximate single-agent tumor activity in SCLC.[13,27,28] This single-agent antitumor activity is based on a compilation of various reports and does not take into consideration either dose or schedule dependency of many of the agents. For example, etoposide, which appears to be both dose and schedule dependent in animal tumor models,[29,30] may be considerably more active than shown in this table. Phase I/II trials of high-dose etoposide in extensive disease by Greco et al[1] clearly suggests such a dose-response phenomenon in humans. Similarly, dose and/or schedule dependency for teniposide, carboplatin, and cisplatin, as well as other agents, may be critical in determining their specific antitumor activity. Furthermore, the activity is highly dependent upon previous treatment. For example, etoposide is highly active as a single agent when used in previously untreated or minimally treated patients, whereas it has marginal antitumor activity in the refractory disease setting.[32] This is a reflection of the emergence of pleiotropic drug resistance. Thus, one potential reason there is not a larger list of active agents for SCLC is the fact that there has been an inability to test many new agents in previously untreated disease.

Despite relatively low orders of activity in refractory disease or incomplete responses as frontline therapy, several agents have the potential for therapeutic synergy when combined. With therapeutic synergy, when two or more agents are combined, there is the potential for a therapeutic effect greater than that expected from the additive effect of either drug used alone. Experiments conducted at the Southern Research Institute examining the interaction of etoposide and cisplatin, doxorubicin and cisplatin, and other combinations have indicated that synergy of up to seven log orders of magnitude (with respect to cell kill) could be achieved when

Table 2. Combination Chemotherapy Containing Cyclophosphamide Used as Treatment for Small-Cell Lung Cancer*

AE	CA	CAV	CAVHNVbP	CCcVP	CVBcPr	EAM
AVB	CAD	CAVD	CAVM	CE	CVM	EPt
AVbP	CAE	CAVE	CAMPt	CMCc	CVMBcPr	HA
BcPMVB	CAMCc	CAVEPt	CAVMPr	CMCcVB	CVMF	HEM
BcVMP	CAMCcV	CAVH	CcVMP	CME	CVMP	
	CAMV	CAVHyMCcP	CCc	CV	CVPPr	
			CCcAP	CVBM	CVPt	

*Acronyms are not necessarily those used in literature.

Abbreviations: A, doxorubicin (Adriamycin); Bc, BCNU, carmustine; C, cyclophosphamide; Cc, CCNU, Lomustine; D, DTIC; E, etoposide (VP-16-213); F, fluorouracil; H, hexamethylmelamine; M, methotrexate; Hy, hydroxyurea; P, procarbazine; N, nitrogen mustard; Pr, prednisone; Pt, platinum; B, bleomycin; V, vincristine; Vb, vinblastine.

the drugs were used in combination.[33] This raises the possibility of multiple synergistic drug combinations derived from the relatively small list of active single agents. These synergistic possibilities have been clearly established in human testicular cancer for the combination of etoposide and cisplatin[34,35] and are strongly suggested by the use of this combination as salvage therapy for SCLC.[36,37] Based in part on the success of combination chemotherapy in other human malignancies, and the identification of multiple active single agents with differing mechanisms of action and nonoverlapping toxicities, a large number of combination chemotherapy regimens have been developed for SCLC (Table 2).

ACE COMBINATION CHEMOTHERAPY

In 1975, a highly active combination chemotherapy regimen containing doxorubicin (Adriamycin [Adria Laboratories, Columbus, Ohio]), cyclophosphamide, and etoposide (ACE), given without adjuvant chest irradiation, was identified at the University of Maryland Cancer Center. This three-drug combination (Table 3) was based on available single-drug activity data in addition to data derived from animal studies that suggested the possibility of multiple synergistic pairs; multiple daily dosing of etoposide was chosen because of available animal and human studies.[29,30,38,39]

All patients seen at the University of Maryland Cancer Center were carefully and aggressively staged for extent of disease and, if found eligible, were stratified and then randomized to one of three sequential studies[14-16] (Fig 1).

The first study compared ACE, plus or minus the methanol-extracted residue (MER) of bacillus Calmette-Guérin. This was based on the concept that nonspecific immune stimulation with MER could offer the potential for increased duration of response and reduced toxicity of chemotherapy. Unfortunately, this study showed that these desired results were not achieved.

The second study was designed, after the identification of a second non–cross-resistant combination,[40] to test the sequential use of two non–cross-resistant regimens *v* an alternation of the two regimens. This study was a prospective

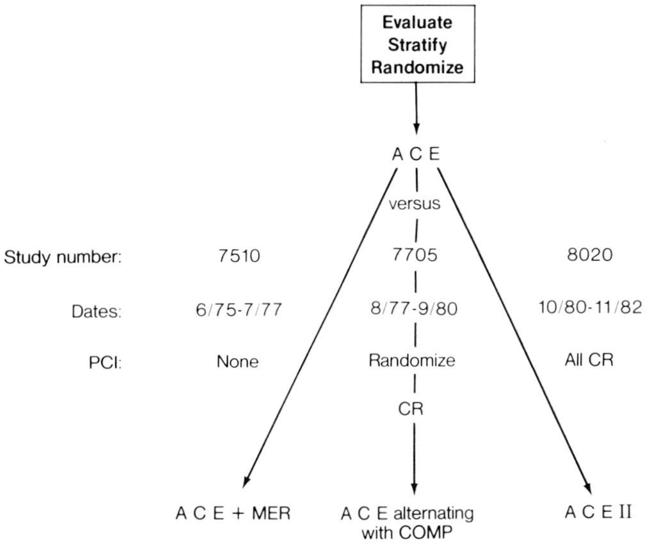

Fig 1. Schema of the randomization of patients to one of three sequential ACE chemotherapy studies for SCLC performed at the University of Maryland Cancer Center (from Tinsley et al[45] with permission). Abbreviations: PCI, prophylactic cranial irradiation; CR, complete response; CAE II, CAE where etoposide = 100 mg/m^2/d by continuous infusion, days 1 through 5.

COMP Therapy

Drug	Dosage and Schedule
Lomustine	75 mg/m^2, day 1, PO
Vincristine	1 mg/m^2 IV, days 1 and 21
Methotrexate	40 mg/m^2 IV, days 1 and 21
Procarbazine	75 mg/m^2 PO, days 1-5 and 21-25

evaluation of the alternating non–cross-resistant hypothesis of Goldie et al.[13,41] In the alternating arm, ACE was given for a minimum of three courses or until the maximum response occurred, and then the second combination was begun on a 42-day cycle. There were no significant differences in the two arms.

The third study began after a maximum tolerated dose of 5-day, continuous, etoposide was established,[42] and sought to determine whether a higher dose of continuous-infusion etoposide might produce a therapeutic advantage. No such advantage could be demonstrated.

The first study did not utilize prophylactic cranial irradiation. The second study sought to determine the value of prophylactic cranial irradiation given to those patients who achieved complete response. The third study included prophylactic cranial irradiation for all patients who achieved complete response, since analysis of the first and second studies demonstrated the value of prophylactic cranial irradiation.[43]

For the first two studies, treatment was delayed if the WBC count had not recovered by the 21st day (first day of the next cycle). In the third sequential study, dosage modifications for the first three courses were not made for leukopenia. For subsequent courses, dosage modifications were made according to the formula of the preceding two studies. All patients were routinely followed on a weekly basis to determine counts and potential toxicities. Patients were completely reevaluated for any change in clinical status. This reevaluation included history and physical examination and, at a minimum, repeat of all tests, in which results were suspicious, including roentgenographic studies, computed tomography (CT) scans, bronchoscopies, isotopic liver and bone scans, bilateral iliac crest-bone-marrow aspirates and biopsies, and CT brain scans. Standard criteria for response assessment were used.

A total of 204 patients (143 males, 61 females; 85 with limited disease) were randomized to the three sequential studies between June 1975 and November 1982 (Table 4). A summary of the patient characteristics has been previously published.[44] In general the median age of the population was 59 years, with a broad range from 29 to 76 years. One hundred six of the patients had a performance status of 0 to 1; 85 had a performance status of 2 to 3; and only 13 patients had a performance status of 4. The overall response to the ACE combination chemotherapy is shown in Table 4. For each of the three studies there was no significant advantage to the addition of MER nonspecific immunotherapy, the use of alternating non–cross-resistant combinations, or the use of a 5-day continuous infusion of etoposide. Nevertheless, there was a high complete response rate (65%, limited disease; 43%, extensive disease). Overall the median duration of survival was 9½ months for extensive disease and 15 months for limited disease (Fig 2).

Table 4. Results of ACE ± Other Treatments

No. of patients	204
Median age (yr)	59
Range (yr)	29–76
Male/female (no. patients)	143/61
Limited/extensive disease (no. patients)	85/119
Performance status (no. patients)	
0–1	106
2–3	85
4	13
Limited CR (%)	55 (65)
Extensive CR (%)	51 (43)
Median no. courses to CR	2
Limited median survival (mo)	15
Extensive median survival (mo)	9.5

Abbreviation: CR, complete response.

Analysis of survival according to response in the various studies has shown clearly that only patients who achieve complete response are candidates for long-term disease-free survival. The median duration of survival for patients achieving complete response was in excess of 18 months for limited disease, and in excess of 14 months for patients with extensive disease. Nearly 40% of the patients with limited disease who achieved complete response were long-term disease-free survivors. Thus, these studies clearly showed that complete response is the only response parameter of any value in determining drug treatment efficacy.

The ACE chemotherapy regimen was highly manageable, with general patient acceptance; >80% of all chemotherapy courses were administered in the outpatient area. Most toxicity was managed by dose modifications. The median lowest WBC count nadir (each patient counted once) was 0.7 x $10^3 \mu L$, and the median WBC count nadir for all courses was $2.0 \times 10^3/\mu L$. The respective median platelet count nadirs were

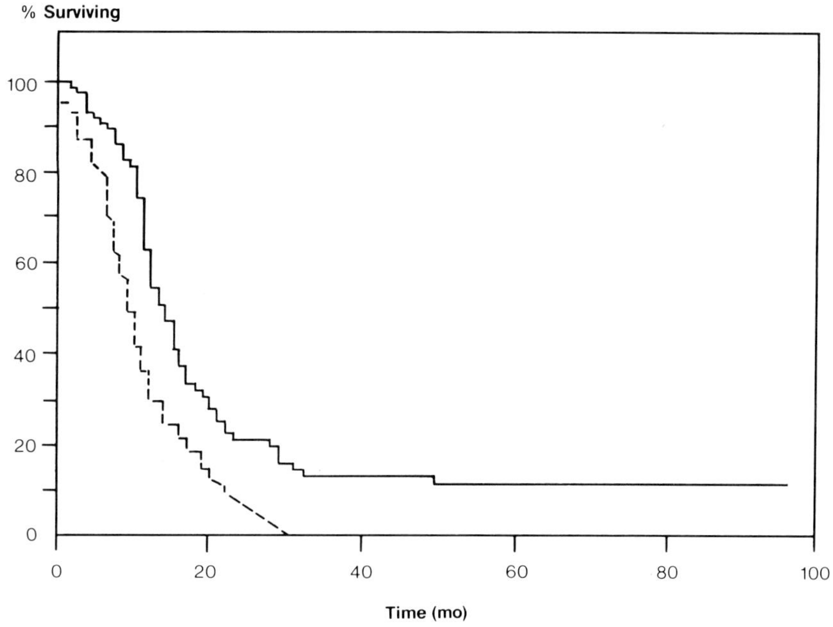

Fig 2. Uncensored cumulative survival curves (limited and extensive disease) for patients treated on three sequential ACE chemotherapy studies for SCLC, performed at the University of Maryland Cancer Center. There were two deaths due to unrelated cardiovascular events (myocardial) without evidence of cancer at postmortem. Two patients died with CNS metastases as the only cancer proven at necropsy. There was one late relapse at 48 months, and the patient died at 51 months. The median duration of survival for limited disease was nearly 15 months, and for extensive disease, nearly 10 months (Reprinted with permission.[44])

$67 \times 10^3/\mu L$ and $>120{,}000 \times 10^3/\mu L$. Nearly 20% of the patients were hospitalized one or more times with febrile neutropenic episodes, and nine patients (eight with performance status 4 and one with performance status 3) died from toxicity as a result of treatment. Although lethal toxicity was seen predominantly in the patients with the worst performance status (levels 3 and 4), some patients with performance status 4 had major objective responses (complete response and partial response) with improvement of performance status. Therefore, aggressive combination chemotherapy should not be denied to patients on the basis of poor performance status, if the deterioration of performance status was due to SCLC.

THE ADDITION OF CISPLATIN TO ACE

A number of studies in animal systems and clinical trials in humans, have demonstrated the synergistic potential of etoposide plus cisplatin (EP).[33-35,45] Subsequently, the combination of EP was studied as a salvage regimen in patients previously treated with cyclophosphamide, doxorubicin, and vincristine (CAV) and as initial treatment for SCLC.[36,37,46,47] These studies showed that EP was active (and therefore probably synergistic) as a salvage regimen, and furthermore, its level of activity as an initial treatment was similar to that of other initial aggressive combination chemotherapy regimens. These observations have led to further testing of alternating non–cross-resistant combination chemotherapies with CAV alternating with EP. To date, no alternating combinations of agents have been shown to be superior to the use of combinations of the most effective drugs, used as primary therapy for as long as possible and for at least six courses.[47]

An alternative approach to incorporating cisplatin into primary therapy of SCLC was the attempt to integrate EP into existing front-line combination chemotherapy. Thus, the addition of cisplatin to the ACE regimen (PACE) was undertaken in an attempt to improve response and duration of survival. Two pilot PACE studies were generated. The first study involved patients with both limited and extensive disease at the University of Maryland Cancer Center and at North Shore University Hospital. The second

Table 5. PACE Combination Chemotherapy

Drug	Dosage and Schedule	
Cisplatin	20 mg/m^2	IV days 1-5
Doxorubicin	45 mg/m^2	IV day 1
Cyclophosphamide	800 mg/m^2	IV day 1
Etoposide	50 mg/m^2	IV days 1-5
Each course	21 days	Cycles 1-3
	28 days	Cycles 4-8

Abbreviations: IV, intravenous.

pilot study was conducted under the auspices of the Cancer and Acute Leukemia Group B (CALGB), but was limited to patients with extensive disease. The preliminary data for both studies were recently reported.[48] The dose and schedule of PACE chemotherapy are shown in Table 5. Courses were repeated every 21 days for the first three courses and adjusted for toxicity. Modification of cisplatin dosages was based on creatinine clearance measurements in the first study, and serum creatinine measurements in the second study. Patient characteristics, response, and current median survivals for the two studies are shown in Table 6. All patients with complete response received prophylactic cranial irradiation. In the University of Maryland Cancer Center study, PACE was moderately tolerated with uniform nausea, vomiting, and alopecia. Aggressive hydration, antiemetics, and hospitalization were required for virtually all courses. The median lowest WBC count nadir was $0.5 \times 10^3/\mu L$, and the median lowest platelet count nadir was $16 \times 10^3/\mu L$. There were 21 infectious episodes among 33 patients and two septic deaths—both among patients with Karnofsky performance status <50%. Serial creatinine clearances and neuropathies required discontinuation of cisplatin in 22 of the 33 patients. Median number of cisplatin-containing courses was five of a planned eight. Toxicities in the CALGB extensive-disease study were similar, with 17% severe and 59% life-threatening toxicities, including 25% leukopenia, 25% thrombocytopenia, and 8% neuropathies. Although the University of Maryland Cancer Center study and the CALGB pilot study were not comparison studies, the complete response frequency in both was higher than previously recorded at the single institution and the cooperative group, respectively. Furthermore, an interim analysis of the survival curves of both studies suggests that there may be an improved median duration of survival and probably an elevated plateau of long-term survivors. Nevertheless, the addition of cisplatin to the ACE combination chemotherapy produced enhanced toxicities when compared historically to ACE combination chemotherapy. Thus, further analysis of the improvement in response and survival is necessary in order to assess whether the increase in toxicity is warranted.

In addition, further studies are necessary to determine the best way to exploit the potential synergy of these four agents. A number of studies are currently in progress that attempt, at least in part, to assess these various drug interactions. One such study in extensive disease conducted by the CALGB is a phase I/II determination of escalating doses of both cisplatin and etoposide, as well as a substitution of the platinum analogs carboplatin and chip for cisplatin. Another study being conducted by the CALGB utilizes ACE for three courses, followed by PCE, (cisplatin substituted for doxorubicin) with concurrent chest irradiation during the PCE chemotherapy administration. Prophylactic cranial irradiation will be administered during this period. In addi-

Table 6. Results of PACE Chemotherapy for Small-Cell Lung Cancer

	Study I		Study II
	LD	ED	ED
No. of patients	15	18	26*
Male/female (no. of patients)	11/14	14/4	18/8
Median age (yr)	58	57	58
Range (yr)	44-76	40-74	—
Performance status (no. patients)			
0	5	6	9
1	8	4	10
2	0	6	4
3	1	1	1
4	1	1	1
CR (%)	9 (60)	7 (39)	7/19 (37)†
Median survival (mo)	14+	15	10.5
% alive at 2 years (projected)	(48)	10	(20)

Abbreviations: LD, limited disease; ED, extensive disease; CR, complete response.

*One patient never received therapy and one had non-small-cell lung cancer.

†Final data not available for five patients.

tion, warfarin sodium will be added in a randomized fashion to this therapy regimen in an attempt to test the suggestions from a prior CALGB study[49] and studies by Zacharski et al[50] that this drug may play a potential role in SCLC therapy. Finally, it is likely that the four-drug PACE combination will need to be reexplored with either dosage modifications or randomizations to determine the role of the various agents within the combination. The careful step-wise application of combination chemotherapy and the identification of highly active and synergistic combinations will improve systemic treatment for this disease, affording the opportunity for improved combined modalities and a greater percentage of long-term disease-free survivors.

REFERENCES

1. Muggia FM, Krezoski SK, Hansen HH: Cell kinetics studies in patients with small cell carcinoma of the lung. Cancer 34:1683–1690, 1974

2. Cohen MH, Matthews MJ: Small cell bronchogenic carcinoma: A distinct clinicopathologic entity. Semin Oncol 5:234–243, 1978

3. Cohen MH: Signs and symptoms of bronchogenic carcinoma. Semin Oncol 1:183–189, 1975

4. Carney D, Broder L, Edelstein M, et al: Experimental studies of the biology of human small cell lung cancer. Cancer Treat Rep 67:27–35, 1983

5. Greco FA, Oldham RK: Small cell lung cancer. N Engl J Med 301:355–358, 1979

6. Hansen HH, Dombernowsky P, Hirsch F: Staging procedures and prognostic features in small cell anaplastic bronchogenic carcinoma. Semin Oncol 5:280–287, 1978

7. Osterlind K, Ihde DC, Ettinger DS, et al: Staging and prognostic factors in small cell carcinoma of the lung. Cancer Treat Rep 67:3–9, 1983

8. Matthews MJ, Kanhouwa S, Pickren J, et al: Frequency of residual and metastatic tumor in patients. Cancer Chemother Rep 4:63–67, 1973

9. Mountain CF: Surgical therapy in lung cancer: Biologic, physiologic and technical determinants. Semin Oncol 1:253–258, 1974

10. Medical Research Council: First report to the Medical Research Council by the working party on the evaluation of different methods of therapy in carcinoma of the bronchus: Comparative trial of surgery and radiotherapy, for the primary treatment of small-celled or oat-celled carcinoma of the bronchus. Lancet 2:979–986, 1966

11. Medical Research Council Lung Cancer Working Party: Radiotherapy alone or with chemotherapy in the treatment of small-cell carcinoma of the lung. Br J Cancer 40:1–10, 1979

12. Aisner J: Is combined modality treatment of small cell carcinoma of the lung necessary? in Wiernik PH (ed): Controversies in Oncology. New York, Wiley and Sons, 1982, pp 155–173

13. Aisner J, Ablert P, Bitran J, et al: Role of chemotherapy in small cell lung cancer: A consensus report of the international association for the study of lung cancer workshop. Cancer Treat Rep 67:37–43, 1983

14. Aisner J, Whitacre M, Van Echo DA, et al: Doxorubicin, cyclophosphamide and etoposide (ACE) by bolus or continuous infusion of small cell carcinoma for the lung (SCCL). Proc Am Soc Clin Oncol 2:196, 1983 (abstr)

15. Aisner J, Whitacre MY, Van Echo DA, et al: Combination chemotherapy for small cell carcinoma of the lung: Continuous vs. alternating non-cross resistant combination. Cancer Treat Rep 66:221–230, 1982

16. Aisner J, Wiernik PH: Chemotherapy vs. chemoimmunotherapy for small cell undifferentiated carcinoma of the lung. Cancer 46:2543–2549, 1980

17. Whitley NO, Fuks JZ, McCrae E, et al: Computerized tomography of the chest in small cell lung cancer: Staging, follow-up and prognostic factors. Am J Radiol 141:885–892, 1984

18. Cohen MH: Is thoracic radiation therapy necessary for patients with limited stage small cell lung cancer? No. Cancer Treat Rep 67:217–221, 1983

19. Mira JG, Livingston RB: Evaluation of radiotherapy implications of chest relapse patterns in small cell lung carcinoma treated with radiotherapy-chemotherapy: Study of 34 cases and review of the literature. Cancer 46:2557–2565, 1980

20. Perez CA, Einhorn LH, Oldham RK, et al: Randomized trial of radiotherapy of the thorax in limited small cell carcinoma of the lung treated with multiagent chemotherapy and elective brain irradiation: A preliminary report. J Clin Oncol 2:1200–1208, 1984

21. Perry MC, Eaton WL, Ware J, et al: Chemotherapy with or without radiation therapy in limited small cell cancer of the lung. Am Soc Clin Oncol 3:230, 1984 (abstr)

22. Fox RM, Woods RL, Brodie GN, et al: A randomized study: Small cell anaplastic lung cancer treated by combination chemotherapy and adjuvant radiotherapy. Int J Radiat Oncol Biol Phys 6:1087–1092, 1983

23. Bunn P, Cohen M, Lichter A, et al: Randomized trial of chemotherapy versus chemotherapy plus radiotherapy in limited stage small cell lung cancer. Am Soc Clin Oncol 2:200, 1983 (abstr)

24. Perez CA, Einhorn L, Oldham RK, et al: Reporting for the Southeastern Cancer Study Group. Preliminary report on a randomized trial of radiotherapy (RT) to the thorax in limited small cell carcinoma of the lung treated with multiagent chemotherapy. Am Soc Clin Oncol 2:190, 1983

25. Catane R, Lichter A, Lee YJ, et al: Small cell lung cancer: Analysis of treatment factors contributing to prolonged survival. Cancer 48:1936–1943, 1981

26. Aisner J, Forastiere A, Aroney R: Patterns of recurrence for cancer of the lung and esophagus. Cancer Treat Symp 2:87–105, 1983

27. Roed H, Vindelow LL, Christensen IJ, et al: Comparison of the potential of the two epipodophyllotoxin derivatives VP16 and VM26 on small cell cancer cell lines. Proc Am Assoc Cancer Res 26:334, 1985

28. Smith IE, Harland SJ, Robinson BA, et al: Carboplatin: A very active new cisplatin analog in the treatment of small cell lung cancer. Cancer Treat Rep 69:43–46, 1985

29. Dombernowsky P, Nissen NI: Schedule dependency of the antileukemic activity of the podophyllotoxin derivative VP16-213 (NSC 141540) in L1210 leukemia. Arch Pathol Microbiol Scand 81:715–724, 1973

30. Venditti JR: Treatment schedule dependency of experimentally active antileukemic (L1210) drugs. Cancer Chemother Rep 2:35–59, 1971

31. Greco FA, Johnson DA, Hande KR, et al: High dose etoposide (VP16) in small cell lung cancer. Semin Oncol 12:42–44, 1985

32. Issell BF, Einhorn LH, Comis RL, et al: Multicenter phase II trial of etoposide in refractory small cell lung cancer. Cancer Treat Rep 69:127–128, 1985

33. Schabel FM Jr, Trader MW, Laster WR, et al: Cis-dichlorodiammine platinum II: Combination chemotherapy and cross resistance studies with tumors of mice. Cancer Treat Rep 63:1459–1473, 1979

34. Williams SD, Einhorn LH: Etoposide salvage therapy for refractory germ cell tumors: An update. Cancer Treat Rev 9:67–71, 1983 (suppl)

35. Bosl GJ, Yogada A, Goldbey RB, et al: Role of etoposide based chemotherapy in the treatment of patients with refractory or relapsing germ cell tumors. Am J Med 78:423–428, 1985

36. Evans WK, Osoba D, Feld R, et al: Etoposide (BP16) and cisplatin: An effective treatment for relapse in small cell lung cancer. J Clin Oncol 3:36–75, 1985

37. Sierocki JS, Hilaris BS, Hopfan E, et al: Cis-diamminedichloroplatinum (II) and VP 16-213: An active induction regimen for small cell carcinoma of the lung. Cancer Treat Rep 63:1593–1597, 1979

38. D'Incalci M, Farina P, Sessa C, et al: Pharmacokinetics of VP16 given by different administration methods. Proceedings of the First International Symposium on Podophyllotoxins in Cancer Therapy, Southampton, Great Britain, July 8–9, 1981, pp 51–60

39. Radice PA, Bunn PA Jr, Ihde DC: Therapeutic trials with VP16-213 and VM26: Active agents in small cell lung cancer, non-Hodgkin's lymphoma and other malignancies. Cancer Treat Rep 63:1231–1239, 1971

40. Poplin EA, Aisner J, Van Echo DA, et al: CCNU, vincristine, methotrexate, and procarbazine treatment of relapsed small cell lung carcinoma. Cancer Treat Rep 66:1557–1559, 1982

41. Goldie JH, Coldman AJ: A mathematic model for relating the drug sensitivity of tumors to their spontaneous mutation rate. Cancer Treat Rep 63:1727–1733, 1979

42. Aisner J, Van Echo DA, Whitacre M, et al: A phase I trial of continuous infusion VP16-213 (etoposide). Cancer Chemother Pharmacol 7:157–160, 1982

43. Aroney RS, Aisner J, Wesley MN, et al: The value of prophylactic cranial irradiation given at complete remission in small cell lung cancer. Cancer Treat Rep 67:675–682, 1983

44. Aisner J, Whitacre M, Van Echo DA, et al: Cyclophosphamide, doxorubicin and etoposide (CAE) for the treatment of small cell lung cancer, in Issell BF, Muggia FM, Carter SK (eds): Etoposide: Current Status and New Developments. Orlando, Fla, Academic, 1984, pp 171–182

45. Tinsley R, Comis R, DiFino S, et al: Potential clinical synergy observed in the treatment of small cell lung cancer with cisplatin and VP16-213. Proc Am Soc Clin Oncol 2:198, 1983 (abstr)

46. Havemann K, Harms V, Gropp C, et al: Randomized trial comparing sequential combination chemotherapy (A) with cyclic alternating chemotherapy (B) in small cell lung cancer. Am Soc Clin Oncol 3:232, 1984 (abstr)

47. Aisner J: Alternating chemotherapy for the treatment of small cell carcinoma of the lung, in Proceedings of the 13th International Congress on Chemotherapy. SY 70/4,205:16–23,1983

48. Aisner J, Whitacre MY, Budman D, et al: Platinum (P), doxorubicin (A), cyclophosphamide (C), and etoposide (E), PACE, for small cell lung cancer (SCLC). Am Soc Clin Oncol 4:181, 1985 (abstr)

49. Chahinian AP, Ware JH, Zimmer B, et al: Update on anticoagulation with warfarin and an alternating chemotherapy in extensive small cell cancer of the lung. Am Soc Clin Oncol 4:191, 1985 (abstr)

50. Zacharski LR, Henderson WG, Rickles FR, et al: Effect of warfarin on survival in small cell carcinoma of the lung. JAMA 245:831–834, 1981

Small-Cell Lung Cancer: A 10-Year Perspective

By Don V. Jackson, Jr and L. Douglas Case

Over the past 10 years, four clinical trials have been conducted with a total of 528 patients with previously untreated small-cell lung cancer. Trials I to III were randomized phase III studies testing the value of prophylactic cranial irradiation, immunotherapy, and etoposide, respectively. They were done in the setting of combined modality treatment with the same local chest radiotherapy (3,000 rad in 10 fractions) and combined agent chemotherapy using a nucleus of CAV (cyclophosphamide, doxorubicin, vincristine). Trial IV was a pilot study evaluating sequential hemibody radiotherapy in a combined modality treatment program with CAV. Overall, the best treatment results to date have been observed following the combination of etoposide with CAV in trial III, particularly for patients with extensive disease. This combination with or without other agents also appears to be a common component of many trials that have reported particularly good survival results in this disease.

DURING THE LAST DECADE, the potential capabilities of chemotherapy and radiotherapy in the treatment of small-cell lung cancer (SCLC) have become widely recognized. Rapid and impressive responses have been seen that are typical of tumors with a high growth fraction. Moreover, durable responses have been observed in some patients and the word "cure" has appeared in the literature dealing with this subject.

However, this optimism has been tempered by the sobering note of late relapses among long-term survivors and the fact that a "cure plateau" has not been reached on survival curves.[1] The median survival of patients with SCLC remains <1 year overall and <2 years in patients with relatively limited disease.[2] Therefore, the management of such patients, although improved, requires further investigation in the setting of carefully designed clinical trials that incorporate information derived from previous studies.

The current report, a review of the SCLC clinical trials done at the Bowman Gray School of Medicine and the Piedmont Oncology Association since 1974, focuses on our most active chemotherapy regimen tested to date in this disease, namely cyclophosphamide, doxorubicin (Adriamycin [Adria Laboratories, Columbus, OH]), vincristine, and etoposide.

MATERIALS AND METHODS

From 1974 through 1984, a total of 528 patients were entered into four prospective clinical trials performed at the Bowman Gray School of Medicine and in collaboration with members of the Piedmont Oncology Association (Table 1). Trials I and IV were done at Bowman Gray and trials II and III were performed within the Piedmont Oncology Association. Trials I to III were randomized to test the value of prophylactic cranial irradiation,[3] methanol extraction residue of Calmette-Guérin bacillus (MER-BCG),[4] and etoposide,[5,6] respectively. Trial IV was a pilot study assessing the addition of hemibody irradiation to chemotherapy and local chest radiotherapy.[7,8]

The basic chemotherapy program in all of these trials has been the three-drug regimen of cyclophosphamide, doxorubicin, and vincristine (CAV) to which was added CCNU (lomustine) and methotrexate in an alternating fashion in trial I and concomitantly in trial II (Table 2). Local chest radiotherapy has been used in each of the trials in both limited- and extensive-disease patients; the same dose and schedule have been used throughout with the exception of trial IV (Table 2). After completing the randomized trial of prophylactic cranial irradiation in trial I, all patients subsequently received prophylactic cranial irradiation.

The term "limited disease" in each of these trials refers to disease confined to one hemithorax, including ipsilateral supraclavicular adenopathy; all else was considered "extensive disease," including pleural effusion. In all of the trials, standard staging and evaluation procedures included hemograms, liver chemistries, chest x-ray, bone marrow, and radionuclide scans of the bone and liver. Evaluation of the brain at diagnosis was routine and was done with radionuclide scanning in trials I, II, and sometimes III. Cranial computed tomography (CT) was employed in trial IV and for most of the patients in trial III.

A complete response (CR) was defined as 100% reduction of all demonstrable tumor and no new areas of malignancy. Reevaluation involving invasive procedures such as bronchoscopy, liver biopsy, and bone marrow aspiration and biopsy were not mandatory. A partial response (PR) was at least a 50% reduction of the product of the longest perpendicular diameters of the indicator lesion(s) since first measured and no new areas of malignancy.

Trials I and II were closed in 1976 and 1979, respectively, and patients have been followed from those dates. At the

From the Oncology Research Center and the Piedmont Oncology Association, Bowman Gray School of Medicine of Wake Forest University, Winston-Salem, NC.

Supported in part by NIH Grants, CA-12197 and CA-33499, National Cancer Institute, Bethesda, Md.

Address reprint requests to Don V. Jackson, Jr, MD, Bowman Gray School of Medicine of Wake Forest University, 300 S Hawthorne Rd, Winston-Salem, NC 27103.

0093-7754/86/1303-3004$05.00/0

Table 1. Bowman Gray School of Medicine/Piedmont Oncology Association Clinical Trials 1974–1984 for SCLC

Trial	Date	Type	No. of Patients	Test (Reference)
I	1974–1976	Randomized	81	Prophylactic cranial irradiation[3]
II	1977–1979	Randomized	142	Immunotherapy (MER-BCG)[4]
III	1980–1984	Randomized	259	Etoposide[5,6]
IV	1981–1983	Nonrandomized	46	Hemibody radiotherapy[7,8]

Abbreviation: MER-BCG, methanol extraction residue of Calmette-Guérin bacillus.

present time, only one patient in trial I and two patients in trial II remain alive. At the time of analysis of trials III and IV (November 1984), which was done in preparation for the Fourth World Conference on Lung Cancer (Aug 1985), the median follow-up times were 26 and 23 months, respectively.

For ease of presentation, the arms of trials I and II have been collapsed and the cumulative data will be given, since there was no statistically significant difference in the response or survival results between the two arms of those studies. The data from both the cumulative and individual arms will be presented for trial III, since there were some interesting differences between these two treatment arms. No statistical comparisons were made between different trials due to the general inappropriateness of historical controls. Within trial III, comparisons were made using the chi-square test for categorical variables and the Wilcoxon rank-sum test for continuous variables. Time-related distributions were estimated using the product-limit method and medians were calculated by interpolation of these estimates. The log rank

Table 3. Patient Characteristics

Trial	No. of Evaluable Patients	Median Age Yr (Range)	Sex (M) (%)	Extensive Disease (%)	Performance Status† (0–2) (%)
I	54*	59 (43–77)	72	65	94
II	102	58 (36–78)	70	65	95
III	242	58 (28–78)	64	47	95
CAV	119	58 (38–73)	66	45	95
VCAV	123	58 (28–78)	63	50	95
IV	46	63 (40–79)	72	48	98

Abbreviations: CAV, cyclophosphamide, doxorubicin, vincristine; VCAV, etoposide, cyclophosphamide, doxorubicin, vincristine.

*Included eight patients who presented with brain metastasis.

†Performance status scale: 0, normal activity; 1, fully ambulatory with symptoms; 2, <50% bedridden and able to care for themselves; 3, >50% bedridden; and 4, 100% bedridden.

test was used to test for differences in distributions unadjusted for pretreatment characteristics. Regression techniques were used to adjust for these factors.

RESULTS

Patient Characteristics

Patient characteristics are given in Table 3. Of the 528 patients entered over a 10-year period into these four clinical trials, 444 (84%) were evaluable for analysis (67%, 72%, 93%, and 100% of patients in trials I to IV, respectively). The median age was 58 to 63 years (range, 28 to 79 years). The male gender predominated and

Table 2. Treatment

Trial	Drug	Doses (mg/m^2) C	A	V	Other	Radiotherapy (Rad/Fractions)	Concurrent RT/CAV
I	CAV alternating with CCNU and M	400	30	1	CCNU–50 M–15*	Local chest (3,000/10)	Yes
II	CAV with concomitant CCNU and M	500	40	1	CCNU–50, M–20 ± MER-BCG†	Local chest (3,000/10) Cranial (3,000/10)	Yes
III	CAV ± etoposide	1,000	50	1.5	±Etoposide –60 × 5d‡	Local chest (3,000/10) Cranial (3,000/10)	No
IV	CAV	1,000	50	1.5	—	Local chest (2,000/10) Cranial (2,000/10) Hemibody (600/1 × 2)§	No

Abbreviations: C, cyclophosphamide; A, doxorubicin; V, vincristine; M, methotrexate; RT, radiotherapy; MER-BCG, methanol extraction residue of Calmette-Guérin bacillus.

*After CAV was given every 2 weeks for 3 months, CCNU 50 mg/m^2 every 4 weeks and methotrexate 15 mg/m^2 twice weekly were given for 3 months alternating with CAV for 3 months, etc.

†CAV was given every 3 weeks with concomitant CCNU every 6 weeks and methotrexate every 3 weeks; MER-BCG 0.4 mg was given every 6 weeks.

‡Induction consisted of CAV plus etoposide given every 3 weeks for 3 cycles; RT was given 2 weeks after the third induction course of chemotherapy; maintenance was begun 2 weeks after completion of RT (≅week 12) and consisted of C, 750 mg/m^2; A, 50 mg/m^2; V, 1.5 mg/m^2 (2.0 mg maximum) ± etoposide 250 mg/m^2 × 1 d every 3 weeks.

§After two cycles of CAV, upper hemibody RT (600 rad) was given and 2 weeks later C and V were given and followed 3 days later by local RT; subsequently two cycles of CAV were given, following which lower hemibody RT (600 rad) was given.

Table 4. Pretreatment Sites of Involvement*

Trial	Patients (%)					
	Nodes	Bone	Liver	Pleural Effusion	Bone Marrow	Brain
I	39	30	22	15	11	11
II	12	28	17	21	11	2
III	23	14	17	9	12	7
CAV	24	14	17	7	10	9
VCAV	22	14	17	11	14	6
IV	22	17	28	7	15	7

*Some patients had more than one site of disease and these data are included in the Table.

accounted for approximately two thirds of the patients. Perhaps a slight increase in the number of women occurred more recently, as observed in trial III. In the first half of this 10-year period, extensive disease was present at diagnosis in two thirds of the patients, but more recently the extent of disease has been equally divided between limited and extensive disease. The performance status at the onset of study appears to have remained constant and has been poor (grade 3 to 4) in only approximately 5% of patients in each of the trials.

The sites of involvement in addition to lung, which were discovered during the pretreatment staging evaluation, are listed in Table 4. As noted above, less extensive disease has been encountered in the more recent trials. The reduction in the percentage of patients with sites of involvement other than lung appears to have occurred across the board with the exception of liver and bone marrow metastases. Pretreatment hepatic and marrow involvement has been present in an average of 21% and 12% of the patients, respectively.

Response

The overall response rate has varied from 63% in trials I and IV to 84% in the etoposide arm of trial III (Table 5). The difference in the overall response rate (64% *v* 84%) between the two treatments arms of trial III (CAV *v* VCAV [etoposide, cyclophosphamide, doxorubicin, vincristine]) was significant ($P = .001$) in favor of the etoposide arm. This difference remained significant after adjustment for pretreatment characteristics (age, performance status, sex, number of disease sites, and others) using logistic regression analysis. The CR rate in patients with limited disease appears to have improved in the last half of this 10-year review. Whereas CRs in patients with limited disease were observed in 32% to 39% of those in trials I and II, this occurred in 52% to 56% of patients in trials III and IV. No difference in the complete or overall response rate was observed between the two arms of trial III in limited-disease patients.

The overall response rate in patients with extensive disease has varied from 35% in trial IV to 84% in trial III, with an average of 54%. The difference in the overall response rate in patients with extensive disease (40% *v* 84%) between the two arms of trial III (CAV *v* VCAV) was statistically significant in favor of the etoposide arm before and after adjustment for covariates ($P < .0001$). The highest CR rate (34%) observed in patients with extensive disease during this 10-year review period has been observed in the etoposide arm of trial III. This was significantly greater than the CR rate (14%) in the nonetoposide arm of trial III ($P = .04$) and remained so after adjustment for pretreatment characteristics ($P = .02$).

Response durations are given in Table 6. Through the years there appears to be a gradual and moderate increase in the duration of overall

Table 5. Response

Trial	% Patients				
	Overall	Limited Disease		Extensive Disease	
	CR + PR	PR	CR	PR	CR
I	63	47	32	29	26
II	65	33	39	36	24
III	74	26	55	39	25
CAV	64	24	54	26	14
VCAV	84	28	56	50	34
IV	63	35	52	20	15

Table 6. Duration of Response*

Trial	Median (mo)			
	Overall CR + PR	Overall CR	Limited Disease CR	Extensive Disease CR
I	4.9	9.9	18.7	8.3
II	7.8	14.0	14.7	13.4
III	8.8	13.6	13.7	10.3
CAV	8.2	11.2	10.7	—†
VCAV	9.4	14.7	17.1	9.7
IV	8.9	14.9	15.3	7.0

*Duration of response was calculated from the first noted response until relapse.

†The median duration of the four patients with extensive disease who had a CR in the CAV arm has not been reached; these response durations are 2.1+, 4.0+, 4.1+, and 5.6+ months.

Table 7. Time to Progression*

Trial	Median (mo)		
	Overall	Limited Disease	Extensive Disease
I	7.6	7.9	6.4
II	8.2	11.0	7.3
III	9.4	12.2	6.8
CAV	8.2	10.7	6.3
VCAV	10.4	13.4	8.4
IV	7.8	10.3	4.4

*Median number of months from the onset of therapy until the time of disease progression.

response (CR + PR), varying from a median of 4.9 months in trial I to 9.4 months in the etoposide arm of trial III. There was no significant difference in overall response duration (8.2 *v* 9.4 months) between the two arms of trial III (CAV *v* VCAV). The differences in duration of CR between the two arms of trial III for limited disease, extensive disease, or overall response were not statistically significant ($P = .3$, .3, and .6, respectively).

The estimated median time to disease progression after the onset of therapy is given in Table 7. Overall, the median time to progression has varied from 7.6 months in trial I to 10.4 months in the etoposide arm of trial III. The overall times to progression for both arms of trial III are shown in Fig 1. The difference in the time to progression distributions (median 8.2 *v* 10.4 months) between the two arms of trial III (CAV *v* VCAV) was significant ($P = .04$) and remained so after adjustment for covariates ($P = .02$). The difference (6.3 *v* 8.4 months) in extensive disease was in favor of the etoposide arm ($P = .008$). However, the latter difference was not statistically significant after adjustment for pretreatment variables. There was a favorable trend but no significant difference (10.7 *v* 13.4 months) in limited disease before ($P = .2$) and after adjustment for covariables ($P = .3$).

The major site of relapse throughout all the trials has been the lung, varying from 38% in trial IV to 55% in the CAV arm of trial III (Table 8). There were no remarkable differences between other sites of initial relapse with the exception of brain. Brain as an initial site of relapse has varied from 2% of patients in trial II

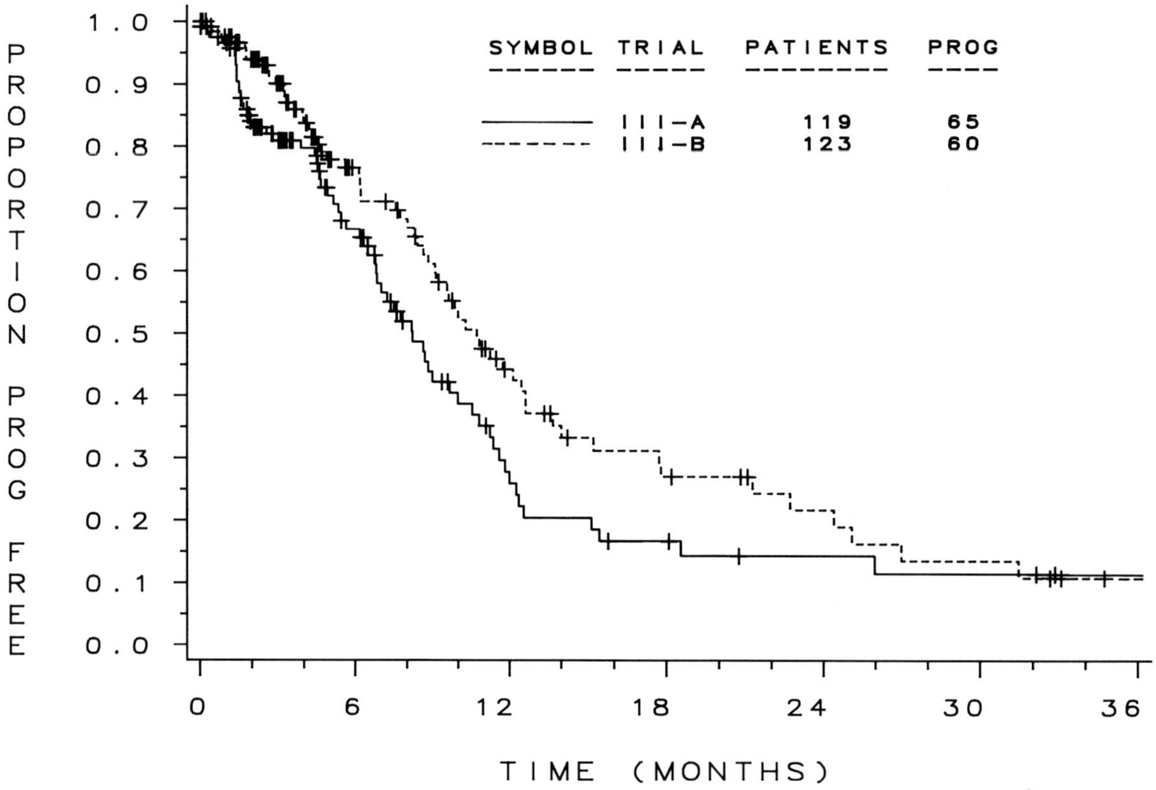

Fig 1. Time to progression in trial III testing chemotherapy with CAV (arm A) in both limited and extensive disease combined *v* CAV plus etoposide (arm B) in both limited and extensive disease combined.

Table 8. Sites of Initial Relapse*

Trial	Patients (%) Lung	Bone	Liver	Nodes	Brain	Pleural Effusion
I	46	23	27	23	23†	8
II	39	37	14	2	2	3
III	48	23	15	14	12	9
CAV	55	23	14	13	9	9
VCAV	39	22	15	15	20	9
IV	38	29	21	17	8	8

*Percentage of patients of those who had documented sites of progression. Some patients relapsed simultaneously in more than one site and these data are included in the Table.

†Includes only one patient who developed brain metastasis following prophylactic cranial irradiation.

to 23% of patients in trial I. In the latter trial only one of 26 evaluable patients (48%) who had been randomized to receive prophylactic cranial irradiation developed brain metastasis, whereas four of 20 evaluable patients (20%) who did not receive this treatment did so; brain relapse was also observed in one patient who received therapeutic cranial irradiation for known brain metastasis at the time of diagnosis. Prophylactic cranial irradiation was given at the onset of treatment in one arm of trial I and all of the patients in trial II, but was delayed until the eighth week of therapy in trial III and the ninth week of therapy in trial IV. Initial relapse occurred in the brain in 9% of patients in the CAV arm of trial III *v* 20% of patients in the VCAV arm. This difference was not significant ($P = .1$), but the numbers are really too small for meaningful comparison.

Survival

Median survival and 2-year survival data are detailed in Tables 9 and 10. Survivorship is shown graphically in Figs 2 and 3. A gradual and modest increase in overall survival is apparent over the 10-year span of this analysis, varying

Table 9. Survival*

Trial	Median (mo) Overall	Limited Disease	Extensive Disease
I	8.1	9.6	5.3
II	9.1	10.0	8.9
III	10.5	14.6	8.3
CAV	9.4	14.0	6.4
VCAV	11.2	15.0	9.4
IV	9.8	14.0	5.4

*Median number of months calculated from time on study until death or last date of contact.

Table 10. Two-Year Survival*

Trial	No. of Patients: Overall Total	Overall CR	Limited Disease Total	Limited Disease CR	Extensive Disease Total	Extensive Disease CR	2-yr Survival (Estimated %)†
I	11	7	7	4	4	3	20.4 ± 5.5
II	14	14	7	7	7	7	13.7 ± 3.4
III	19	17	16	14	3	3	17.4 ± 3.2
CAV	9	7	9	7	0	0	13.9 ± 4.0
VCAV	10	10	7	7	3	3	21.4 ± 4.8
IV	3	3	3	3	0	0	31.5 ± 7.9

*Total number of patients surviving 2 or more years and number of those patients in CR at that point are given.

†Estimated percentage (±SE).

from 8.1 months in trial I to 11.2 months in the etoposide arm of trial III. The difference in overall survival (9.4 *v* 11.2 months) between the two arms of trial III (CAV *v* VCAV) is not significant ($P = .3$).

A moderate increase in survival of patients with limited disease has been observed ranging from 9.6 months in trial I to 15 months in the etoposide arm of trial III. There was no significant difference in the survival of patients with limited disease between the CAV and VCAV arms (14.0 and 15.0 months, respectively) of trial III ($P = .8$).

There has also been a moderate increase in survival of patients with extensive disease varying from 5.3 months in trial I to 9.4 months in the etoposide arm of trial III. The median survival for a small group of 22 patients was only 5.4 months in trial IV. The difference in the survival of patients with extensive disease (6.4 *v* 9.4 months) between the two arms of trial III (CAV *v* VCAV) was significant ($P = .02$) in favor of the etoposide arm. However, this difference was not significant after adjustment for pretreatment characteristics ($P = .20$). This can be explained in part by the imbalance in the distributions of age and sex. There was a greater proportion of younger patients (24% *v* 12%, age <50 years) and females (43% *v* 30%) in the etoposide arm. Cox regression analysis indicated the following covariables to be significantly associated with survival when all extensive-disease patients in trial III were taken into account: age ($P = .0048$), sex ($P = .0002$), performance status ($P = .0407$), and number of sites of disease ($P = .0317$); younger age, female sex, performance status of grade 0 to 1, and fewer sites of disease were the favorable pretreatment characteristics.

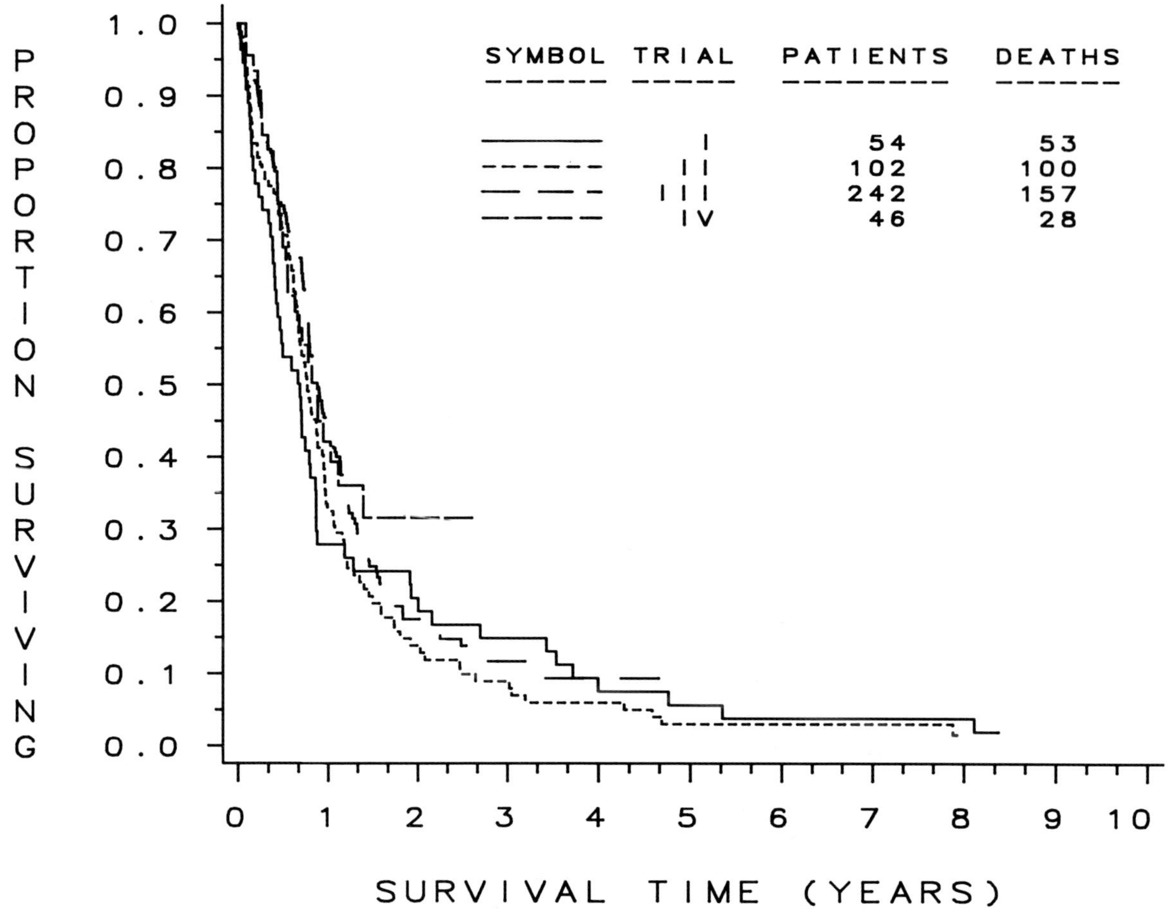

Fig 2. Survival distribution by combining the arms of trial I, trial II, and trial III, which were randomized studies testing the value of prophylactic cranial irradiation, immunotherapy, and etoposide, respectively. The survival of patients in trial IV, which evaluated hemibody radiotherapy, is also shown.

Overall 2-year survival estimates (Table 10) have been between 13.7 ± 3.4% in trial II and 31.5 ± 7.9% in trial IV (although a number of patients were censored in trial III and IV at the time of this analysis). The number of patients with limited disease surviving 2 years with or without active disease was similar in the two arms of trial III. At the time of this analysis, there have been three 2-year survivors among patients with extensive disease in the etoposide arm and none in the CAV arm of trial III. Only one patient in trial I and two patients in trial II remain alive at 8.4, 6.3, and 7.9 years, respectively.

Toxicity

The principal toxicities observed during these trials are listed in Table 11. Myelosuppression of a moderate to severe nature has been common in each of the trials. Grade 3 to 4 WBC count toxicity varied from 23% in trial II and the CAV arm of trial III to 49% in the etoposide arm of trial III ($P = .0001$). The frequency of moderate to severe thrombocytopenia has been observed in 10% of the patients in each of the trials, except in trial IV in which a platelet count $<50{,}000/\mu L$ occurred in 27% of the patients following hemibody radiotherapy in combination with multiagent chemotherapy. Esophagitis was observed most frequently (60% of patients) in the latter trial as well, but was generally mild to moderate; only 4% of patients had grade 3 esophagitis, and none had grade 4. The most severe episodes of esophagitis have been observed during concurrent administration of doxorubicin-containing chemotherapy and chest radiotherapy in trials I

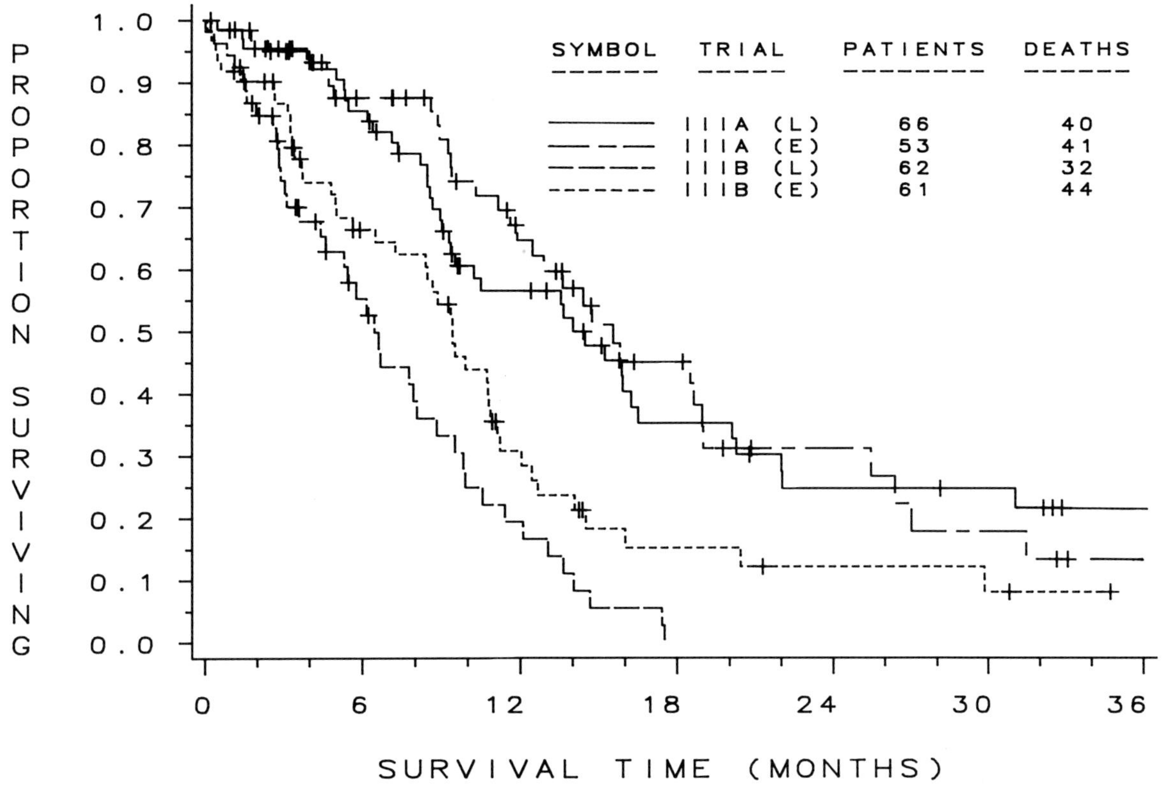

Fig 3. Survivorship in trial III, which tested the value of etoposide by randomizing patients to receive chemotherapy with CAV (arm A) for limited disease or extensive disease *v* chemotherapy with CAV plus etoposide (arm B) for limited disease or extensive disease.

and II. In trial III, in which only vincristine was given during radiotherapy, the frequency and severity of esophagitis was markedly reduced (15% of patients overall, 7% with grade 3, and none with grade 4). The frequency of probable therapy-related deaths has been less than 5% in each of the trials.

DISCUSSION

Although statistical comparisons of the results between these four studies spanning a 10-year period would not be valid, there are a number of interesting observations worthy of comment. In terms of patient characteristics, there has been no change in the median age of the patient or the pretreatment performance status. There may be a slight increase in the proportion of female patients, which is consistent with the trend in the United States of increasing incidence of lung cancer in women.[9]

Most striking is the trend toward presentation with less advanced disease. Perhaps this is a reflection of a greater awareness of lung cancer in our region, which has been associated with both earlier diagnosis and recognition of the availability of potentially effective treatment, particularly for the small-cell variant of lung cancer. An example of this phenomenon, perhaps, is the finding of fewer patients with brain metastasis at the time of diagnosis or during pretreatment staging evaluation. This trend has been apparent even though more patients with asymptomatic brain involvement have been dis-

Table 11. Toxicity

	Patients (%)			
Trial	WBC <2,000/μL	Platelets <50,000/μL	Esophagitis	Probable Therapy-Related Death
I	33	7	Common	3
II	23	4	39	1
III	36	8	15	2
CAV	23	7	12	2
VCAV	49	10	17	4
IV	27	27	60	4

covered through the routine use of CT rather than scanning with the less sensitive radionuclide technique.[10] Currently, however, we seem to be witnessing a trend of increasing extent of disease at presentation, perhaps as a consequence of abdominal CT scanning.[11] The value of routine abdominal CT scanning is underscored by three recently reported studies evaluating this staging procedure.[12–14] Among a total of 166 patients, adrenal involvement was observed in 20% (range, 15% to 31%) of patients and enlarged nodes were present in 7% (range, 3% to 12%).

In each of the four trials, an objective response was observed in the majority of patients. However, little change in the response rate occurred overall during this 10-year period, with about two thirds to three fourths of the patients evidencing a response. The most active regimen in this series has been the etoposide arm of trial III, in which an objective response occurred in 84% of the patients, significantly greater than that in the arm containing identical chemotherapy but without etoposide. This is largely attributed to the greater responsiveness in patients with extensive disease in whom a 34% CR rate and 50% PR rate were noted. These were the highest CR and PR rates for patients with extensive disease seen in any of these trials. Otherwise, the objective response rate in extensive-disease patients has been largely static over the past 10 years. The modest increase in CR in limited disease over this period from about 30% to 50% may be a reflection of the more aggressive chemotherapy dosages used in later years as seen in Table 2. The radiotherapy dose schedule was constant in trials I to III, and the overall dosage to the chest in the hemibody radiotherapy protocol (trial IV) was approximately 3,000 rad or less (2,000 rad conventional plus 600 rad upper hemibody).

The overall response duration and time to progression have improved but only to a modest degree, with the best results observed in the etoposide arm of trial III, particularly among patients with extensive disease. Overall, a significantly longer time to the appearance of disease progression was observed in patients receiving etoposide in addition to the CAV combination.

As found in the majority of reports in SCLC, the chest remains the major site of relapse in each of these trials despite thoracic irradiation. However, the radiation dosage used in these trials (3,000 rad in ten fractions) is currently under question, since higher doses (≥4,000 rad) appear to be correlated with better local control.[15–17] Currently, a dose of 4,800 rad delivered in 24 fractions is being used in patients with limited disease.[11]

Prophylactic cranial irradiation, used routinely since the randomized trial of 1974 to 1976,[3] has reduced the expected frequency of brain mestastasis during the course of the disease from approximately 20% to an average of approximately 7%. The best results using this technique have been observed when it was given at the start of therapy. This was done for some patients in trial I and all in trial II; <5% of patients relapsed in the brain, whereas approximately 10% to 20% did so when prophylactic cranial radiotherapy was given in a delayed fashion (beginning week 8 to 9 in trials III and IV). This suggests the need to reassess the timing of prophylactic cranial irradiation.

Serial CT scanning of the brain over a course of several years following prophylactic cranial irradiation has shown some bothersome results.[18] Among 13 patients examined with cranial CT scans at 6- to 9-month intervals posttreatment all had evidence of cerebral atrophy, which often worsened with time; and white-matter changes were observed in 15%. These changes may correlate with the neurologic difficulties sometimes observed in the minority of patients following prophylactic cranial irradiation.[19–22] The optimal radiation dose schedule to reduce the frequency of these problems and still prevent the common occurrence of brain metastasis needs to be determined. In all of the previous trials, a dose of 3,000 rad given in ten fractions has been used. A dose of 2,400 rad delivered in 12 fractions is being used in the current trial.[11]

It is a humbling experience to review the overall survival results attained in a decade of one's clinical trials; there has been no major increase in survival over this time period. Perhaps some minor progress to this end can be seen (Table 9), especially with comparison of the last three trials to the first one. Quite clear is the fact, however, that there is a continuum of relapse and death (Fig 2). Less than 2% of the patients in trials I and II remain alive. Indeed, there is no apparent survival plateau, as recently pointed out by Bergsagel and Feld.[1]

Overall, the most active regimen among these trials has been that of CAV plus etoposide, particularly in extensive disease. At the time of this analysis, there has been approximately a 3-month survival advantage for patients with extensive disease compared with the CAV-alone arm. This difference may in part be due to the chance occurrence of a greater proportion of patients with more of the favorable pretreatment characteristics (younger age and female sex) as determined by logistic regression analysis. No survival advantage has been demonstrated for limited disease.

Three other randomized trials have compared the regimen of CAV with varying modifications of it that have included etoposide.[23–25] As in our results, the potential benefits associated with inclusion of etoposide appear to occur primarily in patients with extensive disease. Messeih et al[23] compared CAV with CAV plus etoposide and found significantly greater CR rates in extensive disease (0% *v* 35%, respectively), but no increase in survival. There have been two preliminary reports from the Bristol Lung Cancer Study Group dealing with this subject that show encouraging survival results in favor of etoposide for patients with extensive disease, but no improvement in patients with limited disease.[24–25] In one trial, CAV, CV (cyclophosphamide, vincristine) plus etoposide, and CV were compared with the finding of objective response (complete and partial) in 51%, 58%, and 43% of patients with extensive disease, respectively.[24] The longest median survival time among these patients was found in the CV plus etoposide group (7.8 months) compared with 4.8 months in the CAV arm and 5.3 months in the CV arm. In the other trial, CAV was compared with CA (cyclophosphamide, doxorubicin) plus etoposide.[25] Again, the results appeared favorable for the etoposide combination, but only in patients with extensive disease. Objective response rates (complete plus partial) among these patients were 50% in the CAV arm compared with 74% in the etoposide combination, with median survival times of 4.7 and 13.5 months, respectively. The latter difference was stated to be significant ($P = .044$).[25]

How do the survival results of our most active regimen (CAV plus etoposide) compare with those of other trials during this 10-year period? Many trials, in fact most, report median survival time <17 months for limited disease and <12 months for extensive disease, especially those conducted in the 1970s.[2,26] Table 12 lists the characteristics of trials in limited disease in which the median survival time was reported to be 15 months or greater.[6,15,27–42] Among 17 such trials, there were 18 regimens that were associated with this range of median survival. All of the chemotherapy regimens contained both cyclophosphamide and doxorubicin. Vincristine was a part of 83% of the regimens and etoposide was present in 72%. About half or less of the regimens contained methotrexate, cisplatin, CCNU, procarbazine, or other drugs (nitrogen mustard, BCNU [carmustine] and BCG in one each). Radiation therapy was used in all but three regimens, and the dosage was about equally split between ≤4,000 rad and >4,000 rad. Continuous rather than split-course radiotherapy was used in all but three trials. Concurrent chemotherapy with radiotherapy was employed in 61% of the regimens, with the drugs used ranging from vincristine only[6] to cyclophos-

Table 12. Summary of Trials in Limited-Disease SCLC Reporting ≥15-Month Median Survival*

No. of Trials	Reference	No. of Patients	Drugs (% of regimens)								Radiation (% of regimens)†			
			C	A	V	VP	M	CP	L	P	0	≤4	>4	CC
17 trials ≥ 15 mo (18 regimens)	6,16,27–42	546	100	100	83	72	56	44	39	39	17	39	44	61
11 trials ≥ 15–20 mo (11 regimens)	6,16,27–35	362	100	100	73	64	64	36	45	45	18	55	27	55
6 trials ≥ 20 mo (7 regimens)	36–42	184	100	100	100	86	43	57	29	29	14	14	71	71

Abbreviations: VP, etoposide; M, methotrexate; CP, cisplatinum; L, CCNU; P, procarbazine.

*Survival times were converted from weeks to months by dividing the reported number of weeks by a factor of 4.3 wk/mo.

†Radiation dosage is listed as: 0, none; ≤4, ≤4,000 rad; >4, >4,000 rad; and CC, concurrent chemotherapy.

phamide, doxorubicin, vincristine, methotrexate, CCNU, and procarbazine.[16] The percentage of treatment-related deaths in these 17 trials was reported to be between 0%[34,38,41] and 16%[16]; it was not stated in three trials.[28,32,42] The characteristics of six trials are also listed in Table 12, with reported median survival times ≥20 months in limited disease after treatment with seven different regimens.[36–42] The drug combination of cyclophosphamide, doxorubicin, vincristine, and etoposide with or without other agents was used in six of the seven regimens, the exception being one that used CAV alone.[36,37] Cisplatin was a part of four (57%) of the regimens. Methotrexate, CCNU, procarbazine, and nitrogen mustard were each a part of <50% of the regimens. Chest radiotherapy was used in six of the seven regimens and was given continuously rather than as a split course in all but one. The radiotherapy dosage was more aggressive than that used in regimens associated with median survivals ≥15 but <20 months; five of seven (71%) employed >4,000 rad. Concurrent chemotherapy was given with radiotherapy in five of the seven regimens and ranged from three drugs (CAV or CV plus etoposide)[36,39] to five drugs (CAV plus etoposide plus methotrexate).[42] The percentage of treatment-related deaths in these seven regimens varied between 0%[38,41] and 10%[36]; it was not stated in one report that involved two regimens.[42] From a review of the trials that have reported particularly long median survival times in patients with limited disease, radiotherapy to the chest employing doses >4,000 rad (usually given in a continuous course) appears to be a key ingredient. Concurrent administration of chemotherapy has also been a common component. Questions concerning radiotherapy dosage, schedule, and interaction with concurrent chemotherapy await further investigation in controlled clinical trials.

Among the 17 trials referred to in Table 12, patients with extensive disease were included in 14. There are three trials involving 56 such patients in which median survival times >1 year were reported. The median survival times (months) were 12.5,[30] 14.0,[39] and 15.0.[35] In each trial the drug combination employed was cyclophosphamide, doxorubicin, vincristine, etoposide, and cisplatin. Additionally, as previously mentioned, the Bristol Lung Cancer Study Group has reported a significantly greater survival (13.5 *v* 4.7 months) in extensive-disease patients who received cyclophosphamide, doxorubicin, and etoposide compared with those who received CAV.[25]

In summary, during the past 10 years a great deal has been learned about the treatment of SCLC. That is not to say, however, that tremendous gains have been attained in survival outcome. Certainly, some progress has been made in this area. A review of our own clinical trials as well as those of others has shown that combined-agent chemotherapy using the combination of cyclophosphamide, doxorubicin, vincristine, and etoposide with or without other drugs has been associated with some of the best treatment results in this disease. This four-drug combination has been especially active in patients with extensive disease. Other than the expected myelosuppression as seen in early phase 1 trials of single-agent etoposide,[43] there has been no unusual or compounding toxicity such as neurotoxicity[44] as previously suggested possible with the combination of vincristine and etoposide.[45] On the contrary, this particular drug combination (vincristine plus etoposide) in an animal model appears to have synergistic antitumor activity.[46,47] This and other leads are worthy of further investigation in a neoplasm such as SCLC, which appears to be highly responsive to treatment, but for which, thus far, there are few cures.

ACKNOWLEDGMENT

The vision and leadership of Dr Charles L. Spurr, and the support of the many physicians, nurses, and personnel in the statistical unit of the Oncology Research Center and the Piedmont Oncology Association, of the physician assistants and support personnel in the respective hospitals and clinics in a five-state area who assisted with these trials during the past 10 years, is appreciated.

REFERENCES

1. Bergsagel D, Feld R: Small-cell lung cancer is still a problem. J Clin Oncol 2:1189–1191, 1984 (editorial)

2. Morstyn G, Ihde DC, Lichter AS, et al: Small cell lung cancer 1973–1983: Early progress and recent obstacles. Int J Radiat Oncol Biol Phys 10:515–539, 1984

3. Jackson DV, Richards F, Cooper MR, et al: Prophylactic cranial irradiation in small cell carcinoma of the lung. JAMA 237:2730–2733, 1977

4. Jackson DV, Paschal BR, Ferree C, et al: Combination chemotherapy-radiotherapy with and without the methanol-

extraction residue of bacillus Calmette-Guérin (MER) in small cell carcinoma of the lung. Cancer 50:48–52, 1982

5. Jackson DV, Zekan PJ, Caldwell RD, et al: VP–16–213 in combination chemotherapy with chest irradiation for small-cell lung cancer: A randomized trial of the Piedmont Oncology Association. J Clin Oncol 2:1343–1351, 1984

6. Zekan P, Jackson D, Muss H, et al: Improvement in treatment results in SCCL with the addition of VP–16–213 to cyclophosphamide, Adriamycin and vincristine (CAV). IV World Conference on Lung Cancer, Toronto, Canada, August, 1985, p 94

7. Powell BL, Jackson DV, Scarantino CW, et al: Sequential hemibody and local irradiation with combination chemotherapy for small cell lung carcinoma: A preliminary analysis. Int J Radiat Oncol Biol Phys 11:457–462, 1985

8. Powell B, Jackson D, Scarantino C, et al: Integration of hemibody radiotherapy (RT), combination chemotherapy (CC) and local RT (LRT) for small cell lung cancer (SCLC). IV World Conference on Lung Cancer, Toronto, Canada, August, 1985, p 111

9. Loeb LA, Ernster VL, Warner KE, et al: Smoking and lung cancer: An overview. Cancer Res 44:4940–4958, 1984

10. Cruz JM, Jackson DV, Muss HB, et al: Detection of brain metastasis at diagnosis of small cell carcinoma of the lung. J Neuroncol 2:67–71, 1984

11. Jackson DV, Olds WW, Zekan PJ, et al: Cis-platinum (CP) in combination chemotherapy for small cell lung cancer: A randomized trial. Proc Am Soc Clin Oncol 5:177, 1986 (abstr)

12. Harper PG, Houang M, Spiro SG, et al: Computerized axial tomography in the pretreatment assessment of small-cell carcinoma of the bronchus. Cancer 47:1775–1780, 1981

13. Vas W, Zylak CJ, Mather D, et al: The value of abdominal computed tomography in the pre-treatment assessment of small cell carcinoma of the lung. Radiology 138:417–418, 1981

14. Norlund JD, Byhardt RW, Foley WD, et al: Computed tomography in the staging of small cell lung cancer: Implications for combined modality therapy. Int J Radiat Oncol Biol Phys 11:1081–1084, 1985

15. Perez CA, Einhorn L, Oldham RK, et al: Randomized trial of radiotherapy to the thorax in limited small-cell carcinoma of the lung treated with muliagent chemotherapy and elective brain irradiation: A preliminary report. J Clin Oncol 2:1200–1208, 1984

16. Lichter AS, Bunn PA, Ihde DC, et al: The role of radiation therapy in the treatment of small cell lung cancer. Cancer 55:2163–2175, 1985

17. Shank B, Scher HI: Controversies in treatment of small cell carcinoma of the lung. Cancer Invest 3:367–387, 1985

18. Craig JB, Jackson DV, Moody D, et al: Prospective evaluation of changes in computed cranial tomography in patient with small cell lung carcinoma treated with chemotherapy and prophylactic cranial irradiation. J Clin Oncol 2:1151–1156, 1984

19. Ellison N, Bernath A, Kane R, et al: Disturbing problems of success: Clinical status of long-term survivors of small cell lung cancer (SCLC). Proc Am Soc Clin Oncol 1:149, 1982 (abstr)

20. Looper JD, Einhorn SA, Garcia NB, et al: Seven neurologic problems following successful therapy for small cell lung cancer (SCLC). Proc Am Soc Clin Oncol 3:231, 1984 (abstr)

21. Sculier JP, Feld R, Evans WK, et al: Neurological complications in patients (Pts) with small cell lung cancer (SCLC). Proc Am Soc Clin Oncol 3:222, 1984 (abstr)

22. Licciardello JTW, Cersosimo RJ, Karp DD, et al: Disturbing central nervous system complications following combination chemotherapy and prophylactic whole-brain irradiation in patients with small cell lung cancer. Cancer Treat Rep 69:1429–1430, 1985

23. Messeih A, Schweitzer JM, Dixon RH, et al: The addition of VP–16–213 to cytoxan, Adriamycin, and vincristine for remission inducation and survival in patients with small cell lung cancer. Proc Am Soc Clin Oncol 2:201, 1983 (abstr)

24. Issell B, Rudolph A, Lawson R, et al: Cytoxan, etoposide and vincristine (CEV) versus cytoxan, Adriamycin and vincristine (CAV) or cytoxan and vincristine (CV) in the treatment of small cell carcinoma of the lung (SCCL). Proc Am Soc Clin Oncol 2:192, 1983 (abstr)

25. Rudolph A, Einhorn L, Wampler G, et al: Cytoxan, Adriamycin and etoposide (CAE) versus cytoxan, Adriamycin and vincristine (CAV) in the treatment of small cell carcinoma of the lung (SCCL). Proc Am Soc Clin Oncol 2:192, 1983 (abstr)

26. Bunn PA, Cohen MH, Ihde DC, et al: Advances in small cell bronchogenic carcinoma. Cancer Treat Rep 61:333–342, 1977

27. Einhorn LH, Bond WH, Hornback N, et al: Long-term results in combined-modality treatment of small cell carcinoma of the lung. Semin Oncol 5:309–313, 1978

28. Fox RM, Woods RL, Brodie GN, et al: A randomized study: Small cell anaplastic lung cancer treated by combination chemotherapy and adjuvant radiotherapy. Int J Radiat Oncol Biol Phys 6:1083–1085, 1980

29. Abeloff MD, Ettinger DS, Order SE, et al: Intensive induction chemotherapy in 54 patients with small cell carcinoma of the lung. Cancer Treat Rep 5:639–646, 1981

30. Shank B, Natale RB, Hilaris BS, et al: Treatment of small cell carcinoma of lung with combined high dose mediastinal irradiation, whole brain prophylaxis and chemotherapy. Int J Radiat Oncol Biol Phys 2:469–475, 1981

31. Aisner J, Whitacre M, Van Echo DA, et al: Combination chemotherapy for small cell carcinoma of the lung: Continuous versus alternating non-cross resistant combinations. Cancer Treat Rep 66:221–230, 1982

32. Shank B, Scher H, Hilaris BS, et al: Increased survival with high-dose multifield radiotherapy and intensive chemotherapy in limited small cell carcinoma of the lung. Cancer 56:2771–2778, 1985

33. Daniels JR, Chak LY, Branimir IS, et al: Chemotherapy of small-cell carcinoma of lung: A randomized comparison of alternating and sequential combination chemotherapy programs. J Clin Oncol 2:1192–1198, 1984

34. Murray N, Hadzic E, Shah A, et al: Alternating chemotherapy and thoracic radiotherapy with concurrent cisplatin for limited stage small cell carcinoma of the lung (SCCL). Proc Am Soc Clin Oncol 3:214, 1984 (abstr)

35. Aisner J, Whitacre MY, Budman D, et al: Platinum

(p), doxorubicin (a), cyclophosphamide (c), and etoposide (e), PACE, for small cell lung cancer (SCLC). Proc Am Soc Clin Oncol 4:181, 1985 (abstr)

36. Johnson RE, Brereton HD, Kent CH: Small cell carcinoma of the lung: Attempt to remedy causes of past therapeutic failure. Lancet 2:289–291, 1976

37. Greco FA, Einhorn LH, Richardson RL, et al: Small cell lung cancer: Progress and perspectives. Semin Oncol 5:323–335, 1978

38. Sieroki JS, Hilaris BS, Hopfan S, et al: Cis-dichlorodiammineplatinum (II) and VP-16–213: An active induction regimen for small cell carcinoma of the lung. Cancer Treat Rep 63:1593–1597, 1979

39. Natale RB, Wittes RE: Combination cis-platinum and etoposide in small cell lung cancer. Cancer Treat Rep 9:91–94, 1982

40. Goodman GE, Miller TP, Manning MM, et al: Treatment of small cell lung cancer with VP-16, vincristine, doxorubicin (Adriamycin), cyclophosphamide (EVAC), and high dose chest radiotherapy. J Clin Oncol 1:483–488, 1983

41. Arrigada R, Chevalier TLE, Baldeyrou P, et al: Alternating radiotherapy and chemotherapy schedules in small cell lung cancer, limited disease. Int J Radiat Oncol Biol Phys 11:1461–1467, 1985

42. Evans T, Jacobs SA, Earle MT, et al: Up-front VP-16/platinum (DCCP) in small cell lung cancer (SCLC). Proc Am Soc Clin Oncol 4:189, 1985 (abstr)

43. Jackson DV, Bender RA: The clinical pharmacology of the vinca alkaloids, epipodophyllotoxins, and maytansine, in Pinedo HM (ed): Clinical Pharmacology of Anti-Neoplastic Drugs. New York, Elsevier, 1978, pp 277–294

44. Jackson DV, Wells HB, White DR, et al: Lack of potentiation of vincristine induced neurotoxicity by VP–16–213. Am J Clin Oncol 6:327–330, 1983

45. Thant M, Hawley RJ, Smith MT, et al: Possible enhancement of vincristine neuropathy by VP–16. Cancer 49:859–864, 1982

46. Jackson DV, Long TR, Trahey TF, et al: Synergistic antitumor activity of vincristine and VP-16–213. Cancer Chemother Pharmacol 13:176–180, 1984

47. Jackson D, Long T, Rice D, et al: Combination vincristine and VP-16–213: Evaluation of drug sequence. Cancer Biochem Biophys (in press)

Oral Etoposide in Small-Cell Lung Cancer

By Robert L. Comis

Etoposide can be administered orally. On the average, the bioavailability of etoposide administered in a soft gelatin capsule is approximately 50%. For both the oral and intravenous (IV) routes, there is a significant amount of inter- and intrapatient variability. In spite of the variability, clinical studies show that oral etoposide is clearly active in small-cell lung carcinoma (SCLC). In addition, combination chemotherapy studies using etoposide have yielded toxicity equivalent to IV administered programs such as CAV (cyclophosphamide, doxorubicin, vincristine). Oral etoposide has been used in several large combination chemotherapy studies safely and with clear efficacy.

CERTAIN chemotherapeutic agents are used orally. Agents such as procarbazine, phenylalanine mustard, busulfan, and chlorambucil are only approved for oral use. Not without their individual difficulties, these oral agents have become important in the treatment of a variety of malignancies, including Hodgkin's disease, multiple myeloma, and both chronic myelogenous and lymphocytic leukemias. Agents that are used both orally and parenterally include drugs such as cyclophosphamide, methotrexate, and 5-fluorouracil. To a certain extent, their activity and the ease of administration of these agents has driven their oral use. The desired ease of administration is counterbalanced by the need to deliver a reproducible and effective concentration to the tumor target site.

ORAL ETOPOSIDE

Administration of etoposide by the oral route has been extensively evaluated. Initial trials used either lipophilic capsules or drink ampules.[1-3] In 1979, Lau et al[4] reported on a phase I study investigating the soft gelatin capsule. In each of these phase I evaluations, the end point was myelosuppression. In fact, significant dose-related myelotoxicity was reported in each of these studies.

We have shown that the absolute bioavailability of etoposide administered in the soft gelatin capsule is 48% with a considerable amount of variability (range, 25% to 74%).[5] On the average, an equivalent AUC can be obtained by administering twice the intravenous (IV) dose via the soft gelatin capsule. Possibly because of the nature of our study, there was no obvious correlation between the various important pharmacokinetic parameters and toxicity, in particular leukopenia. Our patients were typical patients entered in phase I trials, ie, with heterogeneous prior therapies and disease and response histories. Other studies that have attempted to estimate the bioavailability of etoposide have yielded similar results.[6] It should be noted that in our hands, IV administration was also associated with considerable variability in measured or estimated pharmacokinetic parameters as well. Variability in absorption has been observed with a variety of antineoplastic agents.

For antineoplastic agents, a minimum measure of effective drug delivery can be inferred from the observation of either toxic or therapeutic events, such as myelotoxicity or objective response. Many of the early trials using oral therapy did not involve pharmacokinetic measurements but did include the more classic approach to phase I evaluation. Fairly characteristic dose-response relationships in two such studies are presented in Table 1 for the ampule and soft gelatin capsule.[3,4]

ORAL ETOPOSIDE IN SMALL-CELL LUNG CANCER

Antitumor activity has been noted in studies using oral etoposide. In particular, activity in small-cell lung cancer (SCLC) has been noted from a variety of trials. The majority of the patients treated in the series presented in Table 2[7-11] were previously untreated. As can be seen, etoposide is clearly capable of inducing objective response in SCLC patients when it is administered by the oral route.

From the Fox Chase Cancer Center, Philadelphia.
Address reprint requests to Robert L. Comis, MD, Medical Director, Fox Chase Cancer Center, 7701 Burholme Ave, Philadelphia, PA 19111.

0093-7754/86/1303-3013$05.00/0

Table 1. Dose Effect of Etoposide Administered in Drink Ampules and Soft Gelatin Capsules

Formulation	Daily Dose (mg/m²/5 times daily)	No. of Patients	Patients with WBC × $10^3/\mu L$		
			>4	2–4	<2
Ampule[3]	60	10	5	5	0
	120	19	11	3	5
	180	4	0	1	3
Capsule[4]	70	5	4	1	0
	100	7	2	4	1
	130	11	1	6	4
	150	3	1	0	2

Table 2. Response to Oral Etoposide in SCLC

Reference	No. of Patients	Extent of Disease (n)	CR	CR + PR (%)
Cavalli[7]	17	Limited (11) Extensive (6)	2	65
Anderson[8]	17	NA	2	58
Cavalli[7]	19	Limited (12) Extensive (7)	2	42
Hansen[9]	10	Limited (6) Extensive (4)	0	40
	30*	Limited (2) Extensive (28)	0	40
Honma[10]	13	NA	0	31
Miyamoto[11]	11	NA	1	27

Abbreviations: CR, complete response; PR, partial response; NA, not available; n, number of patients.

*Previously treated with CMC ± V.

COMBINATION SCLC STUDIES USING ORAL ETOPOSIDE

A number of studies have been performed that have included oral etoposide used in combination with other agents. The details of these trials are outlined in Table 3.[12-16] As might be expected, it is difficult to totally isolate the contribution of oral etoposide in these programs. In addition, the number of evaluable patients in each category is relatively small, with the exception of the study by Osterlind et al.[16] The latter study did not directly address the value of oral etoposide. Rather, a second combination of doxorubicin (Adriamycin [Adria Laboratories, Columbus, Ohio]) (30 mg/m²) with oral etoposide (100 mg/m²/three times a day) was administered as part of a fixed alternating scheme, or upon relapse from primary treatment with CCNU, cyclophosphamide, methotrexate, and vincristine (CCMV). There was no difference in objective response or survival in this group of extensive-disease patients. On the other hand, the investigators indicated that a significant increase in response duration and survival occurred with the alternating approach. Although unlikely, it is possible that the alternation of doxorubicin accounted for this difference, but the implication is that the combination including oral etoposide led to the effect.

A more conclusive indication of the activity of oral etoposide is derived from the Bristol study 210, which randomized patients to three treatment options as outlined in Table 4. As can be seen, the first dose of etoposide was administered IV, then the next four doses were given at twice the orally administered dose. As discussed in an accompanying article in this journal supplement,

Table 3. Small-Cell Lung Cancer—Combination Chemotherapy

Reference	Regimen	No. of Patients: Evaluable	LD	ED	PC	CR	CR + PR (%)	Median Survival (Weeks)
Cortes Funes[12]	VP-16-CPA-DDP	24	10	14	0	6	75	24
	VP-16-CPA-Radiotherapy	31	16	15	0	10	81	33
Schilcher[13]	VP-16-Ifos	29	20	9	15	1	34	—
Estape[14]	VP-16-CPA	16	2	14	0	5	75	40
	VP-16-CPA-MTX	12	1	11	0	1	50	20
	VP-16-CPA-ADM	7	1	6	0	1	71	—
Madrigal[15]	VP-16-DDP	12	—	—	7	5	67	—
Osterlind[16]	CCNU-CPA-VCR-MTX Alternate with ADM-VP-16 Versus	70	0	70	0	15	72	38
	CCNU-CPA-VCR-MTX followed at progression by ADM-VP-16	76	0	76	0	11	68	36

Abbreviations: LD, limited disease; ED, extensive disease; PC, prior chemotherapy; VP16, etoposide; Ifos, Ifosfamide; CPA, cyclophosphamide; MTX, methotrexate; ADM, doxorubicin; DDP, cisplatin; CCNU, lomustine; VCR, vincristine.

Table 4. Treatment Plan

Drug	Dose (mg/m^2)	Route	Schedule
CEV			
Cyclophosphamide	1,000	IV	Day 1
Etoposide	50	IV	Day 1
Etoposide	100	orally	Days 2–5
Vincristine*	1.4	IV	Day 1
CAV			
Cyclophosphamide	1,000	IV	Day 1
Doxorubicin	50	IV	Day 1
Vincristine*	1.4	IV	Day 1
CV			
Cyclophosphamide	2,000	IV	Day 1
Vincristine*	1.4	IV	Day 1

*Maximum total dose per injection: 2 mg.

Table 5. Bristol Study 210—Hematologic Toxicity

	CEV	CAV	CV	P
Course 1				
No. of patients	70	71	52	
WBC × $10^3/\mu L$				
Median	2.0	2.2	1.5	.003
% < 1.0 × $10^3/\mu L$	13	15	29	.059
All Courses				
No. of patients	78	75	55	
Median	1.2	1.1	1.0	
% < 1.0 × $10^3/\mu L$	31	37	40	

preliminary data indicate that response duration and survival are superior for the cyclophosphamide plus etoposide plus vincristine (CEV) program. It is unlikely that this effect was from the single IV dose of etoposide. An analysis of the toxicity observed for cyclophosphamide plus doxorubicin plus vincristine (CAV) and CEV indicate that this predominantly oral route of administration yielded toxicity equivalent to that seen with the IV doxorubicin-containing program. An analysis of these data are presented in Table 5. This study indicates that oral etoposide can be incorporated into treatment programs for SCLC and yield therapeutic and toxologic effects comparable to the more commonly used IV CAV program.

As discussed above, investigators from Copenhagen have reported that an alternating regimen including IV doxorubicin and oral etoposide increased response duration and survival in responding patients. More recently, they have conducted a randomized, controlled study that compares the use of oral methotrexate with oral etoposide in combination with CCNU, cyclophosphamide, and vincristine (H. Hansen, personal communication, March 1985). As shown in Table 6, an additional question relates to the timing of the etoposide. This study was performed in 288 patients with extensive disease in whom there were no significant differences in important prognostic variables such as sex, age, and performance status.

No significant differences in complete or overall response rates were noted in the entire group or within specific prognostic categories. On the other hand, a significant increase in response duration, survival, and 2-year disease-free survival occurred in patients who received oral etoposide on days 3 through 6. These differences could not be accounted for by differences in prognostic factors. Treatment with the regimen containing early etoposide therapy was statisti-

Table 6. Treatment Plan

Regimen	Drug	Dose (mg/m^2)	Route	Schedule*
A	Cyclophosphamide	1,000	IV	Day 1
	Lomustine	70	Orally	Day 1
	Vincristine	1.3	IV	Day 1
	Methotrexate	20	Orally	Days 14 and 17
B	Cyclophosphamide	1,000	IV	Day 1
	Lomustine	70	Orally	Day 1
	Vincristine	1.3	IV	Day 1
	Etoposide	280	Orally	Divided days 14–17
C	Cyclophosphamide	1,000	IV	Day 1
	Lomustine	70	Orally	Day 1
	Vincristine	1.3	IV	Day 1
	Etoposide	280	Orally	Divided days 3–6

*Repeated every 4 weeks.

cally significant in a stepwise Cox regression analysis for survival. More complete details of this study will be presented in a future publication.

DISCUSSION

Oral etoposide has a bioavailability of approximately 50%. Although there is considerable interpatient and intrapatient variablility, the drug can be safely and effectively administered by the oral route. As with any other chemotherapeutic program, the effectiveness and safety of drug administration is dependent upon appropriate monitoring of hematologic parameters and indicators of disease response. It is interesting that a considerable amount of variability has been encountered in pharmacokinetic studies of IV administered etoposide as well.

Many of the early trials using etoposide in the treatment of SCLC used the oral route of administration, and clear-cut activity was demonstrated for this route. Recently, there have been additional trials performed using orally administered etoposide in combination chemotherapy programs. Unfortunately, no trials have been designed to test specifically the efficacy of the oral *v* the IV route of etoposide administration. Therefore, only inferences from the results of studies that evaluate the drug in combination with other agents can be drawn. It appears from such studies that oral etoposide can be easily and effectively used in combination chemotherapy programs. Two studies, Bristol study 210 and the recent study performed by the Finsen Institute and their collaborators have shown that regimens using oral etoposide can yield statistically significant advantages over other conventional programs such as CAV or the CCMV regimen, respectively.

REFERENCES

1. Falkson G, van Dyk JJ, van Eden EB, et al: A clinical trial of the oral form of 4'-demethyl-Epipodophyllotoxin- -D ethylidene glucoside (NSC 141540) VP16-213. Cancer 35:1141–1144, 1975

2. Nissen NI, Hansen HH, Pedersen H, et al: Clinical trial of the oral from of a new podophyllotoxin derivative, VP-16-213 (NSC 141540), in patients with advanced neoplastic disease. Cancer Chemother Rep 59:1027–1029, 1975

3. Nissen NI, Dombernowsky P, Hansen HH, et al: Phase I clinical trial of an oral solution of VP16-213. Cancer Treat Rep 60:943–945, 1976

4. Lau ME, Hansen HH, Nissen NI, et al: Phase I trial of a new form of an oral administration of VP16-213. Cancer Treat Rep 63:485–487, 1979

5. Smyth RD, Pfeffer M, Scalzo A, et al: Bioavailability and pharmacokinetics of etoposide (VP-16). Semin Oncol 12:48–51, 1985 (suppl 2)

6. D'Incalci M, Farina P, Sessa C, et al: Pharmacokinetics of VP16-214 given by different administration methods. Cancer Chemother Pharmacol 7:141-145, 1982

7. Cavalli F, Sonntag RW, Jungi F, et al: VP16-213 monotherapy for remission induction of small cell lung cancer: A randomized trial using three dosage schedules. Cancer Treat Rep 62:473–475, 1978

8. Anderson G, Peel ET, Cheong CMB, et al: Etoposide—an effective single drug for treating bronchogenic carcinoma. Clin Oncol 8:215–218, 1982

9. Hansen M, Hirsch F, Dombernowsky P, et al: Treatment of small cell anaplastic carcinoma of the lung with the oral solution of VP16-213 (NSC 141540, 4'-demethylepopodophyllotoxin 9'(4,6-0-ethylidene- -D-glucopyranoside). Cancer 40:633–637, 1977

10. Honma T, Ogawa M, Yoshida S, et al: Phase II study of VP16 (capsule) in patients with solid tumors—a cooperative study. Jpn J Cancer Chemother. 12:309-13, 1985

11. Miyamoto H, Ito M, Araya Y, et al: Effects of oral etoposide in small cell carcinoma of the lung. Jpn J Cancer Chemother 11:1244–1247, 1984

12. Cortes Funes H, Dominguez P, Perrez Torrubia A, et al: Treatment of small cell lung cancer with a combination of VP16-213 and cyclophosphamide with cisplatin or radiotherapy. Cancer Chemother Pharmacol 7:181–186, 1982

13. Schilcher RB, Seeber S, Scheulen ME, et al: Etoposide and ifosfamide in combination for inoperable carcinoma of the bronchus. Cancer Treat Rev 9:107–110, 1982

14. Estape J, Milla A, Agusti A, et al: VP-16 plus cyclophosphamide in the treatment of advanced lung cancer. Cancer 51:385–389, 1983

15. Madrigal PA, Manga GP, Palomero I, et al: VP16-213 combined with cis-platinum (CDDP) in the treatment of small cell carcinoma of the lung. Cancer Chemother Pharmacol 7:203–204, 1982

16. Osterlind K, Sorenson S, Hansen HH, et al: Continuous versus alternating combination chemotherapy for advanced small cell carcinoma of the lung. Cancer Res 43:6085–6089, 1983

Outpatient Administration of VP-16 and Cisplatin

By Terry L. Evans

THE EPIPODOPHYLLOTOXIN etoposide (VP-16) has emerged as one of the most active agents in previously untreated patients with small-cell lung cancer (SCLC) with response rates of 20% to 60%.[1-3] Cisplatin (CDDP), on the other hand, appears to have little activity in this disease when used alone. However, the combination of these drugs has been shown to have synergistic activity both in animal models[4-5] and clinical trials.[6-8] The group from Toronto,[9] using VP-16 and CDDP as frontline therapy, has reported response rates comparable with those achieved with standard induction chemotherapy regimens. In addition, several recent studies, using the Goldie-Coldman mathematical model for tumor cell drug resistance,[10-11] have suggested that response rates, duration of responses, and perhaps even overall survival are increased in SCLC with non–cross-resistant drug regimens including VP-16 and CDDP.[6,12-14]

With this in mind, it would seem pertinent to discuss the administration of these agents in an outpatient setting, since chemotherapy regimens traditionally used in this disease—including cyclophosphamide, doxorubicin (Adriamycin [Adria Laboratories, Columbus, OH]), and vincristine (CAV); cyclophosphamide, CCNU, and methotrexate; and VP-16, doxorubicin, and methotrexate (VAM)—readily lend themselves to being administered in this manner. There appears to be a reluctance on the part of practicing oncologists to use platinum-based regimens outside the hospital environment. Some of the factors to be considered in safely administering VP-16 and CDDP in an office or outpatient facility are shown in Table 1. These include (1) convenient and well-equipped facility, (2) effective antiemetic and hydration regimens, (3) experienced nursing personnel, (4) patient selection, and (5) cost considerations.

The facility itself should be a pleasant, comfortable area removed from the mainstream of activity. It should include infusion chairs or beds, bathroom facilities, equipment for dealing with emergencies, and television or radios to aid in relaxation.

Cisplatin is a potent emetogenic agent. However, in recent years, several more effective antiemetic regimens have been used to control the nausea and vomiting induced by cisplatin. The most notable of these is high-dose metoclopramide (1 to 3mg/kg) administered intravenously (IV). In a prospective randomized trial comparing metoclopramide with prochlorperazine or placebo, Gralla et al[15] observed fewer episodes, reduced volume, and shortened duration of nausea and vomiting in patients who received metoclopramide. Similar results were noted by Strum et al[16] using metoclopramide at a dose of 1 mg/kg for six doses. Several agents have been added to metoclopramide in an attempt to improve antiemetic efficacy, including dexamethasone, diphenhydramine, diazepam, lorazepam, and thiethylperazine.[17] Kris et al[18] found that combinations of metoclopramide plus dexamethasone and diphenhydramine were more efficacious and had fewer side effects than metoclopramide used alone in controlling nausea and vomiting induced by CDDP at a dose of 120 mg/m^2. They further showed that "short-course" regimens consisting of metoclopramide, 3 mg/kg IV for two doses, dexamethasone 20 mg IV for one dose, and diphenhydramine 50 mg IV for one dose were as effective as more prolonged administration of the agents. The implications for patient comfort, outpatient administration, and cost containment are obvious. In spite of recent reports questioning the efficacy of these agents,[19-21] they remain an important part of our antiemetic armamentarium.

Early clinical trials using cisplatin were hampered by dose-limiting nephrotoxicity. Numerous studies have shown that adequate pretreatment hydration and diuresis can exhibit a protective effect on the kidneys in a majority of instances.[22,23] However, even with vigorous hydration and diuresis with mannitol or furosemide, subclinical reductions in renal function do occur. A recent study[24] in patients with testicular

From the University of Pittsburgh School of Medicine.
Address reprint requests to Terry L. Evans, MD, Mercy Hospital, 1400 Locust St, Suite 400, Pittsburgh, PA 15219.

0093–7754/86/1303–3012$05.00/0

Table 1. Considerations for Outpatient Chemotherapy

1. Convenient and well-equipped facility
2. Effective antiemetic and hydration regimen
3. Experienced nursing personnel
4. Patient selection
5. Cost factors

cancer using CDDP in a dose of 20 mg/m^2 days 1 through 5 used a 15% mannitol solution and 4 L of normal saline per 24 hours. Although no difference was noted in pre- and posttreatment creatinine levels, glomerular filtration rate and renal plasma flow decreased by more than 20%. Similar findings were noted by Dentino et al.[25] In this study, plasma creatinine and BUN increased significantly, and creatinine clearances decreased from a pretreatment value of 112 ± 12 mL/min to a posttreatment value at 6 months of 68.5 ± 12 mL/min. Furthermore, light and electron microscopic studies demonstrated changes suggesting cellular injury and death in the collecting ducts as well as in the proximal and distal tubules.

Although the exact mechanism of the protective effect of physiologic saline is not clear, it seems to be related to the process seen in Fig 1.[26] In a high-chloride environment, such as that seen with isotonic or hypertonic saline, cisplatin retains its neutral structure and can cross cell membranes readily. Once inside the cell in which chloride concentrations are lower, the equilibrium is shifted in favor of positively charged species thought to be responsible for cytoxicity. If these structures are formed extracellularly, as might be seen if hypotonic saline or dextrose were used, platinum dimers and trimers, which are felt by some to be responsible for the agent's toxicity, can occur. Likewise, the beneficial effects of mannitol and furosemide on platinum-induced renal injury need further clarification. In a rat model, the partial preservation of function observed with these agents was not related to increased excretion of platinum in the urine or to faster plasma clearance of or decreased renal levels of platinum.[27]

In the office or outpatient clinic, two recent reports seem to be pertinent to the safe administration of cisplatin. In a study by Chary et al,[28] patients were hydrated with 1 L of D5NSS and received platinum, either 1 mg/kg or 60 mg/m^2 twice weekly in 2 L of D5⅓NSS with 37.5 g mannitol preceded by furosemide IV. Transient declines in creatinine clearance were noted in 21% of patients, but BUN and creatinine values remained normal in all but one patient. The dose-limiting toxicity in this study was hematologic, and the investigators felt this type of regimen could be adapted to outpatient use. A separate study[29] analyzed the frequency of azotemia development in patients with a variety of tumors using a dose of cisplatin of 50 mg/m^2 every 3 weeks. Their pretreatment regimen consisted of a 2-L infusion of D5½NSS administered over two hours preceded by furosemide 40 mg IV. Mannitol (12.5 g) was administered just before the administration of CDDP. Azotemia developed after 15 courses (1.3%) in 11 patients (4.5%). Peak serum creatinine was >2 mg/dL in only four patients, and azotemia lasted more than 12 weeks in only one patient. Thus, it would appear that the vast majority of patients can avoid clinically significant renal impairment with adequate hydration and diuresis, and that such regimens can be safely administered in an outpatient facility. A regimen that could be used is shown in Fig 2.

The need for experienced nursing personnel is self-explanatory. In selecting patients for outpatient chemotherapy, certain general guidelines should be followed. The patients should be well nourished, with a relatively good performance status, and free of significant cardiopulmonary

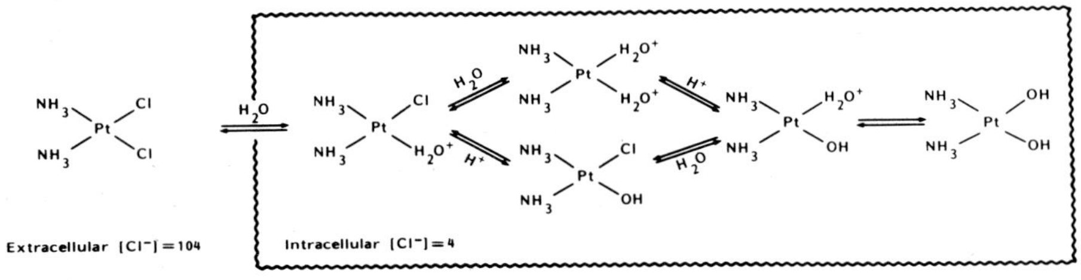

Fig 1. The aquation reaction of cisplatin.

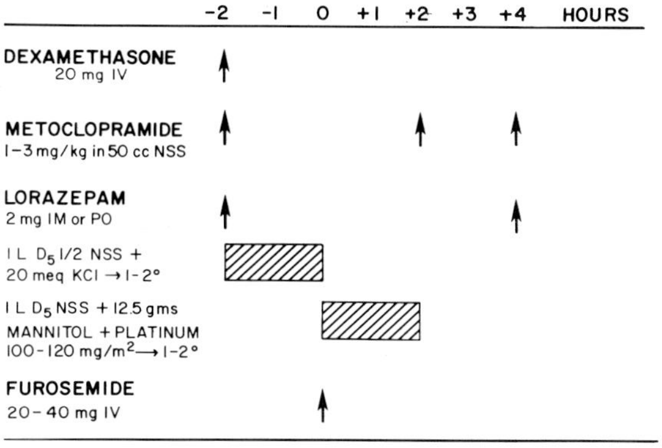

Fig 2. Antiemetic and hydration regimen for outpatient cisplatin.

or renal diseases. The family situation and ease of transportation need to be considered. Finally, although it is said that younger patients tolerate this type of outpatient chemotherapy better, we have one 75-year-old man who walks five miles to the outpatient department every month, receives his chemotherapy, and walks home after he is finished. He has been doing this for nearly 2 years now.

One final consideration is the cost to the system involved in administering chemotherapy in the hospital *v* the office or clinic. Precious little is contained in the medical literature concerning the subject. In a pilot program, sponsored by Pennsylvania Blue Cross and Blue Shield and involving four private oncology practices and four community hospitals in eastern Pennsylvania,[30] Prager found that chemotherapy administered in an outpatient facility was approximately one third as expensive as that given in the hospital. However, he appropriately noted that a decrease in hospital use did not necessarily translate into a decrease in Blue Cross reimbursement for hospital services, since decreased use with no corresponding decrease in operating costs could lead to an increase in reimbursement for other service. Overall patient satisfaction with office chemotherapy in this study was good.

Thus, outpatient administration of VP-16 and CDDP is not only feasible but desirable. Of the protocols discussed in these proceedings, only the platinum, doxorubicin (Adriamycin), cyclophosphamide, etoposide (PACE) regimen described by Aisner et al and the very high-dose VP-16, cyclophosphamide, and CDDP utilized by Greco at Vanderbilt University Medical Center, Nashville, Tenn require hospitalization. The others, employing various combinations of the antiemetic and hydration schedules described previously, are readily adaptable to outpatient administration.

REFERENCES

1. Pederson AG, Hansen HH: Etoposide (VP16) in the treatment of lung cancer. Cancer Treat Rev 10:245–264, 1983

2. Cavalli F, Sonntag RW, Jungi F, et al: VP-16-213 monotherapy for remission induction of small cell lung cancer: A randomised trial using three dosage schedules. Cancer Treat Rep 62:473–475, 1978

3. Tucker RD, Ferguson A, Van Wyck C, et al: Chemotherapy of small cell carcinoma of the lung with VP-16-213. Cancer 41:1710–1714, 1978

4. Mabel JA: Therapeutic synergism in murine tumors for combination of cis-diammine-dichloroplatinum with VP-16-213 or BCNU. Proc Am Assoc Cancer Res 20:230, 1979 (abstr)

5. Dombernowsky P, Nissen NI: Combination chemotherapy with 4'-dimethyl-epipodophyllotoxin 9-(4,6-0-ethylidene-B-D-glucopyranoside), VP-16-213 (NSC 141540) in L-210 leukemia. Eur J Cancer Clin Oncol 12:181–188, 1976

6. Sierocki JS, Hilaris BS, Hopfan S, et al: Cis-diammine-dichloroplatinum (II) and VP-16-213: An active induction regimen for small cell carcinoma of the lung. Cancer Treat Rep 63:1593–1597, 1979

7. Evans WK, Feld R, Osoba D, et al: VP-16 alone and in combination with cisplatin in previously treated patients with small cell lung cancer. Cancer 53:1461–1466, 1984

8. Lopez JA, Mann J, Grapski RT, et al: Etoposide and cisplatin salvage chemotherapy for small cell cancer. Cancer Treat Rep 69:369–371, 1985

9. Evans WK, Shepherd FA, Feld R, et al: VP-16 and cisplatin as first-line therapy for small-cell lung cancer. J Clin Oncol 3:1471–1477, 1985

10. Goldie JH, Coldman AJ: A mathematical model for relating the drug sensitivity of tumors to their spontaneous mutation rate. Cancer Treat Rep 63:1727–1733, 1979

11. Goldie JH, Coldman AJ, Gudauskas GA: Rationale for the use of alternating non–cross-resistant chemotherapy. Cancer Treat Rep 66:439–449, 1982

12. Natale RB, Wittes RE: Combination cis-platinum and etoposide in small-cell lung cancer. Cancer Treat Rev 9:91–94, 1982

13. Daniels JR, Chak LY, Sikic BI, et al: Chemotherapy of small-cell carcinoma of lung: A randomized comparison of alternating and sequential combination chemotherapy programs. J Clin Oncol 2:1192–1199, 1984

14. Natale RB, Shank B,Hilaris BS, et al: Combination cyclophosphamide, Adriamycin, and vincristine rapidly

alternating with combination cisplatin and VP-16 in treatment of small cell lung cancer. Am J Med 79:303–308, 1985

15. Gralla RJ, Itri LM, Pisko SE, et al: Antiemetic efficacy of high-dose metoclopramide: Randomized trials with placebo and prochlorperazine in patients with chemotherapy-induced nausea and vomiting. N Engl J Med 305:905–909, 1981

16. Strum SB, McDermed JE, Opfell RW, et al: Intravenous metoclopramide: An effective antiemetic in cancer chemotherapy. JAMA 247:2683–2686, 1982

17. Plezia PM, Alberts DS, Kessler J, et al: Immediate termination of intractable vomiting induced by cisplatin combination chemotherapy using an extensive five-drug antiemetic regimen. Cancer Treat Rep 68:1493–1495, 1984

18. Kris MG, Gralla RJ, Tyson LB, et al: Improved control of cisplatin-induced emesis with high-dose metoclopramide and with combinations of metoclopramide, dexamethasone, and diphenhydramine: Results of consecutive trials in 255 patients. Cancer 55:527–534, 1985

19. Roemeling RV, Christiansen NP, Hrushesky WJM: Lack of antiemetic effect of high-dose metoclopramide. J Clin Oncol 3:1273–1276, 1985

20. Carr BI, Bertrand M, Browning S, et al: A comparison of the antiemetic efficacy of prochlorperazine and metaclopramide for the treatment of cisplatin-induced emesis: A prospective, randomized, double-blind study. J Clin Oncol 3:1127–1132, 1985

21. D'Olimpio JT, Camacho F, Chandra P, et al: Antiemetic efficacy of high-dose dexamethasone versus placebo in patients receiving cisplatin-based chemotherapy: A randomized double-blind controlled clinical trial. J Clin Oncol 3:1133–1141, 1985

22. Hayes DM, Cvitkovic E, Golbey RB, et al: High dose cis-platinumdiamminedichloride: Amelioration of renal toxicity by mannitol diuresis. Cancer 39:1372–1381, 1977

23. Weiss RB, Poster DS: The renal toxicity of cancer chemotherapeutic agents. Cancer Treat Rev 9:37–56, 1982

24. Meijer S, Sleijfer DT, Mulder NH, et al: Some effects of combination chemotherapy with cisplatinum on renal function in patients with nonseminomatous testicular carcinoma. Cancer 51:2035–2040, 1983

25. Dentino M, Luft FC, Yum MN, et al: Long term effect of cis-diamminedichloride platinum (CDDP) on renal function and structure in man. Cancer 41:1274–1281, 1978

26. Loehrer PJ, Einhorn LH: Diagnosis and treatment. Drugs five years later: Cisplatin. Ann Intern Med 100:704–713, 1984

27. Pera MF, Zook BC, Harder HC: Effects of mannitol or furosemide diuresis on the nephrotoxicity and physiological disposition of cis-dichlorodiammineplatinum-(II) in rats. Cancer Res 39:1269–1278, 1979

28. Chary KK, Higby DJ, Henderson ES, et al: Phase I study of high-dose cis-dichlorodiammineplatinum (II) with forced diuresis. Cancer Treat Rep 61:367–370, 1977

29. Vogl SE, Zaravinos T, Kaplan BH, et al: Safe and effective two-hour outpatient regimen of hydration and diuresis for the administration of cis-diamminedichloroplatinum (II). Eur J Cancer 17:345–350, 1981

30. Prager D: Chemotherapy in the physician's office. Penn Med 87:50–52, 1984

St Thomas Consensus on the Treatment of Small-Cell Lung Cancer

Dr L. Einhorn (Indianapolis): We are now seeing a patient Monday when we get back to work and we have all the data from what we've listened to and, for whatever reason, we don't have the luxury—or the patient refuses—to enter a randomized trial, so we have to decide how we're going to treat a patient off protocol. We have two patients, they're both good performance status patients, one patient with limited small cell, one patient with extensive small cell. Dr Terry Evans, I'll have you participate in this, too, if you don't mind, and Dr Natale, I'll start with you. How would you treat this patient with limited and how would you treat this patient with extensive disease?

Dr R. Natale (Ann Arbor, Mich): For the patient with limited disease, my approach would be to give an intensive treatment program consisting of chemotherapy and concurrent radiotherapy with curative intent. I would use CAV [cyclophosphamide, doxorubicin, and vincristine] alternating with cisplatin/VP-16 for six courses, three of each, and would administer 5,000 rad radiotherapy to the primary disease complex, mediastinum, and supraclavicular regions concurrently with the second course of cisplatin/VP-16. At our institution, we are fortunate to have very good treatment planning using CT scans for simulation, which helps to avoid the problems of geographic misses and excessive toxicity. So, we would plan a radiation therapy course that would use from three to six fields for radiation therapy delivery. For the patient with the extensive disease, on the other hand, I have a different approach. I don't believe I've seen cures. I've only seen a handful of long-term survivors and consequently would treat that patient with something that has a good chance of achieving a remission, that can limit the number of hospitalizations that that patient is going to have, so that the patient will enjoy improved survival duration and quality on an outpatient basis. My approach would be to use CAV alternating with platinum/VP-16 in that setting, without involved field radiotherapy or with hemibody radiotherapy.

Dr L. Einhorn: Okay, Dr McCracken?

Dr J. McCracken (San Antonio, Tex): I think we have to consider the quality as well as the quantity of survival. Using an effective program up front and avoiding the long-term maintenance programs, should be a goal of our treatment. In limited stage disease, I'm very comfortable using concurrent platinum/VP-16 with radiotherapy. I have had excellent success with this program, and it is my preference. The only concern I have is with a patient with superior vena cava syndrome with whom you're worried about the hydration factors associated with platinum. For that patient, I'm a little bit nervous; however, I've been able to avoid problems in most patients. In extensive disease patients, I like the Canadian approach of doxorubicin, cyclophosphamide, vincristine alternating with VP-16/platinum. On occasion I've used a few modifications of this regimen. Sometimes I'll use three or four rounds of doxorubicin, cyclophosphamide, vincristine, and then switch to three or four rounds of VP-16 and platinum.

Dr L. Einhorn: Dr Evans?

Dr T. Evans (Pittsburgh): Since I'm the liaison to the community oncologist, I'd like to preface my response with a few comments. I believe all of the data presented at this meeting is very pertinent to oncologists in the community. For day-to-day experience, most of the oncologists I know, however, give CAV in the office because they find it very easy to administer. And I believe a question on their minds is whether or not sufficient data now exist to warrant the use of front-line therapy with VP-16 and platinum, a regimen which is administered over two or three days, often in a hospital setting, if adequate outpatient facilities are not readily available.

In limited disease, what we have tended to do has been to give the VP-16/platinum as front-line therapy. If the patients are of good performance status and can tolerate it and all the other factors that I mentioned yesterday are operative, we try to do that as an outpatient. However, for any one of a number of reasons, this occasionally is impossible and patients are not very happy about having to come into the hospital 5 or 6 months in a row for their therapy. They'd much rather be treated in the office or the outpatient clinic. What we've been doing to date has been giving two cycles of VP-16/platinum followed by four cycles of CAV. But after hearing some of the data here, I'm not so sure that I wouldn't be inclined just to go with the VP-16/platinum for four cycles in limited disease along with concurrent chest radiation therapy. Quite frankly, I think with extensive disease, you can pick and choose whatever you want to use. Dr Aisner's data with PACE [cisplatin, doxorubicin, cyclophosphamide, and etoposide] are impressive but I think Dr McCracken's comments about quality of life are most appropriate. Some patients, after a few cycles of VP-16/platinum, for whatever reason, just don't do well and don't want any more chemotherapy. Thus, for those who can't tolerate it, CAV may be the next choice.

Dr L. Einhorn: Dr Greco?

Dr F. A. Greco (Nashville, Tenn): In the extensive stage patient, I would use the alternating combination but, for a patient off protocol, I would modify it somewhat. The VP-16 I would administer as one dose, not over three days. And I would use a higher dose of VP-16, probably 400 to 500 mg/m^2. If oral VP-16 were available that would be a major advantage. I might use a slightly lower dose on day 1, and then, on days 2 and 3, use the oral capsules. I would use platinum at 40 to 60 mg/m^2 on days 1 and 8. Therefore, the regimen would be given as an outpatient. I would stop after four courses. So, it's CAV, VP-16, platinum, CAV, VP-16, platinum, then stop. In the limited stage patient, I would use delayed radiotherapy, giving chemotherapy upfront for two courses. The question is, what chemotherapy? Off protocol, a limited stage patient has a potential for cure. I would rely upon the schedules that have been studied more widely and probably use a three day VP-16/platinum schedule for two courses, or a CAV schedule for two courses, then radiation therapy, ie, either the CALGB [Cancer and Acute Leukemia Group B] approach or the SEG [Southeastern Cancer Study Group] approach, and then two or four more cycles after that, then stop therapy.

Dr L. Einhorn: Dr Bunn?

Dr P. Bunn (Denver): For extensive stage, I'd use CAV alternating with VP-16/platinum. The VP-16/platinum would be 80 mg/m^2 times one of platinum, and then 80 mg/m^2 times three of VP-16, all given as an outpatient. We haven't had any trouble doing that as an outpatient and find this very easy to give as an outpatient. For limited stage, I would use four cycles of VP-16/platinum with radiation therapy starting on day 1.

Dr L. Einhorn: Dr Comis?

Dr R. Comis (Philadelphia): In extensive disease, I would use an alternation approach as well. I would try to make it as flexible in this sense as possible. Basically treat with CAV and consider the CAV as a sort of primer for VP-16/platinum therapy. But treat with CAV to maximal response or till the rate of response changes and then switch to VP-16/platinum and probably give the VP-16/platinum for three or four cycles and then stop. In limited disease, I think I would come up with some form of cytoreductive chemotherapy first. I think that in the beginning, cyclophosphamide, VP-16, and vincristine could be considered and I would add the radiation, give the drug concomitantly and then directly after that, switch to VP-16/platinum, and probably stop it after 6 months of total therapy.

Dr L. Einhorn: Dr Aisner?

Dr J. Aisner (Baltimore): In the Baltimore community, many, if not most, of the practitioners are using the combination of doxorubicin, cyclophosphamide, and VP-16 in a day 1 through 5 schedule. Some of the oncologists are using it with chest radiation for limited disease, and alone for patients with extensive disease. I think my approach would be to use the PACE regimen as I presented for extensive disease because, so far, that is clearly the best survival I have seen. Although there is an enhancement of the toxicity, I believe the toxicity is probably worthwhile. It is of relatively short duration. For limited disease, I believe that I would probably start with something similar to the CALGB regimen I described, that is an ACE (doxorubicin, cyclosphosphamide, VP-16) regimen for cytoreduction and then a substitution of platinum for doxorubicin to give the chest irradiation. I would follow the chest irradiation and PCI [prophylactic cranial irradiation] with one or two more courses of chemotherapy.

Dr L. Einhorn: Dr Evans?

Dr W. Evans (Ottawa, Ontario): Based on our Canadian data, I would treat an off study patient with extensive disease with the alternation of CAV and VP-16/cisplatinum for six cycles. I would also give some thought, if the patient was a long distance from the center and it meant considerable hardship for them to get to the center, to the use of four cycles of VP-16/cisplatinum alone. I currently do this and make use of the community physician to give the day 2 and day 3 VP-16/platinum. I must say that we've had very, very little trouble using this approach. It is not a difficult regimen for family physicians to administer with some direction. In my experience, patients who've been on the alternating program have generally preferred the VP-16/cisplatinum chemotherapy from the point of view of the GI toxicity compared with the GI toxicity you get with CAV. For patients with limited disease, the goal is cure. So, carrying forward the information from the Canadian study on extensive disease, I would say that we should employ the alternation of CAV and VP-16/platinum for six cycles. I would give locoregional radiotherapy in a dose of either 3,750 cGy in 15 fractions, or 4,000 cGy in 15 fractions at the end of the treatment program, so as not to reduce the amount of chemotherapy that could be given. I would use this approach until we see something from our current NCI-Canada limited disease study that would indicate that radiotherapy should be used up-front, early in the treatment program. At present, I would delay the radiotherapy to the end of the chemotherapy program for the limited disease patient.

Dr L. Einhorn: So you would give the radiotherapy as a single modality after completion of all the chemotherapy then?

Dr W. Evans: Actually, I would give it concurrently with the last course of chemotherapy which would be VP-16/cisplatinum.

Dr L. Einhorn: Okay. Dr Murray?

Dr. N. Murray (Vancouver, British Columbia): The treatment goal for limited stage disease is cure, and I would treat with a vigorous but short combined modality regimen. The chemotherapy would consist of an alternation of cyclophosphamide, doxorubicin, and vincristine with VP-16/cisplatin given for three courses of each regimen or six cycles in total. Thoracic radiotherapy using 4,000 cGy in 10 fractions would be given concurrently with the first cycle of VP-16/cisplatin chemotherapy. The extensive stage patient would receive the same chemotherapy prescription as the limited stage patient. Alternating CAV and VP-16/cisplatin can easily be given as an outpatient, and the brevity of the treatment program is consistent with the objective of maximizing treatment-free and progression-free survival. We do not routinely recommend radiotherapy for extensive stage patients unless it is required for palliative purposes.

Dr L. Einhorn: Well, before I give my comments, the score card over here is actually almost a consensus. Out of the nine people we cleared around the table, seven of the nine would give CAV alternating with platinum/VP-16 in extensive disease, and the same seven of the nine would give platinum/VP-16 and chest radiotherapy, although in different time sequences, for limited disease patients. So, that's 77%; that's not bad for a consensus. As far as what I would do, I would join the majority for limited disease if I were treating someone off protocol. I'm treating people for curative intent but I don't think duration of therapy is proven, and four courses of platinum/VP-16 and somewhere between 5,000 and 6,000 rad would be attractive to me, based upon my prejudice, not based upon any data. For extensive disease, I think there are a variety of viable options. I am impressed by the limited disease data with CAV followed by two late intensification courses of platinum/VP-16 and I probably would be more likely to give that rather than alternating it, a la Goldie-Coldman. But in reality, if this were an equitable world, which it isn't, and I had easy access to CBDCA [carboplatin], which I don't, and easy access to oral VP-16 capsules, which I don't, I would probably give one day of CBDCA and then follow it with three days of oral capsule VP-16. That may or may not be an easier or better way of doing things. Any other questions or comments from the panel, the audience, or anyone else?

Dr N. Murray: We have not mentioned prophylactic brain irradiation today. Dementia and chronic brain syndromes in long-term survivors are serious problems. Most of the attention has focused on the dose of brain radiotherapy, but it is possible that radiotherapy-chemotherapy interaction is responsible. Brain irradiation disrupts the blood-brain barrier and subsequent cycles of chemotherapy may damage the neurons and/or the oligodendrocytes. Cisplatin, a heavy metal, may be particularly damaging in this regard as other heavy metals like lead and mercury are well-known central nervous system poisons. In Vancouver, we have used prophylactic brain radiation only after the completion of all chemotherapy treatments when hopefully the metastatic process has been controlled. We have not observed an obvious problem with chronic brain syndrome in our long-term survivors. We have not yet completed a careful psychological and brain imaging reassessment of this patient population. I suggest that other groups consider radiotherapy-chemotherapy interactions when they analyze risk factors for chronic brain toxicity.

Dr L. Einhorn: We don't really have much nausea and vomiting. There's a letter to the editor in the *New England Journal of Medicine* which I tend to agree with, since we have a large VA population, many of whom are chronic alcoholics. You probably burn out the Chemotherapy Trigger Zone (CTZ) and Emetic Centers when you have chronic alcoholism. Our VA patients hardly ever need any antiemetics at all. That's vastly different from a VA patient who's a 25-year-old major in the military and gets platinum for testicular cancer, and has profound nausea and vomiting if not prevented by antiemetics. At University Hospital, our nurses give the antiemetics and there are a variety of things they use. Dexamethasone and thorazine have worked very well. Certainly platinum/VP-16 is not a terribly emetogenic regimen in older patients compared to a younger patient with testis cancer.

NON–SMALL-CELL LUNG CANCER

Brief Overview of Combination Chemotherapy in Non–Small-Cell Lung Cancer

By Philip Bonomi

OPINIONS REGARDING treatment of advanced non–small-cell lung cancer (NSCLC) range from recommendations for aggressive chemotherapy to recommendations for supportive care only. The failure to confirm earlier response rates and to clearly show improved survival as a result of treatment have raised doubts about the usefulness of combination chemotherapy in this group of patients. Despite these considerations, during the past 10 years,[1–6] there are data showing that a variety of combination chemotherapy regimens produce responses in NSCLC. Some of these regimens are listed in Table 1.

Two of the earlier regimens, cyclophosphamide, doxorubicin (Adriamycin [Adria Laboratories, Columbus, Ohio]), methotrexate, and procarbazine (CAMP)[1] and methotrexate, doxorubicin, cyclosphosphamide, and CCNU (lomustine) (MACC),[2] contained a common group of drugs: cyclophosphamide, doxorubicin, and methotrexate. Shortly after results from the CAMP and MACC regimens were published, Eagan et al[3] reported results from a regimen in which cisplatin was used rather than methotrexate and the "fourth drug," CCNU or procarbazine. The 38% regression rate observed with the CAP (cyclophosphamide, doxorubicin, cisplatin) regimen[3] provided evidence that cisplatin used in combination with other chemotherapeutic agents produced modest activity in NSCLC.

Since that time a number of the relatively active and more extensively tested regimens have included cisplatin combined either with a vinca alkaloid[4,5,7,8] or with VP-16 (etoposide).[6,8] The initial response rates reported for cisplatin- and noncisplatin-containing regimens were 28% to 53%.[1–6] However, subsequent evaluation of each of these regimens in Eastern Cooperative Oncology Group (ECOG) trials involving larger groups of patients has shown response rates of 12%[7] and 17%[8] for the non–cisplatin-containing regimens, and 23%[8] to 31%[9] for the cisplatin-containing regimens (Table 1). None of these regimens has produced a significantly better response rate.

Results from the initial trials[1–6] have demonstrated that the median survival duration was longer for responding patients than for nonresponding patients. Subsequent studies conducted by Ruckdeschel et al[8,9] confirmed this observation, with a median survival of approximately 40 weeks being observed for responders *v* approximately 20 weeks for nonresponders. However, it is difficult to determine whether there is a relationship between response and survival. In an attempt to elucidate the relationship between response and survival, Ruckdeschel et al have used the "landmark" technique.[9] With this method of analysis, patients who survived < 3 months were excluded from survival analysis because a period of 3 months was required in order to observe a response in most patients. Therefore, most responders would have a "guaranteed" 3-month period of survival. Using this method of analysis, comparison of responders and nonresponders still showed a statistically significant difference. However, even these results do not provide clear evidence that response to combination chemotherapy produces prolongation of survival.

Many investigators believe that a more reliable way of evaluating the impact of treatment on survival is comparison of survival durations in a randomized trial comparing treatment with chemotherapy to supportive treatment only. There are two studies that indicate that treatment did not affect median survival of NSCLC patients.[10,11] In one of these randomized studies, immediate treatment with the CAMP regimen was compared with delayed treatment with this regimen. Results from this study revealed no difference in median progression-free interval or in median survival.[10] More recently, preliminary analysis of a randomized study comparing supportive treatment only to treatment with vindesine-cisplatin has shown no difference in median survival durations.[11] There is an ongoing ran-

From the Rush Medical College, Chicago.

Address reprint requests to Philip Bonomi, MD, Room 830, 1725 W Harrison, Chicago, IL 60612.

0093–7754/86/1303–3014$05.00/0

Table 1. Combination Chemotherapy for NSCLC

Investigator	Regimen	Response Rate (%)
Bitran[1]	CAMP	48
Ruckdeschel[8]	CAMP	17
Chahinian[2]	MACC	46
Vogl[7]	MACC	12
Eagan[3]	CAP	39
Ruckdeschel[9]	CAP	23
Gralla[4]	VP	43
Ruckdeschel[8]	VP	25
Longeval[6]	EP	28
Ruckdeschel[8]	EP	25
Mason[5]	MVP	53
Ruckdeschel[8]	MVP	31

Abbreviations: CAMP, cyclophosphamide, doxorubicin, methotrexate, and procarbazine; MACC, methotrexate, doxorubicin, cyclophosphamide, and CCNU (lomustine); CAP, cyclophosphamide, doxorubicin, and cisplatin; VP, vindesine and cisplatin; EP, etoposide and cisplatin; MVP, mitomycin-C, vinblastine, and cisplatin.

domized study comparing supportive treatment only, treatment with vindesine-cisplatin, and treatment with cyclophosphamide-doxorubicin-cisplatin. A more definitive answer concerning the effect of combination chemotherapy on median and 1-year survival awaits the maturation of these recent prospective studies.

In the meantime, many investigators are studying new single agents in patients with metastatic NSCLC. As an example, the ECOG plans to study new agents and some new combination regimens in a series of phase II trials. This study will include VP-16–cisplatin as a reference arm against which new treatments will be compared. VP-16–cisplatin has been selected as the reference arm because it produced the highest 1-year survival rate (25%) in recent ECOG trials that included the regimens listed in Table 1.[12]

Table 2. Stage Related to Response

Investigator	Stage	Regimen	Response Rate (%)
Ruckdeschel[9]	III_{M1}	MVP	28
Wagner[15]	III_{MO}	MVP	53
Ruckdeschel[9]	III_{M1}	CAP	23
Fram[14]	III_{MO}	CAP	47
Ruckdeschel[8]	III_{M1}	EP	25
Longeval[6]	III_{M1}	EP	28
	III_{MO}	EP	56

Abbreviations: MVP, mitomycin-C, vinblastine, and cisplatin.

In contrast to the results from chemotherapy trials involving NSCLC patients who have distant metastases, an advantage in progression-free survival for patients receiving combination chemotherapy as adjuvant treatment for NSCLC metastatic to hilar or to mediastinal lymph nodes has been recently reported.[13] Also, there is increasing evidence that combination chemotherapy produces higher response rates in patients who do not have distant metastases[6,14,15] (Table 2). These clinical observations suggest that additional combined modality trials should be evaluated in patients who have less advanced disease. A number of the presentations in this symposium describe new combined modality approaches in this group of patients.

REFERENCES

1. Bitran JD, Desser RK, DeMeester TR, et al: Cyclophosphamide, Adriamycin, methotrexate, and procarbazine (CAMP)—Effective four drug combination chemotherapy for metastatic non-oat cell bronchogenic carcinoma. Cancer Treat Rep 60:1225–1230, 1976

2. Chahinian AP, Arnold DJ, Cohen JM, et al: Chemotherapy for bronchogenic carcinoma—Methotrexate, doxorubicin, cyclosphosphamide, and lomustine. JAMA 237:2392–2396, 1977

3. Eagan RT, Ingle JN, Frytak S, et al: Platinum-based poly chemotherapy versus dianhydrogalactitol in advanced non-small cell lung cancer. Cancer Treat Rep 61:1339–1345, 1977

4. Gralla RJ, Casper ES, Kelson DP, et al: Cisplatin and vindesine combination chemotherapy for advanced carcinoma of the lung: A randomized trial investigating two dosage schedules. Ann Intern Med 95:414–420, 1981

5. Mason BA, Catalano RB: Mitomycin, vinblastine, and cisplatin combination chemotherapy in non-small cell lung cancer. Proc Am Soc Clin Oncol 21:477, 1980 (abstr)

6. Longeval E, Klastersky J: Combination chemotherapy with cisplatin and etoposide in bronchogenic squamous cell carcinoma and adenocarcinoma—A study for the EORTC lung cancer working party (Belgium). Cancer 50:2751–2756, 1982

7. Vogl SE, Mehta CR, Cohen MH: MACC chemotherapy for adenocarcinoma and epidermoid carcinoma of the lung. Cancer 44:864–868, 1979

8. Ruckdeschel JC, Finkelstein DM, Ettinger DS: Chemotherapy of metastatic non-small cell lung cancer (NSCLC): The Eastern Cooperative Group experience, in Proceedings of the Fourth World Conference on Lung Cancer. 1985, p 39

9. Ruckdeschel JC, Finkelstein DM, Mason BA, et al: Chemotherapy for metastatic non-small cell bronchogenic carcinoma: EST 2575, generation V—A randomized comparison of four cisplatin-containing regimens. J Clin Oncol 3:72–79, 1985

10. Lad TE, Nelson RB, Diekamp U, et al: Immediate versus postponed combination chemotherapy (CAMP) for

unresectable non-small cell lung cancer: A randomized trial. Cancer Treat Rep 65:973–978, 1981

11. Woods RL, Levi JA, Page J, et al: Non-small cell cancer: A randomized comparison of chemotherapy with no chemotherapy. Proc Am Soc Clin Oncol 4:177, 1985 (abstr)

12. Finkelstein DM, Ettinger DS, Ruckdeschel JC: Long-term survivors in metastatic non–small-cell lung cancer: An Eastern Cooperative Group study. J Clin Oncol 4:702–709, 1986

13. Holmes EC, Hill LD, Gail M: A randomized comparison of the effects of adjuvant therapy on resected stages II and III non-small cell carcinoma of the lung. Ann Surg 202:335–341, 1985

14. Fram R, Skarin A, Balikian J, et al: Combination chemotherapy followed by radiation therapy in patients with regional stage III unresectable non-small cell lung cancer. Cancer Treat Rep 69:587–590, 1985

15. Wagner H, Ruckdeschel J, Bonomi P, et al: Treatment of locally advanced non-small cell lung cancer (NSCLC) with mitomycin-C, vinblastine, and cisplatin (MVP) followed by radiation therapy: An ECOG pilot study. Proc Am Soc Clin Oncol 4:183, 1985 (abstr)

Rationale for Chemotherapy for Patients With Advanced Non–Small-Cell Lung Cancer

By F. Anthony Greco

Patients with advanced non–small-cell lung cancer (NSCLC) are difficult to treat effectively. There is a strong rationale to continue clinical investigation, since this approach has been useful for other groups of patients with "resistant" tumors. This report reviews the major reasons to consider chemotherapy in these patients, and discusses several other important auxiliary issues.

THE PURPOSE of this report is to outline briefly the rationale for the use of chemotherapy for patients with advanced non–small-cell lung cancer (NSCLC). I believe there are two major reasons to consider chemotherapy for these patients: first, to continue our search for more effective therapy in the context of an organized clinical study; and second, to attempt to provide palliation for the patient of several of the distressing symptoms and signs of advanced carcinoma.

In reference to the first reason, Table 1 outlines the historical development of more effective chemotherapy for advanced neoplasms. All of the "responsive" neoplasms that are treated successfully today were at one time considered "unresponsive." A sequence of events has usually led to the improved therapy. A similar sequence has occurred in the past for patients who now have treatable malignancies. Of course, the timing occurred much faster for some neoplasms than for others because not all neoplasms share the same responsiveness to therapy that has been available and developed over the past three decades. The sequence usually started with a patient with advanced and relatively unresponsive neoplasm. Active single agents were identified after appropriate phase I and II studies. Responses to single agents were usually partial, but in rare instances complete responses were observed. After the identification of several active single agents, combination chemotherapy was devised and the response rates were often improved. Complete responses were seen and some were durable. Further phase III studies were often necessary to try to extend the duration of remission. The result of these investigations was an improvement in the overall therapy for these patients, often with very good palliation or even cure in selected patient groups.

The current "position" for patients with advanced NSCLC in this developmental scheme is illustrated in Table 2. Several single agents have been identified with low levels of activity (12% to 20%), and usually only partial responses are seen in a small minority of patients. Combination regimens have been developed from these single drugs and have improved the activity, but response rates have not been >50% (30% to 45%). A small number of these responses have been complete responses (<5%). It appears that some real progression along the scheme, as outlined in Table 1, has already occurred. The clinical investigations required to continue the progress offer the potential of clinical benefit to participating patients.

The search for more effective therapy involves the traditional approach of clinical investigation. Not only should the search for single active agents continue, but appropriate trials of combination chemotherapy are necessary to confirm improvements in overall response rates. The experimental design of phase II and III studies should allow one to confidently interpret the effects of various therapies with respect to response rate, palliation, quality of life, and survival. Our search for more effective therapy also involves basic investigation. More knowledge about the cellular biology of lung cancer is certainly a high priority. Possible clues or leads for therapy can result from a better understanding of the growth requirements and biochemical composition of malignant cells.

Approximately 100,000 patients with unresectable advanced NSCLC will be seen in the United States in 1986. I estimate that approximately 80,000 patients would be suitable for

From the Division of Oncology, Vanderbilt University Medical Center, Nashville.

Address reprint requests to F. Anthony Greco, MD, Division of Oncology, Vanderbilt University Medical Center, Nashville, TN 37232.

0093–7754/86/1303–3019$05.00

Table 1. Historical Development of More Effective Chemotherapy for Advanced Neoplasms

Unresponsive neoplasm.
Active single agents found in phase II study.
Responses are usually partial, but depends on the neoplasm.
Combination chemotherapy with active agents produces increased response rate.
Complete responses are seen; some may be durable; phase III required.
Good palliaiton, prolongation of survival, or cure follow with increasing complete response rates.

clinical trials. A gross estimate of all the cooperative group activity, as well as independent studies from various cancer centers, is that only approximately 4,000 patients per year are entered in organized clinical studies. Therefore, the overwhelming majority of patients are not being treated in a study and do not contribute to the search for more effective therapy. I encourage physicians to enroll more patients in clinical studies, since this may be clinically beneficial and will eventually result in better therapy for all patients. However, even though chemotherapy for advanced NSCLC is in the early development phase, I believe there is a rationale for treating selective patients in an effort to palliate their distressing symptoms and signs.

There are limited options for patients with advanced NSCLC. They can be enrolled in an organized clinical trial, or they may be considered for symptomatic and supportive care only. In selected circumstances, "standard" radiotherapy and/or chemotherapy off protocol should be considered. The source of uncertainty regarding the usefulness of chemotherapy is outlined in Table 3. The response rate to most regimens is <50%, and these responses are usually partial and of relatively short duration. Toxicity is a major concern and there is a considerable amount of pessimism from past experience. In addition, randomized studies have not yet proven a survival advantage for all treated patients *v* those who receive only symptomatic and supportive care.[1]

Table 2. The Current "Position" of NSCLC in Developmental Therapy

Several active single agents identified, but with low levels of activity.
Partial responses observed, 12% to 20%.
Several combinations developed with improved activity, but total response <50%.
Complete responses occur, but are rare (<5%).

Table 3. The Source of Uncertainty Regarding the Usefulness of Chemotherapy

Response rate is <50%.
Toxicity is a major concern.
Large studies have not yet proved a survival advantage for *all* treated patients.
Pessimism from past experience.

Controversy has centered around what I term the "response rate, survival, quality of life dilemma" (Table 4). In patients with good performance status, the response rate to several platinum-based combination regimens average approximately 35%.[2] The responders to therapy live longer than the nonresponders. Is this really the effect of the therapy? Is the quality of life of responding patients improved? Since the total response rate is <50% with only rare complete responders, it will be very difficult to show improvement in the survival of all treated patients compared with untreated control patients, even if such a difference is present for the responding patients. Many oncologists believe that the quality of life of many of the responding patients is improved. This issue is currently being tested in phase III studies. Survival certainly is not the only useful end point to evaluate, particularly if patients who respond experience useful palliation. Advanced NSCLC does not run an indolent course untreated in most patients and there is considerable "toxicity" to the patient from the untreated disease.

There are several clinical factors that have now been relatively well confirmed as prognostic factors for these patients. Patients are very

Table 4. The Response Rate, Survival, Quality of Life Dilemma

In good performance status patients, response rates average approximately 35% for platinum-based regimens.
Responders live longer, but is this really the effect of the therapy?
Is the quality of life improved?
Since the total response rate is <50%, it will be very difficult to show improvement in survival compared with untreated controls (even if it is present).
Quality of life of many responders appears to be improved. This issue is being tested.
Survival is not the only useful endpoint to evaluate.
The neoplasm does *not* run an indolent course untreated and has "toxicity" to the patient.

Table 5. The Case for Chemotherapy for NSCLC

There are unequivocal responses, and even a low order of complete response.
Reduction or disappearance of symptoms and signs definitely occurs in many responding patients.
One can determine response early (6 to 8 wk).
A brief course of induction chemotherapy for responders appears to be as useful and less toxic than prolonged therapy.

unlikely to respond to chemotherapy if they have a poor performance status (Eastern Cooperative Oncology Group [ECOG] 3 to 4); weight loss >10% of previous body weight, poor general medical condition, with concurrent heart disease, liver disease, or kidney disease; and extensive hepatic or bony metastasis. These features are certainly important to consider when making a decision regarding the possible usefulness of chemotherapy for the individual patient.

The psyche of the patient is also an important factor. The patient's feelings regarding this disease and possible treatments are not a minor issue. When a patient is referred to me in Nashville from Florida, he usually does not come to see me to hear a discussion on the advantages of not receiving treatment. This does not mean I should definitely tell him he should receive treatment, but he usually comes with the idea of receiving treatment. This is an important issue in a patient's mind, and an open discussion with the patient and family about what can and cannot be expected from chemotherapy should be undertaken.

Can I make a case for administering palliative chemotherapy for patients with advanced NSCLC? As previously mentioned, there is a strong rationale for entering patients in investigational studies. However, the majority of patients are not placed in studies, and we need to encourage this activity. What about those patients who otherwise have relatively good features (good performance status, no large weight loss, young, and healthy) but will not accept protocol therapy, or for one reason or another will not be entered in a protocol? A case can be made to treat these patients with chemotherapy with palliative intent (Table 5). There are certainly unequivocal responses to chemotherapy, even a low order of complete responses. There is often a reduction or even disappearance of symptoms and signs in many of the responding patients. This may not be appreciated unless the patient is followed carefully. I have noticed a

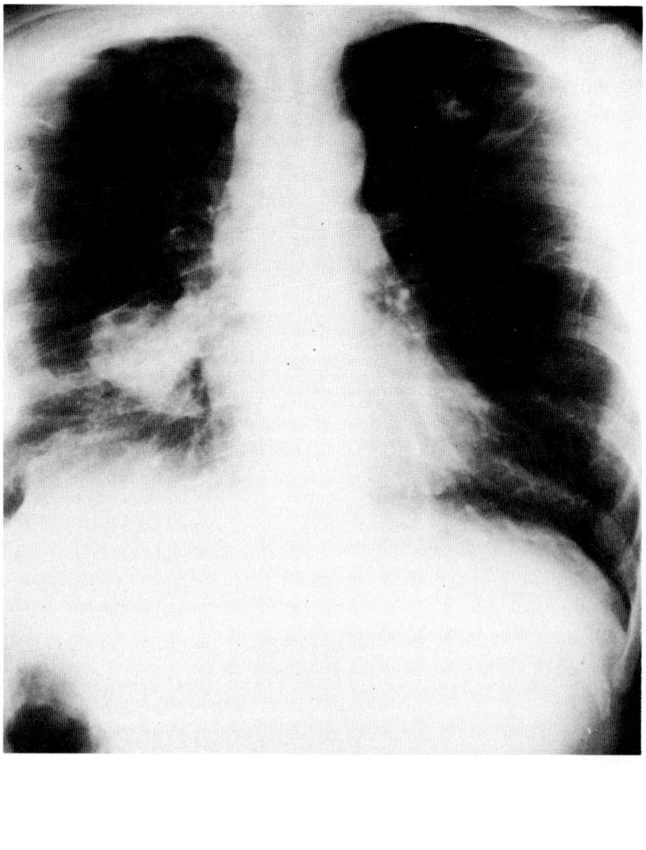

Fig 1. X-ray showing large lung and pleural masses.

tendency for some physicians to ignore or not appreciate the symptomatic benefit in some responding patients. This may arise from the attitude that these patients would be just as well off with morphine and other symptomatic treatment and can be seen at 2- or 3-month intervals. An important feature about a response to chemotherapy is that it can be determined quite early, often within the first month or two. Patients can receive one course of chemotherapy, and if they are clinically stable or improved after a few weeks, a second course may be administered. This is a classic trial of therapy. However, if progressive tumor occurs after one course, the treatment can be stopped. There is no reason to continue to expose a patient who has not responded after two courses of treatment to the same chemotherapy. In addition, in those patients who respond objectively, there is currently no evidence that continuing treatment beyond several induction courses (four to six courses) is any more useful for the patient than stopping treatment. I have the impression that several physicians think that when you treat a patient with chemotherapy you are locked into the treatment for as long as the patient is alive.

Since palliation is the major goal, therapy does not necessarily need to be started when a patient is relatively asymptomatic or has very few signs. Patients can be followed carefully, and the pace of their disease can be estimated. Therapy can be started when symptoms become worse or when the tumor becomes larger. This is an individual decision that is often made after considering many of the clinical features and discussion with the patient.

I will now briefly present a patient with advanced NSCLC to illustrate useful palliation and clinical benefit from currently available chemotherapy.

CASE REPORT

A 58-year-old white man complained of cough, chest pain, and recent hemoptysis. He was a heavy smoker and had lost approximately 20 pounds in the previous 3 months. His physical examination showed him to be cachexic. He had a localized wheeze in the right lung base. His performance status was 2 on the ECOG scale. Chest x-ray is shown in Fig 1. Fiberoptic bronchoscopy showed partial obstruction of the right lower lobe bronchus with a mass. Biopsy of this showed squamous-cell carcinoma. This man did not wish to participate in a phase II evaluation of a new agent. However, he was interested in some form of chemotherapy. The limitations and toxicity of chemotherapy for this type of advanced cancer were discussed in some detail. He received one cycle of VP-16 and platinum, each on a three-day schedule. At the end of one

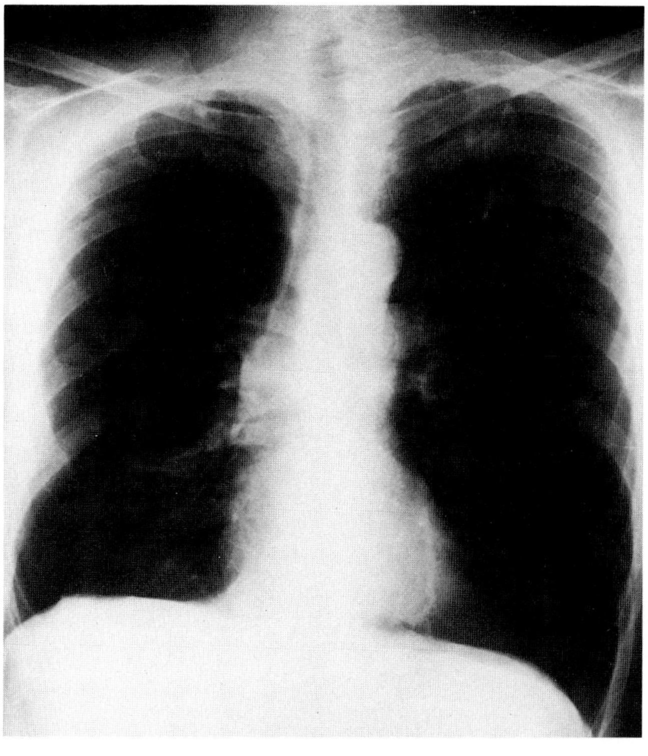

Fig 2. X-ray showing a good reduction in tumor masses.

course of treatment (3 weeks), he had had nearly a 50% reduction in the pleural masses as well as the right lung mass. He received a second course of VP-16 and platinum; his x-ray after two courses is illustrated in Fig 2. There was still a small right pleural-based mass, but he had approximately a 90% shrinkage of evaluable tumor. He was treated with a total of six courses of VP-16 and platinum. His cough, hemoptysis, and chest pain resolved after the first course of therapy; he regained lost weight during the course of treatment despite some intermittent anorexia from the chemotherapy. His performance status was 0 and he returned to work. The remission lasted for approximately 18 months. He developed progressive disease and decided not to receive further therapy and died one month later.

This patient had the type of palliation that unequivocally occurs in some of the responding patients who are treated with chemotherapy. This type of clinical turnabout does not happen, in my opinion, in patients who are not treated. Certainly, some of the pain and other problems related to this neoplasm can be palliated with analgesics, but an overall dramatic improvement in clinical status with weight gain and improvement in performance status is not to be expected. If this particular patient were entered into a randomized comparison with VP-16 and platinum *v* no treatment, and received VP-16 and platinum, his response might not extend the *survival* of the whole group that was treated even if a minority of treated patients showed similar responses. Perhaps a quality-of-life evaluation would favor the treated group.

Table 6. Chemotherapy Off Protocol

Open discussion with the patient.
Evaluation of important patient factors: performance status, weight loss, extent of metastasis, general medical condition, psyche.
Goal is to palliate and perhaps extend useful survival.
Therapy can be delayed or the disease paced.
Use of only one or two courses to determine response; subjective and objective.
Use of maximum of four to six courses of chemotherapy.

In summary, patients can often be best served by participating in a clinical study, and I encourage this approach. If patients are treated with palliative intent off protocol I think some general guidelines are useful (Table 6). Hopefully, treatment will soon be improved, and the controversy about the usefulness of chemotherapy will be resolved.

REFERENCES

1. Wood RL, Levi JA, Page J, et al: Non small cell cancer: A randomised comparison of chemotherapy with no chemotherapy. Proc Am Soc Clin Oncol 4:177, 1985 (abstr C-691)

2. Klastersky J, Sculier JP: Chemotherapy of non-small cell lung cancer. Semin Oncol 12:38–48, 1985 (suppl 6)

A Multicenter Phase II Trial of Cisplatin and Oral Etoposide (VP-16) in Inoperable Non–Small-Cell Lung Cancer

By Ted Splinter, Tjebbe Kok, Siangh Kho, Han Lameris, Fiebo ten Kate, Otilia Dalesio, Bram Dolman, Fernand Palmen, Jaap Bouvy, Jos Burghouts, Frank Simonis, Peter Harper, Elaine Rankin, Ineke van Reijswoud, and Jan van Hoogenhuijze

Sixty patients with inoperable non–small-cell lung cancer (NSCLC) were entered into a phase II study that tested the combination of cisplatin (80 mg/m², day 1), etoposide intravenously (IV) (100 mg, days 1 and 2), and etoposide orally (200 mg/m², days 3 and 5). The regimen was repeated every 28 days for six courses, after which patients were allowed to receive additional treatment at the discretion of their physician. Overall objective response rate in 51 evaluable patients was 69% (95% confidence interval: range, 56% to 81%), with 16% sustaining complete remission (CR), 53% partial remission (PR), 17% stable disease (SD), and 14% progressive disease (PD). CR was pathologically confirmed by bronchoscopy and biopsy. One patient with a clinical PR underwent surgery and was shown to have a pathologic CR. Median survival of all evaluable patients was 52 weeks, greater than 75 weeks for CR patients, 52 weeks for PR patients, 42 weeks for SD patients, and 13 weeks for PD patients. Eleven patients (21.5%) developed CNS metastases, which resulted in the deaths of ten. Survival was significantly correlated with extent of disease, performance status, and albumin level, but not with histology or weight loss. Tumor response was significantly correlated only with histology (squamous-cell and large-cell undifferentiated carcinoma greater than adenocarcinoma). Side effects were nausea, vomiting, anorexia, alopecia, bone marrow suppression, and nephrotoxicity. One patient died from leukopenia and sepsis. Pharmacokinetic studies in ten patients showed the continuous presence of etoposide in plasma for six days at a level of at least 220 to 480 ng/mL. In order to investigate whether this very effective combination of cisplatin and etoposide can prolong survival in NSCLC, it will be tested as preoperative chemotherapy in a randomized trial in operable patients with T_1N_1 and T_2N_{0-1} disease.

SEVERAL STUDIES have been performed with cisplatin and etoposide in patients with advanced non–small-cell lung cancer (NSCLC). The objective response rate in 14 studies comprising 585 patients was 34%, with 31% achieving partial remission (PR), and 3%, complete remission (CR).[1] These studies were based on the synergistic action of both drugs in vitro[2] and in vivo.[3,4] However, no explanation has been offered for the drugs' in vivo synergism. Recently, in vitro experiments have shown that the probable mechanism of cytotoxic action of etoposide is inhibition of the enzyme topoisomerase II. This inhibition leads to interference of the breakage-reunion reaction of topoisomerase II and thereby to DNA single-strand breaks,[5,6] which occur very soon after exposure to etoposide. Similarly, repair of these breaks commences quickly after discontinuance of the drug.[6,7]

Assuming that the synergism of cisplatin and etoposide may depend on continuous inhibition of the DNA strand-rejoining activity of the topoisomerase II by etoposide (which thereby may increase the cytotoxic effect of cisplatin-induced DNA damage), we again tested the combination of cisplatin and etoposide in NSCLC patients. The major difference of this regimen compared with the usual regimens[1] was timing and route of etoposide administration (intravenously [IV] on days 1 and 2 and orally in three divided doses on days 3 and 5). This schedule was designed to obtain continuous plasma levels of etoposide for at least six days from the start of cisplatin infusion. To obviate the variable bioavailability (29% to 100%) of etoposide capsules,[8] the dose of oral etoposide was increased, depending on the leukocyte and platelet nadir. Interestingly, the treatment schedule of cisplatin and etoposide achieving the highest response rate in NSCLC (52%), as published in the literature,[9] consisted of cisplatin (90 mg/m²) on day 1 and etoposide (50 mg/m²) on days 1 through 5.

MATERIALS AND METHODS

Patients were eligible for this study if they had cytologically or histologically proven NSCLC (stage III); measur-

From the Department of Oncology, University Hospital, Dijkzigt, Rotterdam, Netherlands; the EORTC data center, Brussels, Belgium; the Elisabeth Hospital, Tilburg, Netherlands; Holy Hospital, Vlaardingen, Netherlands; Groot Ziekengasthuis, Den Bosch; Guy's Hospital, London; and the University Hospital of the Free University, Amsterdam.

Address reprint requests to T.A.W. Splinter, MD, Department of Oncology, University Hospital, Dijkzigt, 3015 GD Rotterdam, Netherlands.

0093-7754/86/1303-3015$05.00/0

able disease; age under 75 years; Eastern Cooperative Oncology Group (ECOG) performance status of 0, 1, or 2; serum creatinine levels of <150 μmol/L (or creatinine clearance >60 mL/min); no symptomatic brain metastases; no life-threatening conditions, such as hemoptysis, superior cava vein syndrome, or spinal cord compression; no pretreatment with chemotherapy; no uncontrolled infection or uncontrolled cardiac disease; and no second malignancy. Staging was performed according to tumor, node, and metastasis (TNM) classification; the T and N classification were assessed by chest x-ray and/or computed tomography (CT) scan of the thorax, whereas M classification was assessed primarily by physical examination. Other procedures, such as isotope bone scan, CT scan of the abdomen, and ultrasound of the liver were performed if indicated clinically by pain, raised alkaline phosphatase levels, abnormal liver functions, and palpable abdominal mass. Patients with M_0 and M_x were staged as limited disease (LD) and with proven M_1 as extensive disease (ED).

The chemotherapy regimen, repeated every 4 weeks, was as follows: day 1—etoposide (100 mg, IV) as a two-hour infusion, followed by cisplatin (80 mg/m^2) as a four-hour infusion; day 2—etoposide (100 mg, IV) as a two-hour infusion; days 3 and 5—etoposide (200 mg/m^2 orally) as capsules of 100 mg each, divided over three doses at 10 AM, and 2 and 6 PM, respectively. In case of a leukocyte nadir > 2×10^9/L and/or a platelet nadir > 75×10^9/L, the dose of oral etoposide was increased until a sufficient nadir was obtained or to a maximum of 500 mg/m^2.

Patients were evaluated for response with standard World Health Organization (WHO) criteria[10] after every two courses of chemotherapy, unless disease progression occurred earlier. Patients went off study after six courses. Patients with a radiologic CR were further evaluated by bronchoscopy and biopsy. Occurrence of CNS metastasis was not evaluated as progressive disease. Bone metastases were not accepted as parameters for response. Toxicity from chemotherapy was graded according to WHO criteria. Etoposide levels were measured by a high-performance liquid chromography (HPLC) method[11] in heparin plasma, obtained from ten patients after the first IV dose on day 1 and 24 hours later, after the first oral dose on day 3 and 24 hours later. Blood was collected in heparinized tubes, and plasma was removed after centrifugation at 10 g for ten minutes. Plasma was frozen immediately at −20°C and stored until assayed.

RESULTS

Sixty patients were entered into the study from August 1983 to August 1984. Five patients were deemed ineligible (two with hypernephroma, one with small-cell lung cancer (SCLC), one with a germ cell tumor, and one with no measurable disease). Four other patients were deemed not evaluable (one refused further treatment after the first course of chemotherapy, one died from hemoptysis during the second course, one died from diabetic coma after the first course, and there was one toxic death due to leukopenia and sepsis after the second course. Characteristics of the remaining 51 evaluable patients are shown in Table 1. The median number of chemotherapy courses was five (range, one to eight). Almost all LD patients received additional treatment after chemotherapy, independent of the response: two received pneumonectomy, two pneumonectomy plus radiotherapy, and 15 radiotherapy alone.

Table 1. Pretreatment Characteristics of 51 Evaluable Patients

	No. Patients
Males/females	45/6
Age (yr)	
<50	10
50–60	21
61–70	18
>70	2
Performance status*	
Grade 0	11
Grade 1	32
Grade 2	8
Weight loss	
<1%	25
1–5%	2
5–10%	3
>10%	4
Unknown	17
Serum albumin	
>35 g/L	9
≤35 g/L	28
Unknown	14
Histology	
Squamous-cell carcinoma	25
Adenocarcinoma	10
Large-cell undifferentiated	16
Stage	
Limited disease (M_0 + M_X)	9 + 13
Extensive disease (M_1)	29
Previous surgery	1
Previous radiotherapy	1

*Eastern Cooperative Oncology Group criteria.

Overall objective response rate was 69% (95% confidence interval: range, 56% to 81%). Eight patients (16%) achieved CR, 27 (53%) PR, nine (17%) stable disease (SD), and seven (14%) progressive disease (PD). One patient with a clinical CR (unconfirmed by bronchoscopy) was evaluated as a PR. Almost all responding patients showed a response after the second course of chemotherapy; maximum response was observed after four courses.

All patients who underwent surgery were initially inoperable because of a T_3 tumor involving the main bronchus. After five courses of chemotherapy they showed a clinical PR, and repeated

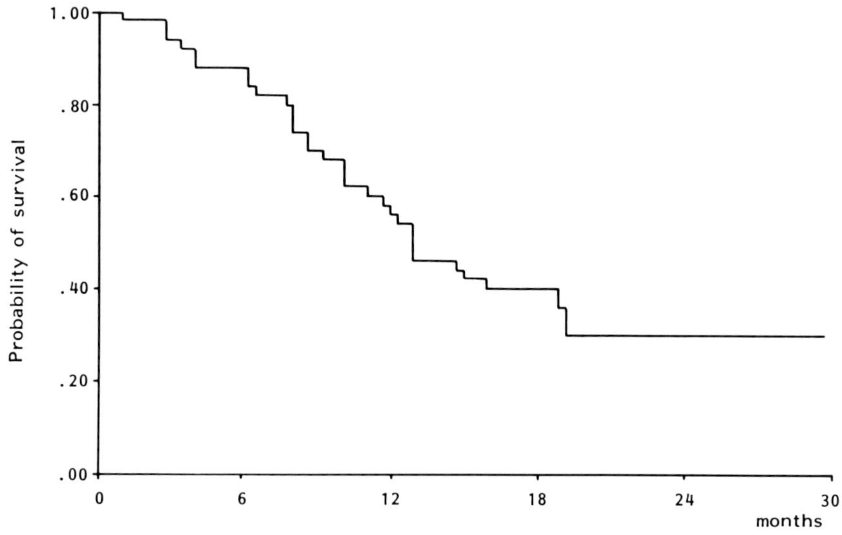

Fig 1. Actuarial survival of 51 evaluable NSCLC patients.

biopsies from the main bronchus were tumor-negative. After surgery, only one patient still had a subepithelial tumor at the resection margin; two patients had become operable with still vital tumor in the intermediate bronchus; in only one patient were necrotic tissue, fibrosis, and inflammatory reaction seen at the site of the former tumor. The first patient died after 81 weeks; the other three patients are alive with no evidence of disease at 79, 80, and 125 weeks.

The median survival (Fig 1) of all evaluable patients was 52 weeks; median follow-up was 54 weeks. Nineteen patients are still alive with a median follow-up of 79 weeks. Median survival of CR patients was greater than 75 weeks; of PR patients, 52 weeks; of SD patients, 42 weeks; and of PD patients, 13 weeks. No significant difference in survival was observed between patients with PR and SD.

Tables 2 and 3 show the relationship between pretreatment characteristics and survival and

Table 2. Relation Between Pretreatment Characteristics and Survival*

	Median Survival (wk)	Log Rank Test *P* Values
Stage of disease		
LD	72	.009
ED	40	
ECOG performance status		
0–1	61	.04
2	33	
Albumin		
>35 g/L	62	.003
≤35 g/L	28	
Weight loss		
<5%	50	NS
≥5%	36	
Histology		
Sq	65	
LCU	51	NS
Ad	35	

Abbreviations: LD, limited disease; ED, extensive disease; ECOG, Eastern Cooperative Oncology Group; NS, not significant; Sq, squamous cell carcinoma; LCU, large-cell undifferentiated carcinoma; Ad, adenocarcinoma.

*Median survival (all patients) equals 52 weeks.

Table 3. Relation Between Pretreatment Characteristics and Response

	Patients (%)				Log Rank Test *P* Value
	CR	PR	SD	PD	
All patients	16	53	17	14	—
Stage of disease					
LD	18	59	14	9	NS
ED	14	48	21	17	
ECOG performance status					
0–1	18	42	24	16	NS
2	25	38	12	25	
Albumin					
>35 g/L	18	43	29	10	NS
≤35 g/L	0	67	11	22	
Weight loss					
<5%	19	46	23	12	NS
≥5%	0	37.5	12.5	50	
Histology					
Sq + LCU	17	58	12	12	.05
Ad	10	30	40	20	

Abbreviations: CR, complete response; PR, partial response; SD, stable disease; PD, progressive disease; LD, limited disease; NS, not significant; ED, extensive disease; ECOG, Eastern Cooperative Oncology Group; Sq, squamous-cell carcinoma; LCU, large-cell undifferentiated carcinoma; Ad, adenocarcinoma.

response, respectively. A significant correlation was observed between survival and stage of disease, performance status, and serum albumin level higher or lower than 35 g/L. No correlation was found between survival and weight loss higher or lower than 5% or between survival and histology. No correlation was found between objective response (CR and PR) and stage of disease, performance status, or serum-albumin level; a trend to significant correlation was observed between objective response and weight loss. In addition, a significant difference was seen between the objective response of squamous-cell and large-cell undifferentiated carcinomas on the one hand and adenocarcinomas on the other.

Ten patients developed symptomatic brain metastases, confirmed by CT scan, and in one patient, leptomeningeal carcinomatosis was confirmed by cytologic examination of cerebrospinal fluid, for an overall incidence of CNS involvement of 21.5%. Ten patients have died from CNS metastases. A comparison of pretreatment characteristics, survival, and response to chemotherapy between patients with and without symptomatic CNS involvement showed that the chance of women developing brain metastases was significantly higher ($P = .02$) than that of men. No other significant differences between patients with and without symptomatic brain metastases were observed.

In Table 4, side effects from chemotherapy are listed. Overall, chemotherapy was tolerated reasonably well. Despite administration of prophylactic antiemetics, such as dexamethasone, domperidone, and lorazepam, all patients experienced at least some degree of cisplatin-induced nausea, vomiting, and/or anorexia. Since these side effects invariably increased with the number of courses, two patients refused further chemotherapy after the fifth course. Most patients did not lose weight, as shown by median weight before and after chemotherapy. Although all patients characterized the large etoposide capsules as "bombs," they did not experience much difficulty in swallowing them. One patient, however, had increasing complaints of stomach pain and nausea due to etoposide and refused further chemotherapy after the fifth course. Five patients had an episode of leukopenia and fever, which had to be treated with antibiotics; one patient died from sepsis during severe leukopenia induced by an increase of the oral etoposide dose from 400 to 600 mg on days 3 and 5 of the second course. Three patients had thrombocytopenia and purpura, which were treated with platelet transfusions. Nineteen patients (38%) developed increased serum creatinine levels as shown by the rise of median serum creatinine levels after chemotherapy in comparison with levels before treatment; three patients went off study because of a creatinine level greater than 150 μmol/L. Figure 2 shows etoposide levels in plasma samples of one patient, obtained at different times during the seventh course of chemotherapy. It can be seen that a plasma level of at least 400 ng/mL of etoposide is maintained for five days (and probably for six days) if the decrease from day 3 to day 5 may be extrapolated to the decrease from day 5 to 7. Etoposide levels measured in the plasma of nine other patients showed very similar curves, with minimal plasma levels varying from 220 to 480 ng/mL.

Table 4. Toxicities of Chemotherapy

	No. Patients
Nausea/vomiting (grades 1 and 2)*	51
Gastrointestinal intolerance	3
Median weight before:after chemotherapy	73.7:74.7
Anemia-alopecia	51
Leukopenia and fever	5
Median leukocyte nadir $\times 10^9$/L (range)	2.1 (0.6–5.8)
Toxic death	1
Thrombocytopenic hemorrhage	3
Median platelet nadir $\times 10^9$/L (range)	92 (6–364)
Nephrotoxicity (grade 1)*	19
Median serum creatinine before:after chemotherapy	80.5:99.3
Neurotoxicity (grades 1 and 2)*	4
Psychologic intolerance	4

*World Health Organization criteria.

DISCUSSION

Much discussion is ongoing regarding the value of chemotherapy for the survival of patients with inoperable NSCLC.[12,13] The main reasons for this discussion are conflicting data from several phase II studies (which by definition cannot prove that chemotherapy causes an improved survival), the statistically invalid method of comparing survival between responders and nonresponders, and lack of a large phase III trial comparing patients randomly

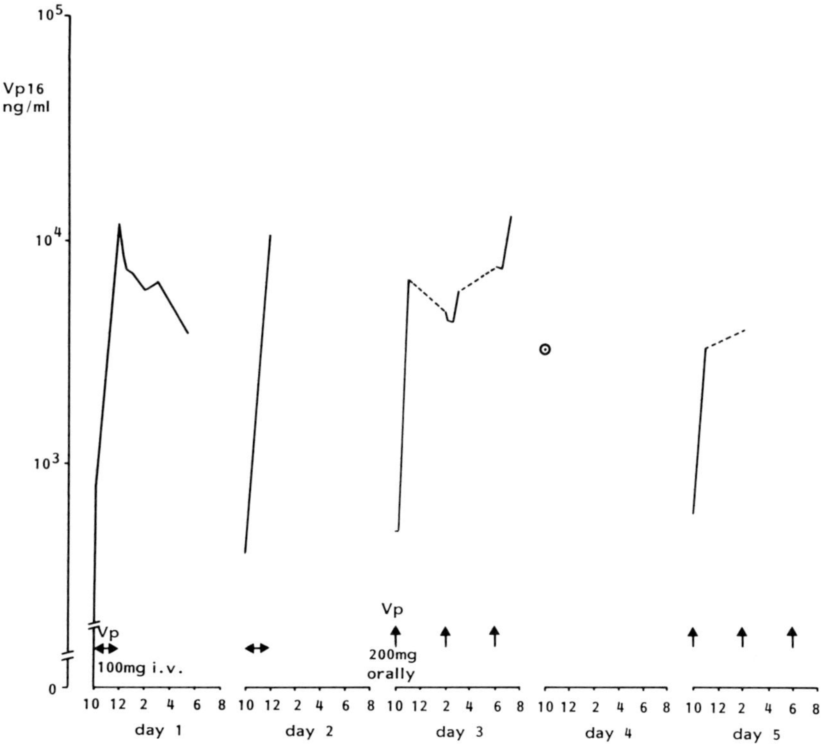

Fig 2. Plasma levels of etoposide in one patient. Plasma samples were obtained on different days and at different times between 10 AM and 8 PM during the seventh course. The patient received a dose of 400 mg/m² of etoposide orally (3 × 200 mg on days 3 and 5).

assigned to treatment with chemotherapy or palliative treatment. However, since response rates of most chemotherapy combinations in NSCLC are well below 50%, it is unlikely that median survival will be affected. Therefore, phase II trials are needed with chemotherapy combinations capable of inducing objective responses in more than 50% of patients and, especially, complete remissions in more than the usual 3%.

In NSCLC, prognostic factors for response and survival are initial performance status, extent of disease, weight loss, previous radiotherapy, histology, sex, abnormal lactic dehydrogenase, number and sites of metastases (eg, subcutaneous, bone, and bone marrow) and probably other factors, which have not yet been defined.[14–17] In our study, a significant correlation was found between survival and extent of disease, performance status, and serum albumin level, respectively, but not between survival and weight loss or histology. The lack of correlation between survival and weight loss may be due to the inaccuracy of evaluating the latter prognostic factor and the large amount of unknown data. Using a cutoff level of 35 g/L, serum albumin is a very significant prognostic factor for survival, as has been observed in SCLC[18] but to our knowledge not in NSCLC.

The combination of cisplatin and etoposide (part IV and part oral) induced a high objective response rate of 69% with 16% CRs, pathologically confirmed by bronchoscopy and biopsy. One patient with a radiologic CR was evaluated as PR, because bronchoscopy was not repeated. Furthermore, one patient with a radiologic PR underwent surgery and was shown to have a pathologic CR. Median survival was 52 weeks with a projected survival at 2 years of 30%. Median survival of CR patients was > 75 weeks. The better survival of CR patients in comparison with PR patients supports the suggestion that achievement of CR may be a more useful criterion of value than overall objective response (CR and PR) in phase II trials in NSCLC.[13] Similarly, the lack of survival difference between PR patients and SD patients suggests that either no difference in survival exists between both groups or that the evaluation of PR is frequently mistaken because of a decrease of atelectasis or inflammatory reaction.

In two recently published studies, high response rates of 85% (CR, 15%)[19] and 57%

(CR, 16%)[20] were obtained with combination chemotherapy. Median survival in the former study was only 24 weeks, despite treating LD patients (60%) additionally with radiotherapy, and 40 weeks in the latter, with a median survival of CR patients of 81 weeks. The major responses in our study were significantly higher in squamous-cell and large-cell carcinomas than in adenocarcinomas, and no correlation was observed between response and extent of disease, performance status, or albumin level. This observation suggests that contradictory to the comments of Aisner and Hansen,[17] prognostic factors for survival and response may be different, and it supports the data of O'Connell et al,[14] which verify that a major response is independently predictive of prolongation of survival.

An important problem encountered in this study was the incidence of CNS metastases (21.5% of patients). Except for a significantly higher incidence in female as compared with male patients, no other correlations could be found between the occurrence of CNS metastases and pretreatment characteristics, survival, and response to chemotherapy. In the future, it may be useful to pay more attention to this problem in NSCLC patients in order to determine whether certain prognostic factors are predictive of the occurrence of brain metastases.

Although the chemotherapy regimen produced a large number of side effects, it was tolerated by most patients. Seven patients refused further treatment: three because of nausea and vomiting, and four because of psychological reasons. Despite nausea and vomiting during chemotherapy and an anorexic period of at least 1 week, patient median weight remained constant during the entire treatment period. The large percentage of patients who developed nephrotoxicity was perplexing. One explanation for this may be that many of the patients who developed nephrotoxicity had prolonged nausea and an incapacity to drink an adequate amount of fluid during the first three days following cisplatin infusion.

In conclusion, the combination of cisplatin and etoposide, as used in this study, produced a high objective response rate and especially a high CR rate in 51 evaluable NSCLC patients. Although median survivals of the whole group and of the different response groups support the observed responses, they do not prove that the induction of a response by chemotherapy leads to a prolongation of survival. In order to investigate the latter very important issue, a randomized trial has been started, in which the effect of preoperative cisplatin and etoposide on tumor response and survival will be compared with the effect of surgery alone on survival in operable T_1N_1 and T_2N_{0-1} patients with NSCLC.

REFERENCES

1. Klastersky J: VP16 and cisplatin in the treatment of non-small cell lung cancer. Semin Oncol 12:17–20, 1985 (suppl 2)

2. Achterrath W, Niederle N, Raettig K, et al: Etoposide—chemistry, preclinical and clinical pharmacology. Cancer Treat Rev 9:3–13, 1982 (suppl A)

3. Evans WK, Osoba D, Feld R, et al: Etoposide (VP16) and cisplatin: An effective treatment for relapse in small cell lung cancer. J Clin Oncol 3:65–71, 1985

4. Williams SD, Einhorn LK: Etoposide salvage therapy for refractory germ cell tumors: An update. Cancer Treat Rev 9:67–71, 1982 (suppl A)

5. Chen GL, Yang L, Rowe TC, et al: Nonintercalative antitumor drugs interfere with the breakage-reunion reaction of mammalian DNA topoisomerase II. J Biol Chem 259:13560–13666, 1984

6. Ross W, Rowe T, Glisson B, et al: Role of topoisomerase II in mediating epipodophyllotoxin-induced DNA cleavage. Cancer Res 44:5857–5860, 1984

7. Long BH, Musial ST, Brattain MG: Single- and double-strand DNA breakage and repair in human lung adenocarcinoma cells exposed to etoposide and teniposide. Cancer Res 45:3106–3112, 1985

8. D'Incalci M, Farina P, Sessa C, et al: Pharmacokinetics of VP16-213 given by different administration methods. Cancer Chemother Pharmacol 7:141–145, 1982

9. Holsti LR, Mattson K, Grohn P, et al: Cisplatinum plus vindesine versus VP16 in combination with radiotherapy in the treatment of non-small cell carcinoma of the lung. Proceedings of the Third World Conference on Lung Cancer, Tokyo, 1982, p 274 (abstr)

10. WHO Handbook for Reporting Results of Cancer Treatment. WHO offset publication No. 48, 1979

11. Holthuis JJM, Römkins FMGM, Pinedo HM, et al: Plasma assay for the antineoplastic agent VP16-213 (etoposide) using high performance liquid chromatography with electrochemical detection. J Pharm Biomed Analysis 1:89–98, 1983

12. Anderson JR, Cain KC, Gelber RD: Analysis of survival by tumor response. J Clin Oncol 1:710–719, 1983

13. Aisner J, Hansen HH: Commentary: Current status of chemotherapy for non-small cell lung cancer. Cancer Treat Rep 65:979–986, 1981

14. O'Connell J, Kris M, Gralla R, et al: A multivariable analysis of clinical factors predictive of survival in 406 stage III non-small cell lung cancer (NSCLC) patients treated

with high-dose cisplatin/vinca-alkaloid regimens. Proceedings of the Fourth World Conference on Lung Cancer, Toronto, 1985, p 17 (abstr)

15. Stanley KE: Prognostic factors for survival in patients with inoperable lung cancer. J Natl Cancer Inst 65:25–32, 1980

16. Lagakos S: Prognostic factors for survival time in inoperable lung cancer, in Straus M (ed): Lung Cancer: Clinical Diagnosis and Treatment. Orlando, Fla, Grune & Stratton, 1977, pp 271–280

17. Ruckdeschel JC, Finkelstein DM, Mason BA, et al: Chemotherapy for metastatic non-small cell bronchogenic carcinoma: EST 2575, generation V—A randomized comparison of four cisplatin-containing regimens. J Clin Oncol 3:72–79, 1985

18. Souhami RL, Bradbury I, Geddes DM, et al: Prognostic significance of laboratory parameters measured at diagnosis in small cell carcinoma of the lung. Cancer Res 45:2878–2882, 1985

19. Cohen MH, Johnston-Early A, Citron ML, et al: An active chemotherapy regimen for squamous cell lung cancer. Cancer Treat Rep 68:475–479, 1984

20. Lindgren D, Cadman E. Erichson R, et al: Use of cisplatin, cyclophosphamide, vincristine and doxorubicin for the treatment of non-small cell lung cancer. Cancer Treat Rep 68:1159–1161, 1984

Therapy With Cisplatin and Etoposide for Non–Small-Cell Lung Cancer

By Jean Klastersky

SURGERY is the principal treatment modality for non–small-cell lung cancer (NSCLC), considered potentially curable. However, favorable results are obtained in only a small fraction of carefully staged patients.

Radiation therapy is an alternative to surgery for patients who are inoperable; treatment with curative intent is associated with an insignificant salvage rate. However, as a treatment for unresectable NSCLC, overall, radiotherapy has been disappointing in prolonging survival, although objective responses can be achieved in many patients.

Systemic dissemination occurs in most patients with NSCLC whose tumors cannot be adequately resected and in many of those with seemingly complete surgery. Systemic therapy, therefore, should play a key role in the management of NSCLC. Unfortunately, until now, chemotherapy in NSCLC patients has been associated with a very low response rate. Although responders live significantly longer than nonresponders, these differences may only indicate patient selection. In addition, since the response rate is low, chemotherapy-induced toxicity must be taken into account: most NSCLC patients will experience toxicity without any benefit from therapy. These issues are further complicated by the failure of most studies to consider the patient's quality of life in order to objectively measure the respective impacts of chemotherapy-induced response and toxicity.

From the Department of Medicine and H.J. Tagnon Laboratory of Clinical Investigation, Jules Bordet Institute, Brussels.

A substantial part of the investigational work of the author has been performed within the EORTC Lung Cancer Working Party and was supported in Belgium by the Fonds de la Recherche Scientifique Médicale (FRSM no. 3.4522.82); Fedetab; Bristol-Myers Laboratories and the Lefevre Foundation.

Address reprint requests to Jean Klastersky, MD, Service de Médicine et Laboratoire d'Investigation Clinique H.J. Tagnon, Institut Jules Bordet, Centre des Tumeurs de l'Université Libre de Bruxelles, 1 Rue Héger-Bordet, 1000 Brussels, Belgium.

0093–7754/86/1303–3020$05.00/0

No such special investigation of the patient's quality of life has been performed so far at our institution. However, it was a common observation that responding patients had a significant decrease in morbid symptoms, and most of them were eager to continue their therapy as long as the response was maintained. A similar experience was reported by Gralla et al,[1] who specifically noted an improvement in symptoms when patients responded; this included relief of pain and dyspnea, improvement in pulmonary function tests and performance status score. Results of a study by the Lung Cancer Group[2] showed that in 151 patients randomized to receive either postoperative radiotherapy alone or postoperative radiotherapy with cyclophosphamide, doxorubicin (Adriamycin [Adria Laboratories, Columbus, OH]), and cisplatin (CAP) after incomplete resection of NSCLC, a statistically significant difference in favor of the chemotherapy arm emerged in both the recurrence and death rates. Morbidity and mortality from cancer could thus be reduced by chemotherapy in that group of NSCLC patients, although the overall significance of such a benefit is still unknown. These considerations stress the need for a comparative evaluation of any new approach, preferably against concurrent controls receiving other treatment, and recognizing that untreated controls are not feasible in most institutions.

Recently, Woods et al,[3] in an ongoing study, compared 50 NSCLC patients receiving vindesine plus cisplatin with 53 similar patients receiving no therapy. Respective response rates were 30% (two complete responses [CR] and 13 partial responses [PR]) and 0%, and survivals were 24 and 21 weeks. Responding patients had a median survival of 35 weeks. Resuls of a placebo-controlled study reported by Cormier et al[4] comparing methotrexate, doxorubicin, cyclophosphamide, and CCNU (lomustine) (MACC) with a placebo "physically comparable to MACC" showed that in 20 patients the response rate was 35% (7/20) in those receiving chemotherapy and 0% in those not receiving it; in addition, the tumor stabilized in five additional patients receiving chemotherapy. The respective median

 Seminars in Oncology, Vol 13, No 3, Suppl 3 (September), 1986: pp 104–114

survivals were 31 and 9 weeks ($P < .0005$). The investigators concluded that polychemotherapy with MACC significantly benefited patients with advanced NSCLC.

In order to understand further the relationship between response to chemotherapy and possible prolonged survival, we analyzed (Table 1) a series of clinical studies performed either with "ineffective" drugs or combinations (defined as treatments with a <10% response rate) and compared them with studies using "effective" regimens (a response rate >25%). All studies had been performed recently (1980 to 1983) as phase II to III trials in previously untreated patients. Patients who entered the studies could be considered reasonably uniform.[5-21] Ineffective regimens were associated overall with a 5.4% response rate and a median survival of 4.0 months (range, 2.8 to 6.1 months); effective regimens, on the other hand, resulted in a 42% response rate and a median overall survival of 8.1 months (range, 4.0 to 13.2 months). In spite of the obvious limitations of this approach, it appears that an increased response rate was associated with a prolonged survival. The proper evaluation of the quality of that increased survival is clearly impossible under the conditions of the present analysis.

CHEMOTHERAPY IN ADVANCED NSCLC

Cytostatic agents given as single-drug therapy for NSCLC (Table 2) do not induce a high rate of objective response[22-24]; these relatively poor response rates suggest that it is unlikely that a combination of these agents will produce much better results. Table 3 shows the results of the so-called best regimens[11,18,25-28] used so far. Objective response rates are between 25% and

Table 1. Response Rate and Survival in Patients With NSCLC Receiving Ineffective and Effective Chemotherapeutic Regimens

Reference	Year	Treatment	Response Rate (%)	Overall Survival (mo)
		Ineffective Regimens		
Ettinger[5]	1980	MTX	4	3.7
Davis[6]	1980	CPA	5	4.6
		CPA + CCNU	8	3.8
		CPA + CCNU + ADR	6	4.2
Creech[7]	1981	CPA + MTX	8	5.0
		Melphalan	0	2.8
		CPA + CCNU	8	3.5
Davis[8]	1981	CPA + ADR + CDDP	4	3.3
		CPA + ADR + CDDP	7	4.8
Luedke[9]	1983	CPA + ADR	5	3.1
Block[10]	1983	CPA + ADR + CNNU + VCR	5	6.1
Mean (range)	1980–1983		5.4	4.0 (2.8–6.1)
		Effective Regimens		
Evans[11]	1981	CDDP + ADR + CPA	27	4.0
Knost[12]	1981	CDDP + ADR + CPA	35	9.5
Takita[13]	1981	CDDP + ADR + 5-FU + MTX + VCR	37	13.2
Eagan[14]	1981	CDDP + VP-16 + ADR + CPA	46	7.5
Eagan[15]	1981	CDDP + ADR + DAG	67	9.5
Rosi[16]	1981	MMC + ADR + 5-FU	33	6.2
Israel[17]	1982	CDDP + BLM	65	9.7
Longeval[18]	1982	CDDP + VP-16	38	7.5
Rinaldi[19]	1983	CDDP + VP-16	37	8.0
Gregor[20]	1983	CDDP + VDS	31	9.5
Woodcock[21]	1983	CDDP + VBL	52	5.5
Mean	1981–1983		42	8.1 (4.0–13.2)

Abbreviations: MTX, methotrexate; CPA, cyclophosphamide; CCNU, lomustine; ADR, doxorubicin; CDDP, cisplatin; VCR, vincristine; 5-FU, 5-fluorouracil; VP-16, etoposide; DAG, dianhydrogalactitol; MMC, mitomycin-C; BLM, bleomycin; VDS, vindesine; VBL, vinblastine.

Table 2. Single-Drug Chemotherapy in NSCLC

	Evaluable Patients (No.)	Objective Response Rate (%)
Ifosfamide	237	26
Mitomycin-C	115	20
Vinblastine	27	20
Vindesine	406	17
Cisplatin	354	14
Doxorubicin	283	12
Hexamethylmelanine	166	11
Etoposide	313	10
Methotrexate	247	10
Dianhydrogalactitol	63	10
Cyclophosphamide	369	8
CCNU (lomustine)	161	7
Methylglyoxalbisguanylhydrazone	183	5

40%, with an overall median survival time of <6 months. For more detailed reviews and discussions, the reader is referred to other recent reports.[22,29–31]

Few investigators have tested single-agent therapy *v* combination chemotherapy: cyclophosphamide *v* cyclophosphamide plus CCNU[32]; cyclophosphamide *v* doxorubicin plus cyclophosphamide *v* doxorubicin plus CCNU[33]; cyclophosphamide plus doxorubicin and methotrexate *v* the sequential administration of these drugs[34]; doxorubicin *v* cyclophosphamide *v* doxorubicin plus cyclophosphamide[35]; vindesine *v* cisplatin plus vindesine.[36] Only one of these studies resulted in improved survival for the patients receiving the combination, probably because relatively ineffective drugs were used. The exception was the trial with cisplatin and vindesine with 105 patients,[36] which resulted in improvement of both response (33% *v* 7%) and survival (median survival, 11 *v* 4 months), especially in patients with limited disease (14 *v* 5 months). Although the trial had an uncommonly high proportion of patients with limited disease (69%), and chest irradiation after chemotherapy was left to the discretion of individual physicians, it suggests again that a chemotherapy that results in a significant response rate might influence survival in NSCLC.

CISPLATIN-CONTAINING CHEMOTHERAPY FOR NSCLC

It should be stressed that no controlled study comparing cisplatin alone with a cisplatin-containing combination has been reported so far. Green et al[37] recently compared cytosine arabinoside (per se ineffective in NSCLC) plus cisplatin with vinblastine plus cisplatin. The response rates were 8% and 15%, and median survivals were 5.6 and 7.5 months ($P = .4$), respectively. Information derived from phase II studies in which many patients had already received some therapy indicates a 14% (48/354) response rate to cisplatin (confidence interval, 10 to 17). In our own study,[38] the response was 26% (confidence interval, 16 to 36): most of the patients were receiving treatment for the first time. Although the overall impression gained from published studies and our own investigations suggests that in NSCLC, cisplatin-containing combinations are more active than cisplatin alone, this has yet to be definitively proven. Our group is presently conducting a study of cisplatin (120 mg/m^2) *v* cisplatin plus etoposide in advanced NSCLC. So far, seven of 19 patients (37%) responded to cisplatin and five of 22 (23%) to the combination. Evaluation of the response rates and their influence on survival is still to come.

Three basic types of cisplatin-containing combinations have been used: those containing cisplatin with doxorubicin and/or an alkylating

Table 3. Main Chemotherapeutic Regimens Investigated in NSCLC

Regimen	Evaluable Patients (No.)	Objective Response Rate (%)	Median Overall Survival (wk)	Median Survival in Responders (wk)
MTX-ADR-CPA-CCNU[25]	101	41	33	59
CPA-ADR-CDDP[11]	131	27	15	33
MMC-VDS[26]	84	28	22	—
CDDP-VP-16[18]	94	38	30	60
CDDP-VDS[27]	81	43	—	52
CDDP-VBL-MMC[28]	104	27	24	41

Abbreviations: MTX, methotrexate; ADR, doxorubicin; CPA, cyclophosphamide; CCNU, lomustine; CDDP, cisplatin; MMC, mitomycin-C; VDS, vindesine; VP-16, etoposide; VBL, vinblastine.

agent (usually cyclosphophamide), combinations of cisplatin with vinca alkaloids, and combinations of cisplatin plus etoposide. Eagan et al[15] summarized their extensive experience at the Mayo Clinic with CAP and suggested that CAP constituted a therapeutic improvement. Several independent studies confirmed these observations. Gralla et al[27] extensively studied cisplatin plus vindesine in NSCLC and found both an impressive response rate of 40% and a survival advantage in patients responding to the high cisplatin dose (120 mg/m^2). Similar response rates were confirmed by several other studies using cisplatin in combination with vinca alkaloids, either vindesine or vinblastine.[39,40] As already mentioned, cisplatin/vindesine has been shown to be superior to vindesine alone for response and survival in a controlled study.[37] Another similar investigation by Fuks et al[41] with a relatively small number of patients compared a combination of cyclophosphamide, doxorubicin, and etoposide with and without cisplatin in NSCLC. It was found that chemotherapy without cisplatin resulted in a response rate of 13% (4/29) and a median survival of 22.5 weeks, whereas the cisplatin-containing regimen was associated with a response rate of 38% (14/36) and a median survival of 34.5 weeks ($P = .04$). Once again, improved response rate was associated with a significantly prolonged survival.

In a study of Block et al,[10] the addition of cisplatin to doxorubicin, cyclophosphamide, CCNU, and vincristine resulted in a significantly increased response rate, but no increased median survival (6.1 *v* 7.6 months); however, twice as many patients survived 1 year after initiation of chemotherapy (18% *v* 10%). In another preliminary study, Briançon et al[42] found a significant difference in response rate for vindesine plus cisplatin as compared with vindesine plus cyclophosphamide (68% *v* 30%), but similar survival (32 weeks).

CISPLATIN AS A RADIOSENSITIZER

By combining chemotherapy with chest irradiation, the therapeutic goal is to achieve simultaneously an optimal control of the local disease and an effect on distant microscopic metastases.[43] Chemotherapy with drugs such as cisplatin can also, at least theoretically, potentiate the effect of the irradiation.

The interaction of cisplatin and irradiation has been investigated mainly in vitro. Results show that cisplatin enhances the radiation response. This has been confirmed by a number of in vivo experiments, and these encouraging results also suggest clinical applicability. From pilot studies[44,45] and radiobiology data, it appears that to obtain maximal therapeutic gain, cisplatin should be administered before irradiation, rather than afterward.

Large-scale prospective clinical studies are currently being performed to test the radiosensitizing effect of cisplatin in NSCLC. So far, three controlled studies have evaluated the concomitant administration of cisplatin-containing regimens and radiotherapy.[2,46,47] The results are summarized in Table 4. Two of these studies showed a modestly improved survival in the patients receiving the combined modality; however, these results neither prove nor disprove the potentiating effect on radiotherapy of cisplatin.

CISPLATIN AND ETOPOSIDE FOR NSCLC

Further interest has been generated in cisplatin-containing combinations by studies using

Table 4. Randomized Studies of Combination Modality Therapy for NSCLC

Reference	Arm	Evaluable Patients (No.)	Stage	Thoracic Irradiation Dose (rads)	Type of Chemotherapy	Timing of Chemotherapy*	Objective Response Rate (%)	Median Survival	Statistical Significance
Wils[46]	A	14	LD	6,000	—	—	50	5 mo	—
	B	19	LD	6,000	CDDP + ADR + VP-16	1 + 3	81	11 mo	S
Lad[2]	A	153	III M_0	4,000	—	—	—	380 d	—
	B		III M_0	4,000	CPA + ADR + CDDP	2 + 3	—	600 d	S
Van Houtte[47]	A	32	LD	5,000	—	—	55	12 mo	—
	B	27	LD	4,500	CDDP + VP-16 + VDS	1	30	9 mo	NS

*1, before radiotherapy; 2, with radiotherapy; 3, after radiotherapy.

Abbreviations: LD, limited disease; CDDP, cisplatin; ADR, doxorubicin; VP-16, etoposide; CPA, cyclophosphamide; VDS, vindesine; S, significant; NS, not significant.

Table 5. Summary of Clinical Studies Using Cisplatin and Etoposide in NSCLC

Reference	Year	Dosage (mg/m²) Cisplatin	Dosage (mg/m²) Etoposide	No. of Evaluable Patients	PR No. (%)	CR No. (%)
Goldhirsch[49]	1981	100	80 × 3	18	7 (39)	0
Longeval[18]	1982	60	120 × 3	94	35 (37)	4
Joss[50]	1982	80	80 × 3	25	7 (28)	1
Holsti[39]	1982	90	50 × 4	25	13 (52)	2
Giaconne[51]	1983	60	100 × 3	28	5 (18)	1
Rinaldi[19]	1983	100	120 × 3	51	19 (37)	0
Scagliotti[52]	1983	100	80 × 3	30	8 (27)	2
Veronesi[53]	1983	100	75 × 5	33	11 (33)	1
Paccagnela[40]	1983	100	100 × 3	26	10 (38)	1
Dhingra[54]	1984	60	120 × 3	37	7 (19)	0
Mitrou[55]	1984	90	100 × 3	46	10 (22)	1
Dhingra[56]	1984	60–80	120 × 3	62	18 (29)	0
Klastersky*	1986	60	120 × 3	114	28 (25)	—
Klastersky*	1986	120	120 × 3	93	27 (29)	—
Total				682	205 (30)	13 (2)

*J. Klastersky, unpublished data, 1986.

etoposide in an effort to duplicate the apparent synergism, evident from animal experiments,[48] between the two drugs. The largest study has been reported by Longeval and Klastersky[18] from the European Organization on Research and Treatment of Cancer (EORTC) Lung Cancer Working Party and has been confirmed by several other investigations, summarized in Table 5.[18,19,39,40,49–56] Response rates varied from 19% to 52%, with an average of 30% and a confidence interval of 30 to 37. A modest proportion (3%) of the responding patients had a CR; as already mentioned, patients with a CR often had a prolonged disease-free survival. The overall median survival in these NSCLC patients was close to 8 months, but all series reported an increased survival in responders, usually in the range of 12 months.

These studies suggest that cisplatin plus etoposide, as well as cisplatin plus vinca alkaloids or etoposide, or CAP, might represent an improvement in the treatment of NSCLC. This conclusion is supported by more recent studies summarized in Table 6. The overall response rate in these investigations was 35%, with 5% CRs.[50,57–59]

Various attempts have been made to improve the results achieved with cisplatin plus etoposide or vindesine. A logical approach was to investigate the triple-drug combination of cisplatin plus etoposide plus vindesine. Such a study was reported by Klastersky et al.[60] In 62 patients with NSCLC, it was found that 40% of the patients responded (five CRs and 20 PRs), but no survival advantage could be found when compared with patients receiving cisplatin plus etoposide, or cisplatin plus vindesine who served as historical controls. On the other hand, toxicity (namely neurotoxicity) was somewhat increased in the group receiving the triple-drug combination.

Table 6. Recent Studies (1985) of Cisplatin Plus Vinca Alkaloids and/or Etoposide in NSCLC

Reference	Regimens*	No. of Patients	No. of Responses, (%) CR	PR	Total	Median Survival (mo) R	NR	Total
Carmichael[57]	CDDP + VDS	63	5	16	21 (33)	14.0	4.8	6.5
Kris[58]	CDDP + VDS	48	2	14	16 (33)	18.4	—	8.5
Kris[58]	CDDP + VBL	49	3	17	20 (41)	16.2	—	12.3
Shinkai[59]*	CDDP + VDS	28	0	12	12 (43)	10.3	3.8	10.1
Joss[50]	CDDP + VP-16	40	1	8	9 (23)	10.0	3.5	8.0
Total		228	11 (5)	67 (29)	78 (34)			

Abbreviations: CDDP, cisplatin; VDS, vindesine; VBL, vinblastine; VP-16, etoposide; R, responders; NR, nonresponders.

*In a controlled study, mitomycin-C plus VDS resulted in a 10% response rate; no difference in survival was found.

Similar experiences have been reported by others: cisplatin plus etoposide has been evaluated in combination with vindesine,[56,61–64] vincristine,[61] doxorubicin plus cyclophosphamide,[15] bleomycin,[65] and to methylglyoxal bisguanylhydrazone (methyl GAG)[66]; cisplatin plus vindesine has been combined with bleomycin[67] and methyl GAG.[68] None of these combinations produced dramatic increases in response rate or survival over that achieved with cisplatin plus etoposide or vindesine (Table 7).

Another potentially promising way to increase the efficacy of cisplatin plus vindesine or cisplatin plus etoposide might be to increase the dose of cisplatin. There are some indications that a dose-response exists for cisplatin in ovarian carcinoma and other tumors. As already discussed in the first part of this review, neither Gralla et al[27] nor ourselves[69] demonstrated a significant difference in response rate among NSCLC patients receiving 120 mg/m^2 or 60 mg/m^2 of cisplatin in combination with vindesine and etoposide, respectively. In our own study, to be published soon, we could not confirm Gralla's observations regarding an improved survival in patients treated with 120 mg/m^2. Thus, there is still no convincing evidence to suggest that therapy with cisplatin-containing combinations should be performed with high-dose cisplatin.

Another approach to improving our present results with cisplatin-containing combinations might be to substitute cisplatin with other derivatives such as carboplatin or iproplatin. Clinical experience with these drugs, either alone or in combination, in previously untreated NSCLC patients virtually does not exist. Evans et al[70] recently published encouraging results with carboplatin plus etoposide in small-cell lung cancer (SCLC) suggesting that the combination is not only active, but reasonably safe regarding hematologic toxicity. Our own group is presently conducting a phase II study in NSCLC using increasing dosages of carboplatin (starting at 300 mg/m^2) and etoposide (3 etoposide × 100 mg/m^2): early results suggest a relatively severe hematologic toxicity in patients with previously untreated advanced-NSCLC.

ALTERNATIVE THERAPIES—MITOMYCIN-C

Mitomycin-C has been shown to be active as a single agent in NSCLC (Table 2), with a 20% response rate reported in phase II studies. Accordingly, mitomycin-C was combined with vinca alkaloids in order to develop active regimens that were "non-cross-resistant" with cisplatin plus etoposide plus vinca alkaloids. The efficacy of such combinations is reviewed in Table 8; the overall response rate in 391 patients was 20%, with few CRs (1.3%).[26,59,71–75] Although these results appear to be less impressive than those obtained with cisplatin plus etoposide or vinca alkaloids, the limited value of comparing data from a retrospective analysis of the literature must be emphasized. Moreover, the median survival in responders, nonresponders, or all patients does not appear to be different whether cisplatin or mitomycin-C is combined with vinca alkaloids or etoposide.

Only one randomized study[59] compared mitomycin-C plus vindesine with cisplatin plus vinde-

Table 7. Effect of Additional Chemotherapeutic Agents on Efficacy of Cisplatin Plus Etoposide or Vindesine

Reference	Combination	Evaluable Patients (No.)	Objective Response Rate (%)	Complete Response (No.)	Median Survival Time (wk)	
					Overall	Responders
Eagan[15]	CDDP-VP-16-ADR-CPA	28	46	—	30	38
Natale[66]	CDDP-VP-16-MGBG	53	58	5	—	53+
Klastersky[60]	CDDP-VP-16-VDS	62	40	5	—	53
Porter[62]	CDDP-VP-16-VDS	72	25	3	—	—
Gropp[63]	CDDP-VP-16-VDS	77	16	1	—	—
Dhingra[56]	CDDP-VP-16-VDS	55	22	1	28	—
Gatzemeier[64]	CDDP-VP-16-VDS	60	40	3	—	—
Bertrand[61]	CDDP-VP-16-VCR	22	27	1	—	16
Osoba[65]	CDDP-VP-16-BLM	48	44	2	35	36
Itri[67]	CDDP-VDS-BLM	52	35	—	—	69
Greenwald[68]	CDDP-VDS-MGBG	32	38	3	—	—

Abbreviations: CDDP, cisplatin; VP-16, etoposide; ADR, doxorubicin; CPA, cyclophosphamide; MGBG, methyl GAG; VDS, vindesine; VCR, vincristine; BLM, bleomycin.

Table 8. Effectiveness of Mitomycin-C Plus Vinca Alkaloids in NSCLC

Reference	Regimens*	No. of Patients	No. of Responses			Median Survival (mo)		
			CR	PR	Total (%)	R	NR	Total
Shinkai[59]	MMC + VDS	30	0	3	3 (10)	—	—	10.2
Weick[71]	MMC + VBL	45	0	11	11 (24)	—	—	4.7
Sculier[72]†	MMC + VDS	47	1	9	10 (21)	10.0	—	5.5
Kris[26]†	MMC + VDS	84	2	23	25 (29)	12.3	4.9	6.1
Ruckdeschel[73]	MMC + VBL	101	2	11	13 (13)	8.8	4.2	4.5
Shah[74]‡	MMC + VCR + (MTX)	21	0	4	4 (19)	—	—	3.0
Miller[75]‡	MMC + VDS + (5-FU)	63	0	13	13 (21)	9.5	5.2	5.7
Total		391	5	74	79 (20)			

Abbreviations: MMC, mitomycin-C; VDS, vindesine; VBL, vinblastine; VCR, vincristine; MTX, methotrexate; 5-FU, 5-fluorouracil; R, responders; NR, nonresponders.

*In a controlled study, cisplatin plus VDS resulted in a 43% response rate of CR + PR; no difference in survival was found.

†Only 6/45 (13%) PRs in previously treated patients.

‡Adenocarcinomas.

sine; the response rate (10% *v* 43%) was greater for the latter regimen, but there was no significant difference in survival (median survival, 10.2 and 10.3 months, respectively). Two studies[26,72] evaluated the response to mitomycin-C plus vindesine in patients who had received cisplatin plus etoposide as first-line therapy. One study reported one PR in 16 patients and the other, five PRs in 29 patients. Although cross-resistance between the two regimens was probably not complete, the response rate to mitomycin-C plus vindesine, when used as second-line therapy, appears to be lower than that of the combination used in untreated patients.

At present, it appears that the combination of mitomycin-C plus vindesine is probably not more active than the combination of cisplatin plus vinca alkaloids or etoposide and is, at least partially, cross-resistant with the latter combination. It is unlikely that these two combinations might be used successfully as alternating regimens in NSCLC. In a limited number of studies, cisplatin was added to the mitomycin-C and vinblastine regimen; in one study,[76] ten (46%) responses (including three CRs) were obtained in 26 patients; in the other,[77] 21 (54%) responses (one CR) were observed in 39 patients who also received methotrexate. In the latter investigation, the median survival time for responders as 11.0 and 8.5 months, respectively, according to extent of disease (stage III M_0, or III M_1); the corresponding figures were 7.0 and 5.5 months for nonresponders. For the two studies, the median duration of response was 6.5 months.

The overall results with mitomycin-C plus vinca alkaloids and cisplatin are summarized in Table 9[26,28,76–80] and appear encouraging. They demonstrate a 48% overall response rate (196 of 405 patients). Controlled studies should assess the value of that combination in comparison with cisplatin plus vinca alkaloids or etoposide.

TOXICITY AND SIDE EFFECTS

Overall, combinations of cisplatin with etoposide or vindesine have been relatively well tolerated. Results from our recent studies showed moderate hematologic toxicity with the regular dose (60 mg/m^2) of cisplatin, but increased toxicity with the higher dose (120 mg/m^2). Severe (grades III and IV) granulocytopenia occurred in 23% and 55% of patients, respectively; as a consequence, serious infection was seen in 5% and 7% of these patients. Severe (grades III and IV) thrombocytopenia was observed in 12% and 23%, respectively; severe bleeding did not occur. Nausea and vomiting occurred in most patients, but did not appear to

Table 9. Response Rate in NSCLC to Mitomycin-C Plus Vinca Alkaloids Plus Cisplatin

Reference	Year	No. of Patients	No. of Responses (%)
Schulman[78]	1983	26	12 (46)
Kris[26]	1985	73	41 (56)
Anderson[78]	1982	25	17 (68)
Folman[79]	1984	45	35 (78)
Niell[77]	1984	45	24 (54)
Ruckdeschel[28]	1985	104	34 (33)
Miller[80]	1984	87	33 (38)
Total		405	196 (48)

be affected in frequency and/or severity by the cisplatin dose. Diarrhea was seen in approximately 20% of patients in both groups, but was rarely severe. Alopecia was observed in about 65% of patients and was severe in 30%. Discrete stomatitis was seen in 12% of patients receiving cisplatin of 120 mg/m^2, but only in 2% of the other group. No differences were seen between the two groups of patients regarding neurologic (peripheral neuropathy), renal, and pulmonary toxicities. These complications were rare and mild, and their relationship to the administration of chemotherapy was unclear. No hearing loss was observed.

The toxic reactions seen with the cisplatin plus vindesine regimen, as exemplified in the study by Gralla et al,[27] were similar to those complicating therapy with cisplatin plus etoposide. Hematologic toxicity was rarely severe, with few infectious or bleeding complications—it was not more pronounced in the patients receiving the higher cisplatin dose (120 mg/m^2); nephrotoxicity was mild and reversible in all patients in whom it occurred. The only important difference in toxicity between the cisplatin plus etoposide and cisplatin plus vindesine regimens was related to peripheral neuropathy. Although reversible, it occurred to some degree in all the patients receiving cisplatin and vindesine; it was mild or moderate in 87%, but severe in 13%. Once again, neurotoxicity was not worse among patients receiving the higher cisplatin dose. Thus, the cisplatin plus vindesine regimen appeared to be more toxic than cisplatin plus etoposide. In our study[62] of cisplatin plus etoposide plus vindesine, we found an increased frequency and severity of leukopenia, febrile episodes, and peripheral neuropathy.

CONCLUSIONS

It appears that the cisplatin-containing regimens (especially if combined with etoposide, vindesine, and/or mitomycin-C) can achieve a reproducible response rate close to 30% to 40% and that responders might benefit from such therapies. Although it seems unjustifiable to deny chemotherapy to patients whose tumors are unresectable, it also is presumptuous to consider the presently available regimens as routine therapy. Current therapies need much improvement, and this is why NSCLC patients, especially those who have a good performance status and thus are more likely to respond, should be invited to participate in clinical studies in which the control regimens are associated with the modest, but significant, response rates that have been analyzed here. Although nonresponding patients achieve little, if any, benefit from chemotherapy—and we do not know exactly what relationship "stabilization" of the disease might have on survival and quality of life—they should probably be offered the possibility of participating in phase I or phase III studies rather than continuing on therapies more likely to provide toxicity than benefit.

The role of combined modalities such as chemotherapy plus radiotherapy or chemotherapy plus surgery is still unclear.[43] Rather than being considered routine, these approaches should be investigated under appropriate clinical conditions, taking into account the delicate balance between the modest benefit possible for some patients and the substantial potential morbidity to which responders as well as nonresponders are exposed.

There is presently no other way for progress than to build on currently available regimens. New drugs might bring further improvement just as cisplatin did, and derivatives of cisplatin should definitely be investigated. Certain older drugs such as ifosfamide and mitomycin-C certainly deserve reevaluation. Finally, more basic research into the biology of NSCLC should be undertaken in order to orient treatment more specifically toward the intrinsic properties and characteristics of these tumors. The recent experience gained in the field of SCLC—to which NSCLC might be more closely related than previously thought—has opened new hopeful concepts and strategies for therapy.

Clearly, today there is no cause for excessive optimism for NSCLC; neither is there reason for pessimism and abstention from therapeutic research. We are hopefully witnessing the first significant steps to more frequent responses, CRs, and prolongation of life. All this will not be achieved easily or rapidly; however, examples of other diseases that can now be cured with chemotherapy indicate that even slowly progressive improvements brought about by dedicated research can in the long run constitute highly effective therapeutic strategies.

REFERENCES

1. Gralla RJ, Cohen EA: Cisplatin plus plant alkaloid chemotherapy in non-small cell lung cancer, in Klastersky J (ed): Lung Cancer. Current Trends and Future Prospects. Bruxelles, Europrint 2000, 1984, pp 119–129

2. Lad T, Weisenburger T: Adjuvant therapy of incompletely resected non small cell bronchogenic carcinoma: A lung cancer study group trial. Proc Am Soc Clin Oncol 4:1985 (abstr C-697)

3. Woods RL, Levi JA, Page J, et al: Non small cell cancer: A randomized comparison of chemotherapy with no chemotherapy. Proc Am Soc Clin Oncol 1985 (abstr C-691)

4. Cormier Y, Bergeron D, La Forge J, et al: Benefits of polychemotherapy in advanced non-small cell bronchogenic carcinoma. Cancer 50:845–849, 1982

5. Ettinger DS, Stanley KE, Nystrom JS: Phase II study of high-dose methotrexate in the treatment of patients with non-small cell carcinoma of the lung: An Eastern Cooperative Oncology Group study. Cancer Treat Rep 64P:1017–1021, 1980

6. Davis S, Pandya MR, Rambotti P: Single-agent and combination chemotherapy for extensive non-small cell carcinomas of the lung. Cancer Treat Rep 64:685–688, 1980

7. Creech RH, Mehta CR, Cohen M, et al: Results of phase II protocol for evaluation of new chemotherapeutic regimens in patients with inoperable non-small cell lung carcinoma. Cancer Treat Rep 65:431–438, 1981

8. Davis S, Rambotti P, Park YK: Combination cyclophosphamide, doxorubicin, and cisplatin (CAP) chemotherapy for extensive non-small cell carcinomas of the lung. Cancer Treat Rep 65:955–958, 1981

9. Luedke DW, Luedke SL, Petruska P, et al: A randomized prospective study of vindesine versus doxorubicin and cylophosphamide in the treatment of epidermoid lung cancer. Cancer 51:778–782, 1983

10. Block JB, Chlebowski RT, Richardson B, et al: Adriamycin, cyclophosphamide, CCNU, and oncovin with or without cisplatin (ACCO vs PACO) for patients with advanced non-small cell lung cancer. Proc Am Soc Clin Oncol 1983 (abstr C-791)

11. Evans WK, Feld R, DeBoer G, et al: Cyclophosphamide, doxorubicin, and cisplatin in the treatment of non-small cell bronchogenic carcinoma. Cancer Treat Rep 65:947–954, 1981

12. Knost JA, Greco FA, Hande KR, et al: Cyclophosphamide, doxorubicin, and cisplatin in the treatment of advanced non-small cell lung cancer. Cancer Treat Rep 65:941–945, 1981

13. Takita H, Edgerton F, Marabella P, et al: Platinum-based combination chemotherapy in non-small cell lung carcinoma. Cancer 48:1528–1530, 1981

14. Eagan RT, Frytak S, Nichols WC, et al: Phase II study of the combination of dianhydrogalactitol, doxorubicin, and cisplatin (DAP) in patients with advanced squamous cell lung cancer. Cancer Treat Rep 65:517–519, 1981

15. Eagan RT, Frytak S, Nichols WC, et al: Evaluation of VP-16-213, cyclophosphamide, doxorubicin and cisplatin (V-CAP) in advanced large cell lung cancer. Cancer Treat Rep 65:715–717, 1981

16. Rosi DR, Gogeire C, Brown B, et al: 5-Fluorouracil, Adriamycin, and mitomycin-C (Hi-FAM) chemotherapy for adenocarcinoma of the lung. Cancer 48:21–25, 1981

17. Israël L, Breau JL, Kerbrat G, et al: Comparison of repeated cis-platinum and bleomycin with repeated cis-platinum, bleomycin and mitomycin C in 96 patients previously untreated with far advanced squamous cell carcinoma of the lung. Proceedings of the 3rd World Conference on Lung Cancer, Tokyo, 1982 (abstr 266)

18. Longeval E, Klastersky J: Combination chemotherapy with cisplatin and etoposide in bronchogenic squamous cell carcinoma and adenocarcinoma. A study by the EORTC Lung Cancer Working Party (Belgium). Cancer 50:2751–2756, 1982

19. Rinaldi M, Venturo J, Tonachella R, et al: Chemotherapy with DDP and VP16-213 in non-small cell lung cancer: Results and toxicity. Proceedings of the 13th International Congress of Chemotherapy, Vienna, 1983 (abstr PS 12.1/15-9)

20. Gregor A, Carmichael J, Cornbleet MA, et al: Active combination chemotherapy with vindesine and cis-platinum in non-small cell lung cancer. Proceedings of the 13th International Congress of Chemotherapy, Vienna, 1983 (abstr PS 12.1/15-14)

21. Woodcock TM, Blumenreich MS, Richman SP, et al: Combination chemotherapy with cis-diamminedichloroplatinum and vinblastine in advanced non-small cell lung cancer. J Clin Oncol 1:247–250, 1983

22. Sculier JP, Klastersky J: Progress in chemotherapy of non-small cell lung cancer. Eur J Cancer Clin Oncol 20:1329–1333, 1984

23. Bakowski MT, Crouch JC: Chemotherapy of non-small cell lung cancer: A reappraisal and a look to the future. Cancer Treat Rev 10:159–172, 1983

24. Hansen HH, Rørth M: Lung cancer, in Pinedo HM, Chalner BA (eds): Cancer Chemotherapy Annual, vol 6. New York, Elsevier, 1984, pp 299–321

25. Chahinian AP, Goldberg J, Holland JF, et al: Chemotherapy versus chemoimmunotherapy with levamisole or *Corynebacterium parvum* in advanced lung cancer. Cancer Treat Rep 66:1291–1297, 1982

26. Kris MG, Gralla RJ, Kelsen DP, et al: Trial of vindesine plus mitomycin in stage-3 non-small cell lung cancer. An active regimen for outpatient treatment. Chest 87:368–372, 1985

27. Gralla RJ, Casper ES, Kelsen DP, et al: Cisplatin and vindesine combination chemotherapy for advanced carcinoma of the lung: A randomized trial investigating two dosage schedules. Ann Intern Med 95:414–420, 1981

28. Ruckdeschel JC, Finkelstein DM, Mason BA, et al: Chemotherapy for metastatic non-small-cell bronchogenic carcinoma: EST 2575, generation V—A randomized comparison of four cisplatin-containing regimens. J Clin Oncol 3:72–79, 1985

29. Hoffman PC, Bitran JD, Golomb HM: Chemotherapy of metastatic non-small cell bronchogenic carcinoma. Semin Oncol 10:111–112, 1983

30. Takasugi BJ, Miller TP: Chemotherapy of advanced non-small cell lung cancer. A review. Invest New Drugs 2:339–347, 1984

31. Klastersky J, Sculier JP: Chemotherapy for non-small-cell lung cancer. Semin Oncol (in press)

32. Edmonson JH, Lagakos SW, Selawry OS, et al: Cyclophosphamide and CCNU in the treatment of inoperable small cell carcinoma and adenocarcinoma of the lung. Cancer Treat Rep 60:925–932, 1976

33. Hyde L, Wolf J, Phillips R, et al: Combined chemotherapy for squamous cell carcinoma of the lung. Chest 73:603–607, 1978

34. Einhorn LH, Williams SD, Stevens EE, et al: Random prospective study of cyclophosphamide, doxorubicin, and methotrexate (CAM) combination chemotherapy versus single-agent sequential chemotherapy in non-small cell lung cancer. Cancer Treat Rep 66:2005–2011, 1982

35. Hoeltgen TM, McIntyre JM, Perlia CP, et al: Adriamycin and cytoxan in the treatment of inoperable lung cancer. Cancer 51:2005–2012, 1983

36. Elliott JA, Ahmedzai S, Hole D, et al: Vindesine and cisplatin combination chemotherapy compared with vindesine as a single agent in the management of non-small cell lung cancer: A randomized study. Eur J Cancer Clin Oncol 20:1025–1032, 1984

37. Green MR, Stoopler M, Anderson JA, et al: Vinblastine (V) and cisplatin (CDDP) chemotherapy in advanced non small cell lung cancer. Proc Am Soc Clin Oncol 1985 (abstr C-686)

38. De Jager R, Longeval E, Klastersky J: High-dose cisplatin with fluid and mannitol-induced diuresis in advanced lung cancer: A phase II clinical trial of the EORTC Lung Cancer Working Party (Belgium). Cancer Treat Rep 64:1341–1346, 1980

39. Holsti LR, Mattson K, Gröhn P, et al: Cis-platinum plus vindesine versus VP16 in combination with radiotherapy in the treatment of non-small-cell carcinoma of the lung. Proceedings of the World Conference on Lung Cancer, Tokyo, 1982 (abstr 274)

40. Paccagnella A, Fiorentino MV, Brandes A, et al: Cis-platin (DDP) plus vindesine (VDS) versus DDP plus VP16-213 (VP) versus doxorubicin (DXR) plus cytoxan (CTX): A randomized study in advanced non-small cell carcinoma of the lung (NSCLC). Proceedings of the 13th International Congress of Chemotherapy, Vienna, 1983 (abstr SE 12.1.15/13)

41. Fuks JZ, Aisner J, Van Echo DA, et al: Randomized study of cyclophosphamide, doxorubicin, and etoposide (VP16-213) with or without cis-platinum in non-small cell lung cancer. J Clin Oncol 1:295–301, 1983

42. Briançon S, Thisse JY, Feintrenie X, et al: Vindesine in stage III non-small-cell carcinoma of the lung: A randomized trial in combination with either cyclophosphamide or cisplatin. Proceedings of the 13th International Congress of Chemotherapy, Vienna, 1983 (abstr SE 12.1/15-3).

43. Klastersky J, Sculier JP: Nonsurgical combined modality therapies in non small cell lung cancer. Chest (in press)

44. Keizer HJ, Karim ABMF, Njo KH, et al: Feasibility study on daily administration of cis-dichlorodiammine-platinum (II) in combination with radiotherapy. Radiother Oncol 1:227–234, 1984

45. Creagan ET, Fauntain KS, Frytal S, et al: Concomitant radiation therapy and cis-diamminedichloroplatinum (II) in patients with advanced head and neck cancer. Med Pediatr Oncol 9:119–120, 1981

46. Wils JA, Utama I, Naus A, et al: Phase II randomized trial of radiotherapy alone vs the sequential use of chemotherapy and radiotherapy in stage III non-small cell lung cancer. Phase II trial of chemotherapy alone in stage IV non-small cell lung cancer. Eur J Cancer Clin Oncol 20:911–914, 1984

47. Van Houtte P, Klastersky J, Nguyen H, et al: Comparative randomized study of chest radiotherapy preceded or not by chemotherapy with cisplatin, etoposide and vindesine for the treatment of non small cell lung cancer (NSCLC). Proc Am Ass Cancer Res 25:785, 1984 (abstr 785)

48. Schabel FM, Trader MW, Laster WR, et al: Cis-dichlorodiammine-platinum (II): Combination chemotherapy and cross-resistance studies of tumors of mice. Cancer Treat Rep 63:1459–1473, 1979

49. Goldhirsch A, Joss RA, Cavalli F, et al: Cis-dichlorodiammineplatinum (II) and VP16-213 combination chemotherapy for non-small cell lung cancer. Med Pediatr Oncol 9:205–208, 1981

50. Joss RA, Alberto P, Obrecht JP, et al: Combination chemotherapy for non-small cell lung cancer with doxorubicin and mitomycin or cisplatin and etoposide. Cancer Treat Rep 68:1079–1084, 1984

51. Giaccone G, Musella R, Bertetto O, et al: DDP-VP16 combination chemotherapy in unresectable non-small cell lung cancer. Proceedings of the 13th International Congress of Chemotherapy, Vienna, 1983 (abstr SE 12.15/14)

52. Scagliotti G, Lodico D, Gozzelino F: Clinical trial with high dose cisplatin and VP16-213 in advanced non small cell lung cancer: Results after two years. Proceedings of the 13th International Congress of Chemotherapy, Vienna, 1983 (abstr PS 12.1/15-5).

53. Veronesi A, Zagonel V, Santarossa M, et al: Cis-platinum and etoposide combination chemotherapy of advanced non-oat cell bronchogenic carcinoma. Cancer Chemother Pharmacol 11:35–37, 1983

54. Dhingra HM, Valdivieso M, Booser DJ, et al: Chemotherapy for advanced adenocarcinoma and squamous cell carcinoma of the lung with etoposide and cisplatin. Cancer Treat Rep 68:671–673, 1984

55. Mitrou PS, Graubner M, Berdel WE, et al: Cis-platinum (DDP) and VP16-213 (etoposide) combination chemotherapy for advanced non-small cell lung cancer: A phase II clinical trial. Eur J Cancer Clin Oncol 20:347–351, 1984

56. Dhingra HM, Murphy WK, Chiuten DF, et al: Chemotherapy with cisplatin (DDP) with vindesine (VDS) and/or VP16 for advanced adeno squamous cell lung cancer (ASCLC) and its effect on P.S. (ECOG) of patients. Proc Am Soc Clin Oncol 1984 (abstr C-861)

57. Carmichael J, Gregor A, Cornbleet MA, et al: Cis-platinum and vindesine in combination in the treatment of non-small cell lung cancer. Eur J Cancer Clin Oncol 21:811–814, 1985

58. Kris MG, Gralla RJ, Kalman LA, et al: Randomized trial comparing vindesine plus cisplatin with vinblastine plus cisplatin in patients with non-small cell lung cancer, with an analysis of methods of response assessment. Cancer Treat Rep 69:387–395, 1985

59. Shinkai T, Saijo N, Tominaga K, et al: Comparison of vindesine plus cisplatin or vindesine plus mitomycin in the treatment of advanced non-small cell lung cancer. Cancer Treat Rep 69:945–951, 1985

60. Klastersky J, Sculier JP, Nicaise C, et al: Combination chemotherapy with cisplatin, etoposide and vindesine in non small cell carcinoma: A clinical trial of the EORTC Lung Cancer Working Party. Cancer Treat Rep 67:727–730, 1983

61. Bertrand M, Multhauf P, Presant C, et al: Phase II trial of etoposide, vincristine and high dose cisplatin in advanced non-small cell lung cancer. Cancer Treat Rep 69:1335–1336, 1985

62. Porter L, Hainsworth J, Hande K, et al: Non-small cell carcinoma of the lung (NSCLC) treated with cisplatinum (DDP), VP-16 and vindesine (VND). Proc Am Soc Clin Oncol 1983 (abstr C-755)

63. Gropp C, Havemann K, Harms V, et al: DDP, vindesine, etoposide and radiotherapy in patients with non resectable non-small cell cancer of the lung. Proceedings of the 13th International Congress of Chemotherapy, Vienna, 1983 (abstr SE 12.1/15-9)

64. Gatzemeier V, Zchaber R, Hossfeld DK, et al: Combination chemotherapy with cisplatinum, vindesine and VP-16 in the treatment of non-small cell carcinoma of the lung. A phase II trial. Proceedings of the 13th International Congress of Chemotherapy, Vienna, 1983 (abstr SE 12.1/15-16)

65. Osoba D, Rusthoven JJ, Turnbull KA, et al: Combination chemotherapy with bleomycin, etoposide and cisplatin in metastatic non-small cell lung cancer. J Clin Oncol 3:1478–1485, 1985

66. Natale RB, Wheeler RH, Long AM, et al: High response rate in non-small cell lung cancer (NSCLC) with combination cisplatin VP-16 and methylglyoxal bis (guanylhydrazone) (MGBG). Proc Am Soc Clin Oncol 1983 (abstr C-759)

67. Itri LM, Gralla RJ, Kelsen DP, et al: Cisplatin, vindesine, bleomycin (CVB) combination chemotherapy of advanced non-small cell lung cancer. Cancer 51:1050–1055, 1983

68. Greenwald E, Vogl S, Berenzweig M, et al: Methylglyoxal bis-guanylhydrazone (MGBG), vindesine and cisplatinum in non-small cell bronchogenic carcinoma (NSCBC). Proc Am Soc Clin Oncol 1983 (abstr C-767)

69. Klastersky J, Sculier JP, Ravez P, et al: High (120 mg/m^2) versus lower (60 mg/m^2) dose of cisplatin (CDDP) in combination with etoposide in the treatment of non-small cell lung carcinoma (NSCLC). Proceedings of the IVth World Conference on Lung Cancer, Toronto, 1985 (abstr)

70. Evans BD, Weston C, Smith IE: Carboplatin (JM8) and VP16 combination chemotherapy for untreated small lung carcinoma: A phase II study. Proc Am Soc Clin Oncol 1985 (abstr C-734)

71. Weick JK, Rainey JM, Livingston RB, et al: Treatment of non–small-cell bronchogenic carcinoma with vinblastine and mitomycin: A Southwest Oncology Group Study. Cancer Treat Rep 69:583–585, 1985

72. Sculier JP, Klastersky J, Dumont JP, et al: Combination chemotherapy with mitomycin and vindesine in advanced non small cell lung cancer. A pilot study conducted by the Lung Cancer Working Party (Belgium). Cancer Treat Rep (in press)

73. Ruckdeschel JC, Day R, Weissman CH, et al: Chemotherapy for metastatic non-small cell bronchogenic carcinoma: Cyclophosphamide, doxorubicin, and etoposide versus mitomycin and vinblastine. Cancer Treat Rep 68:1325–1329, 1984

74. Shah A, Klimo P, Murray N: Phase II study of mitomycin, methotrexate and vincristine combination chemotherapy in advanced adenocarcinoma of the lung. Cancer Treat Rep 68:1299–1300, 1984

75. Miller TP, Weick JK, Grozea PN, et al: Extensive adenocarcinoma and large cell undifferentiated carcinoma of the lung treated with 5-FU, vindesine, and mitomycin (FEMi): A Southwest Oncology Group Study. Cancer Treat Rep 66:553–556, 1982

76. Schulman P, Budman DR, Weiselberg L, et al: Phase II trial of mitomycin, vinblastine and cisplatin (MVP) in non-small cell bronchogenic carcinoma. Cancer Treat Rep 67:943–945, 1983

77. Niell HB, Griffin JP, West WH, et al: Combination chemotherapy with mitomycin C, methotrexate, cisplatin, and vinblastine in the treatment of non-small cell lung cancer. Cancer 54:1260–1263, 1984

78. Anderson P, Spain R, Speer J: Mitomycin C, cisplatinum and vinblastine infusion in combined modality therapy of III non small cell lung cancer. Proc Am Soc Clin Oncol 3:217, 1982 (abstr)

79. Folman R, Rosman M, Auerbach S: Mitomycin C, vinblastine and cisplatinum in the combined modality treatment of non–small-cell lung cancer. Proc Am Soc Clin Oncol 3:232, 1984 (abstr)

80. Miller TP, Vance RB, Tong TC: Treatment of advanced non–small-cell lung cancer with mitomycin C plus cisplatinum plus vindesine: comparisons to other mitomycin C plus vinca-containing combinations. Proc Am Soc Clin Oncol 3:230, 1984 (abstr)

Phase II Trial of Etoposide, Cisplatin, Continuous Infusion 5-Fluorouracil, and Simultaneous Split-Course Radiation Therapy in Stage III Non–Small-Cell Bronchogenic Carcinoma

By Philip Bonomi, Kendrith Rowland, Samuel G. Taylor, IV, Salitha Reddy, Myung-Sook Lee, L. Penfield Faber, and William Warren

Survival in patients with locally advanced, non-small-cell lung cancer (NSCLC) is relatively short, despite treatment with surgery or radiation. A phase II study of simultaneous continuous infusion 5-fluorouracil and split-course radiation with or without surgery has shown possible impovement in median survival compared with that observed in trials of radiation alone. Past success with etoposide plus cisplatin in NSCLC has led to the addition of etoposide to the 5-fluorouracil plus cisplatin plus radiation combination. Twenty-four stage III NSCLC patients were treated with this three-drug regimen, and a 74% clinical partial remission rate was observed. Thoracotomy was done in eight of these patients; subsequent histologic examination of the resected specimen revealed no residual tumor in four patients (50%) and only microscopic foci of tumor in two patients (25%). Major toxicities were leukopenia, nausea, and vomiting. Median leukocyte nadir was 2,900/mm^3. A leukocyte count <1,000/mm^3 was observed in two of 24 patients (8%), one of whom expired from progressive pneumonia. All patients experienced nausea and vomiting, which were classified as moderate in three patients (12%) and severe in four (16%). Moderate to severe esophagitis, dermatitis, and pneumonitis were not observed. Median progression-free interval and median survival were not reached after a median follow-up of 163 days.

THE INCIDENCE of lung cancer continues to increase, with an estimated 144,000 new cases in 1985.[1] Of these patients, approximately one third will present with locally advanced disease and no apparent distant metastases. Few patients will be cured by radiation[2,3] (although thoracic radiation provides palliation for many) or by pulmonary resection.[4]

Recent reports show that in patients with locally advanced disease, response rates for combination chemotherapy regimens range from 47% to 56%,[5-7] approximately double the rate observed in patients with distant metastases.[8] At least two prospective randomized trials comparing thoracic radiation alone to thoracic radiation preceded by combination chemotherapy are being conducted in patients with locally advanced disease. Although assessment of efficacy of sequential chemotherapy/radiation therapy will depend on results of such randomized trials, the median survival observed in nonrandomized trials[6,7] of sequential chemotherapy/radiation therapy shows no apparent advantage over the 9- to 12-month median survival obtained with thoracic radiation alone.[3,4]

Preliminary survival data for sequential chemotherapy/radiation therapy led to our trying a variation of the combined modality approach initially developed by Taylor et al[9] in head and neck cancer. In this treatment design, chemotherapeutic agents with radiation-sensitizing potential are given simultaneously with split-course radiation. The cisplatin plus continuous-infusion 5-fluorouracil regimen[10] was chosen for this purpose.[11,12] When this combined modality study was initiated, the activity of the cisplatin plus 5-fluorouracil regimen in non–small-cell lung cancer (NSCLC) had not been evaluated. However, since that time, Weiden et al[13] have shown that cisplatin and 5-fluorouracil alone produce a 37% response rate in previously untreated NSCLC patients.

Analysis of 64 clinical stage III M_0, NSCLC patients treated with simultaneous 5-fluorouracil, cisplatin, and radiation (5-FU–DDP–RT) suggests that this treatment might be better than radiation alone; such patients had a 16-month median survival[14] compared with 9- to 12-month median survival for radiation alone.[3,4] Similarly, 38% of patients treated with the combined modality regimen survived for 2 years, compared with 15% to 20% of patients treated with radiation alone.[3,4] Approximately two thirds of

From the Section of Medical Oncology, Rush Medical College, Chicago; Section of Medical Oncology, Carle Clinic, Urbana, Ill; Department of Radiation Therapy, Rush Medical College, Chicago; and the Department of Cardiovascular/Thoracic Surgery, Rush Medical College, Chicago.

Address reprint requests to Philip Bonomi, MD, Section of Medical Oncology, Rush Medical College, Room 830, 1725 W Harrison, Chicago, IL 60612.

0093–7754/86/1303–3017$05.00/0

patients initially treated with 5-FU–DDP–RT had subsequent pulmonary resection.[14]

Encouraged by these initial observations, etoposide was added to this regimen for the following reasons: (1) Etoposide/cisplatin had produced a 56% response rate in patients with limited NSCLC.[5] (2) Several trials in small-cell lung cancer (SCLC) had demonstrated acceptable toxicity with simultaneous administration of etoposide, cisplatin, and radiation.[15,16] (3) Both 5-fluorouracil and etoposide appear to act synergistically with cisplatin.[17] (4) Although the differences were not statistically significant, etoposide/cisplatin has produced the longest median survival (26.6 weeks)[18] and highest 1-year survival rate (25%)[19] in Eastern Cooperative Oncology Group (ECOG) lung studies evaluating combination regimens in patients with distant metastases. (5) There is an anecdotal report suggesting that podophyllin might be a radiation sensitizer.[20]

In the 5-FU–DDP–RT trial,[14] patients were reevaluated after four courses (4,000 rad) and surgery was performed if possible. Thirty-nine patients underwent thoractomy; nine patients (23%) had no residual tumor, and eight (21%) had only microscopic foci in the resected specimen. Fifty-nine percent of these patients have not had recurrent tumor compared with 41% of patients whose resected specimen contained gross residual tumor.

The immediate objective of the current trial was to determine whether the addition of etoposide to the 5-FU–DDP–RT regimen would improve combined histologic complete response and microscopic foci response rates by 50%. The ultimate goal was to determine whether the median survival and 2-year survival rates could be increased by 50%. Preliminary results observed with etoposide, 5-fluorouracil, cisplatin, and radiation (VP-16–5-FU–DDP–RT) are described in this report.

MATERIALS AND METHODS

Patients with NSCLC confirmed either histologically or by cytology (obtained by bronchial brushing or by lung or lymph node needle biopsy) were eligible for this study; sputum cytology specimens were not considered adequate. Either histologic or clinical evidence of stage III disease was required for inclusion in this trial. Criteria for classifying disease as clinical stage III included computed tomography (CT) scan depiction of tumor invasion of the mediastinum or chest wall, and/or the presence of mediastinal nodes >2 cm. Evidence of distant metastases (with the exception of supraclavicular lymph node metastases) excluded such patients from this study. Before starting treatment, each patient had a nuclide bone scan, CT brain scan with Hypaque infusion, and CT scan of the chest and upper abdomen. Also, each patient was initially classified by a thoracic surgeon as potentially resectable or nonresectable, regardless of response to treatment. All patients selected gave informed written consent.

Other eligibility requirements include ECOG performance status ≤3; leukocyte count ≥4,000/μl; platelet count ≥100,000/μL; BUN ≤25 mg/dL; serum creatinine ≤1.5 mg/dL; and bilirubin ≤1.5 mg/dL. Physical examination, complete blood cell (CBC) count, platelet count, SMA-18, and chest x-ray were done before each course of treatment.

Patients considered potentially resectable were reevaluated after the fourth course of treatment. Reevaluation consisted of CBC count, platelet count, SMA-18, CT scan of the chest and upper abdomen, bone scan, CT scan of the brain with infusion, and pulmonary function tests. Bronchoscopy was optional at the time of reevaluation.

The chemotherapy regimen was as follows: cisplatin (60 mg/m^2 intravenously [IV]) over one hour on day 1; etoposide (60 mg/m^2 IV), over one hour on days 1 to 4; and 5-fluorouracil (800 mg/m^2 IV), over 24 hours for four consective days. The infusion of 5-fluorouracil was interrupted to give etoposide. Immediately before and after cisplatin, 500 mL of 5% D/0.45 NS was administered IV over one hour. Also, mannitol (12.5 g) was administered immediately before starting cisplatin. Patients were also treated with diphenhydramine, dexamethasone, and metoclopramide on day 1 in an effort to prevent nausea and vomiting. Treatment was repeated every 21 days if toxicity permitted.

The doses of 5-fluorouracil and etoposide, but not cisplatin, were reduced by 25% for a leukocyte count between 3,000 and 4,000 μL, and by 50% for a leukocyte count between 2,000 and 3,000/μL. Neither chemotherapy nor radiation was given if the leukocyte count was <2,000/μL or platelet count was less than 100,000/μL. The dose of each drug was reduced by 25% for moderate nausea and vomiting and by 50% for severe nausea and vomiting.

The cisplatin dose was reduced by 50% for a serum creatinine level >1.5 mg/dL, and cisplatin was not administered if serum creatinine was >2 mg/dL. Treatment was not

Table 1. Patient Characteristics

	No. Patients (%)
Age (median/range) 57/37–71 yr	
Males/females	14/10
ECOG performance status	
0–1/2–3	18/6
Previous weight loss	
0 < 5%	14 (58)
>5 < 10%	3 (13)
>10%	7 (29)
Type of tumor	
Squamous cell	12 (50)
Adenocarcinoma	6 (25)
Large-cell	6 (25)

administered if patients had oral or esophageal mucositis. No dose reduction was made for grade 1 mucositis, but a 25% reduction was required in subsequent courses if grade 2 or 3 mucositis was observed. Radiation therapy was administered on days 1 to 5 of each 21-day cycle. Patients classified as potentially resectable received radiotherapy in 200-rad fractions in a single daily treatment on days 1 to 5. Treatment was stopped after a total dose of 4,000 rad. Patients initially classified as nonresectable received two 116-rad fractions per day on days 1 to 5 of each cycle. Nonsurgical patients received a total dose of 6,000 rad.

Radiation was delievered with megavoltage equipment with effective photon energies higher than 1 MeV Co-60, 2 MeV x-rays, or 4 MeV linear accelerator. Minimal treatment distance to the skin or isocenter was at least 80 cm. Treatment included the primary tumor, the mediastinum, and bilateral supraclavicular areas, and the primary target volume included a minimum 1-cm margin around the mass. Responses were defined according to ECOG criteria.[21]

RESULTS

All 24 patients entered on this protocol were evaluable for toxicity; 23 were evaluable for response. It was too early to determine response in one patient who required a repeat CT scan of the chest to determine tumor size. Two patients who died before completing therapy were classified as having progressive disease.

Patient characteristics are summarized in Table 1. The tumor, node, and metastasis (TNM) grading system for classifying patients as having stage III disease is shown in Table 2. Thirteen patients were not considered surgical candidates at initial evaulation for the following reasons: tumor extending up trachea (three patients); supraclavicular nodal metastases (two patients); inadequate pulmonary function (three patients); bilateral mediastinal lymphadenopathy (three patients); and compression of major blood vessels (two patients).

The number of courses given was as follows: one course (one patient); two courses (one patient); three courses (two patients); four courses (12 patients); five courses (four patients); and six courses (five patients). Clinical responses were determined from chest x-ray and from thoracic CT scan measurement. Seventeen patients (74%) were classified as having a partial response. Although there was no definite mass apparent in some patients, clinical response was not classified as complete unless the CT scan was completely normal.

Median follow-up was 163 days with a range of eight to 320 days. Three patients had progressive disease (two patients developed osseous metastases as the only site of progression while receiving treatment, whereas the third patient had progression of local disease 60 days after completing five courses of therapy). No patient experienced progression of local disease during treatment. Four patients died (one from treatment-related infection, one from progressive osseous metastases, and two from aspiration pneumonia).

Eleven patients were initially classified as potential surgical candidates. Two patients refused surgery at reevaluation, and surgery is pending for one patient. Eight thoracotomies were performed and resulted in three pneumonectomies, three lobectomies, and two segmental pulmonary resections with simultaneous chest wall resection. Margins of resection were negative in all patients. Two patients had tumor in mediastinal nodes. Histologic responses in the primary tumor site were as follows: no residual tumor (four patients); microscopic foci only (two)/ and persistent gross disease (two).

Hematologic toxicity is summarized in Table 3. Median leukocyte count and platelet count nadirs were 2,900/μL and 239,000/μL, respectively. Severe hematologic toxicity (leukocyte count <1,000/μL and platelet count less than 30,000/μL) was observed in two patients. Both of these patients developed infections. One patient had *Staphylococcus aureus* wound infec-

Table 2. Pretreatment Staging

	No. Patients (%)	
TNM Classification	Histologic	Clinical
$T_3N_2M_0$	7 (29)	7 (29)
$T_3N_0M_0$	4 (16)	1 (4)
$T_{1-2}N_2M_0$	2 (8)	1 (4)
$T_{1-3}N_{1-2}M_1$*	2 (8)	—

*Biopsy-proven supraclavicular nodal metastases.

Table 3. Hematologic Toxicity

Type	No. Patients (%)
Leukopenia	
<1,000 μL	2 (8)
>1,000 < 2,000/μL	2 (8)
>2,000 < 3,000/μL	11 (46)
>3,000/μL	9 (38)
Thrombocytopenia	
<30,000/μL	2 (8)
>30,000 < 100,000/μL	1 (4)
>100,000/μL	21 (88)

tion from which she recovered, whereas the other had bilateral pneumonitis (no specific organism cultured), from which he died despite treatment with antibiotics and return of his leukocyte count to 6,100/μL five days after a nadir of 500/μL. This was classified as a treatment-related death.

The two patients with severe hematologic toxicity were classified as ECOG performance status 2 to 3 before starting treatment; one had lost more than 10% of his usual body weight immediately before diagnosis. Similarly, one of the two patients whose leukocyte nadir was between 1,000/μL and 2,000/μL was classified as ECOG performance status 3 and had lost >10% of her usual body weight. Because of the severe hematologic toxicity observed in these patients, the protocol has since been amended as follows: in patients whose ECOG performance status is 2 to 3 or who have lost more than 10% of their body weight, the initial etoposide and 5-fluorouracil doses should be reduced by 25% (or to 45 mg/m^2 and 600 mg/m^2, respectively).

All patients experienced some degree of anorexia, nausea, or vomiting, which were categorized as moderate if vomiting persisted for three days and severe if weight loss >5 lb was noted. Nausea and vomiting were classified as moderate in three patients (12%) and severe in four patients (16%) who lost from 10 to 15 lb during treatment (Table 4). Two of the patients who had severe nausea and vomiting returned to their pretreatment weight within 4 weeks of completing chemotherapy and radiation therapy. Comparison of initial weight and weight observed 4 weeks after completion of chemotherapy/radiation therapy for 22 patients who completed three or more courses of treatment is shown in Table 5. Ten (45%) patients gained more than 5 lb during this interval, whereas ten others (45%) remained stable despite anorexia, nausea, and vomiting during treatment.

Table 4. Gastrointestinal Toxicity

Type	No. Patients (%)
Nausea and vomiting	
Mild	17 (71)
Moderate	3 (12)
Severe	4 (17)
Esophagitis	
None	14 (58)
Mild	10 (42)
Moderate/severe	0

Table 5. Weight Change After Completion of Chemotherapy/Radiotherapy

Weight Change*	No. Patients (%)†
<5-lb loss	2 (10)
5-lb loss to 5-lb gain	10 (45)
>5-lb gain	10 (45)

*Weight 4 weeks after completion of chemotherapy/radiation therapy minus weight at start of treatment.

†Included are patients who completed three or more courses of treatment.

During the five-day treatment period, two patients experienced hiccoughs, which responded to administration of chlorpromazine. Ten patients had mild esophagitis, none had moderate or severe esophagitis, and there were no reports of stomatitis. All patients had significant alopecia and experienced fatigue during treatment. Serum creatinine levels rose to 1.7 mg/dL in two patients; no other patient experienced a serum creatinine level greater than 1.5 mg/dL.

Cough, mild dyspnea, and radiographic findings consistent with radiation pneumonitis were observed in two patients, one of whom subsequently developed a lung abscess which is responding to antibiotics. All patients had erythema in the radiation portal, but none had moist desquamation.

Dense fibrous tissue was encountered at surgical resection, which frequently made identification of surgical planes difficult. One of the surgica patients developed empyema. No other postoperative complications have been observed.

DISCUSSION

Although the 74% clinical response rate observed with 5-FU–VP-16–DDP–RT is higher than the 50% response rate reported for radiation alone,[22] the results are similar to those reported for other sequential chemotherapy/radiation therapy trials.[6,7] Perhaps the combined histologic complete and microscopic foci only response rates are better early indicators of the efficacy of this combined modality treatment. In the 5-FU–DDP–RT trial, surgical patients whose resected specimen contained either no tumor or only microscopic foci of tumor have had a lower recurrence rate than patients whose surgical specimen contained tumor (41% *v* 59%, respectively).[14] Although the number of patients is small, the four (50%) histologic complete responses and two (25%) microscopic-foci–only responses in the VP-16–5-FU–DDP–RT patients compare favorably with the 23% histologic complete response (CR) rate and the 44% combined histologic CR and microscopic disease only observed with 5-FU–DDP–RT.[14] Additional data are needed to determine if the initial complete and microscopic-foci–only response rates are confirmed and, more importantly, to determine median survival, 2-year survival, and sites of failure in this group of patients.

One of the two major toxicities observed with this treatment was leukopenia. Although leukopenia may have been somewhat underestimated because midcycle counts were not done routinely, the median leukocyte count of 2,900/μL at the start of each treatment course shows that, in general, leukopenia was not severe. Two patients experienced febrile episodes while their leukocyte counts were less than 1,000/μL, one of whom died despite treatment with antibiotics and an increase of leukocyte count to 6,100/μL within five days. ECOG performance status in these two patients was 2 to 3, and one had lost more than 10% of his usual body weight. These observations have resulted in our reducing the doses of etoposide and 5-fluorouracil to 75% of the usual starting doses in patients whose ECOG performance status is 2 to 3 or whose weight is 10% lower than usual. Ruckdeschel et al[23] observed similarly severe toxicity from combination chemotherapy in lung cancer patients whose performance status was 2.

Comparison of myelosuppression observed with VP-16–5-FU–DDP–RT and that observed in our previous trial with 5-FU–DDP–RT shows that 5% of patients had a WBC count of $<2{,}000/\mu$L with the two-drug regimen *v* 16% with three drugs, and that 29% of patients had a WBC count of $<3{,}000/\mu$L with the two-drug regimen *v* 62% with three drugs.[15]

Although the addition of etoposide to 5-FU–DDP–RT increased myelosuppression, it was not severe in most patients and was less severe than the myelosuppression observed with the cyclophosphamide plus doxorubicin plus vincristine regimen used simultaneously with radiation (CAV-RT) in the treatment of SCLC.[24] In the CAV-RT trial,[24] 34% of patients experienced bacterial infections during treatment compared with 8% of our patients.

Anorexia, nausea, and vomiting were major toxicities during treatment with VP-16–5-FU–DDP–RT; four patients (16%) lost from 10 to 15 lb during treatment. Despite gastrointestinal side effects during each five-day course of treatment, by the end of four to six courses 45% of patients had not lost weight and 45% had gained more than 5 lb.

Unlike the simultaneous use of doxorubicin and radiation, which produced moderate to severe esophagitis in 56% of patients,[24] none of our patients experienced moderate to severe esophagitis. Similarly, although all of our patients had skin erythema in the radiation portal, none experienced moist desquamation.

Two (8%) of our patients developed mild radiation pneumonitis following treatment, and of eight patients undergoing lung resection, none developed respiratory complications. This is in contrast to a 20% rate of radiation pneumonitis after CAV-RT[24] and three out of four patients developing adult respiratory distress syndrome after pulmonary resection following treatment with mitomycin/cisplatin.[25] Three of the CAV-RT–treated patients (6%) had fatal radiation pneumonitis[24] and two of four mitomycin/cisplatin-treated patients had fatal respiratory insufficiency following lung resection.[25]

In conclusion, the combined modality of VP-16–5-FU–DDP–RT produced a relatively high local response rate in patients with locally advanced NSCLC. Toxicity from combining VP-16–5-FU–DDP and simultaneous thoracic radiation is moderate, with leukopenia, anorexia, nausea, and vomiting being the major toxic effects. Esophagitis and radiation pneumonitis were not significant problems. Similarly, although pulmonary resection is difficult because of dense fibrous tissue, surgery following four courses (4,000 rad) of radiation therapy and a 4-week rest period does not appear to be associated with an increased rate of postoperative complications. More data are needed to determine histologic response rate, median survival, and 2-year survival for patients receiving this treatment.

REFERENCES

1. Cancer Facts and Figures. New York, American Cancer Society, 1985, p 9

2. Perez CA, Stanley K, Rubin P, et al: A prospective randomized study of various irradiation doses and fractionated schedules in the treatment of inoperable non-oat cell carcinoma of the lung. Cancer 45:2744–2753, 1980

3. Petrovich Z, Stanley K, Cox JD, et al: Radiotherapy in the management of locally advanced lung cancer of all cell types. Cancer 48:1335–1349, 1981

4. Mountain CF: Assessment of the role of surgery. Ann Thorac Surg 24:365–373, 1977

5. Longeval E, Klastersky J: Combination chemotherapy with cisplatin and etoposide in bronchogenic squamous cell carcinoma and adenocarcinoma. Cancer 50:2751–2756, 1982

6. Fram R, Skarin A, Balikian J, et al: Combination chemotherapy followed by radiation therapy in patients with regional stage III unresectable non-small cell lung cancer. Cancer Treat Rep 69:587–590, 1985

7. Wagner H, Ruckdeschel J, Bonomi P, et al: Treatment of locally advanced non-small cell lung cancer (NSCLC) with mitomycin C, vinblastine, and cisplatin (MVP) followed by radiation therapy: An ECOG pilot study. Proc Am Soc Clin Oncol 4:183, 1985 (abstr)

8. Ruckdeschel JC, Finkelstein DM, Mason BA, et al: Chemotherapy for metastatic non-small cell bronchogenic carcinoma: EST 2575: generation V—a randomized comparison of four cisplatin containing regimens. J Clin Oncol 3:72–79, 1985

9. Taylor SG IV, Murthy AK, Showel JL, et al: Improved control in advanced head and neck cancer with simultaneous radiation, cisplatin, 5-FU chemotherapy. Cancer Treat Rep 69:933–939, 1985

10. Kish J, Dreilichman A, Jacobs J, et al: Clinical trial of cisplatin and 5-FU infusion as initial treatment of advanced squamous cell carcinoma of the head and neck. Cancer Treat Rep 66:471–474, 1982

11. Byfield JE, Calabro-Jones PM, Klisak I, et al: Pharmacologic requirements for obtaining sensitization of human tumor cells in vitro to combined 5-fluorouracil and ftorafor and x-rays. Int J Radiat Oncol Biol Phys 8:1923–1933, 1982

12. Murthy A, Rossof AH, Anderson KM, et al: Cytotoxicity and influence on radiation dose response curve of cis-dichlorodiammineplatinum. Int J Radiat Oncol Biol Phys 5:1411–1415, 1979

13. Weiden PL, Einstein AB, Rudolph RH: Cisplatin and 5-FU infusion chemotherapy for non-small cell lung cancer. Proc Am Soc Clin Oncol 3:215, 1984 (abstr)

14. Taylor SG IV, Trybula M, Bonomi PD, et al: Simultaneous cisplatin/5-FU infusion and radiation followed by surgical resection in regionally localized non-small cell lung cancer. Ann Thorac Surg 1986 (in press)

15. Murray N, Jadzic E, Shah B, et al: Alternating chemotherapy and thoracic radiotherapy with concurrent cisplatin for simultaneous small cell carcinoma of the lung. Proc Am Soc Clin Oncol 3:214, 1984 (abstr)

16. Woods RL, Levy JH: Chemotherapy for small cell lung cancer: A randomized study of maintenance therapy with cyclophosphamide, Adriamycin, and vincristine (CAV) after remission induction with cisplatinum, VP-16, and radiotherapy. Proc Am Soc Clin Oncol 3:214, 1984 (abstr)

17. Schabel FM Jr, Trader MW, Laster WR, et al: Cis-dichlorodiammineplatinum (II): Combination chemotherapy and cross-resistance studies with tumors of mice. Cancer Treat Rep 63:1459–1473, 1979

18. Ruckdeschel JC, Finkelstein DM, Ettinger DS: Chemotherapy of metastatic non-small cell lung cancer. Proceedings of the Fourth World Conference on Lung Cancer, Toronto, 1985, p 39

19. Finkelstein DM, Ettinger DS, Ruckdeschel JC: Long-term survivors in metastatic non–small-cell lung cancer: An Eastern Cooperative Oncology Group Study. J Clin Oncol 4:702–709, 1986

20. Swartz MR, Rosenman J, Gunderson L, et al: Podophyllin increases tumor radioresponsiveness. Cancer Chemother Pharmacol 7:238, 1982

21. Oken MM, Creech RH, Tormey DC, et al: Toxicity and response criteria of the Eastern Co-operative Oncology Group. Am J Clin Oncol 5:649–655, 1982

22. Salazar OM, Rubin P, Brown JC, et al: Predictors of radiation response in lung cancer: A clinico-pathobiological analysis. Cancer 37:2636–2650, 1976

23. Ruckdeschel JC, Finkelstein DM, Ettinger DS, et al: Predictors of improved response and survival in metastatic non-small cell bronchogenic carcinoma. Proc Am Soc Clin Oncol 4:187, 1985 (abstr)

24. Brereton HD, Kent HC, Johnson RE: Chemotherapy and radiation therapy for small cell carcinoma of the lung: A remedy for past therapeutic failure, in Muggia FM, Rosenczweig M (eds): Progress in Cancer Research and Therapy, volume 11, Lung Cancer: Progress in Therapeutic Research. New York, Raven, 1976, pp 575–586

25. Bonomi P, Trybula M, Sandler SG, et al: Comparison of neoadjuvant chemotherapy to simultaneous chemotherapy-radiotherapy in locally advanced squamous cell bronchogenic carcinoma. Proceedings of the First International Congress on Neo-Adjuvant Chemotherapy, Paris, 1985, p 29

Combined Chemotherapy and Radiation Therapy for Non–Small-Cell Lung Cancer

By David Osoba, J.J. Rusthoven, W.K. Evans, and K.A. Turnbull

In a previous study of patients with recurrent or disseminated non–small-cell lung cancer (NSCLC), the combination of bleomycin, etoposide, and cisplatin (BEP) produced objective responses in ten of 17 (59%) patients with large-cell anaplastic carcinoma and in 14 of 35 (40%) with squamous-cell carcinoma. These results prompted a pilot study of combined modality therapy in which two cycles of BEP were administered prior to split-course radiation therapy. Thirty patients with surgically unresectable stage II or III squamous- or large-cell cancer, were entered into the study, of whom 25 were evaluable for response to chemotherapy. One patient (4%) had a complete response (CR), ten (40%) with measurable disease had a partial response (PR), and four (16%) with evaluable disease had significant disease regression prior to radiotherapy (overall response rate, 60%). After radiotherapy, six of 22 (27%) evaluable patients achieved a CR, and six (27%) a PR, for an overall response rate of 55%. Symptom control was achieved with chemotherapy in the majority of patients. The median survival time after the initiation of BEP had not been reached at 52 weeks. The results of this pilot study suggest that a phase III study comparing BEP plus radiation therapy with radiation therapy alone should be undertaken in this subgroup of patients with NSCLC.

THE IDEA of combining bleomycin, etoposide, and cisplatin (BEP) in the treatment of non–small-cell lung cancer (NSCLC) originated with observations made from European studies using either bleomycin plus cisplatin or etoposide plus cisplatin.[1,2] The three drugs were combined as their toxicities are largely non–overlapping. Other favorable results with this combination were the observed clinical activity of bleomycin and cisplatin in squamous-cell lung cancer arising in the oropharyngeal region,[3] the synergistic effects of bleomycin and cisplatin in cell culture studies,[4] and the additive effects of etoposide and cisplatin in clinical trials with small-cell lung cancer (SCLC)[5] and in cell culture studies.[6]

The initial trial of BEP was with 53 patients with NSCLC who presented with recurrent or disseminated disease after initial therapy with surgery and/or radiation, or whose disease was disseminated (M_1) at presentation.[7] Since then, an additional 26 patients with recurrent or disseminated disease have been treated, making a total of 79 patients available for analysis.

Seventy-four patients were evaluable for response; the overall response rate (complete response [CR] and partial response [PR]) was 38%. Although the response rate in 22 patients with adenocarcinoma was only 18%, it was 59% in 17 patients with large-cell carcinoma and 40% in 35 patients with squamous-cell carcinoma. The response rates in the subgroups with large-cell and squamous-cell carcinomas are not significantly different from each other (P = .24), but the difference in response rates of the combined subgroups of large-cell and squamous-cell carcinoma (46%) and the subgroup of adenocarcinoma (18%) is statistically significant (P = .03).

In this study, performance status (ECOG [Eastern Cooperative Oncology Group] 0, 1 *v* 2, 3) was not associated either with response to BEP or with the median survival time (24 weeks and 23 weeks, respectively).

However, previous therapy (with radiation particularly) was associated with a lower response rate (31% in 26 patients) and a tendency toward shorter survival (median, 22 weeks) than the response rate (62% in 26 patients, P = .05) and survival (median, 27 weeks) in previously untreated patients. Although there was an association between responsiveness to BEP and survival, with responders living significantly longer (median, 38 weeks) than nonresponders (median, 20 weeks, P = .00001), we cannot conclude that a cause-effect relationship exists.

There was a strong positive correlation

From the Toronto-Bayview Regional Cancer Centre, Ontario Cancer Treatment and Research Foundation, Toronto; the Sunnybrook Medical Centre, Toronto; the Toronto General Hospital, Toronto; and the University of Toronto.

Address reprint requests to David Osoba, MD, Department of Medicine, Health Sciences Centre Hospital, University of British Columbia, 2211 Wesbrook Mall, Vancouver, British Columbia, Canada V6T-1W5.

0093–7754/86/1303–3018$05.00/0

between complete relief of symptoms and tumor response when comparing the symptoms in 20 patients with responsive disease to 13 patients with progressive disease ($P = .001$).

Toxicity from BEP was primarily integumentary (alopecia), gastrointestinal (nausea and vomiting in approximately 50% of patients), and hematologic (a neutropenia of $< 0.5 \times 10^9/L$ after 21% of the cycles and a thrombocytopenia of $< 25 \times 10^9/L$ in 3% of the cycles). There were two treatment-related deaths in 79 patients (one from sepsis and one from acute renal tubular necrosis). Only three patients experienced pulmonary toxicity, which was judged to be minor.

These observations suggest that squamous-cell and large-cell tumors respond to BEP more frequently than adenocarcinoma, and that previous radiation therapy is associated with a lower response rate than if no previous treatment has been given.

The combined response rate of 46% in patients with squamous-cell and large-cell carcinoma suggested that BEP might be used profitably with radiation therapy in a combined modality treatment protocol if the BEP was administered before the radiation therapy. Thus, a protocol was designed for patients with previously untreated and surgically unresectable squamous-cell and large-cell lung cancer still limited to the thorax and supraclavicular lymph nodes (stage II or III, any T, N_1-N_2, M_0).

The objectives of this pilot study were to determine the response rate to BEP alone, response rate after the addition of radiation therapy, the length of survival, and to assess clinically the degree of pulmonary toxicity with the combined use of radiation and bleomycin.

MATERIALS AND METHODS

Eligibility requirements included age of < 75 years, histologically proven squamous-cell or large-cell lung cancer, surgically unresectable stage II or III (any T, N_1-N_2, M_0) disease, no previous treatment by either radiation therapy or chemotherapy, lung function studies not indicative of severe obstructive pulmonary disease and DLCO more than 50% of predicted value, and adequate renal, hematologic, and hepatic function.

The chemotherapy schedule was designed for outpatient use and included bleomycin (10 U/m^2), etoposide (100 mg/m^2), and cisplatin (25 mg/m^2) administered intravenously (IV) daily for three days and repeated 28 days later if there was no undue toxicity and no tumor progression.

Four weeks after the second cycle, the patient received the first part of a split course of radiation therapy (2,000 cGy in five fractions per week) with a 4-week off-treatment interval and, in the absence of progression, the second part of the radiation schedule (a further 2,000 cGy in five fractions per week). The field size was dependent on the original extent of disease as measured radiographically and by physical examination. Standard pulmonary function tests were performed before chemotherapy, before radiation therapy, and at intervals after the completion of treatment.

In patients with measurable disease the response to treatment was assessed by standard criteria and designated as CR, PR, stable disease, and progressive disease.[6] In patients who had evaluable but not measurable disease, a regression required reduction in the size of visible disease on chest radiograph or physical examination (equivalent to a PR as evaluated by two independent evaluators); stable disease was any situation less than a regression; and progressive disease was a clear increase in the size of the visible mass.[6]

RESULTS

Thirty patients were entered in the study; 25 were evaluable for response after chemotherapy, and 22, for response after radiation therapy. There were 14 men and 11 women, ranging in age from 50 to 73 years (median, 62 years). The Eastern Cooperative Oncology Group (ECOG) performance status was 0 in three patients, 1 in 21 patients, and 3 in one patient. Three patients received only one cycle of BEP because of disease progression after the first cycle; 21 patients received two cycles as planned; and one patient inadvertently received a third cycle (a total of 48 cycles were given). After completion of chemotherapy, ten patients received a split course of radiation therapy as planned, whereas ten patients received only the first part of the split course because of subsequent disease progression. One patient did not receive radiation because of intercurrent pneumonia, and the remaining four patients received between 3,000 and 5,000 cGy (as a split course in three of the four patients).

There were no treatment-related deaths; two patients (8%) had intercurrent pneumonia; one patient (4%) developed mild respiratory symptoms (dyspnea on exertion), and five patients (20%) were found to have a >25% decrease in the pretreatment DLCO but were asymptomatic. All patients developed some degree of alopecia. Nausea and vomiting were difficult to control after five of the 48 cycles, but were absent after 19 of the 48 cycles. The only noteworthy hematologic toxicity was neutropenia with neutrophil counts of $<0.5 \times 10^9/L$ after six (12.5%) of the 48 cycles. There was no renal toxicity (Table 1).

Table 1. Toxicity After BEP

Toxicity	Percent of Patients (n = 25)	Percent of Cycles (n = 48)
Treatment-related deaths	0	—
Pneumonia	8	—
Alopecia (varying degrees)	100	—
Pulmonary		
DLCO drop > 25% only	20	—
Mild symptoms	4	—
Myelosuppression		
Neutrophils < 0.5×10^9/L	16	12.5
Platelets < 25×10^9/L	0	0
Hemoglobin decrease > 30 g/L	0	0
Renal		
Creatinine > 120 μmol/L	0	0
Gastrointestinal		
Nausea and vomiting		
None	28	40
Controllable	56	50
Intractable	16	10
Diarrhea	4	4
Mucositis	4	2

After chemotherapy in the 25 evaluable patients, one patient (4%) with measurable disease had a CR, ten patients (40%) with measurable disease had a PR, and four patients (16%) with evaluable but unmeasurable disease had regression. The overall response rate was 60%. Seven patients (28%) had stable disease and three patients (12%) had progressive disease (Table 2).

After radiation therapy in 22 evaluable patients, six patients were judged to have a CR (27%) and six patients had a PR (27%), giving an overall response rate of 55% (Table 3). Two patients were not yet evaluable, and one was not treated by radiation because of development of an intercurrent pneumonia. The median survival time after initiation of BEP has not been reached at 52 weeks.

Symptom control was achieved in the majority of patients after chemotherapy only, with all symptoms being controlled in 16 of 25 patients (64%) and relief of at least some symptoms in eight of the nine remaining patients. Only one patient did not have relief of any pretreatment symptoms.

Table 2. Response After BEP

Status	No. of Patients (%)	Total (%)
CR (measurable disease)	1 (4)	60
PR (measurable disease)	10 (40)	
Regression (evaluable disease)	4 (16)	
Stable disease	7 (28)	40
Progressive disease	3 (12)	

Table 3. Summary of Disease Status After Radiation Therapy

Status	No. of Patients (%)	Total (%)
CR	6 (27)	55
PR	6 (27)	
Stable disease	2 (9)	9
Progressive disease	8 (36)	36

DISCUSSION

Attempts to cure surgically unresectable NSCLC have been unsuccessful, and the current form of management is largely palliative. Radiation therapy is frequently used to control localized symptoms, and chemotherapy is still experimental. Many chemotherapy regimens for widely disseminated disease (M_1) have been reported, but the response rates have been low in large series of patients (in the 30% range), and survival times have not been lengthened appreciably.[8-10] The use of BEP in our studies was effective in producing PRs and CRs in about half of patients with squamous-cell and large-cell lung cancer, but was relatively ineffective in those with adenocarcinoma. A similar histology-dependent responsiveness was observed by the ECOG in 121 patients treated with etoposide plus cisplatin, ie, the response rate in 67 patients with squamous- and large-cell cancer was 30%, whereas it was only 7% in 54 patients with adenocarcinoma.[11] However, the response rates reported in all three histologic types of lung cancer were lower than those in our patients. Whether this difference represents the variance in results reported from multi-institution studies as compared with a largely single-institution study, or whether the difference represents an effect of the different drug scheduling in these studies or the addition of bleomycin to etoposide plus cisplatin is unknown.

Our results in recurrent and disseminated squamous-cell and large-cell lung cancer prompted us to embark on a pilot study of combined modality therapy using two cycles of

BEP followed by split-course radiation therapy for previously untreated stage II and stage III squamous-cell and large-cell disease. The response rate after chemotherapy in 25 patients was 60%, and only one patient experienced possible pulmonary toxicity. We feel that the results of this pilot study make it feasible to propose a phase III study comparing BEP plus radiation with radiation alone in this subgroup of patients with lung cancer.

ACKNOWLEDGMENT

The authors acknowledge the contributions made to the study by Drs I. Ackerman, M. Berry, P. Catton, G. Davies, H. Miller, N. Mountifield, F. Shepherd, G. Taylor, and P. Webster. They also thank M. McKenna-Forkin for her assistance.

REFERENCES

1. Israel L, Aguilera J, Breau JL: Treatment des cancers epidermoides par bleomycine et platine en administration continue prolongee. Serie preliminaire de 80 cas avec 75 p. 100 de responses objectifes. Nouv Press Med 10:1817–1824, 1981

2. Longeval E, Klastersky J: Combination chemotherapy with cisplatin and etoposide in bronchogenic squamous cell carcinoma with adenocarcinoma. Cancer 50:2751–2756, 1982

3. Penacchio JL, Hong WK, Shapshay S, et al: Combination of cis-platinum and bleomycin prior to surgery and/or radiotherapy compared with radiotherapy alone for the treatment of advanced squamous cell carcinoma of the head and neck. Cancer 50:2795–2801, 1982

4. Drewinko B, Green C, Loo TL: Combination chemotherapy in vitro with cis-dichlorodiammineplatinum (II). Cancer Treat Rep 60:1619–1625, 1976

5. Evans WK, Osoba D, Feld R, et al: VP-16 alone and in combination with cisplatin for relapse in small cell lung cancer. Cancer 53:1461–1466, 1984

6. Eagan RT, Fleming TR, Schoonover V: Evaluation of response criteria in advanced lung cancer. Cancer 44:1125–1128, 1979

7. Osoba D, Rusthoven JJ, Turnbull KA, et al: Combination chemotherapy with bleomycin, etoposide and cisplatin in metastatic non–small-cell lung cancer. J Clin Oncol 3:1478–1485, 1985

8. Bakowski MT, Crouch JC: Chemotherapy of non-small cell lung cancer: A reappraisal and a look to the future. Cancer Treat Rev 10:159–172, 1983

9. Carter SK: Chemotherapy of lung cancer. Semin Oncol 9:40–55, 1983

10. Hoffman PC, Bitran JD, Golomb HM: Chemotherapy of metastatic non-small cell bronchogenic carcinoma. Semin Oncol 10:111–122, 1983

11. Ruckdeschel JC, Finkelstein DM, Ettinger DS, et al: A randomized trial of the four most active regimens for metastatic non–small-cell lung cancer. J Clin Oncol 4:14–22, 1986

Seminars in Oncology
will publish in future issues

Breast Cancer

Head and Neck Cancer

Tumor Markers

Endocrine Malignancies

VOL XIII, NO 4, SUPPL 4 DECEMBER 1986

Seminars in Oncology

Management of Hormone Responsive Diseases Proceedings of the Third International Conference held June 7, 1986 in Rotterdam, The Netherlands

Contributors

John H. Glick • J.G.M. Klijn • Daniel G. Haller
D.S. Ettinger • J. Allegra • J.R. Bertino
Philip D. Bonomi • H. Browder • P. Byrne • J. Carpenter
R. Catalano • R. Creech • B. Dana • H. Durivage • L. Einhorn
F. Anthony Greco • E. Greenwald • I. Henderson • F. Holmes
J. Keller • B. Kinzbrunner • M. Losada • S. Luedke
H. Muss • N. Nimeh • G. Wampler • N. Weinreb
J. Weisberg • R. Wheeler • P.H. Wiernik • Patricia A. Johnson
Kenning M. Anderson • Janet M. Wolter • S.G. Economou
N. Simon Tchekmedyian • Nancy Tait • Joseph Aisner
Branimir I. Sikic • Sidney A. Scudder • Samuel C. Ballon
Olive M. Soriero • J. Eric Christman • Lily Suey • Mohamed N. Ehsan
Alan E. Brandt • Thomas L. Evans • David Gal • Mark Moody

GRUNE & STRATTON
Harcourt Brace Jovanovich, Inc.

Seminars in Oncology

Seminars in Oncology (ISSN 0093–7754) is published quarterly by Grune & Stratton, Inc., 6277 Sea Harbor Dr, Orlando, FL 32821. Months of issue are March, June, September, and December. Second class postage paid at Duluth, MN, and at additional mailing offices.

POSTMASTER: Send change of address to *Seminars in Oncology,* c/o Grune & Stratton, Inc., PO Box 6280, Duluth, MN 55806.

Editorial correspondence should be addressed to John W. Yarbro, MD, PhD, School of Medicine, University of Missouri at Columbia, Columbia, MO 65212.

Business correspondence (subscriptions, change of address) should be addressed to the Publisher, Grune & Stratton, Inc., PO Box 6280, Duluth, MN 55806.

Change of address notices, including both the old and new addresses of the subscriber, should be sent to the Publisher at least one month in advance.

Customer Service: 1-800-654-2452.

Subscription rates: one volume of four issues, \$58.00 in the United States and Canada; elsewhere, \$83.00. Libraries and institutions: \$75.00 in the United States and Canada; elsewhere, \$83.00. Single copies, \$19.50 in the United States and Canada; elsewhere, \$22.50. Students, fellows, interns, and residents in the United States, Canada, and Australia may subscribe at a discount rate of \$34.00 per year (a letter giving qualifying data must accompany order). Subscriptions are accepted on a calendar year basis. Prices are subject to change. Current prices are in effect for back volumes and back issues. Single issues, both current and back, exist in limited quantities and are offered for sale subject to availability. Journal orders are payable in advance. *Checks* should be sent to Grune & Stratton, Inc., PO Box 6209, Duluth, MN 55806.

Advertising representative: Cunningham Associates, PO Box 308, Park Ridge, NJ 07656, telephone (201) 767-4170.

Agents for Great Britain: Grune & Stratton Limited, 24–28 Oval Rd, London NW1 7DX, England. Agents for Australia and New Zealand: Grune & Stratton Australia, PO Box 300, North Ryde, NSW 2113, Australia.

 G&S **Orlando, FL**

Harcourt Brace Jovanovich, Inc.

Seminars in Oncology

Seminars in
Oncology

Management of Hormone Responsive Diseases

Proceedings of the Third International Conference held June 7, 1986 in Rotterdam, The Netherlands, and sponsored under an educational grant from Mead Johnson Oncology Products, Bristol-Myers Oncology Division, and Bristol-Myers International Group.

VOL XIII, NO 4, SUPPL 4 **DECEMBER 1986**

Table of Contents

Introduction .... *John H. Glick and J.G.M. Klijn* 1

Progestational Agents in Advanced Breast Cancer: An Overview .... *Daniel G. Haller and John H. Glick* 2

Megestrol Acetate *v* Tamoxifen in Advanced Breast Cancer: Correlation of Hormone Receptors and Response .... *D.S. Ettinger, J. Allegra, J.R. Bertino, P. Bonomi, H. Browder, P. Byrne, J. Carpenter, R. Catalano, R. Creech, B. Dana, H. Durivage, L. Einhorn, F.A. Greco, E. Greenwald, I. Henderson, F. Holmes, J. Keller, B. Kinzbrunner, M. Losada, S. Luedke, H. Muss, N. Nimeh, G. Wampler, N. Weinreb, J. Weisberg, R. Wheeler, and P.H. Wiernik* 9

Megestrol Acetate: First-Line Therapy for Advanced Breast Cancer ...... *Patricia A. Johnson, Philip D. Bonomi, Kenning M. Anderson, Janet M. Wolter, and S. G. Economou* 15

High-Dose Megestrol Acetate in the Treatment of Postmenopausal Women With Advanced Breast Cancer .... *N. Simon Tchekmedyian, Nancy Tait, and Joseph Aisner* 20

High-Dose Megestrol Acetate Therapy of Ovarian Carcinoma: A Phase II Study by the Northern California Oncology Group........ *Branimir I. Sikic, Sidney A. Scudder, Samuel C. Ballon, Olive M. Soriero, J. Eric Christman, Lily Suey, Mohamed N. Ehsan, Alan E. Brandt, and Thomas L. Evans* 26

Hormonal Therapy for Lesions of the Endometrium .... *David Gal* 33

Appetite Stimulation With Megestrol Acetate in Cachectic Cancer Patients *N. Simon Tchekmedyian, Nancy Tait, Mark Moody, F. Anthony Greco, and Joseph Aisner* 37

Seminars in Oncology

Management of Hormone Responsive Diseases
Proceedings of the Third International Conference
June 7, 1986
Rotterdam, The Netherlands

Supported by an education grant from
Mead Johnson Oncology Products
and Bristol-Myers Oncology Division, Evansville, Indiana;
and Bristol-Myers International Group, New York, New York.

Dosages, indications, and methods of use for products that are referred to in the supplement by the authors are not necessarily the same as indicated in the package insert for the product and may reflect the clinical experience of the authors or may be derived from the professional literature of other clinical sources. Because of differences between in vitro and in vivo systems and between laboratory animal models and clinical data in humans, in vitro and animal data may not necessarily correlate with clinical results.

Seminars in Oncology

Vol XIII, No 4, Suppl 4 **December 1986**

Introduction

IN 1984, almost 900,000 new cancer diagnoses were made in the United States (excluding carcinoma in situ of the cervix and skin cancer), and approximately half of those patients died. Tumors considered hormone responsive, which include breast, prostate, uterine, ovarian, and endometrial cancers, accounted for approximately 30% of this total, with a mortality of about 17%. Thus, the importance of hormonal therapy used as primary or adjuvant therapy, or for palliation of recurrent or metastatic disease, is clear, both from a research point of view and for practicing oncologists.

The following articles represent new and updated results with progestational agents as therapy for a variety of tumors. The stimulating effect of these agents on the appetite will also be discussed. It is hoped that, in the future, hormonal manipulation with progestins will further improve survival and quality of life for patients with hormone-responsive tumors.

John H. Glick, MD
Professor of Medicine and Director
University of Pennsylvania Cancer Center
Philadelphia, PA

J.G.M. Klijn, MD
Head, Department of Endocrine-Oncology
The Dr Daniel den Hoed Cancer Center
Rotterdam, The Netherlands

Progestational Agents in Advanced Breast Cancer: An Overview

Daniel G. Haller and John H. Glick

Progestational agents, such as megestrol acetate and medroxyprogesterone acetate, are effective hormonal treatments for metastatic breast cancer in postmenopausal women. Clinical trials of these agents have demonstrated that 30% to 60% of patients will experience objective tumor response, depending on pretreatment prognostic variables. Although optimal doses and schedules have not been fully defined, current studies are investigating the therapeutic effectiveness of high-dose progestins. Toxicity of these drugs is mild and generally limited to weight gain related to their anabolic activity. Progestins are active second-line agents for metastatic breast cancer in postmenopausal women. In selected patients, they appear to be equivalent to tamoxifen as first-line therapy for metastatic disease. As more patients are exposed to prolonged adjuvant tamoxifen therapy, the role of progestins as first-line hormonal therapy at the time of relapse is likely to expand.

ALMOST A CENTURY has passed since the initial observations were made concerning the hormone responsiveness of advanced breast cancer. Many treatment variations have evolved, including ablative hormonal modalities (oophorectomy, adrenalectomy, hypophysectomy), additive hormonal therapy (estrogens, androgens, progestins), and antiestrogens. Each, in its turn, has been evaluated relative to reported benefits and toxicities, with the popularity of various therapies waxing and waning over time. Currently, the antiestrogen tamoxifen is considered by many to be the best first-line hormonal therapy for metastatic breast cancer because of its effectiveness and low incidence of side effects.[1] Many hormone-responsive patients, however, will be eligible for more than one hormonal manipulation, and much investigation has resulted in attempts to determine the optimum sequence of such therapies.

From the The Hematology-Oncology Section, Department of Medicine, University of Pennsylvania Cancer Center, Philadelphia.

Address reprint requests to Daniel G. Haller, MD, Hospital of the University of Pennsylvania, Hematology-Oncology Section, 3400 Spruce St, Philadelphia, PA 19104.

0093–7754/86/1304–4001$05.00/0

Progestational agents have been available for 40 years, but initial positive reports of the potential use of such agents in advanced breast cancer did not appear until 1967.[2] Since that time, sufficient information has accumulated on two progestins (megestrol acetate [MA] and medroxyprogesterone acetate [MPA]) to permit investigators to define proper roles for these agents in patients with breast cancer.

Megestrol acetate and MPA are both synthetic derivatives of progesterone.[3] Both are usually administered orally (PO), although MPA also has been given intramuscularly (IM). Megestrol acetate exhibits both antiestrogenic and anovulatory activity, whereas MPA has androgenic, anabolic, and gonadotropin inhibitory effects. In spite of these observations, relatively little information is available concerning the exact mechanisms by which progestins exert their antitumor effect. Allegra and Kiefer[4] performed laboratory studies to determine whether the predominant mechanism is a direct cytotoxic effect on tumor cells, or a modulating influence on the action of other steroid hormones. Results of studies utilizing both MA and progesterone in MCF-7 breast cancer cell lines show direct cytotoxicity. In addition, these drugs were capable of abolishing the stimulating effects of estrogen on the same experimental tumor cells.[4]

Hormone receptor assays have proven useful in predicting remissions with endocrine therapy in hormone-responsive tumors.[5] Studies of the relationships between progestins and hormone receptors in breast cancer have demonstrated that MA may interact with progesterone receptors as well as androgen and glucocorticoid sites.[6] The overall effect of progestins in advanced breast cancer may, in fact, represent a combination of direct cytotoxic effects on the cell via the receptor mechanism and indirect effects on the hypothalamo-pituitary-adrenal axis leading to estrogen deprivation.[7,8] It has also been observed that different dose levels of progestins may exert diverse effects on the endocrinologic environment of breast cancer cells.[9] Ultimately, this may lead to complex patterns of response among patient populations treated with various dose levels of progestins.

Table 1. Megestrol Acetate in Advanced Breast Cancer

Reference	Dose/Schedule	No. of Evaluable Patients	CR + PR (%)
Tchekmedyian[10]	480-1,600 mg/d	18	50
Johnson[23]	40 mg q.i.d.	39	44
Ross[21]	40 mg q.i.d.	48	31
Alexieva-Figusch[18]	60-180 mg/d	160	30
Ansfield[19,27]	40 mg q.i.d.	160	30
Carpenter[28]	160 mg/d	20	30

Abbreviations: CR, complete response; PR, partial response.

CLINICAL RESULTS

A number of trials (Table 1) have reported the benefits of MA in patients with advanced measurable breast cancer. These trials have generally used MA in patients who had had previous hormonal manipulations. In the majority of studies, MA has been utilized in conventional doses of 160 mg/d, although some investigators have escalated to doses as high as 1,600 mg/d.[10] Although few dose-response studies have been performed with MA, a small study from the University of Maryland demonstrated that seven of nine patients failing with standard-dose MA (160 mg/d) subsequently responded to high-dose MA (1,600 mg/d), suggesting a steep dose-response curve for this drug.[10] In general, overall response rates of 30% to 45% are observed in postmenopausal women with advanced breast cancer treated with MA.

In randomized trials of MA *v* tamoxifen as first-line therapy, MA appears equivalent to tamoxifen in overall response rates (Table 2). The study from the Mayo Clinic reported by Ingle et al[11] demonstrated small but statistically insignificant differences in response rates for both agents in perimenopausal women, who typically are not highly hormone responsive. Larger studies by Muss and co-workers[12] and Morgan[13] both demonstrate nearly identical first-line response rates of 29% to 36% for MA and tamoxifen, consistent with previously reported single-agent trials of each of these drugs. Ongoing large-scale studies comparing MA and tamoxifen will further define the role of MA as a first-line treatment for advanced breast cancer.

Studies of MPA in advanced breast cancer have utilized broader dose ranges than similar studies of MA (Table 3). Doses ranging from 500 mg IM twice a week to 4,000 mg/d PO have resulted in response rates ranging from 15% to 67% in both previously treated and untreated patients. A review by Mattson[9] of studies of MPA in doses of at least 500 mg/d given to 696 patients demonstrated a combined objective response rate of 41% (range, 28% to 66%). Several random-design dose evaluations of MPA have been performed, including a large study by Cavalli et al[14] (see Table 3). Patients treated at the higher dose of MPA had a significantly better response rate than those treated at the low dose (33% *v* 15%). The high-dose regimen also demonstrated responses in 23% of patients who were considered to be unresponsive to previous hormonal therapy. However, no benefits were observed with high-dose MPA therapy with regard to time to disease progression and survival. Conclusions based on dose-response data from noncomparative trials utilizing MPA are difficult because of the extreme heterogeneity of prognostic variables in patients with postmenopausal advanced breast cancer.

At least one randomized trial compared the combination of MPA (100 mg/d) plus tamoxifen (30 mg/d) with tamoxifen alone (30 mg/d).[15] In 46 patients randomly assigned to receive tamoxifen, a response rate of 45% was seen, compared with 26% for 55 patients who received the combi-

Table 2. Megestrol Acetate (MA) *v* Tamoxifen (TAM) in Advanced Breast Cancer

Reference	Dose/Schedule	No. of Patients	CR + PR (%)	Comment
Ingle[11]	MA 150 mg/m^2/d	28	14	Difference in response not significant;
	TAM 10 mg b.i.d.	27	26	survival for MA (520 d) longer than for TAM (398 d) (*P* = .02)
Muss[12]	MA 40 mg q.i.d.	63	29	No significant differences between regi-
	TAM 10 mg b.i.d.	62	31	mens in time to progression or survival
Morgan[13]	MA 40 mg q.i.d.	46	31	Median duration of remission not dif-
	TAM 10 mg b.i.d.	48	36	ferent between treatment arms

Abbreviations: CR, complete response; PR, partial response.

Table 3. Medroxyprogesterone Acetate in Advanced Breast Cancer

Reference	Dose/Schedule	No. of Patients	CR + PR (%)	Previous Hormone Therapy
Hortobagyi[22]	400 mg/d PO	10	67	
	800 mg/d PO	29	37	
		39	44	30/39
Hedley[29]	600 mg/d PO	105	20	78/105
Haller[30]	400 mg/d PO	32	47	13/32
Cavalli[14]	500 mg IM biw × 4 wk → 500 mg IM qw	93	15	76/93
	v			
	1,000 mg IM qd × 4 wk → 500 mg IV qw	91	33	75/91
Falkson[31]	1,400 mg/m²/d PO × 6 mo → 500 mg/m² qd	23	22	23/23
Guarnieri[32]	4,000 mg PO qd × 30 d → 1,000 mg PO qd	26	27	8/26

Abbreviations: CR, complete response; PR, partial response; biw, twice per week; qw, once per week; qd, every day; PO, orally, IM, intramuscularly; IV, intravenously.

nation. Although this difference in response was not statistically significant, it is unclear why the patients treated with tamoxifen alone did better than those in the combination arm. Although the authors hypothesize that one agent could interfere with the pharmacodynamics of the other, there are no rational explanations based on experimental models for this apparent detrimental effect seen with the combination.

Based on the ability of tamoxifen to induce the synthesis of progesterone receptors in hormone-responsive breast cancers, new studies utilizing sequential tamoxifen and MPA have been reported. Preliminary results of two small studies are presented in Table 4. The pilot study by Ayme et al[16] of women with postmenopausal, good-prognosis, metastatic disease demonstrated an overall response rate of 56%. However, a randomized trial comparing sequential tamoxifen-MPA therapy to tamoxifen (followed by MPA at relapse), failed to demonstrate a difference in initial response between the sequential combination (24%) and tamoxifen (26%).[17] Although the duration of response for the sequential treatment was longer than for tamoxifen alone (32 *v* 20 weeks), this apparent benefit disappeared when MPA was administered to the tamoxifen patients at failure or relapse. Larger trials of sequential therapy are currently under way to define further the activity of this regimen and to determine whether any subset of patients is more likely to benefit from sequential therapy.

Table 4. Sequential Tamoxifen (TAM) and Medroxyprogesterone Acetate (MPA) in Advanced Breast Cancer

Reference	Dose/Schedule	No. of Patients	CR + PR (%)
Ayme[16]	TAM 30 mg/d, d 1-15 → MPA 500 mg/d, d 16-30	30	56
Mauriac[17]	TAM 30 mg/d, d 1-15 → MPA 1,000 mg/d, d 16-30	25	24
	v		
	TAM 30 mg/d to failure → MPA 1,000 mg/d	23	26

Abbreviations: CR, complete response; PR, partial response.

Based on response data alone, MA at a dose of 160 mg/d and MPA at doses of 400 to 1,500 mg/d appear to be equally effective in producing objective remissions in postmenopausal women with advanced breast cancer. Responses are seen with both progestins as first- and second-line hormonal treatments. Dose-escalation studies of MA and MPA suggest that high-dose therapy may be warranted, but further randomized studies are necessary to determine the optimal dose and schedule.[9] Sequential therapy, based on the modulating ability of tamoxifen on progesterone receptors, also remains to be fully evaluated.

PREDICTION OF RESPONSE

It has been well documented in clinical cancer trials that patient and tumor characteristics are powerful predictors of response to therapy. The following clinical characteristics must be kept in mind when interpreting results of trials of hormonal therapies and when choosing therapy: receptor status, menopausal status, disease-free interval, sites of metastatic disease, and previous response to hormonal therapy. As with other hormonal manipulations, results of progestin therapy are highly dependent on these prognostic variables.

Receptor Status

It has been well documented that levels of estrogen receptor (ER) and progesterone receptor (PgR) are powerful determinants for response to tamoxifen therapy.[5] Many older trials of hormonal therapy, including those utilizing progestins, were undertaken prior to the general availability of receptor assays. Newer studies, however, which include receptor status in the reporting of results, offer conflicting data about the ability of ER and PgR status to predict for hormone responsiveness to progestin therapy.[5,6,12] A summary of the impact of ER and PgR status on response to MA is illustrated in Table 5; PgR appears to be most predictive. Results of other studies, however, have failed to show a significant correlation between either ER or PgR level and response.[6,12]

Menopausal Status

Most studies utilizing hormonal therapy require that patients be clearly postmenopausal, since menopausal status has a direct correlation with response. The study done by Ingle et al[11] of MA and tamoxifen in perimenopausal and castrated women showed responses of only 14% and 26%, respectively. In contrast, women who are more than 5 to 10 years postmenopausal have a better chance of good response: The trial done by Alexieva-Figusch et al[18] of MA given to 155 women demonstrated a response rate of only 9% in those who were less than 5 years postmenopausal, compared with 40% in those more than 5 years postmenopausal.[18] Similarly, the large series of MA-treated patients in another study by Ansfield et al[19] demonstrated response rates of 20% and 43%, respectively, in women who were less than 10 years and more than 10 years postmenopausal.[19]

Table 5. Objective Response to Megestrol Acetate as a Function of ER and PgR Status

ER and PgR Status	CR + PR (%)
ER+/PgR+	61–70
ER+/PgR−	20–25
ER−/PgR+	33
ER−/PgR−	<12
Unknown ER and PgR	30

Abbreviations: ER, estrogen receptor; PgR, progesterone receptor; CR, complete response; PR, partial response.

Disease-Free Interval

In general, a prolonged disease-free interval (more than 2 years) from the primary diagnosis of breast cancer to recurrence predicts for a higher response rate and longer survival. In a study of MPA in doses of 1,000 to 1,500 mg/d, conducted by DeLena et al,[20] response rates were 47% in previously treated patients who had disease-free intervals of longer than 2 years, compared with 19% for those with intervals of less than 2 years. A similar result was observed in the study done by Cavalli et al[14] of high-dose MPA, in which only 11% of patients with a disease-free interval of less than 12 months responded, compared with 63% of those with intervals longer than 60 months.

Sites of Metastatic Disease

Most trials suggest a strong trend toward better response rates to progestins if the dominant site of disease is soft tissue and a trend toward lower response rates in visceral-dominant disease. Although Alexieva-Figusch et al[18] noted a 42% response rate in patients with visceral-dominant disease (chiefly lung), other studies[12,14,21] reported response rates ranging from 0% to 24%. There is general disagreement concerning the effectiveness of progestins in osseous metastases, possibly because of the great difficulty in assessing objective responses in patients with bone-dominant metastases. Alexieva-Figusch and co-workers[18] reported only a 3% response rate with MA in patients with bone metastases. Cavalli and co-workers[14] reported a 44% response rate to high-dose MPA in patients with bone metastases, compared with 18% in patients treated with low-dose MPA in the same study ($P = .03$), suggesting a dose-related effect on response.

Previous Hormonal Therapy

Tables 1 and 3 describe results of MA and MPA therapy, respectively, in large series of patients, the majority of whom had received hormonal therapy previously. Individual series which describe in detail responses after previous hormonal therapy emphasize two important factors: First, responses to progestins are generally highest if they are utilized as first-line therapy, but response rates are also quite high (30% to

Table 6. Side Effects of Progestin Therapy

Common
Weight gain
Occasional
Vaginal bleeding
Nausea
Edema
Hot flashes
Depression
Rare
Hypertension
Thromboembolism
Skin rash
Euphoria
Diabetes

50%) if patients had responded to previous hormonal treatment(s).[11,13,14,21,22] Second, failure to respond to previous hormonal therapy (including tamoxifen) does not negate the possibility of response to MA or MPA: Response rates up to 32% have been noted in patients who initially failed to demonstrate response to tamoxifen.[14,20,22] Objective responses to MPA or MA have been reported in patients who clearly had progressed while taking tamoxifen, indicating a lack of complete cross-resistance between antiestrogens and progestins.[20,21]

SIDE EFFECTS

In general, toxicity from both MA and MPA is modest (Table 6).[3,9] Anecdotal reports of edema, hot flashes, euphoria, glucose intolerance, exacerbation of hypertension, and vaginal bleeding have been reported after treatment with both MA and MPA.[3,9,18,23] Adrenocortical side effects may be seen in 10% to 15% of patients on long-term high-dose MPA.[9] Although the risk of thromboembolism has been considered to be increased in patients on progestin therapy, this association is not well documented in the literature. The most common side effect of progestin therapy is weight gain. Studies of sodium and water metabolism in patients on high-dose MPA have failed to demonstrate fluid retention as a cause for weight gain, suggesting that the anabolic effects of progestins are chiefly responsible.[24] Most studies report weight gains of at least 2 kg in 75% of patients treated, with MA or MPA equally capable of causing this side effect.

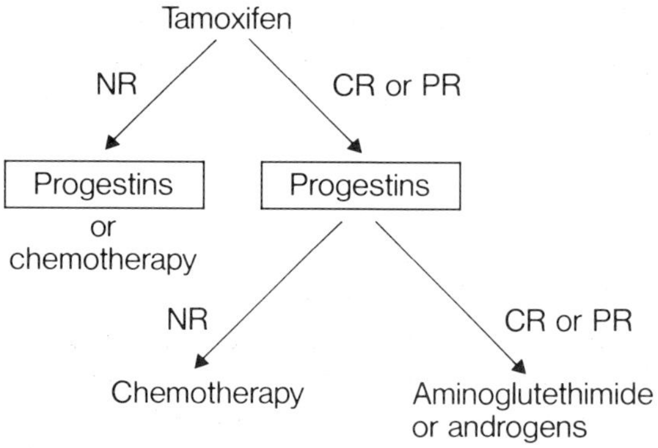

Fig 1. Traditional sequence for administering endocrine therapy to postmenopausal patients with metastatic breast cancer. CR, complete response; PR, partial response; NR, no response.

THE ROLE OF PROGESTINS IN CLINICAL PRACTICE

Figure 1 describes the traditional sequence for administering endocrine therapy to postmenopausal patients with metastatic breast cancer and suggests that progestins are generally considered second-line hormonal therapy. Importantly, the data support the use of MA or MPA not only in patients who have previously responded to tamoxifen but also in selected patients who have failed to respond to tamoxifen. Such patients are likely to be older postmenopausal women who have longer disease-free intervals and soft-tissue sites of dominant disease. A limited number of trials suggest that MA may be considered equivalent to tamoxifen for first-line therapy of selected patients with advanced breast cancer.[12,13] However, we must await the results of current large randomized trials to fully establish MA as first-line therapy. The relatively low incidence of significant side effects with progestins supports this usage in patients who are unable to tolerate tamoxifen therapy.

In 1985, the National Institutes of Health (NIH) Consensus Development Conference on the Adjuvant Therapy of Breast Cancer recommended that postmenopausal women with node-positive, hormone receptor-positive, primary breast cancer should be treated with adjuvant antiestrogen therapy.[25] In addition, although the optimum duration of tamoxifen therapy is not known, some studies have suggested that prolonged therapy (more than 2 years) may be indicated, based on the presumed cytostatic mechanism of action of tamoxifen.[25,26] Based on

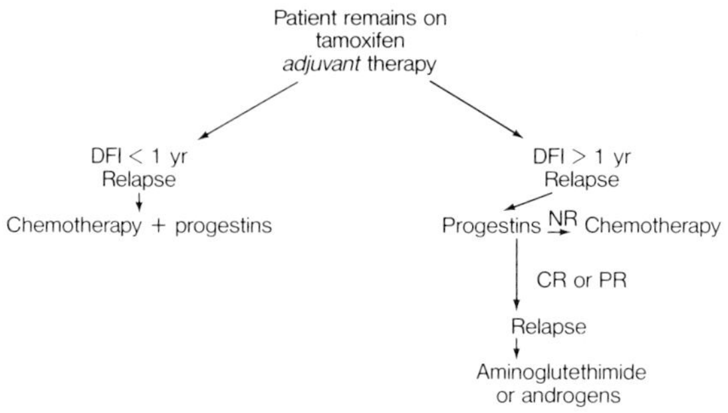

Fig 2. Impact of National Institutes of Health (NIH) Consensus Conference on sequence of administering endocrine therapy in postmenopausal patients with metastatic breast cancer. DFI, disease-free interval; NR, no response; CR, complete response; PR, partial response.

these recommendations, it may be anticipated that many women will experience their first relapse of breast cancer while on adjuvant tamoxifen maintenance therapy. Given the lack of cross-resistance between progestins and tamoxifen and the data concerning the influence of previous therapy on response, it would appear that progestins should be the initial treatment of choice in most of these patients (Fig 2). In general, the same clinical considerations that would dictate the choice of hormonal therapy (favorable sites of disease, long disease-free interval) would also favor the institution of MA or MPA over immediate chemotherapy.

SUMMARY

Progestins are generally underutilized in the therapy of postmenopausal women with metastatic breast cancer. Since the therapeutic goal for palliative therapy is to maintain or improve quality of life in these patients, progestins offer the opportunity of tumor control without excessive side effects. The extensive use of adjuvant tamoxifen therapy in postmenopausal patients suggests that physicians consider progestins at first relapse for this subset of patients.

REFERENCES

1. Kiang DT, Kennedy BJ: Tamoxifen (antiestrogen) therapy in advanced breast cancer. Ann Intern Med 87:687–690, 1977

2. Stoll BA: Progestin therapy of breast cancer: Comparison of agents. Br Med J [Clin Res] 3:338–341, 1967

3. Blumenschein GR: The role of progestins in the treatment of breast cancer. Semin Oncol 10:7–10, 1983

4. Allegra JC, Kiefer SM: Mechanisms of action of progestational agents. Semin Oncol 12:3–5, 1985 (suppl)

5. McGuire WL: Hormone receptors: Their role in predicting prognosis and response to endocrine therapy. Semin Oncol 5:428–433, 1978

6. Teulings FAG, Van Glise HA, Henkelman MS: Estrogen, androgen, glucocorticoid and progesterone receptors in progestin-induced regression of human breast cancer. Cancer Res 40:2557–2561, 1980

7. McGuire WL, Cavalli F, Bonomi P: Progestin therapy for breast cancer: A panel discussion. Breast Cancer Res Treat 6:213–220, 1985

8. Blossey HC, Wander HE, Koebberling J: Pharmocokinetic and pharmocodynamic basis for the treatment of metastatic breast cancer with high-dose medroxyprogesterone acetate. Cancer 54:1208–1215, 1984

9. Mattsson W: Current status of high dose progestin treatment in advanced breast cancer. Breast Cancer Res Treat 3:231–235, 1983

10. Tchekmedyian NS, Tait N, Aisner J: Phase I/II trial of high dose (HO) megestrol acetate (MA) in breast cancer. Proc Am Soc Clin Oncol 5:72, 1986

11. Ingle JN, Ahmann DL, Green SJ: Randomized clinical trial of megestrol acetate versus tamoxifen in paramenopausal or castrated women with advanced breast cancer. Am J Clin Oncol 2:155–160, 1982

12. Muss HB, Paschold EH, Black WR: Megestrol acetate v. tamoxifen in advanced breast cancer: A phase III trial of the Piedmont Oncology Association (POA). Semin Oncol 12:55–61, 1985 (suppl)

13. Morgan LR: Megestrol acetate v. tamoxifen in advanced breast cancer in postmenopausal patients. Semin Oncol 12:43–47, 1985 (suppl)

14. Cavalli F, Goldhirsch A, Sungi F: Randomized trial of low versus high-dose medroxyprogesterone acetate in the induction treatment of postmenopausal patients with advanced breast cancer. J Clin Oncol 2:414–419, 1984

15. Van Veelen H, Willemse PH, Sliejfer DT: Adrenal suppression by oral high-dose medroxyprogesterone acetate in breast cancer patients. Cancer Chemother Pharmacol 12:83–86, 1984

16. Ayme Y, Brandone H, Brandone JM: Antiestrogenothérapie cyclique dans les cancers du sein en phase avancee. Association sequentielle tamoxifen-medroxyprogesterine. Cancerologie 44: 1984

17. Mauriac L, Durand M, Bonichon F: Sequential hormone therapy (tamoxifen-MPA) vs. tamoxifen in metastatic breast cancers. Preliminary results. Bull Cancer (Paris) 72:11, 1985

18. Alexieva-Figusch J, Van Glise HA, Hop WCJ: Progestin therapy in advanced breast cancer. Cancer 46:2369–2372, 1980

19. Ansfield FJ, Kallas GJ, Singson JP: Clinical results with megestrol acetate in patients with advanced carcinoma of the breast. Surg Gynecol Obstet 155:888, 1982

20. De Lena M, Brambilla C, Valagussa P: High dose MPA in breast cancer resistant to endocrine and cytotoxic therapy. Cancer Chemother Pharmacol 2:175–189, 1979

21. Ross MB, Buzdar AV, Blumenschein GR: Treatment

of advanced breast cancer with megestrol acetate after therapy with tamoxifen. Cancer 49:413–417, 1982

22. Hortobagyi GN, Busdar AV, Frye D: Oral medroxyprogesterone acetate in the treatment of metastatic breast cancer. Breast Cancer Res Treat 5:321–326, 1985

23. Johnson PA, Bonomi PD, Anderson KM: Megestrol acetate (MA) in advanced breast cancer: Response rate related to estrogen receptor (ER) and progesterone receptor (PR) levels. Proc Am Soc Clin Oncol 1:89, 1982

24. Lelli G, Angelleli B, Zanichelli L: The effect of high dose medroxyprogesterone acetate on water and salt metabolism in advanced cancer patients. Chemioterapia 3:327–329, 1984

25. National Institutes of Health: Consensus development conference statement: Adjuvant chemotherapy for breast cancer. JAMA 5:3461–3463, 1985

26. Tormey DC, Jordan VC: Long-term tamoxifen adjuvant therapy in node positive breast cancer: A metabolic and pilot clinical study. Breast Cancer Res Treat 5:297–302, 1984

27. Ansfield FJ, Davis HL, Ramirez G: Further clinical studies with megestrol acetate in advanced breast cancer. Cancer 38:53–55, 1976

28. Carpenter JT, Peterson L: Use of megestrol acetate in advanced breast cancer on a single daily-dose schedule. Semin Oncol 12:40–42, 1985 (suppl)

29. Hedley D, Dalgleish A, Raghavan D: Advanced breast cancer: Response to high dose oral medroxyprogesterone acetate. Aust NZ J Med 14:251–254, 1984

30. Haller DG, Glick JG, Ettinger NA: High dose oral Provera in the treatment of recurrent breast cancer. J Steroid Biochem 19:865, 1983

31. Falkson G, Falkson HC: A phase II study of high-dose medroxyprogesterone acetate in advanced breast cancer. Cancer Chemother Pharmacol 11:16–18, 1983

32. Guarnieri A, Tucci E, D'Aniello C: Oral route administration of medroxyprogesterone acetate (MPA) at high doses in the treatment of advanced breast cancer: Clinical results. Chemioterapia 3:320–323, 1984

Megestrol Acetate *v* Tamoxifen in Advanced Breast Cancer: Correlation of Hormone Receptors and Response

D.S. Ettinger, J. Allegra, J.R. Bertino, P. Bonomi, H. Browder, P. Byrne, J. Carpenter, R. Catalano, R. Creech, B. Dana, H. Durivage, L. Einhorn, F.A. Greco, E. Greenwald, I. Henderson, F. Holmes, J. Keller, B. Kinzbrunner, M. Losada, S. Luedke, H. Muss, N. Nimeh, G. Wampler, N. Weinreb, J. Weisberg, R. Wheeler, and P.H. Wiernik

This report describes the preliminary results from a randomized study comparing megestrol acetate with tamoxifen in the treatment of postmenopausal women with advanced breast cancer, correlating estrogen receptors (ER) and progesterone receptor (PgR) status with response. Patients received megestrol acetate (40 mg) orally four times daily or tamoxifen (10 mg) orally twice daily. If the initial therapy failed, patients were crossed over to the alternate treatment. Of 197 patients entered in the study, 190 were considered evaluable. The overall response rates were 35% with megestrol acetate and 42% with tamoxifen. Twenty-three percent (7/30) of patients responded to megestrol acetate after being crossed over from tamoxifen, while 22% (6/27) responded to tamoxifen after being crossed over from megestrol acetate. Response did not correlate significantly with combined receptor (ie, ER plus PgR) levels. A significant trend was seen between ER level and response only in the tamoxifen group. There was no association between PgR levels and response for either tamoxifen or megestrol acetate.

THE PRESENCE of estrogen receptors (ER) in tumor tissue from patients with breast cancer has been used to predict response to hormonal therapy.[1] McGuire et al[1] reported a 60% response rate to hormonal therapy in patients with ER-positive tumors, compared with an 8% response rate in patients with ER-negative tumors. Response to hormonal therapy has been shown to improve with increasing levels of ER in the tumor tissue.[2,3]

It has been demonstrated that progesterone receptor (PgR) status may also be of value in predicting response to hormonal manipulation in the treatment of breast cancer.[4,5] Moreover, the determination of PgR in addition to ER status increases the accuracy of predicting whether or not a patient with breast cancer will respond to hormonal therapy.[6,7] This improved accuracy from utilizing both receptors is consistent with the hypothesis that PgR synthesis in breast tumor tissue is induced by ER binding to the genome, which indicates a functionally intact cell.[8]

With the development of hormonal receptor assays to predict the probability of hormonal responsiveness more accurately in patients with advanced breast cancer, the use of additive hormonal therapy has become an important palliative therapy for advanced breast carcinoma.[9] The most commonly used additive hormones are tamoxifen and megestrol acetate (Megace, Bristol-Myers Oncology Division, Evansville, IN). Tamoxifen is a synthetic antiestrogen, which is administered orally and causes few side effects.[10,11] Megestrol acetate is a synthetic derivative of progesterone, which is administered orally and also has been associated with minimal toxicity.[12,13] Although tamoxifen is the most frequently used additive hormonal therapy in the treatment of advanced breast cancer, megestrol acetate has been shown to be equally effective.[14]

This report describes the preliminary results from a randomized study comparing megestrol acetate with tamoxifen in the treatment of postmenopausal women with advanced breast cancer, correlating ER and PgR status with response.

PATIENTS AND METHODS

Patients with histologically proven advanced breast cancer whose tumors were ER positive, and who had measurable disease, were eligible for the study. Patients had to be at least 1-year post-spontaneous menopause or over age 53 years, have known ER and PgR receptor levels from the primary tumor or the metastasis, and had to be at least partially ambulatory (Eastern Cooperative Oncology Group [ECOG] performance status 0, 1, or 2). Patients who had responded to previous ablative or additive hormonal therapy were eligible if 12 or 6 weeks, respectively, had elapsed prior to study entry. All patients gave informed, written consent to participate in the study.

Patients were ineligible for the study if they had received previous treatment with a progestational agent or an anties-

---

D.S. Ettinger, MD, is an American Cancer Society, Maryland Division, Professor of Clinical Oncology.

Address reprint requests to D.S. Ettinger, MD, Johns Hopkins Oncology Center, 600 N Wolfe St, Baltimore, MD 21205.

0093–7754/86/1304–4003$05.00/0

trogen, or if they had evidence of CNS lesions that required immediate therapy or were the only evidence of measurable disease. Patients were also excluded if they were pregnant, had thrombophlebitis, thromboembolic disorders, or evidence of another primary cancer except superficial nonmelanomatous skin cancer or carcinoma in situ of the cervix. Patients who had liver involvement of greater than 25%, lymphangitic pulmonary disease, or inflammatory breast carcinoma, or other complications for which radiation therapy or chemotherapy was deemed more appropriate, were excluded.

Prior to entry into the study, all patients had a history and physical examination, evaluation of symptoms, performance status, measurement of indicator lesions, complete blood cell count (CBC), serum chemistries (SMA-12), and chest x-ray, as well as staging for metastases. The history and physical examination, evaluation of symptoms, performance status, and measurement of indicator lesions were repeated every 6 weeks. All patients had to have ER-positive tumors.

Patients were stratified as follows: (1) PgR status (positive *v* negative [ie, > 10 fmol/mg *v* < 10 fmol/mg cytosol protein]); (2) site of disease (local/soft tissue *v* visceral *v* osseous); and (3) previous hormonal therapy (additive or ablative, with or without other therapy *v* chemotherapy, including adjuvant chemotherapy with or without other therapy *v* radiation, surgery, or no therapy). Following stratification, patients were randomly assigned to receive megestrol acetate (40 mg orally four times each day) or tamoxifen (10 mg orally twice each day). When disease progressed, the treatment was withheld for 6 weeks. If a withdrawal response was not observed after 6 weeks, the patient was given the alternate therapy. If a withdrawal response occurred, the patient remained off therapy and was reevaluated every 6 weeks until disease progression. At that time, the patient was given the alternate therapy. Criteria for response were defined by the UICC (Union Internationale Contre Cancer) criteria.[15]

Patient responses were analyzed using a global chi-square (χ^2) for comparisons between groups and the chi-square test for trend for assessing ordered categories (χ^2_T). In addition, another analysis correlating receptors and response utilized Spearman rank correlation statistics. Time to progression and time to recurrence were calculated as time from initial treatment to progression or last date of contact. Patients removed from treatment for reasons other than progression were considered censored on the day of removal. Deaths during the study were considered progressions.

RESULTS

Pretreatment characteristics of the patients are presented in Table 1. There were no significant differences between the treatment groups with respect to age, site of dominant disease, performance status, or previous therapy. The ER and the PgR values for the two groups were not significantly different, although the ER values were slightly higher in the megestrol acetate group.

The distribution of ER and PgR status in each of the patient groups is shown in Table 2. The steroid receptor levels were divided into the following categories: high, greater than or equal to 90 fmol/mg cytosol protein; intermediate, 30 to

Table 1. Patient Characteristics

	Megestrol Acetate	Tamoxifen
Total no. of patients entered	94	103
No. of evaluable patients	91	99
Median age, yr (range)	63 (37–89)	67 (38–82)
	No. of Patients (%)	
Site dominant disease		
Local/soft tissue	43 (46)	48 (47)
Bone	32 (34)	36 (35)
Viscera	19 (20)	19 (18)
Performance status		
0 or 1	76 (81)	88 (85)
2	18 (19)	15 (15)
Previous therapy		
Hormone or ablative	4 (4)	2 (2)
Chemotherapy (including adjuvant)	26 (28)	30 (29)
None or radiation	64 (68)	71 (69)
Receptor status*		
ER		
Mean (SE	207.4 (32.6)	168.4 (26.3)
Median (range)	96 (10–2,000)	77 (7–1,647)
PgR		
Mean (SE)	113.3 (23.7)	110.0 (19.0)
Median (range)	22 (0–1,331)	28 (0–950)

*fmol/mg cytosol protein.

Table 2. Distribution of Steroid Receptors

Receptor Level*	No. of Patients† Megestrol Acetate	Tamoxifen
ER high, PgR high	18	22
ER high, PgR inter	11	7
ER high, PgR low	10	4
ER high, PgR neg	10	15
ER inter, PgR high	6	4
ER inter, PgR inter	6	6
ER inter, PgR low	5	5
ER inter, PgR neg	8	11
ER low, PgR high	2	2
ER low, PgR inter	2	8
ER low, PgR low	4	7
ER low, PgR neg	10	10

Abbreviations: ER, estrogen receptor; PgR, progesterone receptor.

*High, ≥90 fmol/mg cytosol protein; inter (intermediate), 30 to 89 fmol/mg cytosol protein; low, 10 to 29 fmol/mg cytosol protein; and neg (negative), ≤10 fmol/mg cytosol protein.

†Includes all except four patients for whom data on ER or PgR levels were not available.

89 fmol/mg cytosol protein; low, 10 to 29 fmol/mg cytosol protein; and negative, less than 10 fmol/mg cytosol protein. The last category applied only to PgR because a positive ER was required for entry in the study. Although the number of patients analyzed was too small to determine statistical significance, the two treatment groups differed in the following categories of receptor levels: ER high/PgR low; ER high/PgR negative; and ER low/PgR intermediate.

The response to the initial treatment, as well as the response by receptor status and site of dominant disease, is presented in Table 3. Of 197 patients entered in the study, 190 were evaluable. Seven patients were not evaluable for the following reasons: two refused the assigned study drug; two were menopausal; receptor values were not available for two; and data were incomplete for one. The overall response rates were 35% with megestrol acetate and 42% with tamoxifen. The complete response (CR) and partial response (PR) rates for 122 evaluable patients with ER+/PgR+ status were 37% with megestrol acetate and 42% with tamoxifen ($P = .68$). For the 62 evaluable patients with ER+/PgR− disease, the response rates (CR and PR) were 26% with megestrol acetate and 40% with tamoxifen ($P = .37$). In both treatment groups, the response rates were higher in patients with soft tissue-dominant disease as compared to patients with bone-dominant or visceral-dominant disease. Table 4 shows that there was no association between combined receptor (ER plus PgR) levels and response (CR and PR) for either the megestrol acetate-treated group ($P = .265$) or the tamoxifen-treated group ($P = .363$). However, Table 5 shows a trend for correlation of ER level and response for the tamoxifen-treated group ($P = .057$), which was not seen in the megestrol acetate-treated group ($P = .293$). There was no association between PgR levels and response for either the tamoxifen ($P = .689$) or megestrol acetate ($P = .639$) group. However, the sample size for analysis of both combined steroid receptor levels and individual steroid receptor levels was too small to offer conclusive results regarding the association of receptor levels and response.

A correlation between steroid receptor levels and a response of stable disease (SD) or better was shown. This correlation for megestrol acetate is demonstrated in Table 6. Of 68 patients with SD or better, ER measurements were available for 66: 40 (61%) had high ER levels. In

Table 3. Response to Megestrol Acetate v Tamoxifen

	Megestrol Acetate (n = 91)					Tamoxifen (n = 99)				
	CR	PR	NC	PD	NE	CR	PR	NC	PD	NE
Overall no. of patients (%)	10 (11)	22 (24)	35 (38)	23 (25)	1	12 (12)	30 (30)	34 (34)	23 (23)	0
Receptor status										
ER+/PgR+	7	15	25	13		9	17	22	14	
ER+/PgR−	2	5	10	10	1	3	11	12	9	
ER+/PgR?	1	2	0	0		0	2	0	0	
Site of dominant disease										
Soft tissue	8	13	10	11		10	18	12	8	
Bone	0	5	19	6	1	0	7	15	12	
Viscera	2	4	6	6		2	5	7	3	

Abbreviations: CR, complete response; PR, partial response; NC, no change; PD, progressive disease; NE, not evaluable; ER, estrogen receptor; PgR, progesterone receptor.

Table 4. Response Related to Combined Receptor Levels*†

	Responses/Total Patients (%)	
	Megestrol Acetate	Tamoxifen
ER high, PgR high	6/18 (33)	9/22 (41)
ER high, PgR intermediate-low	8/19 (42)	7/10 (70)
ER high, PgR negative	3/10 (30)	6/13 (46)
ER intermediate-low, PgR high	2/7 (29)	1/4 (25)
ER intermediate-low, PgR negative	4/19 (21)	6/18 (33)
	(χ^2_T = 1.24, *df* = 1, *P* = .265)	(χ^2_T = .828, *df* = 1, *P* = .363)

Abbreviations: ER, estrogen receptor; PgR, progesterone receptor.

*This table does not include patients with ER intermediate-low, PgR intermediate-low receptor status.

†Response = complete (CR) plus partial (PR) responses.

contrast, among 26 patients with progressive disease, only nine (35%) had high ER levels. Response of SD or better correlated with ER status in general (*P* = .021) and more specifically with ER levels (ie, high to low) (*P* = .011). For tamoxifen, SD or better correlated with ER status (*P* = .039); however, correlation with ER levels only approached a .05 probability. Table 7 demonstrates the relationship between response and ER levels for all patients who had SD or better. In the 141 patients, SD or better correlated with ER (*P* = .002) and ER levels (*P* = .003).

Preliminary results of the crossover data are shown in Table 8. Twenty-three percent (7/30) of patients responded to megestrol acetate after being crossed over from tamoxifen, while 22% (6/27) responded to tamoxifen after being crossed over from megestrol acetate. Fifty percent of patients were doing as well on crossover treatment as on initial therapy. However, at present the majority of patients who responded to the initial hormonal therapy are still on the initial treatment. For patients who initially received megestrol acetate, only 9/32 patients who had a PR or CR have crossed over to the alternate treatment, whereas among those who initially received tamoxifen, only 7/42 patients who had a PR or CR have crossed over.

The median time to disease progression was 41 weeks for all patients receiving megestrol acetate and 52 weeks for the tamoxifen group (NS).

For all responding patients who received megestrol acetate, ER level had no significant prognostic value for longer time to recurrence, whereas the PgR level did (*P* = .024). The median time to recurrence was 27 weeks for PgR-negative patients and 41 weeks for PgR-positive patients receiving megestrol acetate. For patients who responded to tamoxifen, ER level had borderline prognostic value for longer time to recurrence (*P* = .086), and PgR levels were

Table 5. Response Related to Individual Receptor Levels*

	Responses/Total Patients (%)	
	Megestrol Acetate	Tamoxifen
ER (fmol/mg cytosol protein)		
>90	17/47 (36)	22/47 (47)
30-89	9/25 (36)	11/26 (42)
10-29	4/19 (21)	6/26 (23)
Unknown	2/3	3/4
	(χ^2_T = 1.11, *df* = 1, *P* = .293)	(χ^2_T = 3.61, *df* = 1, *P* = .057)
PgR (fmol/mg cytosol protein)		
>90	8/26 (31)	11/27 (41)
30-89	8/20 (40)	6/22 (27)
10-29	6/17 (35)	9/16 (56)
<10	7/27 (26)	14/35 (40)
Unknown	3/4	2/3
	(χ^2_T = .22, *df* = 1, *P* = .639)	(χ^2_T = .16, *df* = 1, *P* = .689)

Abbreviations: ER, estrogen receptor; PgR, progesterone receptor.

*Response = complete (CR) plus partial (PR) responses.

Table 6. Distribution of Estrogen Receptor Levels in Patients Who Received Megestrol Acetate, by Response

Response	ER Level			
	Low	Medium	High	Total
CR, PR, SD*	9	17	40 (61%)	68
PD	9	8	9 (35%)	26

Abbreviations: SD, stable disease; PR, partial response; CR, complete response; ER, estrogen receptor; PD, progression of disease.

*Sixty-eight patients had SD or better; 32 had PR or better; ten had CR.

†Two patients—ER missing.

not significant. The median time to recurrence was 52 weeks for PgR-negative patients and 61 weeks for PgR-positive patients receiving tamoxifen.

Among the tamoxifen and megestrol acetate groups, variables such as CR and PR, site of dominant disease, ER+/PgR+, and ER+/PgR− were found not to be significant in predicting time to recurrence, although ER+/PgR− clearly favored tamoxifen. However, the majority of patients who responded had not yet had recurrence of disease.

DISCUSSION

This study showed similar response rates for patients with advanced metastatic breast cancer who received either megestrol acetate (35%) or tamoxifen (42%) as the initial treatment. In a similar study, Muss et al[14] found the response rates for both drugs to be the same: 29% with megestrol acetate and 31% with tamoxifen.

Response rates in patients with soft tissue-, bone-, and visceral-dominant disease were similar for both hormone treatments; the highest response rate occurred in patients with soft tissue-dominant disease. With megestrol acetate, response rates for patients with soft tissue-dominant, bone-dominant, and visceral-dominant disease were 50%, 17%, and 33%, respectively. With tamoxifen, response rates for patients with soft tissue-dominant, bone-dominant, and visceral-dominant disease were 58%, 21%, and 41%, respectively.

Table 7. Distribution of Estrogen Receptor Levels for All Patients, by Response

Response	ER Level			
	Low	Medium	High	Total
CR, PR, SD*	24	39	78 (55%)	145†
PD	21	12	19 (36%)	52

Abbreviations: SD, stable disease; PR, partial response; CR, complete response; ER, estrogen receptor; PD, progression of disease.

*One hundred forty-five patients had SD of better; 74 had PR or better; 22 had CR.

†Four patients—ER missing.

Table 8. Response to Crossover Treatment

	Tamoxifen (TMX) Crossed From MA					Megestrol Acetate (MA) Crossed From TMX				
	CR	PR	NC	PD	NE	CR	PR	NC	PD	NE
All*	1	5	11	10	3	0	7	11	12	4
6-wk washout†	0	4	9	7	2	0	7	8	8	2

Abbreviations: CR, complete response; PR, partial response; NC, no change; PD, progression of disease; NE, not evaluable.

*All patients crossing without regard to washout times.

†A drug-free period of 6 weeks was initiated to allow for washout of initial hormone and to observe for withdrawal response.

Response rates in this study were similar to those reported by Bonomi et al[13] for megestrol acetate patients with soft tissue-dominant disease, but lower for patients with bone-dominant and visceral-dominant disease. For soft tissue-, bone-, and visceral-dominant disease, Bonomi et al[13] reported a 47%, 37%, and 50% response rate, respectively. These differences between studies may be explained by the small numbers of patients entered in each dominant site category, or differences in patient selection or evaluation.

Preliminary crossover results with megestrol acetate or tamoxifen produced similar response rates: 23% and 22%, respectively. Thus far, the response rate for megestrol acetate has been lower than that reported by Ross et al,[16] who reported a 31% partial response rate with megestrol acetate after therapy with tamoxifen. In the present study, however, 83% of patients who had responded to tamoxifen had not been crossed over to megestrol acetate.

In this study, response did not correlate (significantly) with combined receptor (ie, ER plus PgR) levels for either treatment. A significant trend was seen between ER level, arbitrarily grouped as high, intermediate, and low (as previously defined), and response only in the tamoxifen group. However, if SD was considered as a "response" to therapy, then response (ie, SD or better) correlated with ER levels for both megestrol acetate and tamoxifen. This difference in correlation between the receptor levels and response to hormonal therapy between the two analyses may be based on the differences in the number of patients used in each particular analysis. Muss et al[14] reported that response to megestrol acetate or tamoxifen did not correlate with the amount of ER or PgR. However, Bonomi et al[13] found that ER and PgR status was significantly related to response and that PgR was the best predictor of response to megestrol acetate. Teulings et al[17] found no correlation between ER and PgR levels and response to megestrol acetate. Detection of a significant correlation of ER and PgR to response likely requires more patients than are commonly used in clinical trials, which could account for these apparently conflicting reports.

CONCLUSIONS

Results of this study indicate that megestrol acetate and tamoxifen have similar response rates in the treatment of postmenopausal women with advanced breast cancer. Although the data are preliminary, crossover response to both hormonal therapies appears to be similar.

A correlation between response to therapy and ER status could be shown, depending on the analysis used. In addition, ER and PgR status had significant prognostic value for time to recurrence.

Further follow-up is needed to determine response to crossover therapy after failure with the initial treatment. Studies with larger numbers of patients are needed to assess the correlation between ER and PgR levels and response and survival rates following hormonal therapy more accurately.

REFERENCES

1. McGuire WL, Carbone PP, Sears MED, et al: Estrogen receptors in human breast cancer: An overview, in McGuire WL, Carbone PP, Vollmer EP (eds): Estrogen Receptors in Human Breast Cancer. New York, Raven, 1975, pp 1–7

2. McGuire WL, Pearson OH, Segaloff A: Predicting hormone responsiveness in human breast cancer, in McGuire WL, Carbone PP, Vollmer EP (eds): Estrogen Receptors in Human Breast Cancer. New York, Raven, 1975, pp 17–29

3. Campbell FC, Elston CW, Blamey RW, et al: Quantitative oestradiol receptor values in primary breast cancer and response of metastases to endocrine therapy. Lancet 2:1371–1319, 1981

4. Horwitz KB, McGuire WL, Pearson OH, et al: Predicting response to endocrine therapy in human breast cancer: A hypothesis. Science 189:726–727, 1975

5. King RJB, Redgrave S, Hayward JL, et al: The measurement of receptors for oestradiol and progesterone in human breast tumours, in King RJB (ed): Steroid Receptor Assays in Human Breast Tumors: Methodological and Clinical Aspects. Cardiff, Wales, Alpha Omega Alpha, 1979, pp 55–72

6. Osborne CK, Yochmowitz MG, Knight WA III, et al: The value of estrogen and progesterone receptors in the treatment of breast cancer. Cancer 46:2884–2888, 1980

7. McCarty KS Jr, Cox C, Silva JS, et al: Comparison of sex steroid receptor analysis and carcinoembryonic antigen with clinical response to hormone therapy. Cancer 46:2846–2850, 1980

8. Horwitz KB, McGuire WL: Estrogen control of progesterone receptor in human breast cancer. J Biol Chem 253:2223–2228, 1978

9. Ingle JN: Additive hormonal therapy in women with advanced breast cancer. Cancer 53:766–777, 1984

10. Mouridsen H, Palshof T, Patterson J, et al: Tamoxifen in advanced breast cancer. Cancer Treat Rev 5:131–141, 1978

11. Wiggans RG, Woolley PV, Smythe T, et al: Phase II trial of tamoxifen in advanced breast cancer. Cancer Chemother Pharmacol 3:45–48, 1979

12. Ansfield FJ, David JL Jr, Ramirez G, et al: Further clinical studies with megestrol acetate in advanced breast cancer. Cancer 38:53–55, 1976

13. Bonomi P, Johnson P, Anderson K, et al: Primary hormonal therapy of advanced breast cancer with megestrol acetate: Predictive value of estrogen receptor and progesterone receptor levels. Semin Oncol 12:48–54, 1985 (suppl 1)

14. Muss HB, Paschold EH, Black WR, et al: Megestrol acetate vs tamoxifen in advanced breast cancer: A phase III trial of the Piedmont Oncology Association (POA). Semin Oncol 12:55–61, 1985 (suppl 1)

15. Haywood JL, Carbone PP, Henson JC, et al: Assessment of response to therapy in advanced breast cancer. Cancer 39:1289–1294, 1977

16. Ross MB, Buzdar AH, Blumenschein GR: Treatment of advanced breast cancer with megestrol acetate after therapy with tamoxifen. Cancer 49:413–417, 1982

17. Teulings FAG, van Gilse HA, Henkelman MS, et al: Estrogen, androgen, glucocorticoid, and progesterone receptors in progestin-induced regression of human breast cancer. Cancer Res 40:2557–2561, 1980

Megestrol Acetate: First-Line Therapy for Advanced Breast Cancer

Patricia A. Johnson, Philip D. Bonomi, Kenning M. Anderson, Janet M. Wolter, and S.G. Economou

Megestrol acetate as initial hormonal therapy produced a 40% objective response rate in 53 patients with advanced breast cancer; another 26% achieved stable disease. For 19 patients with visceral-dominant disease, the response rate was 42%. To investigate the effect of the order of sequential hormonal therapy, records of 66 patients treated with tamoxifen before megestrol acetate or with megestrol acetate before tamoxifen were reviewed retrospectively. Of the 24 patients who were given megestrol acetate first, nine (38%) had objective response to primary therapy, and four (17%) to secondary therapy. Among the 42 patients treated with tamoxifen first, there were nine (21%) objective responses to primary therapy and eight (19%) responses to secondary therapy. Results show that megestrol acetate is effective first-line hormonal therapy for advanced breast cancer. Megestrol acetate can be used as primary hormonal therapy and tamoxifen as secondary hormonal therapy, as an alternative to the more usual reverse order. One may also consider megestrol acetate for some advanced breast cancer patients with visceral-dominant disease.

SINCE Ingle et al[1] demonstrated that tamoxifen is as effective as estrogen for the treatment of advanced breast cancer but less toxic, tamoxifen has been widely used as first-line hormonal therapy for this disease. Megestrol acetate (Megace, Bristol-Myers Oncology Division, Evansville, IN), a semisynthetic progestational agent, is more commonly used as second-line therapy; it is often used for patients who initially responded to tamoxifen and subsequently failed to respond, or who have estrogen receptor (ER)-positive cancer but failed to respond to tamoxifen or other first-line hormonal therapy.[2–5]

However, the response rate to the two agents is similar in randomized studies, ranging from 15% to 55% for both drugs, depending on the receptor status of the patients and other prognostic variables.[6–9] In addition, both drugs are relatively well tolerated, with the primary adverse effect of tamoxifen being hot flashes and the primary toxicity of megestrol acetate, weight gain.

Since some laboratory data suggest that progestins might interfere with the replenishment of cytoplasmic ER,[10] one might predict that the best use of the two drugs is tamoxifen as first-line and megestrol acetate as second-line therapy for advanced breast cancer. However, there is a paucity of clinical data to support this contention. Since the response rates are similar and both agents are well tolerated, it seems reasonable to question whether megestrol acetate should always be used as secondary rather than primary hormonal therapy. We examined the records of breast cancer patients treated with megestrol acetate to establish the response rate to megestrol acetate as first-line hormonal therapy and to investigate the effect of the order of sequential hormonal therapy in patients treated with both tamoxifen and megestrol acetate.

MATERIALS AND METHODS

The records of 53 consecutive patients treated with megestrol acetate (40 mg four times daily) as first-line hormonal therapy for advanced breast cancer were reviewed retrospectively. Responses were defined according to Eastern Cooperative Oncology Group (ECOG) criteria,[11] and duration of response was measured from the beginning of treatment in accordance with criteria defined by Hayward et al.[12] Complete response was defined as disappearance of all known disease. In the case of bone metastases, radiologic evidence of recalcification was required. Partial response was defined as a 50% or greater decrease in measurable lesions, and objective improvement judged by two independent observers in evaluable but nonmeasurable lesions, without progression of any lesions. Stable disease was defined as less than a 50% decrease or 25% increase in the size of measurable lesions. A response was classified as stable, partial, or complete only if its duration was 12 weeks or more. Receptor levels were determined with a dextran-coated charcoal assay,[13] and the progesterone receptor level was determined with R5020 in the presence of 20 mmol sodium molybdate.[14] A receptor level of 10 femtomoles/mg was considered positive.

We also reviewed the records of 66 patients with advanced breast cancer treated with sequential additive hormonal therapy. Forty-two patients were treated with tamoxifen (10 mg twice daily) first, and then given megestrol acetate (40 mg four times daily) when they developed progressive disease; 24 patients had megestrol acetate as their initial therapy and were treated with tamoxifen as second-line hormonal therapy.

From the School of Medicine, University of Illinois, Urbana, IL, and Rush Medical College, Chicago.

Address reprint requests to Patricia A. Johnson, MD, Carle Clinic, 602 W University, Urbana, IL, 61801.

0093–7754/86/1304–4002$05.00/0

Table 1. Megestrol Acetate as First-Line Therapy

Receptor Status*	No. of Patients
ER+/PgR+	31
ER+/PgR−	6
ER−/PgR+	8
ER−/PgR−	6
ER+	1
Unknown	1

Abbreviations: ER, estrogen receptor; PgR, progestogen receptor.

*Receptor level of 10 femtomoles/mg considered positive.

RESULTS

The median age of 53 patients (50 women, three men) who received megestrol acetate as first-line hormonal therapy was 64 years. Nineteen had visceral disease as the dominant site, 20 had soft tissue-dominant disease, and 14 had bone-dominant disease. Their receptor status is shown in Table 1. Overall, the complete response rate was 19% and the objective (complete plus partial) response rate was 40% (Table 2). An additional 26% had stable disease. Considering only the 38 ER-positive cases, 24% had complete responses and 20% had partial responses, with 29% achieving disease stabilization. Response according to dominant site of disease was as follows: For visceral-dominant disease, there were 16% complete and 26% partial responses, with another 16% achieving stable disease. For soft-tissue disease, 35% had complete response, 10% had partial response, and 25% had stable disease. Among those patients with bone-dominant disease, there were no complete responses, 29% had partial responses, and 43% had stable disease. The median duration of megestrol acetate first-line therapy was 8 months.

Among the 66 patients treated with sequential additive hormonal therapy, the median age of the "tamoxifen first" group was 57.5 years, and of the "megestrol acetate first" group, 63.5 years. In the patients receiving tamoxifen first, the dominant site of disease was visceral in ten, soft tissue in 12, and bone in 20. In those treated with megestrol acetate first, nine had visceral-dominant disease, eight had soft tissue-dominant disease, and seven had bone-dominant disease. Receptor status of these patients is shown in Tables 3 and 4.

Table 2. Megestrol Acetate as First-Line Therapy: Response by Receptor Status

	No. of Patients (N = 53)			
Receptor Status	CR	PR	SD	PD
ER+/PgR+	9	8	10	4
ER+/PgR−	0	1	1	4
ER−/PgR+	0	1	3	4
ER−/PgR−	0	0	0	6
ER+	0	1	0	0
Unknown	1	0	0	0
Totals (%)	10 (19)	11 (21)	14 (26)	18 (34)

Abbreviations: CR, complete response; PR, partial response; SD, stable disease; PD, progressive disease; ER, estrogen receptor; PgR, progestogen receptor.

Table 3. Tamoxifen as First-Line Therapy, Then Megestrol Acetate

Receptor Status	No. of Patients
ER+/PgR+	23
ER+/PgR−	1
ER−/PgR+	5
ER−/PgR−	6
ER+	3
Unknown	4

Abbreviations: ER, estrogen receptor; PgR, progestogen receptor.

Of 42 patients treated with tamoxifen first and then given megestrol acetate at the time of disease progression, there were four complete and five partial responses to tamoxifen, giving an objective response rate of 21%. An additional 20% had disease stabilization. When these patients were given megestrol acetate as their secondary hormonal therapy, there were three complete and five partial responses, giving an objective response rate of 19%; another 31% had stable disease. Response by receptor category is given in Tables 5 and 6. If only the 27 ER-positive cases are considered, there were six objective responses to tamoxifen (22%), followed by six objective responses to megestrol acetate (22%).

In the group of 24 patients treated with megestrol acetate first and then with tamoxifen, there were four partial and five complete responses, and nine had stable disease, giving an objective

Table 4. Megestrol Acetate as First-Line Therapy, Then Tamoxifen

Receptor Status	No. of Patients
ER+/PgR+	18
ER+/PgR−	1
ER−/PgR+	3
ER−/PgR−	1
Unknown	1

Table 5. Tamoxifen First, Then Megestrol Acetate: Response to Tamoxifen

	No. of Patients (N = 42)			
Receptor Status	CR	PR	SD	PD
ER+/PgR+	0	2	13	8
ER+/PgR−	0	1	0	0
ER−/PgR+	1	0	2	2
ER−/PgR−	0	0	4	2
ER+	1	2	0	0
Unknown	2	0	1	1
Totals (%)	4 (10)	5 (12)	20 (48)	13 (31)

Abbreviations: CR, complete response; PR, partial response; SD, stable disease; PD, progressive disease; ER, estrogen receptor; PgR, progestogen receptor.

Table 7. Megestrol Acetate First, Then Tamoxifen: Response to Megestrol Acetate

	No. of Patients (N = 24)			
Receptor Status	CR	PR	SD	PD
ER+/PgR+	4	3	7	4
ER+/PgR−	0	0	0	1
ER−/PgR+	0	1	2	0
ER−/PgR−	0	0	0	1
Unknown	1	0	0	0
Totals (%)	5 (21)	4 (17)	9 (38)	6 (25)

Abbreviations: CR, complete response; PR, partial response; SD, stable disease; PD, progressive disease; ER, estrogen receptor; PgR, progestogen receptor.

(complete plus partial) response rate to megestrol acetate of 38% (Tables 7 and 8). When these patients were given tamoxifen as their second hormonal therapy, there were two partial and two complete responses (objective response rate, 17%), and six had stable disease. If only the 19 ER-positive cases are considered, there were seven objective responses to megestrol acetate (37%), followed by four objective responses to tamoxifen (21%).

The group given tamoxifen before megestrol acetate received a median of 10 months of therapy with the two hormones; those given megestrol acetate before tamoxifen were treated with the two hormones for a median of 12.5 months. In both cases, patients spent approximately 70% of the total hormone-therapy time taking their first-line drug.

DISCUSSION

The objective response of 40%, seen in our series of 53 patients treated with megestrol acetate as initial hormonal therapy, exceeds that found by Ansfield et al,[2] Alexieva-Figush et al,[4] Morgan,[7] Muss et al,[8] and Allegra et al,[9] all of whom reported a response rate of 29% to 31%. Our group was heavily weighted with receptor-positive patients. In addition, the series by Ansfield et al[2] and Alexieva-Figush et al[4] included patients with previous hormonal therapy, whereas our series was limited to patients receiving megestrol acetate as initial hormonal treatment. A group with many receptor-positive cases with no prior hormonal therapy might reasonably be expected to show a higher response rate to megestrol acetate than series that lack these characteristics.

The objective response rate for cases with visceral-dominant disease was 42%, with another 16% achieving stable disease. While conventional wisdom suggests that patients with visceral disease should be administered cytotoxic chemotherapy rather than hormonal therapy, our results show that nearly half of such patients received some benefit from megestrol acetate as initial hormonal therapy. This observation implies that megestrol acetate might be considered as an alternative to chemotherapy even in

Table 6. Tamoxifen First, Then Megestrol Acetate: Response to Megestrol Acetate

	No. of Patients (N = 42)			
Receptor Status	CR	PR	SD	PD
ER+/PgR+	1	4	9	9
ER+/PgR−	0	0	0	1
ER−/PgR+	0	0	2	3
ER−/PgR−	0	0	1	5
ER+	1	0	1	1
Unknown	1	1	0	2
Totals (%)	3 (7)	5 (12)	13 (31)	21 (50)

Abbreviations: CR, complete response; PR, partial response; SD, stable disease; PD, progressive disease; ER, estrogen receptor; PgR, progestogen receptor.

Table 8. Megestrol Acetate First, Then Tamoxifen: Response to Tamoxifen

	No. of Patients (N = 24)			
Receptor Status	CR	PR	SD	PD
ER+/PgR+	2	2	4	10
ER+/PgR−	0	0	0	1
ER−/PgR+	0	0	1	2
ER−/PgR−	0	0	0	1
Unknown	0	0	1	0
Totals (%)	2 (8)	2 (8)	6 (25)	14 (58)

Abbreviations: CR, complete response; PR, partial response; SD, stable disease; PD, progressive disease; ER, estrogen receptor; PgR, progestogen receptor.

patients with visceral-dominant advanced breast cancer.

Our retrospective cross-over data show no advantage to starting with tamoxifen as opposed to megestrol acetate. Among the 24 patients who were given megestrol acetate prior to tamoxifen, there were nine (38%) objective responses to the primary therapy and four (17%) responses to the secondary therapy. Among the 42 patients treated with tamoxifen first and then with megestrol acetate at the time of disease progression, there were nine (21%) objective responses to the primary therapy and eight (19%) responses to the secondary therapy. These data and those obtained when only receptor-positive cases were included slightly favor the group whose initial therapy was megestrol acetate. In this retrospective study, the groups are not exactly comparable; the "tamoxifen first" group was slightly younger and had more bone-dominant and less visceral-dominant disease than the "megestrol acetate first" group.

There are two series in the literature from which relevant cross-over data can be gleaned. Morgan[7] conducted a study in which patients were randomly assigned to tamoxifen or megestrol acetate treatment. At the time of disease progression, the participants were offered treatment with the alternative hormone. In 48 advanced breast cancer cases receiving tamoxifen as first additive hormonal therapy, 17 (35%) had an objective response; four of 24 (17%) in this group subsequently responded to megestrol acetate. In the 46 patients given megestrol acetate first, 14 (30%) had an objective response; 12 of these patients later received tamoxifen but none responded. In a similar study connected by the Piedmont Oncology Association,[8] 17 (31%) of 54 patients responded objectively to tamoxifen as initial hormonal therapy; 24 of these patients were later treated with megestrol acetate and only one (4%) responded. Eighteen of 56 (24%) responded objectively to megestrol acetate as first-line therapy; 24 of these patients had subsequent treatment with tamoxifen and 3 of 24 (12.5%) had complete or partial response. Our series showed a higher response rate to secondary hormonal therapy than that reported by Morgan and the Piedmont Oncology Association.[7,8] Data from both of these published studies are taken from preliminary reports. Early cross-over data suffer from inclusion of many cases representing early failures on primary therapy. One would expect a low response rate to secondary hormonal therapy in a group of patients who progressed rapidly on primary hormonal therapy. In contrast, Ross et al[3] reported that 15 (31%) of 48 patients treated with megestrol acetate as second-line therapy had complete or partial response; most (45/48) of these patients had initially responded favorably to tamoxifen.

We conclude that megestrol acetate is an effective first-line hormonal therapy for advanced breast cancer. It is reasonable to use megestrol acetate as first-line therapy and tamoxifen as second-line therapy, as an alternative to the conventional use of tamoxifen first and megestrol acetate second. It is also reasonable to consider the use of megestrol acetate in some patients with visceral-dominant disease.

REFERENCES

1. Ingle JN, Ahmann DL, Green SG, et al: Randomized clinical trial of diethylstilbestrol versus tamoxifen in postmenopausal women with advanced breast cancer. N Engl J Med 304:16–21, 1981

2. Ansfield FJ, Davis HL, Ramierez G, et al: Further clinical studies with megestrol acetate in advanced breast cancer. Cancer 38:53–55, 1976

3. Ross MB, Buzdar AH, Bumenschern GR: Treatment of advanced breast cancer with megestrol acetate after therapy with tamoxifen. Cancer 49:413–417, 1982

4. Alexieva-Figush J, Van Gilse HA, Hopwich J, et al: Progestin therapy in advanced breast cancer. Megestrol acetate—An evaluation of 160 treated cases. Cancer 46:2369–2377, 1980

5. Johnson PA, Bonomi PD, Wolter JM, et al: Megestrol acetate as secondary hormonal therapy in advanced breast cancer. Proc Am Soc Clin Oncol 3:122, 1984

6. Ingle JN, Ahmann DL, Green SL, et al: Randomized clinical trial of megestrol acetate versus tamoxifen in postmenopausal or castrated women with advanced breast cancer. Am J Clin Oncol 5:155–160, 1982

7. Morgan LR: Megestrol acetate versus tamoxifen in advanced breast cancer in postmenopausal patients. Semin Oncol 12:43–47, 1985 (suppl 1)

8. Muss HB, Paschold EH, Black WR, et al: Megestrol acetate versus tamoxifen in advanced breast cancer: A phase III trial of the Piedmont Oncology Association. Semin Oncol 12:55–61, 1985 (suppl 1)

9. Allegra JC, Bertino J, Bonomi PD, et al: Metastatic breast cancer: Preliminary results with oral hormonal therapy. Semin Oncol 12:61–64, 1985 (suppl 6)

10. Hsueh AJW, Peck EL, Clark JU: Progesterone antagonism of the estrogen receptor and estrogen-induced uterine growth. Nature 253:337, 1975

11. Oken MM, Creech RH, Tormey DC, et al: Toxicity and response criteria of the Eastern Cooperative Oncology Group. Am J Clin Oncol 5:649–655, 1982

12. Hayward JL, Carbone PC, Heusen JC, et al: Assessment of response to therapy in advanced breast cancer. Cancer 39:1289–1294, 1977

13. Anderson KM, Bonomi P, Marogil M, et al: Comparison of dextran-coated charcoal and sucrose density gradient analysis of estrogen and progesterone receptors in human breast cancer. Cancer Res 40:4127–4130, 1980

14. Anderson KM, Marogil M, Bonomi P, et al: Stabilization of human breast cancer progesterone (5020) receptor by sodium molybdate. Clin Chim Acta 103:367–373, 1980

High-Dose Megestrol Acetate in the Treatment of Postmenopausal Women With Advanced Breast Cancer

N. Simon Tchekmedyian, Nancy Tait, and Joseph Aisner

The optimal dose of progesterone compounds for the treatment of breast cancer is unknown, but there is evidence to suggest a dose-response curve. We are testing the tolerability and efficacy of megestrol acetate administered orally and continuously in doses three to ten times higher than the standard dose of 160 mg/d. We have so far treated 33 patients with metastatic breast cancer and positive or unknown tumor hormone receptor status. Thirty patients had had documented disease progression with previous hormonal therapy, and 22 had failed with previous chemotherapy. Twenty-five patients had objectively measurable metastases. In this heavily pretreated group, the objective response rate was 40%; in addition, 32% of patients had stabilization of disease. Interestingly, ten of 12 patients who had developed disease progression while on standard-dose megestrol acetate therapy had objective response or stabilization on the higher dose. Toxicity was acceptable and reversible and included mild elevations of blood pressure and weight gain. Our results indicate that high-dose megestrol acetate is well-tolerated and highly active in advanced refractory breast cancer, and suggest a dose-response curve for the drug in the treatment of breast cancer.

HORMONAL AGENTS are active in the treatment of breast cancer. Progesterone compounds, particularly megestrol acetate (Megace, Bristol-Myers Oncology Division, Evansville, IN), can be used as front-line systemic therapy for hormone-sensitive tumors in postmenopausal patients. Although the optimal dose of progesterone compounds has not yet been defined, a considerable body of evidence suggests a dose-response relationship. For example, results of a number of clinical trials,[1-10] most of which were conducted in Europe, have suggested a dose-response curve for medroxyprogesterone acetate in breast cancer (Table 1). The data suggest that increases in the orally administered doses yielded considerably higher response rates, which ranged from 9% for doses of 100 mg/d to 37% for doses of 2,000 mg/d. Wide variations in the bioavailability of the drug administered orally have remained a significant problem. However, large intramuscular (IM) doses of medroxyprogesterone acetate were also tested, and again there seemed to be a trend toward higher response rates with higher doses (Table 1). However, severe local toxicity at injection sites with abscess formation precluded long-term administration of higher-dose IM medroxyprogesterone acetate, thus limiting the potential of this therapy.

Comparisons among different studies are difficult because the patient populations vary substantially regarding the extent of disease and previous treatment. In addition, the receptor status in the majority of the patients' tumors in these studies was unknown, and this further confounds the evaluation of a dose-response relationship. Although dosage is considered important, the basis for higher response rates remains unclear. It has been suggested that the differences in activity with higher doses may be secondary to different endocrine effects.[11]

Another progesterone compound that has been evaluated is megestrol acetate. Standard dosages of this agent of 160 mg/d in divided oral doses result in blood levels five to ten times higher than medroxyprogesterone acetate given at high doses either orally or IM,[12] and it has been suggested that there are substantial differences in the intestinal absorption between the two compounds.[13] Megestrol acetate in doses of 160 mg/d has been reported by several investigators[12,14-17] to produce response rates comparable to any other front-line hormonal therapy for advanced postmenopausal breast cancer. The optimal dose of megestrol acetate for the treatment of breast cancer, however, remains unknown, despite small studies

From the Division of Medical Oncology, University of Maryland Cancer Center, Baltimore.
Supported in part by a grant from Bristol-Myers Oncology Division, Evansville, IN.
Address reprint requests to N. Simon Tchekmedyian, MD, University of Maryland Cancer Center, University of Maryland School of Medicine, 22 South Greene St, Baltimore, MD 21201.

0093-7754/86/1304-4007$05.00/0

Table 1. Dose-Response Relationships With Medroxyprogesterone Acetate: A Literature Review

Author, Year	Dose (mg/d)	Route	Duration	No. of Patients	Objective Response (%)
Goldenberg, 1969[1]	100	PO	Continuous	108	9
Hedley, 1984[2]	600	PO	Continuous	105	20
Hortobagyi, 1982[3]	800	PO	Continuous	20	28
Izuo, 1982[4]	1,200	PO	Continuous	20	35
Pannuti, 1982[5]	2,000	PO	30 d	27	37
Cavalli, 1982[6]	500*	IM	28 d	76	11
	1,000	IM	28 d	76	31
Della Cuna, 1978[7]	500	IM	30 d	50	44
	1,000	IM	30 d	51	41
Mattsson, 1978[8]	1,000	IM	30 d	25	28
DeLena, 1979[9]	1,000	IM	40 d	53	32
	1,500	IM	27 d	28	21
Pannuti, 1979[10]	500	IM	30 d	50	43
	1,500	IM	30 d	50	46

Abbreviations: PO, orally; IM, intramuscularly.
*Twice weekly only.

that have addressed the issue.[18] Our questions were, therefore, whether megestrol acetate given at higher than the standard dose would be well tolerated and whether such doses would be associated with increased efficacy.

We designed a phase I/II study of escalating doses of megestrol acetate in patients with advanced breast cancer with the objective of establishing the tolerability at the different dose levels as well as obtaining preliminary information about efficacy.

This report is based on an interim analysis of the data generated in our current phase I/II study of megestrol acetate at doses that are between three and ten times higher than the standard dose. A preliminary report has been published.[19]

PATIENTS AND METHODS

To qualify for this study, patients had to have histologically confirmed advanced breast cancer. Additional eligibility criteria included postmenopausal status, positive or unknown estrogen and progesterone receptor status, and measurable or evaluable disease. Patients who were refractory to previous hormonal therapy, including standard-dose megestrol acetate, were eligible for the study. A Karnofsky performance status of 50% or greater was required. Patients with uncontrolled heart failure or history of thromboembolism were excluded.

Table 2. High-Dose Megestrol Acetate Dose Levels

Dose (mg/d)*	No. of Patients
480	3
800	3
1,280	3
1,600	24

*160-mg tablets (three to four daily doses).

Patients were seen in the outpatient clinic every other week. History and physical examination, tumor measurements when applicable, and evaluation of performance status and body weight were performed before beginning therapy and every other week throughout the treatment period. Complete blood cell (CBC) count with differential and platelet count, serum blood urea nitrogen (BUN), creatinine, electrolytes, glucose, aspartate aminotransferase (SGOT), alanine aminotransferase (SGPT), and bilirubin measurements were obtained at each visit. Coagulation tests, chest roentgenograms, ECGs, and computerized tomography (CT) scans as needed for tumor measurement were obtained every 8 weeks.

Drug dose and schedule of administration are described in Table 2. Megestrol acetate was supplied in specially designed 160-mg tablets by Bristol-Myers Oncology Division, Evansville, IN. Initially, the oral megestrol acetate dose was escalated in cohorts of three patients, with each subsequent cohort receiving 480, 800, 1,280, or 1,600 mg/d, respectively. Since no dose-limiting toxicity was encountered, all subsequent patients were treated with 1,600 mg/d in the phase II part of the study. Further dose escalations were not pursued, mainly because of such reasons as the large number of tablets that would be required on a daily basis and the potential cost. It should be noted, however, that a maximum tolerated dose was not reached.

Standard response criteria were used. Complete response was defined as disappearance of all clinical evidence of tumor for at least 4 weeks; partial response was defined as a 50% or greater decrease in size of measured lesions for at least 4 weeks. Stable disease was defined as insufficient regression to qualify as response, or an increase by less than 25% in the size

Table 3. Patient Characteristics (N = 33)

Females (all postmenopausal)	32
Males (postcastration)	1
Median age, yr (range)	57 (40–83)
Median Karnofsky performance, % (range)	80 (50–100)
Median disease-free interval, mo (range)	24 (0–132)
Dominant disease site	
Soft tissue	4
Bone	15
Viscera	14
Measurable disease	25
Evaluable nonmeasurable disease	8
Receptor status	
ER and PgR positive	12
ER or PgR positive	15
ER and PgR unknown	6
Evaluable for response	33
Evaluable for toxicity	33

Abbreviations: ER, estrogen receptor; PgR, progesterone receptor.

of measured lesions. Durations of response were calculated from the time of maximum response.

The investigational nature of the treatment was explained and an informed consent, approved by the institutional review board, was obtained from each patient.

RESULTS

Patient Characteristics

The characteristics of the 33 patients entered in the study so far are described in Table 3. Most patients were ambulatory and only four had soft tissue–dominant disease. Most of the patients with visceral disease had intraabdominal or lung metastases; only three had liver metastases. All patients were evaluable for response and toxicity.

Previous systemic therapy given to the patients is shown in Table 4. Virtually all of the patients had been previously treated with hormonal therapy or chemotherapy. Thirty (90%) of the 33 patients had had documented disease progression during the previous course of hormonal therapy. Of note is that of the 25 patients with measurable disease, all but one had failed previous chemotherapy or hormonal therapy. Twenty-three (92%) of the 25 patients had had documented disease progression during the previous hormonal treatment.

Table 4. Previous Therapy for Patients on High-Dose Megestrol Acetate

	All Patients (N = 33)	Measurable-Disease Patients (n = 25)
Previous hormonal and/or chemotherapy	33	24
Disease progression while receiving hormonal and/or chemotherapy	32	24
Disease progression while receiving hormonal therapy	30	23
Disease progression while receiving chemotherapy	22	14

Response

Response to therapy for the 25 patients with measurable disease is shown in Table 5. Five patients had complete response, five had partial response, eight had stabilization of disease, and seven had disease progression. The median duration of objective response at the time of this interim analysis is 4+ months (range 2+ to 8+ months). However, the median time on study is 10+ months for patients with a complete response and 8+ months for those with a partial response. Rapid initial responses were seen in several patients, sometimes with almost immediate symptomatic improvement, especially in those with bone pain. The time to maximum response, however, was usually several months. Of the eight patients with evaluable but nonmeasurable cancer, two have had progression and six have had stabilization of disease for a median of 5 months. Some of these patients are still improving, however, and their response may need to be upgraded.

The results of therapy by dominant metastatic site are shown in Table 6. Three of the five complete remissions occurred in patients with soft tissue–dominant disease. Responses were not seen in the three patients with liver metastases. Two complete responses occurred in patients with visceral metastases with the predominant site of disease in the abdominal cavity and pelvis; these responses were documented clinically and by CT scan. In addition, three patients with visceral disease, one with symptomatic (decreased blood counts) bone marrow involvement, one with pulmonary metastases, and one with both pulmonary and bone marrow involvement, had partial remissions. The patients with bone marrow involvement had marked improvement

Table 5. Response to High-Dose Megestrol Acetate in Patients With Measurable Breast Cancer

Response	No./Total (%)	Duration* mo (median [range])	Time on Study† mo (median [range])
Complete response	5/25 (20)	4+ (2+ to 8)	10+ (6+ to 12+)
Partial response	5/25 (20)	4+ (2+ to 6+)	8+ (4+ to 13+)
Stable disease	8/25 (32)	2.5+ (2+ to 4+)	4+ (3+ to 12+)
Progressive disease	7/25 (28)‡	—	—

*From time of maximum response.

†From day 1 of therapy.

‡Five patients had therapy for less than 4 weeks and rapidly progressive disease.

in hematologic parameters, decrease in blood transfusion requirements, and decrease by 50% or more in the measurements of metastases in other sites. In addition, four patients with nonhepatic visceral disease had stabilization for 2 or more months.

Response in Previous Megestrol Acetate Failures

Of particular importance is the analysis of response among 12 patients who had had documented disease progression while receiving megestrol acetate at the standard dose of 160 mg/d orally. The maximum responses seen among the 12 patients with the standard dose were as follows: Six had primary treatment failure, five had stabilization of disease, and one had a partial response. After documentation of disease progression, six of the patients (who had had partial response or stabilization) were observed for a withdrawal response or stabilization during a washout period. The 12 patients were then treated with high-dose megestrol acetate. Two patients had progressive disease on the high-dose regimen, one had a complete response, two had partial responses, and seven had stabilization of disease. These results suggest that there is a dose-response curve for megestrol acetate in the treatment of breast cancer.

Table 6. Results With High-Dose Megestrol Acetate by Dominant Lesion (all patients, N = 33)

	No. of Patients	CR	PR	SD	PD
Soft tissue	4	3	0	1	0
Bone	15	0	2	9	4
Visceral, liver	3	0	0	0	3
Visceral, other	11	2	3	4	2
Total	33	5	5	14	9

Abbreviations: CR, complete response; PR, partial response; SD, stable disease; PD, progressive disease.

Toxicity

Toxicity was tolerable and reversible, as depicted in Table 7. The most frequently occurring side effects were weight gain and appetite stimulation. This was, in fact, a favorable effect in many profoundly underweight and cachectic patients. (A description of weight changes of these patients has been published[20]; another is presented elsewhere in this issue.[21]) Mild edema occurred in seven patients and was reversible with diuretics and reduction in salt intake. Two patients developed mild hypertension and required medication with diuretics and beta blockers. In addition, four patients who had previously had hypertension needed adjustments in their antihypertensive medications. Constipation, exertional dyspnea, hyperglycemia, and

Table 7. Toxicity With 1,600 mg/d Megestrol Acetate (n = 24)

	No. of Patients (%)
Weight gain (>1 kg)	21 (88)
Edema (mild)*	7 (29)
Hypertension†	6 (25)
Constipation	3 (13)
Exertional dyspnea	2 (8)
Chest pressure‡	2 (8)
Hyperglycemia	2 (8)
Heart failure	1 (4)
Urinary frequency	1 (4)

*Reversible with diuretics.

†Requiring new antihypertensive medication (n = 2) or adjustment of previous medication (n = 4).

‡Both patients developed hypertension.

		Megestrol Acetate Dose (mg/d)
Breast cancer		160
No prior hormonal therapy	Randomize	800
Positive or unknown receptors		1600

Fig 1. Proposed protocol of study of megestrol acetate for the treatment of breast cancer (Cancer and Acute Leukemia Group B).

worsening of heart failure were uncommon and reversible side effects (Table 7).

DISCUSSION

Results of this study indicate that high-dose (480 to 1,600 mg/d) oral megestrol acetate given continuously is highly effective therapy for patients with metastatic breast cancer refractory to previous hormonal therapy, including standard-dose megestrol acetate. In addition, a dose-response relationship was inferred because patients refractory to previous standard-dose megestrol acetate had an unexpectedly high rate of response to high-dose megestrol acetate.

These data are in concordance with results seen with medroxyprogesterone acetate in humans and animals, suggesting a dose-response relationship for progestins. This study did not address either the maximally tolerated dose or the optimal dose with consideration of cost and ease of administration.

Treatment with high-dose megestrol acetate was well tolerated. The main side effects seen in patients who received 1,600 mg/d were weight gain and increased appetite.

Further studies are needed to determine which dose of megestrol acetate has the best therapeutic index. This question can be answered only with prospective, random-design studies that contain adequate numbers of patients. One such study has been proposed by the Cancer and Acute Leukemia Group B (CALGB). This would be a random-design trial with patients who have not received hormonal therapy previously and who have positive or unknown receptor status. Patients would be randomized to three dose levels as shown in Fig 1, ie, 160 mg/d (standard dose), 800 mg/d (five times the standard dose), and 1,600 mg/d (ten times the standard dose).

Such carefully designed and conducted studies may answer the question of the optimal dose of megestrol acetate for the treatment of advanced breast cancer, and may allow for a more rational use of this important and active anticancer hormone.

REFERENCES

1. Goldenberg IS: Clinical trial of Δ^1E-testolactone (NSC 23759), medroxyprogesterone acetate (NSC 26386), and oxylone acetate (NSC 47438) in advanced female mammary cancer: A report of the cooperative breast cancer group. Cancer 23:109–112, 1969

2. Hedley D, Dalgleish A, Raghavan D, et al: Advanced breast cancer: Response to high dose oral medroxyprogesterone acetate. Aust NZ J Med 14:251–254, 1984

3. Hortobagyi G, Frye D, Buzdar A, et al: High dose oral medroxyprogesterone acetate for the treatment of metastatic breast cancer. Proc Am Assoc Can Res: 582, 1982 (abstr)

4. Izuo M, Ina Y, Tominaga T, et al: Oral high-dose medroxyprogesterone acetate therapy in advanced breast cancer: Clinical and endocrine studies, in Proceedings of the International Symposium on Medroxyprogesterone Acetate. Amsterdam, Excerpta Medica, 1982, pp 250–263

5. Pannuti F, Martoni A, Fruet F, et al: Oral high-dose medroxyprogesterone acetate versus tamoxifen in postmenopausal patients with advanced breast cancer, in Iacobelli S, Lippman ME, Robustelli, et al (eds): The Role of Tamoxifen in Breast Cancer. New York, Raven, 1982, pp 85–92

6. Cavalli F, Goldhirsch A, Jungi WF, et al: Low- versus high-dose medroxyprogesterone acetate in the treatment of advanced breast cancer, in Proceedings of the International Symposium on Medroxyprogesterone Acetate. Amsterdam, Excerpta Medica, 1982, pp 224–233

7. Della Cuna GR, Calciati A, Strada M, et al: High dose medroxyprogesterone acetate treatment in metastatic carcinoma of the breast: A dose-response evaluation. Tumori 64:143–149, 1978

8. Mattsson W: High-dose medroxyprogesterone acetate treatment in advanced mammary carcinoma: A phase II investigation. Acta Radiol Oncol 17:387–400, 1978

9. DeLena M, Brambilla C, Valagussa P, et al: High-dose medroxyprogesterone acetate in breast cancer resistant to endocrine and cytotoxic therapy. Cancer Chemother Pharmacol 2:175–180, 1979

10. Pannuti F, Martoni A, DiMarco AR, et al: Prospective, randomized clinical trial of two different high dosages of medroxyprogesterone acetate in the treatment of metastatic breast cancer. Eur J Cancer 15:593–599, 1979

11. Blossey HC, Wander HE, Koebberling J, et al: Pharmacodynamic basis for the treatment of metastatic breast cancer with high-dose medroxyprogesterone acetate. Cancer 54:1208–1215, 1984

12. Caneeta R, Florentine S, Hunter H, et al: Megestrol acetate. Cancer Treat Rev 10:141–157, 1983

13. Martin F, Adlercreutz H: Aspects of megestrol acetate and medroxyprogesterone acetate metabolism, in Garattini S, Brendes HW (eds): Pharmacology of Steroid Contraceptive Drugs. New York, Raven, 1977, pp 99–115

14. Ingle JN, Ahmann DL, Green SJ, et al: Randomized clinical trial of megestrol acetate versus tamoxifen in paramenopausal or castrated women with advanced breast cancer. Am J Clin Oncol 5:155–150, 1982

15. Ingle JN: Additive hormonal therapy in women with advanced breast cancer. Cancer 53:766–777, 1984

16. Ansfield FJ, Kallas GJ, Singson JP: Clinical results with megestrol acetate in patients with advanced carcinoma of the breast. Surg Gynecol Obstet 155:888–890, 1982

17. Alexieva-Figusch J, van Gilse HA, Hop WCJ, et al: Progestin therapy in advanced breast cancer: Megestrol acetate—An evaluation of 160 treated cases. Cancer 46:2369–2372, 1980

18. Alexieva-Figusch J, Blankenstein MA, Hop WCJ, et al: Treatment of metastatic breast cancer patients with different dosages of megestrol acetate: Dose relations, metabolic and endocrine effects. Eur J Cancer Clin Oncol 20:33–40, 1984

19. Tchekmedyian NS, Tait N, Aisner J: Phase I/II trial of high dose megestrol acetate in breast cancer. Proc Am Soc Clin Oncol 5:72, 1986 (abstr)

20. Tchekmedyian NS, Tait N, Moody M, et al: Weight gain with high dose megestrol acetate: A possible treatment for cachexia. Proc Am Assoc Cancer Res 27:209, 1986 (abstr)

21. Tchekmedyian NS, Tait N, Moody M, et al: Appetite stimulation with megestrol acetate in cachectic cancer patients. Semin Oncol 1986 (suppl)

High-Dose Megestrol Acetate Therapy of Ovarian Carcinoma: A Phase II Study by the Northern California Oncology Group

Branimir I. Sikic, Sidney A. Scudder, Samuel C. Ballon, Olive M. Soriero, J. Eric Christman, Lily Suey, Mohamed N. Ehsan, Alan E. Brandt, and Thomas L. Evans

The activity of high-dose megestrol acetate was studied in 47 patients with epithelial ovarian cancers after failure of initial chemotherapy. The dose of megestrol acetate was 800 mg/d orally (PO) for 4 weeks and then 400 mg/d until tumor progression. Patients generally had far-advanced disease. Prior therapy included cisplatin, doxorubicin, and cyclophosphamide (PAC) or other cisplatin-containing regimens in 37, other combinations in eight, and single agents in only two patients. Seventeen patients (36%) developed intestinal obstructions within the first 2 months on study. Tumor histology was serous in 37, endometrioid in six, and clear-cell in two. Two thirds of the tumors were histologic grade 3, and the others were grade 2. Complete remission was obtained in one patient, with time to progression of 4 months. There were three partial remissions, with times to progression of 4, 5, and 18 months. The overall response rate (complete and partial) was 8%. Three additional patients had minor remissions (3, 5, and 8 months), and five had stable disease, for 3, 4, 5, 6, and 9 months. There was no correlation of response with grade, histologic type, or site of disease, but responding patients had a longer survival from diagnosis to protocol entry and from protocol failure to death than did nonresponding patients. The major side effect of megestrol acetate was increased appetite, which caused one patient to withdraw from the study, and resulted in a 10- to 20-kg weight gain in five patients. Plasma levels of megestrol acetate averaged 600 ng/mL in the first month of therapy and decreased to approximately 400 ng/mL at 8 and 12 weeks, after the drug dosage had been reduced. Serum follicle-stimulating hormone (FSH) and luteinizing hormone (LH) levels were markedly lower during megestrol therapy compared with pretreatment values. Megestrol acetate at 1 μg/mL in vitro inhibited soft agar colony formation from one of 17 specimens of ovarian carcinomas. We conclude that megestrol acetate in high doses has modest, but definite, palliative effects in some patients with advanced ovarian carcinoma in whom chemotherapy has failed. A controlled trial of megestrol plus combination chemotherapy as first-line treatment of advanced ovarian carcinoma should be considered.

From the Divisions of Medical and Gynecologic Oncology, Departments of Medicine and Obstetrics-Gynecology, Stanford University School of Medicine, Stanford, CA; and SRI International, Menlo Park, CA.

Supported by National Institutes of Health Grant No. 5U10 CA 21744 and the Bristol-Myers Company.

Address reprint requests to Dr Branimir I. Sikic, Stanford University Medical Center, Oncology Division, Department of Medicine, Room M-211, Stanford, CA 94305.

0093–7754/86/1304–4006$05.00/0

THERE HAVE BEEN several reports of therapeutic trials of progestins in patients with epithelial ovarian cancer.[1–12] Remission rates in these studies range from 0% to 65%. It is likely that this variability reflects differences in both patient selection and response criteria. Nonetheless, even in studies with low rates of remission,[5–7] occasional patients have been observed to have objective remissions of greater than 1 year. Recently, high doses of megestrol acetate have been reported to have considerable palliative activity in patients who failed initial chemotherapy.[1,2] Ten of 22 patients with ovarian carcinomas reported by Geisler[2] obtained a remission, including five complete responders, with a median duration of response of 1 year. Most patients had previously received chemotherapy with a single alkylating agent. We sought to confirm these findings in a population of patients with advanced ovarian carcinoma who had failed more extensive chemotherapy, which in most cases consisted of cisplatin, doxorubicin, and cyclophosphamide (PAC).

MATERIALS AND METHODS

Patient Eligibility

The criteria for patient eligibility for the Northern California Oncology Group (NCOG) protocol 50-83-1 were as follows: biopsy-proven epithelial carcinoma of the ovary; failure of standard curative therapy; life expectancy greater than 2 months; Karnofsky performance score greater than or equal to 50%; at least 4 weeks elapsed since previous therapies; and a measurable or evaluable tumor mass. Patients were ineligible if they had a previous malignancy in the preceding 7 years in addition to ovarian carcinoma or if they had received treatment previously with a progestin after the diagnosis of ovarian cancer had been established.

Megestrol Acetate Dosage and Administration

Megestrol acetate (Megace, Bristol-Myers Oncology Division, Evansville, IN) was provided for this study as 40-mg tablets by Bristol-Myers Oncology Division. The dosage for the first 4 weeks of the study was 800 mg/d orally (PO) in four divided doses of 200 mg. Thereafter, in accordance with

Geisler,[1,2] the dose was reduced to 400 mg/d until progression of disease was observed.

Megestrol Acetate Serum Levels

Serum was obtained from patients prior to study entry and at 2, 4, 8, and 12 weeks for determination of megestrol acetate levels by the high-performance liquid chromatography (HPLC) method of Gaver et al.[13] Serum (0.5 mL) was mixed with 0.5 mL of HPLC-grade water. 2,3-Diphenyl-l-indenone (Aldrich Chemical Co) was added as an internal standard and the mixture was extracted with 7.0 mL of hexane. A sample of 5 mL of the upper hexane layer was transferred to a clean glass tube and evaporated under nitrogen. The residue was resuspended in 0.1 mL of methanol, and 0.05 mL of this was injected into the column. Samples were chromatographed at room temperature, with a solvent system of acetonitrile/methanol/water/acetic acid (41:23:36:1), at a flow rate of 2.2 mL/min, using a Bondapak C_{18} column (Waters Co). Megestrol acetate was detected by UV absorbance at 280 nm, and serum levels were determined by peak height ratios using the internal standard and comparison with a standard curve. The lower limit of sensitivity of the assay was 100 ng/mL under these conditions, which is considerably higher than that reported by Gaver et al[13] but well below that required for measurement of megestrol acetate levels in our patients.

Study Parameters

Required tests at study entry included patient history and physical examination, complete blood count, urinalysis, serum chemical tests (including BUN, creatinine, calcium, uric acid, bilirubin, alkaline phosphatase, albumin, lactic acid dehydrogenase, and glutamate oxalate transaminase), chest x-ray, and either an ultrasound or computerized tomogram of the abdomen and pelvis. Interval history, body weight, tumor measurements, blood count, and serum chemical tests were repeated at 2 and 4 weeks after initiation of therapy and every 4 weeks thereafter.

The response criteria were the standard criteria of the NCOG. A complete remission is defined as the disappearance of all evidence of the tumor. A partial remission requires at least a 50% regression in the products of the perpendicular measurements of each tumor mass. A minor response is a reduction in the product of the perpendicular diameters of the tumor of at least 25% but less than 50%. Pleural effusions and ascites are considered evaluable sites of disease if the cytology of the effusions is confirmed to be malignant. A complete remission requires disappearance of these effusions, and a partial remission is an estimated 50% decrease in fluid volume without paracentesis or the use of diuretics. The time to progression of tumor is the interval from study entry to the first recorded progression of tumor growth after a remission is achieved.

CA-125 Serum Assays

The CA-125 assay was performed using a kit supplied by Centocor, Inc (Malvern, PA). Serum samples or standards were incubated with ^{125}I-OC-125 antibody and polystyrene beads to which unlabeled antibody was adsorbed. The mixture was incubated for 20 hours, and the radioactivity associated with the beads (solid phase) was counted after washing the beads. The results are expressed as arbitrary units per milliliter of serum, with 35 units/mL considered to be the upper limit of normal.[14,15]

Serum FSH and LH Levels

Serum levels of follicle-stimulating hormone (FSH) and luteinizing hormone (LH) were measured in nine patients by radioimmunoassay (Pacific Biotech Inc, San Diego) before and 4 and 8 weeks after beginning megestrol acetate therapy.

In Vitro Clonogenic Assays

Specimens of ovarian carcinoma were obtained from patients both on and off this study to examine possible direct in vitro effects of megestrol acetate on tumor colony formation in soft agar culture. The methodology has been described previously.[16] Solid tumor specimens were minced mechanically, digested with an enzyme mixture consisting of Pronase (0.5 mg/mL), collagenase type I (0.2 mg/mL), and DNAase (0.2 mg/mL), and filtered to obtain a single-cell suspension. Cells from malignant effusions were counted and plated without further attempts at cell dissociation into a single-cell suspension, or separation of tumor from nontumor cells. The cells were plated in 24-well plates, in a two-layer agar matrix, with a top layer of Waymouth's and McCoy's media (1:1), containing 15% newborn calf serum, 5 μg/mL porcine insulin, and 0.3% agar, in a volume of 0.5 mL containing 5×10^5 cells/mL. The bottom layer was similar except that there were no cells present and the agar concentration was 0.5%. The concentrations of megestrol acetate were 1 and 10 μg/mL, in triplicate, with continuous drug exposure from the time of plating. The plates were examined on the day after plating to determine the quality of the single cell suspension and to establish a background "colony count," which was subtracted from subsequent counts at 14 to 21 days.

RESULTS

Patient Characteristics

A total of 51 patients entered this study between October 1983 and August 1985. Two of the patients were declared ineligible upon review of histologic slides and operative findings. In one case the primary tumor was determined to be colorectal carcinoma, while in the other case the primary tumor was an ovarian granulosa cell (stromal) carcinoma. Of the remaining 49 patients, two were declared nonevaluable: one had received concurrent 5-fluorouracil from another physician without the knowledge of the investigators; a presumed pelvic tumor mass in the second patient proved to be matted intestine when the patient underwent an operation for intestinal obstruction within 2 weeks of study entry.

Table 1. Patient Characteristics at Study Entry

Total patients eligible	49
Age (yr)	
Range	40–84
Median	57
Karnofsky performance status (%)	
80–100	39
50–70	10
Histologic type (no. of patients)	
Serous	37
Endometrioid	6
Mucinous	3
Clear cell	2
Undifferentiated or unspecified	1

The characteristics of the 49 eligible patients are summarized in Table 1. Histologic grading of the tumor was available in 33 cases, of which 21 were poorly differentiated (grade 3) and 12 were moderately differentiated (grade 2), with no well-differentiated tumors noted among these 33.

Although most patients had a good performance status at entry, their disease was far advanced, and 17 of the 47 evaluable patients (36%) developed intestinal obstruction within the first 2 months of study. These patients were all considered fully evaluable and counted as failures of therapy, even when the obstruction occurred within the first month after protocol entry.

All patients had undergone previous chemotherapy, which in 37 cases was a drug combination including cisplatin (most commonly cisplatin, doxorubicin, cyclophosphamide [PAC]), and in eight cases, doxorubicin plus cyclophosphamide (ACe). Only two patients had been treated primarily with a single alkylating agent, and 12 had received previous pelvic or abdomino pelvic radiation therapy.

The major sites of measurable or evaluable disease were abdominal and pelvic tumor masses in 32 patients, palpable lymph nodes in eight, pleural masses or effusions in five, liver metastases in two, and a paraspinous mass in one patient.

Tumor Response

The number of remissions and time to progression are shown in Table 2. One patient achieved a complete remission of a large pelvic mass for 4 months, and there were three partial responses, for an overall response rate of 8%. The longest remission, 18 months, occurred in a patient with a large pelvic mass (10 × 12 cm), which regressed to a 1 × 2-cm nodule within 3 months of initiation of megestrol acetate. The other two partial responses occurred in supraclavicular and inguinal lymph node metastases. An additional three patients demonstrated minor regressions (greater than 25% but less than 50% reduction in the product of the tumor diameters). Five other patients had stabilization of disease lasting from 3 to 9 months. There was no correlation of response with histologic type or grade. Estrogen and progesterone receptor data were not available for these tumors to correlate with response. One partial and one minor response occurred in the two patients who had received only a single alkylating agent prior to megestrol.

Table 2. Response Data for High-Dose Megestrol Acetate Therapy of Ovarian Carcinoma

	No. of Patients	Duration (mo)
Complete response (CR)	1	4
Partial response (PR)	3	4, 5, 18
Minor response (MR)	3	3, 5, 8
Stable, 3 mo	5	3, 4, 5, 6, 9
Overall		
PR + CR rate	4/47 (8%)	
MR + PR + CR	7/47 (14%)	

Survival

The survival of patients in the study is presented in Table 3: first (A) as months from

Table 3. Survival (mo) of Responding *v* Nonresponding Patients*

	Responders (CR + PR + MR; n = 7)	Nonresponders (n = 40)	*P* Value†
A			
Mean ± SE	39 ± 18	21 ± 16	$P < .05$
Median	26	17	
B			
Mean ± SE	12 ± 13	3 ± 1	$P < .001$
Median	8	2	
C			
Mean ± SE	57+/−20	26 ± 3	$P < .001$
Median	47	21	

*(A) From diagnosis of ovarian cancer to study entry; (B) from failure of megestrol to death or last follow-up; (C) from diagnosis of ovarian cancer to death or last follow-up.

†Unpaired *t* test, responding *v* nonresponding patients.

CR, complete response; PR, partial response; MR, minor response.

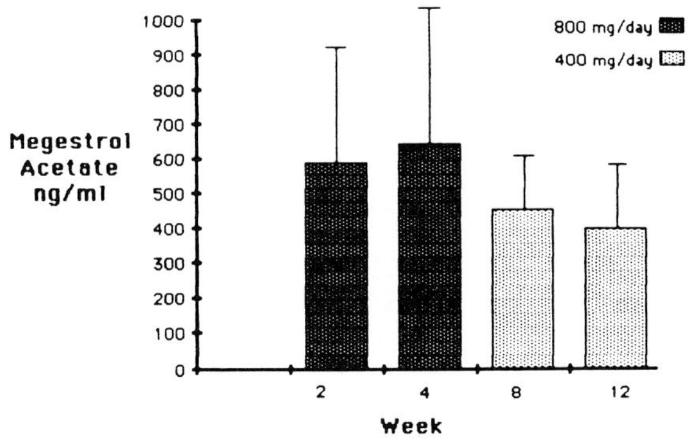

Fig 1. Serum levels of megestrol acetate during the first 3 months of therapy.

diagnosis to study entry, then (B) as survival after failure of megestrol, and finally (C) as total survival from diagnosis of ovarian cancer to death or last follow-up. By every measure, patients who achieved a response (complete, partial, or minor) had significantly longer survivals, even excluding the period of megestrol therapy (A and B). Thus, although response was not well predicted by histologic grade, patients who responded appeared to have a more indolent natural history of their disease.

Toxicities

The major side effect of high doses of megestrol acetate was increased appetite, with a gain in body weight of 10 to 20 kg in five patients and 5 to 10 kg in eight patients. This increase in appetite was not generally regarded as objectionable. Most patients reported an improved sense of well-being while receiving megestrol.

Elevated liver function tests (serum transaminase and alkaline phosphatase) developed in one patient but normalized after cessation of megestrol. This patient also developed dependent edema and a large increase in body weight during 3 months of treatment and refused to continue megestrol despite a minor regression of her tumor mass.

One patient developed a thromboembolism to her popliteal artery, which required operative removal. This was the only thromboembolic event noted in these 47 patients during high-dose megestrol therapy and cannot definitely be attributed to the drug rather than to the underlying malignancy.

Table 4. Feedback Inhibition of Serum Follicle-Stimulating Hormone (FSH) and Luteinizing Hormone (LH) Levels by Megestrol Acetate

	Baseline (mean ± SD; n = 7)	During Megestrol Acetate Therapy* (mean ± SD; n = 40)
Serum FSH, ImU/mL	121 ± 28	28 ± 18†
Serum LH, ImU/mL	88 ± 16	15 ± 10†

*Pooled data at 4 and 8 weeks.

†Significantly lower than baseline, $P < .001$.

Serum CA-125 Levels

Serum CA-125 levels were above the upper limit of normal (35 units/mL) in 32 of 34 patients (94%) at the time of study entry. In 11 of 34 patients (32%), the serum CA-125 was greater than 1,000 units/mL. Serial measurements were made in only seven patients but correlated well with clinical status in two patients with remissions and in four of five patients with tumor progression. In two patients with partial remissions, the CA-125 decreased in one case from 528 to 128 units/mL, and in the other case, from 3,749 to 2,660 units/mL.

Serum Megestrol Acetate Levels

Megestrol acetate levels were measured in the sera of 20 patients and are shown in Fig 1. Blood samples were drawn within a few hours of a drug dose. Since the elimination half-life of megestrol acetate is 30 to 40 hours,[17] these samples can be considered to represent steady-state levels of the drug. Two weeks after initiation of treatment, the mean serum megestrol acetate concentration was 562 ng/mL (SD = 352 ng/mL, n = 20). At 4 weeks, on a dose of 800 mg/d the mean drug level was 601 ng/mL (SD = 417 ng/mL, n = 15). The dose was reduced to 400 mg/d after the first month on study. Megestrol acetate levels at 8 weeks fell to 455 ng/mL (SD = 174 ng/mL, n = 8) and to 344 ng/mL at 12 weeks (SD = 242 ng/mL, n = 7). Only one patient had undetectable drug levels while on study, indicating excellent compliance for the group as a whole, although bioavailability may have been affected in some of these patients because of intermittent intestinal obstructions due to tumor and adhesions. There was wide variability in serum megestrol levels from patient to patient, the range at 4 weeks being 152 to 1,389 ng/mL.

Serum FSH and LH Levels

Marked decreases in serum FSH and LH levels were observed during megestrol therapy, compared with baseline levels (Table 4). There were no significant differences in FSH and LH levels at 4 *v* 8 weeks of megestrol therapy; therefore, these data were pooled.

In Vitro Clonogenic Assays

Ascites was available from six patients enrolled in the high-dose megestrol clinical protocol, and adequate plating efficiency (greater than 0.01%) was achieved in five of these. Tumor specimens, 12 of which grew in vitro, were obtained from an additional 17 patients with ovarian carcinoma not registered on this protocol. A greater than 30% inhibition of tumor colony formation by megestrol acetate at 1 μg/mL was observed in only one (6%) of 17 specimens, which was obtained from a patient who did not respond to megestrol in vivo. At a megestrol acetate concentration of 10 μg/mL, not achievable in vivo, inhibition of colony formation was observed in two specimens, and stimulation in one.

DISCUSSION

Hormonal factors have been implicated in several aspects of the epidemiology and biology of the common epithelial cancers of the ovary.[18] There is an increased risk for the development of ovarian carcinomas in women who are nulliparous or infertile,[18,19] while both multiparity and oral contraceptive use are associated with a decreased risk.[20] Most ovarian carcinomas (50% to 75%) contain estrogen or progesterone receptors, or both.[21-29] Thus it is not surprising that these tumors are occasionally responsive to various hormonal therapies, including progestins, antiestrogens, and gonadotropin antagonists.[1-12,18,30-32]

The results with progestin therapy of ovarian carcinomas from several studies are summarized in Table 5. Remission rates in these reports range from 0% to 65%.[1-12] Differences in response criteria and extent of previous treatments may account for some of the variation in response rates in these reports, several of which stated that occasional patients with advanced ovarian carcinoma obtained long-lasting (greater than 1 year) remission with progestin therapy.

We were particularly interested in the recent series from Geisler,[1,2] which reported a 45% rate of remission, including several complete responses in patients treated with high doses of megestrol acetate. The response rate in our study (8%, partial plus complete, and an additional 6% minor remissions) is considerably lower than that of the previous report. A major difference between our patients and those of Geisler was the extent of previous cytotoxic therapy. The large majority of our patients received combination chemotherapy with three or four agents, whereas most patients in Geisler's series were treated with a single alkylating agent prior to megestrol.[1,2] Both patients in our series previously treated with a single agent obtained tumor regressions with megestrol (one partial and one minor). Other recent studies of progestin therapy in

Table 5. Progestin Therapy of Ovarian Carcinoma: Summary of Literature

Drug	No. of Patients	No. of Responses (%)	Response Duration (mo)	References
Megestrol acetate	47	4 (8)	4–18	This study
Megestrol acetate	22	10 (45)	4–65+	1, 2
Medroxyprogesterone	41	1 (2)	5	12
Medroxyprogesterone	27	1 (4)	5	10
Medroxyprogesterone	19	0	—	9
Medroxyprogesterone	19	1 (5)	4	8
Dehydro-dimethyl progesterone	9	2 (22)	30, 40	7
Hydroxyprogesterone	23	15 (65)	—	6
Hydroxyprogesterone	11	1 (9)	18+	5
Hydroxyprogesterone	6	1 (17)	3	4
Hydroxyprogesterone	10	4 (40)	—	3
Total	234	40 (17)		

patients who had extensive prior chemotherapy also report a low response rate (Table 5).[9,10,12] This suggests that cross-resistance may exist between steroidal hormones and certain cytotoxic drugs.

There was no correlation of the responses in our patients with histologic type or grade. However, it should be noted that none of the 33 tumors that were histologically graded were well differentiated, and two thirds were poorly differentiated. Estrogen and progesterone receptor data were not available for the tumors in our study. Since the majority of these tumors would be expected to be receptor positive and only a small fraction of patients obtained a remission, a prospective correlation of receptor status and response would require large numbers of patients.

The survival of patients who responded to megestrol was longer than survival of nonresponding patients, even after failure of megestrol and before study entry (Table 3, A and B). Thus, the prolonged survival of these responding patients is in large part due to a more indolent natural history of their cancers.

The major side effects of high-dose megestrol in this trial were increased appetite and weight gain, which were acceptable to the vast majority of patients. In fact, these side effects were considered beneficial by some patients and might counteract some of the deleterious effects of cytotoxic drugs if megestrol acetate were administered with combination chemotherapy. A controlled trial of chemotherapy alone *v* chemotherapy plus megestrol as first-line therapy of advanced ovarian carcinoma would be of interest. The combination of a progestin with cyclophosphamide as first-line therapy has been reported to produce a 76% remission rate in 54 patients with ovarian carcinomas.[33]

We observed little direct effect of megestrol acetate on ovarian tumor colony formation in vitro. Others have observed direct inhibition by both progestins and antiestrogens on ovarian carcinomas in clonogenic assays.[29] The feedback inhibition by megestrol acetate of FSH and LH may be of therapeutic relevance in light of the recent report of a remission induced by the LH-RH agonist *D*-Trp-6-LH-RH in a patient with ovarian carcinoma.[32] The mechanism of action of megestrol in ovarian carcinomas may involve both direct inhibition of tumor cell growth and inhibition of gonadotropin production.

We conclude that megestrol acetate has modest but definite palliative activity in patients with advanced ovarian carcinomas in whom chemotherapy has failed. Future clinical trials that should be considered include correlations of response with hormone receptor status, determination of the optimal dose of megestrol, and its addition to initial combination chemotherapy.

ACKNOWLEDGMENT

We thank John Hannigan of NCOG for his statistical advice, the staff of NCOG for their support of this study, and Carolyn Wells for preparation of the manuscript.

REFERENCES

1. Geisler HE: Megestrol acetate for the palliation of advanced ovarian carcinoma. Obstet Gynecol 61:95–98, 1983

2. Geisler H: The use of high-dose megestrol acetate in the treatment of ovarian adenocarcinoma. Semin Oncol 11:20–22, 1985

3. Jolles B: Progesterone in the treatment of advanced malignant tumors of breast, ovary, and uterus. Br J Cancer 16:209–221, 1962

4. Varga A, Henriksen E: Effect of 17-alpha-hydroxyprogesterone-17-n-caproate on various pelvic malignancies. Obstet Gynecol 23:51–62, 1964

5. Kaufman RJ: Management of advanced ovarian carcinoma. Med Clin North Am 50:834–856, 1966

6. Ward HW: Progestogen therapy for ovarian carcinoma. J Obstet Gynecol 79:555–559, 1972

7. Malkasian GD Jr, Decker DG, Jorgenson EO, et al: 6-Dehydro-6,17-alpha-dimethyl-progesterone (NSC-123018) for the treatment of metastatic and recurrent ovarian carcinoma. Cancer Chemother Rep 57:241–242, 1973

8. Malkasian GD Jr, Decker DG, Jorgenson EO, et al: Medroxyprogesterone acetate for the treatment of metastatic and recurrent ovarian carcinoma. Cancer Treat Rep 61:913–914, 1977

9. Slayton RE, Pagano M, Creech RH: Progestin therapy for advanced ovarian cancer: A phase II Eastern Cooperative Oncology Group trial. Cancer Treat Rep 65:895–896, 1981

10. Aabo K, Pedersen AG, Hald I, et al: High-dose medroxyprogesterone acetate (MPA) in advanced chemotherapy-resistant ovarian carcinoma: A phase II study. Cancer Treat Rep 66:407–408, 1982

11. Kauppila A: Progestin therapy of endometrial, breast and ovarian carcinoma. Obstet Gynecol 63:441–450, 1984

12. Hamerlynck JVThH, Maskens AP, Mangioni C, et al: Phase II trial of medroxyprogesterone acetate in advanced

ovarian cancer: An EORTC gynecological cancer cooperative group study. Gynecol Oncol 22:313–316, 1985

13. Gaver RC, Movahhed HS, Farmen RH, et al: Liquid chromatographic procedure for the quantitative analysis of megestrol acetate in human plasma. J Pharm Sci 74:664–667, 1985

14. Bast RC, Klug TL, St John E, et al: A radioimmunoassay using a monoclonal antibody to monitor the course of epithelial ovarian cancer. N Engl J Med 309:883–888, 1983

15. Klug TL, Bast RC Jr, Niloff JM, et al: Monoclonal antibody immunoradiometric assay for an antigenic determinant (CA 125) associated with human epithelial ovarian carcinomas. Cancer Res 44:1048–1053, 1984

16. MacKintosh FR, Evans TL, Sikic BI: Methodologic problems in clonogenic assays of spontaneous human tumors. Cancer Chemother Pharmacol 6:205–210, 1981

17. Gaver RC, Pittman KA, Reilly CM, et al: Bioequivalence evaluation of new megestrol acetate formulations in humans. Semin Oncol 12:17–19, 1985

18. Waxman J: Hormonal aspects of ovarian malignancy. J R Soc Med 77:172–175, 1984

19. Casagrande JT, Pike MC, Ross RK, et al: "Incessant ovulation" and ovarian cancer. Lancet 2:170–173, 1979

20. Cramer DW, Hutchinson GB, Welck WR, et al: Factors affecting the association of oral contraceptives and ovarian cancer. N Engl J Med 307:1047–1052, 1982

21. Friberg LG, Kullander S, Persijn JP, et al: On receptors for estrogens (E_2) and androgens (DHT) in human endometrial carcinoma and ovarian tumours. Acta Obstet Gynecol Scand 57:261–264, 1978

22. Holt JA, Caputo TA, Kelly KM, et al: Estrogen and progestin binding in cytosols of ovarian adenocarcinomas. Obstet Gynecol 53:50–58, 1979

23. Galli MC, De Giovanni C, Nicoletti G, et al: The occurrence of multiple steroid hormone receptors in disease-free and neoplastic human ovary. Cancer 47:1297–1302, 1981

24. Farley AL, O'Brien T, Moyer D, et al: The detection of estrogen receptors in gynecologic tumors using immunoperoxidase and the dextran-coated charcoal assay. Cancer 49:2153–2160, 1982

25. Gronroos M, Kangas L, Maenpaa J, et al: Steroid receptors and response of ovarian cancer to hormones in vitro. Br J Obstet Gynaecol 91:472–478, 1984

26. Quinn MA: Is endocrine status relevant to treatment planning in patients with gynaecological cancer? Aust NZ J Obstet Gynaecol 24:153–157, 1984

27. Lantta M: Estradiol and progesterone receptors in normal ovary and ovarian tumors. Acta Obstet Gynecol Scand 63:497–503, 1984

28. Schwartz PA, Merino MJ, Livolsi VA, et al: Histopathologic correlations of estrogen and progestin receptor protein in epithelial ovarian carcinomas. Obstet Gynecol 66:428–433, 1985

29. Runge HM, Teufel G, Neulen J, et al: In vitro responsiveness of ovarian epithelial carcinomas to endocrine therapy. Cancer Chemother Pharmacol 16:58–63, 1986

30. Myers AM, Moore GE, Major FJ: Advanced ovarian carcinoma: Response to antiestrogen therapy. Cancer 48:2368–2370, 1981

31. Shirey DR, Kavanagh JJ Jr, Gershenson DM, et al: Tamoxifen therapy of epithelial ovarian cancer. Obstet Gynecol 66:575–578, 1985

32. Parmar H, Nicoli J, Stockdale A, et al: Advanced ovarian carcinoma: Response to the agonist D-Trp-6-LHRH. Cancer Treat Rep 69:1341, 1985

33. Guthrie D: The treatment of advanced cystadenocarcinoma of the ovary with gestronol and continuous oral cyclophosphamide. Br J Obstet Gynaecol 86:497–500, 1979

Hormonal Therapy for Lesions of the Endometrium

David Gal

Megestrol acetate, 20 to 40 mg/d, was given continuously to 70 postmenopausal women with a variety of endometrial hyperplastic changes. All patients were followed up with periodic endometrial biopsies. The study was conducted for 14 years with mean patient follow-up of more than 5 years. In 65 patients (93%), surgery was avoided due to this protocol. No patient developed endometrial carcinoma, and there were no major side effects. This regimen proved to be most effective in preventing hysterectomy in postmenopausal patients who presented with surgical risk factors and endometrial hyperplasia.

ENDOMETRIAL HYPERPLASIA has long been recognized as a cancer precursor. In 1947, Gusberg[1] found that 18% of patients with all types of endometrial hyperplasia developed carcinoma within 1 to 30 years after the inital diagnosis. He was also the first to suggest a grading system for endometrial hyperplasia. Others[2–6] reported that 26% to 75% of patients with various grades of endometrial hyperplasia may develop carcinoma within months or up to 20 years from the initial diagnosis. The higher the grade of endometrial hyperplasia, the higher the percentage of patients who develop endometrial cancer and the shorter the transition time. Vellios[7] and others suggest that only few patients with cystic hyperplasia will progress to develop carcinoma. They feel that most lesions of cystic hyperplasia will revert spontaneously and require no treatment. Many gynecologists suggest that abdominal hysterectomy should be the treatment of choice for other than cystic endometrial hyperplasia (ie, adenomatous, atypical, and carcinoma in situ) in the postmenopausal patient.

However, many postmenopausal women with endometrial hyperplasia present with risk factors (ie, diabetes, cardiopathy, hepatic disease, and morbid obesity) which make surgery hazardous.

Table 1. Distribution of Diagnoses*

	No. of Patients
Adenomatous hyperplasia (with or without cystic changes)	38
Atypical hyperplasia	26
Carcinoma in situ	6

*The diagnostic classification of Vellios[7] was used in all cases.

Table 2. Medical Disorders in 70 Patients With Endometrial Hyperplasia

Disorder	No. of Patients
Cardiac	28
Diabetes	19
Hypertension	14
Endocrinopathy	4
Gastrointestinal	5
Epilepsy	2
Asthma	4
Lupus erythematosus	2
Osteoarthritis	4
Chronic anemia	3
Psychosis	3
Obesity (80–190 kg)	51

Therefore a medical alternative to the surgical approach is desired.

Progestins have been used successfully in the treatment of endometrial cancer for more than 30 years. Various protocols of therapy with different progestative agents have been advocated.[8,9] However, many of these studies have been criticized because of the small number of patients, short duration of treatment, and short periods of follow-up observation.

We previously presented evidence that megestrol acetate (Megace, Bristol-Myers Oncology Division, Evansville, IN) used continuously (40 mg/d) is efficacious in controlling endometrial hyperplasia and may prevent surgery in many patients with high-risk factors.[10] We have since decreased the amount of megestrol acetate to 20 mg/d and obtained similar results. Our experience with megestrol acetate for endometrial hyperplasia is presented.

METHODS

Seventy postmenopausal women who had a histologic diagnosis of endometrial hyperplasia, excluding those with cystic hyperplasia (Table 1), and who had medical disorders

From the Department of Obstetrics and Gynecology B, Rambam Hospital Medical Center, Technion School of Medicine, Haifa, Israel.

Address reprint requests to David Gal, MD, Department of Obstetrics and Gynecology B, Technion School of Medicine, Rambam Hospital Medical Center, Haifa, Israel.

0093–7754/86/1304–4004$05.00/0

Table 3. Study Methods (1971–1985)

1. Postmenopausal with endometrial hyperplasia and poor surgical risk
2. Megestrol acetate (Megace) 20 mg b.i.d., daily, continuously*
3. 3 mo reexaminations
4. Endometrial biopsy q 6 mo
5. Abnormal bleeding or stopped therapy—endometrial biopsy
6. Inadequate response or persistent bleeding—total abdominal hysterectomy and bilateral salpingo-oophorectomy

*From 1981, only 10 mg megestrol acetate b.i.d.

Table 4. Weight of Patients

Diagnosis	No. of Patients	Mean (kg)	Range (kg)
Adenomatous	38	114	54–196
Atypical	26	101	60–156
Carcinoma in situ	6	88	68–107
All groups	70	104	54–196

which made surgey hazardous (Table 2), were offered continuous therapy with megestrol acetate according to our protocol (Table 3). During the last 4 years of the study, 18 patients received only 20 mg/d of megestrol acetate. In cases of uterine bleeding or recurrence of the hyperplasia according to the biopsy specimen, patients were hospitalized and underwent formal fractional curettage of the uterine cavity. If endometrial hyperplasia persisted or progressed beyond the original or last biopsy, a hysterectomy was recommended. The distribution of patient weight according to degree of hyperplasia is presented in Table 4.

All histologic diagnoses were based on the most significant change observed as per the classification of Vellios.[7]

RESULTS

The study was conducted over a period of 14 years, with mean follow-up for patients in each hyperplasia group of more than 5 years (Table 5).

Patient compliance was excellent. No patient discontinued follow-up. There were seven patients who temporarily discontinued the megestrol acetate therapy. They had recurrent bleeding ten to 18 months after discontinuation of megestrol acetate, and therefore underwent a repeat endometrial biopsy, which showed a recurrent state of hyperplasia (Table 6). These patients were reinitiated on megestrol acetate therapy and had nonhyperplastic endometrial biopsies thereafter.

The effectiveness of megestrol acetate was evaluated by endometrial biopsies every 6 months, the results of which are presented in Table 7. Five women had persistent or progressive hyperplasia of the endometrium. All five underwent hysterectomy and bilateral salpingo-oophorectomy. None had invasive carcinoma of the endometrium. The histologic evaluation of the surgical specimens was not different from the diagnosis obtained by endometrial biopsy prior to surgery in any of these patients.

Megestrol acetate was well tolerated, with only occasional complaints of mild nausea, which was controlled with change of diet or antiemetics. None of the 18 patients who received 10 mg of megestrol acetate twice daily (as of 1981) had any complaints.

Eight patients died of intercurrent disease while under our surveillance. No endometrial pathology was found at autopsy of five of these patients. No autopsy was permitted on the other three.

The results of this study are summarized in Table 8. In 65 (93%) of 70 patients, megestrol acetate satisfactorily controlled endometrial hyperplasia and prevented the need for hazardous surgery. There were no major side effects with this regimen, and no patient developed endometrial adenocarcinoma during the study.

DISCUSSION

Progestins are used widely for various carcinomas of the genital tract.[11–13] Kistner[14] has used progestins successfully to treat endometrial

Table 5. Length of Therapy With Megestrol Acetate

Type of Hyperplasia	No. of Patients	Length of Therapy (mo)		
		Mean	SD*	Range
Adenomatous hyperplasia	38	62	23	32–142
Atypical hyperplasia	6	65	25	29–128
Adenocarcinoma in situ	6	88	25	26–150
All groups	70	69	29	26–150

*SD, standard deviation.

Table 6. Recurrence of Hyperplasia*

Grade of Initial Hyperplasia (No. of Patients)	Grade of Recurrent Hyperplasia (No. of Women)		
	Adenomatous	Atypical	CIS
Adenomatous (5)	5	—	—
Atypical (2)	1	1	—

*Recurrence was 10 to 18 months from discontinuation of megestrol acetate; all patients responded to reinitiation of megestrol acetate and required no surgery.

CIS, carcinoma in situ.

Table 7. Status of Endometrium After Megestrol Acetate Therapy

Pretreatment Histology	No. of Patients	Histology During Therapy		
		Nonhyper-plastic	Worse	Same
Adenomatous hyperplasia	38	35	2	1
Atypical hyperplasia	26	25	0	1
Carcinoma in situ	6	5	0	1

hyperplasia. Wentz[8] used progestins for only 6 weeks to control endometrial hyperplasia; however, his observation period was too short to conclude that the disease was controlled. Eichner and Abellera[9] found that the disease progressed or recurred when progestin therapy was discontinued. Although the etiology of endometrial hyperplasia is not fully understood, endometrial exposure to unopposed estrogen is usually blamed. The source of these estrogens in most postmenopausal women is adipose tissue.[15] Thus, it makes sense to continue progestin therapy indefinitely, since the treatment is aimed at opposing the estrogenic effect at the level of the endometrium and does not abolish the continuous extraglandular estrogen production.

There are several ways by which progestins oppose the mitogenic stimuli of estrogen (Table 9). Janne et al[16] found that hyperplastic endometrium contained more progesterone receptors than carcinomatous, proliferative, or secretory endometrium. Progesterone receptors seem to be mandatory for progestin action; however, their existence is dependent on intracellular estrogen action. One of the main effects of progestin is to decrease the cellular content of estrogen receptors and thus their intracellular action. There is a theory that intracellular progesterone receptors decrease after short exposure to progestin and, therefore, their effectiveness diminishes. Our results disprove that theory: Throughout many years of treatment and follow-up, the progesterone effect was maintained, as evidenced by repeated biopsies.

Progestins affect estrogen metabolism via two other pathways. They increase the rates of conversion of 17-beta estradiol to the less potent estrone[17] and stimulate inactivation of estrogen through sulfurylation.[18]

In summary, these results show that for postmenopausal patients with endometrial hyperplasia and medical contraindications for surgery, megestrol acetate is an effective and safe alternate management approach.

Table 8. Summary of Results

	No. of Pts	(%)
Patients studied	70	100
Adequate response	65	93
Inadequate response (hysterectomy)	5	7
Developed adenocarcinoma	0	0
Major side effects	0	0

Table 9. Cytochemical Effects of Progestins

1. Decrease of available estrogen receptors
2. Induction of estradiol dehydrogenase ($E_2 \longrightarrow E_1$)
3. Induction of estradiol sulfurylation
4. Secretory histology (giant mitochondria, basal glycogen, etc)

REFERENCES

1. Gusberg SB: Precursors of corpus carcinoma: Estrogens and adenomatous hyperplasia. Am J Obstet Gynecol 54:905–927, 1947

2. Campbell PE, Barter RA: The significance of atypical endometrial hyperplasia. J Obstet Gynecol Br Commonw 68:668–672, 1961

3. Wentz WB: Treatment of persistent endometrial hyperplasia with progestin. Am J Obstet Gynecol 96:999–1004, 1966

4. Gusberg SB, Chen SY, Cohen CJ: Endometrial cancer: Factors influencing the choice of treatment. Gynecol Oncol 2:308–321, 1974

5. Hall KV: Irregular hyperplasia of the endometrium. Acta Obstet Gynecol Scand 36:306–321, 1957

6. Sherman AI, Brown S: The precursors of endometrial carcinoma. Am J Obstet Gynecol 135:947–954, 1979

7. Vellios F: Endometrial hyperplasia and carcinoma in situ. Gynecol Oncol 2:152–161, 1974

8. Wentz WB: Effect of a progestational agent on endometrial hyperplasia and endometrial cancer. Obstet Gynecol 24:370–375, 1964

9. Eichner E, Abellera M: Endometrial hyperplasia treated by progestins. Obstet Gynecol 38:739–742, 1971

10. Gal D, Edman CD, Vellios F, et al: Long term effect of

megestrol acetate in the treatment of endometrial hyperplasia. Am J Obstet Gynecol 146:316–322, 1983

11. Geisler EH: The use of high dose megestrol acetate in the treatment of ovarian adenocarcinoma. Semin Oncol 12:20–28, 1985 (suppl 1)

12. Gusberg SB: Hormone-dependence of endometrial cancer. Obstet Gynecol 30:287, 1967

13. Bonte J: Medroxy progesterone in the management of primary and recurrent metastatic uterine adenocarcinoma. Acta Obstet Gynecol Scand 51:21–43, 1972 (suppl)

14. Kistner RW: Histological effects of progestins on hyperplasia and carcinoma in situ of the endometrium. Cancer 12:1106–1110, 1959

15. Macdonald PC, Edman CD, Hemsell DL, et al: Effect of obesity on conversion of plasma androstenedione to estrone in postmenopausal women with and without endometrial cancer. Am J Obstet Gynecol 130:448–465, 1978

16. Janne O, Kauppila A, Kontula K, et al: Female sex steroid receptors in normal, hyperplastic and carcinomatous endometrium. The relationship to serum steroid hormones and gonadotropins and changes during medroxyprogesterone acetate administration. Int J Cancer 24:545–554, 1979

17. Tseng L, Gurpide E: Induction of human endometrial estradiol dehydrogenase by progestins. Endocrinology, 97:825–833, 1975

18. Pack PB, Tovar R, Booth E, et al: The cyclic relationships of estrogen sulfurilation to the nuclear receptor level in human endometrial curettings. J Clin Endocrinol Metab 48:420–434, 1979

Appetite Stimulation With Megestrol Acetate in Cachectic Cancer Patients

N. Simon Tchekmedyian, Nancy Tait, Mark Moody, F. Anthony Greco, and Joseph Aisner

Cachexia is often a severe problem in the management of cancer and other illnesses because it adds to the morbidity of the underlying disease and complicates its treatment. Megestrol acetate has been observed anecdotally to produce weight gain. A review of our experience, and our ongoing phase I/II study of high-dose megestrol acetate for breast cancer, revealed that weight gain occurred in nearly one third (27%) of patients at conventional doses (160 mg/d), and that a marked weight gain (median, 5.1 kg; range, 0.9 to 20.1 kg) occurred in 27 of 28 patients with breast cancer during treatment with high doses of megestrol acetate. Subjective improvement in appetite occurred in most patients at low doses and in most patients at high doses. Further, nearly one half (48%) of patients at conventional doses and virtually all patients at high doses experienced an increased sense of well-being. Our data suggest that megestrol acetate has a potential role in producing subjective improvement, sense of well-being, and increase in appetite and weight, and that the effect may be dose related. Further research is necessary to understand the mechanism of appetite stimulation and/or anabolic effect.

CANCER CACHEXIA is a complex problem facing both patients and physicians. The loss of appetite and severe wasting, coupled with catabolic activities, deplete body stores of essential compounds, including proteins, carbohydrates, and caloric reserves. The result is muscle wasting, weakness, and progressive weight loss.[1,2] This catabolic process further lowers tolerance to infections, slows healing, and aggravates the toxicities of many treatments. The cachectic state usually occurs in the setting of advancing disease and is thus a severe complication in the overall management of the patient. Furthermore, the decrease in appetite, wasting, and associated weakness produce considerable stress to both patients and their families, physically and emotionally.

The etiology of the cachexia associated with cancer is probably multifactorial, and to a great extent is still obscure. Loss of appetite with decreased caloric intake,[3] increase of the basal metabolic rate,[4] and decreased efficiency in the utilization of energy compounds[5] have been postulated as contributing factors. Recently, metabolic effects of tumor-related products, such as cachectin or tumor necrosis factor, have been added to the list of contributing etiological agents.[6,7] Physical obstruction to food ingestion is an important factor in some diseases; however, in most cases the weight loss is associated with anorexia in an ever-increasing process of undernutrition and loss of tissue mass.

Weight loss and appetite tend to improve with the control of the underlying process. Therefore, the primary approach to treatment of cancer cachexia is to attempt to treat the underlying disease. Many patients, however, have refractory underlying illness, so that anorexia and weight loss continue unabated despite the use of all therapeutic modalities. An approach to reversal of cachexia is thus potentially important for the quality of survival, even in the absence of control of the underlying disease process.

The reversal of cachexia, however, can be a significant problem. Past attempts to remedy undernutrition in cancer patients have focused on either the use of anabolic steroids, such as androgens, or alimentation, either enteral or parenteral.[8–10] Prospective studies in responsive diseases, such as small-cell lung cancer, have not demonstrated an effective role for hyperalimentation.[8,9,11] In general, attempts at alimentation or hyperalimentation have met with some success, ie, improvement of weight status and catabolic state, when the patient had a physical barrier to food ingestion (for example, patients with head and neck cancer or esophageal cancer, in whom chewing or swallowing was difficult). In cases in which no such barrier existed, there has been no conclusive evidence that alimentation by either enteral or parenteral route has made any significant impact on the catabolic state or the toxicity of treatment. Similarly, there is no con-

---

From the Division of Medical Oncology, University of Maryland Cancer Center, Baltimore; and the Division of Medical Oncology, Vanderbilt University Cancer Center, Nashville, TN.

Address reprint requests to Joseph Aisner, MD, University of Maryland Cancer Center, 22 South Greene St, Baltimore, MD 21201.

0093-7754/86/1304-4005$05.00/0

vincing evidence that the use of anabolic steroids or androgens has been of any benefit in patients with cachexia.

Weight gain has been recognized as a side effect, frequently felt to be undesirable, of megestrol acetate in multiple studies, including studies of breast cancer, prostate cancer, and others.[12-16] In addition, our anecdotal experience suggested an increased sense of well-being, an increase in appetite, and an increase in weight for patients treated with megestrol acetate at conventional and higher doses. Pronounced appetite stimulation and weight gain were seen in a phase I/II study of high-dose megestrol acetate (Megace, Bristol-Myers Oncology Division, Evansville, IN) for breast cancer. Both the anecdotal experience and the prospective phase I/II study were therefore reviewed to assess the degree and the rate of weight gain in order to make an assessment of the potential use of megestrol acetate to reverse or inhibit cachexia process.

METHODS

Anecdotal experience at the Vanderbilt University Cancer Center was reviewed for patients given 160 mg of megestrol acetate daily (40 mg four times daily) for the treatment of anorexia. All patients had histologically confirmed metastatic cancer refractory to conventional treatment. All had experienced greater than 10% loss of previous body weight, and all were receiving only symptomatic care (ie, the underlying cancer was not being treated). At the University of Maryland Cancer Center, patients with histologically confirmed metastatic breast carcinoma entered in a dose- and efficacy-seeking study (phase I/II) of megestrol acetate were reviewed for degree and rate of weight gain. In the high-dose study, patients with a history of thromboembolism or uncontrolled heart failure were excluded. In this study, patients were seen for an initial observation and then weekly; at each visit a history and physical examination were obtained, together with tumor measurements, body weight, and an assessment of performance status. Other tests included a complete blood count, and measurements of blood urea nitrogen and serum creatinine, serum electrolytes, serum glucose, and liver function tests (SGOT, SGPT, and alkaline phosphatase). Body weights, measured weekly, were compared with the Metropolitan Life Insurance (New York) health insurance charts and were classified according to deviations from the ideal body weights listed. Overweight was defined as >5% above ideal body weight, underweight, as >5% below ideal body weight, and normal body weight as ideal body weight ±5%. Changes in body weight were calculated from the weekly measurements.

Extent of disease was categorized according to site of involvement as either visceral disease (liver, lung, or other visceral organs) or nonvisceral disease (soft tissue, lymph nodes, pleural effusion, or bone disease). Patients were also categorized according to response to treatment as having an objective response (complete or partial response), stable disease (no progression for at least 2 months), or disease progression (>25% increase in disease or the appearance of new disease). Standard response criteria were used.

Weight changes were subjected to a linear least-squares regression analysis for the first 26 weeks of therapy.[17] Each patient contributed multiple data points, one for each weighing. Comparisons among categories described above and within subsets of the categories were accomplished by the Fisher R-to-Z comparisons of slopes of the regression equations.[17] Comparisons of the frequencies were made by Fisher's Exact Test. In the phase I/II studies patients received doses ranging from 480 to 1,600 mg/d of megestrol acetate in three or four oral daily doses (Table 1). For these studies, megestrol acetate was provided in specially prepared 160-mg tablets through the courtesy of Bristol-Myers Company.

Because of the need for serial evaluations of weight for the high-dose megestrol acetate study, all patients who received therapy for longer than 6 weeks were considered evaluable for weight gain. All patients were considered evaluable for response and toxicity, as reported in detail in a separate paper in this issue by Tchekmedyian et al.[18]

RESULTS

Thirty-three patients, as shown in Table 2, received megestrol acetate at 160 mg daily. There were 15 patients with lung cancer, ten with colon cancer, and eight with other malignancies. All patients were anorectic and had lost more than 10% of their previous body weight; all 33 were on symptomatic care alone. Among the 15 patients with lung cancer, eight (53%) had a

Table 1. Treatment Levels of High-Dose Megestrol Acetate for Breast Cancer

No. of Patients	Dose (mg/d)
3	480
3	800
3	1,280
24*	1,600

*Five patients not evaluable for weight gain: All had rapidly progressive visceral disease within the first 6 weeks of therapy.

Table 2. Anecdotal Experience With Megestrol Acetate for Weight Gain at Vanderbilt University Cancer Center

	No. of Cases (%)			
	Lung Cancer (n = 15)	Colon Cancer (n = 10)	Other Malignancies (n = 8)	Total (n = 33)
Improved sense of well-being	8 (53)	4 (40)	2 (25)	14 (42)
>2.3 kg weight gain	5 (33)	2 (20)	2 (25)	9 (27)
Sustained subjective effect (2 mo)	9 (60)	5 (50)	2 (25)	16 (48)

subjective improvement in their sense of well-being; four of ten patients with colon cancer and two of eight patients with other malignancies also experienced this improvement in sense of well-being. Five of the 15 (33%) patients with lung cancer, two of the ten (20%) with colon cancer, and two of the eight (25%) with other malignancies gained more than 2.3 kg. Thus, 27% of all the patients experienced a significant weight gain at this dose. The subjective effect was sustained for more than 2 months in nine of the 15 patients with lung cancer, five of the ten patients with colon cancer, and two of the eight patients with other malignancies.

In the dose- and efficacy-seeking trial of high-dose megestrol acetate for advanced breast cancer, 33 patients were entered on study at various dose ranges, as shown in Table 1. There were three patients treated at each of the first three dosage levels (480, 800, and 1,280 mg/d) and 24 patients were entered on 1,600 mg/d. Five of the 24 patients treated at 1,600 mg/d were not considered evaluable for weight gain because they had rapidly progressive visceral disease within the first 6 weeks of therapy. None of these patients lost weight, but there were too few weighings for meaningful analysis. Twenty-eight patients received high-dose megestrol acetate for more than 6 weeks; their characteristics are shown in Table 3. Their median age was 58 years, and they were generally ambulatory and had positive estrogen or progestrone receptors (23/28). All patients had received either hormonal therapy or chemotherapy, or both.

Weight gain from the high-dose megestrol acetate is shown according to subsets in Table 4. Twenty-seven of the 28 patients gained weight, with a median weight gain of 5.1 kg and a range of 0.9 to 20.1 kg. Since weight gain was a function of time on study, we analyzed the weight gain by time (ie, rate). For the entire population, there was a consistent time-dependent weight gain (Fig 1). Subgroup comparisons according to weight (underweight *v* overweight *v* normal weight), according to response to treatment (response, stable, or progression), and according to extent of disease (visceral and nonvisceral) are shown in Figs 2 to 4, respectively. These figures show a consistent weight gain in all patients regardless of subgroupings. There were no significant differences in the rate of weight gain between groups according to pretreatment weight or extent of disease. Patients with objective response, however, gained weight significantly faster than those with disease stabilization ($P = .002$). There were too few patients in the group with disease progression to make any statistically meaningful comparisons.

Table 3. High-Dose Megestrol Acetate for Breast Cancer: Patient Characteristics (n = 28)*

Median age (range)	58 (40–83)
Median Karnofsky performance status (%)	80 (50–100)
Estrogen or progesterone receptor	
Positive	23
Unknown	5
Prior therapy†	
Hormonal	27
Chemotherapy	18

*Includes 1 male.

†Patients may have received multiple therapies.

Table 4. Weight Gain From Megestrol Acetate According to Subsets (n = 28)

Category	Gained Weight (No.)	Median Gain (kg)	Range (kg)
All patients	28	5.1	0.9–20.1
Underweight	13	9.1	0.9–17.2
Overweight	11	5.8	2.6–6.9
Normal weight	4	4.3	0–20.1
Response	10	11.9	4.4–17.2
Stable	12	4.4	0.9–20.1
Progression	6	3.0	0–6.9
Visceral	10	5.1	0–17.2
Nonvisceral	18	5.0	2.6–20.1

DISCUSSION

These combined data show that megestrol acetate is capable of inducing weight gain in patients with advanced cancer irrespective of response to therapy or extent of disease. Used at conventional doses (160 mg/d), nearly 30% of patients who were receiving only symptomatic care achieved a weight gain of 2.3 kg (5 lb) or more; a greater percentage experienced an improved sense of well-being. Although not comparable, at higher doses, up to 1,600 mg/d, 27 of 28 patients with advanced breast cancer had a weight gain of at least 0.9 kg, with a median weight gain of 5.1 kg. The breast cancer patients were a group of patients with less advanced disease and were being actively treated for therapeutic gain. Nevertheless, the greater preponder-

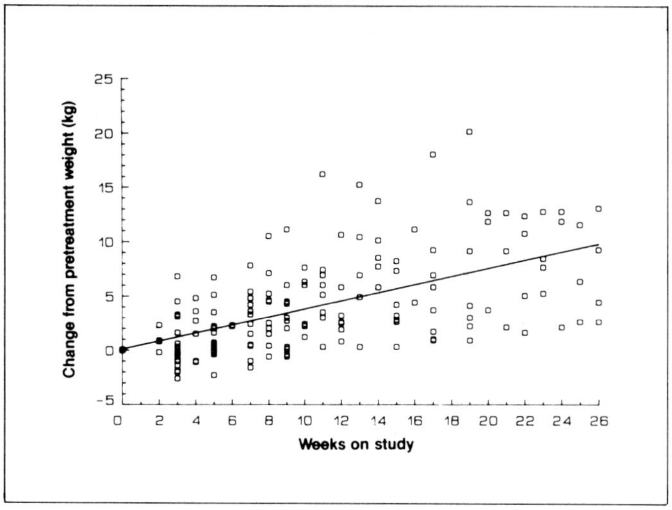

Fig 1. Least-squares regression (LSR) analysis for weight gain for all 28 patients with breast cancer during first 26 weeks of therapy with high-dose megestrol acetate. Each weighing contributed one data point. Slope y and intercept are defined by $y = mx + b$: $y = 0.371x + 0.107$. Correlation coefficient: $r = 0.63$ (196 data points).

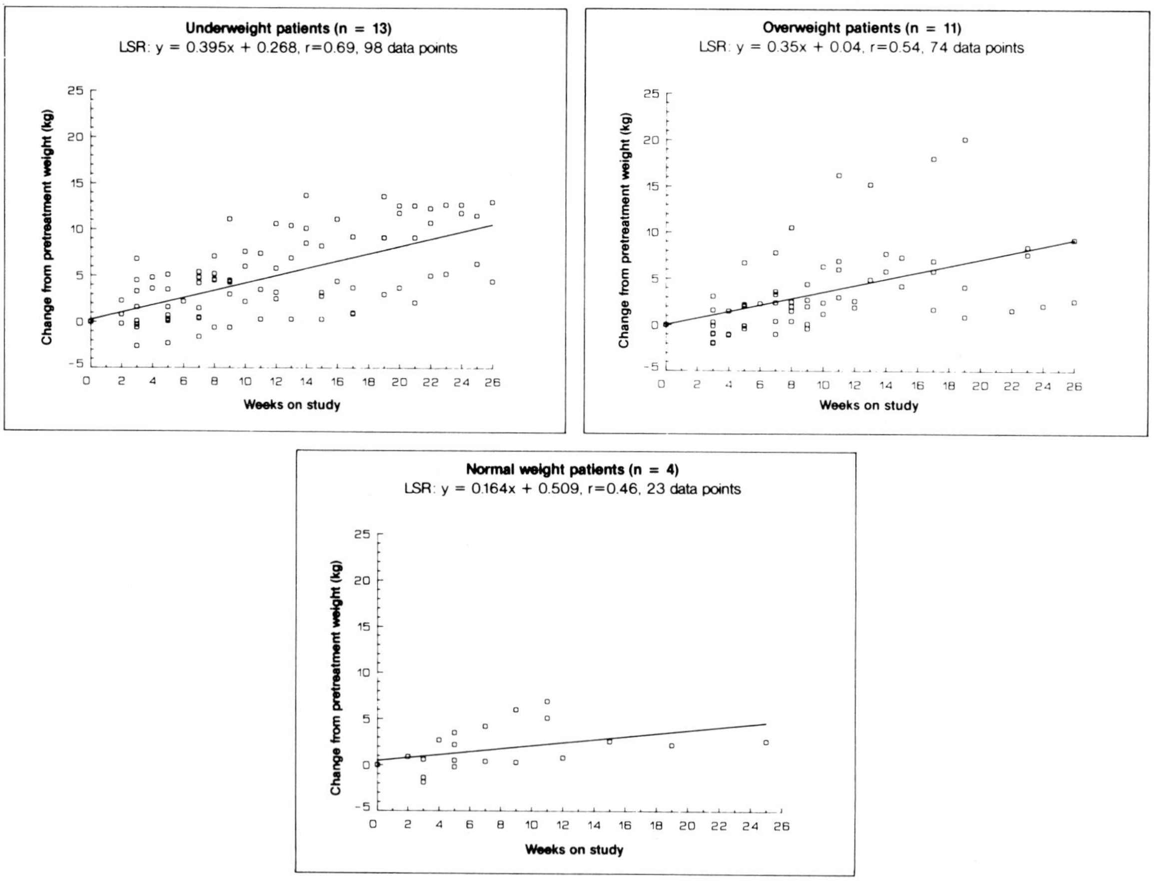

Fig 2. Least-squares regression (LSR) analysis according to pretreatment weight category subsets: underweight, overweight, and normal weight, respectively. Slope intercepts and correlation coefficients as shown.

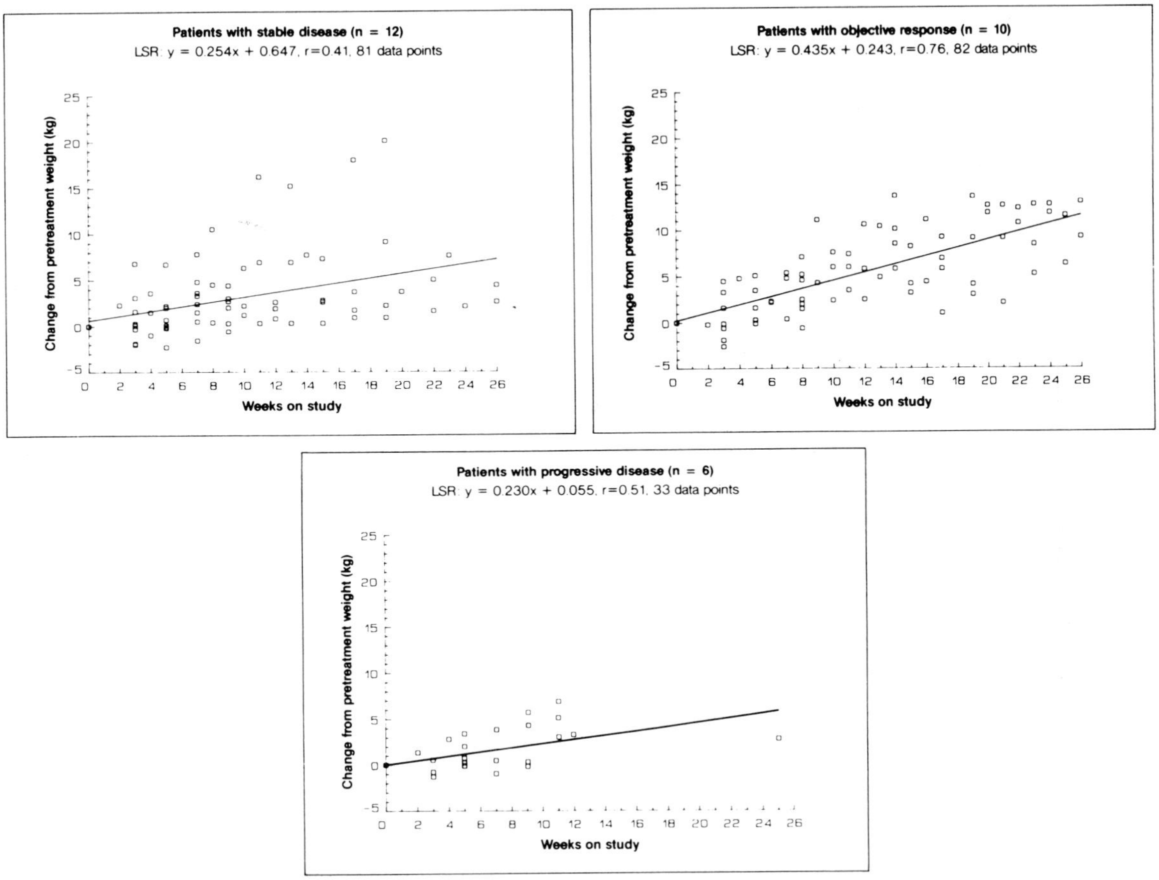

Fig 3. Least-squares regression (LSR) analysis according to response to therapy subsets: stable disease, objective response (complete + partial), and progressive disease, respectively. Slopes, intercepts, and correlation coefficients as shown.

ance of weight gain in the group treated with high-dose megestrol acetate and the striking difference (27/28 *v* 9/33) between the groups suggest a possible dose-response relationship with megestrol acetate for weight gain. There were too few patients at the intermediate doses in the dose-seeking study to ascertain whether a true dose-response relationship exists. Further studies are needed to define an optimal dose for this purpose.

Weight gain has been previously reported as a side effect in patients treated with megestrol acetate for breast cancer.[12-14] Weight gain of at least 2.7 kg was noted in 14 of 22 patients with prostate cancer when treated with 160 mg/d.[19] Weight gain of 4.5 kg or more was also reported in 30 of 54 patients receiving conventional doses of megestrol acetate.[20] This effect, however, has been dismissed as an undesirable side effect in the past and has not been sufficiently studied. The data from the current review suggest that megestrol acetate has a potential for producing subjective improvement and increase in weight as a desirable event, thereby improving the quality of survival, even when specific anticancer therapy is not administered.

Detailed metabolic studies were not done in any of the patients. Most of these patients, however, were seen by multiple physicians and nurse evaluators, whose goal was to observe complications of treatment, including edema. No patient developed cushingoid features, striae, muscle weakness, opportunistic infections, hypokalemia, or psychosis, which suggests that glucocorticoid effect and edema were minimal contributors to the weight gain. The feeling of all the

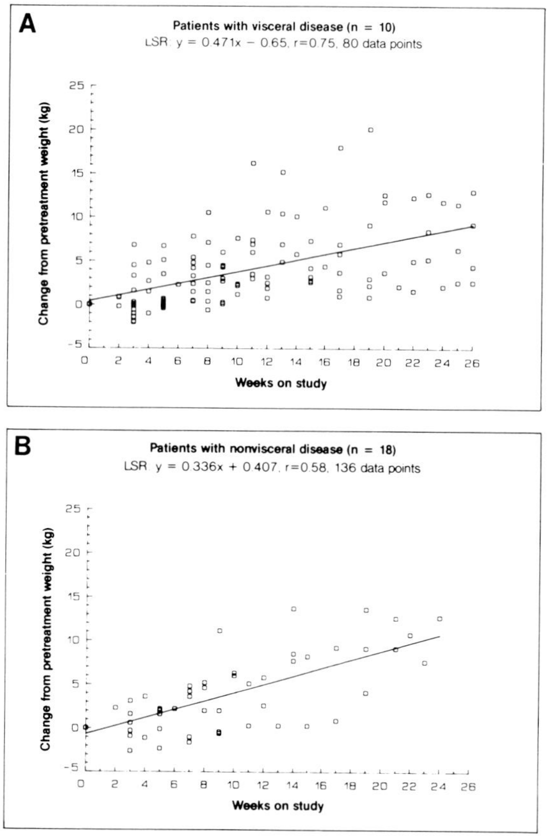

Fig 4. Least-squares regression (LSR) analysis according to the extent of disease subsets: visceral disease (A) and nonvisceral disease (B). Slopes, intercepts, and correlation coefficients as shown.

clinical evaluators was that there was a marked increase in appetite and acquisition of body mass.

The mechanisms of weight gain remain unknown. Further studies are necessary to define the frequency and magnitude of the weight gain in a patient population with nonhormonally dependent tumors, as well as to determine the mechanisms by which appetite is stimulated or catabolism is inhibited, or both. Several questions remain regarding the utilization of megestrol acetate for patients with advanced disease. First, can megestrol acetate improve appetite, and how frequently will it induce weight gain? If megestrol acetate improves symptomatic care, at what dose would it be optimally used? In order to answer these questions, we have developed a prospective, randomized, double-blind study of megestrol acetate given at 1,600 mg/d for a period of up to 6 weeks. The eligibility criteria for this study will include metastatic cancer not considered hormonally sensitive (ie, excluding breast, endometrial, and prostate cancers), anorexia, and a body weight >5% below ideal body weight, or weight loss of >10% of the previous body weight. Life expectancy must be >12 weeks, and the Karnofsky performance status >60%. Although patients might be on active therapy for cancer, they will be stratified according to whether they are receiving active therapy or supportive care only.

The evaluation of this trial will include scales for quality of life assessment, appetite scales, caloric counts, and relative change of weight. If the study shows a significant improvement in weight and quality of survival, a subsequent study will be planned to analyze the minimal dose by which these parameters might be obtained. The potential practical and theoretical implications of the answers to these questions should stimulate further basic and clinical research on weight control and appetite stimulation.

REFERENCES

1. Nixon D, Heymsfield SB, Cohen AE, et al: Protein-calorie undernutrition in hospitalized cancer patients. Am J Med 68:683–690, 1980

2. Brennan MF, Burt ME: Nitrogen metabolism in cancer patients. Cancer Treat Rep 65:65–77, 1981 (suppl)

3. DeWys WD: Anorexia as a general effect of cancer. Cancer 43:2013–2019, 1979

4. Knox LS, Crosby LO, Feurer ID, et al: Energy expenditure in malnourished cancer patients. Ann Surg 197:152–162, 1983

5. Young VR: Energy metabolism and requirements in the cancer patient. Cancer Res 37:2336–2347, 1977

6. [Editorial]: Cachectin. Lancet 2:312–313, 1985

7. Peutler B, Greenwald D, Hulmes JD, et al: Identity of tumor necrosis factor and the macrophage-secreted factor cachectin. Nature 316:352–354, 1985

8. Brennan MF: Total parenteral nutrition in the cancer patient. N Engl J Med 305:375–382, 1981

9. Burt ME, Gorschboth CM, Brennan MF: A controlled prospective, randomized trial evaluating the metabolic effects of enteral and parenteral nutrition in the cancer patient. Cancer 49:1092–1105, 1982

10. Greenspan EM: Hormone anabolic mineral nutritional support (HAMN), in: Innovative Cancer Chemotherapy for Tommorrow. New York, The Chemotherapy Foundation, 1982, p 98 (abstr)

11. Clamon GH, Feld R, Evans WK, et al: Effect of adjuvant central IV hyperalimentation on the survival and

response to treatment of patients with small cell lung cancer: A randomized trial. Cancer Treat Rep 69:167–177, 1985

12. Ross MB, Buzdar AU, Blumenschein GR: Treatment of advanced breast cancer with megestrol acetate after therapy with tamoxifen. Cancer 49:413–417, 1982

13. Alexieva-Figusch J, Van Glise HA, Hop WC, et al: Progestin therapy in advanced breast cancer: Megestrol acetate—An evaluation of 160 treated cases. Cancer 46:2369–2372, 1980

14. Gregory EJ, Cohen SC, Oines DW, et al: Megestrol acetate therapy for advanced breast cancer. J Clin Oncol 3:155–160, 1985

15. Keller J, White JM, Browder H, et al: A phase III randomized comparative trial of megestrol acetate vs diethylstilbestrol in stage D2 prostate cancer: Preliminary results. Proc Am Soc Clin Oncol 5:421, 1986

16. Tchekmedyian NS, Tait N, Moody M, et al: Weight gain with high dose megestrol acetate: A possible treatment for cachexia. Proc Am Assoc Cancer Res 27:209, 1986

17. Bailey DE: Probability and Statistics: Models for Research. New York, Wiley, 1971, pp 532–597

18. Tchekmedyian NS, Tait N, Aisner J: High dose megestrol acetate in the treatment of postmenopausal women with advanced breast cancer. Semin Oncol (in press)

19. Bonomi P, Pessis D, Bunting N, et al: Megestrol acetate used as primary hormonal therapy in stage D prostate cancer. Semin Oncol 12:36–39, 1985 (suppl 4)

20. Morgan LR: Megestrol acetate vs tamoxifen in advanced breast cancer in postmenopausal patients. Semin Oncol 12:43–47, 1985 (suppl 1)

Seminars in Oncology will publish in future issues

Breast Cancer

Part II

March 1987

Scientific Basis for Adjuvant and Primary (Neoadjuvant) Chemotherapy .... *J.H. Goldie*
Current Status of Adjuvant Chemotherapy for Resectable Breast Cancer .... *G. Bonadonna and P. Valagussa*
Current Status of Adjuvant Endocrine Therapy for Resectable Breast Cancer .... *K.I. Pritchard*
New Agents and Medical Treatments for Advanced Breast Cancer .... *I.C. Henderson, D.F. Hayes, S. Come, J.R. Harris, and G. Canellos*
Average Relative Dose Intensity and the Impact on Design of Clinical Trials .... *W.M. Hryniuk*
Psychological Issues in Breast Cancer .... *L.M. Sinsheimer and J.C. Holland*

Head and Neck Cancer

Tumor Markers

Endocrine Tumors

Acute Leukemia

Lung Cancer

Gastrointestinal Cancer

Genital Urinary Cancer

Cancer Biology

VOL XIII, NO 4, SUPPL 5 DECEMBER 1986

Seminars in Oncology

Hematologic Malignancies: Present Status and Future Prospects

Contributors

Joseph R. Bertino
Elaine S. Jaffe • Arthur Skarin
David J. Straus • Kenneth A. Foon • Paul A. Bunn, Jr
Walter J. Urba • Dan L. Longo • Ayad Al-Katib
Ellin Berman • Pat Black
Benjamin Koziner • Carol S. Portlock

GRUNE & STRATTON
Harcourt Brace Jovanovich, Inc.

Seminars in Oncology

Seminars in Oncology (ISSN 0093–7754) is published quarterly by Grune & Stratton, Inc., 6277 Sea Harbor Dr, Orlando, FL 32821. Months of issue are March, June, September, and December. Second class postage paid at Duluth, MN, and at additional mailing offices.

POSTMASTER: Send change of address to *Seminars in Oncology,* c/o Grune & Stratton, Inc., PO Box 6280, Duluth, MN 55806.

Editorial correspondence should be addressed to John W. Yarbro, MD, PhD, School of Medicine, University of Missouri at Columbia, Columbia, MO 65212.

Business correspondence (subscriptions, change of address) should be addressed to the Publisher, Grune & Stratton, Inc., PO Box 6280, Duluth, MN 55806.

Change of address notices, including both the old and new addresses of the subscriber, should be sent to the Publisher at least one month in advance.

Customer Service: 1-800-654-2452.

Subscription rates: one volume of four issues, $58.00 in the United States and Canada; elsewhere, $83.00. Libraries and institutions: $75.00 in the United States and Canada; elsewhere, $83.00. Single copies, $19.50 in the United States and Canada; elsewhere, $22.50. Students, fellows, interns, and residents in the United States, Canada, and Australia may subscribe at a discount rate of $34.00 per year (a letter giving qualifying data must accompany order). Subscriptions are accepted on a calendar year basis. Prices are subject to change. Current prices are in effect for back volumes and back issues. Single issues, both current and back, exist in limited quantities and are offered for sale subject to availability. Journal orders are payable in advance. *Checks* should be sent to Grune & Stratton, Inc., PO Box 6209, Duluth, MN 55806.

Advertising representative: Cunningham Associates, PO Box 308, Park Ridge, NJ 07656, telephone (201) 767-4170.

Agents for Great Britain: Grune & Stratton Limited, 24–28 Oval Rd, London NW1 7DX, England. Agents for Australia and New Zealand: Grune & Stratton Australia, PO Box 300, North Ryde, NSW 2113, Australia.

G&S

Orlando, FL

Harcourt Brace Jovanovich, Inc.

Seminars in Oncology

Seminars in Oncology

Vol 13, No 4, Suppl 5 **December 1986**

Advances in the Treatment of Lymphoid Malignancies

IN THIS SYMPOSIUM, information dealing with the biology and treatment of human lymphoid malignancies is presented.

Dr Jaffe presents data linking the classification of these diseases with biological behavior. With improved chemotherapy regimens, the "unfavorable" or aggressive lymphomas are now curable in as many as 50% to 60% of patients, even those presenting with advanced disease. Thus, the adjectives "favorable" or "unfavorable" should probably not be used to describe lymphoma, but the terms low grade, intermediate, and high grade or "aggressive" should be retained. As Dr Skarin points out, it is important now to define prognostic factors in the intermediate and high grade lymphomas so that these patients may be approached differently in regards to treatment.

The treatment of Hodgkin's disease, another curable lymphoid malignancy, is reviewed by Dr Straus. The issues here are more focused on developing therapy that is still curative, but has less risk of long-term side effects that include sterility and carcinogenesis. In addition, there is still a subset of patients that may be identified a priori, who do not do well with conventional mechlorethamine, vincristine, procarbazine, and prednisone (MOPP), or doxorubicin, bleomycin, vinblastine, and dacarbazine (ABVD). It is still not clear if alternating regimens with or without low dose irradiation will benefit these patients. What to offer patients who relapse after first-line chemotherapy for either aggressive lymphomas or Hodgkin's disease is not clear; treatment with autologous marrow with intensive chemotherapy and irradiation is encouraging, but older patients and extensively treated patients are difficult to treat with these demanding regimens. Monoclonal antibodies, alone or "armed," are potential new approaches. Lymphokine therapy, especially interferon, has not been effective; the value of other lymphokines (gamma interferon, interleukin II ± LAK cells) remains to be studied.

In contrast, the "favorable" or low grade lymphoid malignancies that include nodular poorly differentiated lymphomas (NPDL), cutaneous T cell lymphoma, and hairy cell leukemia, now generally believed to be a B cell neoplasm also, are both sensitive to the effects of alpha interferon as described by Drs Urba and Longo, Foon and Bunn, and Al-Katib et al, respectively. Studies are in progress that evaluate combined chemotherapy and interferon treatment of NPDL. Scheduling, sequencing, and dose intensity will all have to be evaluated to determine if the natural history of this disease can be altered.

The major new success story of recent years is the beneficial effects of alpha interferon as well as pentostatin in the treatment of hairy cell leukemia. This disease, benefited previously only by splenectomy (except for a few patients reported improved with chemotherapy), now is effectively treated in a majority of patients with alpha interferon. The advantage of this therapy is the improvement of peripheral blood cell counts without the risk of severe marrow compromise that occurred with alkylating agent or anthracyline treatment. The recent reports of the effectiveness of pentostatin, an adenosine deaminase inhibitor, provides an additional agent for the treatment of this disease, and the relative effectiveness of each, as well as the possible use of these drugs in combination or in sequence, are for future studies to determine, as pointed out by Dr Portlock.

Other lymphoid malignancies were not discussed in any detail in this symposium, eg, acute lymphocytic leukemia and Burkitt's lymphoma, because of space limitations. As a group of diseases, the lymphoid neoplasms are important, since they demonstrate what can be accomplished when the biology of the tumor is understood, and accurate diagnosis and staging, both clinical and histopathologic, may be accomplished. Perhaps not the least important factor in the progress noted is the unusual susceptibility of these cells to both irradiation and chemotherapy. One might point out as reasons for chemotherapy susceptibility the screens for development of new drugs for lymphoid malignancies (L1210, P-388), as well as the high growth fraction of most of these "aggressive" subtypes. The responsiveness of the less aggressive subtypes to the interferons remains to be explained.

Joseph R. Bertino, MD
Yale University School of Medicine
New Haven, CT

Relationship of Classification to Biologic Behavior of Non-Hodgkin's Lymphomas

Elaine S. Jaffe

The classification of non-Hodgkin's lymphomas (NHLs) is an important factor in treatment. Most clinical protocols divide these tumors into two broad categories—indolent, or low-grade, and aggressive, or high-grade. Patients with low-grade NHLs usually have a relatively long survival, with or without the use of aggressive therapy. Although the tumors can be controlled with conventional chemotherapeutic approaches, they are rarely cured. Patients with high-grade tumors usually die within 1 to 2 years without therapy. However, with aggressive treatment, many patients can be cured if complete remissions can be sustained for at least 2 years. Several types of NHLs represent distinct clinicopathologic entities—lymphoblastic lymphoma, adult T cell leukemia/lymphoma, true histiocytic lymphoma, Burkitt's lymphoma, and hairy cell leukemia. Immunologic concepts are now used to classify NHLs. Identifying the cell of origin of a malignant lymphoma has important therapeutic implications, since malignant cells retain phenotypic and functional properties of their precursors. It is possible, therefore, to predict both the sites of involvement and the patterns of dissemination. Clinical applications are beginning to be developed. These include the use of monoclonal antibodies, monoclonal antibodies coupled to a toxin, alpha interferon, and monoclonal anti-idiotype antibodies. Human leukocyte interferon has been used experimentally to induce spontaneous regressions. Excellent results have been achieved so far only for patients with low-grade lymphomas.

MOST CLINICAL PROTOCOLS for the non-Hodgkin's lymphomas (NHLs) divide tumors into two broad categories: indolent, or low-grade, and aggressive, or high-grade (Table 1).[1]

CLINICAL CLASSIFICATION OF NON-HODGKIN'S LYMPHOMAS

Low-Grade NHL

Using the "Working Formulation" classification system recently developed to supercede the Rappaport and other classification systems (Table 2), the indolent, or low-grade, lymphomas include the small lymphocytic lymphomas and follicular lymphomas of both the small-cleaved cell type and mixed, small-cleaved and large cell type.[2] Probably ≥99% of low-grade lymphomas are of B cell origin. In most cases, these lesions have an indolent clinical course. While patients usually present with disseminated disease, the disease is compatible with a relatively long survival, with or without aggressive therapy. With conventional chemotherapeutic approaches, these tumors may be controlled; however, they are rarely, if ever, cured.

Aggressive NHL

The aggressive lymphomas include those subtypes included under the intermediate and high-grade categories of the working formulation. In contrast to low-grade lymphomas, these have an aggressive natural history and, without therapeutic intervention, will cause the patient's death within 1 to 2 years. Paradoxically, these tumors may have a better prognosis than indolent lymphomas if they are aggressively and appropriately treated. A complete remission may be obtained, and if the remission is sustained for at least 2 years, many affected patients will be cured.[3]

Although there is a statistical trend indicating a more aggressive clinical course for those lesions in the high-grade, as opposed to intermediate-grade, category, the natural history of all of these lesions is aggressive.[4] In general, aggressive therapeutic approaches are required. Moreover, all these lesions share a potential for long-term remission and cure. Thus, in clinical terms, there is little reason to separate lymphomas into intermediate and high grades.

One possible exception to this observation is the intermediate-grade category, malignant lymphomas—diffuse small cleaved cell, which has been correlated with uncertain clinical behavior. Many clinical studies in the United States have indicated that this type of tumor behaves more like a low-grade than a high-grade lymphoma.[5]

From the National Cancer Institute, National Institutes of Health, Bethesda, MD.

Address reprint requests to Elaine S. Jaffe, MD, Chief, Hematopathology Section, Laboratory of Pathology, National Cancer Institute, National Institutes of Health, Bethesda, MD 20892.

0093-7754/86/1304-5002$05.00/0

Table 1. A Clinical Approach to the Classification of the Non-Hodgkin's Lymphomas

Indolent non-Hodgkin's lymphomas
Diffuse, small lymphocytic*
Follicular, small-cleaved cell
Follicular, mixed, small-cleaved and large cell
Diffuse, small-cleaved cell
Aggressive non-Hodgkin's lymphomas
Follicular, large cell
Diffuse, mixed, small and large cell
Diffuse, large cell, immunoblastic
Diffuse, small noncleaved cell
Lymphoblastic

Adapted from Rosenberg.[1]

*Terminology employed is that of the Working Formulation of Non-Hodgkin's Lymphomas for Clinical Usage.

Table 2. Working Formulation for Clinical Usage

Working Formulation	Rappaport Equivalent
Low-grade	
Malignant lymphoma, small lymphocytic	Well-differentiated lymphocytic
Malignant lymphoma, follicular predominantly small-cleaved cell	Nodular poorly differentiated lymphocytic
Malignant lymphoma, follicular mixed, small-cleaved and large cell	Nodular mixed cell type
Intermediate-grade	
Malignant lymphoma, follicular predominantly large cell	Nodular histiocytic
Malignant lymphoma, diffuse small-cleaved cell	Diffuse, poorly differentiated lymphocytic
Malignant lymphoma, diffuse mixed, small and large cell	Diffuse, mixed cell type
Malignant lymphoma, diffuse large cell	Diffuse, histiocytic
High-grade	
Malignant lymphoma, large cell, immunoblastic	Diffuse, histiocytic
Malignant lymphoma, lymphoblastic	Lymphoblastic
Malignant lymphoma, small noncleaved cell	Diffuse, undifferentiated Burkitt's Non-Burkitt's
Miscellaneous	
Composite	
Mycosis fungoides/Sezary syndrome	
Histiocytic	
Extramedullary plasmacytoma	
Adult T cell leukemia/lymphoma	
Hairy cell leukemia	

Although such tumors appear to have a more aggressive clinical course than follicular lymphomas of the small-cleaved cell type, it is uncertain if they share with other aggressive lymphomas a potential for long-term cure.

The aggressive lymphomas included in the intermediate-grade and high-grade categories are histologically and immunologically heterogenous.[6,7] Approximately 70% of these tumors are of B cell origin, and in many cases they appear to be derived from low-grade B cell lymphomas. In fact, multiple biopsies performed at the time of initial patient presentation demonstrate diverse histologic types in different anatomic sites: for example, a high-grade, or diffuse large cell, lymphoma in one site and a low-grade, or follicular, lymphoma in another site.[8] This finding has clinical relevance because although the high-grade component may be successfully treated, the low-grade component is more resistant to therapy. As a result, the patient may subsequently relapse with a low-grade lymphoma.[7] For this reason, it is important to note such histologic distinctions.

About 15% to 20% of the aggressive lymphomas are of the T cell type.[6,9] These are histologically heterogenous and, in the Working Formulation, fall predominantly into the categories of diffuse, mixed small and large cell lymphoma, and large cell immunoblastic lymphoma.[9] These so-called peripheral T cell lymphomas commonly have different patterns of involvement, such as more frequent involvement of the skin, lungs, or certain extranodal sites. However, at least in the experience of the National Cancer Institute (NCI), these lesions are susceptible to aggressive chemotherapy, and the clinical responses of the high-grade lymphomas of the T cell type have been equivalent to those of the B cell type.[6] Thus, immunologic phenotype alone has not been useful in predicting whether or not a patient will respond to aggressive therapy.

There are several categories of NHL that represent distinct clinicopathologic entities and should be considered separately.

Lymphoblastic Lymphoma

Lymphoblastic lymphoma, which is included in the Working Formulation under high-grade NHL, is immunologically, biologically, and clinically very closely related to acute lymphoblastic leukemia (ALL).[10,11] This lesion should be treated with the clinical approaches appropriate for ALL rather than those ordinarily used for NHL. Most lymphoblastic lymphomas are of T-cell type and are phenotypically very similar to T cell ALL; they are also associated with a similar clinical course to T cell ALL, and patients have a high risk of central nervous system relapse.[12] Although this disease used to have a dismal prognosis, recent treatment with protocols developed for T-cell ALL have resulted in long-term remissions.

Approximately 10% to 20% of cases of lymphoblastic lymphoma have a phenotype comparable to that of precursor B lymphocytes and are closely related to the common type of ALL.[12] These patients usually do not present with mediastinal masses. They may present with genralized peripheral adenopathy, or in some cases localized lytic bone lesions. These patients appear to have an excellent prognosis, comparable to patients with common ALL. Lymphoblastic lymphoma occurs most often in children and young adults. In his clinical approach to the classification of NHL, Rosenberg[1] stressed the importance of segregating lymphoblastic lymphoma (Table 1).

Adult T Cell Leukemia/Lymphoma

Another distinct clinicopathologic entity is adult T cell leukemia/lymphoma.[13] The etiology of the disease is thought to be associated with human T cell leukemia virus, type I (HTLV-I). This retrovirus is tropic to T4 or helper T lymphocytes and can transform them in vitro. The disease was first described in southwestern Japan, where it is endemic.[14] Subsequently, it has been identified in other parts of the world and appears to cluster in specific geographic areas. In such areas of high prevalence, a significant percentage of the normal population (generally 12% to 15%) carries antibodies to HTLV-I. Only a small number of patients with antibodies to HTLV-I ever acquire the disease. However, the retrovirus has been isolated from the tumor cells of all patients with the disease who have been studied. This disease is associated with a very aggressive clinical course; the median survival, even with aggressive therapy, generally has been less than 1 year. Patients present with generalized lymphadenopathy, hepatosplenomegaly, hypercalcemia, skin lesions, and peripheral blood involvement. More recently, a subacute, or smoldering form of the disease has been identified in Japan.[15] Patients with this form of adult T cell leukemia/lymphoma seem to have small numbers of circulating abnormal cells in the peripheral blood over a period of several years.

Histiocytic Lymphoma

True histiocytic lymphoma, also called histiocytic sarcoma, is another distinct clinicopathologic entity.[16] This lymphoma is difficult to recognize histologically; without the benefit of immunologic and enzyme cytochemical testing, most of the lesions would probably be classified as diffuse large-cell immunoblastic NHL. This is a very rare form of NHL, representing no more than 2% of NHL cases. In addition to lymph node involvement, patients may show involvement of skin and bone. In our limited clinical experience with true histiocytic lymphoma, patients have not had the syndrome of hepatosplenomegaly, lymphadenopathy, fever, pancytopenia, and a rapidly progressive course, formerly described for malignant histiocytosis or histiocytic medullary reticulosis. Most such cases may have represented hemophagocytic syndromes rather than true histiocytic malignancies.[17]

Burkitt's Lymphoma

In the Working Formulation, Burkitt's lymphoma is categorized as a subtype of undifferentiated or small noncleaved cell lymphoma. It is a distinct clinicopathologic entity with unique epidemiologic, clinical, and pathologic features.[18] Burkitt's lymphoma should be distinguished from small noncleaved cell non-Burkitt's lymphoma. Although there is no difference in survival that correlates with the minor histologic differences between Burkitt's and non-Burkitt's lymphoma, there are significant clinical distinctions.[19]

Classic Burkitt's lymphoma occurs most commonly in children; it usually presents in extranodal sites. In Africa, where the disease is endemic, frequent sites of involvement include the jaw and the bones of the face. In the United States and other areas where Burkitt's lymphoma is not endemic, intra-abdominal presentations are most frequent, involving either the ileocecal region or the ovaries or testes. Lymph node presentations are very rare.

In contrast, most non-Burkitt's lymphoma affects adults, commonly involves lymph node presentations, and more closely resembles diffuse aggressive NHL.

Burkitt's lymphomas are associated with specific cytogenetic translocations involving the immunoglobin gene loci on chromosomes 14, 2, and 22 and chromosome 8 at the site of the cellular oncogene, c-myc.[20] It is postulated that this translocation results in the activation, and constitutive expression, of the c-myc oncogene, resulting in the neoplastic transformation of the cell.[21,22] Similar translocations have been identified in small, noncleaved cell lymphomas of the non-Burkitt's type. These lymphomas have been identified frequently in immunosuppressed individuals, particularly those with the acquired immunodeficiency syndrome.[23,24]

Hairy Cell Leukemia

Hairy cell leukemia is generally not included with NHL since it represents a form of leukemia. Both immunologic and molecular genetic studies have demonstrated a B cell origin for virtually all cases of hairy cell leukemia.[25] Patients usually present with marked splenomegaly, leukopenia, anemia, and a diffusely replaced bone marrow. The cells in the bone marrow are associated with reticular fibrosis usually resulting in dry tap, so that the diagnosis usually has to be established with a bone marrow biopsy.[26] A common, but not universally specific, feature of the malignant cells is the presence of tartrate-resistant acid phosphatase activity. Generally, the number of cells circulating in the peripheral blood at presentation is small—less than 10% of the peripheral WBC count. However, following splenectomy, the degree of peripheral blood involvement may increase.

Hairy cell leukemia has a very indolent course. When studied kinetically, the disease shows a very low rate of DNA synthesis or proliferation for the malignant cells.[27] As a result, conventional cytotoxic therapy has not been effective in controlling the disease. In fact, in some case studies therapy has been harmful since it may create a greater potential for infectious complications. Until recently, splenectomy has been the primary mode of therapy for this disease.[28] Following splenectomy, patients usually achieve an improvement in their RBC and WBC levels.

Alpha interferon has recently been found to be very efficacious in the treatment of hairy cell leukemia.[29] The mechanism of action of this form of therapy is not well understood. Alpha interferon does not appear to act as an immunomodulator and may have a direct antitumor cell effect.

RELATION OF NHL TO THE NORMAL IMMUNE SYSTEM

Over the past 15 years, it has become apparent that the malignant lymphomas are tumors of the immune system. As a result, it has become possible to apply immunologic concepts to the classification of NHL.[30]

This development has had significant practical consequences. First, it has become possible to precisely identify the cell of origin of an individual lymphoma, thereby establishing an objective basis for classification. Second, and more importantly, it has been determined that the malignant cells not only retain the phenotypic properties of their precursors, enabling the use of phenotypic markers to identify them, but also often retain the functional properties of their precursors.

The phenotypic and functional continuity of malignant cells and their precursors has a direct impact on the features of the diseases encountered in clinical practice. For example, NHLs of B cell origin involve those areas of the lymphoid system normally populated by B lymphocytes; that is, the tumor disseminates in a pattern that mimics the migration pattern of normal B cells. This allows us to predict both sites of involvement and dissemination patterns of malignant lymphomas. Similarly, for tumors of T cell origin, the tumor cells tend to follow unique patterns of dissemination with frequent involvement of specific extranodal sites, such as skin and lung, allowing accurate clinical prediction of patterns of spread.

The functional similarity between tumor cells and their precursors is also evident. For example, B cell lymphomas produce immunoglobulin and patients with B cell lymphomas have abnormalities of immunoglobulin secretion. These include monoclonal gammapathy, an excess accumulation of a single immunoglobulin moiety, or hypogammaglobulinemia that may lead to a functional defect in the patient's humoral immune system and susceptibility to particular infections.[31]

Similarly, in T cell systems, the tumor cells may retain the ability to secrete products elaborated by normal T cells, and these lymphokines can cause striking clinical effects. For example, adult T cell leukemia/lymphoma is frequently associated with marked hypercalcemia and lytic bone lesions[32]; it is likely that the hypercalcemia is due to the elaboration of lymphokine by the neoplastic cells.[33]

The angiocentric immunoproliferative lesions include lymphomatoid granulomatosis and angiocentric lymphomas. These lesions frequently involve the lung and other extranodal sites. The proliferating cells, which are mature T cells, have an angiocentric and angiodestructive growth pattern. In the angiocentric immunoproliferative lesions, the tumor cells appear to be capable of elaborating a lymphokine that can stimulate the cells of the mononuclear phagocytic system. This can lead to marked activation of normal histiocytes throughout the body and a hemaphagocytic syndrome resulting in anemia, thrombocytopenia, leukopenia, and possibly death.[17,34]

Therapeutic Approaches

Overall, these observations underscore the importance of the tumor cell type in understanding the clinical consequences of NHL. Indeed, the phenotypic and functional characteristics of the tumor cells may also prove to be of significance in developing new forms of therapy for lymphomas. The clinical possibilities of these new approaches are just beginning to be developed.

One significant therapeutic implication is that the characteristic phenotypic markers retained by tumor cells may be used as targets for therapy with monoclonal antibodies. For example, T cell lymphomas that express the p65 antigen (CD5) Tl have been treated with monoclonal antibodies against Tl.[35] This treatment modality has been used in mycosis fungoides/Sezary syndrome, and low-grade B cell lymphomas that also express this antigen, such as chronic lymphocytic leukemia.[35,36] Thus far, these approaches have resulted in transient responses with immediate elimination of some of the malignant cells but no long-term effect.

Another therapeutic approach now under study is the use of monoclonal antibodies coupled to a toxin, such as ricin or pseudomonas exotoxin. This approach is expected to have greater efficacy since the malignant cell expressing the antigen can be definitively eliminated.[37] Without coupling, the monoclonal antibody may bind to the antigen on the surface of the cell, causing the antigen to modulate off the surface without killing the cell.[38] By coupling the monoclonal antibody with a toxin, the malignant cell will be destroyed. This approach is currently being used for the treatment of adult T cell leukemia, a disease in which the malignant cells express tac, an antigen associated with the IL-2 receptor.[39]

Attempts to modulate the immune system in order to control malignant lymphomas represent still other ways of relating the treatment of malignant tumors to the normal immune system. There is substantial evidence that many of the malignant lymphomas, particularly the low-grade malignant lymphomas, are capable of responding to immunoregulation. This is in contrast to the high-grade lymphomas, which are consistently autonomous (Table 3).[40] Many patients with low-grade, and particularly follicular, lymphomas have a history of lymph nodes that wax and wane in size over many years. There are also reports of spontaneous regression of such tumors, in some cases following what appears to be a bacterial or viral infection.[41]

It has been postulated that host immunity may be involved in these spontaneous clinical regres-

Table 3. Pathologic and Experimental Characteristics of Low-Grade and High-Grade Malignant Lymphomas

Low-Grade	High-Grade
Nondestructive growth pattern	Destructive growth pattern
Absence of cellular atypia	Presence of cellular atypia/anaplasia
Respect privileged sites	Invade privileged sites
Respond to regulatory influences	Autonomous
Fail to grow in culture	Immortalized in culture
Nontransplantable	Transplantable in immunodeficient host

sions, since the infectious episode might result in an activation of the immune system. In an attempt to test this hypothesis, human leukocyte interferon has been used experimentally to induce spontaneous regressions.[42] Excellent results have been obtained in patients with low-grade lymphomas; however, patients with high-grade, apparently more autonomous, lymphomas have not responded to alpha interferon.[43]

The recent therapeutically successful use of monoclonal anti-idiotype antibodies is an additional attempt to capitalize on the susceptibility of the tumors to be modulated or regulated, or both, by the immune system.[44,45] In Levy's studies, anti-idiotype antibodies have been prepared against the specific surface idiotype secreted by a B cell lymphoma. Thus, the anti-idiotypic antibody reacts only with the surface immunoglobulin of the neoplastic cells, not with the surface immunoglobulin of normal cells. The first patient treated with this approach had a dramatic clinical remission, and is still in remission.[44] However, subsequent trials with a larger number of patients have produced inconsistent results. In some cases, there has been partial remission; in other cases there has been no remission.[46]

In an attempt to predict responsiveness to this treatment modality, Meeker et al[46] studied the effect of infiltrating normal cells into the follicular lymphomas. They found that the likelihood of a tumor responding to anti-idiotypic therapy is most closely associated with the number of normal T cells infiltrating the tumor.[46] This finding further supports the concept that the anti-idiotype antibody is acting not by simple lysis of tumor cells but probably by activating immunoregulatory circuits. For this reason, the host T cells are probably crucial to the efficacy of this form of therapy. Indeed, it has been shown in studies of follicular lymphomas that the lesions may contain numerous T cells and that the T cells may be present not only in between the nodules as residual lymphoid elements, but also within the neoplastic nodules themselves, in intimate association with the tumor cells.[7] Moreover, patients with extensive infiltration of their B-cell tumors by normal T cells appear to pursue a more indolent clinical course than patients lacking such infiltrates.[47] Thus, it is likely that the presence of T cells represents significant host response to disease. If it were possible to effectively capitalize on the presence of these T cells, remission might be achieved.

Still other experimental approaches to the therapy of malignant lymphomas are now being studied. One promising development is the use of other biologicals to stimulate the host T cells. IL-2 or IL-2 in combination with lymphokine-activated T cells or LAK cells are among the biologicals that have been tried.[48] Findings are as yet too preliminary to evaluate the efficacy of these approaches.

REFERENCES

1. Rosenberg SA: Current concepts in cancer: Non-Hodgkin's lymphoma—selection of treatment on the basis of histologic type. N Engl J Med 301:924–928, 1979

2. Rosenberg SA, Berard CW, Brown BS, et al: National Cancer Institute sponsored study of classification of non-Hodgkin's lymphomas: Summary and description of a working formulation for clinical usage. Cancer 49:2112–2135, 1982

3. DeVita VT, Canellos GP, Chabner BA, et al: Advanced diffuse histiocytic lymphoma: A potentially curable disease. Lancet 1:248–250, 1975

4. Fisher RI, Hubbard SM, DeVita VT, et al: Factors predicting long-term survival in diffuse mixed, histiocytic or undifferentiated lymphoma. Blood 58:45–51, 1981

5. Garvin AJ, Simon R, Young RC, et al: The Rappaport Classification of non-Hodgkin's lymphomas: A closer look using other proposed classifications. Semin Oncol 7:234–243, 1980

6. Cossman J, Jaffe ES, Fisher RI: Immunologic phenotypes of diffuse aggressive non-Hodgkin's lymphomas: Correlation with clinical features. Cancer 54:1310–1317, 1984

7. Jaffe ES: Non-Hodgkin's lymphomas as tumors of the immune system, in Berard CW (moderator): A multidisciplinary approach to non-Hodgkin's lymphomas. Ann Intern Med 94:218–235, 1981

8. Fisher RI, Jones RB, DeVita VT, et al: Natural history of malignant lymphomas with divergent histologies at staging evaluation. Cancer 47:2022–2025, 1981

9. Jaffe ES: Pathologic and clinical spectrum of post-thymic T-cell malignancies. Cancer Invest 2:413–426, 1984

10. Nathwani BN, Diamond LW, Winberg CW, et al: Malignant lymphoma, lymphoblastic. Cancer 38:964–983, 1976

11. Jaffe ES, Berard CW: Lymphoblastic lymphoma, a term rekindled with new precision. Ann Intern Med 89:415–417, 1978

12. Cossman J, Chused T, Fisher R, et al: Diversity of immunologic phenotypes of lymphoblastic lymphoma. Cancer Res 43:4486–4490, 1983

13. Blayney D, Jaffe E, Blattner W, et al: The human T cell leukemia/lymphoma virus (HTLV) associated with American adult T cell leukemia/lymphoma (ATL). Blood 62:401–405, 1983

14. Uchiyama T, Yodoi J, Sagawa K, et al: Adult T-cell

leukemia: Clinical and hematologic features of 16 cases. Blood 41:4738–4739, 1977

15. Kawano F, Yamaguchi K, Nishimura H, et al: Variation in the clinical courses of adult T-cell leukemia. Cancer 55:851–856, 1985

16. Jaffe ES: Malignant histocytosis and true histiocytic lymphomas, in Jaffe, ES (ed): Surgical Pathology of Lymph Nodes and Related Organs. Philadelphia, Saunders, 1985, pp 381–411

17. Jaffe ES, Costa J, Fauci AS, et al: Malignant lymphoma and erythrophagocytosis stimulating malignant histiocytosis. Am J Med 75:741–749, 1983

18. Arseneau JC, Canellos GP, Banks PM, et al: American Burkitt's lymphoma: A clinicopathologic study of 30 cases. I. Clinical factors relating to prolonged survival. Am J Med 58:314–321, 1975

19. Miliauskas JR, Berard CW, Young RC, et al: Undifferentiated non-Hodgkin's lymphomas (Burkitt's and non-Burkitt's types). The relevance of making this histologic distinction. Cancer 50:2115–2121, 1982

20. Taub R, Kirsch I, Morton C, et al: Translocation of the c-myc gene into the immunoglobulin heavy chain locus in human Burkitt's lymphoma and murine plasmacytoma cells. Proc Natl Acad Sci USA 79:7837–7841, 1982

21. Robertson M: Paradox and paradigm: The message and meaning of *myc*. Nature 306:733–736, 1983

22. Croce CM, Tsujimoto Y, Erikson I, et al: Biology of disease: Chromosome translocations and B cell neoplasia. Lab Invest 51:258–269, 1984

23. Magrath I, Erikson I, Whang-Peng J, et al: Synthesis of kappa light chains by cell lines containing an 8;22 chromosomal translocation derived from a male homosexual with Burkitt's lymphoma. Science 222:1094–1096, 1983

24. Chagante RSK, Jhanwar SC, Koziner B, et al: Specific translocations characterize Burkitt's-like lymphoma of homosexual men with acquired immunodeficiency syndrome. Blood 61:1269–1278, 1983

25. Korsmeyer S, Green W, Cossman J, et al: Rearrangement and expression of immunoglobulin genes and expression of TAC antigen in hairy cell leukemia. Proc Natl Acad Sci USA 80:4522–4526, 1983

26. Burke JS: The value of the bone-marrow biopsy in the diagnosis of hairy cell leukemia. Am J Clin Pathol 70:876–884, 1978

27. Braylan RC, Fowlkes BJ, Jaffe ES, et al: Cell volumes and DNA distributions of normal and neoplastic human lymphoid cells. Cancer 41:201–209, 1978

28. Golomb HM, Vardiman JW: Response to splenectomy in 65 patients with hairy cell leukemia. An evaluation of spleen weight and bone marrow involvement. Blood 61:349–352, 1983

29. Quesada JR, Reuben J, Manning JT, et al: Induction of remission in hairy cell leukemia with alpha interferon. N Engl J Med 310:15–18, 1984

30. Mann RB, Jaffe ES, Berard CW: Malignant lymphomas: A conceptual understanding of morphologic diversity. Am J Pathol 94:105–192, 1979

31. Callihan TR, Holbert JM, Berard BW: Neoplasms of terminal B-cell differentiation: The morphologic basis of functional diversity, in Malignant Lymphomas: A Pathology Annual Monograph. Norwalk, Appleton-Century-Crofts, 1983, pp 169–268

32. Blayney DW, Jaffe ES, Fischer RI, et al: The human T-cell leukemia/lymphoma virus (HTLV), lymphoma, lytic bone lesions, and hypercalcemia. Ann Intern Med 98:144–150, 1983

33. Grossman B, Schecter GP, Horton JE, et al: Hypercalcemia associated with T-cell lymphoma-leukemia. Am J Clin Pathol 75:149–155, 1981

34. Simrell CR, Margolick JB, Crabtree GR, et al: Lymphokine induced phagocytosis in angiocentric immunoproliferative lesions (AIL) and malignant lymphoma in AIL. Blood 65:1469–1476, 1985

35. Miller RA, Levy R: Response of cutaneous T cell lymphoma to therapy with hybridoma monoclonal antibody. Lancet 2:226–230, 1981

36. Dillman RO, Shawler DL, Sobol RE, et al: Murine monoclonal antibody therapy in two patients with chronic lymphocytic leukemia. Blood 59:1036–1045, 1982

37. Vitetta ES, Krolick KA, Uhr JW: Neoplastic B cells as targets for antibody-ricin A chain immunotoxins. Immunol Rev 62:159–183, 1982

38. Pesando JM, Ritz J, Lazarus H, et al: Fate of a common acute lymphoblastic leukemia antigen during modulation by monoclonal antibody. J Immunol 126:540–544, 1981

39. Waldman TA: Use of anti–IL-2 receptor antibodies in the therapy of HTLV-1–induced adult T-cell leukemia, in Green WC (moderator): Normal and abnormal expression of interleukin-2 receptor cells in T-cell and HTLV-induced leukemias. Ann Intern Med (in press)

40. Jaffe ES: Follicular lymphomas: Possibility that they are benign tumors of the lymphoid system. J Natl Cancer Inst 70:401–403, 1983

41. Krikorian JG, Portlock CS, Cooney DP, et al: Spontaneous regression of non-Hodgkin's lymphomas. A report of nine cases. Cancer Res 46:2093–2099, 1980

42. Merigan TC, Sikora K, Breeden JH, et al: Preliminary observations of the effect of human leukocyte interferon in non-Hodgkin's lymphoma. N Engl J Med 299:1449–1453, 1978

43. Foon KA, Sherwin SA, Abrams PG, et al: Treatment of advanced non-Hodgkin's lymphoma with recombinant leukocyte A interferon. N Engl J Med 311:1148–1152, 1984

44. Miller RA, Maloney CG, Warnke R, et al: Treatment of B-cell lymphoma with monoclonal anti-idiotype antibody. N Engl J Med 306:517–522, 1982

45. Lynch R: Immunoregulation of malignant lymphoma. N Engl J Med 306:543–544, 1982

46. Meeker TC, Lowder J, Maloney DG, et al: A clinical trial of anti-idiotype therapy for B cell malignancy. Blood 65:1349–1363, 1985

47. Jaffe ES, Longo DL, Cossman J, et al: Diffuse B cell lymphomas with T cell predominance in patients with follicular lymphoma or "pseudo T cell lymphoma." Seventy-Third Annual Meeting of the International Academy of Pathology, San Francisco, March 12–16, 1984. Lab Invest 50:27–28, 1984 (abstr)

48. Rosenberg SA, Lotze MT, Muul LM, et al: Observations on the systemic administration of autologous lymphokine-activated killer cells and recombinant interleukin-2 patients with metastatic cancer. N Engl J Med 313:1485–1492, 1985

Diffuse Aggressive Lymphomas: A Curable Subset of Non-Hodgkin's Lymphomas

Arthur T. Skarin

The diffuse aggressive lymphomas are a major group of non-Hodgkin's lymphomas characterized by diffuse disease, in most cases, and a rapidly progressive clinical course. Until recently, the disease was fatal. Over the last 10 years, use of intermittent high-dose combination chemotherapy with non–cross-resistant drugs has significantly increased the survival time for patients with both local and advanced disease. For those with advanced disease, the most recent studies show complete response rates of 85%, complete-response relapse rates of 10%, and a 73% rate of survival for more than 3 to 5 years. The role of radiation therapy is also important, particularly in the early stages of disease. Salvage treatment with single-agent chemotherapy has achieved often impressive, but brief, responses usually of <1 year. Not all patients can tolerate these intensive regimens, however, and new avenues of therapy are being investigated. Various types of biologic response modifiers have been tried in patients who have been heavily pretreated. Monoclonal antibodies initially produced responses in patients with low or intermediate grade tumors, but overall results are still disappointing. Recent trials with interferons show promise especially in patients with low-grade, indolent B cell lymphomas and cutaneous T cell lymphoma. Because antitumor effects are generally of short duration, however, there is probably only a minimal role for biologic therapy in patients with aggressive lymphomas.

THE DIFFUSE AGGRESSIVE lymphomas represent a major subgroup of non-Hodgkin's lymphomas that are characterized by disseminated disease in most cases, and a rapidly progressive clinical course. About half of the patients present with classic B symptoms as seen in Hodgkin's disease, and a small subset may have a poor performance status as assessed by criteria used in nonhematologic malignancies.

Histologically, these "aggressive" lymphomas show a diffuse replacement of normal lymph node architecture by mainly large malignant cells, giving rise to the term diffuse large cell lymphoma (DLCL). While, in the past, DLCL has been called diffuse histiocytic lymphoma (DHL) by Rappaport, use of surface marker studies as pioneered by Lukes and Collins has resulted in more accurate terminology (and also more subsets). About 60% to 70% of DLCL cases in adults arise from B cells, while about 20% are of T cell origin, with only 5% or less of histiocyte (monocyte) origin. Depending upon the number and sophistication of marker studies available, 1% to 10% of cases may be unclassifiable.

In the United States, the term "DLCL" includes the following morphologic diagnoses: DHL, large cleaved follicular center cell lymphoma, large noncleaved follicular center cell lymphoma, B-immunoblastic sarcoma, T-immunoblastic sarcoma, large hyperlobated T or B cell lymphoma, and true-histiocytic (monocytic) lymphoma. In the International Panel Working Formulation classification of non-Hodgkin's lymphomas, DLCL generally refers to category II (intermediate grade), G-diffuse large cell, cleaved/noncleaved, and category III (high grade), H-diffuse large cell, immunoblastic.[1] In addition to the above histologic subgroups, the term "diffuse aggressive lymphoma" has been interpreted by some investigators to include diffuse undifferentiated lymphoma (non-Burkitt's type), nodular histiocytic lymphoma, and diffuse poorly differentiated lymphocytic and mixed lymphomas. Lymphoblastic T cell lymphoma and Burkitt's lymphoma are high grade tumors seen mainly in pediatric patients and will not be considered in this review.

Use of modern DNA molecular probes makes it possible to define monoclonal B cell lymphomas by immunoglobulin gene rearrangement studies and T cell lymphomas by T cell receptor gene rearrangement studies.[2,3] These latter studies allow for diagnosis of a malignant lymphoma in tissue specimens that may otherwise lack histologic features of a malignancy. In addition, cell lineage can be traced or followed during transition from one phase of lymphoma to another, which can differentiate between development of a new or unrelated malignancy.

The first report of long-term survival in

From the Dana-Farber Cancer Institute, Boston, MA.
Address reprint requests to Arthur T. Skarin, MD, Associate Professor of Medicine, 44 Binney St, Dana-Farber Cancer Institute, Boston, MA 02115.

0093-7754/86/1304-5003$05.00/0

patients with advanced DHL was published by DeVita et al[4] in 1975. Using MOPP (nitrogen mustard, vincristine, procarbazine, and prednisone) or C-MOPP (cyclophosphamide plus MOPP) combination chemotherapy, 11 (41%) of 27 patients achieved a complete response (CR), and only one relapsed. For all study patients, a survival plateau of 37% was reached from 2 to 9 years, with median survival of CR patients exceeding 48 months. Five of the 11 CR patients had single extranodal sites of disease, now recognized as a favorable prognostic factor. These encouraging results in a disease that was previously rapidly fatal despite use of available treatment regimens stimulated a number of subsequent combination chemotherapy trials that incorporated new chemotherapeutic agents as they became available. The initial regimens, often termed the first-generation studies,[5] led to the development of second-generation and third-generation studies as experimental rationales became available that defined the optimal use of alternating non–cross-resistant chemotherapy, based on the hypothesis of Goldie et al.[6] This somatic mutation hypothesis predicted that the early introduction of all active agents in a treatment regimen reduced the probability of resistant clones and would thus increase the response rate and ultimate cure rate. Also, important concepts concerning the intensity, timing, and placement of drugs in the design of treatment schedules were developed, mainly by Norton and Simon.[7]

The evolution of treatment strategy has emphasized the importance of intermittent high-dose combination chemotherapy with use of non–cross-resistant drugs. The role of radiotherapy remains important, particularly in early-stage disease. The value of radiotherapy in disseminated disease remains to be determined.

TREATMENT OF ADVANCED DLCL

First Generation Treatment Regimens

It became evident in the early- and mid-1970s that COP (cyclophosphamide, vincristine, prednisone) or CVP (cyclophosphamide, vincristine, prednisone) combination chemotherapy programs provided inadequate treatment for DLCL. Complete remission rates were only 30%, and rapid relapse and death occurred. With the use of four-drug programs (MOPP and C-MOPP) and the availability of new agents (doxorubicin and bleomycin) that could be added to the existing COP regimens, CR rates increased and survival significantly increased. Results of the National Cancer Institute (NCI) MOPP-C-MOPP regimen described above are summarized in Table 1, together with other combination chemotherapy programs (a listing and definition of selected regimens appear in the appendix). The CR rates, relapse rates, and long-term survival rates of all treated patients are quite similar to these programs. The popular CHOP (cyclophosphamide, hydroxydaunorubicin, vincristine, prednisone) regimen, devised by the Southwest Oncology Group (SWOG) in 1972, was used alone or in combination with bleomycin, BCG, and levamisole in several sequential protocols. A recent detailed analysis of all of the programs reported that none of the combinations substantially changed the treatment outcome when compared with CHOP alone.[8] The SWOG randomized trials have the longest follow-up of any study, up to 12 years. Of interest, continuous relapse occurred up to 9 years, when a plateau was reached on the survival curve. Similar overall results were noted by a single institution study of CHOP.[9] Addition of bleomycin to CHOP (CHOP-Bleo) at the M.D. Anderson Hospital[10] or use of slightly different dose schedules of the same five drugs (BACOP) at the Dana-Farber Cancer Institute,[11] NCI,[12] or University of Southern California,[13] led to almost identical results. A slightly lower relapse rate was noted in the CHOP-Bleo regimen[10] with a higher survival

Table 1. Results of Selected First Generation Regimens for DLCL

Regimen	No. of Patients	% CR	% Relapse	% Long-term Survival >3-5 Years (All Patients)
MOPP-C-MOPP[4]	27	41	9	37
CHOP, CHOP-Bleo CHOP-BCG, CHOP-Levamisole[8]	418*	53	44	30
CHOP[9]	75	51	30	35
BACOP[11]	22	56	31	30
BACOP[12]	32	48	13	37
BACOP[13]	57	47	33	30
COMLA[16]	72	40	28	30

*Combined studies.

rate, but the follow-up was relatively short compared with the BACOP programs.

The COMLA regimen, utilized intitially at Yale,[14] and then at the University of Chicago, differed from the above regimens because cyclophosphamide was administered infrequently (one dose every 85 days) while methotrexate/leucovorin (MTX/LV) rescue and cytosine arabinoside were given weekly. The initial results in 42 patients treated at Chicago were quite encouraging, with a projected survival rate of 65% for all patients, and 96% for patients in their first or second CR.[15] Accrual of more patients, however, with long-term follow-up to 10 years showed a lower CR rate and decrease in disease-free survival and overall survival, as noted in Table 1. Patients over age 65 and those with prior curative radiation therapy or minimal chemotherapy faired particularly poorly.[16] A modified COMLA (cyclophosphamide, vincristine, methotrexate, leucovorin, cystosine arabinosine) regimen has been recently utilized by clinicians in Nashville, TN wherein cyclophosphamide is given twice as frequently, cytosine arabinoside is given by continuous infusion, and the total duration of therapy is reduced to 16 weeks.[17] A CR was achieved in 12 of 15 patients with DLCL (80%) with only three relapses to date.

It is apparent from Table 1 that the first-generation regimens give similar results— namely, a CR rate of about 50%, CR relapse rate of about 30%, and a 3-year to 5-year survival rate of 30% to 35%. A valid comparison of results between the selected studies, however, is not possible owing to a variety of factors, including a wide range of eligibility requirements for each study, selection factors for entrance onto a protocol, bias related to institutional *v* cooperative group study, and variation in individual prognostic factors among the patient populations.

At least three prospective randomized studies have been carried out in patients with DLCL (Table 2). In the largest study, conducted by the Southeastern Cancer Study Group, patients received either conventional CHOP (doxorubicin plus COP) or BCOP (carmustine plus COP).[18] The survival of all patients was significantly increased with CHOP, related to a higher CR rate. Toxicity of both regimens was similar except for less alopecia with BCOP. Significant granulocytopenia occurred in only 40% of

Table 2. Selected Randomized First Generation Studies in DLCL

Regimen	No. of Patients	% CR	% Relapse	% Survival at 3 Years (All Patients)	
CHOP[18]	90	54	42	48	P = .03
BCNU-COP	80	34	42	37	
C-MOPP[19]	43*	49	52	37	
BACOP	49*	51	32	37	
CHOP-Bleo[20,21]	28	71	14	63	
ACOMLA	20	65	28	63	

*Includes 11 patients with diffuse mixed lymphomas.
†Includes eight patients with diffuse mixed lymphomas.

patients in both arms, suggesting that dose escalation may have been tolerable and perhaps have improved the results.

In a cooperative study between Buenos Aires and Georgetown, C-MOPP was compared with BACOP (bleomycin and doxorubicin plus COP).[19] The CR rates were identical, but patients treated with C-MOPP had a higher relapse rate (Table 2). This trend, however, has not yet translated into any difference in overall survival.

At Yale, CHOP-Bleo was prospectively compared with ACOMLA. With use of doxorubicin in ACOMLA, the dose of cyclophosphamide was reduced from 1.5 g/m^2 to 1.0 g/m^2. Results of both regimens were similar (Table 2). Long-term follow-up (median of 49 months) shows no major differences between the two regimens in regard to response, response duration, survival, or toxicity.[21]

A four-arm randomized study was conducted by the Eastern Cooperative Oncology Group (ECOG) comparing COP plus doxorubicin (COPA), COP plus carmustine (BCVP), or COP plus two different bleomycin dose schedules (COPB or CPOB).[22] Survival advantages were shown for COPA and COPB. Of interest, CPOB utilized vincristine and bleomycin on day 15 of each 21-day cycle, which resulted in a therapeutic advantage over use of the two drugs on day 1 as in the COPB regimen. No advantage for maintenance therapy with BCVP was observed when compared with a control group.

In a randomized SWOG study comparing CHOP to CHOP-levamisole or CHOP-levamisole-BCG, patients with unfavorable histology

Table 3. Selected Second Generation Regimens for DLCL

Regimen	No. of Patients	% CR	% Relapse	% Survival at 3 Years (All Patients)
M-BACOD[24,25]*	101	72	26	59
Pro-MACE/MOPP[26,27]†	81	74	18	65
COP-BLAM-I[28]	33#	72	12	70
Modified COP-BLAM[29]	51	73	33	53 (estimate)
ACOMLA[21]	24	75	33	63
NHL-3[30] "ACOMLA"§	44	50	NA	48‖
CHOP/HOAP-Bleo[31]/IMVP-16[28]¶	56	82	20	92 (stages I–III) 50 (stage IV)
F-MACHOP[32]‡	46	81	23	71

*Includes DU (13 cases).
†Includes DPDL (two cases) and DM (14 cases).
‡Includes lymphoblastic and undifferentiated lymphoma.
§Selected patients received radiotherapy.
‖Includes eight patients with nonevaluable disease.
¶Includes stage I patients.
#Previously untreated patients only.

receiving levamisole had a shorter CR duration.[23] Survival for the three treatment arms was similar, thus abrogating any advantage to this type of immunotherapy.

Thus, two of the randomized studies of basically first-generation regimens (Table 2) show an advantage for doxorubicin-containing combinations, with some improvement in overall survival[18] and disease-free survival.[19]

More recent treatment programs, often referred to as second-generation regimens, are listed in Table 3. These regimens contain more agents often administered in alternating cycles, and are considered as moderately intensive treatment programs. The M-BACOD regimen conducted at the Dana-Farber Cancer Institute and Brigham and Women's Hospital, utilized high-dose methotrexate (3 mg/m^2) with leucovorin rescue (M = MTX/LV) administered on day 14 between cycles of BACOD agents (bleomycin, doxorubicin, cyclophosphamide, vincristine, dexamethasone).[24] Previous studies had shown the therapeutic efficacy of MTX/LV as a single agent in relapsed malignant lymphomas and the rationale for use in the M-BACOD regimen.[33,34] The results were far superior to the previous

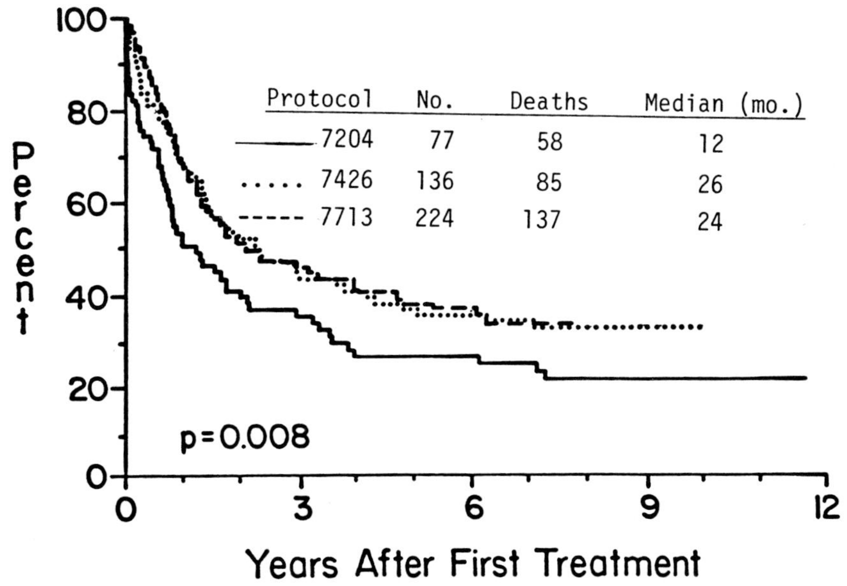

Fig 1. Overall survival of DLCL patients on CHOP arms of SWOG protocols 7204, 7406, and 7713. (Reprinted with permission.[8])

Table 4. Comparison of High Dose M-BACOD and Moderate Dose m-BACOD in DLCL

	M-BACOD[24] (95 Patients) 5-Year Results (%)	m-BACOD[25] (80 Patients) 3-Year Results (%)
CR rate	77	75
Relapse free survival	74	77
Overall survival	59	65
CNS relapse*	4/95	4/80

*No. of relapses of CR patients/total number of evaluable patients.

BACOP regimen (Fig 1). The overall survival for all patients treated with M-BACOD was 59%, projected to 6 years, compared with 23% for BACOP ($P = .001$).

In order to allow for greater use of the M-BACOD regimen, the dose of methotrexate was decreased to 200 mg/m^2 (moderate-dose MTX/LV), which reduced potential serious renal toxicity, avoided a need for urinary alkalinization as well as pharmacologic studies, and lowered the cost. The moderate-dose methotrexate (m) was administered on days 8 and 15 of each cycle. Leucovorin factor (LV = 10 mg/m^2) was started 24 hours after each dose of m and given orally every 6 hours for eight doses. If any vomiting occurred, the LV was given intravenously (IV). The results of m-BACOD are identical to those for M-BACOD.[25] As noted in Table 4, CNS relapse occurred in both programs in approximately 5% of patients. While high-dose MTX/LV may have reduced the CNS relapse rate, no randomized studies have been carried out to support this conclusion. Moderate dose MTX/LV was not utilized with prophylaxis of CNS disease in mind, owing to the nontherapeutic levels achieved in cerebral spinal fluid. Toxicity of the two regimens was similar, although more mucositis occurred with m-BACOD compared with M-BACOD (40% *v* 10% of patients). With greater hydration, and mouth care, this problem should lessen. Also, leukopenia with fever was more common with m-BACOD (28% *v* 8%). Reversible pulmonary infiltrates related to bleomycin occurred in both programs (20% and 12%).

The ProMACE-MOPP (prednisone, methotrexate, doxorubicin, cyclophosphamide, etoposide) regimen (Table 3) developed at the NCI, alternates two non–cross-resistant combinations. As compared with other regimens, a flexible number of courses of treatment was administered, depending on the degree of tumor regression.[26] Late intensification with ProMACE therapy was given to patients in complete remission. Results are noted in Table 3, and long-term survival compared with previous treatment programs at the NCI (C-MOPP/BACOP) is illustrated in Fig 2.[27] The survival curves are almost identical to the results achieved at the Dana-Farber Cancer Institute (Fig 3).

The COP-BLAM regimen utilized at the New York Hospital[28] consisted of the addition of procarbazine to five active chemotherapeutic agents (BACOP or CHOP-Bleo). Drug dosages were escalated according to patient tolerance, with treatment cycles administered every 3 weeks. Results are noted in Table 3. More recently, results of a modified COP-BLAM regi-

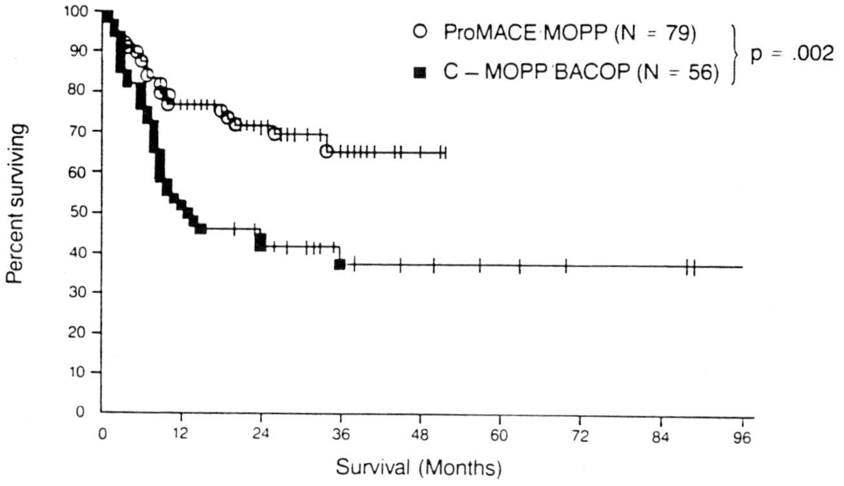

Fig 2. Overall survival of patients with mainly DHL treated with C-MOPP at the National Cancer Institute. (Reprinted with permission.[27])

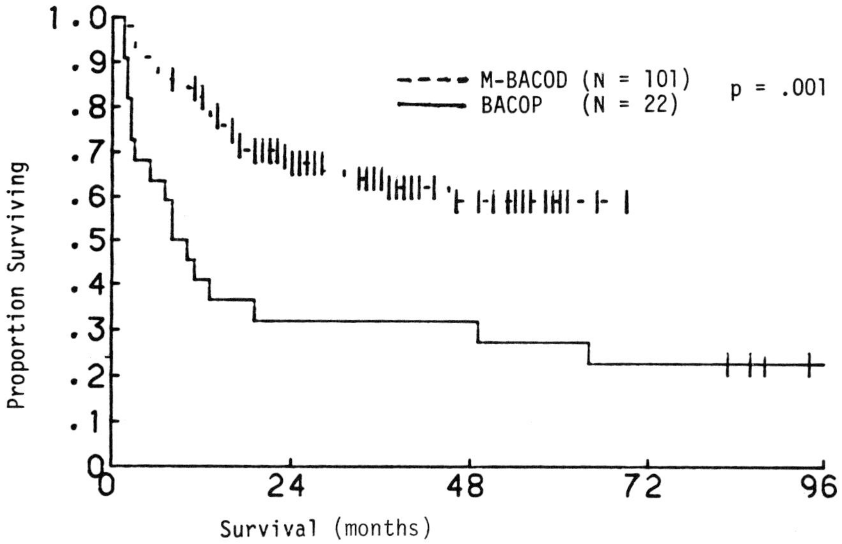

Fig 3. Overall survival of patients with mainly histiocytic lymphoma treated with BACOP or M-BACOD at the Dana-Farber Cancer Institute and Brigham and Women's Hospital. (Data from Skarin et al.[11,24])

men employed at the University of Nebraska Medical Center were reported.[29] Treatment duration was based upon the time required to achieve complete remission. After CR was achieved, two additional cycles of chemotherapy were administered, similar to the original MOPP program for Hodgkin's disease.

Overall results of the Nebraska modified COP-BLAM regimen are noted in Table 3. Of importance is the fact that rapidly responding patients did not require prolonged treatment (ie, as few as five cycles) and had a better prognosis than did patients achieving a CR more slowly. Thus, the speed of CR significantly affected survival.

Updated results of the Yale ACOMLA (doxorubicin plus COMLA) regimen[21] are noted in Table 3. The same ACOMLA agents were utilized by the Memorial Sloan-Kettering Cancer Center in the NHL-3 protocol.[30] The doses of doxorubicin (25 mg/m^2) and methotrexate (10 mg/m^2 × 3) were somewhat reduced, and leucovorin was not required. Prophylactic intrathecal MTX was given to patients under age 40 and/or with bone marrow involvement. Treatment duration was 10 months. Tumor masses that were initially bulky or resistant to treatment were irradiated; a dosage of 2,000 rad was planned, but varied from 500 to 3,000 rad. Patients were also randomized to receive pseudomonas vaccine or immunotherapy. The latter did not affect prognosis. Overall results are noted in Table 3.

Three sequential treatment regimens with late intensification were utilized at M.D. Anderson Hospital and Tumor Institute.[31] Three cycles of CHOP were administered, followed by further CHOP if CR was achieved, and then late intensification with OAP-Bleo (vincristine, Ara-C, prednisone, bleomycin). If CR did not occur, three cycles of HOAP-Bleo (doxorubicin plus OAP-Bleo) were given followed by IMVP-16 (ifosfamide, methotrexate, VP-16). Patients with a partial response (PR) or no response on HOAP-Bleo received IMVP-16 only. The results (Table 3) were much improved over previous doxorubicin-containing regimens used at M.D. Anderson Hospital and Tumor Institute, particularly in patients with stage I–III disease.

A recently completed study at the University of Rome utilized high doses of ara-C (1,000 mg/m^2 over six hours) and moderate-dose MTX/LV (500 mg/m^2), combined with CHOP agents and also 5-fluorouracil (15 mg/m^2 over six hours). The resultant F-MACOP regimen was conceptually designed to exploit cell kinetic and synergistic principles.[32] Cycles were administered every 3 to 4 weeks, for a total of six courses. The results are noted in Table 3. The F-MACOP regimen is unique since 5-fluorouracil is utilized (only limited data is available for efficacy). Also, the high dose ara-C and moderate-dose methotrexate may reduce CNS relapse, especially since both drugs are also given intrathecally in patients with advanced stage, marrow involvement, or age under 30 years. Patients with lymphoblastic and undifferentiated lymphoma are also eligible for treatment. Only one patient subsequently relapsed in the CNS at the time of the report.[32]

The second generation intensive treatment regimens all result in an improved prognosis for patients with DLCL compared with the original first-generation protocols (Table 3). CR rates average about 75%, with relapse rates of 25% and 3-year survival rates of approximately 65%. Longer follow-up in some of the studies is required to determine the durability of complete remissions.

Results of recently introduced, third-generation regimens are noted in Table 5. The original NCI ProMACE-MOPP flexible induction regimen was changed to a randomized study comparing alternating half cycles of two regimens: ProMACE (day 1) - MOPP (day 8) (P-M), or ProMACE (day 1) - CytaBOM (day 8) (P-C). The dose of MTX was reduced to 500 mg/m^2 in P-M and to 120 mg/m^2 in P-C. Both regimens resulted in high CR rates, but toxicity was greater with P-C, owing to pneumocystis pneumonia, which was fatal in three of seven patients.[35] With the addition of prophylactic trimethoprimsulfamethoxazole, no further serious infection was encountered.[36]

The New York Hospital COP-BLAM III regimen differed from the earlier protocol by use of infusional vincristine and bleomycin alternated with bolus vincristine.[37] Dose escalation of doxorubicin and cyclophosphamide was carried out, but a less degree than COP-BLAM-I. Results (Table 5) show a higher CR rate and projected overall survival rate compared with the first regimen, but longer follow-up is required before definitive conclusions can be made. Of significance, 18 patients (33% of all patients) developed bleomycin pulmonary-toxicity, which was fatal in two patients. The COP-BLAM-III regimen is mainly administered in a hospital setting, compared with COP-BLAM-I which can be easily given on an outpatient basis. The dose of bleomycin is reduced in a new regimen called COD-BLAM-IV which also incorporates high-dose MTX/LV, etoposide, and ara-C.[38]

Table 5. Selected Third-Generation Studies for DLCL

Regimen	No. of Patients	% CR	% Relapse	% Survival at 2 Years (All Patients)
ProMACE[35]-CytaBOM	37	89	12	NA
COP-BLAM-III[37,38]	43	86	8	70
MACOP-B[39]	61	84	10	76

The MACOP-B regimen, developed at the University of British Columbia, is different from other programs, since chemotherapy is administered every week along with daily corticosteroids and antibiotic prophylaxis.[39] The duration of MACOP-B is also short, requiring only 12 weeks of 12 IV treatments. Most other regimens are administered over four to 10 months, with 16 to 33 IV injections. Results of MACOP-B (Table 5) are similar to the other two intensive regimens. Major toxicity proved to be moderate mucositis, occurring in 56% of patients or severe mucositis in 26% of patients. The incidence of mucositis decreased after several measures were introduced, including substitution of bleomycin for MTX/LV on weeks 4, 8, and 12; use of bicarbonate loading; prophylactic use of oral nystatin or ketoconazole; prompt treatment of herpes simplex infection with acyclovir; and extension of leucovorin rescue to 12 doses when mucositis occurred. Other side effects included granulocytopenia of less than 500 cells/mm^2 in 21% of patients and requirement for red blood cell transfusions in 20% of patients. With rigorous supportive care, only one toxic death occurred. The MACOP-B regimen must not be undertaken lightly, however, and should only be administered by experienced oncologists and hematologists. A recent update of MACOP-B administered to 94 patients showed a CR rate of 84%, relapse rate of 16%, and actuarial survival for all patients of 78% beyond two years.[41] Toxicity has remained modest with serious infection in less than 10% of patients and only three treatment-related deaths.

The best single indicator of the efficacy of a treatment program is the product of the CR rate multiplied by the relapse-free survival rate. This product tends to correct for errors in assessment of response, impact of salvage treatment on survival, and deaths due to unrelated causes. As an example, for MACOP-B, the figure is 66%, indicating that about two thirds of patients may be cured by a 12-week treatment program.

The third-generation regimens result in the highest CR rates reported to date (about 85%).

With low CR relapse rates, the actuarial 2-year survival rates for all patients are impressive: 70% to 76% (Table 5). These regimens are the newest, however, and still need greater patient accrual and longer follow-up to determine whether the high predicted cure rates will be realized. The protocols also originate from single institutions, which introduces some bias in patient selection. Many patients may not tolerate such intensive treatment, particularly older individuals and those with a poor performance status. For example, with MACOP-B, only 28% of patients were older than 60 years. Patient characteristics at the time of treatment also vary considerably and can significantly affect therapeutic results. Features that have been found to adversely affect prognosis include presence of bulky disease, B symptoms, certain histologic subtypes such as immunoblastic sarcomas, increased lactate dehydrogenase levels, and stage IV disease (especially bone marrow and CNS involvement).[41] Prognostic factors will be discussed in more detail below.

Prospective randomized trials are now being carried out to evaluate second-generation and third-generation regimens compared with a standard CHOP control arm. The largest study is being conducted by the SWOG, which compares m-BACOD *v* ProMACE-CytaBOM *v* MACOB-P *v* CHOP. The ECOG is currently randomizing between m-BACOD and CHOP, and in Milan, ProMACE-MOPP is being compared with CHOP. It will be critically important to properly stratify patients in these prospective studies, owing to differences in results that might occur because of variability in prognostic factors such as prior therapy, stage of disease, bulky disease, and other features noted below.

TREATMENT OF LOCALIZED DLCL

Management of localized DLCL, defined as stage I, I_E, II, and II_E disease, varies considerably, from use of chemotherapy or radiotherapy only to combined modality treatment programs. While one third of patients present with early-stage disease, complete evaluation will detect other sites of disease in most patients. Thus, treatment programs usually employ chemotherapy with or without radiotherapy. A summary of various treatment approaches is outlined in Tables 6 and 7.

Table 6. Treatment of Stage I/IE DLCL

Center	Treatment	No. of Patients	% CR	% Relapse	% RFS at 5 Years	% Actuarial Survival (yr) 5	10
Chicago[42]	RT†	17*	17 (100)	1 (6)	94 (DFS)	94	70
Minneapolis[43]	RT‡	16*	16 (100)	3 (19)	NA	77	77
Boston[44]	RT§	17‡‡	NA	NA	52	61	NA
Boston[44]	RT + CT‖	23‡‡	NA	NA	81	96	NA
Tucson[45]	CHOP	8	8 (100)	1 (13)			
Tucson[45]	CHOP + RT¶	7	7 (100)	1 (14)	75	100	NA
Houston[46]	CT#	11**	11 (100)	1 (9)	83	100	68
Milan[47] (randomized)	CVP + RT	83††	NA	NA	69	87	NA
	BACOP + RT	76††	NA	NA	81	100	NA

Abbreviations: RFS, relapse-free survival; DFS, disease-free survival; NA, not applicable.

*Laparotomy staged patients.

†RT (radiotherapy) includes involved field (IF), extended mantle, or other; total dose = 4,000 rad + 1,000 to 1,500 rad boost.

‡RT = variable but extended field to a dose of 5,000 rad + boost of 1,000 rad in some cases.

§RT = involved or required 3,500–5,600 rad.

‖CT (chemotherapy) variable = CHOP, C-MOPP, BACOP, M-BACOD.

¶RT = involved field 3,600–6,000 rad.

#CT = COP, CHOP ± bleomycin, or other multiple agents.

**Eleven patients only (category G Working Formulation).

††Includes stage II/II_E patients CT × 3 before and after RT. RT = IF 4,000–4,000 rad plus 3,500–4,000 rad uninvolved field.

‡‡Stage I/II minimal disease (1 or 2 contiguous sites <10 cm). Table 7 patients had stage I/II extended disease (>2 sites of discontiguous sites and/or >10 cm).

Table 7. Treatment of Stage II/II$_E$ DLCL

Center	Treatment	No. of Patients	% CR	% Relapse	RFS (5 yr)	Actuarial Survival (yr) 5	10
Chicago[42]	RT†	14*	12 (86)	4 (33)	56 (DFS)	62	45
Minneapolis[43]	RT‡	3*	3 (100)	1 (33)	2 relapse-free	3 alive	NA
Boston[44]	RT§	11‡‡	NA	NA	9	18	NA
Boston[44]	RT + CT‖	23‡‡	NA	NA	44	56	NA
Tucson[45]	CHOP	20	20 (100)	4 (20) }			
Tucson[45]	CHOP + RT¶	10	9 (90)	0 (0) }	86	85	85
Houston[46]	CT#	28	24 (86)	7 (29)	75	77	70
Milan[47] (randomized)	CVP + RT	83††	NA	NA	49	NA	NA
	BACOP + RT	76††	NA	NA	78	NA	NA

Abbreviations: RFS, relapse-free survival; DFS, disease-free survival; NA, not applicable.
*Laparotomy staged patients.
†RT (radiotherapy) includes involved field (IF), extended mantle, or other; total dose = 4,000 rad + 1,000 to 1,500 rad boost.
‡RT = variable but extended field to a dose of 5,000 rad + boost of 1,000 rad in some cases.
§RT = involved or required 3,500–5,600 rad.
‖CT (chemotherapy) variable = CHOP, C-MOPP, BACOP, M-BACOD.
¶RT = involved field 3,600–6,000 rad.
#CT = COP, CHOP ± Bleo, or other multiple agents.
**Eleven patients only (category G Working Formulation).
††Includes stage II/II$_E$ patients CT × 3 before and after RT. RT = IF 4,000–4,000 rad plus 3,500–4,000 rad uninvolved field.
‡‡Stage I/II minimal disease (1 or 2 contiguous sites <10 cm). Table 7 patients had stage I/II extended disease (>2 sites of discontiguous sites and/or >10 cm).

While most centers do not carry out staging laparotomy, this approach was followed by at least two institutions. At the University of Chicago[42] and University of Minnesota Hospitals,[43] patients subjected to staging laparotomy with pathologically confirmed stage I or II disease received radiotherapy only. The results in stage I or I$_E$ disease show 5-year survival rates of 77% to 94%, indicating a high cure rate (Table 6). In Boston, a retrospective review of clinically evaluated stage I/II minimal disease patients treated by radiotherapy alone showed a lower survival rate of 61% at 5 years.[44] Addition of chemotherapy (various regimens) increased the survival rate to 96% (relapse-free, 81%). Chemotherapy with CHOP was used in all clinically staged patients treated at Tucson,[45] but involved-field radiotherapy was also employed in those patients failing to achieve a CR within three courses, or in patients who required a reduction in the dose-rate of chemotherapy due to poor marrow reserve (generally over age 65 years). All patients with stage I/I$_E$ disease were alive at 5 years, with an actuarial relapse-free survival of 75%. Equally good results with chemotherapy only were reported from Houston.[46] The only prospective randomized trial to date, from Milan, compared CVP to BACOP, given before and after radiotherapy.[47] The five-year survival rate is significantly higher for BACOP (Table 6).

In patients with laparotomy-proven stage II/II$_E$ disease treated by radiotherapy only, survival drops off at 5 and 10 years (Table 7). Survival after radiotherapy is particularly low in the retrospective review from Boston, but use of chemotherapy and radiotherapy improves the prognosis. In patients with state II/II$_E$ disease treated at Tuscon with CHOP or CHOP plus radiotherapy, results are somewhat similar to the chemotherapy programs employed at Houston. The randomized Milan study shows an increased relapse-free survival rate for patients receiving BACOP compared with the non–doxorubicin-containing regimen.

All of the above studies show increased survival for patients with stage I/I$_E$ disease compared with stage II/II$_E$ disease. Analysis of sites of relapse does not show any obvious patterns, since decrease may develop at distant sites or within previously involved areas, particularly if bulky disease was initially present. In DLCL, unlike Hodgkin's disease, there may not be a clear dose-response relationship to radiotherapy. Furthermore, large tumor masses will have drug-resistant cell populations. In the Boston study,[44] patients were subclassified as stage I/II minimal disease if only one or two contiguous sites were involved and were less than 10 cm. Patients with disease exceeding these limitations or with discontiguous sites were categorized as stage I/II extended disease and had a much worse prognosis.

A reasonable therapeutic approach to patients with localized DLCL can be summarized as follows. For clinical stage I/I_E patients, surgical staging can be offered if the patient strongly desires to avoid chemotherapy and related side effects and is willing to risk the morbidity or complication of a laparotomy. If no other sites of disease are found (PS I/I_E), then modern radiotherapy results in a high cure rate. If staging laparotomy is not considered feasible or justified, then the cure rate from radiotherapy alone is lowered, although use of chemotherapy at the time of relapse may be successful. For CS II/II_E or PS II/II_E disease, chemotherapy alone is quite effective, although many centers utilize combined modality treatment. Poor prognostic features include tumor masses greater than 10 cm, discontiguous sites of disease, and three or more lesions. Patients having these features should receive chemotherapy and radiotherapy. The precise role of radiotherapy, however, has not been evaluated prospectively in a randomized fashion. Also, second-generation and third-generation chemotherapy regimens have not been generally employed for localized DLCL. Future studies should address these issues.

SALVAGE TREATMENT PROGRAMS

Treatment failure in DLCL is generally associated with rapidly progressive disease that is refractory to secondary chemotherapy. If the patient relapses after a CR that lasted for a year or more, occasional brief responses can be achieved with use of conventional regimens that had not been previously used, such as C-MOPP or COMLA. However, since most intensive regimens employ the most active agents, there are very few salvage regimens available (Table 8). Single agents that have resulted in impressive but brief responses include high-dose methotrexate with leucovorin rescue,[53] high-dose ara-C,[54] cisplatinum,[55] VP-16,[56] and amsacrine.[57] The salvage regimens listed in Table 8 all utilize VP-16 plus other drugs that show some activity in non-Hodgkin's lymphoma (NHL). Response rates are variable, with CRs ranging from 5% to 37% and PRs from 13% to 47%. The response durations also vary considerably, but are gener-

Table 8. Salvage Regimens in Non-Hodgkins Lymphomas

Institution	Drugs	Dose (mg/m^2)	No. of Pts.	Response (%)	Duration (mo)
Royal Marsden[47]	VP-16	100 IV d 1–3	17	CR (29)	4–12
	Platinum	50 IV d 1		PR (24)	
SAKK[48]	VP-6	120 PO d 3–5	17	PR (29)	3
	Platinum	60 IV d 1			
	Prednisone	60 PO d 1–5			
Sheffield University[49]	Vindesine	3 IV d 1 and 8	20	CR (20)	9–13+
	VP-16	100 IV d 1		PR (20)	1.5–5
	Prednisone	200 PO d 2,3			
		25 PO d 1–7			
Christie[50]	Hydroxyurea	1 g total q6h × 8	19	CR (5)	2–19
	Ifosfamide	3 g IV d 1		PR (47)	
	VP-16	80 IV d 5			
		160 PO d 6			
M.D. Anderson[51]	Ifosfamide	1 g d 1–5	52	CR (37)	13
	Methotrexate	30 IV d 3 and 10		PR (25)	
	VP-16	100 IV d 1–3			
University of Florida[52]	VP-16	100 IV d 1–3	15	CR (27)	4–32
	BCNU	100 IV d 1		PR (13)	4
	Bleomycin	10 IV d 1,8,15,22			
	Methotrexate	50 IV d 1			
	Leucovorin	5 q6h × 6 d2			

ally under 6 or 12 months. The data must be interpreted with caution, since it is derived from patients with a variety of histologic subgroups, different prognostic factors, and previous treatment programs.

The most encouraging results of salvage chemotherapy were reported by M.D. Anderson Hospital and Tumor Institute.[51] The factor that best predicted for response to IMVP-16 was the quality of the remission achieved from front-line therapy. The median relapse-free survival of the responding patients was 12 months, while median survival of all patients was 15 months. Of 18 patients who achieved CR, 10 remained disease-free at the time of the report.

Recently introduced single agents that show activity in failed patients include mitoxantrone,[58] methyl-GAG,[59] gallium nitrate,[60] and VM-26.[61] The role of these agents in future chemotherapy regimens is beginning to be explored, but at least one study reports the same activity of the single drug (VM-26) as when combined with two other drugs.[62]

NEW TREATMENT APPROACHES

The role of bone marrow transplantation in the therapy of non-Hodgkin's lymphoma has been recently reviewed.[63,64] Most studies have been carried out in patients failing standard treatment regimens. The results of syngeneic transplantation have been most encouraging, with a long-term survival rate of about 60%.[64] In contrast, results of allogeneic transplantation have been disappointing, with only 10% to 20% of patients cured. With improvements in technology, it has been demonstrated that bone marrow can be cryopreserved and reinfused safely, allowing for successful autologous bone marrow transplantation (ABMT). Unfortunately, the fatal complication rate is high and about 75% of patients have relapsed after ABMT. It is impossible to distinguish between relapses due to failure to eradicate the lymphoma and relapses due to infused tumor cells.

At the Dana-Farber Cancer Institute, a different approach to ABMT has been carried out. Bone marrow has been rendered free of tumor cells in vitro by the B cell specific monoclonal antibody anti-B1 and rabbit complement.[65] Thirteen patients with relapsed B1 positive lymphoma received intensive chemoradiotherapy followed by ABMT with processed marrow.[66] Eight patients remain disease-free in an unmaintained remission up to 2 years. Further patient accrual and longer follow-up are necessary to fully evaluate this unique treatment of failed lymphoma patients. Current and future studies are evaluating the role of ABMT in patients at high risk of relapse when they are in remission. With a minimal tumor burden, an overall improvement in survival is expected.

Various biologic response modifiers have been utilized in NHL patients who have been heavily pretreated. Monoclonal antibodies, including highly specific antiidiotypic antibodies, initially caused disease regression in patients with low or intermediate grade lymphomas, but overall results have been disappointing. Recent studies employing interferons have demonstrated significant activity, especially in patients with low grade indolent B cell lymphomas and cutaneous T cell lymphomas, with response rates of 54% and 45%, respectively.[67] However, in patients with aggressive or high grade lymphomas, response rates have been much lower, averaging 18% in combined trials.[68] Since antitumor effects are of short duration, there appears to be a minimal role for the new biologic agents in aggressive lymphomas.

PROGNOSTIC FACTORS

Most studies show that prognosis is adversely affected by extensive prior therapy, advanced disease (ie, stage IV *v* I), and failure to achieve a CR. A variety of other pretreatment features, however, also affect response and survival, but there is no uniformity among institutional or group studies as to the ranking of these prognostic parameters. There are numerous reasons for this discrepancy, varying from patient referral patterns to the intensity of treatment. Furthermore, factors that are significant by univariate analysis may not be important by multivariate analysis. A detailed analysis of these factors is beyond the scope of this report and the reader is referred to a recently published review.[69]

A retrospective review of pretreatment characteristics of patients with DLCL treated by M-BACOD or m-BACOD at the Dana-Farber Cancer Institute was recently carried out.[70] Only patients with all clinical, laboratory, radiological, and histopathological material available for

Table 9. Prognostic Risk Groups of Patients Treated With M-BACOD and m-BACOD[70]

Risk Group	% of Patients	Categories*			5-Year Survival (%)
		PS	Mass	ENS	
Low	42	0,1	<10	0	68
		0,1	<10	1	
Moderate	41	0,1	>10	0	
		0,1	<10	≥2	55
		0,1	>10	1	
High	17	0,1	>10	2	
		2-4	<10	0	
		2-4	<10	1	
		2-4	<10	0	24
		2-4	<10	≥2	
		2-4	<10	1	
		2-4	>10	≥2	

*PS, Performance status; Mass, Size of largest mass in cm; ENS, Extranodal sites of disease.

review were analyzed. Factors evaluated for potential prognostic significance included age, sex, stage, performance status, presence of constitutional symptoms, pathologic subtype by both the Rappaport and Lukes and Collins classifications, sites of disease involvement, number of extranodal sites, location and largest dimension of the largest site of bulk disease, serum lactate dehydrogenase (LDH), time to complete response, and prior therapy. Since clinical features, response rates, and survival curves for the two treatment regimens were identical, the data from both programs were consolidated. In a multivariate analysis, only two characteristics, poor performance status and massive bulky disease, adversely affected the response rate. These same two factors, plus increasing numbers of extranodal sites of disease, negatively affected survival in a multivariate analysis (proportional hazards regression analysis). These three pretreatment variables were then used to construct a model containing 12 categories of patients at increasing risk for relapse and decreased survival. The categories divided naturally into three broad groups of patients with decreasing five-year survival rates as noted in Table 9.

It is apparent from Table 9 that more intensive treatment is required for patients with moderate-risk and high-risk features. Some of these patients may be ideal candidates for initial ABMT. The role of regional radiotherapy also remains to be explored, particularly in patients with bulky disease. On the other extreme, patients in the low risk group may have an equally good prognosis with regimens less intense or of shorter duration than m-BACOD. These questions form the basis of future studies. The optimal treatment programs will require prospective randomized studies with careful stratification by prognostic features. If the risk groups as defined by the Farber study are confirmed in additional studies of patients treated by other current regimens with similar response rates, then treatment strategy can be developed that will be more precisely tailored to individual patient needs.

REFERENCES

1. Rosenberg S: Non-Hodgkin's lymphoma pathologic classification project. National Cancer Institute sponsored study of classification of non-Hodgkin's lymphomas: Summary and description of a working formulation for clinical usage. Cancer 49:2112, 1982

2. Arnold A, Cossman J, Bakhshi A, et al: Immunoglobulin-gene rearrangements as unique clonal markers in human lymphoid neoplasms. N Engl J Med 309:1593, 1983

3. Bertness V, Kirsch I, Hollis G, et al: T-Cell receptor gene rearrangements as clinical markers of human T-cell lymphomas. N Engl J Med 313:534, 1985

4. DeVita VT, Chabner B, Hubbard SP, et al: Advanced diffuse histiocytic lymphoma, a potentially curable disease. Lancet 1:248, 1975

5. Coleman M: Chemotherapy for large-cell lymphoma: optimism and caution. Ann Intern Med 103:140, 1985

6. Goldie JH, Goldman AJ, Gudauskas GA, et al: Rationale for the use of alternating non-cross-resistant chemotherapy. Cancer Treat Rep 66:439, 1982

7. Norton L, Simon R: Tumor size, sensitivity to therapy, and design of treatment schedules. Cancer Treat Rep 61:1307, 1977

8. Coltman CA, Dahlberg S, Jones SE, et al: CHOP is curative in thirty percent of patients with large cell lymphoma. A twelve year Southwest Oncology Group follow-up. Advances in Chemotherapy: Update on Treatment for Diffuse Large Cell Lymphoma. New York, Wiley, 1986, pp 71–77

9. Armitage JO, Fyfe MAE, Lewis J: Long-term remission durability and functional status of patients treated for diffuse histiocytic lymphoma with CHOP regimen. J Clin Oncol 2:898, 1984

10. Rodriguez V, Cabanillas F, Burgess MA, et al: Combination chemotherapy ("CHOP-Bleo") in advanced (Non-Hodgkin) malignant lymphoma. Blood 49:325, 1977

11. Skarin AT, Rosenthal DS, Moloney WC, et al: Combination chemotherapy of advanced non-Hodgkin's lymphoma with bleomycin, Adriamycin, cyclophosphamide, vincristine, and prednisone (BACOP). Blood 49:759, 1977

12. Schein PS, DeVita VT, Hubbard S, et al: Bleomycin,

Adriamycin, cyclophosphamide, vincristine, and prednisone (BACOP) combination chemotherapy in the treatment of advanced diffuse histiocytic lymphoma. Ann Intern Med 85:417, 1976

13. Levine AM, Goldstein M, Meyer PR, et al: Heterogeneity of response and survival in diffuse histiocytic lymphoma after BACOP therapy (bleomycin, doxorubicin, cyclophosphamide, vincristine, prednisone). Hematol Oncol 3:87, 1985

14. Berd D, Cornog J, DeConti RC, et al: Long-term remission in diffuse histiocytic lymphoma treated with combination sequential chemotherapy. Cancer 35:1050–1054, 1986

15. Sween DL, Golomb HM, Ultmann JE, et al: Cyclophosphamide, vincristine, methotrexate with leucovorin rescue, and cytarabine (COMLA) combination sequential chemotherapy for advanced diffuse histiocytic lymphoma. Ann Intern Med 92:785, 1980

16. Gaynor ER, Ultmann JE, Golomb HM, et al: Treatment of diffuse histiocytic lymphoma (DHL) with COMLA (cyclophosphamide, Oncovin, methotrexate, leucovorin, cytosine arabinoside): A 10-year experience in a single institution. J Clin Oncol 3:1596, 1985

17. Baer MR, Stein RS, Greer JP, et al: Modified cyclophosphamide, vincristine, methotrexate, leucovorin, and cytarabine (COMLA) in intermediate and high grade lymphoma: An effective short course regimen. Cancer Treat Rep 70:785–777, 1986

18. Gams RA, Rainey M, Dandy M, et al: Phase III study of BCOP vs CHOP in unfavorable categories of malignant lymphoma: A Southeastern cancer study group trial. J Clin Oncol 3:1188, 1985

19. Dupont J, Caray G, Scaglione C, et al: A randomized comparison of two chemotherapy regimens: BACOP vs COPP in the treatment of diffuse histiocytic and mixed lymphoma, in Second International Conference on Malignant Lymphoma. Lugano, Switzerland, 1984, p 475

20. Todd M, Cadman E, Spiro P, et al: A follow-up of a randomized study comparing two chemotherapy treatments for advanced diffuse histiocytic lymphoma. J Clin Oncol 2:986, 1984

21. Todd MB, Cadman EC, Newcomer LN, et al: ACOMLA and COMLA for malignant lymphoma. Advances in Cancer Chemotherapy: Update on Treatment for Diffuse Large Cell Lymphoma. New York, Wiley, 1986, pp 53–61

22. Johnson GJ, Costello WG, Oken MM, et al: Sequential cyclophosphamide-prednisone and vincristine-bleomycin (CPOB). Cancer 52:1133, 1983

23. Jones SE, Grozea PN, Miller TP, et al: Chemotherapy with cyclophosphamide, doxorubicin, vincristine, and prednisone alone or with levamisole or with levamisole plus BCG for malignant lymphoma: A Southwest Oncology Group study. J Clin Oncol 3:1318, 1985

24. Skarin AT, Canellos GP, Rosenthal DS, et al: Improved prognosis of diffuse histiocytic and undifferentiated lymphoma by use of high dose methotrexate alternating with standard agents (M-BACOD). J Clin Oncol 1:91, 1983

25. Skarin AT, Canellos GP, Rosenthal DS, et al: Moderate dose m-BACOD in advanced diffuse large cell lymphoma—an interim report. Advances in Cancer Chemotherapy: Update on treatment of diffuse large cell lymphoma. New York, Wiley, 1986, pp 23–29

26. Fisher RI, DeVita VT, Hubbard SM, et al: Diffuse aggressive lymphomas: Increased survival after alternating flexible sequences of ProMACE and MOPP chemotherapy. Ann Intern Med 98:304–309, 1983

27. Fisher RI, Young RC, DeVita VT: ProMACE-MOPP combination chemotherapy for diffuse lymphomas. Semin Oncol 12:29, 1985

28. Laurence J, Coleman M, Allen SL: Combination chemotherapy of advanced diffuse histiocytic lymphoma with the six-drug COP-BLAM regimen. Ann Intern Med 97:190, 1982

29. Armitage JO, Weisenburger DD, Hutchins M, et al: Chemotherapy for diffuse large-cell lymphoma: Rapidly responding patients have more durable remissions. J Clin Oncol 4:160, 1986

30. Koziner B, Sklaroff R, Little C, et al: NHL-3 Protocol: Six-drug combination chemotherapy for non-Hodgkin's lymphoma. Cancer 53:2592, 1984

31. Cabanillas F, Burgess MA, Bodey GP, et al: Sequential chemotherapy and late intensification for malignant lymphomas of aggressive histologic type. Am J Med 74:382, 1983

32. Amadori S, Guglielmi C, Anselmo AP, et al: Treatment of diffuse aggressive non-Hodgkin's lymphomas with an intensive multi-drug regimen including high-dose cytosine arabinoside (F-MACHOP). Semin Oncol 12:218, 1985

33. Skarin AT: High dose methotrexate/leucovorin factor rescue (HDMTX/LF) in diffuse large cell lymphoma (DLCL): Development of folates and folic acid antagonists in cancer chemotheapy. (in press)

34. Canellos GP, Skarin AT, Rosenthal DS, et al: Methotrexate as a single agent and in combination chemotherapy for the treatment of non-Hodgkin's lymphoma of unfavorable histology. Cancer Treat Rep 65:125, 1981

35. Fisher RI, DeVita VT, Hubbard SM, et al: Randomized trial of ProMACE-MOPP vs ProMACE-CytaBOM in previously untreated advanced stage, diffuse aggressive lymphomas. Proc Am Soc Clin Oncol 3:242, 1984

36. Browne MJ, Hubbard SM, Longo DL, et al: Excess prevalence of pneumocystis carinii pneumonia in patients treated for lymphoma with combination chemotherapy. Ann Intern Med 104:338, 1986

37. Coleman M, Boyd DB, Bernhardt B, et al: COPBLAM III: Combination chemotherapy for diffuse large cell lymphoma (LCL) with cyclophosphamide (C), infusional Oncovin (O), prednisone (P), infusional bleomycin (BL), Adriamycin (A) and Matulane (M). Proc Am Soc Clin Oncol 3:246, 1984

38. Coleman M, Boyd DB, Beshevkin M, et al: COP-BLAM treatment of large cell lymphoma: A status report, in Advances in Cancer Treatment for Diffuse Large Cell Lymphoma. New York, Wiley (in press)

39. Klimo P, Connors JM: MACOP-B chemotherapy for the treatment of diffuse large-cell lymphoma. Ann Intern Med 102:596, 1985

40. Connors JM, Klimo P: MACOP-B chemotherapy for the treatment of diffuse large cell lymphoma: 1985 update: Advances in Cancer Chemotherapy: Update on Treatment

for Diffuse Large Cell Lymphoma, New York, Wiley, (in press)

41. Jagannath S, Velasquez WS, Tucker SL, et al: Stage IV diffuse large-cell lymphoma: A long-term analysis. J Clin Oncol 3:39, 1985

42. Vokes EE, Ultmann JE, Golomb HM, et al: Long-term survival of patients with localized diffuse histiocytic lymphoma. J Clin Oncol 3:1309, 1985

43. Levitt SH, Lee CKK, Bloomfield CD, et al: The role of radiation therapy in the treatment of early stage large cell lymphoma. Hematol Oncol 3:33, 1985

44. Mauch P, Leonard R, Skarin AT, et al: Improved survival following combined radiation therapy and chemotherapy for unfavorable prognosis stage I-II non-Hodgkin's lymphomas. J Clin Oncol 3:1301, 1985

45. Miller TP, Jones SE: Initial chemotherapy for clinically localized lymphomas of unfavorable histology. Blood 62:413, 1983

46. Cabanillas F: Chemotherapy as definitive treatment of stage I-II large cell and diffuse mixed lymphomas. Hematol Oncol 3:25, 1985

47. Bonadonna G: Chemotherapy of malignant lymphomas. Semin Oncol 12:1, 1985

48. Cavalli F: VP-16 in the treatment of malignant lymphomas: A report from the Swiss Group for clinical cancer research (SAKK). Semin Oncol 12:33, 1985

49. Hancock BW: Vindesine, etoposide (VP-16), and prednisone (VEP) in relapsed patients with grade II non-Hodgkin's lymphoma. Semin Oncol 12:26, 1985

50. Gasser AB, Steward WP, Wagstaff J, et al: Treatment of relapsed non-Hodgkin's lymphoma with a combination of hydroxyurea, ifosfamide, and etoposide. Cancer Treat Rep 69:225, 1985

51. Cabanillas F, Hagemeister FB, Bodey GP, et al: IMVP-16: An effective regimen for patients with lymphoma who have relapsed after initial combination chemotherapy. Blood 60: 693, 1982

52. Helms SR, Oblon DJ, Braylan RC, et al: Etoposide, carmustine, bleomycin, and methotrexate with leucovorin rescue as re-treatment for unfavorable non-Hodgkin's lymphoma. Cancer Treat Rep 69:783, 1985

53. Skarin AT, Zukerman KS Pitman SW, et al: High-dose methotrexate with folinic acid in the treatment of advanced non-Hodgkin's lymphoma including CNS involvement. Blood 50:1039, 1977

54. Shipp MA, Takvorian RC, Canellos GP: High-dose cytosine arabinoside. Active agent in the treatment of non-Hodgkin's lymphoma. Am J Med 77:845, 1984

55. Cavalli F, Jungi WF, Nissen NI, et al: Phase II trial of cisdichlorodiammineplatinum (II) in advanced malignant lymphoma: A study of the cancer and acute leukemia group B. Cancer 48:1927, 1981

56. Jacobs P, King HS, Dent DM, et al: VP-16–213 in the treatment of stage II and IV diffuse large cell lymphoma. Cancer 56:1006, 1985

57. Case DC: m-AMSA: Phase II trial in advanced lymphoma and leukemia. Am J Clin Oncol 7:357, 1984

58. Case D, Jones S, Stein R, et al: Mitoxantrone in refractory malignant lymphoma. Proc Am Soc Clin Oncol 4, 210, 1985

59. Warrell RP, Lee BJ, Kempin SJ, et al: Effectiveness of Methyl-GAG (Methylglyoxal-bis[Guyanylhydrazone]) in patients with advanced malignant lymphoma. Blood 57:1011, 1981

60. Warrell RP, Coonley CJ, Straus DR, et al: Treatment of patients with advanced malignant lymphoma using gallium nitrate administered as a seven-day continuous infusion. Cancer 51:1982, 1983

61. Tirelli U, Carbone A, Crivellari D, et al: A Phase II trial of teniposide (VM 26) in advanced non-Hodgkin's lymphoma, with emphasis on the treatment of elderly patients. Cancer 54:393, 1984

62. O'Connell MJ, Anderson J, Merrill JM, et al: Comparative trial of two teniposide-based combination chemotherapy regimens for the treatment of advanced malignant lymphomas. Cancer Treat Rep 66:2021, 1982

63. Applebaum FR, Thomas ED: Review of the use of marrow transplantation in the treatment of non-Hodgkin's lymphoma. J Clin Oncol 1:440, 1983

64. Champlin RE, Gale RP: Role of bone marrow transplantation in the treatment of hematologic malignancies and solid tumors: Critical review of syngeneic, autologous, and allogeneic transplants. Cancer Treat Rep 68:145, 1984

65. Nadler LM, Botnick LB, Rinberg R, et al: Anti-B1 monoclonal antibody and complement treatment in autologous bone-marrow transplantation for relapsed B-cell non-Hodgkin's lymphoma. Lancet 2:427, 1984

66. Takvorian T, Nadler LM, Anderson KC, et al: Autologous bone marrow transplantation (ABMT) in B-cell malignancy: Anti-B1 monoclonal antibody treated autologous bone marrow. Proc Am Soc Clin Oncol 4, 204, 1985

67. Bunn PA, Ihde DC, Foon KA: The role of interferon Alfa-2a in the therapy of cutaneous T-cell lymphoma. Cancer 57:1689, 1986

68. Canellos GP: Interferon in the treatment of malignant lymphoma. Semin Oncol 12:25, 1985

69. Canellos GP, Shipp M, Harrington DP, et al: Prognostic factors in diffuse large cell lymphoma. Advances in Cancer Chemotherapy: Update on Treatment for Diffuse Large Cell Lymphoma. New York, Wiley, 1986, p 11

70. Shipp MA, Harrington DP, Klatt MK, et al: Identification of Major Prognostic Subgroups of Patients with large-cell lymphoma treated with m-BACOD or M-BACOD. Ann Intern Med 104:757, 1986

APPENDIX

Selected Regimens in Non-Hodgkin's Lymphoma

Regimen	Drugs	Dosage (mg/m^2)	Days of Treatment	Frequency
1. C-MOPP:	cyclophosphamide	650 IV	1 and 8	q 28 days
	vincristine (Oncovin*)	1.4 IV	1 and 8	
	procarbazine	100 PO	1 to 14	
	prednisone	40 PO	1 to 14	
2. CHOP	cyclophosphamide	750 IV	1	q 21 days
	doxorubicin (Adriamycin†)	50 IV	1	
	vincristine (Oncovin*)	1.4 IV	1 and 5	
	prednisone	100 PO	1 to 5	
3. CHOP-Bleo	cyclophosphamide	750 IV	1	q 21 days
	doxorubicin (Adriamycin†)	50 IV	1	
	vincristine (Oncovin*)	1.4 IV	1 and 5	
	prednisone	100 PO	1 to 5	
	bleomycin	4 IV	1 and 5	
4. BCVP	carmustine (BCNU)	60 IV	1	q 21 days
	cyclophosphamide	1,000 IV	1	
	vincristine (Oncovin*)	1.4 IV	1	
	prednisone	100 PO	1 to 15	
5. BACOP	cyclophosphamide	650 IV	1 and 8	q 28 days
	doxorubicin (Adriamycin†)	25 IV	1 and 8	
	vincristine (Oncovin*)	1.4 IV	1 and 8	
	bleomycin	5 IV	15 and 21	
	prednisone	60 PO	15 to 28	
6. COMLA	cyclophosphamide	1,500 IV	1	q 21 days
	vincristine (Oncovin*)	1.5 IV	1, 8 and 15	
	methotrexate	120 IV	22, then weekly × 7	
	leucovorin	25 PO	q 6 hr × 4, 24 hr after MTX	
	cytosine arabinoside	300 IV	22, then weekly × 7	q 21 days
7. m-BACOD	methotrexate	200 IV	8 and 15; LV 10mg/m^2 po q6h × 8; 9 and 16	
	bleomycin	4 IV	1	
	doxorubicin (Adriamycin†)	45 IV	1	
	cyclophosphamide	600 IV	1	
	vincristine (Oncovin*)	1.0 IV	1	
	dexamethasone	6 PO	1 to 5	
8. ProMACE-MOPP (flexitherapy)	cyclophosphamide	650 IV	1 and 8	q 28 days
	doxorubicin (Adriamycin†)	25 IV	1 and 8	
	epipodophyllotoxin (VP-16)	120 IV	1 and 8	
	prednisone	60 PO	1 to 14	
	methotrexate	1,500 IV	14 (LV 50mg/m^2 q6h × 5 day 15)	
	standard MOPP		after remission	q 28 days
9. COP-BLAM-I	cyclophosphamide	400 IV	1	
	vincristine (Oncovin*)	1 IV	1	
	prednisone	40 PO	1 to 10	q 21 days
	bleomycin	15 IV (total)	14	
	doxorubicin (Adriamycin†)	40 IV	1	
	Matulane	100 PO	1 to 10	
10. ACOMLA	doxorubicin (Adriamycin†)	40 IV	1	
	cyclophosphamide	1,000 IV	1	
	vincristine (Oncovin*)	2 IV total	1, 8, 15	q 3 months
	methotrexate	120 IV	22, 29, 35, 43, 50, 57, 64, 71	
	leucovorin	25 PO total	24 hrs after MTX, q6h × 6	
	Ara-C	300 IV	1 hr after MTX on same days	
11. Pro-MACE (day 1)	ProMace	see above	1 (no MTX)	
Cytaboma (day 8)	cytarabine	300 IV	8	q 21 days
	bleomycin	5 IV	8	
	methotrexate	120 IV	8	
	leucovorin	25 PO	9 q6h × 4 24 hrs after MTX	

APPENDIX (Cont'd)

Regimen	Drugs	Dosage (mg/m^2)	Days of Treatment	Frequency
12. COP-BLAM-III	cyclophosphamide	350 IV (escalate to 500	1 and 22	
	vincristine (Oncovin*)	1 IV	1 to 2; 22 to 23 (con't IV infusion)	q 6 weeks
	prednisone	40 IV	1 to 5; 22 to 27	
	bleomycin	7.5 IV	1 (IV push) 1 to 5; 22 to 23 (con't IV infusion)	
	doxorubicin (Adriamycin†)	35 IV (escalate to 50)	1 and 22	
	Matulane	100 PO	1 to 5; 22 to 27	
13. MACOP-B	methotrexate	400 IV	weeks 2, 6, 10	
	doxorubicin (Adriamycin†)	50 IV	weeks 1, 3, 5, 7, 9, 11	
	cyclophosphamide	350 IV	weeks 1, 3, 5, 7, 9, 11	
	vincristine (Oncovin*)	1.4 IV	weeks 2, 4, 6, 8, 10, 12	
	bleomycin	10U IV	weeks 4, 8, 12	
	prednisone	75 PO	daily, dose tapered over the last 15 days	
	co-trimoxazole	2 tablets PO	twice daily throughout	

Abbreviations: IV, intravenously; LV, leucovorin; MTX, methotrexate; PO, orally.

*Manufactured by Eli Lilly and Company, Indianapolis.

†Manufactured by Adria Laboratories, Columbus, OH.

Strategies in the Treatment of Hodgkin's Disease

David J. Straus

The current treatment methods for the four stages of the four histologic subtypes of Hodgkin's disease are described. In the last several years, the use of radiotherapy and combination chemotherapy has dramatically improved the prognosis of patients with even the most advanced stages of disease. However, toxicity remains a problem. Gonadal function is adversely affected in many patients, and the risk of subsequent acute leukemia or myelodysplastic syndrome is about 10% at 10 years after treatment. There have been few trials of biologic response modifiers in Hodgkin's disease, and the results show no advantage over chemotherapy and radiotherapy. Newer therapeutic approaches will need to be devised, both to reduce toxicity and to improve the response of the relatively small number of patients who do not achieve a durable remission with present treatment.

THE USE of radiotherapy (RT) and chemotherapy for Hodgkin's disease has been one of the major success stories in medical oncology in the last 20 years. This success has been aided by an understanding of the clinical features and course of the disease.

HISTOPATHOLOGY

Currently the Rye modification of the Lukes and Butler classification is in use throughout the world.[1] Lymphocyte predominance is characterized by an abundance of small lymphocytes and with occasional, often atypical, Reed-Sternberg cells of "lymphocytic-histiocytic" variety. The classic presentation is in a high cervical node in a young asymptomatic male. It carries the most favorable prognosis of the four histologic subtypes. Nodular sclerosis is the most common subtype in North America. There is often abundant fibrosis in the node dividing tumor nodules containing inflammatory cells and the "lacunar cell" variant of Reed-Sternberg cells. The classic presentation would be in a young female with mediastinal involvement with or without symptoms. Although it has classically been felt to carry a relatively favorable prognosis, this seems to be dependent on the stage of the disease, the bulkiness of the tumor masses, and the presence or absence of systemic symptoms. Mixed cellularity is characterized by a pleomorphic cellular infiltrate of plasma cells, eosinophils, lymphocytes, histiocytes, and Reed-Sternberg cells. Subdiapharagmatic and extranodal presentations and the presence of B symptoms may be somewhat more frequent than with the nodular sclerosis subtype. It is the second most common histologic subtype in North America and is more common in the poorer parts of the world and among older patients. It has been associated with a worse prognosis than is nodular sclerosis, but this may be due to the association of this subtype with unfavorable clinical prognostic features. The lymphocyte depletion subtype has a paucity of cellular elements and an increased reticular network. It is associated with advanced age, systemic symptoms, retroperitoneal node, and extranodal involvement, and has the worst prognosis of the four histiologic subtypes.

STAGING

The current staging classification was established by the Ann Arbor Workshop in 1981.[2] Clinical staging (CS) refers to all staging procedures short of staging laparotomy. Pathologic staging (PS) refers to the findings at staging laparotomy during which liver biopsies, splenectomy, and excisional biopsies of retroperitoneal nodes are performed. An attempt is made by the surgeon to biopsy nodes that are suspicious on lymphangiogram. Some centers also perform open bone marrow biopsies from the iliac crest.

Staging procedures include chest X-ray, bipedal lower extremity lymphangiogram, liver-spleen scan, complete blood counts with platelet and differential counts, bone marrow aspiration and biopsy, serum liver biochemistries including alkaline phosphatase and 5′ nucleotidase, and erythrocyte sedimentation rate. The latter test has been shown to carry prognostic significance.[3] Computerized tomography of the abdomen will

From the Department of Hematology/Oncology, Memorial Sloan-Kettering Cancer Center, New York.

Address reprint requests to David J. Straus, MD, Associate Attending Physician, Department of Hematology/Oncology, Memorial Sloan-Kettering Cancer Center, 1275 York Ave, New York, NY 10021.

0093-7754/86/1304-5004$05.00/0

show enlarged retroperitoneal and pelvic lymph nodes. There may be nodes involved by disease that are not enlarged, but that may show abnormalities on the filling pattern of lymphangiogram contrast material. Mesenteric node involvement at presentation in Hodgkin's disease is much less common than in the non-Hodgkin's lymphomas. The accuracy of lymphangiography in determining the presence or absence of Hodgkin's disease in retroperitoneal and pelvic nodes approaches 90% in experienced hands.

If there are abnormalities of the liver-spleen scan, gross abnormalities of serum liver biochemical studies, a lymphangiogram indicating retroperitoneal or pelvic nodal disease, or systemic B symptoms, a liver biopsy should be performed. Slight elevations of serum alkaline phosphatase may be seen without liver involvement. Laparoscopy with direct visualization of the surface of the liver and biopsy of suspicious areas increases the yield of this procedure over blind percutaneous needle biopsy.[4] Gallium scanning may be a useful procedure for following mediastinal disease, but it is associated with a significant number of false negatives and false positives. Computerized tomography of the chest may show disease, particularly retrosternal disease, missed by a plain chest X-ray. Although traditional RT treatment planning seems rarely to be affected by these findings, computerized tomography may allow for refinements in RT treatment planning in the future.

The necessity for surgical staging is controversial.[5,6] There is general agreement that it is only performed if it makes a difference in treatment, either alone or in combination with chemotherapy. As a consequence, it is also generally agreed that it is not necessary when treatment of even early stage patients involves combination chemotherapy. It is controversial as to whether or not it is necessary to use RT treatment for supradiaphragmatic stage IA or IIA disease in the mantle port (cervical, supraclavicular, mediastinal, and axillary regions), or in para-aortic nodes including the spleen or splenic pedicle if the spleen has been removed—subtotal nodal irradiation (SNI). A large study using this type of treatment with either surgical staging or CS showed no difference in overall survival, relapse-free survival, or pelvic recurrence rate between CS, patients and those surgically staged.[7]

The major finding at staging laparotomy has been that 20% to 30% of patients who are CS IA or IIA have occult disease in the spleen and will hence increase their stage to $IIIA_s$.[5,8] There has been controversy as to whether disease in the spleen or high para-aortic nodes carries a better prognosis following treatment with RT only, than does disease in the lower para-aortic nodes or pelvis.[9] The Stanford group has found that minimal disease in the spleen (four or fewer tumor nodules) carries a more favorable prognosis than does more extensive disease in the spleen (five or more tumor nodules) following treatment with RT only.[10]

The problems associated with staging laparotomy must also be considered in the decision of whether or not it is to be performed. The overall mortality is 1.5% and has been as high as 3%. The overall mortality is in the range of 6% including wound infection, subphrenic abscess, intestinal obstruction from adhesions, and pulmonary embolus.[6] Late sepsis with pneumococcus or Hemophilus influenzae has also been reported. Pneumococcal vaccine may reduce the risk of pneumococcal sepsis. The discomfort caused by the surgery to the patient and its expense should also be considered.

In summary, staging laparotomy is indicated only when a potential treatment choice must be made between RT alone and combination chemotherapy with or without RT. Even if subtotal nodal RT is contemplated for supradiaphragmatic CS IA or IIA disease, the necessity for staging laparotomy is not completely clear.

TREATMENT

Stages IA and IIA

The work of Gilbert, Peters, and later Kaplan[11] demonstrated that recurrences rarely occur within the treated areas with doses of RT to 3500 rad. The use of the linear accelerator made it possible to deliver these doses to large fields. The mantle port (cervical, supraclavicular, mediastinal, and axillary regions—an area like the mantle on a suit of armor), the "inverted Y" (para-aortic nodes, spleen—depending on whether or not it was removed, and iliac, inguinal, and femoral nodes), and combinations of the two were developed in the 1960s. Total nodal irradiation (TNI) refers to combinations of the two, which have also at times included low-dose irradiation of the liver and lung. SNI includes the mantle port with irradiation of the para-aortic nodes and the spleen, if it was not removed, sparing the pelvis.

Local irradiation is probably adequate for high cervical stage IA disease with a single tumor mass and lymphocyte predominant or nodular sclerosis histology in a young patient.

There is also general agreement that bulky mediastinal disease, with a mediastinal mass over one-third of the chest diameter, should be treated with combination chemotherapy or combined modality treatment with chemotherapy and RT.[12]

The prognostic importance of extension of disease from the hilar nodes into the lung parenchyma is controversial. Some centers employing RT only, generally with low-dose irradiation also administered to the entire affected lung, report good results.[13] Others have had better success with combined modality treatment.[14]

There are several treatment options for the bulk of patients with stages IA and IIA Hodgkin's disease: SNI, which can include the spleen to doses of at least 3500 rad in 3½ weeks, has resulted in complete remission (CR) rates in excess of 90% with a 20% to 40% relapse rate, probably depending upon RT technique and patient selection. The salvage rate of these patients into second durable CRs may be in excess of 50%. The risks of leukemia and sterility are less than with combination chemotherapy. Long-term potential side effects of RT include radiation lung fibrosis, pericarditis, premature coronary artery disease, and second solid tumor malignancies, particularly sarcomas.

Combination chemotherapy alone and combined with RT has resulted in a CR rate of >90% with a relapse rate of <10%. This is achievable with six cycles of chemotherapy with the MOPP (nitrogen mustard, vincristine, procarbazine, and prednisone) or similar type of regimen. (Table 1). One randomized trial suggested that RT may not be necessary with six cycles of CVPP (cyclophosphamide, vinblastine, procarbazine, and prednisone).[16] When RT is also used, fewer cycles of chemotherapy may give similar results.[17,18] The current protocol at Memorial Hospital randomized patients to four cycles of either MOPP or TBV (ThioTEPA), bleomycin,

Table 1. MOPP and C-MOPP Regimen for Treatment of Patients With Stages IA and IIA Hodgkin's Disease[22]

Attentuation of Doses		
WBC	Platelets	Doses
≥4,000	150,000	Full doses
3,000–3,900	100,000–149,000	100% VCR, Pred; 50% HN_2, Pro
2,000–2,900	50,000–100,000	100% VCR, Pred; 25% HN_2, Pro
1,500–1,999		50% VCR; 25% HN_2, Pro
<1,500	50,000	Hold therapy, re-evaluate in 1 week.
Days 1 and 8	HN_2 (mustargen) 6 mg/m^2. Cyclophosphamide 650 mg/m^2 IV could be given instead, if nausea and vomiting are intolerable. VCR 1.4 mg/m^2 IV (maximum 2 mg).	
Days 1–14	Pro 100 mg/m^2 orally (maximum 150 mg) Pred 40 mg/m^2 orally (cycle 1 and 4).	

Abbreviations: VCR, vincristine; Pred, prednisone; Pro, procarbazine.

vinblastine). An interruption is made between the second and third cycle for RT to the involved regions to 3500 rad over 3½ weeks. The involved regions consist of the mantle port, para-aortic nodes and spleen, and pelvic nodes. Every effort is made to avoid or limit RT to the pelvis, since it may be associated with considerable morbidity. The results with follow-up extending to 4 to 5 years are similar in both arms of the trial to results achieved with six cycles of MOPP and involved region RT.[15] Two French studies suggest that three cycles of MOPP may be sufficient in combination with RT.[17,18]

Azospermia occurs in approximately 80% of men with six cycles of MOPP, and another 10% are rendered oligospermic.[19] Sperm banking with cryopreservation is encouraged for men who may wish to have children in the future. Unfortunately, pretreatment sperm from male Hodgkin's disease patients may be qualitatively and quantitatively abnormal, possibly related to the degree of their systemic symptoms. As many as 18% of male patients may be oligospermic before treatment (Dr John Redman, personal communication). However, successful inseminations have been achieved with pretreatment cryopreserved sperm in spouses of male Hodgkin's disease patients following treatment. Women <30 years of age are less likely to become permanently infertile than those >30 years of age. Trials are in progress to attempt gonadal suppression in women with estrogens and progestins and in men with androgens in an attempt to preserve gonadal function.

The actuarial risk of acute leukemia or myelodysplastic syndrome has been estimated to be approximately 10% at 10 years.[20] At Memorial Hospital only one patient of approximately 200 stage IA, IIA, or IIIA patients treated during the past 10 years with either six or four cycles of chemotherapy and involved region RT developed a myelodysplastic syndrome. This patient died of sepsis and hemorrhage. No protocol patients have developed acute leukemia.

Stage IIIA

As mentioned in the section on staging, it has been proposed that patients with high retroperitoneal nodal or splenic disease ($IIIA_s$, $IIIA_1$) fare better with TNI than those with disease in lower para-aortic or pelvic nodes ($IIIA_2$). This was true with respect to relapse-free survival.[9] With longer follow-up, other groups noted increased survival and relapse-free survival with combined modality treatment for $IIIA_1$ patients as compared with that achieved with TNI.[21] The only possible exception is in patients with minimal splenic involvement only (<5 nodules).[10,21]

Good results have been reported with six cycles of MOPP or modifications of MOPP alone without RT, although the numbers of patients studied are too small for definitive conclusions. Currently, the combined modality protocol for stage IIIA Hodgkin's disease at Memorial Hospital is the same as that for stage IA- and IIA-disease. Patients are randomized to four cycles of MOPP or four cycles of TBV. An interruption is made between the third and fourth cycles for RT: 3,500 rad to a mantle port for supradiaphragmatic disease; 3,500 rad to a subtotal nodal port for supradiaphragmatic and high abdominal disease; and 3,500 rad to a subtotal nodal port and 2,000 rad to iliac and inguinal ports for supradiaphragmatic and pelvic or inguinal node involvement.

Stages IIB, IIIB, and IV

The major advance for patients with advanced Hodgkin's disease came from the use of MOPP by DeVita et al.[22] A total of 80% of 198 patients achieved a CR, and 68% of these were free of disease 10 years later. A total of 90% of these patients had stage IIIB or IVB disease.[23]

There have been many modifications of the MOPP regimen. One of these, carmustine (BCNU), cyclophosphamide, vinblastine, procarbazine, and prednisone (BCVPP), achieved CR rates similar to MOPP (76% *v* 73% in a randomized trial); the duration of CR and the survival of patients achieving a CR was longer for patients on BCVPP than those on MOPP. Neurologic and gastrointestinal toxicity was also reduced with BCVPP.[24]

The optimum treatment of stage IIB disease is still not settled. The Stanford group reported a 79% survival rate for PS IB and IIB patients treated with TNI, which often included irradiation of liver and lung. There was no increase in survival with combined modality treatment.[25] Others have suggested that patients with PS IIB without bulky mediastinal masses (less than one-third the thoracic diameter) fare well with SNI, although the numbers of patients are small.[26]

Combined modality treatment of stage CS IIB using alternating potentially non–cross-resistant drug combinations and low-dose RT as described below has also been successful.[27] Between January 1975 and October 1985, 55 CS IIB patients were treated with either two or three alternating drug combinations and low-dose RT. Forty-six (83.5%) achieved CR, seven (13%) a partial remission (PR), and two (3.5%) progressed. Five patients relapsed from a CR, and eight died. Fourteen patients failed to achieve a durable CR (PRs, progressions, and relapses from CR), and most of these had bulky mediastinal presentations. It should be recalled that the favorable RT results for stage IIB were in PS patients, while the combined modality results are for CS IIB patients, approximately 30% of whom would have disease below the diaphragm at laparotomy.[5] The excellent results in CS patients would seem to obviate the need for staging laparotomy for CS IIB patients if combined modality treatment is used.

Bonadonna et al[28] demonstrated that a drug combination differing from MOPP in the pharmacology and mechanism of action of the components could result in a CR rate similar to that achieved with MOPP. It was also demonstrated that at least some patients relapsing after MOPP could be put into second remissions, although the duration of these remissions were not as long as with primary treatment.[29] This combination was doxorubicin, bleomycin, vinblastine, and dacarbazine (ABVD). Bonadonna et al[28] suggested that this combination might be potentially non–cross-resistant with MOPP in that tumors resistant to MOPP might be sensitive to ABVD. Following this suggestion, we reasoned that the use of both regimens together in alternating months might be more successful in eradicating tumor than either combination alone. We also thought that the addition of adjuvant low-dose RT to the initially involved lymph node areas might prevent relapses in these areas. This had been suggested by Farber et al[30] at Yale, who employed low-dose RT with a five-drug combination of nitrogen mustard, vincristine, vinblastine, procarbazine, and prednisone (MVVPP) for patients with stage IIIB and IV Hodgkin's disease. A protocol was started in January 1975, in which MOPP and ABVD were alternated monthly for eight cycles. An interruption was made between cycles four and five for low-dose RT to the involved lymph node regions, 2000 rad in 2 weeks, with an additional boost of 1000 rad of bulky disease. The fifth cycle was resumed after a rest of 2 to 3 weeks.[27] In 1979 a new trial was started in which MOPP/ABVD/RT (eight-drug regimen) was randomized against three alternating potentially non–cross-resistant combinations (10-drug regimen). The third combination was lomustine (CCNU), melphalan (Alkeran), and vindesine (DVA), following phase II trials with vindesine alone and in this combination for relapsed patients. Dacarbazine was dropped from ABVD, since it was most troublesome for patients because of its association with severe nausea and vomiting. Also, the phase II data supporting its use in Hodgkin's disease were scanty. All patients received six cycles of chemotherapy with either two or three combinations. The same low-dose RT was administered as in the initial protocol, and, following a rest of 2 to 3 weeks, an additional three cycles of chemotherapy were given (Table 2). The results for the initial eight-drug/RT protocol and the subsequent 8- *v* 10-drug/RT protocol are the same. Less nausea and vomiting have been seen with the 10-drug protocol, although transient myelosuppression has been somewhat greater with the eight-drug protocol.[31] Sepsis associated with neutropenia, hemorrhage associated with thrombocytopenia, and prolonged myelosuppression have been comparable and rare with both the 8- and 10-drug/RT regimens.

Fifty-nine of 68 patients with CS IIIB, treated since 1975 on both protocols, have achieved a CR (87%), seven a PR (10%), and two have progressed (3%). There have been 16 deaths. Eleven patients have relapsed from a CR, and thus slightly less than 80% of the patients remain in CR at 10 years. There have been 14 failures (PRs, progressions, relapses from CR) and, as with CS IIB, patients with bulky nodal disease remain a challenge.

Since 1975, 50 patients with stage IV disease have received these treatments. Thirty-eight (76%) achieved a CR, 11 (22%) a PR, and one (2%) progressed. Approximately 70% of the patients are remaining in CR at 10 years. Thirteen patients have died. Nineteen patients failed to achieve a durable CR as defined above.

The recurrence rate within the RT treatment portals was only 7% for low-dose RT in combination with MOPP/ABVD or CAD/MOPP/ABV, which is comparable to that reported for full-dose RT used as a single modality for early stage Hodgkin's disease.[11] Low-dose RT in combination with MVVPP resulted in a 74% relapse-free survival at 5 years for advanced stage patients in the Yale study with a similar low recurrence rate within the low-dose RT treatment portals.[30] These two studies and those of the Stanford group, who employed low-dose RT in combination with chemotherapy in pediatric patients,[32] suggest that doses of RT between 1500 and 3000 rad may be adequate in combined modality treatment. As with early stage Hodgkin's disease, the question of whether the RT adds anything to the chemotherapy has not been answered as yet.

Bonadonna et al[33] reported similar results to those achieved at Memorial Hospital in a randomized trial comparing 12 cycles of MOPP/ABVD with 12 cycles of MOPP for patients with stage IV Hodgkin's disease. The 8-year disease-free survival rate was 72.6% for MOPP/ABVD, compared with 45.1% for MOPP, a difference that was statistically significant.

There have been three acute leukemias and one non-Hodgkin's lymphoma in 209 previously untreated patients at risk for up to 11 years in the

Table 2. Eight- v 10-Drug Protocol for Advanced Hodgkin's Disease: Stages IIB, IIIB, and IV[30]

Dose	Schedule	
Group 1		
MOPP	Days 1 and 8	HN_2 (mustargen), 6 mg/m^2. Cyclophosphamide 650 mg/m^2 IV may be substituted if nausea and vomiting are intolerable.
		VCR 1.4 mg/m^2 IV (maximum 2 mg).
	Days 1–14	Pro 100 mg/m^2 orally (maximum 150 mg).
		Pred 40 mg/m^2 orally, (cycles 2 and 5 in group 1; cycle 1 and 5 in group 2).
	Days 15–30	Rest
ABV	Days 1 and 15	Adriamycin 25 mg/m^2 IV.
		VBL 6 mg/m^2 IV (maximum 10 mg).
	Days 4–10 and 18–24	Bleomycin 2 mg/d, subcutaneously.
	Days 26–30	Rest
CAD	Day 1	CCNU 100 mg/m^2 po.
		DVA 3 mg/m^2 IV. VBL 4 mg/m^2 IV if DVA not available.
		Alkeran 6 mg/m^2 po day 1–4.
	Day 8	DVA 3 mg/m^2 IV.
		Rest 4–5 wk.
Group 2		
MOPP	Days 1 and 8	HN^2 (mustargen) 6 mg/m^2 IV. Cyclophosphamide 650 mg/m^2 IV may be substituted if nausea and vomiting are intolerable.
		VCR 1.4 mg/m^2 IV (maximum 2 mg).
	Days 1–14	Pro 100 mg/m^2 orally (maximum 150 mg).
		Pred 40 mg/m^2 orally (cycles 2 and 5 in group 1; cycle 1 and 5 in group 2).
	Days 15–30	Rest
ABVD	Days 1 and 15	Adriamycin 25 mg/m^2 IV.
		VBL 6 mg/m^2 IV (maximum 10 mg).
		DTIC 250 mg/m^2 IV.
	Days 4–10	Bleomycin 2 mg/d, subcutaneously.
Attenuation of Doses		
WBC (μL)	Platelet (μL)	
$\geq$4,000	150,000	
3,000–3,900	100,000	149,000, 100% VCR, bleomycin, pred, DTIC
		50% VBL, DVA, Alkeran, HN_2, Adriamycin, CCNU
2,000–2,999	50,000	100,000, 100% bleomycin, pred, VCR
		50% DTIC
		25% DVA, VBL, Alkeran, HN_2, Adriamycin, Hold CCNU
1,500–1,999		100% bleomycin
		50% VCR
		25% DVA, VBL, Alkeran, HN_2, Adriamycin, DTIC, hold CCNU
1,500		50,000 hold therapy, re-evaluate in 1 wk.

Abbreviation: VBL, vinblastine.

Radiation therapy was administered in both groups. Regional radiation therapy to critical or bulky areas of disease (Dose 2,000 rad in 2½ wk; 200 rad/d, 4/wk). Boost of 1,000 rad to areas of bulky disease permissible, if possible (may not be possible for pelvic disease). If there is indirect extension into an extranodal site (IIB), this area will be included with an adequate margin. In cases of emergencies, ie, cord compression, superior vena cava syndrome, etc, RT is given initially at a minimum dose of 3,000 rad in 3 wks. Treatments should be given to anterior and posterior fields even if adjacent nodal region is not involved.

original 8-drug/RT and the more recent 8- *v* 10-drug/RT protocols.

Salvage Treatment

As previously mentioned, approximately 50% of patients relapsing after RT can be successfully put into durable CR with combination chemotherapy. Localized nodal relapses outside the irradiated portals may be treated with RT alone. Although second CR rates with ABVD following primary chemotherapy range from 4% to 59% due to patient selection, only ≤20% of these patients remain in ongoing unmaintained CR in even the best series. Results are similar with other salvage drug combinations. We have had our best success with MOPP/ABVD (8-drug) or CAD/MOPP/ABV (10-drug) in patients relapsing after other combination chemotherapy, with 40% to 50% of patients achieving a CR. With the unavailability of vindesine (3 mg/m^2), we have successfully substituted vinblastine (4 mg/m^2 IV) in CAD (Table 2). Factors predicting a favorable response include limited nodal sites of relapse, treatment in first as opposed to subsequent relapse, high performance status, absence of B symptoms, and, most importantly, a disease-free interval of at least 11 to 12 months.[34] Because of dissatisfaction with high relapse rates following salvage chemotherapy after primary chemotherapy, some groups are using supralethal doses of chemotherapy with autologous bone marrow rescue. The results are mixed and preliminary, as discussed below.[35]

Future Directions

There have been few trials employing biologic response modifiers in Hodgkin's disease. No dramatic results have as yet been reported. In our own original 8-drug/low-dose RT protocol, we tested levamisole *v* no levamisole in a randomized comparison, along with a chemotherapy maintenance; in our subsequent 8-drug/low-dose RT *v* 10-drug/low-dose RT trial, we randomized patients to levamisole maintenance or no maintenance. Levamisole showed no benefit with respect to prolongation of remission or survival in either trial.[27,31]

A new approach was recently suggested by Lenhard et al,[36] who employed 131_I-labeled antiferritin antibody, and demonstrated responses in 15 of 37 relapsed Hodgkin's disease patients, one of which was complete. Unfortunately, there was no proof that the 131_I-labeled antibody was targeted to the tumor and that the effect was not one of systemic irradiation. If an appropriate monoclonal antibody reacting with Hodgkin's disease tissue could be found, clinical trials with antibody alone, or antibody conjugated with radioisotopes, chemotherapeutic agents, or toxins might be possible in the future.

Allogeneic bone marrow transplantation has been employed for relapsed Hodgkin's disease patients. The toxicity has been extreme and the results disappointing. Among eight patients reported recently from Seattle, only two survived.[37] Autologous bone marrow transplantation seems to have some promise. In a literature review by Canellos,[38] 21 of 51 relapsed Hodgkin's disease patients (51%) treated with bone marrow-ablative doses of chemotherapy followed by autologous bone marrow rescue achieved a CR, and 10 relapsed. Follow-up time is too short to draw any conclusion as to the duration of most of these remissions. If this approach continues to show promise, it might be applied as part of the initial treatment for patients initially presenting with advanced Hodgkin's disease and features predicting a poor prognosis. Such an analysis of prognostic factors is underway for patients treated with the 8-drug/low-dose RT and 10-drug/low-dose RT protocols at Memorial Hospital.

For the earlier stages of Hodgkin's disease, the focus is currently on achieving the same excellent results with less toxicity, even using combined modality treatment. The ABVD regimen may be less leukemogenic than MOPP[39] and may cause less sterility, although it is associated with severe unpleasant nausea and vomiting. There is also theoretic concern about cardiac toxicity, which may occur as a late complication, particularly when this doxorubicin-containing regimen is combined with mediastinal RT. Preliminary results are promising with another regimen, vinblastine, bleomycin, and methotrexate (VBM), in combination with RT. This regimen also omits alkylating agents, the probable major culprit with respect to leukemogenesis and sterility.[40] The role of methotrexate, a drug with limited single-agent activity in Hodgkin's disease, is unclear. Further follow-up with a larger number of patients will be necessary. There are indications that four or even three cycles of MOPP may achieve the same results in combination with RT as six cycles of MOPP.[17,18]

Thus the challenges for the future are somewhat different for Hodgkin's disease than for other types of malignancy where RT and chemotherapy are less effective. Newer approaches will be necessary for the relatively small number of patients who are still not achieving durable remission with present treatment. The second challenge is to devise less toxic treatment for the patients who do achieve durable remissions with present treatment. Ultimately, it would be desirable for new, as yet unknown, less toxic approaches based on a better understanding of the biology of Hodgkin's disease to replace RT and chemotherapy.

REFERENCES

1. Lukes RJ, Craver LF, Hall TL: Report of the nomenclature committee. Cancer Res 26:1311, 1966

2. Carbone PP, Kaplan HS, Mushoff K, et al: Report of the committee on Hodgkin's disease classification. Cancer Res 31:1860–1861, 1971

3. Tubiana M, Henry-Amar M, Burgers MV, et al: Prognostic significance of erythrocyte sedimentation rate in clinical stages I-II of Hodgkin's disease. J Clin Oncol 2:194–200, 1984

4. DeVita VT, Bagley CM, Goodell B, et al: Peritoneoscopy in the staging of Hodgkin's disease. Cancer Res 31:1746–1750, 1971

5. Kinsella TJ, Glatstein E: Staging laparotomy and splenectomy for Hodgkin's disease: Current status. Cancer Invest 1:87–91, 1983

6. Lacher MJ: Routine staging laparotomy for patients with Hodgkin's disease is no longer necessary. Cancer Invest 1:93–99, 1983

7. Tubiana M, Hayat M, Henry-Amar M, et al: Five-year results of the EORTC randomized study of splenectomy and spleen irradiation in clinical stages I and II of Hodgkin's disease. Europ J Cancer 17:355–363, 1981

8. Glatstein E, Guernsey JM, Rosenberg SA, et al: The value of laparotomy and splenectomy in the staging of Hodgkin's disease. Cancer 24:709–718, 1969

9. Stein RS, Golomb HM, Wiernik PH, et al: Anatomic substages of stage IIIA Hodgkin's disease: Follow-up of a collaborative study. Cancer Treat Rep 66:733–741, 1982

10. Hoppe RT, Cox RS, Rosenberg SA, et al: Prognostic factors in pathologic stage III Hodgkin's disease. Cancer Treat Rep 66:743–749, 1982

11. Kaplan HS: Hodgkin's Disease (ed 2). Cambridge, MA, Harvard University Press, 1980

12. Mauch P, Gorshein D, Cunninham J, et al: Influence of mediastinal adenopathy on site and frequency of relapse in patients with Hodgkin's disease. Cancer Treat Rep 66:809–817, 1982

13. Lee CK, Bloomfield CD, Levitt SH: Results of lung irradiation for Hodgkin's disease patients with large mediastinal masses and for hilar disease. Cancer Treat Rep 66:819–825, 1982

14. Wiernik PH, Slawson RG: Hodgkin's disease with direct extension into pulmonary parenchyma from a mediastinal mass: A presentation requiring special therapeutic considerations. Cancer Treat Rep 66:711–716, 1982

15. Koziner B, Myers J, Cirrincione C, et al: Treatment of stages I and II Hodgkin's disease with three different therapeutic modalities. Am J Med 80:1067–1078, 1986

16. Pavlovsky S, Dupont J, Jimenez E, et al: Combination chemotherapy with cyclophosphamide, vinblastine, prednisone and procarbazine (CVPP) alone vs CVPP plus radiation therapy in clinical stage I-IIA Hodgkin's disease. Proc Am Soc Clin Oncol 2:233, 1983 (abstr)

17. Ferme C, Teillet F, D'Agay MF, et al: Combined modality in Hodgkin's disease. Comparison of six versus three courses of MOPP with clinical and surgical restaging. Cancer 54:2324–2329, 1984

18. Anrieu JM, Montagnon B, Asselain B, et al: Chemotherapy-radiotherapy association in Hodgkin's disease, clinical stage IA, IIA: Results of a prospective clinical trial with 162 patients. Cancer 46:2126–2130, 1980

19. Redman J, Bajorunas D, Goldstein M, et al: Semen cryopreservation and artificial insemination in Hodgkin's disease. Proc Am Soc Clin Oncol 2:219, 1983

20. Petersen-Bjergaard J, Larsen SO: Incidence of acute nonlymphocytic leukemia preleukemia and acute myeloproliferative syndrome up to 10 years after treatment of Hodgkin's disease. N Engl J Med 7:965–971, 1982

21. Mauch P, Goffman T, Rosenthal DS, et al: Stage III Hodgkin's disease: Improved survival with combined modality therapy as compared with radiation therapy alone. J Clin Oncol 3:1166–1173, 1985

22. DeVita VT, Serpick AA, Carbone PP: Combination chemotherapy in the treatment of advanced Hodgkin's disease. Ann Intern Med 73:881–895, 1970

23. DeVita VT, Simon RM, Hubbert SM, et al: Curability of Hodgkin's disease with chemotherapy. Long-term follow-up of MOPP-treated patients at the National Cancer Institute. Ann Intern Med 92:587–595, 1980

24. Bakemeier RF, Anderson JR, Costello W, et al: BCVPP chemotherapy for advanced Hodgkin's disease: Evidence for greater duration of complete remission, greater survival, and less toxicity than with a MOPP regimen. Ann Intern Med 101:447–456, 1984

25. Rosenberg SA, Kaplan HS: The evolution and summary results of the Stanford randomized clinical trials of the management of Hodgkin's disease: 1962–1984. Int J Radiat Oncol Biol Phys 11:5–22, 1985

26. Leslie NT, Mauch PM, Hellman S: Stage IA-IIB supradiaphragmatic Hodgkin's disease: Long-term survival and recurrence frequency. Cancer 55:2072–2078, 1985

27. Young CW, Straus DJ, Myers J, et al: Multidisciplinary treatment of advanced Hodgkin's disease by an alternating chemotherapeutic regimen of MOPP/ABVD and low-dose radiation therapy restricted to originally bulky disease. Cancer Treat Rep 6:907–914, 1982

28. Bonadonna G, Zucali R, Monfardini S, et al: Combination chemotherapy of Hodgkin's disease with adriamycin, bleomycin, vinblastine and imidazole carboximide versus MOPP. Cancer 36:252–259, 1975

29. Santoro A, Bonfante V, Bonadonna G: Salvage chemotherapy with ABVD in MOPP-resistant Hodgkin's disease. Ann Intern Med 96:139, 1982

30. Farber LR, Prosnitz LR, Cadman EC, et al: Curative potential of combined modality therapy for advanced Hodgkin's disease. Cancer 40:1509–1517, 1980

31. Straus DJ, Myers J, Lee BJ, et al: Treatment of advanced Hodgkin's disease with chemotherapy and irradiation: Controlled trial of two versus three alternating potentially non-cross resistant drug combinations. Am J Med 76:270–278, 1984

32. Donaldson SS, Kaplan HS: A survey of pediatric Hodgkin's disease at Stanford University: Results of therapy and quality of survival, in Rosenberg, SA, Kaplan HS (eds): Malignant Lymphomas: Etiology, Immunology, Pathology, Treatment. New York, Academic Press, 1982, pp 571–596

33. Bonadonna G, Valagussa P, Santoro A: Alternating non-cross-resistant combination chemotherapy or MOPP in stage IV Hodgkin's disease. Ann Intern Med 104:749–759, 1986

34. Straus DJ, Myers J, Koziner B, et al: Combination chemotherapy for the treatment of Hodgkin's disease in relapse. Results with lomustine (CCNU), melphalan (Alkeran), and vindesine (DVA) alone (CAD) and in alternation with MOPP and doxorubicin (Adriamycin), bleomycin and vinblastine (ABV). Cancer Chemother Pharmacol 11:80–85, 1983

35. Carella AM, Stantini G, Giordano D, et al: High-dose chemotherapy and non-frozen autologous bone marrow transplantation in relapsed advanced lymphomas or those resistant to conventional chemotherapy. Cancer 54:2826–2839, 1984

36. Lenhard RE, Order SE, Spunberg JJ, et al: Isotopic immunoglobulin: A new systemic therapy for advanced Hodgkin's disease. J Clin Oncol 3:1296–1300, 1985

37. Appelbaum FR, Sullivan KM, Thomas ED, et al: Allogeneic marrow transplantation in the treatment of MOPP-resistant Hodgkin's disease. J Clin Oncol 3:1490–1494, 1985

38. Canellos GP: Editorial: Bone Marrow transplantation as salvage therapy in advanced Hodgkin's disease: Allogeneic or autologous. J Clin Oncol 3:1451–1454, 1985

39. Valagussa P, Santora A, Fossati-Bellani F, et al: Second acute leukemia and other malignancies following treatment for Hodgkin's disease. J Clin Oncol 4:830–837, 1986

40. Horning SJ, Hoppe RT, Rosenberg SA: VBM chemotherapy: An effective adjuvant to involved field irradiation in favorable Hodgkin's disease (HD). Proc Am Soc Clin Oncol 5:198, 1986 (abstr)

α-Interferon Treatment of Cutaneous T Cell Lymphoma and Chronic Lymphocytic Leukemia

Kenneth A. Foon and Paul A. Bunn, Jr

The interferons represent an important first member of a family of biological response modifiers used in treating human malignancies. Activities associated with the interferons include inhibition of viral replication, influence on cellular protein production, direct antiproliferative effects, and a variety of modulatory effects on the immune response. These regulatory functions of interferon underlie the interest in its use as an anticancer agent. α-interferon is the most extensively studied interferon species. While antitumor activity has been seen both in vivo and in vitro in some solid malignancies, the most impressive responses have occurred in the hematologic malignancies. For patients with cutaneous T cell lymphoma (CTCL) (mycosis fungoides and the Sezary syndrome), a response rate of 45%, with 10% complete responses, was seen in patients treated with recombinant α-interferon at the National Cancer Institute (NCI). Interferon appears to be one of the most effective single agents for cutaneous T cell lymphoma. Current trials include further phase II trials to determine whether lower doses of α-interferon will be as effective as the high doses used in the previously reported studies. Additional trials include phase III trials where interferons are included in combination with chemotherapy agents, as well as using interferon in the adjuvant setting. Results for patients with chronic lymphocytic leukemia (CLL) were not as encouraging. A response rate of 15% was reported for crude and recombinant α-interferon in studies outside the NCI, and in our trial, only two of 18 patients (11%) had brief partial responses to recombinant α-interferon.

INTERFERON was the term originally applied to a soluble factor that was recognized by its ability to induce interference against viral infection of chick chorio-allantoic membrane by influenza A virus.[1] It has subsequently been shown to be a family of closely related proteins and glycoproteins that, in addition to having antiviral activity, are potent regulators of cellular function and structure and possess direct antiproliferative activities. These latter properties underlie the current interest in interferon as an anticancer agent.

Three major species of human interferon are recognized and are designated as α-, β-, and γ-interferon.[2] α-Interferon is produced by leukocytes, (B cells, T cells, and macrophages) on exposure to B cell mitogens, viruses, foreign cells, or tumor cells. β-Interferon is produced by fibroblasts on exposure to viruses or foreign nucleic acids. γ-Interferon is produced by T lymphocytes on stimulation with T cell mitogens, specific antigens, or interleukin 2.[3] By use of recombinant DNA techniques, complete nucleotide sequences for all three types of interferon are defined, and amino acid sequences derived.

The genes recognized to code for α-interferon have been assigned to chromosome 9.[4] Sixteen distinct sequences for α-interferon have been described. Each is approximately 166 amino acids in length, with an additional 20 amino acid secretory peptides present on the aminoterminal end. The human genes differ by approximately 10% in nucleotide sequence, and 15% to 20% in amino acid sequence.[5] Two recombinant human interferons, α-A and α-D, make up only 60% of interferons present after buffy coats stimulation and have been extensively studied.[6] While they possess different antiviral and antiproliferative activity in vitro, similar in vivo effects on immune effector cells have been observed.[6] The α-interferon used in the first human clinical trials was obtained from Sendai-virus–stimulated buffy coat leukocytes and represented 1% purity (10^6 U/mg protein).[7] Refinement in purification methods using high performance liquid chromatography, two-dimensional polyacrylamide gel electrophoresis, and immunoaffinity chromatography has allowed purification to homogeneity (10^8 U/mg protein).[8–10] The use of recombinant DNA techniques with splicing of the α-interferon gene into *Escherichia coli* has further allowed for pure single-species α-interferon in larger quantities.

Industrial scale production of β- and γ-interferon has only recently been accomplished, and clinical trials are limited in number. On the other hand, α-interferon has been extensively studied

---

From the Department of Hematology/Oncology, Memorial Sloan-Kettering Cancer Center, New York.

Address reprint requests to David J. Straus, MD, Associate Attending Physician, Department of Hematology/Oncology, Memorial Sloan-Kettering Cancer Center, 1275 York Ave, New York, NY 10021.

0093-7754/86/1304-5005$05.00/0

for the past decade in both basic science and clinical research, and it is among the most potent biologic agents ever administered to humans. While antitumor activity has been seen both in vitro and in vivo, and in some solid malignancies (breast cancer, renal cell cancer, Kaposi's sarcoma, bladder cancer, ovarian cancer, and melanoma),[11,12] the most impressive responses have occurred in the hematologic malignancies.[13] This report presents a summary of the results for patients with cutaneous T cell lymphoma (CTCL) and chronic lymphocytic leukemia (CLL).

CUTANEOUS T CELL LYMPHOMA

The CTCLs, comprising primarily mycosis fungoides and the Sezary syndrome, are indolent T cell non-Hodgkin's lymphomas.[14]

Phenotypic and functional studies have shown that the malignant cells in these disorders are the helper T cells.[15,16] These lymphomas are characterized by initial symptoms in the skin and subsequent spread to peripheral blood, lymph nodes, and other organs. The prognosis is highly dependent on the stage, as determined by the type of skin lesions and the presence or absence of peripheral blood, lymph node, and visceral involvement. Overall, the CTCLs are indolent in nature, with median survivals of approximately 8 to 10 years, similar to the B cell indolent non-Hodgkin's lymphomas. Systemic spread is nearly universal and can be documented by light microscopic examination in as many as 50% of patients at the time of diagnosis.[17] Initial therapies developed for these disorders were directed at the skin. These included the use of topical nitrogen mustard applied daily to the skin,[18] the three-times-weekly administration of psoralen plus UV A light irradiation (PUVA),[19] and the total body application of electron beam irradiation.[20] These treatment approaches effectively alleviate skin lesions and produce skin clearing in the majority of patients. For all three treatments, the complete response rate is directly related to the disease stage and occurs in the majority of patients with plaque lesions, but in a minority of those with tumors or erythroderma. The median duration of response for these therapies is 1 to 2 years, and 10% to 20% of patients remain disease-free at 3 years. This long disease-free interval occurs exclusively in patients with early plaque lesions. Relapses after 3 years were reported with topical nitrogen mustard, but were not observed with total skin electron irradiation. This observation suggests that some of these patients may be cured of this malignant neoplasm. Long-term data are not available for PUVA therapy, but late relapses appear to be common.

Patients with more advanced disease stages have been treated with chemotherapy, either with single drugs or in multiagent combinations.[21,22] These treatments produced objective remissions in the majority of patients, but complete remissions in only 20% to 25% of the patients. Furthermore, relapse is universal; there have been no suggestions of cures reported to date. Because of the propensity for early systemic spread and the lack of cure with known treatments, new systemic approaches are clearly needed. For these reasons, the maximally tolerated doses of recombinant leukocyte A interferon were studied in these neoplasms in our National Cancer Institute (NCI) trial. All of the patients entered in this trial had failed multiple therapies.

As shown in Table 1, objective antitumor responses were noted in nine of the 20 patients in this study, representing the response rate of 45%, with 95% confidence interval of 25% to 69%.[23] The objective responses were all noted within 1 month, and lasted a minimum of 3 months to a maximum of more than 36 months. At 3 months, none of the remissions were complete; however, normal skin biopsy results were later obtained in two patients, who were scored as complete responders. Thus, the complete response rate is 10%, and the partial response rate is 35%. Responses were seen in extracutaneous and cutaneous sites and did not correlate with prior therapy. Eight of nine responders had previously received systemic chemotherapy. Extracutaneous responses were documented by a decrease in the size of palpable lymph nodes in eight of 16 patients with adenopathy, and by a >50%

Table 1. Results of α-Interferon Trials of CTCL and CLL

	No. of Patients	Complete Response	Partial Response	Percent Response	Reference
CTCL					
NCI study	20	2	7	45	23
CLL					
NCI study	18	0	2	11	28
Published literature	39	0	6	15	24-27, 34

decrease in the number of circulating malignant cells in two patients documented by cytologic study and DNA content analysis. The median duration of response was 5.5 months. Notably, three patients, representing one third of the responders and 15% of all patients, have responded for more than 2 years.

Mixed or minor responses were noted in five patients, and three others remained stable for 3 months; therapy was discontinued in these eight patients at 3 months. Another three patients progressed during the initial 3 months of therapy; one patient received only the initial dose of therapy, and two others progressed after 1 and 2 months, respectively.

CHRONIC LYMPHOCYTIC LEUKEMIA

CLL is a hematologic malignancy characterized by proliferation and accumulation of relatively mature-appearing lymphocytes.[24] Most cases involve a clonal proliferation of B lymphocytes. CLL typically occurs in persons over 50 years (median age, 60 years) and affects males more than females at a ratio of 2:1.[24] The disease is usually stable over months to years, but transformation to a more aggressive disease state does occur. Alkylating agents, radiation therapy, and corticosteroids are commonly used to treat patients, although few data show that survival is substantially increased. Crude and purified α-interferon preparations were reported to be moderately active in patients with advanced CLL,[25–27] but this was controversial.[28–30] In our phase II trials at the NCI, 19 patients were treated with both high-dose (50×10^6 U/m^2 of body surface area [BSA] intramuscularly [IM]) and low-dose (5×10^6 U/m^2 BSA IM) recombinant α-interferon three times weekly.[30] As noted in Table 1, 18 patients were evaluable for response, and only two brief partial responses were seen. Five patients appeared to have an acceleration of disease while receiving recombinant α-interferon. This finding is in marked contrast to responses in patients with chemotherapy-refractory, low-grade non-Hodgkin's lymphoma, and hairy cell leukemia.[31]

TOXICITY OF INTERFERON

The major dose-limiting toxicity of interferon was a flu-like syndrome consisting of malaise, fatigue, anorexia, and in rare cases, mental confusion. These were clearly dose-dependent toxic effects, since they were relieved by a dose reduction. In our NCI studies, the average duration of therapy was 4 weeks at the 100% dose of 50×10^6 U/m^2 BSA, and 9 weeks at the 50% dose. Fatigue was the most common reason for dose reduction, and all except one patient required at least 50% reduction. Febrile responses were noted in all patients, but were almost always most severe after the first dose and were rarely a problem after the first week of therapy. The peak temperatures ranged from 38 °C to 42 °C. Hematologic toxicity was not dose limiting. One patient with extensive pulmonary involvement had the adult respiratory distress syndrome after receiving 50×10^6 U/m^2 BSA of recombinant leukocyte interferon; he responded rapidly to corticosteroids. Since the patient had previously responded to interferon and had not responded to a number of chemotherapy regimens, interferon was carefully reinstituted, and he had an excellent partial response. One patient with underlying coronary artery disease had a massive myocardial infarction and died after the first dose of interferon.[32] Reversible elevations in hepatic enzyme levels occurred in a minority of patients. The dose was reduced in all of these patients, and the hepatic enzyme levels returned to normal. One patient developed a reversible nephrotic syndrome and renal failure with minimal-change glomerulonephritis.[33] This syndrome disappeared after discontinuation of the interferon. One patient with the Sezary syndrome developed acute monocytic leukemia after 11 months on interferon therapy; therapy was discontinued at this time. The patient had been heavily pretreated with alkylating agents and electron beam irradiation. The patient was then treated with high-dose cytosine arabinoside, which produced a complete remission; he has been in remission from the leukemia and the Sezary syndrome for more than 16 months since completion of therapy.

For patients with CLL, an unexpected toxicity was seen in seven of the 19 patients where reactivation of perioral herpes simplex lesions were seen during treatment, two of sufficient severity to require discontinuation of interferon therapy and treatment with acyclovir.[30] One other interesting and unusual side effect was uncontrolled growth of eyelashes, and axillary and pubic hair in two of the patients with low-grade B cell non-Hodgkin's lymphoma.[34] This hair growth ceased when the interferon was discontinued.

DISCUSSION

Much of the initial enthusiasm for interferon as an anticancer agent has been dampened by disappointing clinical results. However, recent clinical studies have shown that interferons do have considerable activity in a limited spectrum of disease. The studies reported here establish the activity of interferon for low-grade non-Hodgkin's lymphoma and CTCL. In the same study, we also reported the activity of interferon for low-grade non-Hodgkin's lymphoma.[32] All of these patients had advanced disease refractory to one or more standard treatments, including systemic chemotherapy, and interferon was more active than any other recently evaluated experimental therapy. The observed high response rate and long duration of response in this study suggested that interferon should be evaluated in earlier stages of disease and added to standard treatment, so that the efficacy of this combined approach can be compared with that of standard agents used alone.

The issue as to whether interferon has any role at all for CLL remains open. In our studies at the NCI, there was minimal response and perhaps even a progression of disease in a number of patients who were treated with either 50×10^6 or 5×10^6 U/m^2 BSA of recombinant leukocyte A interferon. Perhaps future studies of CLL should include patients with earlier stages of disease and different doses of interferon that have been proven to have biological response modifying effects.

The toxicities with interferon at high doses have been troublesome. The flu-like syndrome and high fever can be alleviated by initiating therapy with low-dose interferon and then escalating the dose. This "tachyphylaxis" appears to be a consistent finding in most patients. However, the severe fatigue following high doses of interferon is not alleviated by these methods. It seems clear from these studies that acetaminophen should be administered routinely to all patients at the institution of interferon therapy to alleviate the fever. Patients with severe cardiac disease and those where high temperature is life-threatening should not be placed on interferon at high doses. Renal and hepatic functions should be monitored routinely, since occasionally patients have a dose-limiting toxicity to one of these organs. Lowering of blood counts did not appear to be due to direct bone marrow suppression, but is important when considering combined chemotherapy and interferon trials because the chemotherapy doses are modified according to the peripheral blood counts. It has been suggested that because chemotherapy is immunosuppressive and interferons may be immunostimulatory, chemotherapy should be administered intermittently and the interferon continuously.

In our studies, there was no correlation between the development of antibodies to interferon, response rate, or response duration. There was no obvious correlation between in vitro laboratory tests, including phytohemagglutinin stimulation and T cell subsets, and clinical responses. There does not appear to be any likelihood that the response was due to the fever, because there was no correlation with the degree of the febrile response, and the responses continued long after the patients ceased having fevers. Direct cytotoxic effects have been proposed as a likely mechanism of interferon activity, particularly in light of the demonstrated effect in patients with CTCL where disease occurred when the dose was lowered, and disease responded when the dose was increased in a number of patients.[23]

Interferons also increase the expression of tumor-associated antigens and histocompatability antigens on malignant cells, suggesting the possibility of combining interferon with monoclonal antibodies or other biological response modifiers. Future phase II trials will also address these issues.

The optimal dose of interferon for any particular malignancy is unknown. The responses observed in our studies were to a high dose of interferon, which was associated with considerable toxicity and required dose reduction in nearly all patients. Lower doses of interferon, such as 3×10^6 U/d,[31] have demonstrated consistent responses in patients with hairy cell leukemia. Whether lower doses of interferon will be effective in the low-grade non-Hodgkin's lymphomas and CTCL is unknown. Randomized trials with low-dose interferon for patients with low-grade non-Hodgkin's lymphoma and CTCL have recently begun. It is too early to review these results, but important information should be forthcoming soon.

REFERENCES

1. Isaacs A, Lindenman J: Virus interference: I. The interferon. Proc R Soc Lond Biol 147:258–267, 1957

2. Stewart WE II, Blalock JE, Burke DC, et al: Interferon nomenclature. J Immunol 125:2353, 1980 (letter)

3. Fleischmann WR, Klimpel GR, Tyring SK, et al: Interferon and cancer: Current use and novel approaches, in Sunkara PS (ed): Novel Approaches to Cancer Chemotherapy. Orlando, FL, Academic, 1984, pp 1–22

4. Sengal PB: The interferon gene. Biochem Biophys Acta 695:17–33, 1982

5. Borden EC: Progress toward therapeutic application of interferons, 1979–1983. Cancer 54:2770–2776, 1984

6. Hawkins MJ, Borden EC, Merritt JA, et al: Comparison of the biologic effects of two recombinant human interferons alpha (rA and rD) in humans. J Clin Oncol 2:221–226, 1984

7. Cantell K, Hirvonen S: Preparation of human leukocyte interferon for clinical use. Tex Rep Biol Med 35:138–144, 1977

8. Pestka S: The purification and manufacture of human interferons. Sci Am 249:37–43, 1983

9. Lin LS, Steward WE II: Purification of human leukocyte interferon by two-dimensional polyacrylamide gel electrophoresis. Methods Enzymol 78:481, 1981

10. Berg K, Heron I: Antibody affinity chromatography of human leukocyte interferon. Methods Enzymol 78:487, 1981

11. Kirkwood JM, Ernstoff MS: Interferons in the treatment of human cancer. J Clin Oncol 2:336–352, 1984

12. Bonnem EM, Spiegel RJ: Interferon-d: Current status and future promise. J Biol Response Mod 3:580–598, 1984

13. Roth MS, Foon KA: Alpha interferon in the treatment of hematologic malignancies. Am J Med (in press)

14. Lutzner M, Edelson R, Schein P, et al: Cutaneous T-cell lymphomas: The Sezary syndrome, mycosis fungoides, and related disorders. Ann Intern Med 83:534–552, 1975

15. Broder S, Edelson RL, Lutzner MA, et al: The Sezary syndrome: A malignant proliferation of helper T cells. J Clin Invest 58:1297–1306, 1976

16. Haynes BF, Metzgar RS, Minna JD, et al: Phenotypic characterization of cutaneous T-cell lymphoma: Use of monoclonal antibodies to compare with other malignant T cells. N Engl J Med 304:1319–1323, 1981

17. Bunn PA, Huberman MS, Whang-Peng J, et al: Prospective staging evaluation of patients with cutaneous T-cell lymphomas: Demonstration of a high frequency of extracutaneous dissemination. Ann Intern Med 93:223–230, 1980

18. Vonderheid EC, Van Scott EJ, Wallner PE, et al: A 10-year experience with topical mechlorethamine for mycosis fungoides: Comparison with patients treated by total-skin electron beam radiation therapy. Cancer Treat Rep 63:681–689, 1979

19. Roenigk HH Jr: Photochemotherapy for mycosis fungoides: Long-term followup study. Cancer Treat Rep 63:669–673, 1979

20. Hoppe RT, Cox RS, Fuks Z, et al: Electron-beam therapy for mycosis fungoides: The Stanford University experience. Cancer Treat Rep 63:691–700, 1979

21. Winkler CF, Bunn PA Jr: Treatment of T-cell lymphomas: Mycosis fungoides and the Sezary syndrome, in HF Conn (ed): Current Therapy. Philadelphia, Saunders, 1985, p 317

22. Bunn PA Jr, Carney DN: Treatment of cutaneous T-cell lymphomas. J Surg Dermatol Oncol 6:383–388, 1980

23. Bunn PA, Foon KA, Ihde DC: Recombinant leukocyte A interferon: An active agent in advanced cutaneous T-cell lymphomas. Ann Intern Med 101:484–487, 1984

24. Gale RP, Foon KA: Chronic lymphocytic leukemia: Recent advances in biology and treatment. Ann Intern Med 103:101–120, 1985

25. Gutterman JU, Blumenschein GR, Alexanian R: Leukocyte interferon-induced tumor regression in human metastatic breast cancer, multiple myeloma, and malignant lymphoma. Ann Intern Med 93:399–406, 1980

26. O'Connell MJ, Colgan JP, Oken MM, et al: Clinical trials of recombinant leukocyte A interferon in initial therapy for favorable histology non-Hodgkin's lymphoma and chronic lymphocytic leukemia. An Eastern Cooperative Oncology Group pilot study. J Clin Oncol 4:128–136, 1986

27. Misset JL, Mathe G, Gastiaburu J, et al: Traitement des leucemies et des lymphomes par les interferons. II Essai phase II de traitement de la leucemie lymphoide chronique par l'interferon d humain. Biomedicine 36:112–116, 1982

28. Horning SJ, Merigan TC, Korwn SE, et al: Human interferon alpha in malignant lymphoma and Hodgkin's disease. Result of the American Cancer Society trial. Cancer 56:1305–1310, 1985

29. Schuloff RS, Lloyd MJ, Stalling JJ, et al: Recombinant leukocyte A interferon in B-cell chronic lymphocytic leukemia: In vivo effects on autologous antitumor immunity. J Biol Response Mod 4:310–323, 1985

30. Foon KA, Bottino G, Abrams PG: Phase II trial of recombinant leukocyte A interferon in patients with advanced chronic lymphocytic leukemia. Am J Med 78:216–220, 1985

31. Foon KA, Maluish AE, Abrams PG, et al: Recombinant leukocyte A interferon therapy for advanced hairy cell leukemia: Therapeutic and immunologic results. Am J Med 80:351–356, 1986

32. Foon KA, Sherwin SA, Abrams PG: Treatment of advanced non-Hodgkin's lymphoma with recombinant leukocyte A interferon. N Engl J Med 311:1148–1152, 1984

33. Averbuch SD, Austin HA III, Sherwin SA, et al: Acute interstitial nephritis with nephrotic syndrome following recombinant leukocyte A interferon therapy for mycosis fungoides. N Engl J Med 310:32–35, 1984

34. Foon KA, Dougher G: Increased growth of eyelashes in a patient given leukocyte A interferon. N Engl J Med 311:1259, 1984 (letter)

α-Interferon in the Treatment of Nodular Lymphomas

Walter J. Urba and Dan L. Longo

Patients with nodular lymphoma initially respond to a number of therapies but relapse is common and inexorable with time, and despite further therapy, most patients will ultimately die of their lymphoma. The recent demonstration of their sensitivity to α-interferon is promising. The importance of this human antitumor effect is that it is presumably based on mechanisms different from conventional agents. Phase I trials of various doses and schedules of recombinant α-interferon have shown that effective serum levels can be obtained by intramuscular (IM), intravenous (IV), or subcutaneous (SC) routes. Virtually all patients experienced some degree of acute toxicity manifested by fever, chills, myalgia, and headache. Tolerance usually developed to acute adverse effects within the first few weeks of therapy, regardless of dose or schedule. Fatigue and anorexia were the most important adverse reactions, occurring during the first two weeks of treatment and generally persisting for the duration of therapy. Occasional adverse effects relating to the central nervous and cardiovascular systems have been reported. Primary laboratory abnormalities observed during treatment include decreases in hematologic parameters and elevations of liver function tests. The clinical efficacy of α-interferon, both natural and recombinant, has been demonstrated in both untreated and heavily pretreated patients with nodular lymphoma. The response rate has approached 50% in recent studies; however, less than half were complete responders. Future directions include combination of interferon with cytotoxic agents or other biological response modifiers and use as adjuvant therapy.

IN 1970 Jones et al[1] related the natural history of minimally treated patients with non-Hodgkin's lymphoma (NHL) to histologic subtypes of the Rappaport scheme and found that NHLs could be divided into good and bad prognostic groups. This division into indolent and aggressive neoplasms has provided the framework for most clinical trials and is currently the major determinant of treatment selection in clinical practice.[2] The Working Formulation has confirmed this relationship between histopathologic diagnosis and clinical behavior.[3]

The indolent lymphomas (Table 1) include diffuse well-differentiated lymphocytic (DWDL), nodular poorly differentiated lymphocytic (NPDL), nodular mixed lymphocytic/histiocytic (NML), diffuse intermediately differentiated lymphocytic (DIDL), and diffuse poorly differentiated lymphocytic of the small cleaved cell type (DPDL-SC). NPDL and NML are by far the most common subtypes. Most patients present with a history of waxing and waning lymphadenopathy. Their treatment is based on accurate staging of the extent of disease. Stage I and II indolent lymphomas are rare and comprise only 10% to 15% of patients after complete staging. Given the current trend toward conservative management of advanced-state indolent lymphoma patients, it is important to recognize the potential curability of stage I and II patients when treated with radiation therapy.[4]

Patients with advanced stage disease may experience prolonged survival even without therapy.[5] Median survival varies from 5 to 10 years depending on the series, and it is unclear whether therapy makes a major impact on survival or is merely palliative. The optimal management of these patients is controversial but generally follows one of two divergent approaches.[6] The aggressive approach may include radiation therapy, combination chemotherapy, or combined modality therapy, while the conservative approach consists of no initial treatment followed by single-agent chemotherapy or involved field radiotherapy, if required for symptom relief (Table 2). This dichotomy is due to the fact that although most forms of systemic therapy will produce high complete-response rates, they fail to induce prolonged disease-free survival in advanced stage patients with indolent lymphomas. Overall response rates approach 90%, with over two-thirds being complete responses, but relapse is common and inexorable with time, and despite further therapy most patients will die of their lymphoma. Preterminally, nearly all patients develop diffuse aggressive lymphomas. The search for curative approaches to patients with indolent lymphomas continues. Since most

---

From the Medicine Branch, National Cancer Institute, Bethesda, MD.

Address reprint requests to Dan L. Longo, MD, Associate Director Biological Response Modifiers Program, NCI-FRCP, Bldg 567, Room 135, Frederick, MD 21701.

0093-7754/86/1304–5006$5.00/0

Table 1. Histologic Classification and Prognosis

Good Prognosis	Poor Prognosis
Nodular poorly differentiated lymphocytic (NPDL)	Nodular histiocytic (NH)
Nodular mixed lymphocytic-histiocytic (NM)	Diffuse histiocytic (DH)
Diffuse well differentiated lymphocytic (DWDL)	Diffuse mixed lymphocytic-histiocytic (DM)
Diffuse poorly differentiated lymphocytic small cleaved cell type (DPDL-SC)	Diffuse undifferentiated (Burkitt's or non-Burkitts)
Diffuse intermediately differentiated lymphocytic (DIDL)	Lymphoblastic

of these patients will develop resistance to conventional chemotherapeutic agents, the recent demonstration of complete and partial responses in these tumors after treatment with interferon is promising. The importance of this human antitumor effect is that it is presumably based on mechanisms different from conventional agents and therefore may be non-cross resistant in its effects on NHL.

Interferon

The interferons comprise a family of hormone-like cellular proteins produced by virtually all eukaryotic cells in response to a wide range of stimuli.[7–9] The interferons have a variety of biologic actions including antiviral, antiproliferative, antitumor, and immunomodulating effects. The major species of interferon and their abbreviations are summarized in Table 3. The interferons are now designated α, β, and γ according to their antigenic type. The natural α-interferons are produced from peripheral blood leukocytes or lymphoblastoid cell lines; β-interferon is from fetal foreskin fibroblasts; and γ- or immune-interferon is produced by T lymphocytes.

The effects of the interferons, whether antiviral, antiproliferative, or immunologic, appear to follow binding of the interferon molecules to a specific cell-surface receptor. Both α and β interferons interact with the same receptor, while γ appears to interact with a distinct receptor.[10] Following interaction with its receptor and subsequent internalization, interferon induces a number of biochemical changes within the cell. One of the first effects is the induction of oligoadenylate synthetase, which is an enzyme capable of generating oligo 2′5′ adenylate, which in turn activates an endoribonuclease that inhibits transcription and translation.[8] The induction of a kinase that phosphorylates peptide elongation factor and a phosphodiesterase that removes the CCA terminus of transfer ribonucleic acid (tRNA) may contribute to the inhibition of protein synthesis in cells. Immune stimulation by interferon has also been demonstrated, including enhancement of the action of sensitized cytotoxic T cells, as well as heightened cytotoxic action of macrophages and natural killer lymphocytes. Interferon also has profound influences on the cell surface structure, including increasing expression of surface antigens (notably major histocompatibility antigens), strengthening the cytoskeleton, and modifying cell surface characteristics.[7]

Interest in interferon as an antitumor substance stemmed from the demonstration by Gresser et al[11] of antitumor effects in both virally induced and virus-unassociated murine tumors. Subsequent studies monitoring the effect of interferon on human cells grown in vitro showed both inhibition of division and subsequent cell death of both normal and malignant cells. These

Table 2. Treatment of Advanced Stage Indolent Lymphomas

Deferred initial therapy
Local field irradiation
Total lymphoid irradiation
Whole body irradiation
Single alkylating agent chemotherapy
Combination chemotherapy
Combined chemotherapy/radiation therapy

Table 3. Interferon Nomenclature

Natural interferon	
Leukocyte interferon	IFN-α (Le)
Lymphoblastoid interferon	IFN-α (Ly); IFN-α-N1
Fibroblast interferon	IFN-β
Immune interferon	IFN-γ
Recombinant interferon	
α-2	rIFN-α 2; IFN-α-2b (Schering Corporation, Kenilworth, NJ)
α-A	rIFN-α; IFN-α-2a (Roche Laboratories, Nutley, NJ)
β	rIFN-β
γ	rIFN-γ

Abbreviation: IFN, interferon.

results led to the initiation of clinical trials with interferon in patients with advanced cancer.

CLINICAL TRIALS

Toxicity

The original clinical trials employed partially purified human leukocyte (α) interferon extracted from Sendai virus-stimulated pooled buffy coats. In retrospect it was determined that this preparation contained at least eight different interferon-like proteins with antiviral activity. These trials were limited by the small quantity, relatively low purity ($<1\%$), and low specific activity of these interferon preparations. Standard Phase I studies were not performed because of the scarcity of interferon and, as a consequence, the dose and schedule were chosen arbitrarily. The early studies demonstrated that α-interferon could be administered safely by the intramuscular (IM) route with predictable toxicity.[12–14] Acute toxicities included fever, rigors, headache, nausea, and hypotension, followed by myelosuppression, elevation of liver enzymes, and general malaise. It was felt that many of these problems were the result of impurities in the preparation, but subsequent studies with highly purified α-interferon ($>90\%$ pure) and eventually recombinant α-interferon found the same spectrum and degree of side effects.

Phase I trials of various doses and schedules of recombinant α-interferon have shown that effective serum levels can be obtained by IM, intravenous (IV), or subcutaneous (SC) routes.[15–18] The maximum tolerated dose (MTD) and dose-limiting toxicity varied depending on route and schedule of administration. IM administration has been most extensively studied and when given in low daily doses interferon was well tolerated. Patients receiving higher doses frequently required dose attentuation to 50% or less of the starting dose to improve clinical tolerance. Toxicity was essentially identical to non-recombinant sources of α-interferon. Dose-related temperature elevation was universal and usually coincided with peak serum levels of interferon, four to six hours after IM injection. The elevated temperature was usually associated with a chill, returned to normal within 24 hours, and was no longer experienced after tachyphylaxis developed during the first week of therapy. Additional dose-related toxicity included a flu-like syndrome with myalgias, arthralgias, headache, nausea, and diarrhea. These symptoms were more prominent at higher doses but resolved in most patients, with only a minority experiencing problems throughout the entire treatment period. Acetaminopen pretreatment was generally useful in ameliorating these symptoms. Fatigue and anorexia were also dose dependent, but since tachyphylaxis did not occur, these symptoms tended to be cumulative, progressive, and a common reason for dose reduction. Dose-dependent leukopenia with granulocytopenia, which often persisted throughout interferon administration, has been observed. It can be a basis for discontinuation or interruption of interferon therapy. The myelotoxicity of interferon appears to be due to a reversible inhibition of myeloid maturation, perhaps with an element of sequestration. Less frequent side effects include alopecia, decreased libido, impotence, confusion, depression, somnolence, EEG changes, paresthesias, cardiac arrhythmias, cardiac ischemic events, hypotension, proteinuria, elevated liver-transaminases, thrombocytopenia, and recurrent herpes simplex lesions.

The potential for antibody formation to exogenous interferon has been a concern during early treatment trials. There have been descriptions of antibody production in early studies employing either leukocyte or recombinant α-interferon. Recently, Spiegel et al[19] retrospectively reviewed the incidence of serum neutralizing factors in patients receiving recombinant interferon-α-2b. Neutralizing factors developed in 13 of 537 (2.4%) patients during systemic therapy. Only 1 of 47 (2.1%) patients with lymphoma developed antibodies. A similar study of recombinant interferon-α-2a[20] found that 153 of 559 (27%) cancer patients developed neutralizing antibodies. Twenty-two percent of lymphoma patients receiving interferon-α-2a developed antibodies. The reason for this disparity is unknown. It could be related to antigenic differences in the recombinant molecules or to variability in assay methods. Continued clinical responses despite antibody production have been observed, and to date no deleterious clinical or laboratory effects have been associated with the development of antibodies to either interferon preparation. In fact, it is possible that antibody binding to interferon (if the antibody is not neutralizing) may be associated with altered clearance and a prolonged serum half-life, an alteration that might even be beneficial.

Clinical Efficacy

Early trials demonstrated the antitumor effects of human leukocyte interferon in patients with NHLs (Table 4). It was appreciated early on that the favorable prognosis of indolent lymphomas responded more readily than the aggressive subtypes. Merigan et al[12] treated six lymphoma patients with α-interferon at a dose of 5×10^6 U IM twice a day for 30 days. Three patients with aggressive lymphoma (DHL) failed to respond, while all three patients with NPDL responded (one complete response [CR] and two partial responses [PR]). This study was updated by Louie et al[13] to include 11 patients; five responses were noted in eight patients with indolent subtypes (1 CR, 2 PR, 2 minimal responses [MR]). Three of five responders were previously untreated, and the duration of response was six to 12 months. The dose-limiting toxicity was leukopenia which exhibited a pattern different from that observed after administration of cytotoxic agents. WBC and platelet counts fell rapidly during the first week, and then leveled off by day 10 even with continued therapy. Gutterman et al[14] treated 11 NHL patients with α-interferon 3×10^6 U daily for 4 weeks and observed three responses in six patients with NPDL and two in four with CLL, and no response in the one with DHL. Responses lasted up to 1 year, with responders receiving maintenance therapy. Horning et al[21] reported the results of the American Cancer Society trial of human α-interferon in malignant lymphoma and Hodgkin's disease. Interferon was administered IM in doses of 1×10^6, 3×10^6, or 9×10^6 U daily for 30 days. Six of 18 patients with nodular lymphoma had partial or minimal responses, four at a dose of 9×10^6 U and two at 3×10^6 U. Five of the six responders were previously untreated, and in one partial responder, the maximum tumor reduction was noted 3½ months after discontinuation of interferon. There were no responses in ten patients with DWDL or chronic lymphocytic leukemia (CLL). The Southeastern Cancer Study Group[22] investigated low and high dose lymphoblastoid α-interferon in 25 patients with indolent lymphoma who had failed previous chemotherapy. Initial treatment consisted of 5×10^6 U/m^2 three times per week for eight weeks, with dose increases to 30×10^6 U/m^2 for 10 days for nonresponders. Responses were noted in six patients (2 CR, 4 PR) at the lower doses, with occasional further responses seen at the higher doses.

The experience with human leukocyte or lymphoblastoid α-interferon suggests modest activity against nodular lymphomas when low doses are given daily for short periods. A CR and PR rate of 25% to 30% was seen in 50 to 60 patients with advanced low grade NHL treated in this manner. Responses were achieved whether or not patients had received previous chemotherapy.

A single European trial has investigated the activity of partially purified human fibroblast β-interferon in patients with low grade NHL.[23] Ten patients received daily IV infusions of 4.5×10^6 U for four weeks followed by 9×10^6 U daily for two weeks. Two patients responded (1 CR; 1 PR) to this treatment.

Table 4. Alpha Interferon Trials in Non-Hodgkin's Lymphoma of Low Grade Histologic Type

					Response			
Trials	Dose ($\times 10^6$)	Schedule	Route	Entered	CR	PR	MR	CR%
Natural inteferon								
Merigan et al[12]	2.5-5	BID × 1 mo	IM	3		3		0
Gutterman et al[14]	3-9	QD × 1 mo	IM	10	2	2	1	20
Louie et al[13]	5-10	BID × 1 mo	IM	7	1	3	3	14
Horning et al[15]	1,3,9	QD × 1 mo	IM	18		3	3	0
Gams et al[21]	5,30	TIW	IM	20	1	4		5
Recombinant interferon								
Quesada et al[23]	3-50	QD	IM	17	2	4		12
Foon et al[24]	50	TIW × 3 mo	IM	24	4	9		16
Wagstaff and Crowther[25]	2	TIW × 3 mo	SC	16	1	3		6
Ozer et al[26]	10-25/m^2	TIW × 3 mo	SC	6		2		0

The development of recombinant α-interferon led to more extensive Phase I-II testing and permitted the treatment of larger numbers of patients with significantly higher doses. Initial Phase I studies confirmed the activity of α-interferon in the nodular lymphomas. They also proved that recombinant α-interferon was biologically active despite the absence of glycosylation resulting from production in bacteria. Quesada et al[24] treated 17 NPDL patients in a Phase I-II study using daily IM injections of α-interferon with dose escalation from 3×10^6 to 50×10^6 U per day. Dose-limiting toxicity (fatigue, asthenia, elevated transaminases) occurred in patients receiving 36×10^6 U or more. There were six responses (2 CR, 4 PR) in the 17 patients (35%). There was no obvious dose-response relationship since responses occurred at 9×10^6, 18×10^6, 36×10^6, and 50×10^6 U, but there were no responses in three patients treated at 3×10^6 U/day. Maintenance therapy (three times a week) was given for one to six months in all responders. The duration of the CRs was 6 and 10 months with both relapses occurring in previously involved sites. The PRs lasted 2, 4, 10, and 12 months, respectively.

At the NCI Biological Response Modifiers Program (BRMP), Foon et al[25] described objective responses in 13 of 24 (54%) heavily pretreated patients with low grade lymphoma. Four CRs and nine PRs were noted during treatment with 50×10^6 U of recombinant interferon-alfa-2a three times a week for 3 months or longer. Initially, patients were to receive recombinant interferon for only 2 months after CR or stable PR; however when it became clear that patients routinely relapsed 2 to 7 months after termination of interferon, maintenance therapy was instituted in the absence of unacceptable toxicity. Most responding patients continued to receive interferon for 4 to 13 months, and the median duration of response was 8 months. Six responding patients were described as having bulk disease and three of four CRs had previous bone marrow involvement. Two patients with a CR relapsed after discontinuation of interferon and achieved another CR upon its reinstitution.

Wagstaff and Crowther[26] described four responses (1 CR, 3 PR) in 16 patients with advanced stage low grade NHL (8 DWDL, 5 NPDL, and 3 NM). Each patient received 2×10^6 U of recombinant α-interferon by SC injection three times per week for 3 months. Ozer et al[27] described five responses in 11 nodular lymphoma patients using recombinant α-interferon at various doses (10×10^6 to 25×10^6 U/m^2) via IV or SC routes.

Interferon α-2a also has demonstrable activity in patients with advanced cutaneous T-cell lymphomas. Bunn et al[28] noted responses in nine (2 CR, 7 PR) of 20 heavily pretreated patients. The median duration of response was less than 6 months, but remission lasted two or more years in three patients.

Early reports suggesting activity of α-interferon in patients with CLL have not been confirmed by recent studies during recombinant interferon. Foon et al[29] noted only two PRs in 19 patients treated with IM interferon at 50×10^6 U three times per week. Responses consisted of a transient reduction in lymphocyte count, and five patients appeared to have acceleration of their disease while receiving recombinant leukocyte α-interferon.

Combination Therapy

Based on preclinical data from clonogenic assay studies and human tumor xenograph studies that demonstrate additive cytotoxicity when human interferons are tested in combination with cytotoxic drugs,[30] Phase I-II trials of combinations of biological response modifiers and chemotherapeutic agents have begun. In a pilot study at the University of Wisconsin, Hawkins et al[31] found that five days of interferon-α-2a at 6×10^6 U/m^2 did not delay recovery from COPA (cyclophosphamide, vincristine [Oncovin], prednisone, doxorubicin [Adriamycin]) chemotherapy-induced leukopenia. The objective responses noted in patients with NHL led to the current ECOG Phase III study that randomizes patients with favorable-prognosis lymphomas between COPA alone every 28 days and COPA plus interferon-α-2a (I-COPA) 6×10^6 U/m^2 IM interposed on days 22 to 26. Trials have been instituted by the CALGB and SWOG for Phase II testing of interferon-α-2b in combination with the alkylating agents cyclophosphamide or chlorambucil. The Northern California Oncology Group is currently treating patients with CVP (cyclophospamide, vincristine, prednisone) to achieve a CR and then randomizing to no maintenance therapy *v* maintenance therapy with intermittent subcutaneous administration of interferon-α-2a 8 $\times$ 10^6 U/m^2 per day for 30 days every 4 months for a total of four cycles.

DISCUSSION

The experience with leukocyte α-interferon antitumor activity against lymphomas of favorable histology with little activity against unfavorable subtypes. Trials of leukocyte and lymphoblastoid cell α-interferon demonstrate 25% to 30% CR and PR rates while Phase II trials of recombinant α-interferon report up to 60% response rates in this group of patients. Among the malignancies most responsive are the nodular lymphomas (NPDL and NML), a subset of the favorable prognosis lymphomas.

Why the beneficial effects of interferon therapy are not found in all the indolent lymphomas is unknown. It is clear that neither DWDL nor CLL respond as well to interferon as do NPDL and NML. There are insufficient data to determine the responsiveness to interferon of neoplasms of the DIDL or DPDL-SC subtypes. There appears to be a spectrum of responsiveness to interferon among the B cell malignancies. Hairy cell leukemia appears to be exquisitely sensitive, the nodular lymphomas less so, and CLL, DWDL, and the aggressive lymphomas the least responsive. This may be related to the unique characteristics of B cells at different stages of differentiation. Responsiveness does not seem to correlate with the number of cell surface interferon receptors.[32] A more complete understanding of the differential sensitivity of these B cell malignancies may provide further insights into the antitumor properties of α-interferon.

Effective serum levels of α-interferon can be achieved by IM, IV, or SC administration. There are no data to indicate superior efficacy of any particular route of administration. Toxicity is similar and includes severe symptoms such as fever, chills, myalgia, fatigue, anorexia, and leukopenia. Less frequent side effects include headache, nausea and vomiting, diarrhea, confusion, depression, somnolence, EEG changes, paresthesias, cardiac arrhythmias, cardiac ischemic events, hypotension, proteinuria, elevated transaminases, thrombocytopenia, and recurrent herpes simplex lesions. Acute toxicity is most pronounced in intermittent dosing schedules when an interval of two to three days is exceeded, and tolerance of the acute toxicity wanes. Acute toxicity appears to be less with continuous or frequent (daily) interferon administration, and it may be possible to minimize toxicity by starting at low doses initially with escalation to higher doses after tolerance is established.[33] Fatigue and asthenia were the most common dose-limiting toxicities and were responsible for dose reductions in nearly all patients treated with high doses. Tumor lysis syndrome,[34] the nephrotic syndrome with acute renal failure,[35] and acute non-lymphocytic leukemia[36] have also been reported in patients with NHL treated with interferon.

Since the interferons have both direct cytotoxic effects on tumor cells and indirect effects via immune modulation, it is difficult to determine in a given case which is responsible for the observed antitumor effects. The inability to determine an optimal immunomodulating dose of interferon despite using a variety of in vitro tests of immune function and the observation that higher response rates are seen at higher dosage are more consistent with a direct cytotoxic or antiproliferative effect of interferon. Gams et al[22] noted occasional responses in patients treated with higher doses after failing on a low dose schedule, and Bunn et al[28] noted that dose escalation resulting in a clinical benefit in four of 10 patients with cutaneous T cell lymphoma. The effect of dose is currently being tested in a prospective randomized fashion at the BRMP of the NCI. Patients with favorable prognosis lymphomas are being randomized betweeen low dose daily interferon-α-2a (3 $\times$ 10^6 U) and twice weekly doses of 50 $\times$ 10^6 U. All patients failing to respond after 3 months of low dose therapy will be treated on the high dose arm.

Current data suggest that α-interferon is not curative since most patients relapse in previous sites of disease within 3 to 6 months of discontinuing therapy. Similar observations have been made in patients with hairy cell leukemia treated with interferon. It is therefore important to determine a dose and schedule of administration that could be continued indefinitely in responding patients. The ability to minimize side effects is also important when one contemplates the use of interferon in combination with other agents or as adjuvant therapy.

While α has been the interferon species most extensively studied, it may not prove to be the most useful clinically. β-interferon has shown minor activity,[23] but does not seem to represent an improvement over α-interferon. Furthermore, α and β interferons appear to use the same cell surface receptor. Although γ-interferon has antiviral, immunomodulating, and antitumor properties that overlap with α, it also has distinct features, including its own cell surface receptor. The two interferons differ slightly in their spectrum of antitumor activity; γ has greater in vitro antiproliferative activity,[7] is a much more potent stimulator of macrophages, and has been shown to exhibit synergy in vitro and in vivo with a number of other cytokines, including α-interferon and tumor necrosis factor, for both antitumor and immunologic effects. Phase I trials of γ-interferon are currently in progress.

Future prospects for the use of α-interferons will include their direct comparison to standard therapy for refractory lymphoma, combination with chemotherapeutic agents, combination with other biological response modifiers (eg, other interferons), and evaluation as adjuvant therapy. The notion of combining interferon with chemotherapuetic agents is particularly attractive since interferons seem to act by a distinct mechanism, and their capacity to inhibit normal cell proliferation (eg, in the GI tract and bone marrow) could conceivably protect these organs from the toxic effects of chemotherapeutic agents (which have some selectivity for dividing cells).[37]

REFERENCES

1. Jones SE, Fuks Z, Bull M, et al: Non-Hodgkin's lymphomas. IV. Clinicopathologic correlation in 405 cases. Cancer 31:806–823, 1973

2. Rosenberg SA: Non-Hodgkin's lymphoma-selection of treatment on the basis of histologic type. N Engl J Med 301:924–928, 1979

3. The non-Hodgkin's lymphoma classification project: National Cancer Institute sponsored study of classifications of non-Hodgkin's lymphomas. Summary and description of a working formulation for clinical usage. Cancer 49:2112–2135, 1982.

4. Glatstein E: Alice revisits lymphoma-land. Int J Radiat Biol 10:571–572, 1984

5. Portlock CS and Rosenberg SA: No initial therapy for stage III and IV non-Hodgkin's lymphomas of favorable histologic types. Ann Intern Med 90:10–13, 1979

6. Longo DL, Young RC, Devita VT: What is so good about the "good prognosis" lymphoma?, in Williams CJ and Whitehouse JMA (eds): Recent Advances in Clinical Oncology, Edinburgh, Churchill-Livingstone, 1982, pp 223–231

7. Kirkwood JM, Ernstoff MS: Interferons in the treatment of human cancer. J Clin Oncol 2:336–352, 1984

8. Lengyel P: Biochemistry of interferons and their actions. Ann Rev Biochem 51:251–282, 1982

9. Yabrov A: Interferon: Anticancer agent having multifarous activity. Prog Clin Cancer 8:99–145, 1982

10. Williams BRG: Mechanisms of interferon action, in Sikora C (ed): Interferon in Cancer. New York, Plenum Press, 1983

11. Gresser I, Maurey C, Brouty-Boye D: Mechanisms of the antitumor effects of interferon. Nature 239:167–169, 1972

12. Merigan TC, Sikora K, Breden JH, et al: Preliminary observations on the effect of human leukocyte interferon in non-Hodgkin's lymphoma. N Engl J Med 299:1449–1453, 1978

13. Louise AC, Gallgher JG, Sikora K, et al: Follow-up observations on the effect of human leukocyte interferon in non-Hodgkin's lymphoma. Blood 58:712–718, 1981

14. Gutterman JU, Blumenshein GR, Alexanien R, et al: Leukocyte interferon induced tumor regression in human metastatic breast cancer, multiple myeloma, and malignant lymphoma. Ann Intern Med 93:399–406, 1980

15. Horning SJ, Levine, JF, Miller RA, et al: Clinical and immunologic effects of recombinant leukocyte A interferon in eight patients with advanced cancer. JAMA 247:1718–1722, 1982

16. Sherwin SA, Knost JA, Fein S, et al: A multiple-dose phase I trial of recombinant leukocyte A interferon in cancer patients. JAMA 248:2461–2466, 1982

17. Gutterman JU, Fine S, Quesada, et al: Recombinant leukocyte A interferon: Pharmacokinetics single-dose tolerance and biologic effects in cancer patients. Ann Int Med 96:549–556, 1982

18. Quesada JR, Gutterman JU: Clinical study of recombinant DNA-produced leukocyte interferon (Clone A) in an intermittent schedule in cancer patients. J Natl Cancer Inst 70:1041–1046, 1983

19. Spiegel RJ, Spicehandler JR, Jacobs SJ, Oden EW: Low incidence of serum neutralizing factors in patients receiving recombinant alfa-2b interferon (Intron A). Am J Med 80:223–228, 1986

20. Jones GJ, Itri LM: Safety and tolerance of recombinant interferon alfa-2a (Roferon®-A) in cancer patients. Cancer 57:1709–1715, 1986

21. Horning SJ, Merigan TC, Krown SE, et al: Human interferon alpha in malignant lymphoma and Hodgkin's disease: Results of the American Cancer Society Trial. Cancer 56:1305–1310, 1985

22. Gams R, Gordon D, Guaspari A, Tuttle R: Phase II trial of human polyclonal lymphoblastoid interferon (Welferon) in the management of lymphoma. Proc Amer Soc Clin Oncol 3:65, 1984

23. Siegert W, Theml H, Fink U, et al: Treatment of non-Hodgkin's lymphoma of low-grade malignancy with human fibroblast interferon. Anticancer Res 2:193–198, 1982

24. Quesada JR, Hawkins M, Horning S, et al: Collabora-

tive phase I-II study of recombinant DNA produced leukocyte interferon (Clone A) in metastatic breast cancer, malignant lymphoma, and multiple meyloma. Am J Med 77:427–432, 1984

25. Foon KA, Sherwin SA, Abrams PG, et al: Treatment of advanced non-Hodgkin's lymphoma with recombinant leukocyte interferon. N Engl J Med 311:1148–1152, 1984

26. Wagstaff J, Crowther D: Human 2 interferon (IFN) (Schering Plough 30500) in the non-Hodgkin's lymphoma (NHL): A report of 2 phase II studies. Br J Cancer 50:244, 1983

27. Ozer H, Ratanatharathorn V, Leavitt R, et al: A phase II trial of rDNA interferon in low-grade non-Hodgkin's lymphoma. Proc Am Soc Clin Oncol 2:215, 1983 (abstr C-840)

28. Bunn PA, Foon KA, Ihde DC et al: Recombinant leukocyte A interferon: An active agent in advanced cutaneous T cell lymphoma. Ann Intern Med 101:484–487, 1984

29. Foon KA, Bottino GC, Abrams PG, et al: Phase II trials of recombinant leukocyte A interferon in patients with advanced chronic lymphocytic leukemia. Am J Med 78:216–220, 1985

30. Clark RH, Dimitrov NV, Axelson JA, et al: Leukocyte interferon as a biological modifier in lymphoproliferative disease resistant to standard therapy. Blood 62:1882, 1983

31. Hawkins MJ, O'Connell MJ, Schiller JH, et al: Phase I evaluation of recombinant A interferon alpha (rIFN-α) in combination with COPA chemotherapy (I-COPA). Proc Am Soc Clin Oncol 4:229, 1985 (abstr C-890)

32. Faltynek C, et al: in press

33. Bunn PA, Jr, Ihde DC, Foon KA: The role of recombinant interferon alfa-2a in the therapy of cutaneous T-cell lymphomas. Cancer 57:1689–1695, 1986

34. Fer M, Bottino GC, Sherwin SA: Atypical tumor lysis syndrome in a patient with T cell lymphoma treated with recombinant leukocyte interferon. Am J Med 77:953–956, 1984

35. Averbuch SD, Austin HA, III, Sherwin SA, et al: Acute interstitial nephritis with nephrotic syndrome following recombinant leukocyte A interferon therapy for mycosis fungoides. N Engl J Med 310:32–35, 1984

36. Warrell RP, Jr, Krown SE, Koziner B, et al: Acute non-lymphoid leukemia after treatment of nodular lymphoma with human leukocyte interferon. Ann Intern Med 98:482–483, 1983

37. Slapak C, Richman C: Interferon protects normal human granulocyte/macrophage progenitors (CFU-GM) from ara-C cytoxicity in vitro. Proc Amer Soc Clin Oncol 5:224, 1986

Hairy Cell Leukemia: A Model for Studying the B Cell Family of Diseases

Ayad Al-Katib, Ellin Berman, Pat Black, and Benjamin Koziner

Nineteen patients with hairy cell leukemia (HCL) were treated with recombinant interferon α-2a/Roche (Roferon) given by daily intramuscular injection of 3 × 10^6 for 6 months followed by three injections per week. Pretreatment and follow-up marker studies were performed on 14 of 16 evaluable patients. Peripheral blood and bone marrow mononuclear cells were analyzed by flow cytometry for reactivity with monoclonal antibodies to B cell associated surface antigens (B1, B2, B4, BL1, BL3, and BL7) and two hairy cell (HC) antibodies, anti-HCL1 and HCL3. B cell monoclonality was determined by clonal excess calculation of immunoglobulin light chains. Right angle scatter analysis showed that HCs are scattered between lymphocytes and monocytes. Nine of the 14 patients achieved a partial remission, three patients achieved a minimal response, and two patients failed therapy. Phenotypically, ten patients had κ clonal excess and four had λ clonal excess. These cases expressed a mature B cell phenotype, ie, $BL1^-$, $BL7^+$, $BL3^+$, $B1^+$, $B2^-$, $B4^+$, $HCL1^+$, $HCL3^+$. All 12 responders became nonreactive with monoclonal antibodies 4 to 8 weeks after therapy; in five of these cases, reactivity with monoclonal antibodies was again detected at the time of maximum clinical response (2 to 8 months), without affecting clinical response status. In four of 12 responders, clonal excess disappeared 4 to 8 weeks after therapy; in three more patients, clonal excess disappeared at the time of maximum clinical response (2 to 4 months); in three patients, clonal excess disappeared from the peripheral blood, but not from the bone marrow at the time of maximum clinical response (3 to 5 months); two patients had persistent cloncal excess. In the two failures, there was persistence of clonal excess and reactivity with monoclonal antibodies. This study shows that phenotypic analysis is a sensitive and objective method of assessing response of HCL to α interferon. This system could be used as a model for the study of other B cell neoplasms.

THERE HAS BEEN considerable controversy about the cellular origin and state of differentiation of the neoplastic cells comprising hairy cell leukemia (HCL).[1–5] Origin from B cells,[4] monocytes,[1] or a hybrid cell has been suggested and well documented cases of T cell HCl were reported.[3] Present evidence suggests that HCL represents a B cell neoplasm.[6] Hairy cells (HC) were found to express B cell phenotype of surface immunoglobulins (SIg) and B cell associated surface antigens detected by monoclonal antibodies[7,8]; these cells were also found to synthesize immunoglobulins.[9,10] In addition to these B cell markers, genotypic analysis of HCs demonstrated rearranged immunoglobulins, heavy and light chain genes consistent with B cell genotype.[11] Analysis of these marker profiles suggests a rather mature stage of B cell differentiation. The neoplastic cells seem to be arrested at a more mature stage than cells of chronic lymphocytic leukemia (CLL).[7,12]

Treatment of HCL has also evolved over the years. Splenectomy and chemotherapy are regarded as the conventional treatment modalities.[13–15] More recently, several groups have reported significant responses of HCL to interferon.[16–18] However, as in other diseases treated with interferon, the selection of dose and schedule of treatment was empirically chosen and variable. Moreover, the length of treatment that represents adequate trial of therapy with interferon is not known. In this communication we present data on patients treated with rα-interferon showing that it may take up to 4 months or more for evidence of B cell monoclonality (as determined by SIg light chain clonal excess (CE) analysis) to disappear. Such phenotypic analysis could also be used to evaluate responses to interferon (or other biologic response modifiers) in other human B cell malignancies.

MATERIALS AND METHODS

Patients

At the time of this interim report, 19 patients are analyzed. This study is still ongoing and open for patient accrual.

Treatment Schedule

Recombinant α-Interferon was provided by Hoffmann-La Roche (Nutley, NJ) for this study. Treatment was given by daily intramuscular (IM) injection of 3 × 10^6 units for 6 months. In those responding, the same dose was given 3 times a week as a maintenance therapy.

From Memorial Sloan-Kettering Cancer Center, New York.

Address reprint requests to Ayad Al-Katib, MD, Wayne State University School of Medicine, Division of Medical Oncology, P.O. Box 02188, Detroit, MI 48201.

0093–7754/86/1304–5007$5.00/0

Definition of Response

Criteria for clinical response were based on changes in the proportion of HCs in bone marrow (BM) aspirate and biopsy, BM granulocytes (BMG) and peripheral blood parameters including hemoglobin (Hb) level, absolute granulocytes and platelet count. Complete remission (CR) is defined by complete absence of HCs in BM aspirate and biopsy, BMG of ≥ 35%; HB ≥ 12 g/dL; absolute granulocytes of ≥ 1500 × 10/L and platelet count of ≥ 100,000/mm^3. A partial remission (PR) is defined by a decrease of HC infiltrate in the BM by at least 50%, BMG ≥ 35%, peripheral blood (PB) parameters like in CR. If there is only improvement in PB parameters; BMG between 25% to 35%, and ≥ 50% reduction in BM hairy cell (BMHC) infiltrate, this is regarded as a minimal response. Stabilization of disease is designated when there is no change in HC infiltrate in BM or increase in BMG.

Marker Studies

Preparation of cells. PB and BM samples were obtained from all patients after signing a consent form and before starting therapy (day 0) and at 4 weekly intervals while on therapy with rα-interferon. Mononuclear cells are then separated by Ficoll-Hypaque density centrifugation (Pharmacia Fine Chemicals, Piscataway, NJ). Cells are then washed and resuspended in Hank's balanced salt solution (HBSS) at 5 × 10^6/mL. These cells are then aliquoted for determination of the phenotype.

Monoclonal Antibodies

To determine the surface phenotype of HCs at a given point during therapy, a number of monoclonal antibodies were selected (Table 1) that reflect different stages of B cell maturation. Anti-BL1, BL3, and BL7 were developed and kindly provided by Dr C.Y. Wang. These antibodies recognize B cell surface antigens associated with early, late, and intermediate stages of differentiation, respectively, as previously reported.[19,20] Anti-HCL1 (Leu-14) and anti-HCL3 (Leu-M5) are useful in confirming the diagnosis of HCL. Although none of them by itself is specific for HCL, when used in combination positive reactivity was seen only in this disease.[21] Other antibodies included were B1, B2 (not shown in Table 1), and B4.[22-24]

Table 1. Methodology—III: Monoclonal Antibodies

Antibody	Target Antigen	Lineage and State of Differentiation
anti-BL1	heat stable antigen	early B cells
anti-BL3	105 KD glycoprotein	mature (Ig secreting) B cells
anti-BL7	heat stable antigen	intermediate B cells
anti-HCL-1 (Leu-14)	94 KD glycoprotein	HCs and B cells
anti-HCL-3 (Leu-M5)	90, 150 KD glycoprotein	HCs and monocytes
B1	35 KD glycoprotein	immature and mature B cells
B4	40, 80 KD protein	immature and mature B cells

Surface Immunoglobulins (SIg)

The test used in this study to determine B cell monoclonality is the SIg light chain clonal excess (CE). This is based on the predominance of κ or λ light chain bearing cells at different channels of immunofluorescence intensity according to the Ligler's method[25] (% K$^+$ to % λ^+ cells)/(% K$^+$ + % λ^+ cells) at each 10 channel units of fluorescence intensity. A positive value (above zero, Fig. 1) of 0.4 or more indicates K CE at that unit while a negative value (below zero) of −0.4 or more indicates λ CE. CE of either light chain in five consecutive channel units or more (above channel 50) is required to label that case as having K or λ CE.

Immunofluorescence Staining (IF) and Flow Cytometric Analysis (FCM)

The monoclonal antibodies, Leu-14 and Leu-M5, and the anti-immunoglobulin antibodies, anti-K, -λ, -A. -M, -D, and -G were obtained from Becton Dickinson (Mountainview, CA). B1, B2 and B4 were obtained from Coulter (Hialeah, FL). To stain for these antibodies, indirect IF method was used as previously described.[20] Briefly, 0.5 × 10^6–1.0 × 10^6 cells were incubated with 100 μL of the corresponding antibody at 4 °C for 35 minutes. Cells are then washed and incubated with the second antibody, which is fluorescin isothiocyanate (FITC) (conjugated goat anti-mouse) antibody, for 35 min at 4 °C. The cells are then washed and resuspended in 0.5 mL of phosphate buffered saline (PBS) and analyzed by FCM on the cytofluorograf system 30-L (Ortho Diagnostics, Westwood, MA). Forward *v* right angle (90°) light scattergram of cells was obtained and regions of interest gated for analysis. A minimum of 10,000 cells per test were analyzed and results expressed as percentage of cells displaying IF. Results were considered positive for a given monoclonal antibody when ≥ 25% of cells were positive.

RESULTS

Table 2 shows the clinical characteristics of the 19 patients. Median age at diagnosis was 53 years (mean 20 to 74). Median age at treatment was 57 years (range 23 to 76). There were 17 men and 2 women. PB parameters at the start of therapy were as follows: Median WBC count 5.42 × 10^3/mm^3 (range 0.4 to 59.6); median neutrophil count 16% (range 0% to 57%); median Hb 9.8 g/dL (range 7.7 to 13.9); median platelet count 65,000/mm^3 (range 27 to 261). Nine patients had received no prior therapy and 10 had received previous therapy including prednisone, CVP (cyclophosphamide, vincristine, prednisone), and oxymethalone. Fifteen patients had splenectomy. The other four patients had enlarged spleens at the time of entry to this study.

Of the 19 patients, 16 are evaluable for clinical response. Of the other three, one had an early

Table 2. Results—Clinical

Total # of patients	19
Age at diagnosis	
median	53 yrs
range	(20–74)
Age at treatment	
median	57 yrs
range	(23–76)
Male: Female	17:2
Total # evaluable	16
pending	2
early death	1
Adequate marker studies	14/16
Clinical responses	
CR	0/14
PR	9/14
MR	3/14
Failure	2/14

Abbreviations: CR, complete response; PR, partial response; MR, minimal response.

death and two have not attained MCR (pending). None of the patients achieved a CR according to our clinical criteria. Nine of 16 achieved a PR for a median duration of 5.0^{+}m (range 2.0^{+} to 8.7^{+}). Three of 16 had an MR for a median of 3^{+}m (range 2.6^{+} to 6.5^{+}m). Two patients had stable disease and two others failed treatment. Further details about the clinical course of these patients will be reported separately. In this report we will focus on the changes of phenotypic markers during therapy. Fourteen of 16 evaluable patients had adequate marker studies. In the remaining two patients, an adequate number of cells could not be consistently obtained from the PB and BM for analysis. The breakdown of the 14 patients by response is shown in Table 2.

All patients, except one, displayed a pretreatment phenotype of mature B cells ($BL1^{-}$, $BL7^{+}$, $BL3^{+}$, $B1^{+}$, $B2^{-}$, $B4^{+}$, $HCL1^{+}$, $HCL3^{+}$). The other patient did not react with these antibodies despite the presence of K CE as evidence of B cell monoclonality (patient AP, Table 3). Ten of 14 cases had K CE and four of 14 had λ CE. A typical phenotype is shown in Fig 1. An important technical aspect in the analysis of HCs by FCM is the gating of the proper cell population. We found that the HC population is located between lymphocytes and monocytes. This population when gated out and analyzed gave the highest proportion of HCL1 + HCL3+ cells in cases with PB and BM involvement with HCL. This is a useful enrichment procedure for HCs, especially when they form only a relatively small proportion of mononuclear cells in the sample tested.

In all responders that had adequate marker studies (12 of 14) reactivity with monoclonal antibodies disappeared within 4 to 8 weeks of therapy (Table 3 and Figure 2, upper panel). In the remaining two patients, who eventually failed, reactivity with monoclonal antibodies did not significantly change in one patient (HE, Table 3 and Figure 3). In the other failure patient (MG, Table 3 and Figure 3) reactivity with monoclonal antibodies decreased by 8 weeks

Table 3. Results—Markers

			Monoclonal Antibodies			Clonal Excess		
Pt	MCR	TMCR	Initial	4–8 wks	at MCR	Initial	4–8 wks	at MCR
DB	PR	5m.	+	–	–	λ	–	–
AD	MR	2m.	+	–	–	κ	–	–
MK	PR	3m.	+	–	–	κ	–	–*
GH	PR	4m.	+	–	+	κ	–	–
AP	PR	4m.	–	–	–	κ	κ	–
RL	PR	4m.	+	–	–	κ	κ	–
MS	PR	2m.	+	–	–	λ	λ	–*
								PB BM
ST	PR	4m.	+	–	–	κ	κ	– κ
AV	MR	3m.	+	–	+	λ	λ	– λ
PD	PR	5m.	+	–	+	λ	λ	– λ
AC	PR	8m.	+	–	+	κ	κ	κ
DM	MR	2m.	+	–	+	κ	κ	κ
HE	F	5m.	+	+	+	κ	κ	κ
MG	F	8m.	+	+#	+	κ	κ	κ

Abbreviations: Pt, patient; MCR, Maximum clinical response; TMCR, time to MCR; initial, pretreatment; F, failure; PB, peripheral blood; BM, bone marrow; #, reactivity with monoclonal antibodies decreased; +, >25% of cells express immunofluorescence.

*Clonal excess subsequently reappeared without affecting clinical response status.

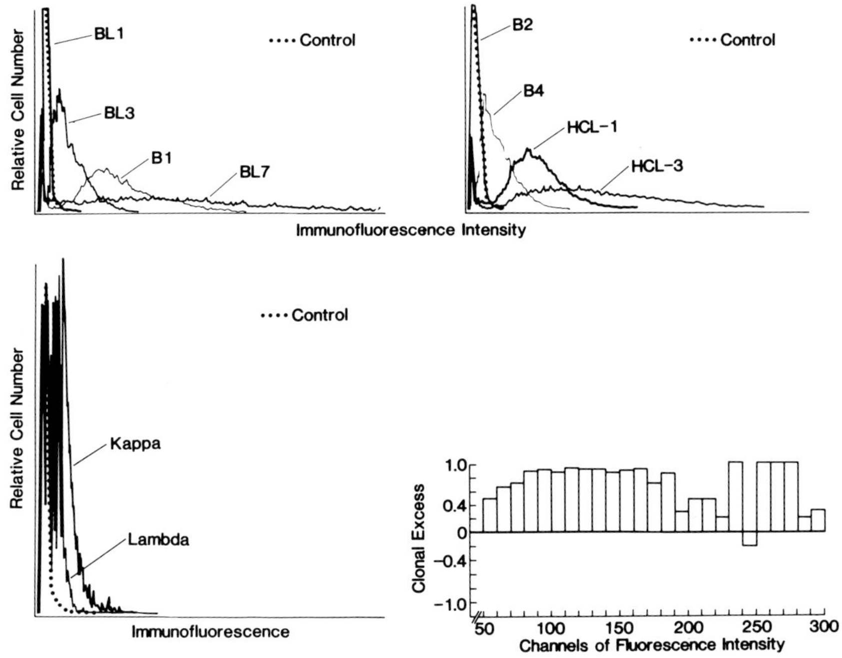

Fig 1. Pre-treatment surface phenotype of a patient (MK). The upper panel shows immunofluorescence profiles of monoclonal antibodies. The dotted line (control) indicates background fluorescence. The horizontal axis represents channels of increasing fluorescence intensity. The lower panel shows the surface immunoglobulins light chain histogram (left) and CE calculation (right) on the same histogram. Note the right shift of κ over λ indicating predominance of κ that is confirmed by CE calculation.

(20% to 30% positive). At the time of maximum clinical response (TMCR shown in Table 3), reactivity with monoclonal antibodies reappeared in five patients (three PRs and two MRs) without affecting their clinical response status.

As compared with monoclonal antibody reactivities, CE took a longer time to disappear in responding patients. According to the pattern of change in CE, patients could be divided into four groups: in the first group, comprised of four patients (top 4, Table 3), CE disappeared 4 to 8 weeks after the initiation of α-interferon therapy and remained negative at the time of MCR. In one of the patients in this group (MK) KCE became detectable on subsequent follow-up. However, the patient remains in PR clinically. In

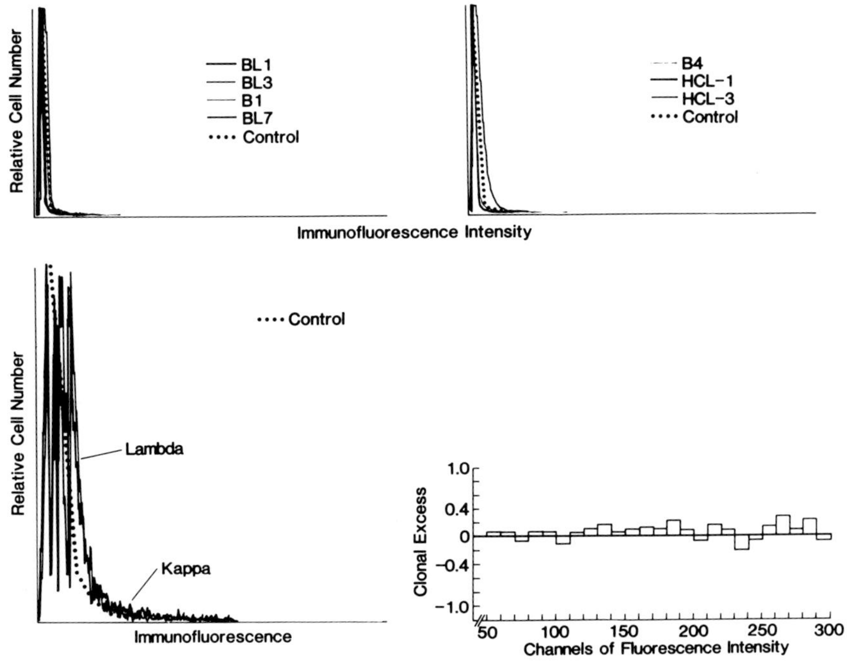

Fig 2. Surface phenotype on the same patient in figure 1 (MK) 4 weeks after treatment with α-interferon. Note the loss of reactivity with all monoclonal antibodies (upper panel) and the disappearance of the difference between κ and λ on histogram (lower left) and the loss of κ CE (lower right).

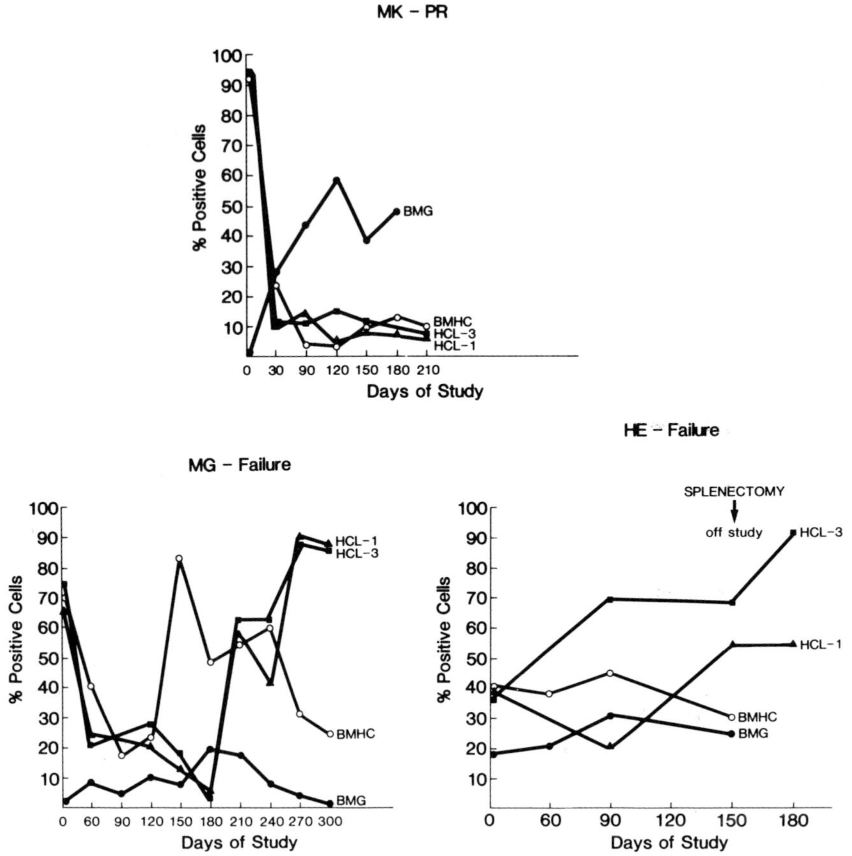

Fig 3. Correlation between BM morphology (BMHC infiltration and BMG) and reactivity with monoclonal antibodies anti-HCL1 and -HCL3. The upper figure is from a responding patient (MK) shown in figure 1 and 2. Note the simultaneous decrease in BMHC and reactivity with anti-HCL1 and -HCL3. At the same time there was a gradual increase in BMG. The lower graphics are from the two failures. The discrepancy between BMHC and the proportion of HCL1 + HCL3 + cells may be due to the subjectivity in determining hairy cells by morphology.

the second group (three patients) CE did not disappear after the initial 4 to 8 weeks of α-interferon therapy, but became undetectable at the time of MCR (4 months). Again, in one of these patients (MS) CE reappeared on subsequent follow-up without affecting the clinical response status. The third group consisted of three patients (Table 3) and like the previous group, CE did not disappear after 4 to 8 weeks of α-interferon therapy. However, at the time of MCR (3 to 5 months), CE was detectable in BM, but not in PB. In the last group (four patients) CE persisted throughout the treatment. Two of the patients among this group were the failures; in these patients reactivity with monoclonal antibodies also persisted. In the other two patients (1 PR and 1 MR) reactivity with monoclonal antibodies disappeared after 4 to 8 weeks, but reappeared at the time of MCR. However, these patients are still in clinical response and are being followed.

Figure 3 presents a correlation between changes in reactivity with monoclonal antibodies (anti-HCL1 and anti-HCL3) and morphologic findings (BMG and BMHC infiltrate) on α-interferon therapy. The upper panel is from patient MK (PR), showing the dramatic reduction in reactivity with anti-HCL1 and anti-HCL3 after 4 weeks of therapy coinciding with reduction in BMHC infiltrate. At the same time there was a gradual increase in the BM granulocytes. The two graphics at the bottom of Figure 3 are from the two failures where reactivity with monoclonal antibodies either remained positive (HE) or transiently decreased (MG). In both cases there was no significant increase in BMG.

DISCUSSION

This study demonstrates the value of surface markers in the evaluation of response of HCL to α-interferon. One technical point that should be emphasized is the proper gating on right angle scattergram. HCL is a disease known to be associated with difficulty in obtaining adequate samples for study. We found that gating the proper area (between lymphocytes and monocytes) helps to obtain an enriched population with HCs. This conclusion is based on patterns of reactivity with HC-associated monoclonal antibodies (anti-HCL1 and HCL3) in the different populations displayed on scattergram. However, we had not sorted these cells out to study their morphologic and histochemical characteristics. Recently, van Bockstaele et al[26] reported a similar observation that was confirmed by cell sorting and morphologic examination.

Generally, reactivity with monoclonal antibodies disappeared before CE (Table 3). This may be because CE is a more sensitive test in detecting B cell monoclonality than monoclonal antibodies. It was reported that CE can detect B cell monoclonality at the level of 1% or less.[27] Since the eventual aim of any anticancer therapy is to eliminate the neoplastic clone, these markers could be used in the future as more stringent criteria for evaluating the effectiveness of therapy with interferon in B cell malignancies. In a group of three patients (Table 3) we observed that CE has disappeared from PB, but not from BM. The significance of this finding is unclear at the present time. In two of those patients, reactivity with monoclonal antibodies reappeared at the time of MCR. Whether the persistent expression of CE in the BM represents resistant disease that will eventually progress or will disappear with further therapy remains to be seen. Our results indicate that it may take up to 4 months or more of therapy with interferon before evidence of B cell monoclonality (as indicated by CE) disappear. Such a finding may help in deciding on the duration of therapy that will represent an adequate clinical trial in the future.

The phenotype of our HCL cases presented in this study agrees with other reports[6,7,28] showing that HCL is a disease of mature B cells. During therapy with α-interferon, the proportion of cells reacting with the monoclonal antibodies decreased gradually in responding patients. There was no change in the surface phenotype of those cells, indicating an antiproliferative rather than a differentiative effect of interferon.

The discrepancy between BMHC proportion by morphology and the reactivity with anti-HCL1 and anti-HCL3 at some time points in the failure patients (Fig 3) is of interest. Such discrepancy could be explained by the fact that it is not always possible to distinguish with certainty on morphologic ground between those neoplastic cells and other mononuclear cells. Therefore, the use of these markers represents an objective and reliable method of measuring changes in the proportion of HCs in PB and BM. However, the significance of the reappearance of reactivity with monoclonal antibodies in some patients (5 of 12 responders, Table 3) remains unknown. This finding did not affect their clinical response status (as defined in materials and methods). However, in four of these patients there was also evidence of persistent CE. Further follow-up is required to assess the significance of these findings.

In summary, analysis of surface markers during therapy with interferon is a valuable adjunct in assessing response. The panel of markers used in this study also has a potential of measuring changes in phenotype to a more mature stage. However, we did not see evidence of differentiation in any of the cases. This study on HCL could be used as a model to study other B cell malignancies.

REFERENCES

1. Scheinberg M, Brenner A, Sullivan A, et al: The heterogeneity of leukemic reticuloendotheliosis, "hairy cell leukemia" evidence for its monocytic origin. Cancer 37:1302–1307, 1976

2. Burns G, Cawley J: A re-examination of the alleged monocytic features of Hairy-cell leukemia. Scand J. Haematol 22:386–396, 1979

3. Cawley J, Burns G, Nash T, et al: Hairy cell leukemia with T cell features. Blood 51:61–69, 1978

4. Utsinger P, Yount W, Randall Fuller C, et al: Hairy cell leukemia: B lymphocyte and phagocytic properties. Blood 49:19–27, 1977

5. Korsmeyer S, Greene W, Waldmann T: Cellular origin of hairy cell leukemia: Malignant B cells that express receptors for T cell growth factor. Semin in Oncology 11:394–400, 1984

6. Jansen J, LeBien T, Kersey J: The phenotype of the neoplastic cells of hairy cell leukemia studied with monoclonal antibodies. Blood 59:609–614, 1982

7. Jansen J, Schuit H, Meijer C, et al: Cell markers in hairy cell leukemia studied in cells from 51 patients. Blood 59:52–60, 1982

8. Posnett D, Chiorazzi N, Kunkel H: Monoclonal antibodies with specificity for hairy cell leukemia cells. J Clin Invest 70:254–261, 1982

9. Reynes M, Tricottet V, Capron F, et al: Immunoglobulin synthesis in hairy cell leukemia: Ultrastructural immunocytochemical study of 3 cases. Scand J Haematol 31:501–506, 1983

10. Cawley J, Burns G, Bevan A, et al: Typical hairy cell leukemia with IgGK paraproteinaemia. British J Haematol 43:215–221, 1979

11. Korsmeyer S, Greene W, Cossman J, et al: Rearrangement and expression of immunoglobulin genes and expression of Tac antigen in hairy cell leukemia. Proc Natl Acad Sci USA 80:4522–4526, 1983

12. Jansen J, den Ottolander G, Schuit H, et al: Hairy cell leukemia: Its place among the chronic B cell leukemia. Semin in Oncology 11:386–393, 1984

13. Golomb H, Schmidt K, Vardiman J: Chlorambucil therapy of twenty-four postsplenectomy patients with progressive hairy cell leukemia. Semin in Oncology 11:502–506, 1984

14. Golomb H, Catovsky D, Golde D: Hairy cell leukemia: A clinical review based on 71 cases. Annals of Internal Medicine 89:677–683, 1978

15. Flandrin G, Sigaux F, Sebahoun G, et al: Hairy cell leukemia: Clinical presentation and follow-up of 211 patients. Semin in Oncology 11:458–471, 1984

16. Jacobs A, Champlin R, Golde D: Recombinant α-2-interferon for hairy cell leukemia. Blood 65:1017–1020, 1985

17. Worman C, Catovsky D, Bevan P, et al: Interferon is effective in hairy cell leukemia. British J Haematol 60:759–763, 1985

18. Quesada J, Reuben J, Manning J, et al: Alpha interferon for induction of remission in hairy cell leukemia. New Engl J Med 310:15–18, 1984

19. Wang C, Azzo W, Al-Katib A, et al: Preparation and characterization of monoclonal antibodies recognizing three distinct differentiation antigens (BL1, BL2, BL3) on human B lymphocytes. J Immunol 133:684-691, 1984

20. Koziner B, Stavnezer J, Al-Katib A: Surface immunoglobulin expression by a "common" acute lymphoblastic leukemia (ALL) cell line (REH). Clin Immunol Immunopath 37:135–141, 1985

21. Schwarting R, Stein H, Wang CY: The monoclonal antibodies α S-HCL 1 (α Leu-14) and α S-HCL3 (α Leu-M5) allow the diagnosis of hairy cell leukemia. Blood 65:974–978, 1985

22. Stashenko P, Nadler L, Hardy R, et al: Characterization of a human B lymphocyte-specific antigen. J Immunol 125:1678–1685, 1980

23. Nadler L, Stashenko P, Hardy R, et al: Characterization of a human B-cell specific antigen (B2) distinct from B1. J Immunol 126:1941–1946, 1981

24. Nadler L, Anderson K, Marti G, et al: B4, a human B lymphocyte-associated antigen expressed on normal mitogen-activated and malignant B lymphocytes. J Immunol 131:244–250, 1983

25. Ligler F, Graham-Smith R, Kettman J, et al: Detection of tumor cell in the peripheral blood of nonleukemic patients with B-cell lymphoma: Analysis of "Clonal Excess". Blood 55:792–801, 1980

26. Van Bockstaele B, Berneman Z, Peetermans M: Flow cytometric analysis of hairy cell leukemia using right-angle light scatter. Cytometry 7:217–220, 1996

27. Ligler F, Vitetta E, Graham-Smith R, et al: An immunologic approach for the detection of tumor cells in the peripheral blood of patients with malignant lymphoma; implications for the diagnosis of minimal disease. J Immunol 123:1123–1126, 1979

28. Koziner B, Kempin S, Passe S, et al: Characterization of B-cell leukemias: A tentative immunomorphological scheme. Blood 56:815–823, 1980

Therapeutic Approaches to the Treatment of Hairy Cell Leukemia

Carol S. Portlock

Although a rare disease, hairy cell leukemia has great biologic and clinical significance. New therapeutic options of α-interferon and pentostatin have challenged the role of splenectomy in the overall management of the disease. α-Interferon can now be considered the treatment of choice for patients who progress after splenectomy, and it may also be considered as initial treatment in selected patients. Future clinical trials will focus on the relative efficacies of α-interferon and pentostatin, their potential for sequential or combined use, and the role of splenectomy.

HAIRY CELL LEUKEMIA (HCL) is a rare, chronic lymphoproliferative disorder originally described by Bouroncle in 1958 and termed leukemic reticuloendothelinosis.[1] The disease has gained increasing interest because of its unusual cellular biology, clinical behavior, and remarkable responsiveness to α-interferon. The focus of this review will be the clinical features, diagnosis, and treatment of HCL.

CLINICAL FEATURES

Because of its rarity (approximately 600 new cases in the United States each year), HCL is often difficult to diagnose, although its clinical presentation is rather characteristic.[2,3] The disease is most often identified in middle-aged or elderly males (the average age is 50 to 60 years, and the male to female ratio is at least 3:1 or 4:1). Symptoms are usually insidious in onset and referrable to pancytopenia or splenomegaly. Approximately one third of patients will present with infection and one third with weakness and fatigue: Left upper quadrant pain and hemorrhage are less frequently found. As many as 25% of patients are identified fortuitously by routine blood and physical examination abnormalities.

Most patients have a good general performance status at diagnosis. However, a subset of approximately one fourth of all patients may have significant clinical deterioration. This patient group is more likely to have massive splenomegaly, serious infection, or bleeding and severe neutropenia.

Physical Findings

Splenomegaly is present in 70% to 80% of all patients at diagnosis. The spleen is at least 3 to 10 cm below the left costal margin in the majority of patients. Hepatomegaly is infrequently detected and correlates with the extent of splenomegaly. Peripheral lymphadenopathy is rare, whereas retroperitoneal adenopathy is more frequent and may be bulky as well as a source of abdominal pain.

Laboratory Findings

Cytopenia is the rule in HCL. Only 16% of all patients had normal blood counts in one series.[3] The majority have at least two if not all three cell counts reduced. Presplenectomy counts may include a median hemoglobin value of 10.4 g/dL (range, 4.9 to 15.7); a median white blood cell (WBC) count of 2,860/μL (range, 100 to 68,200), with a mean neutrophil count of 552/μL; a median platelet count of 57,000/μL (range, 10,000 to 752,000). The degree of splenomegaly appears to have no significant effect on the blood counts, although with spleens larger than 10 cm neutropenia and thrombocytopenia are more pronounced.[2]

In addition to cytopenia, most patients will have some circulating hairy cells and 15% to 20% of patients will be frankly leukemic.

DIAGNOSIS AND DIFFERENTIAL DIAGNOSIS

The peripheral smear may demonstrate characteristic hairy cells: Mononuclear cells with abundant cytoplasm and hairy-like cytoplasmic projections (best seen with phase contrast microscopy). The nucleus is ovoid or kidney shaped and nucleoli are not prominent. The cell

---

From Yale University School of Medicine, New Haven, CT.

Address reprint requests to Carol S. Portlock, MD, Associate Professor of Medicine, Yale School of Medicine, New Haven, CT 06510.

0093-7754/86/1304-5008$05.00/0

size is intermediate between lymphocyte and monocyte, approximately 10 to 20 μm.

Bone marrow core biopsy establishes the diagnosis in the majority of patients.[4] Bone marrow aspiration is usually unsuccessful, yielding only dilute and frequently inadequate marrow particles. Marrow hypercellularity is found in the majority of core biopsies, while approximately 10% will have marked hypocellularity. The mononuclear infiltrate is composed of widely spaced cells in a web-like meshwork, most apparent at low power. The wide separation of cells is secondary to abundant pale or water-clear cytoplasm. The nuclei are ovoid and cytologically bland, with occasional indentation or reniform configuration. Normal marrow elements are markedly decreased and scattered throughout the specimen. Among hypocellular specimens, marrow fat is prominent and few malignant cells as well as normal elements are seen. Stromal reticulin is increased in all core biopsies, regardless of marrow cellularity. Fibrosis is not seen. Dilated marrow sinuses and extravasated red blood cells have also been described. The cytochemical presence of tartrate resistant acid phosphatase (isoenzyme 5) in the hairy cells of peripheral smears or bone marrow may be very useful in establishing the diagnosis of HCL.

The pathology of the spleen is also a characteristic feature of HCL, although splenectomy should not be necessary to establish the diagnosis. The spleen is homogeneously involved with diffuse infiltration of the red pulp and sinuses by mononuclear hairy cells. The white pulp is often obliterated. The dilated sinuses are filled with red cells and lined by hairy cells forming pseudosinuses or blood lakes.

Disorders that may be confused with HCL include chronic lymphocytic leukemia, low grade non-Hodgkin's lymphomas, prolymphocytic leukemia, and malignant histiocytosis.[4]

HCL is a B cell neoplasm, as established by the presence of cell surface immunoglobulin and Fc receptors for IgG or IgM as well as the presence of clonal immunoglobulin gene rearrangements[5] of the light chains and heavy chains. These B cells also have Tac antigen (T cell growth factor receptor) on their cell surface. The antigen is present in small quantities as compared with normal T cells, and its pathophysiologic role is uncertain. Rarely, HCL may be found to be of T cell origin, and human T-lymphotropic virus II (HTLV-II) has been isolated from one such T cell HCL cell line.[6]

CLINICAL PROBLEMS

Complications of hairy cell leukemia fall into two broad classes: Cytopenias/splenomegaly and paraneoplastic.[7]

Infection in the setting of cytopenia is the most frequent morbidity and the major cause of death in HCL. The most prominent pathogens are gram-negative bacteria, although other bacteria, viruses, protozoa, fungi, and other opportunistic infections have been reported. Up to 10% of patients may have atypical mycobacterial infections with 5% to 7% mycobacterium tuberculosis. Predisposing factors to infection are neutropenia and immunosuppressive treatment. Fever in HCL must always be considered secondary to infection and not a constitutional symptom of the disease. In the setting of absolute neutropenia and immunosuppressive therapy, the institution of broad spectrum antibiotics is required when fever develops.

Rare paraneoplastic complications include an autoimmune syndrome manifested by vasculitis and/or arthritis sometimes responsive to steroid or splenectomy, paraproteinemia, amyloidosis, and lytic bone lesions.

TREATMENT

Because HCL is a chronic disorder and no curative therapy has yet been established, the goal of management is palliation. Approximately 15% of all patients will require no specific therapy following diagnosis and may remain untreated for as long as 10 years.[3]

For the majority of patients, however, complications of pancytopenia or splenomegaly require intervention. In the past, this has required splenectomy. However, more recently interferon and pentostatin have each been used in this setting and are currently being evaluated as potential primary treatment modalities.

Splenectomy

Splenectomy results in excellent hematologic improvement in the majority of cases, regardless of the degree of splenomegaly. It does not, however, have any effect upon the status of bone marrow involvement.

Progressive normal blood count deterioration postsplenectomy often dictates additional therapeutic interventions. The median time to postsplenectomy treatment was 8.3 months in Golomb's series, with a range of 1 to 164 months.[3] Approximately one half of patients with progressive disease became leukemic and half pancytopenic.

Treatment approaches that have been used postsplenectomy include chemotherapy, leukapheresis, bone marrow transplantation, and interferon.

Chemotherapy

Low-dose daily chlorambucil results in clinical hematologic improvement in the majority of patients. Objective improvement of bone marrow disease is also seen in some patients. Among 11 leukemic patients, Golomb et al[8] reported six complete and two partial hematologic responses, with two demonstrating objective bone marrow response; and among 13 leukopenic patients, two achieved a complete and five achieved a partial response, with objective marrow responses in three. Infectious complications were prominent during therapy, with four deaths.

Joosten et al[9] have recently reported their experience with high-dose methotrexate and leucovorin rescue in six patients. Five achieved hematologic improvement without exacerbation of neutropenia. Responses were transient in all but two patients, with remissions of 14+ and 44+ months.

Combination chemotherapy has resulted in occasional prolonged remissions; however, toxicity has been severe and fatalities common. Calvo et al[10] reported the use of rubidazone, cytosine arabinoside, and cyclophosphamide in seven patients. Three achieved durable remissions of 23 to 44+ months after an average of 37 days of aplasia. Three patients died during induction, and one achieved a partial response.

Pentostatin (2′-deoxycoformycin) is an inhibitor of adenosine deaminase and recently has been reported to have activity in HCL. Spiers et al[11] reported complete hematologic and bone marrow responses in two patients, and these responses have remained durable for 36+ and 33+ months.[12] Moreover, Spiers et al[12] have treated an additional 20 evaluable patients, and thus far 15 have achieved complete bone marrow remissions and five partial responses. The complete remissions have all been durable to date, with the longest follow-up at 22+ months. In general, toxicity has been acceptable in carefully selected patients with good performance status, no active infection, and adequate renal function, using low-dose therapy (4 mg/m^2 intravenously [IV] every 2 weeks).

Johnson et al[13] have preliminarily confirmed these findings. They have treated ten patients for longer than 2 months, and three have achieved a complete hematologic and bone marrow response, as well as four obtaining partial responses. Using low-dose therapy (4 mg/m^2 IV every week × 3 repeated every 8 weeks), toxicity has been acceptable.

Leukapheresis

Leukapheresis has been reported to be an effective means of controlling leukemic HCL in young patients. Yam et al[14] have reported their results in seven patients as well as nine from the literature. Sustained responses from leukapheresis alone were documented in five (12 to 54 months).

Bone Marrow Transplantation

A case report of successful and durable (5+ years) bone marrow transplantation from an identical twin emphasizes the use of this technique in the rare circumstance of HCL and an identical twin donor.[15]

α-Interferon

α-Interferon is an active agent in several B cell neoplasms including the low-grade non-Hodgkin's lymphomas and multiple myeloma.[16] In 1984, Quesada et al[17] first reported the successful treatment of seven HCL patients with partially purified human leukocyte α-interferon. A follow-up report[18] confirmed these preliminary findings in 22 patients receiving 3×10^6 U/d intramuscularly (IM). Five complete, 13 partial, and four minor responses were observed, with a median response duration of 20+ months.

The same authors[18] have also treated 30 patients with α-2a recombinant interferon at doses of 3×10^6 to 12×10^6 U/d IM. Five complete, 17 partial, and six minor responses were observed in this study, with no relapses for 12+ months. Toxicity was considered minor:

Influenza-like symptoms were experienced on first exposure, but rapidly disappeared with continued therapy; approximately 5% complained of moderate to severe fatigue requiring dose modification.

Golomb et al[19] have recently reported a multiinstitutional prospective study of 64 patients. α-2b Recombinant interferon (2×10^6 U) was administered subcutaneously three times per week. Three patients achieved a complete response (5%), 45 achieved a partial response (70%), and nine achieved a minor response (14%).

In these and other reports,[20-30] improvement in hemoglobin, neutrophil, and platelet counts occurred promptly within the first month of therapy. Normal blood counts were maintained for at least 1 year of continued interferon treatment. As expected, transfusion requirements and infectious complications were dramatically reduced with the onset of therapy.

Bone marrow involvement with HCL also improves with interferon treatment. Golomb et al[19] noted a continuous fall in the HCL index during the first nine months of treatment, and complete responders had normalization of bone marrow findings.

Most results with α-interferon are reported in patients with prior splenectomy and often prior chemotherapy. Quesada et al[18] have described six previously untreated patients with splenomegaly who received α-2a interferon as primary treatment. Resolution of splenomegaly began within 2 weeks of therapy in all patients, and five of six achieved a complete response. These results contrast with those patients with prior splenectomy in whom only four of 24 achieved a complete response with interferon α-2a.

The remarkable effectiveness of α-interferon in HCL has raised many questions: (1) What is interferon's mechanism of action? Quesada et al[18] have speculated a direct antitumor effect, induction of tumor cell differentiation, and immunomodulation. (2) What is the optimal dose and duration of α-interferon therapy? Most studies have administered 2×10^6 to 10×10^6 U daily or three times weekly for a minimum period of 1 year. (3) Is maintenance therapy necessary after maximal interferon response? A prospective trial is underway to answer this question. (4) What is the role of interferon in previously untreated patients before splenectomy? The preliminary data of Quesada et al[18] are encouraging and suggest that interferon may be considered as first-line therapy in selected patients. Prospective studies are currently underway to answer this important question.

REFERENCES

1. Bouroncle BA, Wiseman BK, Doan CA: Leukemia reticuloendotheliosis. Blood 13:609–630, 1958

2. Flandrin G, Sigaux F, Sebahoun G, et al: Hairy cell leukemia: Clinical presentation and follow-up of 211 patients. Semin Oncol 11:458–471, 1984 (suppl 2)

3. Golomb HM, Ratain MJ, Vardiman JW: Sequential treatment of hairy cell leukemia: A new role for interferon, in Devita VT Jr, Hellman S, Rosenberg SA (eds): Important Advances in Oncology. Philadelphia, Lippincott, 1986, pp 311–321.

4. Burke JS, Rappaport H: The diagnosis and differential diagnosis of hairy cell leukemia in bone marrow and spleen. Semin Oncol 11:334–346, 1984

5. Korsmeyer SJ, Green WC, Waldmann TA: Cellular origin of hairy cell leukemia: Malignant B cells that express receptors for T cell growth factor. Semin Oncol 11:394–400, 1984

6. Wachsman W, Golde DW, Chen ISY: Hairy cell leukemia and human T cell leukemia virus. Semin Oncol 11:446–450, 1984

7. Westbrook CA, Golde DW: Clinical problems in hairy cell leukemia: Diagnosis and management. Semin Oncol 11:514–522, 1984 (suppl 2)

8. Golomb HM, Schmidt K, Vardiman JW: Chlorambucil therapy of twenty-four postsplenectomy patients with progressive hairy cell leukemia. Semin Oncol 11:502–506, 1984 (suppl 2)

9. Joosten P, Hagenbeek A, Lowenberg B, et al: High-dose methotrexate with leucovorin rescue: Effectiveness in relapsed hairy cell leukemia. Blood 66:241–242, 1985

10. Calvo F, Castaigne S, Sigaux F, et al: Intensive chemotherapy of hairy cell leukemia in patients with aggressive disease. Blood 65:115–119, 1985

11. Spiers ASD, Parekh SJ, Bishop MB: Hairy-cell leukemia: Induction of complete remission with pentostatin (2'-deoxycoformycin) J Clin Oncol 2:1336–1342, 1984

12. Spiers ASD: Personal communication, 1986

13. Johnston JB, Eisenhauer E, Barr R, et al: 2'-deoxycoformycin (DCF) in hairy-cell leukemia: A Canadian phase II trial. Proc Am Soc Clin Oncol 5:159, 1986 (abstr)

14. Yam LT, Klock JC, Mielke CH: Therapeutic leukapheresis in hairy cell leukemia: Review of literature and personal experience. Semin Oncol 11:493–501, 1984 (suppl 2)

15. Cheever MA, Fefer A, Greenberg PD, et al: Identical twin bone marrow transplantation for hairy cell leukemia. Semin Oncol 11:511–513, 1984 (suppl 2)

16. Kirkwood JM, Ernstoff MS: Interferons in the treatment of human cancer. J Clin Oncol 2:336–352, 1984

17. Quesada JR, Reuben J, Manning JT, et al: Alpha interferon for induction of remission in hairy cell leukemia. N Engl J Med 310:15–18, 1984

18. Quesada JR, Gutterman JU, Hersh EM: Treatment of hairy cell leukemia with alpha interferons. Cancer 57:1678–1680, 1986

19. Golomb HM, Jacobs A, Feder AM, et al: Alpha-2-interferon therapy of hairy cell leukemia; a multicenter study of 64 patients. J Clin Oncol 4:900–905, 1986

20. Ratain MV, Golomb HM, Vardiman JW, et al: Treatment of hairy cell leukemia with recombinant alpha-2-interferon. Blood 65:644–648, 1985

21. Jacobs AD, Champlin RE, Golde DW: Recombinant α-2-interferon for hairy cell leukemia. Blood 65:1017–1020, 1985

22. Hofmann V, Scheel A, Schwarzmeier J, et al: Wirksamkeit von Interferon-α-2 (*E. coli*) bei der Haarzell-Leukamie Schweiz Med Wochenschr 7:115, 1985

23. Flandrin G, Sigaux F, Castaigne S, et al: Quantification of bone marrow changes in hairy cell leukemia treated by interferon alpha, in Stewart WE, Schellekens H (eds): The Biology of the Interferon System. Amsterdam, Elsevier, 1985 (in press)

24. Thompson JA, Brady J, Kidd P, et al: Recombinant interferon alpha-2 in the treatment of hairy cell leukemia. Cancer Treat Rep 69:791–793. 1985

25. Gastl G, Denz H, Abbrederis C, et al: Treatment with low dose human recombinant interferon alpha-2 ARG induces complete remission in patients with hairy cell leukemia. Onkologie 8:143–144, 1985

26. Worman CP, Catovsky D, Bevan PC, et al: Interferon is effective in hairy cell leukaemia. Br J Haematol 70:759–763, 1985

27. Duhrsen U, Meusers P, Gries E, et al: Long-lasting remission of hairy cell leukemia after eight weeks' therapy with low-dose alpha-(leukocyte-) interferon. Blut 51:297–298, 1985

28. Castaigne S, Sigaux F, Cantell K, et al: Interferon alpha in the treatment of hairy cell leukemia. Cancer 57:1681–1684, 1986

29. Quesada JR, Hersh E, Gutterman JU: Treatment of hairy cell leukemia with recombinant DNA-derived interferon alpha. Proc Am Soc Clin Oncol 4:222, 1985 (abstr)

30. Quesada JR, Hersh EM, Reuben J, et al: Treatment of hairy cell leukemia with alpha interferon. Proc Am Soc Clin Oncol 3:207, 1984 (abstr)

Seminars in Oncology will publish in future issues

Breast Cancer

Part II

March 1987

Scientific Basis for Adjuvant and Primary (Neoadjuvant) Chemotherapy............................ *J.H. Goldie*
Current Status of Adjuvant Chemotherapy for Resectable Breast Cancer........................ *G. Bonadonna and P. Valagussa*
Current Status of Adjuvant Endocrine Therapy for Resectable Breast Cancer .... *K.I. Pritchard*
New Agents and Medical Treatments for Advanced Breast Cancer........... *I.C. Henderson, D.F. Hayes, S. Come, J.R. Harris, and G. Canellos*
Average Relative Dose Intensity and the Impact on Design of Clinical Trials................. *W.M. Hryniuk*
Psychological Issues in Breast Cancer..*L.M. Sinsheimer and J.C. Holland*

Head and Neck Cancer

Tumor Markers

Endocrine Tumors

Acute Leukemia

Lung Cancer

Gastrointestinal Cancer

Genital Urinary Cancer

Cancer Biology